The **Nursing Assistant**

Essentials of Holistic Care

by

Sue Roe
Phoenix, Arizona

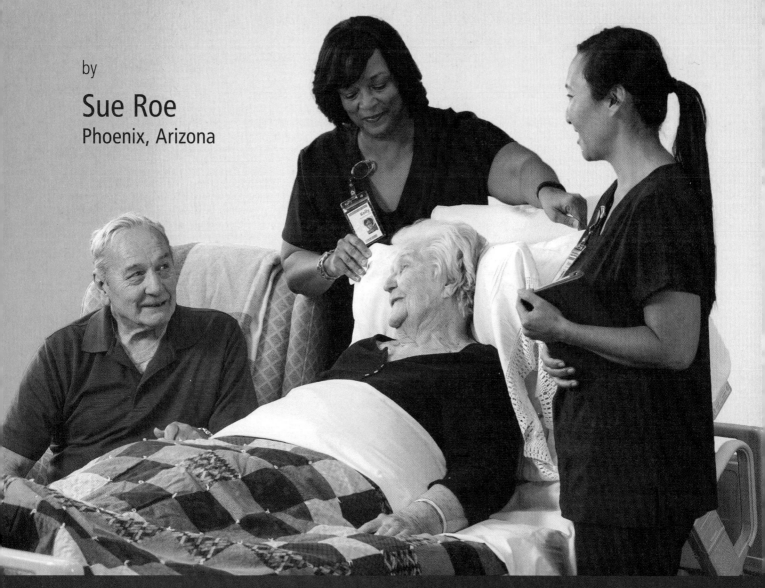

Publisher
The Goodheart-Willcox Company, Inc.
Tinley Park, IL
www.g-w.com

The Goodheart-Willcox Company, Inc. Brand Disclaimer: Brand names, company names, and illustrations for products and services included in this text are provided for educational purposes only and do not represent or imply endorsement or recommendation by the author or the publisher.

The Goodheart-Willcox Company, Inc. Safety Notice: The reader is expressly advised to carefully read, understand, and apply all safety precautions and warnings described in this book or that might also be indicated in undertaking the activities and exercises described herein to minimize risk of personal injury or injury to others. Common sense and good judgment should also be exercised and applied to help avoid all potential hazards. The reader should always refer to the appropriate manufacturer's technical information, directions, and recommendations; then proceed with care to follow specific equipment operating instructions. The reader should understand these notices and cautions are not exhaustive.

The publisher makes no warranty or representation whatsoever, either expressed or implied, including but not limited to equipment, procedures, and applications described or referred to herein, their quality, performance, merchantability, or fitness for a particular purpose. The publisher assumes no responsibility for any changes, errors, or omissions in this book. The publisher specifically disclaims any liability whatsoever, including any direct, indirect, incidental, consequential, special, or exemplary damages resulting, in whole or in part, from the reader's use or reliance upon the information, instructions, procedures, warnings, cautions, applications, or other matter contained in this book. The publisher assumes no responsibility for the activities of the reader.

The Goodheart-Willcox Company, Inc. Internet Disclaimer: The Internet resources and listings in this Goodheart-Willcox Publisher product are provided solely as a convenience to you. These resources and listings were reviewed at the time of publication to provide you with accurate, safe, and appropriate information. Goodheart-Willcox Publisher has no control over the referenced websites and, due to the dynamic nature of the Internet, is not responsible or liable for the content, products, or performance of links to other websites or resources. Goodheart-Willcox Publisher makes no representation, either expressed or implied, regarding the content of these websites, and such references do not constitute an endorsement or recommendation of the information or content presented. It is your responsibility to take all protective measures to guard against inappropriate content, viruses, or other destructive elements.

Image Credits: Front cover   *Top image*: © Tori Soper Photography; *Bottom images left to right*:
© Tori Soper Photography, michaeljung/Shutterstock.com, © Tori Soper Photography

Library of Congress Cataloging-in-Publication Data

Names: Roe, Sue C. DPA, author.
Title: The nursing assistant : essentials of holistic care / Sue Roe.
Description: Tinley Park, IL : The Goodheart-Willcox Company, Inc., [2020] |
   Includes index.
Identifiers: LCCN 2018008257 | ISBN 9781619609747
Subjects: | MESH: Nurses' Aides | Holistic Nursing | Nursing Care
Classification: LCC RT84 | NLM WY 193 | DDC 610.7306/98--dc23 LC record
available at https://lccn.loc.gov/2018008257

Brief Contents

Preface

How exciting to think about becoming a nursing assistant and starting a career in nursing. Perhaps you have been thinking about this endeavor for as long as you can remember because you have always wanted to help others. Perhaps you know someone who is a nurse and would like to be like him or her. Perhaps you had a memorable nurse take care of you when you were ill, and you knew that was the kind of work you wanted to do someday. Whatever your reason for embarking on this career path, this textbook will provide you with the knowledge and skills you need to be successful.

In this textbook, you will learn fundamental and important content and procedures to guide you in delivering safe, quality care. You will also learn about the importance of holistic care; interactions between the body, mind, and spirit; and the profound effect that interactions between the body, mind, and spirit have on the way people maintain wellness and respond to illness. Interactions between the body, mind, and spirit create the connection and harmony people need to live their lives as "whole" human beings.

As a holistic nursing assistant, you will make a difference in the lives of others by

- being sensitive to and respectful of yourself and fully understanding your own body, mind, and spirit so you can do the same for others;
- being strong, but gentle, and using a caring manner;
- focusing on the unique needs and desires of others to help them be as independent as possible;
- being positive and using supportive communication;
- paying close attention to the way you walk into a room, the tone of your voice, and the way you interact with others;
- sensing when others are stressed and helping them understand the importance of maintaining their health and wellness; and
- creating trust, being attentive, and showing appropriate concern and respect.

> *When you touch a body, you touch the whole person, the intellect, the spirit, and the emotions.*
> Jane Harrington, American author

The goal of this textbook is to assist you in becoming an effective and successful nursing assistant. As you study the information and detailed procedures in this text, you will learn how to provide holistic care that is memorable for patients, residents, and their families. Note that the procedures in this book reflect the best general practices. The exact guidelines for procedures in your state may vary, and new knowledge is always shaping the field of nursing, so always check your state's or facility's regulations.

I wish you the best as you embark on this life-changing journey.

Sue Roe

About the Author

Dr. Sue Roe has taught and designed academic courses and training programs in the fields of nursing, allied health, and health administration for more than 35 years. She has served in many academic settings, including public and private universities and colleges. During her years of experience, she has used a variety of delivery formats.

Dr. Roe is the executive editor of *Wholistic Now!*, which is an online newsletter focusing on the areas of holistic health, wellness, leadership, and education. She is also a co-leader for the Arizona Holistic Nurses chapter of the American Holistic Nurses Association.

Dr. Roe is both the manager and a member of The Roe Group Enterprises, LLC. The Roe Group Enterprises, LLC, is a resource for educational materials about the subject of holistic health. Dr. Roe has a doctorate in public administration, with an emphasis in administration and health policy. She has completed graduate-level work in educational administration and instructional development.

Dr. Roe has extensive experience in nursing and nursing education. She holds a master of science degree and a bachelor of science degree in nursing.

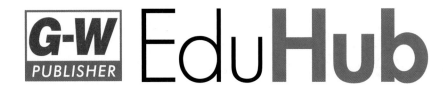
G-W PUBLISHER EduHub

Be Digital Ready on Day One with EduHub

EduHub provides a solid base of knowledge and instruction for digital and blended classrooms. This easy-to-use learning hub delivers the foundation and tools that improve student retention and facilitate instructor efficiency. For the student, EduHub offers an online collection of eBook content, interactive practice, and test preparation. Additionally, students have the ability to view and submit assessments, track personal performance, and view feedback via the Student Report option. For instructors, EduHub provides a turnkey, fully integrated solution with course management tools to deliver content, assessments, and feedback to students quickly and efficiently. The integrated approach results in improved student outcomes and instructor flexibility.

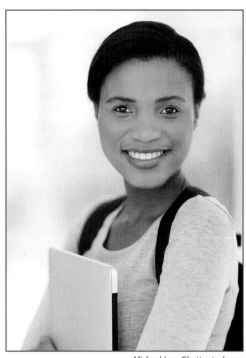

Michael Jung/Shutterstock.com

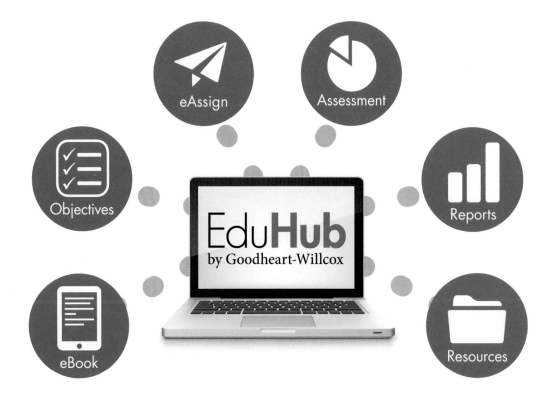

eBook

The EduHub eBook engages students by providing the ability to take notes, access the Text-to-Speech option to improve comprehension, and highlight key concepts to remember. In addition, the accessibility features enable students to customize font and color schemes for personal viewing, while links to videos and animations bring content to life.

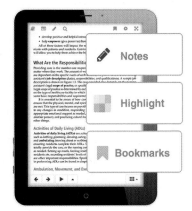

Objectives

Course objectives at the beginning of each eBook chapter help students stay focused and provide benchmarks for instructors to evaluate student progress.

eAssign

eAssign makes it easy for instructors to assign, deliver, and assess student engagement. Coursework can be administered to individual students or the entire class.

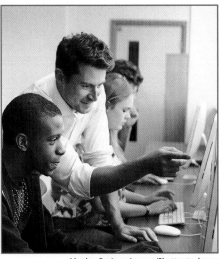

Monkey Business Images/Shutterstock.com

Assessment

Self-assessment opportunities enable students to gauge their understanding as they progress through the course. In addition, formative assessment tools for instructor use provide efficient evaluation of student mastery of content.

Reports

Reports, for both students and instructors, provide performance results in an instant. Analytics reveal individual student and class achievements for easy monitoring of success.

	🖨 Print	⬇ Export
Score	**Items**	
100%	●	●
80%	●	●
100%	●	●
80%	●	●
100%	●	●
100%	●	●

Instructor Resources

Instructors will find all the support they need to make preparation and classroom instruction more efficient and easier than ever. Lesson plans, answer keys, and PowerPoint® presentations provide an organized, proven approach to classroom management.

Learn more about EduHub at www.g-w.com/eduhub

TOOLS FOR STUDENT AND INSTRUCTOR SUCCESS

EduHub

EduHub provides a solid base of knowledge and instruction for digital and blended classrooms. This easy-to-use learning hub provides the foundation and tools that improve student retention and facilitate instructor efficiency.

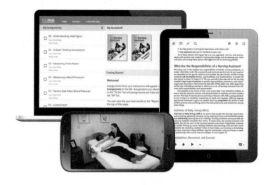

For the student, EduHub offers an online collection of eBook content, interactive practice, and test preparation. Additionally, students have the ability to view and submit assessments, track personal performance, and view feedback via the Student Report option. For the instructor, EduHub provides a turnkey, fully integrated solution with course management tools to deliver content, assessments, and feedback to students quickly and efficiently. The integrated approach results in improved student outcomes and instructor flexibility. Be digital ready on day one with EduHub!

- *eBook content:* EduHub includes the textbook in an online, reflowable format. The eBook is interactive, with highlighting, magnification, note-taking, and text-to-speech features.
- *Procedure Videos:* Using EduHub, students can access **dozens of professional videos** that demonstrate important procedures in the text. These videos clarify steps and aid students in visualizing important skills.
- *Reflection and Practice:* Additional activities for reflection and practice are available on EduHub. Reflective journals offer students the opportunity to reflect on each chapter and apply the principles of holistic care to each nursing content area. These opportunities to journalize will encourage prospective nursing assistants to develop the habit of recording their thoughts, feelings, and assessments regarding their care. EduHub also provides practice through vocabulary games and e-flash cards to help with mastering key nursing terms.
- *Assignments:* In EduHub, students can complete the text review questions as online assignments. Instructors can assign activities, procedural checklists, and practice certification competency exam questions from the Study Guide. Many activities are autograded for easy class assessment and management.

Student Tools

Student Textbook

The Nursing Assistant: Essentials of Holistic Care introduces the field of nurse assisting and outlines the procedures needed to deliver care that meets the physical and socioemotional needs of patients and residents. This text focuses on the holistic care of patients and residents—that is, care that attends to all the needs of a person. Topics covered include nursing assistant responsibilities, legal and ethical standards, healthcare teamwork, cultural humility, ways to promote mobility, and ways to assist with hydration and elimination. Infection control, anatomy and disease, personal hygiene procedures, and care for people with disabilities are also covered in this text. At the end of each chapter, practice questions for the certification competency examination assess knowledge and skills gained.

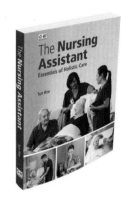

Study Guide

The Study Guide that accompanies *The Nursing Assistant: Essentials of Holistic Care* includes instructor-created activities to help students recall, review, and apply concepts introduced in the book. The Study Guide also includes procedural checklists and two full practice tests for the certification competency examination.

Instructor Tools

LMS Integration

Integrate Goodheart-Willcox content in your Learning Management System for a seamless user experience for both you and your students. Contact your G-W Educational Consultant for ordering information or visit www.g-w.com/lms-integration.

Instructor Resources

The Instructor Resources provide all the support needed to make preparation and classroom instruction easier than ever. Included are time-saving preparation tools such as answer keys, editable lesson plans, chapter outlines, and other teaching aids. In addition, presentations for PowerPoint® and assessment software with question banks are provided for your convenience. These resources can be accessed at school, at home, or on the go.

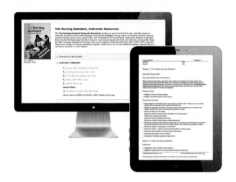

Instructor's Presentations for PowerPoint® Instructor's Presentations for PowerPoint® provide a useful teaching tool for presenting concepts introduced in the text. These fully customizable, richly illustrated slides help you teach and visually reinforce the key concepts from each chapter. Slides include the list of Learning Objectives for each section; discussion, review, and activity slides; and slides with practice questions for the certification competency examination.

Assessment Software with Question Banks Administer and manage assessments to meet your classroom needs. The test banks that accompany this textbook include hundreds of matching, true/false, completion, multiple choice, and short answer questions to assess student knowledge of the content in each chapter. Using the assessment software simplifies the process of creating, managing, administering, and grading tests. You can have the software generate a test for you with randomly selected questions. You may also choose specific questions from the question banks and, if you wish, add your own questions to create customized tests to meet your classroom needs.

G-W Integrated Learning Solution

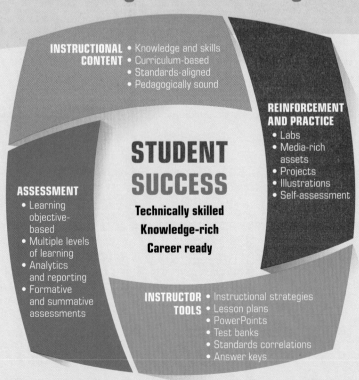

INSTRUCTIONAL CONTENT
- Knowledge and skills
- Curriculum-based
- Standards-aligned
- Pedagogically sound

REINFORCEMENT AND PRACTICE
- Labs
- Media-rich assets
- Projects
- Illustrations
- Self-assessment

STUDENT SUCCESS
Technically skilled
Knowledge-rich
Career ready

ASSESSMENT
- Learning objective-based
- Multiple levels of learning
- Analytics and reporting
- Formative and summative assessments

INSTRUCTOR TOOLS
- Instructional strategies
- Lesson plans
- PowerPoints
- Test banks
- Standards correlations
- Answer keys

The G-W Integrated Learning Solution offers easy-to-use resources that help students and instructors achieve success.

▶ **EXPERT AUTHORS**
▶ **TRUSTED REVIEWERS**
▶ **100 YEARS OF EXPERIENCE**

EMPLOYABILITY SKILLS · TECHNICAL SKILLS · ACADEMIC KNOWLEDGE · INDUSTRY RECOGNIZED STANDARDS

Guided Tour

Emphasis on Holistic Care

The Nursing Assistant: Essentials of Holistic Care takes a holistic approach to nursing assistant information, skills, and procedures. At the beginning of each chapter, a *Providing Holistic Care Framework* helps prospective nursing assistants visualize the aspects of holistic care and identify the areas they will learn. *Becoming a Holistic Nursing Assistant* features also introduce important skills and considerations for delivering holistic care. These features cover such topics as providing care in isolation, answering call lights, and caring for a patient in a coma.

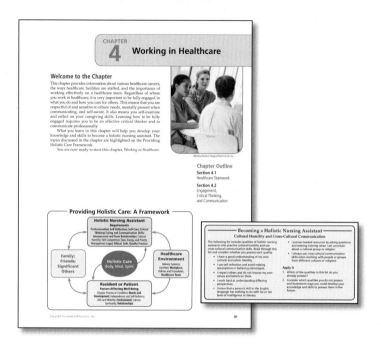

Practice Questions for the Certification Competency Examination

After studying this text, prospective nursing assistants will be prepared to take the certification competency examination in their state. At the end of each chapter, practice test questions similar to those found on certification competency examinations across the United States provide an opportunity for students to practice answering exam questions and apply their test-taking skills. Exam questions are multiple choice and assess understanding of the topics covered in each chapter. Two full practice exams are also provided in the Study Guide that accompanies this text. *The Nursing Assistant: Essentials of Holistic Care* covers all of the information assessed on the certification competency exam and also includes reinforcement, application, and critical thinking questions at the end of each section to solidify learning. The last chapter of this text presents information about study skills and test-taking strategies.

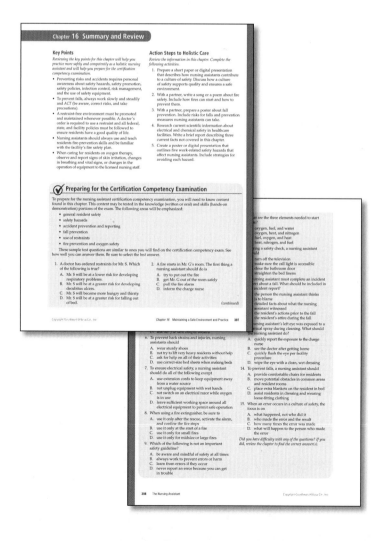

Procedures

Throughout *The Nursing Assistant: Essentials of Holistic Care*, numerous detailed procedures outline the steps prospective nursing assistants need to follow to pass the certification competency examination and practice in healthcare. Every procedure contains a rationale, preparation instructions, procedure steps, follow-up actions, and information for reporting and documentation. Procedures are easy to follow and are richly illustrated with numerous, professionally photographed images and illustrations. **Best Practice** notes advise prospective nursing assistants about safety precautions and ways to provide care holistically. **Step-by-step videos** are also available on EduHub to help students visualize the tasks involved in each procedure.

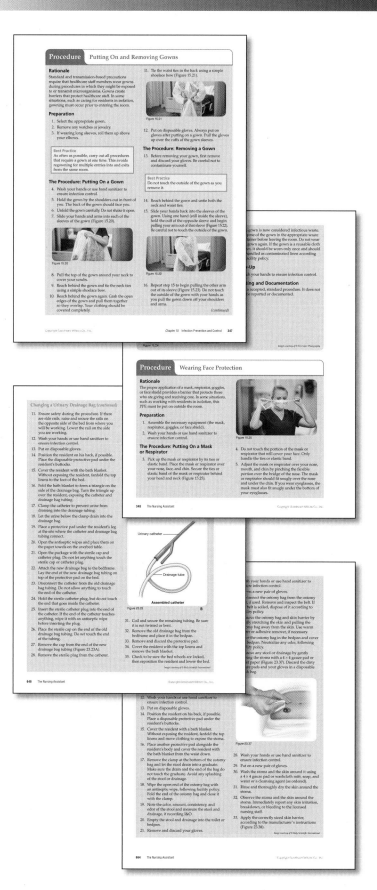

Best Practice
A resident may feel dizzy for the first few minutes of dangling, but this feeling should pass. If it doesn't, return the resident to a lying position with the head raised and immediately notify the charge nurse.

Best Practice
Arrange your equipment on the overbed table so you do not have to reach over or turn your back on your work area.

Best Practice
Avoid allowing the patient to see the soiled side of the dressing, as this may make the patient feel uncomfortable.

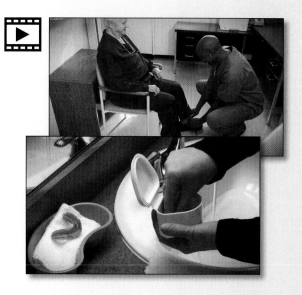

Features

In addition to *Becoming a Holistic Nursing Assistant*, the text contains other features that address topics of interest in nurse assisting. *Culture Cues* prompt prospective nursing assistants to examine cultural considerations for improved care. Some examples include cultural considerations about personal space, food traditions, and communication. *Healthcare Scenarios* introduce concepts using lifelike situations and ask students to analyze and apply knowledge to dilemmas. These address topics ranging from intergenerational teamwork to observation skills to surgically implantable hearing aids. *Think About This* features throughout each chapter provide additional information about healthcare topics of interest, and *Remember* features share motivating quotes related to nursing to hold student attention.

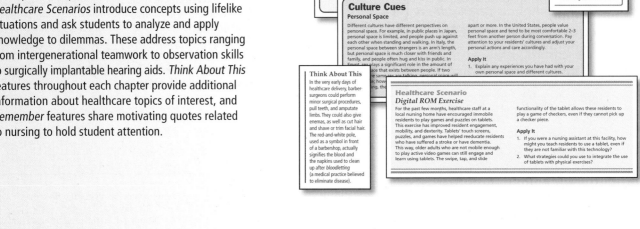

Photographs and Illustrations

Numerous colorful photographs demonstrate important care guidelines. These images help students visually understand the concepts being presented.
Detailed illustrations bring anatomical concepts to life, helping students comprehend body positions and the complex structure of the human body.

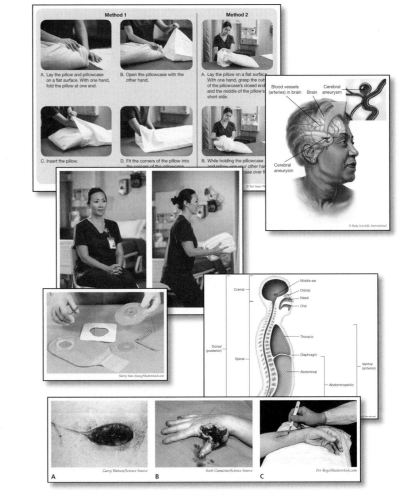

Organization

The Nursing Assistant: Essentials of Holistic Care is divided into 11 parts and 28 chapters. The first few parts introduce foundational knowledge prospective nursing assistants need to know as they provide care. Later parts introduce important procedural skills and information about working with specific populations. The following provides a brief overview of concepts covered in these parts:

- Part 1 explains the role of the nursing assistant and the meaning of holistic care. It provides information about the healthcare environment, legal and ethical standards, the nursing process, and procedures for admission, transfer, and discharge.

- Part 2 introduces necessary information about the human body, health and wellness, and diseases and conditions. This part discusses human development and needs, basic anatomy and physiology, types of diseases and conditions, and pain relief.

- Part 3 describes the interpersonal skills prospective nursing assistants need to practice effectively. Communication skills and cultural humility are discussed in these chapters.

- Part 4 discusses the details of planning, observing, and reporting care. It also introduces skills for keeping records and documenting care. Different types of health records, including paper charts, electronic health records, and electronic medical records, are discussed in this part.

- Part 5 explains immunity and the chain of infection and covers important infection control procedures. These chapters introduce the body's defenses to infection and steps for putting on and taking off personal protective equipment such as gloves, face protection, and gowns.

- Part 6 outlines procedures for maintaining a safe environment and promoting mobility in residents. It explains how to prevent falls and position, lift, and turn residents.

- Part 7 introduces procedures for measuring vital signs, height, and weight and collecting specimens. In this part, prospective nursing assistants learn how to take blood pressure and pulse and collect sputum, urine, and stool samples for examination.

- Part 8 discusses the fundamentals of creating a safe, restful environment for residents. It explains how to make beds, answer call lights, and assist with personal hygiene.

- Part 9 describes the fundamentals of healthy eating, hydration, and elimination. In this part, prospective nursing assistants learn to assist with eating, care for feeding tubes, ensure hydration, and assist with elimination.

- Part 10 addresses care for specific populations. It includes information about caring for people with disabilities and cognitive disorders, mothers and newborns, and surgical patients. It also discusses emergency and end-of-life care.

- Part 11 concludes the book by explaining the best methods for taking the certification competency examination, seeking employment, and advancing in a healthcare career. It teaches study skills and avenues of finding employment.

Reviewers

Goodheart-Willcox Publisher and the author would like to thank the following professionals who reviewed selected chapters and provided valuable input into the development of this textbook program.

Theresa Bloom
Technical Instructor of Medical Preparation
Western Colorado Community College
Grand Junction, CO

Renae Boydston
RN/Nurse Aide Instructor
Blackhawk Technical College
Janesville, WI

Kimberly Budd
Health Technology Instructor
Delaware Area Career Center
Delaware, OH

Lisa Carrigan
RN Program Coordinator
Applied Technology Center
Rock Hill, SC

Sally Christiansen
Nursing Assistant Coordinator
Waukesha County Technical College
Pewaukee, WI

Christine Curry
CNA Classroom Coordinator
Granite Technical Institute
Salt Lake City, UT

Sheryl Diglia
Health Science Instructor
Apollo Career Center
Lima, OH

Michael Donahue
RN/CNA Instructor
North Shore Community College
Danvers, MA

Laura Eser
Health Professions Instructor
Caroline Career and Technology Center
Ridgely, MD

Ines Lovio Estrado
Career and Technical Education Instructor
Imperial Valley Regional Occupational Program
El Centro, CA

Robin Finney
Nursing Faculty
Southwestern Oregon Community College
Coos Bay, OR

Deborah Grubb
Health Professions Teacher
Carroll County Career and Technology Center
Westminster, MD

Betty Gruber
Nurse Aide Coordinator
Panola College
Carthage, TX

Patty Hawley
Nursing Educator
Ferris State University
Big Rapids, MI

Brittany Hendrix
CNA Instructor
Ogeechee Technical College
Metter, Georgia

Shelly Holt
Medical Assisting Program Director
Chattahoochee Valley Community College
Phenix City, AL

Cassandra Howard
Health Occupations Methods Teacher
Essex County Vocational Technical Schools
Newark, NJ

Heidi Janowicz
STNA Instructor
Owens Community College
Perrysburg, OH

Mia Jones
Instructor
Lone Star College
Conroe, TX

Wanda King
NAHAA Instructor
Minneapolis Community and Technical College
Minneapolis, MN

Deb Kupecz
Affiliate Faculty
Community College of Denver
Denver, CO

Pat Lawton
Nursing Instructor
Central Nine Career Center
Greenwood, IN

Pam Logalbo
Nursing Assistant Program Faculty
Clackamas Community College
Portland, OR

Donna Mathias
CNA Program Coordinator
Bartow County College and Career Academy
Cartersville, GA

Billi McClintock
Nursing Assistant Instructor
Orange-Ulster BOCES
Goshen, NY

Korrie McFarlane
RN/CNA Instructor
Kent Career Technical Center
Grand Rapids, MI

Victor Palmer
CNA/Student Success Specialist
Hawkeye Community College
Waterloo, IA

Jennifer Sayler
Director of Professional Development
Spaulding Nursing and Therapy Center North End
Boston, MA

Rene Stark
Professional Faculty
Washtenaw Community College
Ann Arbor, MI

Karen Sullivan
Nursing Instructor
Carroll County Career and Technology Center
Westminster, MD

Glenna Texler
Pre-Nursing Instructor
Tolles Career and Technical Center
Plain City, OH

Sandra Ukah
Health Science Instructor
Atlanta Technical College
Atlanta, GA

Kristen Woods
Nurse Assisting Program Coordinator
Gateway Community College
Phoenix, AZ

Acknowledgments

Goodheart-Willcox Publisher and the author would like to thank Rasmussen College for the use of the college's simulation lab for a photoshoot. The author would also like to thank Dina J. Capek, RN, MSN, LNHA, Director of Health Services, Royal Oaks Retirement Community, in Sun City, Arizona, who generously shared her expertise and experience with long-term care and at-risk geriatric populations and provided some needed supplies for the photoshoot. The author is also grateful to Sherry Zumbrunnen, BSN, MN, RN, HNBC, Certified Yoga Instructor, and Reiki Master, for her helpful insights and perspectives about holistic nursing care.

Contents

Identified features include:
Becoming a Holistic Nursing Assistant
Culture Cues   Healthcare Scenario

The Holistic Nursing Assistant

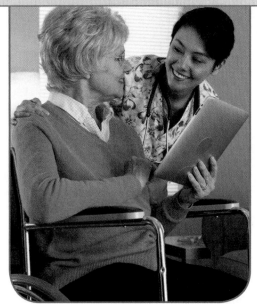

Rocketclips, Inc./Shutterstock.com

Chapter Outline

Section 1.1
Role and Responsibilities

Section 1.2
Professionalism
and Boundaries

Welcome to the Chapter

This chapter provides information you will need to understand your role and demonstrate your responsibilities as a holistic nursing assistant. You will learn about the qualities, behaviors, and professionalism expected of a successful holistic nursing assistant. Further, you will explore the personal and professional boundaries within which a nursing assistant must work. These boundaries are important, as they define what a nursing assistant can and cannot do as a caregiver.

When you become a holistic nursing assistant, you will care for many different people. You may deliver care to **patients**. Patients are people who receive care in a healthcare facility, such as a hospital. Patients need immediate care due to illness or disease and often can expect recovery. A patient's stay in a hospital is usually short. You may also deliver care to **residents**. Residents are people who need ongoing care over a longer period of time. Residents are older and reside in long-term care facilities due to age, illness, or inability to care for themselves at home. During your career as a nursing assistant, you may work in many different healthcare facilities and therefore will likely care for both patients and residents. The terms *patients* and *residents* will both be used throughout this textbook. The quality of care you provide to each will be the same.

You are now ready to start this chapter, *The Holistic Nursing Assistant*.

Objectives

To provide the best possible holistic care, you will need to understand the role, responsibilities, and requirements of a nursing assistant. To achieve the objectives for this section, you must successfully

- **describe** the role of a holistic nursing assistant;
- **explain** the requirements for nursing assistants to become certified; and
- **discuss** the typical responsibilities of a holistic nursing assistant.

Key Terms

Learn these key terms to better understand the information presented in the section.

activities of daily living (ADLs)
ambulating
certification
certified nursing assistant (CNA)
compassion
contaminated
empower
holistic care
hospice
infection control
job description
licensed nursing staff
licensed practical/vocational nurse (LPN/LVN)
patients
registered nurse (RN)
residents
scope of practice
vital signs

Questions to Consider
- Have you ever taken care of someone? Maybe you took care of your mother, friend, younger brother or sister, or even your pet. How did you feel about the responsibility of providing care? What did you do to ensure that person or pet was cared for properly?
- How would you describe the caregiving role you took or what you had to do? What daily responsibilities, abilities, and attitudes helped you do the best job possible?

What Is a Nursing Assistant's Role?

Becoming a nursing assistant gives you a special opportunity to make a difference in someone else's life. It is also an excellent way to grow personally by gaining knowledge and skills as you journey into the exciting career pathway of nursing.

A **certified nursing assistant (CNA)** is a person who has successfully completed the education and training needed to take and pass a state certification competency examination. The certified nursing assistant helps deliver care and is supervised by licensed practical/vocational nurses (LPNs/LVNs) and registered nurses (RNs). In some states, a CNA is known as a *nurse aide, registered nursing assistant,* or *licensed nursing assistant.*

Pursuing a role as a certified nursing assistant (CNA) may be your first step toward becoming a licensed practical/vocational nurse (LPN/LVN) or a registered nurse (RN). A **licensed practical/vocational nurse (LPN/LVN)** is a licensed nursing staff member who is supervised by a registered nurse (RN). The duties of LPNs/LVNs vary by state, but typically include monitoring and reporting, preparing and giving medications, and inserting catheters. A **registered nurse (RN)** is a licensed nursing staff member who delivers nursing care that includes assessment; providing nursing diagnoses; and planning, implementing, and evaluating care.

Pursuing a role as a nursing assistant can also help you decide if you would like a long-term career providing care to others. Whether or not you advance to other nursing or healthcare delivery roles, the knowledge you learn and the skills you acquire during your education and experience as a nursing assistant can be used throughout your life.

A nursing assistant is an important member of the healthcare team and provides care to both patients and residents (Figure 1.1). Nursing assistants work under the supervision of **licensed nursing staff**, which consists of LPNs/LVNs and RNs. Healthcare facilities such as hospitals, community clinics, skilled nursing facilities, residential care or long-term care facilities, **hospices** (healthcare facilities that care for people who are terminally ill), and home healthcare services employ nursing assistants.

Working as a nursing assistant requires much more than just meeting the basic needs of those in your care. Nursing assistants are often the first to communicate with residents and their families. This is because nursing assistants spend more time with residents than LPNs/LVNs or RNs, who may be involved in other procedures and tasks. As a result, nursing assistants may be the first ones who observe changes in resident behavior and function or who become aware of residents' specific needs. This information is then reported to the licensed nursing staff for follow-up. The role of the nursing assistant is important and essential and has many responsibilities.

How Do You Become a Nursing Assistant?

Becoming a nursing assistant requires specialized education and training and the use of knowledge and skills learned to deliver safe, quality care.

Education and Training

In 1987, the US Congress passed the *Omnibus Budget Reconciliation Act (OBRA)*, which standardized the minimum requirements for certified nursing assistant training programs and evaluation. OBRA is specific to nursing assistants working in nursing homes that receive federal funding. Today, nursing assistant education and training courses that lead to **certification** (a credential indicating that a person has completed required education and training) must meet OBRA standards. Since OBRA was passed, states have taken the responsibility of making sure nursing assistant education and training programs meet these standards. States also determine how nursing assistant certification is granted, what certification competency examination will be used, and when and where the exam will occur.

The minimum age requirement for entering a nursing assistant education and training program differs from state to state. Instruction ranges from a minimum of 75 hours to more than 150 hours. Requirements for supervised clinical training include at least 24 hours or more in long-term care facilities. Some programs also include hospital and other related clinical experiences.

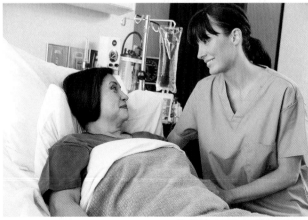 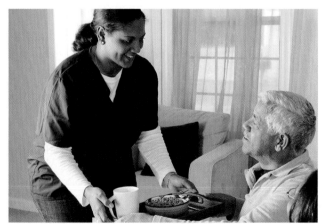

Monkey Business Images/Shutterstock.com   *Rob Marmion/Shutterstock.com*

Figure 1.1 Nursing assistants work in a variety of settings, including hospitals and long-term care facilities.

The Certification Competency Examination

On completion of a state-approved nursing assistant education and training program, graduates are expected to take the certification competency examination required by the states in which they reside. The examination tests an individual's knowledge (in a written or oral exam) and skills (as part of a hands-on demonstration). The written exam usually consists of 50 or more multiple-choice questions and is timed. The skills demonstration requires applicants to show how well they can perform specified procedures (for example, hand washing, providing oral care, dressing a resident, or performing a partial bed bath). To become certified, a graduate must pass both parts of the examination with a state-determined score. Many resources, including this textbook, provide practice questions similar to those found on the examination.

When a nursing assistant becomes certified, he or she may use the legal title *certified nursing assistant (CNA)*. Using this title means you have met the requirements to practice as a nursing assistant within the regulations, or *rules*, determined by your state.

Registration as a Nursing Assistant

Federal law requires every state to maintain a *registry*, or list, of nursing assistants. Individuals who successfully complete an approved nursing assistant education or training program and pass the certification competency exam are listed on the registry. The registry also has information about nursing assistants who have findings of abuse, neglect, and theft.

To work as a nursing assistant, a person must maintain an *active status* on the registry. This means that a person's information is up-to-date and that a person has no charges of abuse, neglect, or the theft or misuse of resident property. Nursing assistants must renew their registration every two years.

Requirements for education or training and the certification competency exam may vary from state to state, as will regulations for nursing assistants. Be sure to check the specific requirements for the state in which you live.

What Do I Need to Know to Become a Holistic Nursing Assistant?

Learning how to be a holistic nursing assistant emphasizes the caring aspect of the nursing assistant's role and strengthens the knowledge and skills needed to provide **holistic care** (care that integrates the body, mind, and spirit). Understanding and using the *Providing Holistic Care Framework*, shown in Figure 1.2 on the next page, will be a helpful guide in this learning process.

The Providing Holistic Care Framework includes the key knowledge and skills you will need to know as a holistic nursing assistant. These knowledge and skills include being professional, using critical thinking, caring and effectively communicating, having cultural humility, and building skills competence. The framework also incorporates the healthcare environment in which you will work. Holistic nursing assistants must be knowledgeable about different healthcare delivery systems and the workplace, familiar with facility policies and procedures, and capable of working effectively as team members.

The framework illustrates the important interactions between residents or patients; families, friends, and significant others; the holistic nursing assistant; and the healthcare facility. The arrows in the framework represent the support each individual or entity gives to the others. For example, family members support a resident, but may also work closely with a holistic nursing assistant to help ensure the resident's needs are met. Similarly, understanding facility policies and effectively demonstrating procedures enable holistic nursing assistants to provide safe, quality care.

> **Remember**
>
> *One person caring about another represents life's greatest value.*
>
> Jim Rohn, entrepreneur and motivational speaker

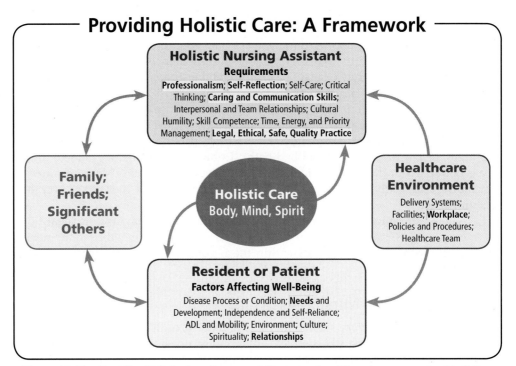

Figure 1.2 The Providing Holistic Care Framework illustrates the different components of holistic care and the support each entity lends to others. Highlighted in this framework are the topics covered in chapter 1.

An effective holistic nursing assistant is aware of a resident's disease process and knows how to respond or take action (for example, by providing assistance with activities of daily living, or ADLs). Holistic nursing assistants are also responsible for responding to patients' or residents' needs, emotions, and feelings.

Of great importance in caregiving is sensitivity to the holistic dimensions of the body, mind, and spirit. To provide care that integrates the body, mind, and spirit, holistic nursing assistants must not only respond to physical needs (body), but must also focus on the mind, which includes the patient's or resident's needs, wants, feelings, and emotions. Understanding the spirit is also essential. The spirit is a person's *higher self*, which includes perceptions, sensations, values, culture, and religion.

By using this holistic approach, caregivers establish an environment that supports the *whole person* and does not just focus on, respond to, and care for a disease. The holistic approach promotes healing and helps patients and residents achieve overall well-being.

As you build your holistic knowledge and skills as a nursing assistant, you will also become aware of how you, as a person, must become sensitive to your *own* body, mind, and spirit. Holistic caregiving should always include this awareness and sensitivity because it is hard to care for others holistically if you do not feel whole yourself. See chapter 6 for more information about holistic care.

This textbook will guide you through the essentials of holistic caregiving. Each chapter will emphasize a different area of the Providing Holistic Care Framework. This information will be identified and highlighted in the Providing Holistic Care Framework at the beginning of each chapter and will serve as your guide to reading the chapter and becoming a holistic nursing assistant. In Figure 1.2, the topics covered in this chapter are highlighted.

In addition, you are encouraged to reflect and journal about what you have learned in each chapter of your textbook. Creating a reflective journal will give you the opportunity to document and reflect on both the knowledge and skills you learned from the chapter and ways you can use them when you begin working as a holistic nursing assistant. It is only through this self-examination and reflection that you can build the confidence and ability to

- be sensitive to special needs and culture;
- understand diseases, conditions, and disabilities;
- use your knowledge and skills competently and safely;
- develop positive and helpful interactions with others; and
- help **empower** (give power to) those in your care.

All of these factors will impact the way you approach, care for, and communicate with patients and residents. Gaining knowledge and developing your skills will allow you to help them achieve the highest levels of well-being possible.

What Are the Responsibilities of a Nursing Assistant?

Providing care is the number-one responsibility of holistic nursing assistants, no matter where they work. The amount of work involved and the type of care required are dependent on the specific needs of each resident, the plan of care, and the nursing assistant's **job description** (duties, responsibilities, and qualifications). A sample job description is shown in Figure 1.3. The care provided also depends on the nursing assistant's legal **scope of practice**, or specific responsibilities, procedures, and actions. Legal scope of practice is determined by each state. While duties may differ depending on the type of healthcare facility in which you work, all nursing assistants have the same basic responsibilities and requirements.

It is essential to be aware of how care is provided. Care should be holistic to ensure that the physical, mental, and spiritual needs of residents and their families are met. This type of care focuses on providing assistance with ADLs, paying attention to any changes in condition, responding to needs and requests, offering ongoing appropriate emotional support as needed, showing **compassion** (the desire to help another person), and practicing *cultural humility* (awareness and sensitivity), among other things.

Activities of Daily Living (ADLs)

Activities of daily living (ADLs) are actions that people take during a typical day, such as bathing, grooming, dressing, eating, toileting (urinary and bowel elimination), and **ambulating** (moving about or walking). Nursing assistants are responsible for ensuring residents complete their ADLs. In some cases, the nursing assistant will totally provide the care, or the nursing assistant may assist independent residents as needed. Setting up meals, feeding residents, documenting what and how much residents ate, recording residents' levels of fluid intake, and assisting with toileting are other important responsibilities. Specific information and procedures to assist in performing ADLs can be found in chapter 21 and chapter 23.

Ambulation, Movement, and Exercise

Older residents and residents who have illnesses that cause them to be weak or bedridden may need assistance with ambulation. This assistance may include lifting, moving, or transferring residents. Some residents may require assistance with *range-of-motion exercises*, which help residents maintain or improve their flexibility. Nursing assistants also work with residents who need help gaining body strength or need assistance with physical exercise to maintain effective muscular function and general well-being. You will learn more about ambulation and range-of-motion exercises in chapter 17.

Certified Nursing Assistant (CNA)
Job Description

Job Summary: Assists licensed nursing staff in the provision of basic care for residents and provides necessary unit tasks and functions in compliance with facility policies, procedures, and applicable healthcare standards.

Duties and Responsibilities: Other duties may be assigned.

- Assist residents to meet daily needs while providing a safe environment and ensuring the dignity and well-being of residents.
- Bathe, dress, and undress residents who need help. Assist with other tasks, including but not limited to shaving, nails, and hair.
- Change linens and towels regularly, straighten room, remove soiled linens, and make residents' beds, ensuring that all residents' rooms look neat and clean.
- Ensure all call lights are in reach of residents and answer call lights within five minutes.
- Serve meals. Assist with eating, if needed.
- Assist with new resident admission.
- Maintain safety and security at all times.
- Report pertinent resident information to licensed nursing staff.
- Complete all forms according to policies and procedures.
- Participate in facility activities, including in-service education and disaster drills.
- Consistently display professional behavior and attitudes and represent the goals and values of the facility.

Qualifications:

- Must have a current and valid Nursing Assistant Certification.
- Must be at least 18 years of age.
- Must be compassionate, mature, sympathetic, and professional at all times.
- Must have good organization and communication skills.
- Must have the ability to read, write, understand, and carry out instructions.
- Must successfully complete all preemployment requirements.
- Must have the physical ability to perform job-related duties, which may require lifting, standing, bending, transferring, stooping, stretching, walking, pushing, and pulling.

Acknowledgement:

I have read this job description and fully understand the requirements for employment. I hereby accept the position of Certified Nursing Assistant (CNA) and will perform all said duties to the best of my ability.

Printed Employee Name: _____

Employee Signature: _____

Date: _____

Figure 1.3 This is an example of a job description for a nursing assistant position.

Measurement and Observation

Among the most important responsibilities of a nursing assistant are measuring, documenting, and reporting information about a patient or resident. Information that nursing assistants measure, document, and report are

- **vital signs**, which include the rates or values of a person's temperature, pulse, respiration, and blood pressure (Figure 1.4);
- height and weight;
- fluid intake and output; and
- changes in condition.

Nursing assistants are often the first to know how well a patient or resident is responding to a medicine or treatment. This is because nursing assistants spend more time at the bedside. Any changes in a patient's or resident's condition should be immediately reported to the licensed nursing staff. See chapter 12, chapter 18, and chapter 23 to learn more about these observations and measurements.

Procedures

Nursing assistants perform numerous procedures when giving care. These procedures may include providing skin and oral care and admitting, transferring, and discharging patients.

Procedures performed are standardized and are found in a healthcare facility policy and procedure manual. Nursing assistants must always perform procedures as defined by the duties and responsibilities of their position and by the healthcare facility. Unless assistance is needed, nursing assistants perform these procedures on their own. They are always, however, under the supervision of licensed nursing staff.

Infection Control

Infection control is another essential part of a nursing assistant's daily responsibilities and is used to minimize the risk of infection. For example, performing *hand hygiene* (washing hands or rubbing hands with sanitizer) helps prevent the spread of infection. Additionally, the appropriate care and handling of **contaminated** (dirty) objects is important for controlling infection in a healthcare facility. Wearing *personal protective equipment (PPE)*, such as a mask, gloves, protective eyewear, and a gown, is sometimes required (Figure 1.5). Infection control also includes observing and reporting environmental situations that might cause the spread of infection. In chapter 15, you will learn how to follow procedures for hand hygiene and how to properly put on masks, gowns, and gloves.

Communication

Nursing assistants are constantly communicating with residents and their families, other visitors, and healthcare team members. Nursing assistants are also responsible for recording necessary information in electronic or paper charts and forms, answering the telephone, and taking messages. Communicating electronically has become significant in healthcare delivery. Electronic communication may include recording resident information in an *electronic medical record (EMR)*, using mobile devices, or using social media

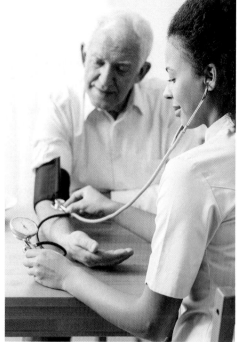

Photographee.eu/Shutterstock.com

Figure 1.4 Nursing assistants measure and record residents' vital signs. This nursing assistant is measuring a resident's blood pressure.

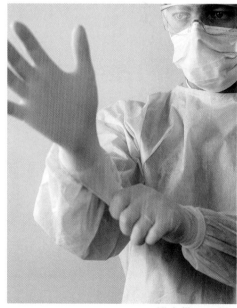

Micolas/Shutterstock.com

Figure 1.5 To ensure infection control, nursing assistants sometimes wear personal protective equipment (PPE).

to educate and inform others. Important information about communication, documentation rules, and the use of electronic communication are described in chapter 10 and chapter 13.

Environmental Care and Safety

It is important to keep resident room conditions as comfortable and safe as possible. To achieve this, nursing assistants must keep rooms clean and neat. Ensuring a comfortable and safe environment includes making beds; adjusting room temperature and lighting; emptying trash; and removing potential safety hazards or sources of personal injury, such as spills or objects left on the floor. Practicing environmental care and safety might also include responding to emergency situations. You may perform emergency procedures, such as responding to fainting or a seizure or evacuating residents in case of a fire or other environmental emergency. See chapter 16, chapter 20, and chapter 26 for more information.

Specimen Collection

When directed, nursing assistants collect specimens from patients or residents. These specimens help in diagnosing illnesses, preparing for a procedure, or evaluating progress. Specimens may include *sputum* (mucus from the respiratory system), urine, or *feces* (stool). After collection, specimens are labeled and delivered to a clinical laboratory for analyses. Details on collecting specimens can be found in chapter 19.

What Is a Typical Day for a Nursing Assistant?

When you work as a holistic nursing assistant, you will find that no two days are exactly the same. While there is no "typical" day for a nursing assistant, there are several major duties nursing assistants perform while giving care to patients or residents:

- answering *call lights*, which alert staff that a resident is in need
- assisting with daily needs while promoting independence
- measuring and recording vital signs
- serving meals and feeding residents when necessary (Figure 1.6)
- transporting residents
- lifting or turning residents
- making beds and helping change soiled linens or gowns
- helping maintain personal hygiene
- assisting with toileting
- recording food intake
- measuring and recording fluid intake and output
- collecting required specimens
- observing and reporting health issues, behaviors, and responses to the licensed nursing staff
- assisting staff with any required tasks involving care
- keeping all lines of communication open

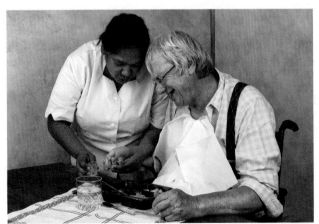

Anneka/Shutterstock.com

Figure 1.6 In a typical day, a nursing assistant might serve meals and feed patients or residents, if necessary.

- protecting rights, privacy, confidentiality, and dignity
- being sensitive to and respectful of diversity
- promoting safety and well-being
- making sure all care provided is of the highest quality

When you work as a nursing assistant, you will often perform the same duties daily. Remember that these duties are very important. They will make a difference in the health and well-being of those in your care.

Section 1.1 Review and Assessment

Using the Key Terms

Complete the following sentences using the key terms in this section.

1. When someone earns a(n) _____, he or she has completed the necessary education or training to work in a specific field or discipline.
2. A nursing assistant's _____ outlines his or her procedures, actions, and responsibilities as determined by the state.
3. The desire to help another person is called _____.
4. To _____ residents is to give them the power to control their own decision making.
5. Care that integrates the body, mind, and spirit is known as _____.
6. Nursing assistants help measure and record _____, such as blood pressure and pulse.
7. _____ refers to policies and procedures that minimize the risk of spreading infection.
8. The appropriate handling of _____, or dirty, objects is important for controlling infection.

Know and Understand the Facts

9. Discuss the role a holistic nursing assistant has when delivering care.
10. Describe four duties a holistic nursing assistant may perform during a "typical day."
11. List three characteristics of a holistic nursing assistant that you possess.

Analyze and Apply Concepts

12. Explain how OBRA affects the role and responsibilities of a nursing assistant.
13. Describe three actions a person must take to become a certified nursing assistant.
14. Provide a detailed list of five responsibilities you will have as a nursing assistant.

Think Critically

Read the following care situation. Then answer the questions that follow.

Jenny is thinking about becoming a nursing assistant. She has spent time talking with her friends, who are already in a nursing assistant program. Jenny recently found out she will need to successfully complete an education and training program and then pass an examination if she wants to work in this field. She really wants to become a nurse one day, but finds the requirements to become a nursing assistant somewhat overwhelming. Not only is she concerned about how well she will do in the program, but she is also afraid to take the certification competency examination.

15. What advice would you give Jenny to help her achieve her dream of becoming a nursing assistant?
16. How might Jenny decrease her fears about the nursing assistant program and competency certification examination?

Questions to Consider

- Being *professional* means having knowledge and skills that show others you are competent to do a particular job. Being professional also means demonstrating behaviors and attitudes that are positive and supportive of others. Have you ever been in a position where you were asked to be professional? Maybe this happened at a job or at a special meeting you attended.
- What was the experience of being professional like? Did you have to act and dress differently?
- What was your comfort level while acting professional? Is acting in a professional manner something you can do every day, even if it feels uncomfortable?

Objectives

Demonstrating professional qualities and behaviors is essential to delivering safe, quality care. As a nursing assistant, you must also understand the importance of recognizing personal and professional boundaries. To achieve the objectives for this section, you must successfully

- **identify** the qualities and professional behaviors needed to deliver safe, quality care;
- **demonstrate** professional behaviors; and
- **describe** the personal and professional boundaries of a nursing assistant.

Key Terms

Learn these key terms to better understand the information presented in the section.

attitudes
boundaries
Centers for Disease Control and
   Prevention (CDC)
competence
culture

integrity
positive regard
professional
unethical
values
work ethic

What Professional Qualities, Attitudes, and Behaviors Are Expected from a Nursing Assistant?

Being **professional** requires the consistent, daily demonstration of very specific qualities, **attitudes** (ways of thinking or feeling), and behaviors. These are essential to delivering safe, quality care. Because working as a nursing assistant can be challenging, maintaining your professionalism is vital. You may work long hours to provide care for ill residents, but the satisfaction of making a difference in someone else's life can make up for feeling tired and frustrated. To know that your professionalism and work are appreciated and valued is priceless (Figure 1.7).

Professional qualities, attitudes, and behaviors that make a difference in providing holistic care are those that show you are a thoughtful, caring person. These qualities, attitudes, and behaviors demonstrate your respect for the healthcare facility where you work and for the staff with whom you work. They also help you support and promote the independence and well-being of residents.

Possessing the qualities, attitudes, and behaviors discussed in this section will help you deliver safe, quality care; keep your skills up-to-date; and ensure

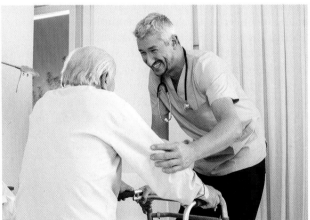

Tyler Olson/Shutterstock.com

Figure 1.7 Being a nursing assistant gives you the opportunity to make a difference in someone's life. Acting professionally allows you to provide the best care possible.

the needs of those in your care are met. The healthcare facility's employee handbook may also include specific expectations and guidelines.

Competence

Competent nursing assistants are able to do their jobs well. When you have **competence**, you have learned everything you need to know to feel comfortable completing required procedures safely and appropriately. You also strive to keep your knowledge and skills up-to-date.

Thoughtful, Caring Approach

Thoughtful, caring holistic nursing assistants are often the most successful. It is important to be aware of your approach, be upbeat, and see the positives in what you do. Having an easygoing attitude and a friendly face sends a message to others that you are open and approachable. It lets others know you can be trusted and may help residents feel more comfortable with you. This approach often decreases resident stress. Remember not to spread rumors, share gossip, or act disrespectfully at work. Those in your care are ill and need a healing environment.

Professional Appearance

It is important to maintain a clean and neat appearance (Figure 1.8). Wearing ironed, clean, wrinkle-free scrubs will help you achieve a professional appearance. Underclothing should not be visible. You can wear a neutral-colored, long-sleeve shirt or sweater under the scrubs if cold.

Hair must be clean. If you have long hair, it must be pulled off your collar and away from your face using an elastic band or clip. If makeup is worn, it should be limited to a simple, neutral application of cosmetics. Fingernails should be clean and trimmed short. If nail polish is worn, healthcare facilities usually require that it be clear. The **Centers for Disease Control and Prevention (CDC)**, a US federal agency that helps prevent and control health threats, has guidelines stating that harmful bacteria may grow under artificial nails. These bacteria may be transferred to residents during care. Therefore, healthcare staff members should not wear artificial nails. Having short, clean nails is not a matter of looks, but rather of safety.

Remember

A professional is someone who can do his best work when he doesn't feel like it.

Alistair Cooke, journalist, author, and broadcaster

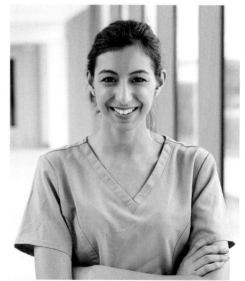

Monkey Business Images/Shutterstock.com

Figure 1.8 Nursing assistants who act professionally look clean and neat. This builds trust with residents and promotes a safe environment.

Body art, such as tattoos, must be covered by clothing. Jewelry should be kept to a minimum—for example, small or stud earrings, a watch, and a simple ring such as a wedding band. Body jewelry, including jewelry in the tongue or eyebrow piercings, must be removed.

Physical Stamina

Being an effective holistic nursing assistant requires that you take care of your own health so you have the *physical stamina*, or strength, to perform the duties of your job. Make sure you eat correctly, exercise, and are mindful of your own well-being.

Respect and Compassion

Holistic nursing assistants understand the importance of treating others with respect and compassion. There are many ways you can show respect for your coworkers and those in your care. A respectful attitude will help you succeed in your position. Having **positive regard**, or an attitude that is supportive and accepting of others, is another way of demonstrating respect.

As a nursing assistant, you may encounter difficult situations that require dignity and compassion. Holistic nursing assistants see residents who are injured, ill, irritable, anxious, lonely, impatient, and depressed. Nursing assistants may also work with residents who are dying. Being compassionate when caring for residents who are dealing with these difficult life events can ease their pain (Figure 1.9). Heartfelt kindness can go a long way.

> ### Remember
>
> *To do what nobody else will do; in a way nobody else can do, in spite of all we go through; that is to be a nurse's aide.*
>
> Anonymous

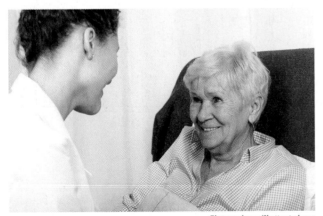

Photographee.eu/Shutterstock.com

Figure 1.9 Nursing assistants promote a healing environment by showing respect and compassion to residents.

Work Ethic, Reliability, and Dependability

It is important to be punctual and arrive to work on time. This demonstrates a positive **work ethic**, or belief in the importance of work. You are responsible to your coworkers and those in your care to be ready for work when you are scheduled. Be thorough, follow policies, immediately let licensed nursing staff know when you observe any changes in a patient's or resident's condition, and be accurate and timely in your reporting and documentation.

Trustworthiness

Both your coworkers and those in your care will appreciate working with someone they can trust. Be trustworthy by keeping information confidential and recording it in the proper place. You must take this part of your role and responsibilities very seriously. It is your legal and ethical responsibility to protect personal and medical information.

Honesty and Integrity

Honesty and **integrity** (strong moral principles) are vital to resident safety. If you make a mistake, you must always tell the truth about what happened. Do not try to cover up the mistake. Residents' health and well-being depend on your honesty. No matter how busy you are or how unimportant you think information is, never leave out details or information about a patient's or resident's condition or about care given when reporting or documenting.

Flexibility

Being able to complete a wide range of duties and being able to work independently, when appropriate, are important qualities for any holistic nursing assistant. You may see different residents every day, so become accustomed to adjusting to change and to working with new people. You should also be flexible about your schedule, as you may have to work different hours every week, long shifts, or odd hours.

Teamwork

Always work toward being a productive, helpful, and supportive member of the healthcare team. Be aware of and sensitive to ways you can assist other staff. Supporting your coworkers will help increase the quality of your care. This also pays off when other staff members reciprocate and help you when you need assistance.

Positive Relationships

When you provide care, you will often have close contact with residents' family members, friends, and significant others. Establishing positive relationships with these people will help you provide quality care and create a positive, healing environment. Be calm, kind, supportive, and ready to help when needed. Remember to enjoy what you are doing. A positive attitude will improve the quality of care you provide.

Communication Skills

As a holistic nursing assistant, seek to understand the differences and diversity of those in your care. Be courteous and communicate clearly and directly when interacting with others in person, on the phone, or by e-mail. Also ensure that documentation is well written and easily understood. *Nonverbal communication*, such as gestures and body language, must be considered and should be appropriate to the people you are speaking with and to the situation. You will learn more about developing strong communication skills in chapter 10.

Being professional means putting the resident first. No matter the circumstances, never let your personal feelings and needs get in the way of providing quality care. Being professional also means maintaining high standards. Nursing assistants who act in a professional manner will earn reputations as being people who seek the best for those in their care. Acting in a professional manner at work will allow you to relax during your free time, knowing you have done a good job.

Residents depend on holistic nursing assistants. When you are a nursing assistant, residents will put their trust in you. Therefore, you must demonstrate the professional qualities, attitudes, and behaviors you would want to see in somebody who was caring for you or your loved one.

What Are Personal and Professional Boundaries?

As a holistic nursing assistant, you will be expected to demonstrate professional behaviors and establish helping and caring relationships with patients and residents. **Boundaries**, or accepted and expected limits on behavior or actions, are a fundamental aspect of all relationships. Both personal and professional boundaries exist for everyone, and particularly for nursing assistants, regardless of the healthcare facility. Therefore, when acting within one's role as a nursing assistant, you must recognize and maintain these boundaries. Maintaining personal and professional boundaries will help you establish appropriate relationships with patients and residents and their families (Figure 1.10).

Personal Boundaries

Personal boundaries allow you to protect and take care of yourself. Some personal boundaries, such as not allowing personal abuse or violence, are rigid and absolute. Other personal boundaries, such as allowing an acquaintance to use your cell phone, are more flexible and often need to be worked out between the people in a relationship. Setting personal boundaries lets others know what is acceptable and what the consequences may be if boundaries are crossed.

Professional Boundaries

Professional boundaries are specific to delivering care and are part of a nursing assistant's legal scope of practice. Professional boundaries distinguish helping behaviors from behaviors that are not helpful. Behaviors that are not helpful, such as focusing on yourself rather than on a resident, cross or violate professional boundaries. When boundaries are crossed or violated, an unhealthy relationship can develop.

Crossing and Violating Boundaries

There is a difference between crossing a boundary and violating a boundary, although both actions are inappropriate. Brief, nonhelpful acts or behaviors *cross* boundaries. An example of crossing a boundary would be doing something thoughtless or saying something inappropriate, such as telling a resident about the details of your date last night. Acts or behaviors that meet your needs, but not the needs

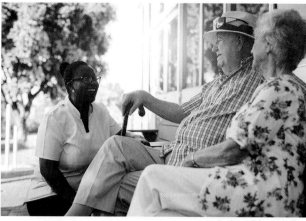

Jacob Lund/Shutterstock.com

Figure 1.10 As a nursing assistant, you will want to establish relationships with both the resident and his or her family.

of those in your care, *violate* boundaries. Boundary violations are **unethical** (not in line with accepted rules of conduct), are harmful, and in some cases, are considered criminal behavior.

Following are some signals that indicate you may be crossing or violating a boundary:

- You think a lot about a patient or resident when you are not at work.
- You choose sides with a patient or resident against his or her family or other staff members.
- You trade assignments with other staff members so you can provide care for a specific patient or resident.
- You share inappropriate personal information.
- You flirt or make sexual comments.
- You share secrets.
- You receive personal gifts after the patient or resident has left the healthcare facility.
- You act in a verbally or physically abusive way.

It is always the holistic nursing assistant's responsibility to maintain both personal and professional boundaries. To do this, use the following guidelines:

- Act and communicate professionally at all times.
- Do not visit or spend extra time with a patient or resident who is not part of your work assignment.
- Do not use offensive language.
- Do not make sexual comments or jokes.
- Use touch appropriately.
- Do not accept gifts, loans, money, or other valuables.
- Do not give gifts, loans, or money.
- Do not share personal or financial information.

Holistic nursing assistants are expected to act in the best interest of those they care for and to always respect the dignity of others. This means that a nursing assistant should never seek personal gain at anyone's expense.

The best way to ensure that your care is within professional boundaries is to be aware of and knowledgeable about appropriate boundaries, to have integrity, and to work as a professional.

Remember

Appropriate boundaries create integrity.

Anonymous

Using the Key Terms

Complete the following sentences using the key terms in this section.

1. Boundary violations, such as the exchange of gifts or money, could be considered _____, or not in line with rules of conduct.

2. A nursing assistant's _____—which is made up of traditions, beliefs, rituals, customs, and values that are learned over time—influences how he or she delivers care and interacts with patients.

3. Showing up on time, maintaining respectfulness, and being reliable and responsible all demonstrate a strong _____.

4. Being supportive and accepting of others, which is known as having _____, is one of the many ways you can show respect for your coworkers and those in your care.

5. A nursing assistant who demonstrates an expected level of excellence in behavior, attitude, and practice, even in challenging and demanding situations, could be described as being _____.

6. Establishing _____ helps nursing assistants determine what is personally and professionally acceptable in their relationships with patients.

7. Omitting details or information about a patient's or resident's condition displays a lack of _____.

Know and Understand the Facts

8. Identify three professional qualities, attitudes, or characteristics that demonstrate a nursing assistant's caring.

9. List two professional behaviors nursing assistants can demonstrate to show they are competent in delivering care.

10. Describe two examples of professional boundary violations.

Analyze and Apply Concepts

11. Discuss three challenges or obstacles a holistic nursing assistant may encounter in demonstrating professional behaviors. Explain how these obstacles can be overcome.

12. Identify three of your personal boundaries and explain how you maintain them.

13. Explain three guidelines that help nursing assistants maintain professional boundaries.

Think Critically

Read the following care situation. Then answer the questions that follow.

Mrs. F has been ill for a long time. Yesterday she was admitted to a long-term care facility because she had pneumonia. Mrs. F had been living with her daughter, who was widowed last year and is still grieving. Mrs. F found it difficult living with her daughter because Mrs. F has always enjoyed her independence. It was also hard for Mrs. F to deal with her daughter's aggressive behavior. Mrs. F's daughter liked to tell her what to do.

When you introduce yourself to Mrs. F, she turns her back to you and speaks in a harsh voice, saying she hates being in this facility. You can tell Mrs. F is not breathing well. When you go to help, Mrs. F says she does not want you to give her any care this morning. She would rather sleep, so she asks you not to touch her and to stay away.

14. What professional qualities, attitudes, and behaviors would you need to demonstrate in this situation to ensure Mrs. F is provided quality care?

15. What should you report to licensed nursing staff about Mrs. F's behavior?

16. What personal or professional boundaries should you be aware of when caring for Mrs. F?

Key Points

Reviewing the key points for this chapter will help you practice more safely and competently as a holistic nursing assistant and will help you prepare for the certification competency examination.

- The nursing assistant is a member of a healthcare team and provides holistic nursing care under the supervision of an LPN/LVN or an RN.

- Nursing assistants must complete a specific education or training program and pass a certification competency exam to practice as certified nursing assistants (CNAs).

- Holistic nursing assistants provide holistic care, which integrates the body, mind, and spirit. The Providing Holistic Care Framework outlines the components of holistic care.

- The primary responsibility of a nursing assistant is to provide safe, quality care to residents.

- Holistic nursing assistants must act in a professional, ethical manner at all times.

- Nursing assistants must recognize and maintain boundaries that establish appropriate limits in their relationships with residents and their families. Behaviors that violate these boundaries are typically considered unethical, harmful, and in some cases, illegal.

Action Steps to Holistic Care

Review the information in this chapter. Complete the following activities.

1. Select two responsibilities of holistic nursing assistants. Prepare a short paper or digital presentation that identifies and describes two challenges a nursing assistant may encounter.

2. With a partner, select one professional boundary. Prepare a poster that illustrates at least three facts other nursing assistants should know about this boundary.

3. Find two pictures in a magazine, in a newspaper, or online that demonstrate professional behavior. Discuss why you believe these images represent professionalism.

4. Research the requirements and scope of practice for nursing assistants in your state. Write a brief report that includes this information and two new facts not discussed in this chapter.

5. With a partner, write a song or poem about holistic care and its impact on residents. Include the reasons why holistic care is important, some of the responsibilities of a holistic nursing assistant, and include information about professionalism and maintaining boundaries.

Preparing for the Certification Competency Examination

To prepare for the nursing assistant certification competency examination, you will need to know content found in this chapter. This content may be tested in the knowledge (written or oral) and skills (hands-on demonstration) portions of the exam. The following areas will be emphasized:

- the nursing assistant's role
- the functions, roles, and responsibilities of nursing assistants
- characteristics of professional behavior

These sample test questions are similar to ones you will find on the certification competency exam. See how well you can answer them. Be sure to select the *best* answer.

1. A nursing assistant who presents a professional appearance
    A. wears a red, printed shirt under her scrubs
    B. keeps her hair below her collar
    C. wears her engagement ring with her wedding band
    D. has short, clean fingernails and wears clear nail polish

2. Nursing assistants who demonstrate caring skills have
    A. an awareness of their strengths
    B. a good exercise plan, which they follow
    C. a habit of reading a great deal
    D. a good diet

(continued)

3. Which of the following must nursing assistants do to become certified?
    A. work in a long-term care facility for a minimum of two years
    B. be in good physical condition
    C. complete an approved education or training program and pass the certification competency exam
    D. receive two positive professional character recommendations

4. What does the term *residents* mean?
    A. people cared for in hospitals
    B. people cared for in hospices
    C. people cared for at home
    D. people cared for in long-term care facilities

5. Which of the following is an example of a boundary violation by a nursing assistant?
    A. taking too much time at a resident's bedside
    B. accepting gifts after a resident has left the facility
    C. putting residents' personal items in the bedside table
    D. helping a resident's family member contact a community resource

6. When nursing assistants provide holistic care, they integrate
    A. body, mind, and spirit
    B. care with medication
    C. therapy with care
    D. culture, ethnicity, and values

7. A nursing assistant with several years of experience has been difficult to work with the last few days. Which of the following approaches could you use to model professional behavior?
    A. tell the nursing assistant that she needs to be more cheerful
    B. ask the nursing assistant if you can help her
    C. report the nursing assistant's behavior
    D. stay away from the nursing assistant

8. Which of the following healthcare staff members supervises nursing assistants?
    A. doctor
    B. therapist
    C. counselor
    D. licensed nurse

9. Which of the following is *not* a professional boundary violation?
    A. visiting with a resident in your care during your shift
    B. accepting a gift from a family member after a resident is discharged
    C. sharing pictures and stories about your family with residents
    D. defending a resident's desires to his or her family members

10. A nursing assistant is really angry at a nurse on his team. What is the most professional way for him to deal with his anger?
    A. He should post his angry feelings on his blog as soon as he can.
    B. He should ask his supervisor if she can meet with him.
    C. He should send an e-mail message to his supervisor and express his anger.
    D. He should do nothing and just avoid the nurse whenever he can.

11. Which of the following behaviors would lead staff at a local long-term care facility to call a new nursing assistant professional?
    A. working many shifts
    B. leaving work early
    C. maintaining high standards of care
    D. working as quickly as possible

12. Mr. J has been a resident at the city's rehabilitation facility for nearly four weeks. During the last week, he has appeared lonely and depressed. What might a holistic nursing assistant do to support him?
    A. increase his activities
    B. give him snacks several times a day
    C. let him stay in his room longer
    D. ask him about the change in his behavior

13. Which of the following describes OBRA?
    A. a rare disease
    B. a law that standardizes nursing assistant training and education requirements
    C. a law that protects nursing assistants from working in unsafe conditions
    D. a procedure used to prevent residents from falling

14. For which of the following is a new nursing assistant *not* responsible?
    A. helping residents with ADLs
    B. assisting residents with ambulation
    C. discussing residents' conditions with their families
    D. documenting care given in residents' charts

15. When holistic nursing assistants are supportive and accepting of others, they exhibit
    A. competence
    B. values
    C. integrity
    D. positive regard

Did you have difficulty with any of the questions? If you did, review the chapter to find the correct answer(s).

Welcome to the Chapter

This chapter provides information about how healthcare is delivered in the United States. Over the past 200 years, US healthcare has advanced greatly. Today, there are a variety of healthcare facilities and ways care is delivered and funded. Understanding healthcare delivery, the types of facilities available, and the services offered, will give you a strong foundation to be successful as a holistic nursing assistant. It will also provide you with important information for determining where you might like to work when you become a nursing assistant. This chapter also provides information about the organizational structures within a healthcare facility and healthcare facility culture.

What you learn in this chapter will help you develop your knowledge and skills to become a holistic nursing assistant. The topics discussed in the chapter are highlighted on the Providing Holistic Care Framework.

You are now ready to start this chapter, *Understanding Healthcare*.

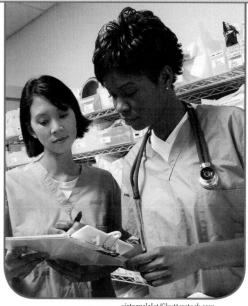

sirtravelalot/Shutterstock.com

Chapter Outline

Section 2.1
Healthcare Delivery

Section 2.2
Structure and Culture in Healthcare Facilities

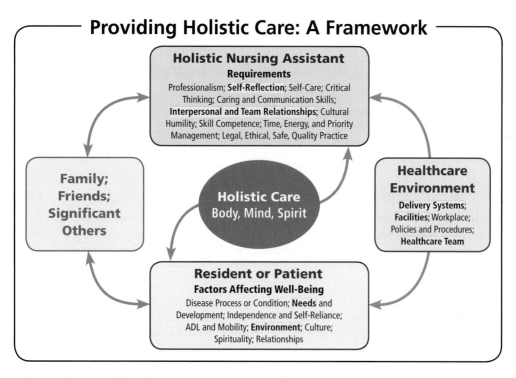

Providing Holistic Care: A Framework

Holistic Nursing Assistant
Requirements
Professionalism; **Self-Reflection**; Self-Care; Critical Thinking; Caring and Communication Skills; **Interpersonal and Team Relationships**; Cultural Humility; Skill Competence; Time, Energy, and Priority Management; Legal, Ethical, Safe, Quality Practice

Family; Friends; Significant Others

Holistic Care
Body, Mind, Spirit

Healthcare Environment
Delivery Systems; Facilities; Workplace; Policies and Procedures; **Healthcare Team**

Resident or Patient
Factors Affecting Well-Being
Disease Process or Condition; **Needs** and Development; Independence and Self-Reliance; ADL and Mobility; **Environment**; Culture; Spirituality; Relationships

Questions to Consider

- Have you, a member of your family, or a friend been a patient in a healthcare facility? If so, what type of facility was it? What was the experience like?
- Describe the services the facility offered. Did the services provided help you or others get well?

Objectives

Understanding how healthcare is delivered is essential to providing the best possible care. Learning how healthcare and different types of healthcare facilities developed over time will enable you to better understand today's healthcare systems and the way healthcare is funded. To achieve the objectives for this section, you must successfully

- **list** important medical milestones and healthcare leaders who influenced US healthcare delivery;
- **describe** the levels or categories of care;
- **identify** a variety of healthcare facilities; and
- **describe** how healthcare is funded.

Key Terms

Learn these key terms to better understand the information presented in the section.

acute care	Medicaid
chronic care	Medicare
co-payment	premium
epidemic	primary care provider (PCP)
deductible	private insurance
dementia	Social Security
diabetes mellitus	stem cell
healthcare	subacute care
healthcare facility	trauma
healthcare services	vaccine
immunization	wellness
managed care	

Think About This

In the very early days of healthcare delivery, barber-surgeons could perform minor surgical procedures, pull teeth, and amputate limbs. They could also give enemas, as well as cut hair and shave or trim facial hair. The red-and-white pole, used as a symbol in front of a barbershop, actually signifies the blood and the napkins used to clean up after *bloodletting* (a medical practice believed to eliminate disease).

How Has History Influenced Healthcare Delivery?

The delivery of **healthcare** in the United States has not always been what we experience today. In fact, it was not until the early part of the twentieth century that healthcare was delivered as part of an organized system. Before this time, healthcare was typically delivered in small communities by family members, some trained doctors, or even the local barber.

The Advancement of Healthcare and Medicine

Over time, phenomenal growth in healthcare was made possible by several remarkable medical discoveries and by the passion of early healthcare leaders, both in the United States and in other countries. These advances allowed the delivery of healthcare to evolve into what we know today.

The 1800s

Increased understanding of disease greatly improved medical care in the 1800s. In the mid-1800s, Hungarian doctor Ignaz Semmelweis introduced the practice of doctors washing their hands between patients. This practice significantly reduced death, particularly during childbirth, where infections were often transferred to previously healthy new mothers (Figure 2.1).

The discovery of germs as the cause of disease by Louis Pasteur furthered Semmelweis's mission to improve hygiene practices in healthcare. Florence Nightingale also advocated for sanitary medical facilities, better hygiene, and proper nutrition, particularly during wartime (Figure 2.2). In the late 1860s, Nightingale established a nursing school in London. Today, she is considered the founder of modern nursing after successfully demonstrating the value of nurses and their positive impact on patient health outcomes.

After English doctor Edward Jenner successfully administered the first vaccine against smallpox in 1796, the development of other vaccines continued throughout the nineteenth century. **Vaccines** are injections or oral medications that introduce a mild form of a disease so the body builds immunity, or *resistance*, to the disease. The vaccines developed in the 1800s provided **immunization**, or protection, against diseases such as cholera, anthrax, rabies, and typhoid fever.

Other healthcare advances made during this time include

- the development of aspirin by Felix Hoffmann;
- the invention of the stethoscope and hypodermic syringe; and
- Wilhelm Röntgen's discovery of X-rays.

The 1900s

Throughout the 1900s, vaccines were developed for diseases such as diphtheria, whooping cough, tetanus, tuberculosis, measles, mumps, rubella, chicken pox, pneumonia, and meningitis. A vaccine was also developed in the mid-1960s by Dr. Jonas Salk to protect children from polio, a life-threatening disease that had previously left many paralyzed. Prior to the development of these vaccines, many of these diseases caused **epidemics**, where a large number of people became very sick or even died.

In addition to these life-saving vaccines, many other medications were developed during the 1900s. Insulin was discovered and used to control **diabetes mellitus**, a disorder characterized by excessive glucose (sugar) in a person's blood. Penicillin was first discovered by Sir Alexander Fleming in 1928, but was not used to treat bacterial infections until the 1940s, when it was made into a powdered form that could be used as a medicine.

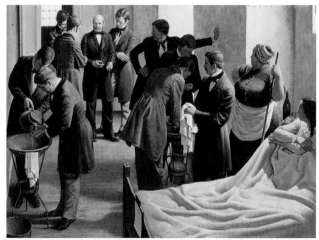

From the collection of Michigan Medicine, University of Michigan, Gift of Pfizer, UMHS. 26

Figure 2.1 Before Ignaz Semmelweis introduced the practice of hand washing between patients, doctors' hands often transferred germs from sick patients to patients who were previously healthy.

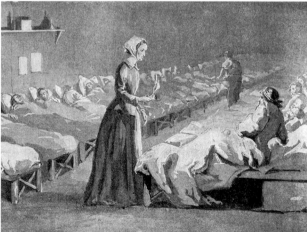

Everett Historical/Shutterstock.com

Figure 2.2 Florence Nightingale served as a nurse during the Crimean War, during which she improved hygiene practices. She also established the first school of nursing and is considered the founder of modern nursing.

Many other healthcare advances occurred during this time:

- Band-Aids® were invented.
- Cardiopulmonary resuscitation (CPR) was developed by Dr. Peter Safar.
- The first iron lung was used for respiratory failure and was powered by two household vacuum cleaners (Figure 2.3).
- The first blood bank was established.
- The artificial kidney dialysis machine was invented.
- Bill Wilson and Dr. Robert Smith founded Alcoholics Anonymous, a 12-step program that helps people overcome problems with alcohol and achieve sobriety.
- The first human heart transplant was performed by Dr. Christiaan Barnard.
- Dr. Henry Heimlich developed the use of an abdominal thrust, now known as the *Heimlich maneuver*, to clear blocked airways.
- The first cases of human immunodeficiency virus (HIV) were identified in the United States.
- The first US child conceived using in vitro fertilization (IVF) was born. IVF is a process in which an egg cell is fertilized outside of the body and then inserted into a woman's uterus (Figure 2.4).

The 2000s

Technology is now commonly used in all healthcare facilities. For example, electronic health records (EHRs), rather than paper-and-pen charting, ensure the standardization of policies and procedures and more accurate documentation. Detailed information about the use of EHRs, EMRs, and documentation can be found in chapter 13.

In addition to these developments, the following also influence healthcare delivery today:

- Robotics are used for many different types of surgery (Figure 2.5).
- Research involving **stem cells** (human cells that can become specific tissues or organ cells) offers new possibilities for treating diseases by replacing diseased cells with healthy cells. This research will also lead to the development of better ways to provide medical therapies such as bone marrow transplants.
- The groundbreaking Human Genome Project mapped approximately 30,000 genes in human deoxyribonucleic acid (DNA). The human genome may help researchers identify damaged genes that cause genetic disorders and possibly eliminate these disorders.

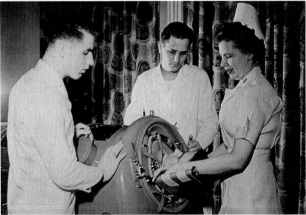

National Library of Medicine

Figure 2.3 The first iron lung was powered by two household vacuum cleaners.

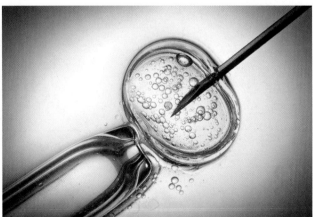

nevodka/Shutterstock.com

Figure 2.4 In vitro fertilization (IVF) is a process in which the female egg cell is fertilized outside of the body and then inserted into a woman's uterus.

- Evidence-based research (actions based on facts) is now used consistently to make medical decisions.

These and many other medical discoveries and leaders forged the path to establish what is known today as modern healthcare.

The Development of Healthcare Facilities

Medical advances have not only influenced *how* healthcare is delivered, but also *where* it is delivered. Starting in the early 1920s, increasing numbers of **healthcare facilities** were established. Hospitals replaced homes, for example, as places to treat the ill.

As time passed, the number of hospitals increased. By the 1940s and 1950s, hospitals were being built across the United States (Figure 2.6). The growth of hospitals was motivated by the Lanham Act of 1941, which provided government assistance money for housing, community facilities, and improvements in communities that had national programs that aided the war effort (World War II).

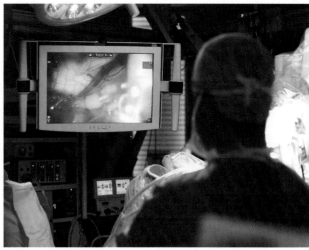

Figure 2.5 Surgeons now use robotic equipment to perform minimally invasive surgeries.

The Hill-Burton Act of 1946 continued the growth of healthcare facilities by providing federal funding to existing hospitals and other healthcare facilities. The goal of the Hill-Burton Act was to determine if these facilities were able to provide the care needed in a certain area, and to build new facilities where there was a need. The Act also required that any services provided be available to anyone who needed care.

By the late 1950s, the number of healthcare facilities had increased so much that better planning was needed. In 1974, a *certificate of need* was required before a healthcare facility could be built. The certificate of need was created to prevent overbuilding of healthcare facilities in areas where services were not needed. Today, some states still require certificates of need, while others do not. Either way, today there are over 5,000 hospitals in the United States (Figure 2.7).

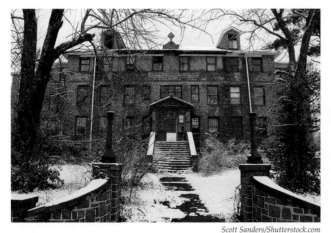

Figure 2.6 This is an example of what the first hospitals looked like. The architecture has certainly changed over time as technology and the needs of patients evolve.

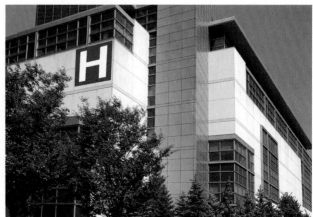

Figure 2.7 Modern hospitals meet the ever-evolving needs of patients. Hospitals today are also built to incorporate new technologies.

What Types of Healthcare Facilities Are Available in the United States?

There are many different types of **healthcare services** available to those who need care; these services are provided by healthcare facilities. Healthcare facilities fall into three levels, or categories, of care:

1. **Primary care:** the initial medical care a person receives at a doctor's office or a medical clinic. Primary care is used to treat an illness or disease.

2. **Secondary care:** care that only focuses on the prevention of disease or the promotion of health and **wellness** (well-being). This might include immunization, health education, or health screening. This care might occur in a community or public health clinic or even in a pharmacy.

3. **Tertiary care:** highly specialized care, such as treating **trauma** (serious injury or shock), burns, or cancer. This type of care is typically found in hospitals or medical centers.

Healthcare delivery may also be categorized as acute, subacute, or chronic. **Acute care** refers to serious, critical, or surgical care. Acute care is typically received in hospitals. **Subacute care** is provided to a person who has a moderate-to-severe illness, injury, or recurrence of a disease, but who does not require the level of care delivered at a hospital. Often subacute care is given in a specialty facility, or in a long-term care or skilled nursing facility, to people who have a serious episode of a chronic illness or who need intense rehabilitation due to a surgery.

Chronic care applies to those who have a long-term disease or illness that may never go away. Examples of chronic diseases include diabetes; heart or respiratory diseases; conditions that occur at birth, such as cerebral palsy; or diseases of older adults, such as **dementia** (severe loss of mental capacity). Chronic care is often provided in doctors' offices, outpatient clinics, rehabilitation centers, long-term care facilities, or even in people's homes.

Hospitals

Hospitals, or *medical centers*, are healthcare facilities that primarily provide acute care. There are three ways to classify hospitals:

1. not-for-profit: do not have to pay taxes

2. for-profit: owned by investors

3. public: funded by federal, state, or local governments. County and veterans hospitals are examples of public hospitals.

Hospitals also vary by size and location. Some hospitals are very small and may be located in rural communities, while others are large and found in cities. Large hospitals may be part of a system of hospitals that spans a state or several states.

Hospitals are typically described according to their inpatient bed capacity. For example, a hospital may have a 150-bed capacity. The state determines how many beds, called *licensed beds*, a hospital is authorized to have. A hospital that has a maximum of 150 licensed beds is only allowed to care for up to 150 patients at one time.

Some hospitals are also educational facilities, training future doctors and nurses to practice, while others focus on research. Specialty hospitals also exist, providing services such as women's health, cancer treatment, surgery, or rehabilitation. Other hospitals may take only certain patients, such as those with mental health disorders, children (as in pediatric hospitals), or prisoners.

Think About This

The American Hospital Association reports that there are 5,564 hospitals in the United States. Approximately 51 percent of these facilities are not-for-profit hospitals, 19 percent are for-profit hospitals, and 18 percent are state or local government hospitals. The remaining facilities are a combination of federal, psychiatric, long-term care, and prison hospitals.

Another type of hospital is a Critical Access Hospital (CAH). This title is given to rural hospitals by the Centers for Medicare and Medicaid Services (CMS) when a hospital meets certain requirements and standards. The purpose is to reduce financial challenges faced by rural hospitals and improve healthcare access. Examples of CAH requirements include a location more than 35 miles from another hospital, 25 or fewer acute-care inpatient beds, and appropriately staffed 24/7 emergency care services.

The primary purpose of hospitals is to provide inpatient, tertiary care for people who have a severe illness or who have experienced trauma that requires surgery or emergency care. When a patient enters the hospital, many services are available to him or her (Figure 2.8). These services may include

- nursing, medical, surgical, and critical care services;
- trauma center services (some are designated as Level 1, providing quick, complex surgery and care for the seriously injured; others may be at a Level 5, providing only assessment and referral);
- laboratory and medical imaging (radiology);
- pharmacy and central services for supplies and equipment;
- rehabilitation services and respiratory therapy; and
- social services, dietary services, and environmental services.

There are a variety of other healthcare facilities that deliver care outside of hospitals or medical centers.

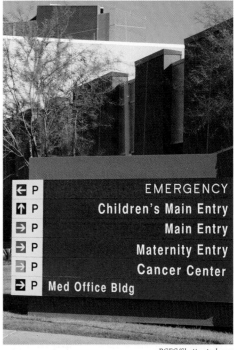

BCFC/Shutterstock.com

Figure 2.8 Many hospitals include multiple areas or buildings, such as specific areas for maternity care, pediatric care, and care for cancer patients.

Doctors' Offices

Doctors' offices are staffed with **primary care providers (PCPs)**. Primary care providers may include family practice doctors, internal medicine doctors, nurse practitioners, or physician assistants. These healthcare providers may practice individually or in an office that has a group of several providers. These offices may also have RNs, LPNs/LVNs, certified medical assistants (CMAs), and laboratory or other diagnostic and supportive care staff.

Outpatient or Community Clinics

Outpatient clinics or centers and community clinics provide preventive and wellness care. These clinics may be a part of a hospital system or funded by a city, county, or state community or government public health organization. Services offered include annual specialized exams for women (called *well-woman exams*); dental care; and care for the chronically ill, such as dialysis (an artificial means of removing waste and excess water from the blood of patients with acute kidney disease or kidney failure).

Some outpatient or community clinics have a specific purpose. There are outpatient public health clinics that provide only health screenings or immunizations, as well as clinics that provide specific care for those in pain, known as *pain management clinics*. Other clinics offer physical or occupational therapy for people who need to relearn lost abilities. Certain other clinics provide special services such as family planning, birthing, or fertility treatments.

Clinics may be fully funded by the government and offer services for free. They may also use a sliding scale so that patients pay what they can afford or they may have set fees in place. Clinics may be freestanding or part of the services provided by a hospital.

Urgent-Care Centers

Urgent-care centers are sometimes known as *convenient* or *immediate-care centers*. These facilities treat people with short-term, acute-care needs such as colds, viruses, fractures, sprains, or other minor injuries. Some of these centers are open 24 hours a day, seven days a week.

Surgical Centers

Surgical centers, or *surgicenters,* offer a limited range of surgical and diagnostic procedures. These services may include cosmetic surgeries, cataract removals, biopsies (surgical excisions of body tissue samples for diagnosis), hernia repairs, or colonoscopies (diagnostic examinations of the small and large intestines). Surgical centers may be freestanding or may be services provided within a hospital.

Skilled Nursing Facilities

People who need around-the-clock care and rehabilitation for conditions such as a stroke, fractured hip, or knee-replacement surgery can be cared for at a skilled nursing facility. Stays at skilled nursing facilities are often short. The goal is to help patients become well enough to return to their homes and function effectively.

Residential Care Facilities

There are a variety of levels of residential care facilities that provide services 24 hours per day, seven days a week. Depending on state laws and the services provided, residential care facilities may need to be licensed by the state and have licensed nursing staff. The levels of residential care facilities include

- **Independent living:** residents must be independent in all ADLs, be ambulatory, be mentally alert, and have bowel and bladder control. Facilities may include apartments, condominiums, or town houses. Some residents enter independent living and then move to a setting that provides additional care due to changes in their ability to function as they age.

    - **Assisted living:** residents may live in their own apartments, which are equipped with emergency devices to alert licensed nursing staff in a central location if help is needed. Services also offered may include dining rooms, recreational activities, transportation, and housekeeping.

    - **Continuing care:** these are retirement communities that offer multilevel care, such as skilled nursing care, assisted living, or independent living. Care depends on residents' needs, which may change over time.

    - **Residential care:** sometimes called *personal care homes, sheltered housing,* or *domiciliary care homes,* these facilities are for people who need ongoing assistance with personal care or medical needs, but who require only moderate assistance and supervision. These facilities range from apartments to shared rooms and provide services such as a central dining room.

    - **Long-term care facilities:** sometimes called *nursing homes,* these facilities are designed to care for residents who can no longer take care of themselves. These residents need medical and nursing care, as well as varying assistance with ADLs, ambulation, feeding, and elimination (Figure 2.9). Some facilities also have memory care units for those residents with dementia. Most people who enter long-term care stay there for the remainder of their lives.

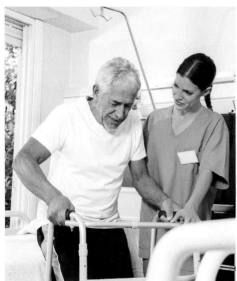

Tyler Olson/Shutterstock.com

Figure 2.9 In long-term care facilities, nursing assistants helps residents with ADLs. This nursing assistant is helping with ambulation.

Hospices

As you learned in chapter 1, hospice provides care for terminally ill people who have a life expectancy of six months or less. Care may be provided at a residential hospice center, in the home, or in a long-term care facility. In addition to general care services, hospices provide pain relief, grief counseling, family caregiver support, and assistance during the grieving process.

Home Healthcare Services

Home healthcare does not provide care in a facility. Instead, care is delivered exclusively in the home. Home healthcare services employ different levels of skilled nursing services, including RNs, LPNs/LVNs, CNAs, caregivers, and home health aides, as well as nonskilled workers. Home healthcare services may offer companion care, which includes reminding patients to take their medications; cooking meals and feeding; performing light housekeeping; running errands; escorting to appointments; assisting with pet care; and providing conversation or entertainment, such as reading or playing games. Home healthcare also offers respite care, which gives family members a break or time off from caring for those who are confined to their beds or dying. All of these services are provided in a person's home (Figure 2.10). In addition, skilled nursing services such as monitoring blood pressure or providing wound care are usually prescribed by doctors, and visits to provide these services may occur daily, weekly, or monthly.

Pharmacies

Pharmacies are responsible for filling, dispensing, and refilling prescriptions (Figure 2.11). In addition, licensed pharmacy staff members also provide information about medications, including any side effects and interaction between different medications.

Laboratories and Medical Imaging Facilities

Laboratories and medical imaging facilities provide assistance with the diagnosis of a disease or condition and help doctors determine if a patient is getting better. The diagnostic procedures these facilities conduct may include checking a patient's blood or taking an X-ray. These facilities may be freestanding or may be services provided within a hospital, a clinic, or a doctor's office.

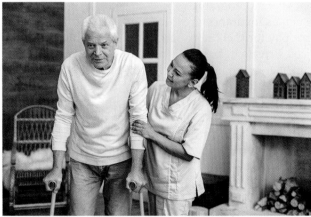

YAKOBCHUK VIACHESLAV/Shutterstock.com

Figure 2.10 Home healthcare services provide healthcare in a person's home, which promotes independence and an environment that is more comfortable.

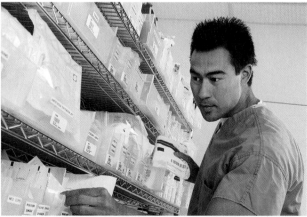

sirtravelalot/Shutterstock.com

Figure 2.11 Pharmacies employ healthcare staff authorized to dispense and explain medications.

How Is Healthcare Funded?

Early in the history of US healthcare, people typically paid cash or bartered (traded goods and services) for their healthcare services. As formal healthcare facilities were developed, how people would pay for healthcare came into question. It was at this time that both public funding and private insurance emerged as options for paying healthcare costs.

Public programs, because they are funded and administered by the federal and state government, are always influenced by changing healthcare needs, the availability of financial resources, and congressional and executive office directions. As a result, how public programs are structured and what healthcare benefits are offered often changes over time. Changes regarding private insurance also occur often, sometimes annually. On an ongoing basis, private insurance companies evaluate the healthcare needs of those they cover and the costs of providing healthcare services. Private insurance companies also take into consideration the financial relationships they have with those who provide healthcare and with employers who offer insurance coverage for employees.

Public funding today includes Medicare, Medicaid, the Children's Health Insurance Program (CHIP), and coverage under the Affordable Care Act (ACA). The Centers for Medicare & Medicaid Services (CMS) is a federal agency that provides the administration, resources, and information for Medicare and the Children's Health Insurance Program (CHIP); works with states to provide administration and support for Medicaid; and provides the resources, standards, and information for the Health Insurance Marketplace (part of the ACA). CMS also develops and sets standards to ensure quality care, provides guidance and education, and tracks and publishes information on specific statistics that inform the users and the public about the usage and effectiveness of its programs.

Private insurance today, such as insurance provided through Blue Cross® Blue Shield® or Aetna®, helps people pay for their care, particularly hospitalization and other related healthcare services. Private insurance is paid ahead of time, ensuring that a person is covered in case he or she needs to use healthcare services. Most employers provide group healthcare insurance as one of their employee benefits. Over the years, the cost of these plans has increased, causing some employers to ask their employees to pay for more of these costs. The amount of money a person is required to pay out-of-pocket to cover healthcare costs is called a **deductible**. Many private insurance plans have **co-payments**, which are fixed amounts that a person pays for specific medical services, such as for a doctor's visit. In these situations, the insurance company pays part of the total fee, but not all of it.

Medicare

In 1965, the US Congress established Medicare and Medicaid, two public programs that help fund healthcare for specific individuals. **Medicare** is a health insurance program for people 65 years and older. The funding for Medicare comes from taxes paid to the federal government. Part of every employee's pay is deducted from his or her paycheck to help fund Medicare.

Medicare is considered a prospective payment system (PPS) because payment to providers for healthcare services is based on a predetermined, fixed amount. This amount is determined by using a classification of services. For example, diagnosis-related groups (DRGs) are categories used when paying for hospital services such as surgeries. The removal of a gallbladder, for example, is priced at a certain amount, and that amount is all that is paid to the hospital by Medicare, even if the hospital charges more than that amount for that service.

The federal government also makes automatic paycheck deductions to fund **Social Security**, a program that provides retirement benefits, disability coverage, dependent coverage, and survivor benefits. Employee contributions to Medicare and Social Security are mandatory, and employers are also required to pay into these programs. As a result, any US citizen who works a minimum of 10 years qualifies for Social Security and Medicare benefits as soon as he or she turns 65 (Figure 2.12).

Medicare Coverage

Medicare is divided into different parts. Part A covers care given in a hospital, skilled nursing facility, nursing home, or hospice, as well as home healthcare services. Part B is medical insurance that covers medically necessary services performed by doctors in their offices or in an outpatient setting. Part B also covers preventive services such as flu shots. Medicare also has a Part C, which is called Medicare Advantage Plans. Part C is a contracted plan between Medicare and a private company; the private company provides both Parts A and B of Medicare and may also offer prescription drug services. Additionally, Medicare has a Part D, which adds prescription drug coverage offered by insurance or private companies approved by Medicare.

Supplementing Medicare Coverage

Medicare will cover most of the cost of a hospital stay. For example, consider the case of a senior who needs to have his arthritic hip replaced. Medicare will cover the cost of the hospital stay, the walker he will need to use after surgery, and any physical therapy or rehabilitation care needed after his hospital stay. If the patient is not well enough to return home after a specified period of time, however, he may need to move to an assisted living or long-term care facility. In that case, only a portion (or possibly none) of the costs of the long-term care may be paid for by Medicare.

Supplemental, or additional, private insurance plans are available to take care of costs not covered by Medicare. Unfortunately, some older adults may not be able to afford this type of insurance, leaving a gap, or hole, in coverage. For example, suppose the older man who had hip surgery chooses to go home for continued recovery after his surgery, instead of going to a skilled nursing facility. If he needs a health-care provider to visit him in his home, this healthcare service would not be covered by Medicare. He would have to pay cash or write a check for this service. If, however, he had supplemental private insurance, that plan might assist in paying for these additional healthcare services.

Medicaid

Unlike Medicare, which is run by the federal government, **Medicaid** funds healthcare at the state level. Medicaid is a program that provides health insurance to people with low incomes, children, pregnant women, seniors, and individuals with disabilities.

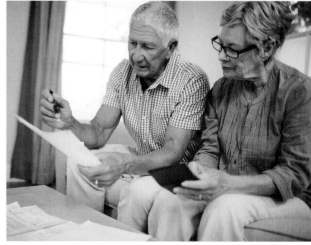

wavebreakmedia/Shutterstock.com

Figure 2.12 After the age of 65, a person who has worked 10 or more years qualifies for Social Security and Medicare.

To receive federal funding for Medicaid, states must cover certain groups. States have flexibility in deciding whether to cover other groups. States can set criteria using the federal minimum standards, which, for example, mandate coverage for people under 65 years of age earning an income at a specified percent below the federal poverty level (FPL). The states can also ask for a waiver to expand coverage for other individuals, such as children. Each state has its own set of requirements for those who qualify for Medicaid.

The Patient Protection and Affordable Care Act (ACA)

The Patient Protection and Affordable Care Act (ACA) was passed into law in 2010. The purpose of this law is to increase the quality of care and healthcare accessibility, while also decreasing healthcare spending and making healthcare affordable for many who do not have adequate coverage. There are several key requirements and healthcare benefits under this law:

- The law expands Medicaid coverage and improves benefits in Medicare.
- Larger employers are required to insure employees.
- Insurance companies cannot drop people who are sick or make unjustified rate hikes.
- Protections exist against gender-based insurance rate discrimination.
- People with preexisting conditions can obtain health insurance.
- Individuals under the age of 26 may be eligible for coverage under a parent's healthcare plan.
- People have the right to request that insurance plans reconsider a denial of payment.
- Lifetime limits on most insurance benefits are banned for all new healthcare plans.
- People may select their primary care doctors from their healthcare plan networks and also seek emergency care outside of their healthcare plan networks.
- People can seek free preventive services and health benefits, such as yearly checkups, immunizations, and screenings.
- An insurance marketplace called an *exchange* exists to provide people with a place to shop for free or low-cost private health insurance.

Managed Care

During the 1970s, health maintenance organizations (HMOs) were developed in the United States. HMO healthcare facilities were the first to offer **managed care**. Managed care, a common practice today, is a form of insurance in which there are contracts with specific healthcare providers who will deliver care at a reduced cost. This group of providers is called the plan's *network*.

In current managed care networks, a person may be enrolled in an HMO where he receives most, or all, of his care from one in-network provider. The HMO requires that a primary care provider be selected to manage and coordinate care. If the patient needs to see a specialist, such as a dermatologist, he must get a referral from his PCP. In an HMO, there are also deductibles and co-payments for visits. If the person goes outside the network, he will have to pay for all, or most, of his care.

Managed care can also be offered as a preferred provider organization (PPO). In this approach, the health plan contracts with a broad network of preferred providers from which a person can choose. A primary care provider is not needed, nor are referrals. There are annual deductibles and co-payments for a doctor's visit, which may be higher than in an HMO. If a person decides to choose a provider not in the PPO, she will pay a higher amount, pay the provider directly, and then request reimbursement by filing a claim.

The most recent step in managing care resulted from a quality and cost-savings development called Accountable Care Organizations (ACOs). Healthcare providers who are part of an ACO integrate the following with the goal of providing safe, quality care to all:

- prevention of disease and promotion of health
- coordination of care, particularly for patients who have more than one condition, such as needing care for both diabetes and heart disease
- easy availability of services, such as services being located in patients' communities
- access to as many services as may be needed for a patient's disease or condition
- use of technology, such as EHRs
- use of health and wellness technology applications
- ability of providers to communicate with their patients who may be living in remote locations (telemedicine)
- evidence-based treatment

Large healthcare facilities see ACOs as an opportunity to promote wellness and expand services so patients have a smooth transition between different healthcare providers and services.

Private Insurance

Private insurance is another way to pay for healthcare. People may have private insurance as a benefit through their work or they may pay for it on their own. Employers typically only pay for a portion of the insurance cost, and the employee is responsible for paying the remainder, called a **premium**. The premium pays for the specified coverage for the employee and, if elected, his or her family.

The insurance company and coverage offered is also determined by the person's employer. Employee benefits may include coverage for a variety of different healthcare services, such as hospitalization, doctor visits, and specialists. Vision or dental plans may also be included in an employee's benefits, as well as prescription drug coverage. These benefits usually change each year, depending on what is available from the private insurance company and how much it will cost the employer.

With increased life expectancies, long-term care insurance has become more prevalent. This type of insurance generally covers home care, assisted living, adult daycare, respite care, hospice, and nursing homes. There are two types of long-term care insurance: private and public. Under the private plan, people pay out-of-pocket costs for specific coverage. The public plan is provided through Medicaid and covers the cost of medically necessary services in long-term care facilities for people with limited financial resources.

While it is important to understand how individuals might pay for their healthcare, it should not matter what insurance arrangements people have. Healthcare staff should treat all residents with the same dignity and respect. Always remember that patients and residents are funding your salary as a nursing assistant, whether it is through federal or state programs, private insurance, or their own out-of-pocket payment.

Section 2.1 Review and Assessment

Using the Key Terms

Complete the following sentences using the key terms in this section.

1. The _____ is the portion of an insurance plan that is not paid for by the employer and that covers specified care for the employee and, if elected, his or her family members.
2. In a(n) _____ plan, a group of providers called a *network* will deliver care to the insured patient at a reduced cost.
3. _____ is care given to those with a long-term disease or illness.
4. A health insurer, program, or employer requires an individual to pay an out-of-pocket expense known as a(n) _____ as his or her share of the cost for health insurance coverage.
5. Patients who have a moderate-to-severe illness, injury, or recurrence of a disease, but who do not require the level of care delivered at a hospital, require _____.
6. A doctor is an example of a(n) _____.
7. Secondary care helps to promote _____, or well-being.
8. Any serious, critical, or surgical care typically received in a hospital could be considered _____.

Know and Understand the Facts

9. Identify three significant medical discoveries that have impacted healthcare today.
10. Identify two healthcare leaders and explain what they did to influence healthcare delivery.
11. Identify the three levels of care.

Analyze and Apply Concepts

12. Define *acute care*, *subacute care*, and *chronic care*. Which types of patients fall into each of these categories?
13. Describe five different types of healthcare facilities and explain the differences among them.
14. Discuss four different ways healthcare is funded.

Think Critically

Read the following care situation. Then answer the questions that follow.

Marion's mother is no longer able to take care of herself at home. She is forgetful and has not been able to get around like she used to. While Marion would like her mother to stay at home or even move into Marion's home, Marion feels that a healthcare facility offers better care for her mother.

15. What care options are available if Marion's mother stays in her own home?
16. If Marion decides that it will not be possible for her mother to stay at home, what type of healthcare facility might work best and why?

Objectives

Understanding the structures of healthcare facilities will provide you with the foundation you need to deliver the best possible care. It will also give you an awareness of how to fulfill your role as a holistic nursing assistant and follow the chain of command. To achieve the objectives for this section, you must successfully

- **describe** the different levels of a healthcare facility's organizational structure;
- **discuss** how the culture of a healthcare facility influences its effectiveness in delivering care; and
- **explain** the chain of command.

Key Terms

Learn these key terms to better understand the information presented in the section.

chain of command
charge nurse
delegate
healthcare team

nursing unit
orientation
shift

Questions to Consider

- Have you or a friend recently started a new job? Did the job and the company turn out as expected? Was the supervisor helpful? If not, how did that affect the job and your (or your friend's) desire to go to work every day?
- Were some people at the job more likeable than others? What did you think of the work environment? Did your (or your friend's) coworkers feel good about where they worked?
- How did the coworkers' attitudes affect their communication? Did their attitudes impact those with whom they worked?

How Are Healthcare Facilities and Nursing Units Structured?

A healthcare facility's organizational structure includes the staff members who work at the facility, the levels at which staff members work, and each person's decision-making authority. This structure is needed to effectively accomplish the facility's mission and goals. The organizational structure outlines the delivery of care and the communication networks that function based on the facility's **chain of command** (levels of authority).

Most healthcare facilities use a similar organizational structure, although no two organizations are exactly the same. A facility's unique mission, vision, values, leadership, and staff all impact how the organization functions.

Every healthcare facility has a chart illustrating its organizational structure and chain of command (Figure 2.13). This chart typically includes four levels that show the facility's organization, positions within the facility, and the names of staff who hold each position. The four different levels shown on the chart will help you navigate the facility and understand who is responsible for different departments.

First Level

As a holistic nursing assistant, you will work at the first level of a facility's organizational structure, and you will deliver care on a **nursing unit**, which is an area within a healthcare facility that serves a group of residents. In some healthcare facilities, such as long-term care facilities, there may be nursing units located in different parts

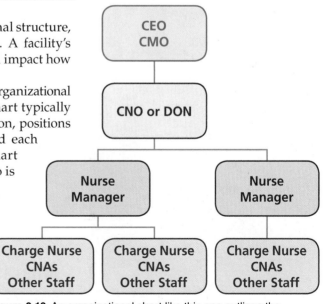

Figure 2.13 An organizational chart like this one outlines the chain of command within a healthcare facility and important communication channels.

of the same building. In hospitals, there may be nursing units that take care of patients on different sides of the same floor.

You will be working as part of a **healthcare team** with the primary goal of delivering safe, quality care. Nursing assistants are supervised by members of the licensed nursing staff (RNs and LPNs/LVNs) who are also working at this first level of organization. For each **shift**, or period of time at work, members of the licensed nursing staff are usually assigned as **charge nurses**. Sometimes the charge nurse is an RN, and other times he or she may be an LPN/LVN. The charge nurse will **delegate** specific duties you need to perform and will provide guidance (Figure 2.14). You should communicate any concerns or resident issues to the charge nurse.

Second Level

The second level of a facility's organizational structure includes the licensed nursing staff to whom the charge nurses report. Licensed nursing staff members at this level are usually called *nurse managers*. The nurse manager is responsible for supervising and monitoring staff, creating schedules, conducting **orientation** (introduction and training for new employees), and creating the budget for the nursing unit. The nurse manager may have an office on the nursing unit. Nurse managers may be responsible for more than one nursing unit.

The nurse manager is concerned with both resident and staff satisfaction. If you feel an issue has not been taken care of appropriately at the first level (with the charge nurse), you should discuss the issue with the nurse manager. People working at this level have more decision-making authority to address problems or concerns than staff members at the first level do.

Third Level

People at the third level of a facility's organizational structure oversee the entire facility and are considered the top level of the chain of command for nursing. This level includes a chief nursing officer (CNO) or a director of nursing (DON). This nurse has the highest authority concerning the nursing staff members who work on the nursing unit, resident care, safety, the nursing budget, nursing unit staffing, and the quality of nursing care delivery. The CNO or DON is ultimately responsible for the facility's nursing *reputation*, or how others view the facility. In some facilities, the CNO may also have responsibility for workers outside the nursing staff, such as those who provide respiratory care or take X-rays. CNOs and DONs are known by other titles in some facilities.

Fourth Level

At the fourth level of a facility is the chief executive officer (CEO) or administrator, who has full authority and responsibility for all staff in the healthcare facility. The CNO or DON reports to the CEO. In many healthcare facilities, there is also a chief medical officer (CMO). The CMO has the same authority as the CEO, but is only responsible for doctors and the care they provide in the facility. The CEO and the CMO, if there is one, are accountable to a Board of Trustees or Directors.

What Is It like Working on a Nursing Unit?

Many healthcare facilities operate 24 hours a day, 365 days a year. Each nursing unit in a given facility has an organizational structure similar to the one described earlier.

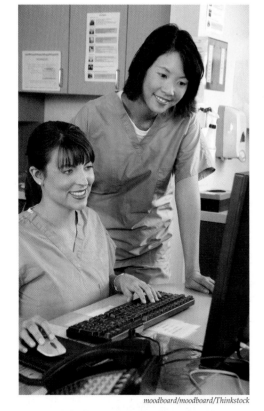

moodboard/moodboard/Thinkstock

Figure 2.14 Charge nurses supervise and instruct nursing assistants in required tasks.

Healthcare facilities divide the 24 hours in a day into shifts. Shifts may be 8, 10, or 12 hours long and often are described as *day, evening,* or *night shifts.* For example, if you worked an eight-hour day shift, you might start work at 7:00 a.m. and work until 3:00 p.m. If you worked a 12-hour day shift, you might start work at 7:00 a.m. and work until 7:00 p.m. The lengths and structures of shifts are determined by facility policy, services provided, and sometimes the types of residents. Healthcare facilities may also have overlapping shifts, where staff members are asked to work shifts that cover the busier parts of the day. An example of an overlapping shift would be a shift that lasted from 11:00 a.m. to 7:00 p.m.

Healthcare delivery is usually a 24-hour responsibility in long-term care facilities and hospitals, so a traditional Monday-through-Friday, 40-hour work-week may not apply (Figure 2.15). For example, you may be assigned to work a 12-hour shift three days a week or for six days in a two-week period. If you work eight-hour shifts, you will probably work five days a week or for 10 days in a two-week period. There are usually requirements for how many weekends and holidays staff must work. For example, often staff are required to work every other weekend and some holidays. Other policies related to scheduling are typically specific to the healthcare facility, the nursing unit, and sometimes the type of care being given.

When nursing assistants are hired by a healthcare facility, an orientation is provided. The orientation typically covers the various skills and regulations required, expectations of staff, the levels of structure in the facility, and an explanation of how work is scheduled. These issues are discussed thoroughly so that new staff members know what is expected of them.

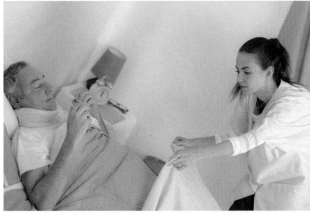

ALPA PROD/Shutterstock.com

Figure 2.15 Healthcare is a 24-hour responsibility. As a nursing assistant, you may have to work unusual shifts, such as night shifts or shifts during the holidays.

Remember

Great organizations demand a high level of commitment by the people involved.

Bill Gates, entrepreneur and philanthropist

How Does the Culture of a Healthcare Facility Affect Care?

A healthcare facility's *culture* includes its mission, vision, values, traditions, languages, and customs. Culture also encompasses the way a facility's staff members feel, think,

---

Becoming a Holistic Nursing Assistant
Contributing to a Positive Culture

Being a holistic nursing assistant means you are a major contributor to your healthcare facility's culture. Your positive attitude and passion for delivering safe, quality care will make a difference in residents' lives and in the facility where you work. The following guidelines can help you contribute to a positive culture:

- Be aware of your feelings and behaviors and how you express them. People will notice if you are approaching them in a positive and supportive way.

- Be sure to take care of yourself. Take your breaks to give yourself the energy you need during a shift and eat healthy snacks.

- Be *mindful*, or mentally present and aware.

When you adopt these behaviors, attitudes, and actions, you will find that having passion for what you do and exhibiting a positive attitude come easily and effortlessly. You can even encourage others to follow in suit by being their role model.

Apply It

1. If asked, would people say you are a positive and supportive person? Explain your answer.

2. Are you mentally present when you work with others? If not, what can you do to be more present?

3. What healthy habits do you have? What could you do to become even healthier?

and behave. Rules and procedures, both official and unofficial, shape the culture of a healthcare facility. For example, in some nursing units, staff birthdays are celebrated at the end of the month and not when they actually occur, laboratory personnel cannot sit in certain areas of a nursing unit when they come to draw blood, or wheelchairs can only be stored according to written policy and procedures.

Culture is developed over time, often by the leadership of the facility or nursing unit and by other staff. Different nursing units within the same healthcare facility may have unique cultures. The culture of a facility or nursing unit might be described as positive or negative. The perception of a particular unit's culture is often dependent on the personal experiences of staff. The charge nurse or nurse manager greatly influences the overall culture.

Culture affects the entire healthcare facility and impacts delivery of care in profound ways. When you begin a new job, it is essential to determine if you fit within the specific culture of the healthcare facility. To do this, ask yourself if your beliefs and values match well with those of the facility and with the way care is being delivered.

Sometimes, you may find you do not fit well with the facility's culture. When this happens, work can become stressful because the facility's culture fails to align with your beliefs and values. Over time, trying to work in a culture that fits poorly with your personality and work style can cause physical and mental fatigue. Since it is unlikely that a facility's culture will change, you will need to make adjustments in your approach and style if you want to stay at the facility or on the nursing unit.

There are some signs that will help you determine if a facility's culture is a good fit for you. For example, if the answers to any of the following questions are not to your liking, then you may not fit well with a facility or nursing unit:

- Are staff members recognized for doing a good job?
- Is communication between shifts open, and does it promote a good working environment?
- Do staff members get along well and generally like each other (Figure 2.16)?
- Are staff members on first-name bases with each other and the charge nurses?
- Are staff members encouraged to ask questions and give input into how a nursing unit is run?
- Do leaders communicate with staff verbally or use written communications?

- Are there any special rules or policies that can never be broken? Are certain subjects or ideas forbidden from being discussed?
- Is the workplace environment attractive? Is it clean and tidy?
- Are the nursing units noisy or quiet?
- Are there quiet areas or places for the staff to take breaks?
- Are there seating areas for families and visitors?

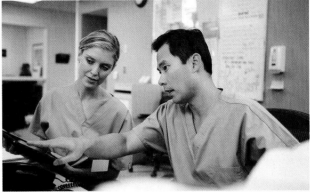

Monkey Business Images/Shutterstock.com

Figure 2.16 Each healthcare facility has a culture. How you align with this culture will impact your job satisfaction.

Section 2.2 Review and Assessment

Using the Key Terms

Complete the following sentences using the key terms in this section.

1. A charge nurse may _____ certain tasks, such as taking a patient's blood pressure, to the nursing assistant.
2. If a nursing assistant is scheduled to work from 7:00 p.m. to 7:00 a.m., he or she is working a 12-hour night _____.
3. Nursing assistants deliver care on a(n) _____, which is an area within a healthcare facility that serves a group of residents.
4. A licensed RN or LPN/LVN is the _____ for each shift.
5. One role of the nurse manager is to conduct introduction and training, known as _____, for new employees.
6. The _____ is a facility's levels of authority.
7. As a nursing assistant, you will work as part of a(n) _____ consisting of other healthcare staff members.

Know and Understand the Facts

8. Identify the staff members who work in the four levels of a healthcare facility's organizational structure.
9. Describe what makes up the culture in a healthcare facility.

Analyze and Apply Concepts

10. Identify how differences in organizational levels influence communication in a facility.
11. What two ways do you think you, as a holistic nursing assistant, could contribute to making a healthcare facility's culture positive?

Think Critically

Read the following care situation. Then answer the questions that follow.

Jake has been a nursing assistant in his county's healthcare facility for 10 years. He has a good relationship with his charge nurse, Joe. Jake and Joe are friends outside of work, which has affected the culture on the nursing unit for years. Jake feels so comfortable with residents that he sometimes calls them by their first names. Jake has also been known to share stories about his kids with the residents in his care.

12. In what ways is the chain of command affected by Jake and Joe's friendship?
13. How do you think the culture of this nursing unit affects the care given by its staff?
14. How would you rate Jake's level of professional behavior? Explain your answer.

Key Points

Reviewing the key points for this chapter will help you practice more safely and competently as a holistic nursing assistant and will help you prepare for the certification competency examination.

- Healthcare services fall into three levels of care: primary, secondary, and tertiary care. Care may also be categorized as acute, subacute, or chronic.

- A variety of healthcare facilities are available in the United States, and each facility specializes in a particular type of care.

- In the United States, people can use both public funding and private insurance to pay for healthcare costs. Public funding includes Medicare, Medicaid, and coverage under the Patient Protection and Affordable Care Act. Private insurance is often available through a person's employer.

- Health maintenance organizations (HMOs) and preferred provider organizations (PPOs) are forms of private insurance that offer managed care. This contracted insurance oversees the relationship between the patient and healthcare providers in an effort to provide high-quality care and reduce costs.

- Healthcare facilities are structured to ensure effective communication and decision making through a chain of command. Additionally, facilities have unique cultures that influence the feelings and behaviors of their staff.

Action Steps to Holistic Care

Review the information in this chapter. Complete the following activities.

1. Select one way healthcare is funded. Prepare a short paper or digital presentation that describes three issues related to healthcare funding not included in this chapter. Discuss one issue that promotes quality and one that ensures a safe environment.

2. With a partner, write a song or poem about a particular type of healthcare facility.

3. Find two pictures in a magazine, in a newspaper, or online that best demonstrate working as a holistic nursing assistant in a healthcare facility. Describe each image and provide a rationale for why it was selected.

4. Research a healthcare facility in your community. Write a brief report describing its organizational structure and where nursing assistants work in the facility. Also discuss the mission and values. Explain whether or not you might like working in this organization.

Preparing for the Certification Competency Examination

To prepare for the nursing assistant certification competency examination, you will need to know content found in this chapter. This content may be tested in the knowledge (written or oral) and skills (hands-on demonstration) portions of the exam. The following areas will be emphasized:

- the variety of available healthcare facilities
- the services provided by healthcare facilities and the differences between facilities
- healthcare facility structure

These sample test questions are similar to ones you will find on the certification competency exam. See how well you can answer them. Be sure to select the *best* answer.

1. A nursing assistant is working in a residential care facility. What type of facility is this?
   - A. a place where people who have had a stroke can regain their function and abilities
   - B. a place where people who have been injured in a car accident can recuperate
   - C. a place where people can get cosmetic or other types of surgery
   - D. a place where people who need 24-hour supervised care can live and receive care

2. What type of care is given to people who are required to stay in a hospital?
   - A. acute care
   - B. chronic care
   - C. subacute care
   - D. trauma care

3. Mrs. G's insurance requires a deductible. What is a deducible?

    A. a type of insurance older adults get
    B. the premium that families pay to cover their children
    C. the cost of private insurance policies
    D. the amount of money paid out-of-pocket for healthcare services

4. A nursing assistant likes his coworkers and appreciates the praise he gets from his charge nurse. He also enjoys the residents in his care. You could say that the nursing assistant's values align well with which of the following?

    A. the facility's structure
    B. the facility's culture
    C. the facility's staffing
    D. the facility's strategy

5. Which of the following best describes a facility's organizational structure?

    A. how people communicate with each other
    B. how people work together as a team
    C. the levels at which people work
    D. the ways in which people do their jobs

6. A nursing assistant works in a skilled nursing facility. What type of facility is this?

    A. a place where people who have had a stroke can regain their function and abilities
    B. a place where people who have been injured in a car accident can receive immediate care
    C. a place where people can get cosmetic or other types of surgery
    D. a place where people who need 24-hour supervised care can live and receive care for an extended period of time

7. When were the benefits of hand washing for removing germs discovered?

    A. 1700s
    B. 1900s
    C. 1800s
    D. 1600s

8. Mrs. D has just turned 65. She has worked full-time since she was 35 and is planning on retiring soon. For what type of public insurance is she eligible?

    A. Medicaid
    B. Medicare
    C. Aetna®
    D. Blue Cross® Blue Shield®

9. What was discovered by Jonas Salk?

    A. the polio vaccine
    B. penicillin
    C. the diphtheria vaccine
    D. insulin

10. A nursing assistant is working in a hospice. What type of facility is this?

    A. a place where people who have had a stroke can regain their function and abilities
    B. a place where people who have been injured in a car accident can recuperate
    C. a place where people who are dying can receive care and comfort
    D. a place where people who need 24-hour supervised care can live and receive care

11. Which of the following helps prevent epidemics?

    A. X-rays
    B. blood tests
    C. capsules
    D. vaccines

12. Which type of care are people provided when there is a contract for healthcare services?

    A. trauma care
    B. managed care
    C. chronic care
    D. acute care

13. Which of the following provides direct services for people who need long-term chronic care?

    A. hospice
    B. hospital
    C. nursing home
    D. pharmacy

14. Which category of care focuses on disease prevention and wellness?

    A. secondary care
    B. tertiary care
    C. acute care
    D. primary care

15. Which of the following describes the culture of a healthcare facility?

    A. the structure and organizational chart
    B. the beliefs, customs, and attitudes
    C. the different types of personnel
    D. the communication levels of the facility

Did you have difficulty with any of the questions? If you did, review the chapter to find the correct answer(s).

CHAPTER 3

Legal and Ethical Practice

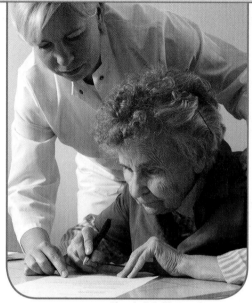

Alexander Raths/Shutterstock.com

Welcome to the Chapter

To gain a better understanding of the role and responsibilities of a nursing assistant, you must know the nursing assistant's scope of practice; regulations that affect healthcare facilities; and the healthcare laws and regulations that you, as a nursing assistant, will need to follow. Legislation and regulations that affect nursing assistants include the Patient Bill of Rights, Nursing Home Resident Rights, and laws related to elder neglect and abuse. In this chapter, you will also learn about why ethical practice is important and how ethical decisions are made.

What you learn in this chapter will help you develop your knowledge and skills to become a holistic nursing assistant. The topics discussed in the chapter are highlighted on the Providing Holistic Care Framework.

You are now ready to start this chapter, *Legal and Ethical Practice*.

Chapter Outline

Section 3.1
Healthcare Laws, Regulations, and Scope of Practice

Section 3.2
Ethics, Problem Solving, and Decision Making

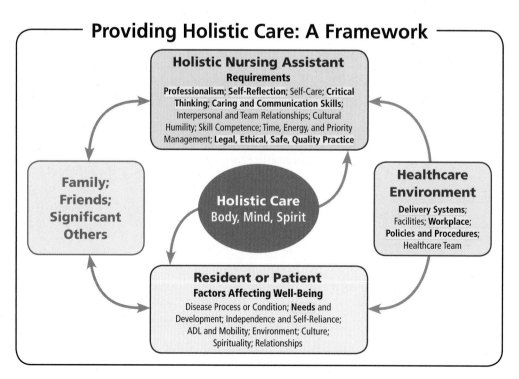

Providing Holistic Care: A Framework

Holistic Nursing Assistant
Requirements
Professionalism; Self-Reflection; Self-Care; **Critical Thinking; Caring and Communication Skills;** Interpersonal and Team Relationships; Cultural Humility; Skill Competence; Time, Energy, and Priority Management; **Legal, Ethical, Safe, Quality Practice**

Holistic Care
Body, Mind, Spirit

Family; Friends; Significant Others

Healthcare Environment
Delivery Systems; Facilities; **Workplace; Policies and Procedures;** Healthcare Team

Resident or Patient
Factors Affecting Well-Being
Disease Process or Condition; **Needs** and Development; Independence and Self-Reliance; ADL and Mobility; Environment; Culture; Spirituality; Relationships

Healthcare Laws, Regulations, and Scope of Practice

Objectives

To provide the best possible care, you must know your legal scope of practice and the laws that guide and regulate healthcare. You must also recognize and abide by the rights of patients and residents and ensure that those you care for are not mistreated, neglected, or abused. To achieve the objectives for this section, you must successfully

- **describe** the laws that influence healthcare and how organizations are regulated;
- **explain** the key laws and regulations nursing assistants must know;
- **follow** the legal scope of practice for a nursing assistant;
- **abide** by patient and resident rights;
- **respond** to any observed mistreatment, neglect, and elder abuse; and
- **identify** ways to avoid negligence and malpractice.

Questions to Consider

- Have you ever watched a television show—perhaps a medical drama—where laws were violated or broken? Maybe the situation had to do with abuse, neglect, or theft.
- What happened to the victim when the law was broken? What feelings or emotions were involved, and how did they affect the victim's life? What happened to the person who violated or broke the law?

Key Terms

Learn these key terms to better understand the information presented in the section.

abuse	liability
accreditation	libel
assault	licensure
battery	malpractice
civil law	neglect
confidentiality	negligence
criminal law	regulation
defamation of character	rehabilitation
elder abuse	self-determination
false imprisonment	slander
informed consent	The Joint Commission (TJC)

What Are Laws and Regulations?

The United States legal system has a long and rich history. *Laws* are formal rules or actions enforced by a legal authority such as the US government, a state, a county, or a city. **Regulations** are rules or requirements that are based on laws and that healthcare facilities and staff must follow. Regulations are usually enforced by an authority, such as the federal or state government.

There are different types of law in the US. *Constitutional law* is a system of laws that governs a nation, such as those laws found in the US Constitution. *Common law,* or *case law,* is a system of laws established as a result of decisions usually made in a court of law.

Federal laws, such as laws regarding income tax, affect everyone in the United States. States also pass laws that must be obeyed. *State laws,* such as traffic laws, affect only those who live in that state. Within a state, there are also county and city governments that pass their own laws, such as laws regarding city sales tax.

There are many federal laws that require healthcare facilities to meet specific regulations and standards. State laws also address areas of healthcare, including patient rights, safety, and licensure (Figure 3.1).

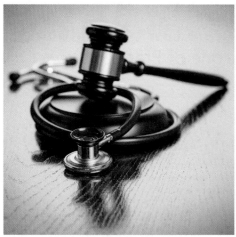

Andy Dean Photography/Shutterstock.com

Figure 3.1 Laws regulate many aspects of healthcare delivery, including licensure of healthcare facilities, scope of practice, and the rights of patients and residents.

How Do Accreditation and Licensure Affect Healthcare?

Delivering healthcare services means making decisions and providing care that can make a difference in the outcome of a resident's life. Therefore, healthcare facilities must adhere to very high standards and always comply with federal and state laws.

Healthcare facilities must also follow accreditation and licensure rules and regulations. **Accreditation** recognizes that a healthcare facility meets predetermined professional and community standards that promote safety and quality. Seeking accreditation is a voluntary decision made by a healthcare facility. **Licensure** recognizes that a healthcare facility meets standards set by law and has the legal permission to deliver care. Unlike accreditation, licensure is mandatory.

Accreditation

Private organizations usually accredit healthcare facilities. For example, **The Joint Commission (TJC)** accredits hospitals, ambulatory healthcare services, behavioral healthcare services, home healthcare services, and nursing and **rehabilitation** (recovery) centers. The majority of healthcare facilities seek accreditation by at least one major accrediting body, such as TJC.

There are other organizations that accredit healthcare facilities or healthcare services. For example, some organizations accredit rehabilitation centers, trauma centers, chest pain centers, and primary stroke centers.

Licensure

Licensure of healthcare facilities usually occurs at the state level. Specific agencies within a state's health department set the standards for licensure. These agencies also oversee healthcare facilities through routine monitoring, site visits, and consultation. An example of a licensing body would be an agency, located in a state's health department, that licenses long-term care facilities such as nursing homes.

What Is the Legal Scope of Practice for Nursing Assistants?

The *legal scope of practice* describes, using laws and regulations, what nursing assistants can and cannot do and who supervises them. In all cases, nursing assistants must be supervised by the licensed nursing staff, which consists of RNs and LPNs/LVNs. Nursing assistants must also have the range of skills and qualifications necessary to perform their responsibilities properly. If using the title *CNA*, they must have a certification.

Understanding Regulations and the Scope of Practice

The legal scope of practice for nursing assistants is defined by regulations. These regulations were established by the Omnibus Budget Reconciliation Act (OBRA), which is a federal law. Since OBRA was passed, each state has determined the legal scope for a nursing assistant's practice in that state. Regulations regarding scope of practice are usually found in a nurse practice act (NPA) or in other forms of regulation, such as those set by a state's department of health. State regulations outline a nursing assistant's responsibilities in that state, including limits on duties and responsibilities and the definition of competent practice.

Determining Your Scope of Practice

To find out if a responsibility is in your scope of practice, always ask yourself these three questions:

1. Do I have the education and training to perform this responsibility?
2. Is the responsibility allowed by my state's regulations or laws?
3. Is the responsibility allowed by my healthcare facility's policies and regulations?

If the answers to all of these questions are *yes*, it is safe to perform the responsibility. If the answer to any one of these questions is *no*, then it is not safe to perform the responsibility. If you don't know the answers to any of these questions, ask the licensed nursing staff (Figure 3.2).

In addition to the responsibilities of a nursing assistant discussed in chapter 1, some states now include the delivery of some medications as part of a nursing assistant's scope of practice. This added responsibility requires additional training and certification. An individual who has this responsibility is often called a *certified medication aide, medication assistant*, or *medication technician*. Review the regulations in your state to determine whether this role is included in the nursing assistant's scope of practice and what requirements a nursing assistant must meet to perform these responsibilities.

Working Outside the Scope of Practice

When you work within the legal scope of practice, you know the limitations of your position and are aware of your **liability** (legal responsibility) when practicing as a nursing assistant. If nursing assistants work outside their legal scope of practice, they may be disciplined by both their healthcare facilities and by the regulatory bodies that oversee certification in their states. Working outside the scope of practice may affect patients, residents, nursing staff, and doctors and may result in disciplinary, criminal, or civil actions.

Disciplinary Actions

The first type of action, *disciplinary action*, is taken when a policy or procedure in a healthcare facility has not been followed appropriately or correctly. Violations that require disciplinary actions can range from being late to work or breaking the dress code to not completing a care assignment or not following a procedure correctly. These violations are usually handled according to a facility's disciplinary policy and procedure. Consequences may include counseling by a supervisor, suspension from duties for a period of time, or termination, depending on the frequency or severity of the violation. Issues that become formal complaints may be reported to the state board of nursing or state department of health.

Criminal Actions

Criminal actions are taken when someone breaks or violates a **criminal law**. Violations of criminal law may be misdemeanors or felonies. *Misdemeanors* are less serious crimes. Examples of misdemeanors include petty theft, trespassing, or public intoxication. Fines, probation, or community service are often the penalties for a misdemeanor.

Felonies are more serious crimes, such as homicide (murder), arson (setting a fire), or robbery. A prison sentence is often the result of a felony if a person is found guilty beyond a reasonable doubt. Felonies committed in a healthcare facility are handled by the state's legal system. When criminal offenses occur, the state board of nursing or department of health may also be involved.

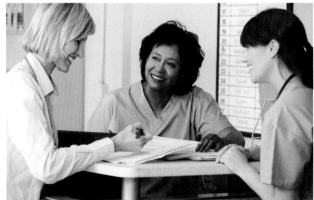

Monkey Business Images/Shutterstock.com

Figure 3.2 As a nursing assistant, you should always ask the licensed nursing staff if you have a question or are uncertain about your scope of practice.

Civil Actions

A *civil action* occurs in response to a violation of a **civil law** (a law that deals with disagreements between individuals and organizations). Negligence and malpractice are two violations of civil law. They are also called *torts* because physical or emotional injury occurs as a result of failing to deliver proper care.

Negligence is the unintentional failure to act or provide care, possibly resulting in injury. An example of negligence might be a busy nursing assistant forgetting to check on a hot compress he or she put on a confused, frail resident's leg. When the nursing assistant returned to the room and removed the compress, the skin on the resident's leg was very red.

Malpractice is more serious, occurs when professional standards are not followed (known as a *breach of duty*), and always results in an injury. An example of malpractice might be the continued failure to properly and regularly turn a frail, immobile resident in bed as ordered. This would cause the resident to spend long periods of time in the same position, resulting in skin breakdown and the formation of decubitus ulcers.

When there is a civil action due to negligence or malpractice, the result is monetary compensation for the extent of injury determined. When civil actions are taken, the state board of nursing or department of health responsible for nursing assistants may also be involved.

To prevent negligence and avoid malpractice,

- give care only within your legal scope of practice;
- know and understand all healthcare facility policies and procedures;
- always ask for instruction if you are not sure how to do a procedure;
- be honest, particularly if you have made a mistake, and inform licensed nursing staff immediately;
- document appropriately and effectively (see chapter 13 for information on documentation); and
- maintain resident privacy and confidentiality of information.

Which Laws and Regulations Affect Nursing Assistants?

Overseeing healthcare laws and regulations is primarily the responsibility of doctors, nursing administrators, quality improvement staff, and people working in finance. While a facility's chief executive officer (CEO), chief nursing officer (CNO), or director of nursing (DON) are ultimately accountable for abiding by these laws and regulations, several important regulations are also the responsibility of nursing assistants.

Healthcare facilities, particularly those receiving Medicare and Medicaid funds, must follow specific guidelines and standards. State laws and requirements for licensing long-term care facilities may place additional regulations. These regulations and standards include important requirements, such as the maintenance of a restraint-free environment. Nursing assistants must learn a facility's specific regulations and understand how these regulations affect the facility's policies; procedures; and delivery of safe, quality care.

Key laws and regulations that holistic nursing assistants must know and follow include the Health Insurance Portability and Accountability Act (HIPAA), the Patient Bill of Rights, and Nursing Home Resident Rights.

Health Insurance Portability and Accountability Act (HIPAA)

In 1996, the US federal government enacted the *Health Insurance Portability and Accountability Act (HIPAA)* to ensure that personal medical information is stored and shared securely, thus maintaining confidentiality. Two parts of HIPAA—the Privacy Rule (2003) and Security Rule (2005)—affect the daily work of nursing assistants. These rules define and protect patient and resident rights regarding their personal health information.

HIPAA states that *health information* is considered any paper, oral, or electronic record shared with a healthcare provider, insurer, or similar entity that can be used to identify a patient. This includes details concerning a patient's past, present, or future physical or mental health; any healthcare received; or payment information related to healthcare. Any information collected that identifies or could potentially be used to identify a patient must be protected. This type of information is called *individually identifiable health information* or *protected health information (PHI)*. The HIPAA Privacy Rule covers protected health information collected by any means, and the HIPAA Security Rule covers any electronic protected health information.

HIPAA is very specific about what types of information can and cannot be shared. For example, a patient may provide a doctor's office a written release that dictates what information can be disclosed to other healthcare providers. This shared information may be needed to provide follow-up care or for insurance purposes. Penalties for disclosing confidential information without a patient's permission range from civil suits to discipline, the loss of a job, and fines (Figure 3.3).

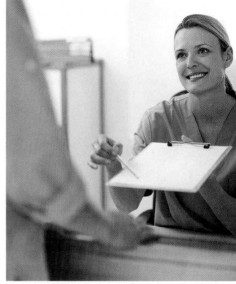

wavebreakmedia/Shutterstock.com

Figure 3.3 Patients must sign forms to grant the release of their health information.

Confidentiality

In addition to complying with HIPAA requirements, maintaining the **confidentiality** of patient or resident information is an essential part of any healthcare provider's responsibility. To maintain confidentiality, healthcare providers must consider any information communicated by a patient or resident to be private. They must also know the limits on and procedures for sharing this information. If healthcare providers share information inappropriately, it can be considered an *invasion of privacy*.

Holistic nursing assistants should always remember the following *never* statements about confidentiality:

- *Never* discuss any patient or resident information, including progress, with anyone who is not directly involved in care.

- *Never* read the chart of a patient or resident who is not in your care.

- *Never* remove any resident information from where it is stored.

- *Never* discuss a resident with another staff member in a public place (for example, a cafeteria or parking lot) where information may be overheard.

- *Never* talk about a patient or a resident in a way that would allow other people, such as your friends, family, or acquaintances, to identify the patient or resident.

Bills of Rights

In addition to maintaining confidentiality, holistic nursing assistants are responsible for supporting and promoting a safe environment and good quality of life for patients and residents. Both a Patient Bill of Rights (used in hospitals) and Nursing Home Resident Rights (used in long-term care) are documents that contain standards that must be posted and shared with patients and residents. The documents outline legal and ethical responsibilities for all healthcare providers and facilities. Typically, a bill of rights guarantees privacy of information, a safe environment, fair treatment, and the ability to make one's own medical decisions, among other rights.

Patient Bill of Rights

A Patient Bill of Rights is shared with every patient admitted to a healthcare facility and is posted in prominent places. Many states have specific laws that determine what a Patient Bill of Rights contains. Some facilities are required to provide their

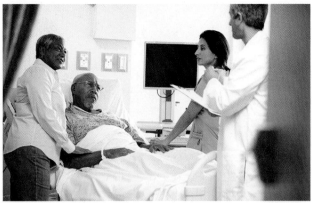
Monkey Business Images/Shutterstock.com

Figure 3.4 Patients have the right to involve their family members in care.

Patient Bill of Rights to receive accreditation. The American Hospital Association (AHA), a large professional trade organization, developed a set of rights used by their member hospitals. These rights are distributed in a brochure called *The Patient Care Partnership*. According to this brochure, a patient should expect the following during hospitalization:

- high-quality care
- a clean and safe environment
- family involvement in care (Figure 3.4)
- protection of privacy
- help when leaving the hospital
- assistance with billing claims

In addition to the AHA, The Joint Commission (TJC) also provides a brochure describing patients' rights. This brochure is provided as a resource to hospitals and other healthcare facilities. While TJC has standards similar to the AHA, it also outlines such rights as

- being informed about the care received;
- knowing the names of the caregivers;
- getting important information about care in a preferred language that also meets any needs resulting from vision, speech, hearing, or mental impairment;
- knowing when something goes wrong with care;
- being able to refuse care; and
- having a personal advocate or representative to support care, ask questions, help make decisions, or request needed care.

Nursing Home Resident Rights

In 1987, Nursing Home Resident Rights were established under OBRA and the Nursing Home Reform Act. Nursing homes must meet these federal resident rights requirements if they receive Medicare or Medicaid funds. OBRA and the Nursing Home Reform Act require that resident rights be protected and promoted and place a strong emphasis on individual dignity and **self-determination** (the ability to make choices based on one's own preferences). Some states also have additional laws or regulations that determine resident rights for long-term care facilities and other residential care centers. Residents must be informed of their rights in a language they understand. These rights are to be provided in writing and signed by residents upon admission and during their stays. Nursing Home Resident Rights include the rights to

- have freedom from abuse (verbal, physical, mental, or sexual), mistreatment, and neglect;
- have freedom from physical restraints;
- have privacy;
- have personal items in one's room, manage one's own money, live with a spouse, and privately send and receive personal mail and e-mail;
- receive accommodation for medical, physical, psychological, and social needs and full disclosure about medical conditions and treatments;
- make one's own schedule and visit with family and friends;
- be treated with respect and dignity;
- exercise self-determination, which includes leaving a healthcare facility temporarily or permanently, with or without a doctor's permission (if this right is not upheld, the resident's stay can be seen as **false imprisonment**);
- communicate freely;

- participate in the review of one's plan of care, access one's health information, and be fully informed in advance about any changes in care, treatment, or status in the facility;
- have an advocate or representative;
- be told in writing about all nursing home services and fees; and
- make complaints without discrimination or reprisal.

Many facilities have *resident councils*. A resident council is provided with a meeting space and a facility representative who must listen and respond to grievances and recommendations of the council.

Informed Consent

When certain medical or surgical procedures are needed, patients and residents must sign an **informed consent** prior to the procedures being performed. These procedures are determined by a doctor and guided by a doctor's order. Patients or residents must understand their treatment choices and the associated risks. Either the patient or resident or the patient's or resident's legal guardian must be given a detailed explanation of each procedure, including the benefits and risks. Doctors may delegate the responsibility of providing this explanation and securing the patient's or resident's signature to licensed nursing staff. When informed consent documents are signed, the resident accepts the risks and grants permission for the specific procedure to be performed.

Healthcare providers must always have a resident's verbal permission to give care. Remember that it is not acceptable to force someone to do something he or she does not want to do. Using threats or force to make someone do something is considered *coercion* and an invasion of privacy. To gain verbal consent, you must follow these steps:

1. Carefully explain what you plan to do.
2. Make sure the resident understands.
3. Provide the resident with opportunities to ask questions.
4. *Never* give care against the resident's wishes. Report any refusals of care to the licensed nursing staff.

Neglect and Mistreatment

One important right of residents is the right to freedom from neglect or mistreatment. Holistic nursing assistants must prevent neglect or mistreatment, be able to recognize it if it does happen, and know how to report it. While it is essential to be aware of neglect and mistreatment in any care delivery environment, it is particularly significant among seniors, who are one of the most vulnerable populations.

Neglect is the failure to provide necessary care that meets a resident's daily needs, such as needs for treatments, medication, food, clothing, hygiene, or shelter. Neglect can be accidental. For example, a healthcare provider may forget to perform treatments or deliver medications. Neglect may also be deliberate. Neglect can cause injury to the resident and may result in sores on the skin, weight loss, dehydration, complaints of hunger or thirst, a body that is not clean, and soiled clothes and bed linens.

If you observe any of these signs of neglect, you must immediately report them to the licensed nursing staff.

Defamation of character, which consists of false statements made about a person that damage his or her reputation, is a form of mistreatment. Defamation of character is categorized as **libel** when the statements are written, or as **slander** when the statements are spoken. Both libel and slander can result in a legal action.

Assault, Battery, and Abuse

While doing harm of any kind to another person is unacceptable, assault and battery are the most serious types of harm and are considered criminal acts. **Assault** refers to any words or actions that a person finds threatening, causing him or her to fear harm. **Battery** is the act of touching a person without his or her permission. If you perform a procedure without a resident's consent, it *may* be considered battery. This is why it is essential to always get permission from residents prior to performing a procedure.

Abuse is a deliberate action, such as assault or battery, that causes harm. There is never an excuse for abusing another person. Abuse can happen to anyone. **Elder abuse**, or deliberate actions that harm seniors, is particularly concerning because seniors may be defenseless due to illness and the loss of cognition and mobility. Seniors' dependence on caregivers and family can make them very vulnerable to the frustrations and anger of others, which can lead to abuse.

Elder abuse may be physical, verbal, financial, or sexual:

- **Physical abuse**: the use of force that causes injury and pain. It includes grabbing, hitting, slapping, pulling hair, shaking, or using a restraint inappropriately.
- **Verbal, mental, or emotional abuse**: the use of words or actions that cause emotional pain or injury. It includes threatening physical harm or abandonment, laughing at or teasing a person, insulting or harassing a person, isolating a person, or keeping a person alone in a room over a long period of time with the door closed.
- **Financial abuse**: the theft or misuse of another person's money or property
- **Sexual abuse**: the touching of a person's body parts in inappropriate ways, suggestive comments or gestures, inappropriate photography, or rape

Signs and symptoms of abuse include

- unexplained bruises or injuries, such as broken bones;
- burns with unusual shapes or bite marks;
- dry, cracked, or bleeding skin or red marks;
- severely poor personal hygiene, such as matted or missing hair, broken and unbrushed teeth, body odor, or skin ulcers;
- changes in personality or fear when being touched;
- attempts to cover abused areas with clothing; and
- statements by a resident that suggest neglect or abuse.

If abuse or neglect is suspected, the licensed nursing staff must be alerted. Nursing assistants are not responsible for determining if a resident is being abused, but *are* responsible for observing and reporting any signs or symptoms of abuse. If signs of abuse are not reported, the nursing assistant can be legally liable, as reporting this information is required by federal and state laws.

If nursing assistants are accused of abuse, they are usually suspended until a full investigation is conducted. Typically, the healthcare facility conducts an investigation; however, state agencies such as adult protective services and the state board of nursing may also be involved.

Think About This

Every year, hundreds of thousands of adults over the age of 60 are abused, taken advantage of, or neglected. Elder abuse is experienced by one out of every 10 people, ages 60 and older, who live at home. This number is likely larger than reported because many who experience this violence are unable or afraid to tell the police, their family, or friends.

Using the Key Terms

Complete the following sentences using the key terms in this section.

1. Sores on the skin and complaints of hunger and thirst may be evidence of the failure to provide necessary care, known as _____.

2. _____ occurs when professional standards of duty are not met, resulting in patient injury.

3. Denying a resident the right to leave a nursing facility, either temporarily or permanently, could be considered _____ and violates Nursing Home Resident Rights.

4. Sharing a patient's or resident's information inappropriately is a breach of _____.

5. _____ occurs when a senior is neglected by a caretaker or family member on whom he or she is reliant.

6. Before certain medical or surgical procedures can be performed, residents must sign a(n) _____ form.

7. OBRA and the Nursing Home Reform Act emphasize the importance of _____, or the ability to make choices based on one's own preferences.

8. Accidentally serving a diabetic patient the wrong meal could be considered _____ because the mistake was an unintentional failure.

Know and Understand the Facts

9. Explain the difference between negligence and malpractice.

10. Describe one similarity and one difference between accreditation and licensure.

11. List the three questions holistic nursing assistants should ask themselves to determine if they're working within their scope of practice.

12. What is the difference between libel and slander?

13. What are five signs of elder abuse?

Analyze and Apply Concepts

14. Describe how Nursing Home Resident Rights affect the kinds of care you will provide as a nursing assistant.

15. What are two ways a nursing assistant can maintain confidentiality?

16. List the steps you would take if you suspected elder abuse was taking place in your healthcare facility.

Think Critically

Read the following care situation. Then answer the questions that follow.

Dominick, a new nursing assistant, has been taking care of Mr. C for the past week. He has become quite friendly with Mr. C and likes Mr. C's family very much. Mr. C and his family are also fond of Dominick. Dominick feels he should do extra for Mr. C, but he sometimes forgets to ask the RN whether what he wants to do is acceptable. For example, Dominick makes sure Mr. C's family brings in vitamins and food supplements so Mr. C can get stronger. He also tries to get Mr. C to ambulate even when Mr. C does not want to. Dominick has started walking out with Mr. C's family when they leave the healthcare facility; he lets them know how Mr. C is doing and what more they can do to help him. Dominick has been invited to dinner with Mr. C's family next week, and he is considering the invitation.

17. In what ways is Dominick acting within his legal scope of practice as a nursing assistant?

18. In what ways is Dominick practicing outside his legal scope of practice?

19. Is Dominick violating confidentiality? Explain your answer.

20. Which resident rights is Dominick supporting, and which may he be violating?

21. Is Dominick doing anything in his care that might be considered abuse?

Questions to Consider

- Have you ever been in a situation in which someone told you to act in a way that made you feel uncomfortable? Perhaps you were told to take something that, while a small item, was not yours to take. You did it because the person who told you to was your friend and said it would be all right.
- Have you been in a situation where you knew you should have helped someone who was struggling, but you chose not to, telling yourself you were too busy when you were not?
- How did you feel about your decisions and actions in these situations? Looking back, should you have made a different decision? Why?

Objectives

It is essential that you practice ethically. This means you understand what is morally right and wrong, act within your legal scope of practice, and follow ethical guidelines. The facility in which you work will provide a framework for ethical practice and when ethical decision making is required. Healthcare providers also have specific codes of ethics to follow. To achieve the objectives for this section, you must successfully

- **identify** ethical principles and their impact on care;
- **explain** the importance of a code of ethics;
- **discuss** the importance of ethical practice;
- **explain** the relationship between problem solving and decision making; and
- **describe** the process that is used for ethical decision making.

Key Terms

Learn these key terms to better understand the information presented in the section.

beneficence	nonmaleficence
dilemma	perception
ethics	prognosis
fidelity	veracity

What Does It Mean to Act Ethically?

You must act ethically to be a professional. **Ethics** are principles that guide our conduct; they help us determine what is the right or wrong thing to do. A person's ethics and values are influenced by his or her parents, significant others, teachers, friends, and experiences. Each person has his or her own set of values. Some people might value education or happiness, while others value earning a lot of money or enjoying leisure time. Values influence a person's attitudes and behavior and are the basis of ethics and a person's ethical practice. It is important for you to know and understand your values so you can determine how they might affect your ability to practice ethical caregiving.

Remember

Ethics is knowing the difference between what you have a right to do and what is right to do.

Potter Stewart, Associate Justice of the US Supreme Court

Principles of Ethical Caregiving

There are several important ethical principles in caregiving. These principles build the framework for how residents should be seen and approached and how healthcare staff should practice ethically:

- **Autonomy**: residents should maintain their own values and uniqueness.
- **Freedom**: residents should function independently and make their own decisions (Figure 3.5).
- **Confidentiality**: residents have the right to privacy and to the expectation that information will not be shared in an unethical or illegal manner.
- **Beneficence**: healthcare staff have a moral obligation to do good.
- **Nonmaleficence**: healthcare staff have the moral obligation to avoid doing harm.

- **Veracity**: healthcare staff must be honest, represent themselves truthfully, and admit if they work outside their legal scope of practice. This honesty will enable residents to make informed decisions.
- **Fidelity**: healthcare staff are faithful and do not abandon those in their care.
- **Justice**: healthcare staff treat all residents fairly.

Codes of Conduct and Ethics

All professions or disciplines have a code for conduct and ethics, called a *code of conduct* or a *code of ethics*. These guidelines set standards for care delivery and practice and direct actions and behaviors. Some codes of conduct or ethics are outlined in a nurse practice act (NPA) or in other regulations. You can check to see if your state's regulations for nursing assistants have a code of conduct or ethics. If a code of conduct or ethics is set out in regulations, this means it is enforced by law. Codes of conduct or ethics can also be set by a discipline's professional association, and the members of that discipline or profession are expected to comply with the code's guidelines.

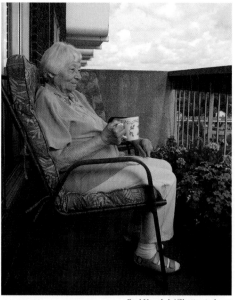

Figure 3.5 Ethical caregiving respects the resident's right to freedom, which includes functioning independently.

Codes of conduct or ethics set high benchmarks for care and practice. The following is a sample code of ethics for nursing assistants:

For my patients and residents:

- I will provide you with competent, high-quality care.
- I will be dependable.
- I will treat you with respect and dignity.
- I will ensure you are in a safe environment.
- I will recognize and follow your bill of rights.
- I will honor your individual choices about your care.
- I will recognize and appreciate that you have your own beliefs and values.
- I will protect your privacy and property.
- I will hold confidential all information I learn about you.
- I will care for you in a positive and approachable manner.
- I will be supportive and encouraging when communicating with your family members and significant others.

For my fellow healthcare staff:

- I will be sensitive to your needs, values, and beliefs.
- I will listen to your opinions and recommendations.
- I will work with you as a cooperating and trustworthy team member.
- I will help you, whenever I am able, to ensure quality care.
- I will be patient and supportive in all of my communications with you.

For the healthcare facility:

- I will follow all policies and procedures.
- I will perform only those duties that are within my legal scope of practice.
- I will follow directions that are given by the licensed nursing staff and that are within my legal scope of practice.
- I will attend all facility and educational meetings requested.
- I will fully and accurately document the care and information I provide.
- I will report errors and incidents immediately and truthfully.

For myself:
- I will know the limits of my role and responsibilities.
- I will perform only those skills that I have the competence and preparation to do.
- I will carry out directions and instructions to the best of my ability.
- I will come to work with a positive attitude.
- I will always be conscientious about my work.
- I will be respectful in all of my relationships.
- I will be accountable for my actions.

In addition, I will be conscious of my responsibilities when using electronic communication and social media. I will abide by the healthcare facility's policy and pay attention to the following rules:
- I will not use my cell phone to make personal calls during my work shift, particularly if I am in a resident's room.
- I will not disclose confidential or private information about the healthcare facility, residents and their families, or staff on social media or in electronic communication.
- I will not use e-mail or social media to broadcast anything that might violate confidentiality or to disclose any information about the healthcare facility, residents and their families, or other staff. I understand that sending an electronic message is more permanent than saying something to another person. Long after, the words will still be there, and a message can be read by others as it travels through the Internet.
- I will ask the licensed nursing staff if I have any questions about the use of electronic communication and social media.

Remember

The problem is not that there are problems. The problem is expecting otherwise and thinking that having problems is a problem.

Theodore Rubin, American psychiatrist and author

Why Are Ethical Problem Solving and Decision Making Important?

Life is full of problems, which can be big or small and simple or complex. Some problems you have experienced before, while others are new. In healthcare, problems are an everyday occurrence. Successful holistic nursing assistants are comfortable with this reality and find ways to identify and solve the problems they encounter. While you will respond to problems on a daily basis, your skills in problem solving will be especially important when you encounter situations that violate principles of ethical caregiving or codes of conduct. Having an awareness and understanding of the problem-solving and decision-making process will help you provide helpful information when resolving ethical issues and dilemmas.

——— Becoming a Holistic Nursing Assistant ———
A Nursing Assistant's Code of Ethics

The principles and guidelines of the sample code of ethics in this section provide excellent guidance for new holistic nursing assistants. Following these principles and guidelines will allow you to become a holistic nursing assistant who practices ethically. Carefully read the sample code of ethics again and then consider the following questions.

Apply It
1. Which of the ethical guidelines discussed in this chapter do you find come naturally to you? Explain your answer.
2. Are there any ethical guidelines that you think will be harder to practice as a holistic nursing assistant? Explain your answer.

Some people believe that a problem is simply an obstacle that gets in the way of a desired goal. The best way to look at a problem, however, is as a question or issue that requires a solution.

Problems rarely go away without attention and effort. This is particularly true in healthcare. It is critical for you to understand, respond to, and identify problems quickly. Then you can determine how the problems will impact a situation and how the problems can be solved.

The strategy used to respond to problems is called the *problem-solving and decision-making process* (Figure 3.6). This process has six steps. The first three steps—identify the problem, examine the problem, and determine alternatives—are considered problem solving. The last three steps—select an alternative, implement, and evaluate—are steps that lead you to decision making.

Problem solving requires you to become aware of a problem, identify and accept it, look at all aspects of the problem, and then list possible alternatives that will lead to a solution. Decision making begins during the next step in the process. To make a decision, you need to determine which alternative will lead to the best solution, implement that solution, and then determine whether the solution was successful. Using your critical thinking skills, which help you examine your thinking and the thinking of others, is one way to begin the problem-solving process. Let's look at the steps of this process more carefully.

Identify the Problem

Identifying the problem is one of the most important steps in the problem-solving and decision-making process. The principal lesson in this step is that problems are based on **perception** (the ability to notice or recognize something using the senses). A problem is not a problem unless you see it as one. Once you are aware of a problem, the identification step allows you to focus on the difference between what *is* happening and what *is supposed to be* happening.

Examine the Problem

To solve a problem, you must have a well-defined understanding of the problem. You must be able to state the problem clearly and identify all aspects of the problem.

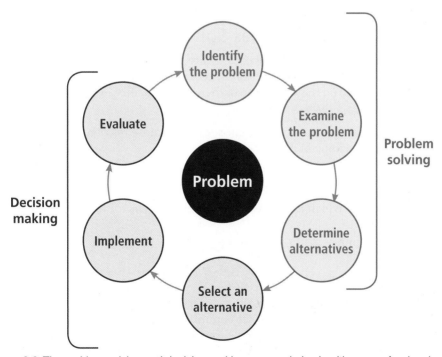

Figure 3.6 The problem-solving and decision-making process helps healthcare professionals make decisions.

To do this, look at the factors that influence the problem, ask others what they see, and search for factual evidence to help you understand what is happening. If a problem is not examined carefully and fully, the alternatives that are identified will likely be faulty, and the decision made will not solve the problem.

Determine Alternatives

Alternatives are possible courses of action that result from the information uncovered during the examination step. Alternatives must be realistic and should respond to the problem as it was identified. Talking to someone else can be useful during this step and provide a broader perspective. It is helpful to have a minimum of two alternatives from which to choose.

Select an Alternative

In this step, select the best alternative. This would be the alternative that best solves the problem. Sometimes a specific alternative is selected based on the resources available, such as time or money. If this is the case, be sure you are not sacrificing the best solution for a quick fix.

Implement

Implementation is an important step. During this step, an alternative should be implemented completely. All aspects of the alternative should be put in place.

Evaluate

Think About This

The more decisions a person makes on a daily basis, the more mentally tired the person can become. This can affect the quality of decision making. By the end of a day (or a shift), after making both large and small decisions, a person can have *decision fatigue*. This type of fatigue is not the same as physical or mental fatigue because people may not be aware of how drained they are becoming. Still, people who have decision fatigue may make critical decisions quickly without sufficient thought because they are tired and simply want to move on to the next task or activity.

This step provides an opportunity to determine if the action taken solved the problem. Evaluation usually occurs right after implementation and can also occur at specific times thereafter. The process of evaluation determines whether the alternative selected was the correct one. If the alternative was not the correct one, then the problem-solving and decision-making process starts again. If starting the process again, it is usually helpful to reexamine the problem. Maybe there are new facts that can be uncovered. Another option is to review the alternatives. Perhaps an alternative that was missed is the very alternative that will solve the problem.

How Are Ethical Dilemmas Solved?

There are many ethical **dilemmas** in healthcare that arise from situations in which there is not a clear right or wrong decision. These are examples of ethical dilemmas that occur in healthcare. You may see some of them in the facility in which you practice.

- a resident who refuses care and treatment;
- a family that requests the ventilator for a comatose resident be turned off, as there is no hope of recovery;
- the performance of procedures that are not medically necessary;
- the covering up of mistakes;
- a situation in which there are too few donor organs for those who need them; and
- a family that requests a resident not be told he or she is dying.

Ethics Committees

To respond to ethical dilemmas, healthcare facilities usually refer specific ethical issues to an *ethics committee*. The ethics committee uses ethical decision making to help assess and resolve ethical problems involving care. The size of the committee is usually consistent with the needs of the facility. Committee members are selected based on their interest in the welfare of others, expertise, integrity, and respect for others. Most members of the committee are doctors, licensed nursing staff, and other healthcare providers. The committee also includes members of the clergy, social workers, and community members (Figure 3.7).

The work of an ethics committee is confidential and deals exclusively with ethical matters. Usually, the facility's code of ethics; other guidelines, such as facility policy and current standard practice; and deep consideration of the facts and issues at hand are used to help make decisions. Recommendations are made with the purpose of educating and providing guidance for the facility and family members.

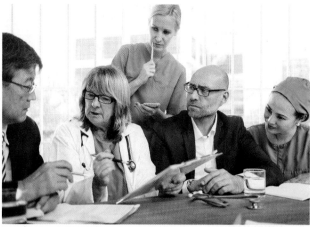

Rawpixel.com/Shutterstock.com

Figure 3.7 Ethics committees meet concerning specific ethical dilemmas. They help advise healthcare staff and families.

The Nursing Assistant's Role in Ethical Practice

As a holistic nursing assistant, you will not typically be part of an ethics committee, although you may be asked by the licensed nursing staff to provide information you learned when caring for residents.

You will be responsible for providing this information, and you are also always responsible for practicing ethically every day. You may be confronted with questions from residents or family members about care delivery, treatments, and the **prognosis** (likely outcome) of a resident's condition. You may even be asked what you would do. It is essential that you always practice ethically by following the code of conduct. If you are unsure how to practice ethically, you must always ask the licensed nursing staff.

Healthcare Scenario
An Ethical Dilemma

It was recently reported in a medical journal that an ethics committee in a local hospital was asked to meet regarding an older patient who was hit by a car last week. The patient was in the critical care unit and on a ventilator. Both of his legs were fractured, he had a severe head injury, and he was in a coma. He was also recently diagnosed with early-stage dementia. The patient's family asked the committee to meet because there was conflict about how to continue the patient's care. The patient's grown children wanted to wait and see if he would recover, but the patient's wife believed he would want to die and was requesting that he be taken off the ventilator. There was no documentation that stated what the patient would prefer.

To address this ethical dilemma, the committee followed its typical protocol:

- clarifying and assessing the facts, issues, and goals to determine if there was enough information to help make a decision

- identifying what steps to take, what the consequences were for each potential action, and if actions violated core ethical values or principles

- making a recommendation and implementing it

- monitoring and evaluating to see if changes were needed

Apply It

1. Which ethical principles would the committee be considering in this situation?

2. According to the sample code of ethics in this section, how should a nursing assistant practice ethically while caring for this patient and communicating with his wife and children?

Using the Key Terms

Complete the following sentences using the key terms in this section.

1. Identifying a problem requires _____, or the use of the senses to assess a situation.
2. A nursing assistant who represents himself or herself as an LPN/LVN to a patient would be violating the ethical principle of _____.
3. The decision about whether or not to continue care for a dying patient with no chance of recovery would be considered a(n) _____.
4. _____ are principles that guide conduct and help determine what is the right or wrong thing to do.
5. The principle of _____ implies that healthcare staff have the moral obligation to avoid doing harm.
6. On the job, nursing assistants may encounter ethical dilemmas when discussing the _____, or likely outcome, of a patient's condition.
7. The moral obligation to do good is called _____.
8. According to the principle of _____, healthcare staff must not abandon those in their care.

Know and Understand the Facts

9. What are ethics?
10. Identify four principles of ethical caregiving.
11. What is a code of ethics?
12. How is an ethics committee used in healthcare?
13. Identify the six steps of the problem-solving and decision-making process. Give an example of each.

Analyze and Apply Concepts

14. List two ways ethics committees help with ethical dilemmas and decision making.
15. Describe how problem solving and decision making influence each other.
16. Identify a recent problem you solved. Describe how you could have applied the six-step problem-solving and decision-making process. Would the outcome have been different?

Think Critically

Read the following care situation. Then answer the questions that follow.

Mr. D, a new resident in the assisted living facility where you work, was hospitalized recently with abdominal pain. He had a series of tests, which revealed he has cancer of the stomach. Mr. D's daughter does not want her father to know that he has cancer. She is very upset and thinks it's better if he knows less. The doctor is concerned, as a treatment plan needs to be made to determine the best course of action. He thinks Mr. D should be making these decisions. Mr. D's daughter thinks she should. While you care for Mr. D, he asks if you have his test results because he really feels that there is something wrong with him.

17. How should you respond to Mr. D?
18. Do you believe that you would be practicing ethically if you checked to find out what was wrong with Mr. D? Explain your answer.
19. What should you do next to show you are practicing ethically?

Key Points

Reviewing the key points for this chapter will help you practice more safely and competently as a holistic nursing assistant and will help you prepare for the certification competency examination.

- Regulations are enforced by state and federal laws. Healthcare facilities follow accreditation and licensure rules and regulations that guarantee safety and quality standards.

- The legal scope of practice dictates what nursing assistants can and cannot do and who supervises them.

- The Patient Bill of Rights and Nursing Home Resident Rights dictate how patients and residents should be treated. These rights include privacy of information, a safe environment, fair treatment, and the ability to make one's own medical decisions.

- Principles of ethical caregiving include autonomy, freedom, beneficence, nonmaleficence, veracity, fidelity, justice, and confidentiality.

- A code of conduct or ethics outlines standards for practice. If ethical problems occur, an ethics committee uses ethical decision making to help assess and resolve the issue.

Action Steps to Holistic Care

Review the information in this chapter. Complete the following activities.

1. Select one ethical principle discussed in the chapter. Prepare a short paper or digital presentation that describes three issues related to this principle when giving care.

2. With a partner, write a song or poem about a nursing assistant's legal scope of practice. Include the three questions nursing assistants should ask themselves about how to stay within the legal scope of practice.

3. With a partner, select one type of elder abuse. Prepare a poster that illustrates at least three facts about this type of abuse and ways to prevent it.

4. Research current scientific information about an ethical dilemma. Write a brief report that describes three current facts about the dilemma.

5. Find two pictures in a magazine, in a newspaper, or online that best represent a selected part of a nursing assistant's code of ethics. Describe the behaviors and attitudes demonstrated in the images.

Preparing for the Certification Competency Examination

To prepare for the nursing assistant certification competency examination, you will need to know content found in this chapter. This content may be tested in the knowledge (written or oral) and skills (hands-on demonstration) portions of the exam. The following areas will be emphasized:

- the nursing assistant's role as outlined in regulatory and professional guidelines
- the legal limits of nursing assistant practice
- healthcare laws and regulations
- the Patient Bill of Rights and Nursing Home Resident Rights
- ways of protecting residents from neglect, mistreatment, and abuse
- types of elder abuse
- ways of reporting neglect, mistreatment, and abuse
- nursing assistant ethics
- the nursing assistant standards of conduct

These sample test questions are similar to ones you will find on the certification competency exam. See how well you can answer them. Be sure to select the *best* answer.

1. If a nursing assistant unintentionally fails to act or provide care, resulting in harm to a resident, this is called which of the following?
   A. liability   C. negligence
   B. malpractice   D. ethics

2. Which of the following is a document that sets and guides nursing practice?
   A. code of behavior   C. code of practice
   B. code of discipline   D. code of ethics

(continued)

3. A nursing assistant has been praised for demonstrating ethical behavior. What behavior may have helped him earn that reputation?
   A. He asks other staff to do some of his work.
   B. He maintains confidentiality.
   C. He spends a lot of time talking with the family.
   D. He likes residents to think he is a friend.

4. Which of the following describes the legal scope of practice for nursing assistants?
   A. the boundaries that define what a nursing assistant can and cannot do
   B. standards of care defined by regulation
   C. the type of holistic care given to residents
   D. how well a nursing assistant does his or her work when practicing

5. A person commits a serious criminal offense and goes to jail. What type of criminal offense did the person commit?
   A. felony   C. misdemeanor
   B. certification   D. due process

6. A nursing assistant wants to determine if a specific responsibility he has been given is part of his scope of practice. Which of the following should he do to make that determination?
   A. He should ask his friend Joe, who is also a nursing assistant.
   B. He should ask his mother, who is an RN.
   C. He should review the regulations for nursing assistants.
   D. He should look at his healthcare facility's procedure manual.

7. When a nursing assistant came to work on Monday, the RN asked her to do a procedure she did not have the training or education to perform as a nursing assistant. If the nursing assistant did the procedure, which of the following would she be violating?
   A. accreditation   C. liability
   B. boundaries   D. scope of practice

8. A nursing assistant needs to perform care for her residents quickly. Mr. A does not want his morning care, but because the nursing assistant is so busy, she performs it anyway. Which resident right was violated?
   A. freedom from coercion and invasion of privacy
   B. freedom from mistreatment and neglect
   C. freedom from verbal abuse and coercion
   D. freedom from physical abuse

9. During morning care, a nursing assistant notices bruises on a resident's body and teeth marks. She should tell the licensed nursing staff that she suspects which of the following?
   A. malpractice   C. abuse
   B. libel   D. slander

10. As Mrs. K is being prepared for a special procedure, the doctor asks her to sign a written permission form that explains the procedure and its risks. What is the name of this document?
    A. informed consent
    B. bill of rights
    C. code of conduct
    D. protected health information

11. What is the major difference between certification and licensure?
    A. Certification is voluntary, and licensure is mandatory.
    B. Certification costs more than licensure.
    C. Licensure takes longer to get than certification.
    D. Unlike certification, licensure does not require the meeting of standards.

12. A nursing assistant made a false, written statement about another nursing assistant. Which of the following did she commit?
    A. slander   C. mistreatment
    B. abuse   D. libel

13. A new nursing assistant is learning about Nursing Home Resident Rights. He knows very little about what is included. Which of the following sentences would best describe it to him?
    A. Nursing Home Resident Rights are a set of requirements that protects residents in nursing homes from harm and empowers residents to make their own healthcare decisions.
    B. Nursing Home Resident Rights are a set of requirements that ensure older people have proper insurance over their lifetimes.
    C. Nursing Home Resident Rights are a set of requirements that protects older people from spending too much money.
    D. Nursing Home Resident Rights are a set of requirements that ensure healthcare staff have good employee benefits.

14. Why is HIPAA an important law in healthcare?
    A. It protects healthcare staff from retaliation.
    B. It protects the families of residents.
    C. It protects the environment in healthcare facilities.
    D. It protects the privacy of healthcare information.

15. What should a nursing assistant do if she suspects that a resident is being abused?
    A. She should ask the family about the abuse.
    B. She should ask the resident about the abuse.
    C. She should tell the licensed nursing staff.
    D. She should call the police.

Did you have difficulty with any of the questions? If you did, review the chapter to find the correct answer(s).

Working in Healthcare

Welcome to the Chapter

This chapter provides information about various healthcare careers, the ways healthcare facilities are staffed, and the importance of working effectively on a healthcare team. Regardless of where you work in healthcare, it is very important to be fully engaged in what you do and how you care for others. This means that you are respectful of and sensitive to others' needs, mentally present when communicating, and self-aware. It also means you self-examine and reflect on your caregiving skills. Learning how to be fully engaged requires you to be an effective critical thinker and to communicate professionally.

What you learn in this chapter will help you develop your knowledge and skills to become a holistic nursing assistant. The topics discussed in the chapter are highlighted on the Providing Holistic Care Framework.

You are now ready to start this chapter, *Working in Healthcare*.

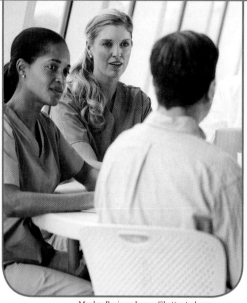

Monkey Business Images/Shutterstock.com

Chapter Outline

Section 4.1
Healthcare Teamwork

Section 4.2
Engagement, Critical Thinking, and Communication

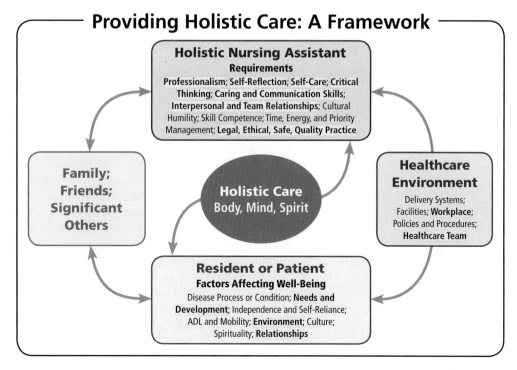

Providing Holistic Care: A Framework

Holistic Nursing Assistant
Requirements
Professionalism; Self-Reflection; Self-Care; Critical Thinking; Caring and Communication Skills; Interpersonal and Team Relationships; Cultural Humility; Skill Competence; Time, Energy, and Priority Management; Legal, Ethical, Safe, Quality Practice

Family; Friends; Significant Others

Holistic Care
Body, Mind, Spirit

Healthcare Environment
Delivery Systems; Facilities; Workplace; Policies and Procedures; Healthcare Team

Resident or Patient
Factors Affecting Well-Being
Disease Process or Condition; Needs and Development; Independence and Self-Reliance; ADL and Mobility; Environment; Culture; Spirituality; Relationships

Questions to Consider

- Have you ever played on a sports team or participated in another group activity? What was the most important factor in how effectively you worked with others to achieve a goal?
- While on the team, did you need to know whom you were working with and what roles your team members played? How did understanding each person's role help you achieve your shared goal?

Objectives

Nursing assistants work with a variety of healthcare staff. Getting to know the different types of staff, staff roles, and nursing unit staffing procedures helps to ensure effective teamwork. Having a good balance of staff and successful teamwork among staff members is essential to providing safe, quality care. Understanding how teams function, what role each team member has, and how you can be an effective team member are important parts of providing holistic care. To achieve the objectives for this section, you must successfully

- **describe** the healthcare staff you will be working with to provide holistic care;
- **identify** the ways facilities ensure there are enough staff members to provide safe, quality care;
- **explain** the functions of a healthcare team and team member roles; and
- **demonstrate** how you can be an effective healthcare team member.

Key Terms

Learn these key terms to better understand the information presented in the section.

census

level of care

ratio

staffing

staffing plan

turnover

What Healthcare Staff Members Work with Nursing Assistants?

One exciting part of working in healthcare is that you will become a member of a healthcare team. Teamwork is of the utmost importance in healthcare because it helps ensure that residents are receiving safe, quality holistic care. To find your place on the healthcare team, you will need to know and understand the different roles and responsibilities of healthcare staff. Several team members are directly involved in the care of residents and work closely with nursing assistants.

Doctor (MD or DO)

The *doctor* has the primary role in patient and resident care. A doctor is often called a *physician, primary care provider (PCP), medical doctor (MD),* or *doctor of osteopathic medicine (DO).* A doctor diagnoses illness or disease based on symptoms and the analysis of laboratory tests, X-rays, and other findings. Doctors also evaluate patients' progress (Figure 4.1). The decisions that doctors make result in orders for medication prescriptions, treatments, laboratory tests, X-rays, or the need for the use of medical equipment. Doctors' orders are also needed for admissions, transfers, and discharges in and out of healthcare facilities.

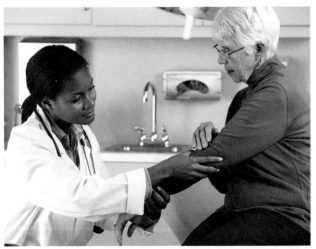

Monkey Business Images/Shutterstock.com

Figure 4.1 Doctors diagnose illnesses and diseases and prescribe treatments.

A doctor usually does not spend as much time with patients or residents as nursing assistants or licensed nursing staff members do. Doctors rely on verbal and written communication from staff to keep them informed.

Registered Nurse (RN)

As you learned in chapter 1, a *registered nurse (RN)* is a licensed professional who leads the nursing team and is accountable for the coordination of healthcare services; for nursing care; and for the assessment and evaluation of treatments, medications, and resident progress. RNs complete specialized education and training that allow them to become licensed and practice their profession. An RN may obtain an associate's degree in nursing (ADN) after completing two years of education and training at an approved community college or technical school. Another way to become an RN is to earn a bachelor's of science degree in nursing (BSN) after completing four years of education and training at a college or university. An RN must pass a licensing exam administered by the state board of nursing to practice.

RNs work in all types of healthcare facilities. In hospitals, RNs are primary care coordinators and work very closely with nursing assistants. In long-term care settings, RNs often work at a higher level—for example, as a director of nursing. The director of nursing has authority and responsibility for all nursing staff.

Licensed Practical/Vocational Nurse (LPN/LVN)

Depending on the state in which you live, this member of the healthcare team will be known as either a *licensed practical nurse (LPN)* or a *licensed vocational nurse (LVN)*. The LPN/LVN is a licensed caregiver who can administer medications, perform treatments (such as applying sterile dressings), and assist with ADLs. LPNs/LVNs work under the supervision of an RN.

To become an LPN/LVN, a person must complete 12–18 months of technical education and training from a school that has been approved by the state board of nursing. After graduating, the person must then pass a licensing exam. LPNs/LVNs typically work in subacute care facilities, skilled nursing facilities, some clinics, home healthcare services, and hospices. LPNs/LVNs work very closely with nursing assistants in healthcare facilities.

Nursing Assistant (NA)

Nursing assistants (NAs) work most frequently in long-term care facilities and hospitals. Some nursing assistants also work in clinics, hospices, and home healthcare services. Nursing assistants work within their legal scope of practice as part of the healthcare team and take directions from licensed nursing staff. Facilities usually require nursing assistants to obtain certification after completing a state-approved education and training program. Certification is obtained by passing the certification competency exam administered by the state in which the nursing assistant resides.

Caregiver

Caregivers typically work in assisted living facilities or in people's homes. In some states, regulatory requirements guide the training, certification, and testing of caregivers. In other states, only training is regulated, and in some states, there are no requirements at all. Training programs can be short or as long as 180 hours. When regulations are present, they are usually monitored by the state department of health services, board of nursing home administrators, or other regulatory boards. Topics covered in training may include basic caregiver skills (assisting with ADLs), nutrition and food management, resident rights, legal and ethical issues, communication and interpersonal skills, restorative care services, safety, infection control, emergency procedures, and medication management.

Health Unit Coordinator (HUC)

A *health unit coordinator (HUC)*, also known as a *unit secretary* or *unit clerk*, is trained to coordinate the administrative and support responsibilities of a nursing unit or healthcare facility (Figure 4.2). HUCs may process doctors' orders to schedule lab testing or X-rays; order dietary trays; and handle orders for admission, discharge, or transfer to another healthcare facility.

HUCs often receive training at a technical school or community college. Some have high school diplomas and are trained on the job. HUCs work closely with nursing assistants in both long-term care facilities and hospitals.

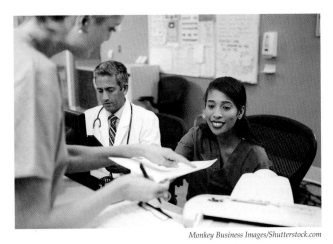

Monkey Business Images/Shutterstock.com

Figure 4.2 The HUC performs administrative and support functions for healthcare staff.

Laboratory, Medical Imaging, and Respiratory Therapy Staff

Laboratory, medical imaging, and respiratory therapy staff are responsible for procedures such as drawing blood, collecting specimens, taking X-rays, and providing breathing treatments. These procedures may be done on a nursing unit, in a designated area of a healthcare facility, in a doctor's office, or in a specialized facility that offers these services.

Laboratory, medical imaging, and respiratory therapy staff have a range of education depending on their scopes of practice. These staff members may be certified, and in some states, they must also be licensed. Nursing assistants are often asked to help these staff, particularly if a resident has a limited range of motion or is not fully conscious.

Care Support Staff

Care support staff, such as housekeeping staff and transport aides, may assist nursing assistants during the transfer or discharge of a patient. Transport aides also provide assistance when patients are taken to other departments for procedures. Care support staff members are trained on the job.

Case Manager

Case managers help provide special resources and support that patients need. For example, a case manager might plan and implement assistance for a patient who is going home. Case managers also help facilitate the process of moving patients from hospitals to long-term care facilities for continued rehabilitation, or from subacute rehabilitation facilities back home. A case manager may also refer patients for state assistance with healthcare insurance or provide other supportive and community resources. Case managers may be RNs or other staff members who have a degree, and possibly certification, in case management.

Social Worker

Social workers are similar to case managers. The difference is that social workers have specialized education, usually including a graduate degree that emphasizes the psychological, social, and economic aspects of healthcare. For example, a patient may be admitted to the hospital with pneumonia and be very worried about who will care for his dog while he is in the hospital. With the patient's permission, a social worker can use community resources to enter the patient's home and temporarily relocate the dog to the care of a relative or an animal care center. The social worker may also assist patients with financial, emotional, or other aspects of their care.

Physical Therapist (PT)

A *physical therapist (PT)* is usually the leader of a team that provides activities and assistance to maintain and improve resident flexibility and mobility. Physical therapists often have a graduate degree in physical therapy and are highly educated, trained specialists. Physical therapists work with residents during recovery to help residents achieve the highest levels of function possible (Figure 4.3). This type of rehabilitation and restoration might include helping a resident walk again after a severe stroke. A physical therapist often oversees resident rehabilitation and restoration under the guidance of a plan of care and with the help of an assistant—either a physical therapy assistant (PTA) or a rehabilitation or restoration aide.

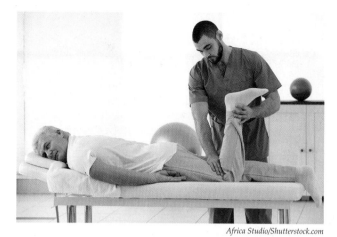

Africa Studio/Shutterstock.com

Figure 4.3 Physical therapists help residents regain flexibility and mobility.

Speech Therapist

A *speech therapist* also helps residents return to their preillness states and restore as much function as possible. For example, a speech therapist might help a resident learn how to swallow and speak again after a stroke. Speech therapists have a graduate degree in speech therapy.

Occupational Therapist (OT)

Occupational therapists (OTs) work with residents who have trouble performing daily tasks due to injury or illness. An occupational therapist promotes restoration by assisting a resident in returning to his or her preillness state and by helping him or her regain the ability to perform ADLs. This role requires a graduate degree in occupational therapy.

Dietitian

Dietitians help patients and residents with their nutritional needs. Dietitians are responsible for creating special diets that are required due to illness or disease. They also help patients and residents adjust to new diets, learn about these diets, and make dietary changes (with a doctor's order) when needed (Figure 4.4).

A dietitian has a degree in nutrition and may specialize in a particular area, such as working with diabetic residents or with those who have cardiovascular diseases. The dietary department in a healthcare facility also has other staff members who help order; cook; and deliver food, drinks, and healthy supplements.

How Are Healthcare Facilities Staffed?

Staffing is the process of determining the numbers and types of healthcare staff needed to care for a group of patients or residents on a nursing unit. Staffing a nursing unit can be complicated because the need for staff and the financial objectives of the healthcare facility must be balanced. The nurse manager of the nursing unit is usually responsible for its staffing. In a healthcare facility, the mix of staff should include

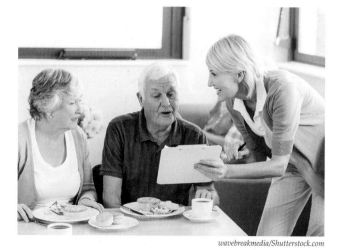

wavebreakmedia/Shutterstock.com

Figure 4.4 A dietitian creates a diet for a resident and explains the diet so the resident understands what is required and the diet's importance.

those with skills that match the nursing unit's **census** (number of residents) and required **levels of care** (types of care). During one shift, staffing needs might change due to fluctuations in

- the number of patients, due to admissions, transfers, and discharges; and
- the levels of care needed, due to changes in condition.

The **ratio** (the number of patients or residents per each healthcare staff member) is also considered when developing the **staffing plan** for a nursing unit. The staffing plan is a formal document that shows the mix and types of staff members who will work on each shift in the nursing unit. In a typical nursing unit, there are usually 10 residents for each nursing assistant. In units where residents have more serious conditions, the ratio may change so there are fewer residents for each nursing assistant.

The actual mix of the types and levels of staff is determined by the healthcare facility. Some hospitals, for example, do not hire nursing assistants; instead, they hire only RNs, LPNs/LVNs, and other healthcare providers. Other facilities may not use LPNs/LVNs. In long-term care facilities, there are usually many nursing assistants and LPNs/LVNs and a smaller number of RNs.

If a census falls below a set level, adjustments must be made. These adjustments might include sending staff home or transferring staff to another nursing unit. If the census increases and there are not enough staff members, staff members may be transferred from another unit or called in from home. Internal or external staffing agencies may also be temporarily used to meet the need. Sufficient staffing has a direct impact on providing safe, quality care. If there are not enough staff members, for example, certain important procedures might not be performed, and this can affect safety and resident well-being.

Staffing can be a challenge because it is always difficult to know in advance what the census will be on a particular shift or over time. Even with this lack of consistency, staffing must always be as accurate as possible. Maintaining the necessary numbers and types of staff needed in each nursing unit is essential to providing safe, quality care.

What Are the Functions of a Healthcare Team?

No matter where you work as a nursing assistant, you will always be delivering care alongside a group of staff members on the nursing unit. This group is called the *healthcare team*. The healthcare team may consist of a combination of RNs, LPNs/LVNs, HUCs, and nursing assistants. In some cases, respiratory therapists, transport aides, and social workers will also be part of the healthcare team. When these healthcare providers are also included, the healthcare team is usually called an *interdisciplinary healthcare team*. Whatever its composition, the healthcare team is always responsible and accountable for delivering safe, quality care.

Successful Teams

The goal of any team is to work well together, or exhibit *teamwork*. The primary goal of a healthcare team is to achieve specific outcomes. In healthcare, the primary outcome for a healthcare team is to deliver safe, appropriate, and effective care to patients and residents so patients and residents achieve their optimal levels of wellness. How well the healthcare team functions can make a difference in this outcome.

For a team to function at its best, its members must

- trust one another and the team leader;
- communicate effectively;
- establish clear goals;
- work together harmoniously;
- make decisions as a group; and
- understand how to handle conflicts.

Team Life Cycle

Successful teamwork does not happen overnight. Teams have a *life cycle*, or a series of developmental stages that influences their ability to achieve their primary outcome. A team's life cycle includes the following stages:

1. **Forming**: the team is established, and team members get to know one another. Team members learn to trust one another and develop positive relationships.
2. **Storming**: effective and ongoing communication becomes increasingly important as conflicts develop between team members. In this stage, learning how to handle conflicts is essential to ensuring optimal teamwork.
3. **Norming**: team members have worked through their differences and determined ways to work together and make effective decisions.
4. **Performing**: team members work together harmoniously and successfully, resulting in the achievement of the team's intended outcomes.

Becoming a Holistic Nursing Assistant
Being an Effective Team Member

The following behaviors and actions will help you be an effective team member and contributor to a successful healthcare team:

- Be dependable. Show up on time and be attentive to the team's efforts.
- Participate by sharing your ideas, unique perspective, and experiences.
- Value the contributions of others.
- Listen and show understanding.
- Speak honestly, but do not blame or judge others.
- Disagree without being rude or argumentative.

- Be positive and open to new ideas.
- Treat everything you hear as an opportunity to learn and grow.
- Show respect and integrity by not sharing confidential information with others.
- Always seek understanding and clarification.

Apply It

1. Examine the behaviors and actions of an effective team member. Which behaviors are good matches for you? Explain your answer.
2. Which behaviors might be challenging for you? Explain your answer.

Establishing a well-functioning and successful team is not always easy. It takes work and practice. Sometimes teams have a hard time moving past the forming stage because of **turnover** (the number of staff members who leave a healthcare facility) on a unit. Other teams may not move out of the storming stage because team members cannot work through differing opinions and successfully handle conflict. Teams are also affected by the characteristics of their members, such as age, gender, and ethnicity. The team leader has a great deal of influence over how well a team will progress through its life cycle (Figure 4.5).

How Can I Be an Effective Member of the Healthcare Team?

Working on a healthcare team is a very important part of daily work as a holistic nursing assistant. Each team member has a unique role. Certain members may help the team function well, while others may interfere with the team's ability to achieve its intended outcomes. One can often observe these roles. The following list describes some common roles you may encounter when working with a team:

- **The clarifier**: the team member who provides further information so everyone understands the issue, problem, or situation
- **The dominator**: the team member who tries to take over the team or meeting with his or her opinions or tries to sway the team with his or her preferences for a certain decision or direction
- **The energizer**: the team member who is always upbeat and finds ways to help others feel uplifted and energized
- **The gatekeeper**: the team member who always wants everyone else to share his or her opinions or give input on issues or problems
- **The harmonizer**: the team member who always tries to keep the peace and avoid conflict
- **The information seeker or giver**: the team member who is either always asking questions or who always gives information, even when not asked
- **The initiator**: the team member who can always be counted on to suggest new ideas
- **The optimist**: the team member who always sees situations in a positive light and tries to help others do the same
- **The skeptic**: the team member who always looks for problems or flaws in an idea, solution, or direction
- **The summarizer**: the team member who is willing to provide a review of what happened in a meeting
- **The timekeeper**: the team member who keeps track of time, even if not asked to do so

These roles are all played on a team at some time or another. You likely have seen some of these roles and will see them all as you gain more experience in your position as a holistic nursing assistant. Remember to be aware of each role and to be sure the roles you play help the healthcare team be successful.

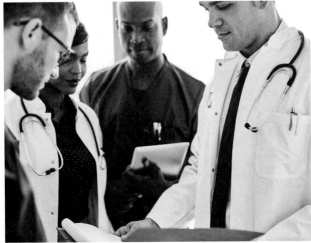

Uber Images/Shutterstock.com

Figure 4.5 Teams have life cycles. It takes work and practice to become an effective and well-functioning team.

Using the Key Terms

Complete the following sentences using the key terms in this section.

1. A patient who is paralyzed would require a higher _____ than a patient who is not paralyzed.
2. The financial objectives of the healthcare facility are one factor affecting the process of _____.
3. The _____, or number of patients or residents on a nursing unit, impacts how many members of staff are required on duty per shift.
4. The average nursing unit maintains a(n) _____ of 10 residents for each nursing assistant.
5. High _____ makes teams difficult to form due to losses of members.
6. A hospital's _____ shows the mix and types of staff members who will work on each shift in the nursing unit.

Know and Understand the Facts

7. Identify three different staff members whom nursing assistants work with on the healthcare team.
8. Describe the responsibilities associated with the healthcare staff members identified in the previous question.
9. What factors need to be considered when staffing nursing units?
10. Explain the life cycle of a healthcare team.

Analyze and Apply Concepts

11. Name two staff members who might be assigned to help patients who have had a stroke recover.
12. Describe what the staff members identified in the previous question do to help patients who have had a stroke recover.
13. In what ways do you think staffing affects the delivery of safe, quality care?
14. Describe two roles in a team you have experienced and how the roles helped or hindered the team.
15. List five ways you can be an effective healthcare team member.

Think Critically

Read the following care situation. Then answer the questions that follow.

A city's rehabilitation center has a special unit for patients who have had a stroke. There are 26 beds on this nursing unit, which is staffed by an LPN and three nursing assistants. Today you are working a day shift. There are 24 patients who have had strokes, and five of these patients were just admitted last week.

16. If the ratio during your shift is eight patients to one nursing assistant, how many nursing assistants will be needed?
17. Besides numbers, are there other factors to be considered when staffing this unit?
18. If one of your patients were discharged, how would this affect the staffing plan?

Engagement, Critical Thinking, and Communication

Questions to Consider

- When was the last time you stopped and took a quiet walk, either by yourself or with a good friend?
- Take a walk today. This time, stop to appreciate what you see. For instance, observe today's sunset, admire its colors, and feel the warmth it brings. Don't think about anything else except for the feelings and emotions you have at that very moment. Stay with this experience for at least two minutes. Were you able to focus on the sunset and let all other thoughts and feelings fade away? How did you feel when you looked away?

Objectives

Providing safe, quality care includes fully engaging people and providing them with the best care possible. Engagement requires being mindful, being self-aware, and practicing self-reflection. It is also essential that you have critical thinking skills and are able to communicate effectively and report concerns to appropriate healthcare staff in a professional manner. These skills are essential to helping you accomplish your daily responsibilities and to ensuring you provide safe, quality care. To achieve the objectives for this section, you must successfully

- **demonstrate** ways to engage residents who receive your care;
- **examine** strategies that will assist you in becoming more mindful and self-reflective when you give care;
- **examine** the characteristics of a critical thinker; and
- **explain** how to communicate effectively.

Key Terms

Learn these key terms to better understand the information presented in the section.

anxiety

bias

deduction

engagement

humility

intuitive

journal

meditation

mindfulness

nonverbal communication

rational

self-reflection

stress

systematic

verbal communication

Why Is Engagement Important?

People enter healthcare facilities because they are ill, are injured, or can no longer care for themselves. When this happens, some people feel **stress**, which is a physical or psychological response to a situation that causes worry or tension. People may also feel **anxiety** (uneasiness and nervousness) or feel lonely or depressed. Some people express these feelings as sadness, hopelessness, withdrawal, or even anger. At this time, attention, support, and care from a holistic nursing assistant can make a huge difference in a person's mental and emotional well-being.

Engagement refers to complete involvement and commitment. In your role as a holistic nursing assistant, being engaged means focusing your attention completely on those in your care. You may engage with residents when you first enter their rooms, while you provide care, or as you prepare to leave their rooms. Engagement can also occur when you are answering a call light. When you are engaged, you take the time to fully address the needs and desires of another. This allows you to give attention that shows others you care about them and provides others with a positive, helpful experience. It has been found that a resident's satisfaction increases when a caregiver takes notice and responds to the resident's needs, answers questions, and acknowledges the resident's presence. Increased satisfaction can decrease a resident's stress and anxiety, which may help the resident heal more rapidly, increase the resident's efforts to follow his or her treatment plan, and improve the resident's cooperation with caregivers.

There are two skills you can learn to achieve engagement—**mindfulness** and **self-reflection**. Possessing these skills allows you to observe the interactions you have with others and analyze the role you play in them. These skills usually need to be learned and then practiced.

Being Mindful of Others

Have you ever driven somewhere and found that, when you arrived, you did not remember the details of the drive? Have you ever been to dinner with your family and afterwards not remembered a word that was said? These situations—in which you are physically, but not mentally, present—may occur because you are preoccupied. When you pay attention, you are mindful and are present in the moment. You can see situations for what they really are. Being mindful also means being open to your thoughts and feelings, as well as the thoughts and feelings of others, without **bias** (unfair beliefs) or judgment.

Mindfulness can be integrated into daily living in two ways—through informal activities or through a more formal approach called **meditation**. Meditation helps you achieve mindfulness by allowing you to free your mind from those thoughts and feelings that may be stressful (Figure 4.6). Meditating daily can provide you with time to truly relax and be with yourself.

Informal mindfulness activities can include taking a few minutes out of each day to pay attention to simple activities such as washing your face. This awareness can make you more conscious of the physical act of washing and of the emotional response to how washing your face feels. This takes just a few minutes and can help you start your day more mindfully.

Sometimes events during the day are stressful and cause you to feel nervous or anxious. You can regain your sense of being present and mindful by stopping what you are doing for just a few minutes and consciously taking five slow, deep breaths without thinking about anything else. It is helpful if you think of the word *strong* when you inhale and the word *calm* when you exhale. This simple action can change your focus from feeling anxious and stressed to being present and mindful.

Whether you become more mindful through informal or formal practice, you will soon find that mindfulness spreads to your interactions and communications with others. Practicing mindfulness will help you become more fully engaged with your patients, residents, coworkers, friends, and family.

Practicing Self-Reflection

Nursing assistants who practice self-reflection are mindful not only of others, but also of themselves. They examine the work they have done and ways it can be improved. Self-reflection is like giving yourself a work performance review. Self-reflection need not occur at a specified time; you can reflect on your performance when it is convenient. The key is to be honest about your performance. You must regularly reflect on your behavior and actions for self-reflection to become a part of your daily routine. One way to accomplish self-reflection is to be self-aware and to keep a **journal** (written record) of your thoughts and feelings about your work performance and experiences.

Remember

Follow effective action with quiet reflection. From quiet reflection will come even more effective action.

Peter Drucker, PhD, management consultant, educator, and author

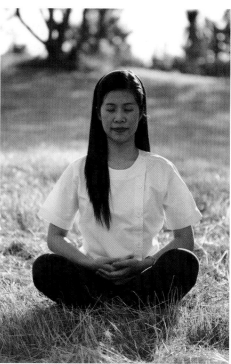

jannoon028/Shutterstock.com

Figure 4.6 Meditation involves emptying your mind of stressors and negative thoughts and instead focusing on the moment.

Journaling is most effective when you write your thoughts and feelings so they can be saved, read again, and compared with later entries. Journaling is not the same as keeping a diary. When you journal, you list specific actions, resulting thoughts and feelings, and further actions that are meant to improve your skills as a nursing assistant.

How Can I Become a Critical Thinker?

Another important skill that you need to be effectively and appropriately engaged, be self-aware, and self-reflect is critical thinking. Critical thinking is helpful in many situations, both personal and professional. As a nursing assistant, you will apply critical thinking to work through specific aspects of care delivery.

Critical thinking is a cognitive process that helps you examine your thinking and the thinking of others. As a critical thinker, you will reflect on what has been done and determine if you are accurate and on target when considering particular situations. The best way to understand and learn critical thinking is to remember its key components. Critical thinking requires the following:

- the ability to be purposeful, **rational** (having clear thinking), and **systematic** (orderly) when examining a situation

- focus and presence

- the ability to form conclusions and make decisions

- an attitude of inquiry

- the capacity to reflect on one's thinking

Experience and knowledge can help a person think critically; however, having little experience or knowledge will not stop you from being a critical thinker. In nursing, critical thinking is an important skill, particularly when you are asked to help solve a problem, observe a resident, or learn something new.

There are several characteristics of an effective critical thinker. Review the following list and consider which of these characteristics you possess:

- stops and thinks carefully about a situation before acting

- is able to see complex situations and work with them

- can use **deduction**, or use specific assumptions to develop reasonable conclusions
- is able to modify judgments when new information is uncovered
- is objective and reasonable
- is **intuitive** (perceptive) and curious
- is creative
- communicates clearly and logically
- is willing to listen
- can consider multiple viewpoints and shows interest in other people's ideas
- demonstrates confidence and perseverance
- is responsible and accountable
- possesses **humility** (modesty) and integrity
- is honest with one's self and recognizes limitations
- can control feelings rather than letting feelings be in control
- regards problems as exciting challenges

Remember

Invest a few moments in thinking. It will pay good interest.

Author Unknown

How Do Staff Members Communicate Effectively?

Along with mindfulness and critical thinking, effective communication is an essential part of working in a healthcare facility. It is important that you learn how staff members in your facility communicate so you can interact effectively with residents and their families, visitors, the leadership team, and others. The goal is always for you to communicate in a way that promotes healing and well-being.

As you learned in chapter 1, nursing assistants are the first line of communication with patients, residents, and their families. Nursing assistants spend the most time with residents. Because of this, it is very important that nursing assistants always share relevant information with licensed nursing staff and clearly and effectively provide resident information verbally, nonverbally, and in writing.

The chain of command, which you learned about in chapter 2, plays an important role in a facility's communication practices. Knowing with whom to discuss your concerns, as well as the concerns of your residents, is part of understanding a facility's chain of command. You should always communicate and work out any issues or problems with your charge nurse first. This maintains the chain of command. If this approach does not work, the next person to communicate with is the nurse manager.

Think About This

Research has found that effective communication in healthcare facilities can increase productivity, decrease employee turnover, and establish and maintain a positive work environment.

Healthcare Scenario
Using Critical Thinking

This morning, a local cable company reported a news story about a 12-year-old boy who helped save a family from perishing in a fire. The boy was walking past the family's house on his way home from school and saw smoke escaping out of the side door. He also saw two small children through the front window. The boy recalled his parents telling him that everyone has a responsibility to help others, especially when others might be in trouble. The boy called 911 using his cell phone.

Apply It

1. What characteristics of critical thinking do you think the boy used to evaluate this situation?

2. What did the boy have to think about to take the action he did?

3. What other alternatives could the boy have considered when deciding how to act? What might have been the consequences of these actions?

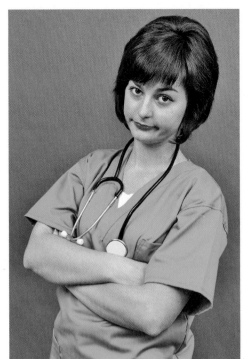

Kristo-Gothard Hunor/Shutterstock.com

Figure 4.7 Some older residents may interpret crossing one's arms as a sign of disrespect. What do you think this nursing assistant's body language communicates?

Verbal and Nonverbal Communication

Properly, effectively, and clearly communicating any concerns and issues can help foster a positive response to and resolution of a potential problem. How you communicate is very important. **Verbal communication**, which includes speaking clearly and using the appropriate words, is important; however, communication is more than the words you say. Nonverbal communication can also make a big difference in how people receive and respond to what you say.

Nonverbal communication includes gestures, facial expressions, body movements, and even your tone of voice. Pay attention to your nonverbal communication and ensure you are accurately expressing your thoughts and feelings. If you are feeling angry, this can come across to others through your nonverbal communication. Therefore, avoid angry facial expressions, such as scowling or frowning. If you are happy, express this appropriately. Do not cross your arms when you want people to feel your concern and openness. Older individuals may think actions such as crossing your arms or leaning on furniture express negativity or are disrespectful (Figure 4.7).

Written Communication

Another type of communication in healthcare facilities is *written communication*, which includes documentation, letters, memorandums (or *memos*), e-mails, reports, policies, and procedures. Communication, particularly written communication, is used to share information between staff in healthcare facilities. This helps establish mutual understanding about a resident's needs, improves decision making, and helps staff members provide the best holistic care possible. You will learn more about communication in chapter 10 and chapter 13.

Professional Communication

In chapter 1, you learned about professional boundaries and behaviors. Maintaining these boundaries is a requirement for all nursing assistants. Professional communication is essential to accomplishing this. To communicate professionally, you should

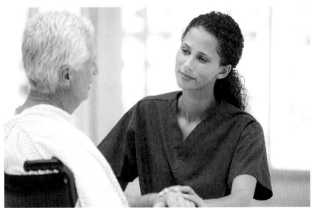

Monkey Business Images/Shutterstock.com

Figure 4.8 Listen carefully to residents' thoughts and concerns so that you can accurately communicate this information to the licensed nursing staff.

- always speak in a courteous and polite manner;
- never use first names when addressing residents and their families, and instead use Mr., Mrs., or Ms. and the resident's last name;
- use only respectful language and never use names such as *sweetie* or *honey*;
- be clear and concise in your directions;
- always take the time to respond to residents and their families;
- let residents communicate their own thoughts and feelings, and then convey this information as accurately as you can to the licensed nursing staff (Figure 4.8);
- never use offensive or slang language;
- never make sexual comments or suggestions;

- never share your own personal problems and information with residents or their families;
- only share your personal information with those who need this information, such as your charge nurse;
- be conscious of your nonverbal communication and how you come across to others;
- never post pictures or comments about your workplace on social media; and
- never send an angry or emotional e-mail or post similar comments on Facebook, Twitter, or other social media websites.

Remember

Communication is a skill that you can learn. It's like riding a bicycle or typing. If you're willing to work at it, you can rapidly improve the quality of every part of your life.

Brian Tracy, motivational speaker and author

Section 4.2 Review and Assessment

Using the Key Terms

Complete the following sentences using the key terms in this section.

1. It is important that nursing assistants remain _____, or think clearly, as they make decisions.
2. A nursing assistant who is _____ could use perception to pick up on a resident's unspoken needs.
3. _____ is a method of achieving mindfulness through relaxation and concentration and can reduce stress when practiced daily.
4. A(n) _____ may contain a nursing assistant's thoughts and feelings about his or her work performance and experiences.
5. The process of using reasonable assumptions to reach a conclusion is called _____.
6. _____, or looking at one's self in an honest and truthful way, can lead to improved interactions with others.
7. Giving a resident undivided attention is one example of _____ and shows dedication to providing quality care.
8. When practicing _____, a nursing assistant focuses on the present, including what is being said, what he or she is doing, or what is happening in his or her environment.

Know and Understand the Facts

9. Discuss what it means to engage residents.
10. Identify one formal and one informal approach to mindfulness.
11. Identify the five components of critical thinking.
12. List three characteristics of a critical thinker.

Analyze and Apply Concepts

13. Describe how mindfulness can contribute to effective caregiving.
14. Describe two informal exercises a person can use to help develop mindfulness.
15. Explain two strategies that can be used to increase engagement.
16. Discuss five ways you can communicate professionally.

Think Critically

Read the following care situation. Then answer the questions that follow.

Lately, it has been difficult to care for Mr. J. Mr. J has not wanted to get up, bathe, or talk with other residents. This behavior is unusual for Mr. J. During the last week, you noticed Mr. J's behavior getting worse. You have been busy and have tried to be helpful and attentive to him, but that does not seem to be working. Each time you walk into Mr. J's room, he turns away.

17. What might be the first action that you, as a holistic nursing assistant, could take the next time you walk into Mr. J's room?
18. What might you say to Mr. J?
19. What engagement strategies could you use to find out what has happened to Mr. J. that is causing this change in behavior?

Key Points

Reviewing the key points for this chapter will help you practice more safely and competently as a holistic nursing assistant and will help you prepare for the certification competency examination.

- Healthcare teams may consist of a combination of RNs; LPNs/LVNs; HUCs; nursing assistants; and in some cases, respiratory therapists, transport aides, and social workers.

- Engagement can be accomplished through mindfulness and self-reflection. Practicing mindfulness means accepting your thoughts and feelings, as well as the thoughts and feelings of others, without bias or judgment. Self-reflection requires you to examine your behaviors and actions and determine if there is a need for improvement.

- In nursing, critical thinking is an important skill for solving a problem, observing a resident, or learning something new.

- Various communication methods, including nonverbal strategies, are used to ensure holistic care. Being able to effectively and professionally communicate and share issues and concerns optimizes the ability to achieve a holistic healing environment.

Action Steps to Holistic Care

Review the information in this chapter. Complete the following activities.

1. Select one of the following aspects of staffing: ratio, census, or staffing plan. Prepare a short paper or digital presentation that describes the aspect of staffing selected in more detail than what is found in the chapter.

2. With a partner, write a short song or poem that expresses the importance of critical thinking.

3. With a partner, prepare a poster that illustrates communication and teamwork among nursing assistants and other healthcare staff.

4. Research current scientific information about either mindfulness or self-reflection. Write a brief report that describes three current facts.

 ## Preparing for the Certification Competency Examination

To prepare for the nursing assistant certification competency examination, you will need to know content found in this chapter. This content may be tested in the knowledge (written or oral) and skills (hands-on demonstration) portions of the competency examination. The following areas will be emphasized:

- healthcare staff and their roles
- the roles and functions of healthcare teams
- ways of communicating and working with members of healthcare teams
- positive, nonthreatening communication with others
- professional communication

These sample test questions are similar to ones you will find on the certification competency examination. See how well you can answer them. Be sure to select the *best* answer.

1. When nursing assistants engage with residents, they are being which of the following?
   A. compliant
   B. present
   C. happy
   D. noticed

2. A nursing assistant prides himself on being an outstanding critical thinker. Which of the following characteristics most confirms that this is true?
   A. He works well with others, and everyone likes working with him.
   B. He is fun to be around, and everyone seeks him out.
   C. He stops and thinks carefully about a situation before acting.
   D. He is a very competent and experienced nursing assistant.

3. When communicating, a nursing assistant should show she understands the chain of command by sharing resident concerns with which staff member first?
   A. her coworkers
   B. the DON
   C. the charge nurse
   D. the nurse manager

4. Which of the following is one way nursing assistants can self-examine and reflect back on the care they deliver?
   A. contemplating
   B. analyzing
   C. reading
   D. journaling

5. When nursing assistants are being mindful, they are doing which of the following?
   A. making a resident's bed
   B. being aware of call lights ringing
   C. being present and focused on residents' needs
   D. keeping residents' rooms tidy and clean

6. Which of the following actions would you recommend a new nursing assistant take to ensure she is an effective member of the healthcare team?
   A. She should let everyone know she is experienced.
   B. She should tell everyone how much she likes them.
   C. She should go out with her team after her shift.
   D. She should be dependable, respectful, and present.

7. Which of the following statements or questions made by a nursing assistant is the most professional and best demonstrates holistic care?
   A. "Are you getting out of bed today? I need to change the linens."
   B. "I have been so busy with other residents that I was not able to give you your bath today."
   C. "I need to help you with a bath today. What would be the best time for us to do that?"
   D. "You need to get up and walk today, and I am busy. Maybe your family can help when they get here."

8. Which healthcare staff member coordinates administrative and support responsibilities such as processing doctors' orders?
   A. RN
   B. HUC
   C. LPN
   D. PTA

9. For a healthcare team to function optimally, its team members need to do which of the following?
   A. know one another well
   B. spend time talking about everyone's experience
   C. have worked on the unit for a long time
   D. make decisions collaboratively

10. Which of the following behaviors demonstrates that a holistic nursing assistant is an effective team member?
    A. sharing only personal opinions and giving advice
    B. disagreeing without being rude or argumentative
    C. declining when asked to participate
    D. reviewing everything said using one's own experience

11. Which healthcare staff member provides activities and assistance to maintain and improve resident flexibility and mobility?
    A. speech therapist
    B. language therapist
    C. physical therapist
    D. occupational therapist

12. There are 32 residents in today's census at a community long-term care center. The ratio of nursing assistants to residents is 1:8 on the day shift. How many nursing assistants will be needed for this shift?
    A. six
    B. three
    C. five
    D. four

13. A nursing assistant always tries to keep peace and avoid conflict during healthcare team meetings. Which team role is she playing?
    A. initiator
    B. optimist
    C. clarifier
    D. harmonizer

14. Which of the following considerations are most important to the staffing of a unit?
    A. census and level of care
    B. level of care and doctor's preferences
    C. census and available resources
    D. staff education and training

15. Which of the following is *not* an example of professional communication?
    A. speaking in a courteous and polite manner
    B. speaking clearly and being concise in your directions
    C. using first names when addressing residents and their families
    D. always taking the time to respond to residents and their families

Did you have difficulty with any of the questions? If you did, review the chapter to find the correct answer(s).

CHAPTER 5

Providing Holistic Nursing Care

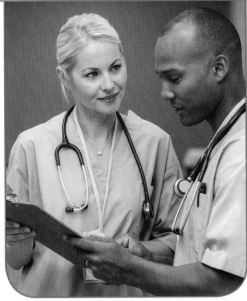

Rido/Shutterstock.com

Chapter Outline

Section 5.1
Levels and Types
of Nursing Care

Section 5.2
The Nursing Process,
Policies, and Procedures

Section 5.3
Admission, Transfer,
and Discharge

Welcome to the Chapter

This chapter discusses the different levels and types of nursing care delivered in healthcare facilities. You will also learn about the role holistic nursing assistants play in the nursing process and about the importance of policies and procedures for safe and competent practice. Members of the licensed nursing staff will delegate work to nursing assistants. It is important that delegated tasks are completed in an accurate and timely manner. Nursing assistants may also perform procedures for patients and residents entering a facility (admission), moving within or to another facility (transfer), and leaving a facility (discharge).

The information and procedures presented in this chapter will help you build the knowledge and skills needed to become a holistic nursing assistant. Check with your instructor to ensure these procedures are within your state's regulations for nursing assistant practice. The topics discussed in the chapter are highlighted on the Providing Holistic Care Framework.

You are now ready to start this chapter, *Providing Holistic Nursing Care.*

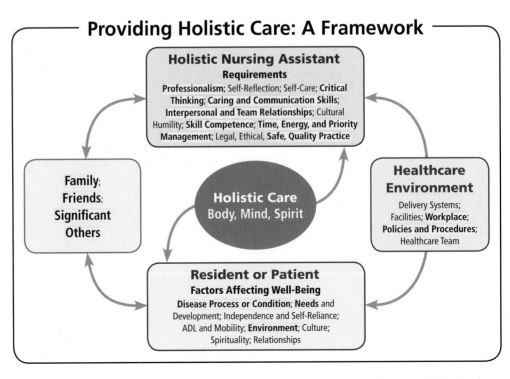

Providing Holistic Care: A Framework

Holistic Nursing Assistant
Requirements
Professionalism; Self-Reflection; Self-Care; **Critical Thinking; Caring and Communication Skills; Interpersonal and Team Relationships;** Cultural Humility; **Skill Competence; Time, Energy, and Priority Management;** Legal, Ethical, **Safe, Quality Practice**

Family;
Friends;
Significant
Others

Holistic Care
Body, Mind, Spirit

Healthcare Environment
Delivery Systems; Facilities; **Workplace; Policies and Procedures;** Healthcare Team

Resident or Patient
Factors Affecting Well-Being
Disease Process or Condition; Needs and Development; Independence and Self-Reliance; ADL and Mobility; **Environment;** Culture; Spirituality; Relationships

78

Objectives

To provide the best possible care, you must recognize the different levels and types of nursing care delivered in healthcare facilities. You must also be knowledgeable about delegation and about the influence this process has on the care you will deliver as a nursing assistant. To achieve the objectives for this section, you must successfully

- **describe** the different levels and types of nursing care delivery; and
- **recognize** the process of delegation and its impact on delivering care.

Key Terms

Learn these key terms to better understand the information presented in the section.

accountable

cognitive status

continuity

philosophy

tracheostomy

Questions to Consider

- Have you ever been asked by a friend or coworker to do something? Maybe you were asked to do a job or task that was part of your friend's responsibilities or to attend a meeting in your coworker's place.
- When your friend or coworker requested your help, did he or she give you the information you needed to decide if you were capable? If he or she did not, what would have helped in your decision making?
- If you did what was asked of you, did your friend or coworker follow up to see how it went?

What Are Levels of Care?

Every healthcare facility provides varying levels of care to meet the unique needs of each patient or resident. As you learned in chapter 4, *levels of care* describe the types and amounts of care that patients and residents require to achieve the best result or outcome. Providing the right level of care helps ensure that a patient improves enough to be discharged from a hospital or that a resident in a long-term care facility remains as independent as possible. For example, the level of care needed by an older adult helps determine whether a healthcare facility has the staff and resources to meet the older adult's needs. Knowing the level of care a resident requires also helps healthcare staff evaluate the resident's insurance to determine what care will be covered.

Determining Levels of Care

For residents, levels of care are usually evaluated prior to the selection of a long-term care facility to ensure the facility will offer the specific care needed. For example, someone with dementia might need special memory care; therefore, a facility that offers this type of care would need to be selected.

Levels of care are also evaluated for patients admitted to a hospital. For example, if a patient were in a car accident, the severity of his or her injury would determine the level of care needed. When the patient arrived at the hospital, a decision would be made about whether to admit him or her to a critical care unit or to a general medical unit on a hospital floor.

Level of care is evaluated again once a patient or resident has spent some time in the healthcare facility. After the information provided by doctors and nurses is reviewed, medical needs are considered, including the level of nursing staff needed for specific care. The nursing staff needed can range from a nursing assistant to an RN. Personal care needs, such as the amount of assistance required to complete ADLs, are a factor in evaluating level of care. A patient's or resident's **cognitive status** (ability to think clearly, make decisions, and remember) is considered. Self-care abilities, such as a patient's or resident's ability to swallow medications, also influence the level of care. Once these factors are considered by the doctor and licensed nursing staff, a *level-of-care assignment* is made.

Assigning Levels of Care

Level-of-care assignments are dynamic because they are based on patient or resident needs and conditions, which change over time. This is especially true for patients who need hospitalization. A patient's care needs are first matched with what services are provided by the facility, such as rehabilitation services or specific surgical procedures. Level of care is evaluated again once the patient is in the hospital. Care needs can change from shift to shift because a patient's condition changes. As a result, level of care needs to be evaluated continually in a hospital.

Levels of care change less frequently in long-term care facilities. Typically, an initial evaluation places residents in facilities that will best meet their care needs. When people seek long-term care, it is often helpful for them to consider both current and future needs and choose a facility that meets both. This way, when residents have more advanced needs, they are able to stay in the facility first selected. Levels of care in a long-term care facility include skilled, intermediate, and supportive care.

Skilled Care

Skilled care requires 24-hour, hands-on care in a healthcare facility. This level of care may also include physical therapy, rehabilitation therapy, speech therapy, or wound care. Skilled care is typically needed for only a short period of time. Depending on the services required, Medicare will regulate, or limit, the number of days it will pay for care in a skilled care facility. The goal of skilled care is to stabilize or improve a resident's medical condition so the level of care can be changed to intermediate.

Intermediate Care

Intermediate care is provided for those who require assistance with ADLs, such as bathing or hygiene. Usually, care is provided by nursing assistants, caregivers, home health aides, or even family members. The assessment of healthcare needs and progress requires monitoring by licensed nursing staff and doctors. Intermediate care can occur in a person's home or in a healthcare facility such as *assisted living*.

Supportive Care

Residents who need *supportive care* may require special rehabilitation. These services could include **tracheostomy** care (care for a surgical opening in the trachea), care for multiple medical problems (called *comorbidity*) that require blood pressure or medications to be monitored, or respiratory therapy (Figure 5.1). This care may be given in a person's home by an RN or LPN/LVN. This level of care also includes *end-of-life care*, which provides for a person's physical, emotional, and spiritual needs.

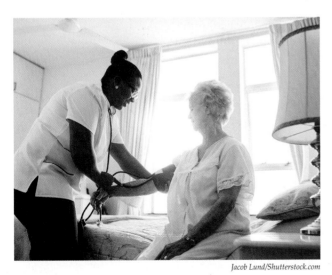

Jacob Lund/Shutterstock.com

Figure 5.1 Supportive healthcare services include monitoring blood pressure.

What Are Different Types of Nursing Care Delivery?

There are different ways nursing care is delivered in healthcare facilities. The type of nursing care delivery selected is usually determined by the healthcare facility's **philosophy**, or beliefs about how care should be delivered. The medical conditions of patients or residents are also considered, as are the numbers and types of nursing staff available. The goal is to match needs with the best, most cost-effective care possible.

When you start to work at a healthcare facility as a holistic nursing assistant, it is essential to identify the type of nursing care delivery used at the facility. Identifying the way care is delivered will allow you to best understand the role you will play. In this section, we will discuss six ways nursing care may be delivered.

Total Patient Care

The first formal type of nursing care delivery used in healthcare facilities was *total patient care*. In total patient care, one licensed nursing staff member provided all required care—from planning to organizing and performing nursing care—for each assigned patient for the shift in which the licensed nursing staff member worked. This licensed nursing staff member was usually an RN, but may have also been an LPN/LVN. This type of care required a large number of licensed nursing staff to care for patients. Because there is often only a limited number of licensed nursing staff in healthcare facilities today, this type of nursing care delivery is not usually seen. An exception would be in critical care units, where an RN can best respond to the demanding care needs of only one or two patients.

Functional Nursing

Since the era of total patient care, several other types of care delivery have emerged. *Functional nursing* requires that available nursing staff members complete all required care tasks needed for an assigned group of patients or residents. In this type of care delivery, medications may be given by an RN, an LPN/LVN might do all treatments, and a nursing assistant might measure vital signs and help residents meet their hygiene needs.

Team Nursing

Team nursing relies on an RN team leader. The RN team leader coordinates a small group of staff (the team) to provide care for a group of patients or residents. The RN team leader is responsible for developing a cooperative environment. Team member cooperation allows the team leader to plan, assign, assist with, teach, coordinate, and delegate care assignments to the staff on the unit.

Primary Nursing

Another way of delivering care is called *primary nursing*. In this type of delivery, one licensed nursing staff member (usually an RN) coordinates and also provides all individualized care during the full length of a patient's medical condition or illness. The goal is to achieve **continuity** (an uninterrupted sequence of events) by having a licensed nursing staff member coordinate and provide direct care. While primary nursing was very popular in hospitals during the late 1970s, it became challenging and too costly to employ sufficient staff to continue this type of care delivery.

Progressive and Patient-Centered Care

In more recent years, progressive care and patient-centered care have become common. In *progressive care*, the delivery of care is determined by the degree of an illness and the level of care needs. For example, a patient receiving progressive care who is well enough to leave a critical care unit may move to a *step-down unit* if he or she is still too sick to be cared for on a general medical unit.

In *patient-centered care*, patients or residents are seen as the center or focus of care. Rather than care being "done" to them, they are the primary sources of information about how care is best delivered. Care delivery is holistic and also individualistic.

In patient-centered care, time is devoted to consistently requesting information from patients or residents. Licensed nursing staff members use this information to identify and act on expressed needs and wants and to inquire about how the care was experienced. These inquiries can range from asking what food residents like to eat to when residents want to rest and sleep. In patient-centered care, patients and residents also learn about their own diseases and conditions and ways they can be involved in their ongoing care. The goal of patient-centered care is to deliver care that is appropriate to individual patients or residents and to create partnerships in care. This allows patients or residents to identify their needs and requirements for achieving well-being. The emphasis is on promoting self-reliance and independence.

For example, in patient-centered care, a patient who requires insulin due to a new diagnosis of diabetes will learn how to balance nutrition, exercise, rest, and relaxation. The patient will learn when to use insulin and how much insulin to use to accommodate his or her lifestyle. The patient will also learn his or her own unique patterns and understand when he or she may need more or less insulin to manage diabetes. Usually, a diabetes educator who may also be a member of the licensed nursing staff will work with a patient to provide this information. This staff member would develop a helping relationship with the patient to teach him or her about this new lifestyle and provide emotional support as the patient works toward achieving a new level of well-being.

How Does Delegation Influence Delivery of Care?

Delegation occurs when licensed nursing staff members ask a nursing assistant to take the responsibility of performing specific tasks. Sometimes the delegated tasks are routine, and other times they may require special knowledge or skill. No matter what the delegated task is, it must always be a part of your scope of practice as a nursing assistant. You must be able to do the task safely and accurately.

An example of delegation would be an RN asking that, during the care you provide Mrs. J today, you monitor her blood pressure, taking it every two hours because it was unusually high this morning. The RN also asked that you report back and document the results each time you take Mrs. J's blood pressure.

When a licensed nursing staff member delegates a task to a nursing assistant, he or she also transfers the responsibility for performing that task. Upon accepting, the nursing assistant becomes responsible for performing the task correctly. A fundamental part of delegation is trust. How much licensed nursing staff members trust a nursing assistant's ability will determine what will be delegated.

Delegation and the Licensed Nursing Staff

Delegation is a legal act within a licensed nursing staff member's scope of practice. Nursing assistants cannot delegate a task. Licensed nursing staff members are always **accountable** (responsible) for the completion of delegated tasks, even if a nursing assistant is giving the care. When delegating tasks, licensed nursing staff members will be aware of the nursing assistant's scope of practice, skill level, and performance. The written policies and procedures of the healthcare facility must also be considered.

When delegating, licensed nursing staff members must observe the five rights of delegation, which are provided in a guide by the National Council of State Boards of Nursing.

According to these guidelines, licensed nursing staff members must ensure

1. the **right task** is delegated;
2. the delegation occurs under the **right circumstance**;
3. the task is delegated to the **right person**;
4. the **right direction and communication** are given; and
5. the **right supervision and evaluation** are provided.

Acceptance of a Delegated Task

When you begin working as a nursing assistant, it is your responsibility to let the licensed nursing staff know if you believe you do *not* have the skill to accomplish a delegated task. Sharing such concerns will enable you to ensure that residents receive safe and accurate holistic care. When you recognize your limitations as a nursing assistant, you act in a professional manner. You are also giving licensed nursing staff members information they need to help you develop your skills and abilities. Doing this strengthens collaboration and will improve your ability to work as a team.

Section 5.1 Review and Assessment

Using the Key Terms

Complete the following sentences using the key terms in this section.

1. A healthcare facility's _____, or beliefs about how care should be delivered, influences the type of nursing care delivery selected.
2. A(n) _____ is a surgical opening in the trachea.
3. Licensed nursing staff members are always _____ for the completion of tasks they delegate to nursing assistants.
4. A patient's or resident's ability to think clearly, make decisions, and remember is known as _____.
5. Primary nursing offers the patient _____ because one licensed nursing staff member provides direct care throughout the entirety of the patient's stay.

Know and Understand the Facts

6. Describe three levels of resident care.
7. Identify two types of nursing care delivery.
8. Explain the five rights of delegation.

Analyze and Apply Concepts

9. Explain the level of care a resident might receive if he or she were provided skilled nursing care.
10. Describe how care would be delivered on a unit that used team nursing.
11. Discuss what you should do if you are delegated a task you do not know how to do.

Think Critically

Read the following care situation. Then answer the questions that follow.

Tasia is assigned to Ms. O, a 78-year-old resident who badly broke her leg. Ms. O was in the hospital for one week before being transferred to an assisted living facility. The doctor has ordered physical therapy as well as daily dressing changes. Ms. O will likely need three weeks of care before she is discharged home. Today, the RN team leader delegated Ms. O's dressing change to Tasia. Tasia learned how to change a dressing, but she is concerned she may not do the procedure well.

12. What level of care is Ms. O receiving?
13. What type of nursing care delivery do you think is being provided in this facility?
14. How would you suggest Tasia deal with her concerns about being delegated a dressing change?

Questions to Consider

- What policies and procedures do you have to follow in your life? Are there policies in your home about how late you can stay out of the house? Are there procedures regarding how a particular room should be cleaned?
- There are also policies and procedures at school or at work. Have you found any of these policies and procedures helpful? If so, how and in what ways have they helped?
- Have you ever encountered policies and procedures that are not helpful or are frustrating? What could you do to make these policies and procedures more helpful and less frustrating?

Objectives

It is important to understand that the nursing process is a set of accepted guidelines that help organize, coordinate, and evaluate care. You will also need to understand, obey, and follow healthcare policies and procedures to ensure you are providing safe, quality care. To achieve the objectives for this section, you must successfully

- **explain** the nursing process and the role of the nursing assistant;
- **discuss** the importance of understanding and obeying healthcare policies;
- **recognize** the differences between policies and procedures; and
- **describe** how following written healthcare procedures ensures safe, quality practice.

Key Terms

Learn these key terms to better understand the information presented in the section.

assessing
evidence-based practice
nursing diagnosis
nursing process

plan of care
priorities
standards of care

One fundamental of delivering care is using a set of criteria and guidelines to direct the care you give. These guidelines are established by the nursing profession and are called **standards of care**. Standards of care are methods, processes, and actions. In nursing, one standard of care is called the **nursing process**. In the 1970s, the American Nurses Association recognized the nursing process as an important standard of care for guiding nursing practice. By the 1980s, state boards of nursing had adopted the nursing process as part of nursing education and the licensing examination for licensed nursing staff.

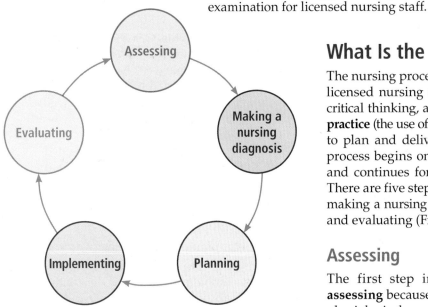

Figure 5.2 The nursing process consists of five steps.

What Is the Nursing Process?

The nursing process is a systematic method in which licensed nursing staff members, led by an RN, use critical thinking, analytical skills, and **evidence-based practice** (the use of research findings to guide decisions) to plan and deliver safe, quality care. The nursing process begins on admission to a healthcare facility and continues for as long as a resident needs care. There are five steps in the nursing process: assessing, making a nursing diagnosis, planning, implementing, and evaluating (Figure 5.2).

Assessing

The first step in the nursing process is called **assessing** because information is gathered about the physiological, psychological, emotional, sociological, economic, lifestyle-related, and spiritual aspects of a resident for the purpose of providing a holistic perspective. This information may be collected through observation, a physical examination, medical history, or an interview with the resident. Assessment is ongoing during care.

Making a Nursing Diagnosis

When making a **nursing diagnosis**, licensed nursing staff members use clinical judgment based on information collected to identify a potential or existing health problem experienced by a resident. The nursing diagnosis describes health *problems*, such as sleep deprivation, that can be helped through nursing care. A nursing diagnosis is *not* the same as a medical diagnosis, in which a disease or medical condition is diagnosed by a doctor. For example, a resident may receive a medical diagnosis of cardiac ischemia (reduced blood flow to the heart due to partial or complete blockage of the arteries) and a nursing diagnosis of chest pain and discomfort radiating to the arm, neck, jaw, or back. Other problems identified by a nursing diagnosis might include impaired mobility or impaired swallowing. NANDA International is an organization and resource that defines, distributes, and integrates standardized nursing diagnoses worldwide.

A resident's risk for developing further problems is also determined during this step. The nursing diagnosis is critical because it is used by licensed nursing staff to develop a plan of care.

Planning

During this step, licensed nursing staff members develop a resident's **plan of care** (also called a *service plan*). The plan of care is a written document that provides directions and serves as a guide to delivering individualized, holistic care. In the plan of care, measurable and achievable goals are written for each identified problem. To work toward the highest level of wellness possible, each problem is written with a positive outcome. It is helpful when the resident and licensed nursing staff agree to the plan's outcomes and set **priorities** (actions of high importance). Others involved in the planning process include the resident's family members and healthcare team members. Resources such as medical and nursing books, research-based articles, and standards of care are available to licensed nursing staff members to guide them through planning.

Implementing

Care is implemented by the healthcare and nursing staff based on the plan of care developed. These actions may include direct care, education and instruction of residents, or referrals for follow-up therapies. Implementation can be completed during several hours or take as long as a few months. Care and any actions taken are always recorded in a resident's chart or EMR.

Evaluating

The evaluating step of the nursing process is ongoing throughout care. Even if all nursing actions have been completed and licensed nursing staff members have evaluated the attainment of stated goals, changes may occur along the way. As a result, new goals may have to be identified. The nursing process will then begin again from the first step. In this case, the care plan will usually be changed to meet the new needs identified.

The Importance of the Nursing Process

The nursing process is always part of the delivery of nursing care. You will hear about the nursing process often during your education and when you begin and during your nursing assistant career. The nursing process will be used when licensed nursing staff members assess a resident and when they determine nursing diagnoses.

Using this information, goals and actions are written in the resident's plan of care to provide guidance for the nursing and healthcare staff as they deliver care.

As a nursing assistant, you will participate in the nursing process when you are asked to provide your observations of a resident's status and information about your ongoing interactions with residents. This information will be very useful during the planning, implementing, and evaluating steps. Be aware that your observations must be timely and accurate and that you should report any changes to the licensed nursing staff. More information about observations and reporting will be discussed in chapter 12.

In addition to plans of care, healthcare policies and procedures are developed to provide a standardized way of accomplishing your work. Policies and procedures are developed by a healthcare facility based on legal and regulatory requirements, medical and nursing standards of care, facility and nursing practice expectations, evidence-based practice findings about particular policies and procedures, and doctors' approaches in caring for patients and residents with specific diseases and conditions.

What Are Policies and Procedures?

All healthcare facilities have written policies and procedures that set mandatory guidelines for the care you deliver as a holistic nursing assistant. In healthcare, policies and procedures are required by several regulatory bodies and by other agencies, such as Medicare, that oversee the quality and safety of healthcare.

Policies and procedures set boundaries, directions, and guidelines that ensure the actions taken by healthcare staff are based on good evidence and best practice. Policies and procedures are usually specific to a healthcare facility, but are based on external rules and standards, research, and factual evidence. Policies and procedures also take into account the way that a healthcare facility delivers care and the facility's resident population.

Policies and procedures are always written. For example, policies and procedures concerning patient care are usually found in a facility's policy and procedure manual or may be accessible online. Policies and procedures related to administrative tasks and employee conduct are found in a facility's employee handbook. Policies and procedures are always recorded in a place that is easily accessible to all healthcare staff.

The goal is to ensure that all staff members are guided by policies and are performing tasks according to set procedures. This helps guarantee accuracy, safety, and consistency to avoid errors.

Policies

Policies are rules or guidelines developed by a healthcare facility and its staff (Figure 5.3). Healthcare facilities may have policies on proper dress, behavior, or benefits (for example, how many vacation days staff members may have). Facilities may also have care-related policies, such as a policy about hand hygiene.

Procedures

Procedures are specific and consistent actions or steps taken to deliver care. Procedures are always based on policies. Procedures are very detailed and tell you exactly how to perform a task. In section 5.3, you will learn the procedures for admitting, transferring, and discharging patients. Step-by-step procedures for providing care are included throughout this textbook.

How Do Policies and Procedures Ensure Safe, Quality Care?

Policies and procedures are developed to guide and assist healthcare staff. All nursing and healthcare staff members are responsible for obeying policies and following

Policy: Using the Chain of Command

Approved by: _____

Effective date: _____

Last revision date: _____

Policy:

Any staff member who identifies a concern, problem, or issue and is unable to resolve it through regular organizational channels of communication can bring the concern, problem, or issue to successively higher levels of authority. This process is essential to providing a timely response to resident care needs, maintaining professional behavior and standards of care, and ensuring resident safety.

Procedure:

1. The use of the chain of command should be initiated in conditions that may endanger resident care and safety and after regular organizational channels of communication have been exhausted. Situations that require use of the chain of command may be unclear or potentially unsafe orders, nonresponsiveness of care providers, or demonstration of unprofessional behavior that may affect the delivery of care.

2. Identify the appropriate levels of authority to contact.

3. Prior to bringing the concern, problem, or issue to the next level of authority, gather factual information that pertains to the situation, the care being endangered, or the employee issue in question.

4. If the concern, problem, or issue remains unresolved, the next levels of authority in the chain of command should be contacted until the concern, problem, or issue is resolved.

5. If after hours, the administrative person with facility authority should be contacted after the regular organizational channels of communication have been exhausted.

6. The date, time, name of the person contacted, information provided, orders received, and actions implemented shall be documented in the appropriate records.

7. Failure to implement the chain of command policy, when needed, may result in disciplinary action.

8. Retaliation against an employee for implementing the chain of command policy will not be tolerated.

Figure 5.3 This is an example of a policy for using the chain of command.

procedures. Policies and procedures are meant to help deliver care, not to block or hinder it. They are also written to be followed. Without policies and procedures in place, errors can be made, and care can be inconsistent, creating anxiety and feelings of being unsafe for both staff and patients or residents. In some cases, ignoring a policy or procedure can lead to harm and a legal or ethical problem for healthcare staff and the healthcare facility. Therefore, when you work as a nursing assistant, it is not appropriate for you to take shortcuts or decide there is a better or easier way to complete a task.

If you change the way a policy is interpreted or do not follow a procedure, this can lead to disciplinary action. A better way of dealing with a challenging or difficult policy or procedure is to bring this information to your charge nurse. When doing this, always identify the specific policy or procedure that needs to be reviewed. Also explain which part of the policy or procedure is not working and include a recommendation for how it can be improved. Always talk about the recommended change as it relates to improving care. The charge nurse can bring this information to members of the facility administration, who have the authority to review and rewrite policies and procedures, if needed.

Section 5.2 Review and Assessment

Using the Key Terms

Complete the following sentences using the key terms in this section.

1. During the nursing process, licensed nursing staff members use _____, which involves using research findings to guide decisions.
2. When the resident and the licensed nursing staff collaborate to set _____, this assures that the most important actions are taken in a resident's plan of care.
3. In the 1970s, the American Nurses Association recognized the _____ as an important standard of care for guiding nursing practice.
4. During the _____ step in the nursing process, information is gathered about the physiological, psychological, emotional, sociological, economic, lifestyle-related, and spiritual aspects of a resident.
5. A patient's _____ lists measurable and achievable goals for each identified health problem.
6. _____ are the methods, processes, and actions that direct the care nursing assistants provide.
7. Sleep deprivation and stomach pains may be included in a patient's or resident's _____.

Know and Understand the Facts

8. What is a standard of care and why is it important?
9. Identify the five steps in the nursing process.
10. Explain the difference between a policy and a procedure. Give an example of each.
11. Describe the importance of a resident plan of care.

Analyze and Apply Concepts

12. Identify two ways nursing assistants participate in the nursing process.
13. What might happen if a policy or procedure is not followed?
14. What should a nursing assistant do if he or she thinks a policy or procedure is not helpful?
15. What influences the development of a facility policy?
16. Identify two ways in which policies and procedures ensure safe, quality care.

Think Critically

Read the following care situation. Then answer the questions that follow.

Over the past year, the unit on which Louis works has twice changed the procedure for putting on gloves before entering an isolation room. The reason for the second change is that, after reading a newly published article on the subject, a member of the nursing administration decided to change the procedure. Louis is frustrated because he had just learned the procedure well when it changed. Louis decides to continue following the old procedure since that is what he knows. After all, he is an experienced nursing assistant, and the procedure has worked in the past. Louis wonders, *Why should I change how I put on gloves?*

17. Is Louis doing the right thing by continuing to use the old procedure? Explain your answer.
18. Why do you think the nursing administration chose to change the procedure?
19. What actions should the charge nurse take to ensure Louis and other staff members follow the new procedure?

Objectives

Patients and residents enter and leave healthcare facilities through the admission, transfer, and discharge processes. To provide the best possible care, you must understand the role and responsibilities of a holistic nursing assistant in the admission, transfer, and discharge procedures so you can ensure the procedures are performed safely and smoothly. To achieve the objectives for this section, you must successfully

- **describe** the procedure for admission to a healthcare facility and the nursing assistant's role;
- **list** the steps that are taken to ensure safe transfer within a facility or to another facility; and
- **explain** the procedure for discharging a patient to his or her home.

Key Terms

Learn these key terms to better understand the information presented in the section.

discharge plan
pulse oximeter
sphygmomanometer

Questions to Consider

- Have you ever had to pack up and leave quickly after a vacation? What actions did you take to ensure you took all your personal belongings? If someone helped you, how did you make sure they took all your belongings?
- When you packed up quickly, did you or your family leave something behind? How did that experience feel? What did you do to retrieve or replace the lost items?

In this section of the chapter, you will learn three procedures you need to know as part of your role and responsibilities as a holistic nursing assistant. These procedures are for admitting a patient or resident to a healthcare facility, transferring a patient within or to another healthcare facility, and discharging a patient from a healthcare facility. You will use these procedures often.

As you review and learn these procedures, remember to

- always ask for help if you need it;
- always follow your facility's policies; and
- consider the safety and comfort of the patient or resident before, during, and after each procedure.

Each procedure is organized so you can clearly understand how to perform it effectively when delivering care. *Best Practice* reminders are included in each procedure to point out important strategies and actions that help ensure safety and quality care. In each procedure, you will find

- the reason for performing the procedure (*Rationale*);
- important steps to take before starting the procedure (*Preparation*);
- the procedure itself (*The Procedure*);
- important steps to take after the procedure is completed (*Follow-Up*); and
- directions for reporting and recording the procedure (*Reporting and Documentation*).

What Is the Procedure for Admitting to a Healthcare Facility?

Admission to a healthcare facility occurs when people have serious illnesses or conditions or can no longer take care of themselves. People are usually *admitted to*, or enter,

Remember

People forget how fast you did a job—but they remember how well you did it.

Howard W. Newton, American advertising executive and author

Think About This

According to the American Hospital Association (AHA), an estimated 35 million admissions occur each year in US registered hospitals. A recent estimate by the Centers for Disease Control and Prevention (CDC) indicates that there are 1.4 million residents in long-term care facilities in the United States.

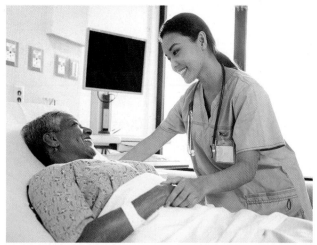
Monkey Business Images/Shutterstock.com

Figure 5.4 Not all patients in a hospital are admitted because of medical emergencies. Some require observation until a condition is diagnosed or treatment begins.

a hospital or long-term care facility. In hospitals, there are two major types of admission: emergency admission and elective admission. *Emergency admission* occurs when someone goes to the emergency room. From there, the person may be admitted to a hospital. *Elective admission* usually occurs if a person has a scheduled procedure or surgery. Sometimes people are admitted to a hospital because they need to be observed for a short period of time until decisions can be made about their conditions or illnesses (Figure 5.4).

Admissions to long-term care facilities are almost always elective. The decision to enter a long-term care facility is made when a person is no longer able to independently live at home. Usually, the person will need some level of assistance with ambulation, eating, or hygiene and may need special treatments or the administration and monitoring of medications.

Specific policies and procedures are used to collect needed information and prepare people for admission. Sometimes healthcare staff members complete the paperwork for admission in the admitting office of the facility. Other times, the paperwork is completed in a patient's or resident's room by a person from the admitting office, a HUC, a member of the licensed nursing staff, or a nursing assistant. Room preparation and the admission process are always the responsibility of the nursing assistant or another assigned healthcare staff member, depending on directions from the licensed nursing staff.

Becoming a Holistic Nursing Assistant
Admission and Anxiety

Admission to any healthcare facility is often hard on patients or residents and their families. This may be the first time a patient is experiencing an illness, or maybe an illness has become so acute that a patient needs to be admitted to a hospital. Illness is not the only reason for admission. Perhaps a patient was severely injured in an accident, and it will be a long time before he or she can walk or talk. It can be very frightening to wake up in a strange room and bed surrounded by whirring medical equipment.

Similar fears, anxieties, and challenges exist for residents who can no longer care for themselves at home and need to live in long-term care facilities. For many residents, there is no hope of returning home. When residents enter a long-term care facility, they leave behind friends, family, and even pets to live in a new, strange place with people they do not know. Many times, the decision was not the resident's, but belonged to the resident's family. Once residents enter a long-term facility, they are being taken care of rather than taking care of themselves. This is even more frightening for residents who are no longer mobile or who have dementia. Needing someone to assist you with every move, when you were once independent, can be a hard reality to accept.

There are several ways holistic nursing assistants can ease fear and anxiety to make a patient or resident more comfortable. These might include

- making eye contact when communicating;
- asking questions or giving instructions slowly and clearly;
- being patient and waiting for an answer to a question before asking another;
- using a pleasant and even tone of voice;
- expressing body language that is open, relaxed, and accepting; and
- smiling and showing concern, when appropriate.

Apply It

1. Which approaches to anxiety do you already take when interacting with people? Are there any approaches that are new and that you would need to learn? How will you go about doing that?

2. What other approaches can you think of that might also help decrease fear or anxiety for a resident?

The information needed for admission usually includes a person's personal information, employment information, closest relatives, insurance carriers, reasons for admission, and medications. Admission documents are used to aid in collecting necessary information. A clothing and personal belongings list is also completed as part of the admission process to safeguard items that remain in the facility. Other forms that require a person's signature include privacy practices and treatment agreements.

Hospitals usually provide a patient with an admission kit that includes a water pitcher, a cup, a basin, toothpaste, a toothbrush, soap, lotion, and other hygiene items (Figure 5.5). In long-term care facilities, the admission kit might not include hygiene items such as a toothbrush or toothpaste since residents often bring their own.

The admission procedure focuses on making sure people are oriented to and made comfortable in the facility and their rooms, are aware of their rights, and have rooms that are prepared with needed supplies and equipment. Once patients or residents are settled into their rooms, treatments ordered by their doctors are started.

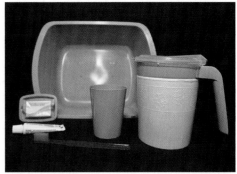

Wards Forest Media, LLC

Figure 5.5 This is an example of a hospital admission kit containing a basin, pitcher, cup, and hygiene items.

Procedure | Admission to a Healthcare Facility

Rationale

The nursing assistant's role and responsibilities during admission are to prepare the room, assist with gathering necessary information, and help with orientation to the healthcare facility and room.

> **Best Practice**
> If you are admitting to a hospital or long-term care facility, there may be an admission coordinator on staff. Therefore, room assignments may be made before the resident arrives to the unit. If not, licensed nursing staff members will have the responsibility to assign a room.

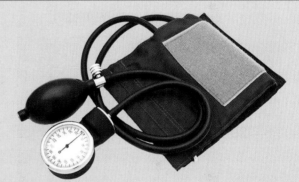

Figure 5.6

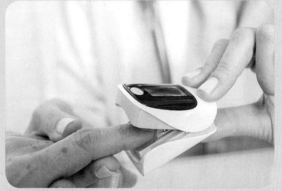

Figure 5.7

Preparation

1. Wash your hands or use hand sanitizer before entering the room.

2. Bring the necessary equipment into the room. Place the following items in an accessible location:

   - instruments for measuring vital signs, such as a thermometer, **sphygmomanometer** for measuring blood pressure, stethoscope (Figure 5.6), and **pulse oximeter** for measuring oxygen in the blood (Figure 5.7)

   - an intravenous (IV) pole, if needed

   - a urine specimen container for collection of a sample, if ordered by the doctor

   - any other items requested by the licensed nursing staff

(continued)

Place the following items on or inside of the bedside stand:

- an admission kit, including a washbasin, a water pitcher and cup, a toothbrush, toothpaste, soap, and other items
- a bed pan and urinal (for men)
- towels and washcloths

3. Prepare the bed by pulling back the bed covers and placing the bed in a low position so the resident can easily enter the bed. Lock the bed wheels so the bed does not roll or move.

4. Ensure the call light is easily accessible and within the resident's reach (Figure 5.8).

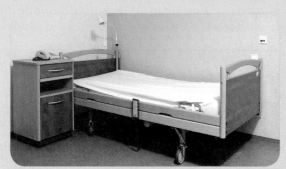

Figure 5.8

The Procedure

5. When the resident arrives at the room, a licensed nursing staff member will check the resident's name with any admission forms.

6. Introduce yourself using your full name and title. Explain that you work with the licensed nursing staff and will be assisting with the admission.

7. If instructed by the licensed nursing staff, place an identification bracelet on the resident's wrist if he or she is not already wearing one.

Best Practice
Some facilities may use alternative methods of identification, such as identifying residents using a photo in the EMR. Check your facility's guidelines for verifying a resident's identify.

8. Use Mr., Mrs., or Ms. and the last name when conversing.

9. Explain the part of the admission procedure you will be doing in simple terms, even if the resident is not able to communicate or is disoriented.

10. Provide privacy by closing the curtains, using a screen, or closing the door to the room.

Best Practice
It is important to provide privacy during the admission process. If a resident's family members or friends are present, determine whether they will stay during admission.

11. Access the approved admission forms for the resident. You may have to ask the licensed nursing staff for these forms. Admission forms are usually filled out electronically using a tablet, laptop, or computer on wheels.

12. As directed by the licensed nursing staff, ask the resident the questions on the admission forms, assuming the admission forms have not already been completed. If the resident is disoriented or unable to answer questions, you may ask an accompanying family member the questions.

13. Additionally, a member of the licensed nursing staff or a social worker may explain to the resident what his or her rights are and provide a booklet on the topic. The resident's photo may also be taken for identification purposes.

14. If the resident has a roommate, make introductions.

15. Let the resident stay dressed, if approved, or help the resident change into a gown or pajamas.

16. Help the resident into bed or into a chair, as directed by the licensed nursing staff.

17. An RN will usually conduct a resident assessment. Assist with the assessment by measuring vital signs, height, and weight.

18. Complete the resident's clothing and personal belongings list (per facility policy). Along with the licensed nursing staff, sign the list to verify which belongings have been left in the room and if any valuables have been put in the facility's safe. If you are in a long-term care facility, label the resident's belongings.

19. Unless a family member or friend wishes to assist, put away the resident's clothes and personal items.

20. Provide the resident with an orientation to the room by doing the following:
   - Identify and explain the purposes of items in the bedside stand.
   - Explain how to use the overbed table.
   - Show the resident how to use the call light, bed controls, TV, and light control.

- Explain how to make a telephone call and place the telephone within reach.
- Show the resident where the bathroom is and how to use the bathroom's emergency call light.

21. Explain the facility's visiting hours and policies, as well as where to find the nurses' station, chapel, dining room or cafeteria, and any other areas specific to the facility. Also explain how to identify different staff. Some facilities have different colored uniforms or different types of identification badges for staff members.
22. Explain any ordered activity limits, such as bed rest or ambulation restrictions.
23. Explain when meals are served and how to request snacks.
24. If fluids are allowed per the doctor's orders, fill the water pitcher and cup in the resident's room.
25. Provide a denture cup, if needed, and label it with the resident's name, room number, and bed number.

> **Best Practice**
> If handling dentures, use disposable gloves. Wash your hands before and after discarding the disposable gloves to ensure infection control.

Follow-Up

26. Wash your hands to ensure infection control.
27. Make sure the resident is comfortable and place the call light and personal items within reach.
28. Conduct a safety check before leaving the room. The room should be clean and free from clutter or spills.
29. Wash your hands or use hand sanitizer before leaving the room.

Reporting and Documentation

30. Report the completion of admission. Communicate any specific observations, complications, or unusual responses to the licensed nursing staff. Record this information, along with the care provided, in the chart or EMR.

Figure 5.6 Sergej Razvodovskij/Shutterstock.com; Figure 5.7 Click and Photo/Shutterstock.com; Figure 5.8 Bildagentur Zoonar GmbH/Shutterstock.com

What Are the Steps for Transfer?

When a patient's condition changes, the patient may be transferred to a different location in the same healthcare facility or to another facility entirely. For example, if a patient were in a serious car accident, the patient's hospital stay may end when his or her condition is stabilized, even if the patient is not yet ready to go home. The patient may lack mobility due to broken bones and a head injury, and he or she may not be able to fully dress or bathe without help. In this case, the patient would likely be *transferred* to a rehabilitation center for physical or occupational therapy to regain limited or lost function.

Transfer is voluntary. Prior to transfer, patients are provided the opportunity to accept or refuse the transfer. If a transfer is refused, the patient is usually discharged with documentation stating that he or she refused the transfer against the recommendation of the healthcare provider.

Like admission, a transfer requires a written doctor's order. Licensed nursing staff members may delegate transfer responsibilities to nursing assistants or HUCs. A staff member from social services often assists patients and their families in locating a facility that will meet treatment needs and is covered by insurance.

Forms are used for the transfer procedure. Transfer forms usually request information about the destination facility, patient diagnosis, medications, treatments, allergies, physical and mental assessments, the patient's level of independence, safety concerns, and personal belongings.

Some patients become frightened during the transfer procedure. This is especially common among older adults, who may not understand the reasons for the transfer. In these situations, it is essential that you stay calm and reassure and reorient the patient as necessary (Figure 5.9). Seek assistance from another staff member to help with the transfer, if needed.

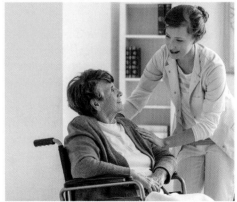

Photographee.eu/Shutterstock.com

Figure 5.9 Some patients may experience anxiety or fear during transfer. You can help by reassuring these patients during the process.

If the transfer occurs between units in a facility, the destination unit is notified about the transfer, and the patient is usually accompanied by a nursing assistant or other assigned healthcare staff member to the new unit. The nursing assistant or other assigned healthcare staff member checks in with the licensed nursing staff on the new unit and transfers the patient's paper chart, assuming the patient's information has not already been shared electronically.

If the transfer is to another facility, a licensed nursing staff member will contact the destination facility about the patient's arrival. A nursing assistant or other assigned healthcare staff member will accompany the patient to the transport vehicle. At the transport vehicle, those responsible for transport will take responsibility for the patient, the patient's documents, and any belongings and valuables not taken by the family.

Procedure — Transfer Within or to Another Facility

Rationale

It is essential that transfers be safe and smooth. The nursing assistant will assist licensed nursing staff as directed with completing paperwork, packing personal belongings, and helping with transport.

Preparation

1. Ask the licensed nursing staff how this procedure fits into the plan of care, if there are doctor's orders for the procedure, if there are any special instructions or precautions, and if the patient can be moved into the positions required for this procedure.

2. Obtain the transfer forms ordered by the doctor. You may have to ask the licensed nursing staff for these forms.

3. Wash your hands or use hand sanitizer before entering the room.

4. Knock before entering the room.

5. Introduce yourself using your full name and title. Explain that you work with the licensed nursing staff and will be assisting with the transfer.

6. Greet the patient and ask the patient to state his or her full name, if able. Then check the patient's identification bracelet.

7. Use Mr., Mrs., or Ms. and the last name when conversing.

8. Explain the part of the transfer procedure you will be doing in simple terms, even if the patient is not able to communicate or is disoriented. Ask permission to perform the procedure.

9. Prepare the patient for transfer by explaining what is about to happen. This can help decrease any anxiety and stress the patient may be feeling.

> **Best Practice**
> Prior to transfer, licensed nursing staff members must provide patients with information about the transfer and give the right to refuse. If the transfer is refused, discharge from the healthcare facility is discussed.

The Procedure

10. Provide privacy by closing the curtains, using a screen, or closing the door to the room.

11. Assist in moving or packing the patient's belongings and any needed equipment. If the patient will be moving to another facility, return any valuables that have been kept in the safe. Check the belongings against the list created during admission.

12. If the patient needs to be transported in a wheelchair, ensure the bed is locked and transfer the patient from the bed to the wheelchair using the appropriate procedure.

13. Assist the patient in changing his or her clothes, if necessary.

14. Manually transport the patient's paper chart with the patient to the new unit or to the transport vehicle. In some facilities, the patient's information may be entered into an EMR and transferred electronically to the new unit or facility.

> **Best Practice**
> Calm, reassure, and reorient the patient as necessary during transfer.

15. Monitor the patient's vital signs during the transfer per the facility's policy and instructions given by the licensed nursing staff.

16. Ensure safety during the transfer process and seek assistance from another staff member, if needed.

17. If transferring the patient to another unit within the same facility, alert the charge nurse at the destination unit that the patient has arrived and provide a verbal report. When you arrive in the new room, make sure that the patient is safe and comfortable, that the bed is in its lowest position, and that the call light is within reach.

18. If transferring the patient to another healthcare facility, make sure the patient is moved safely into the transport vehicle.

Follow-Up

19. Wash your hands to ensure infection control.

Reporting and Documentation

20. Report the completion of the transfer to the licensed nursing staff on your unit. Communicate any specific observations, complications, or unusual responses to the licensed nursing staff.

How Are Patients Discharged from a Healthcare Facility?

Patients are *discharged from* (leave) a healthcare facility and can go home when their health has improved enough that they have the ability, support, and resources to take care of themselves. Discharge from a facility can only occur when there is a written doctor's order. Sometimes patients decide to terminate treatments or care prescribed by a doctor while in a healthcare facility. Patients may also decide to leave a healthcare facility earlier than when a doctor believes is best. If patients leave a healthcare facility against a doctor's wishes, they are making these decisions *against medical advice (AMA)*. If this situation occurs, the patient is asked to sign a release indicating that the healthcare facility and those providing care are not liable for any harm resulting from discontinuance of care or early discharge.

A nursing assistant or HUC may assist with discharge by following doctors' orders and completing tasks delegated by the licensed nursing staff. Sometimes a transport aide or volunteer will take the patient to a waiting vehicle once discharge is completed in the room (Figure 5.10).

A discharge form must be completed before a patient can leave the healthcare facility. Discharge forms ensure all of the necessary information is retrieved, including patient personal information, medical diagnoses, insurance carriers, and a clothing and personal belongings list.

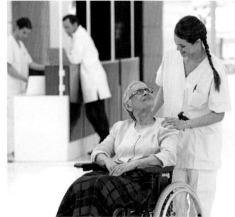

Blend Images/Shutterstock.com

Figure 5.10 Nursing assistants and other healthcare staff members escort patients to their vehicles upon discharge.

Healthcare Scenario
Admission and Discharge Concerns

Today, at 9 p.m., the news shared that a local healthcare facility reported higher-than-expected numbers of admissions and discharges. This had an impact on the patient experience and on staffing. A reporter interviewed the facility administration, doctors, nurses, and several patients. During the interviews, it was clear that the healthcare staff and patients were concerned about whether the high numbers of patients moving in and out of the facility would affect safety and the delivery of quality care.

Apply It

1. What can nursing assistants do during admission and discharge to ensure safety?

2. Identify steps in the admission and discharge procedures where quality of care might be compromised. Discuss how this compromise can be prevented.

In addition to discharge forms, discharge also requires a **discharge plan**. The discharge plan provides instructions concerning medications, activity levels, treatments to continue at home, and follow-up appointments with the doctor. These instructions are shared with the patient and family members by the licensed nursing staff.

Be sure to practice safety during discharge. Make sure the patient does not trip or fall when getting ready to leave, and safely move the patient from the discharge wheelchair to the patient's transport vehicle. Get assistance from another staff member, if needed.

Procedure   Discharge from a Healthcare Facility

Rationale

During the discharge process, the nursing assistant assists the licensed nursing staff as directed with completing paperwork, packing personal belongings, and helping with transport. This helps ensure that patients safely and efficiently leave a healthcare facility.

Preparation

1. Ask the licensed nursing staff how this procedure fits into the plan of care, if there are doctor's orders for the procedure, if there are any special instructions or precautions, and if the patient can be moved into the positions required for this procedure.

2. Obtain the discharge forms ordered by the doctor. You may have to ask the licensed nursing staff for these forms.

3. Wash your hands or use hand sanitizer before entering the room.

4. Knock before entering the room.

5. Introduce yourself using your full name and title. Explain that you work with the licensed nursing staff and will be assisting with discharge.

6. Greet the patient and ask the patient to state his or her full name, if able. Then check the patient's identification bracelet.

7. Use Mr., Mrs., or Ms. and the last name when conversing.

8. Explain the part of the discharge procedure you will be doing in simple terms.

The Procedure

9. Provide privacy by closing the curtains, using a screen, or closing the door to the room.

10. Help the patient get dressed. Then help collect and pack the patient's belongings and any needed equipment.

11. Return any valuables that have been kept in the facility's safe to the patient. Check the patient's belongings against the list created during admission.

> **Best Practice**
> Family members may want to assist with the patient's discharge. Include the patient's family members, as directed by the licensed nursing staff and as appropriate. Take care that the family's involvement does not interfere with the safe discharge of the patient.

12. During discharge, observe and report any issues regarding the patient's ability to complete ADLs, as well as any of his or her concerns or fears, to the licensed nursing staff.

> **Best Practice**
> Practice safety during the discharge process. Get assistance from another staff member, if needed.

13. Notify the licensed nursing staff when the patient is ready for final discharge instructions. At this time, an RN will usually
    - provide the patient with prescriptions ordered by the doctor;
    - communicate discharge instructions; and
    - have the patient sign clothing and personal belongings forms.

14. Help escort the patient in a wheelchair from the unit to the transport vehicle.

15. Lock the patient's wheelchair and assist the patient into the transport vehicle.

16. Help move the patient's belongings into the transport vehicle.

Follow-Up

17. Return the wheelchair and cart (if used) to the storage area for cleaning.

18. Put on disposable gloves and practice infection control to prevent transmission of any possible pathogens (bacteria or viruses).

19. Clean the patient's room and prepare it for a new occupant. The housekeeping staff may share some of the following duties:
    - stripping the bed and cleaning the room
    - disposing of dirty linen
    - making the bed using clean linen

20. Wash your hands to ensure infection control.

Reporting and Documentation

21. Report the completion and time of discharge, the staff who assisted with the discharge, the way in which the patient was transported, the people who accompanied the discharged patient, the patient's destination, and any observations and responses to the licensed nursing staff. Also record this information in the chart or EMR.

Section 5.3 Review and Assessment

Using the Key Terms

Complete the following sentences using the key terms in this section.

1. A(n) _____ is a medical device used to measure blood pressure.
2. Instructions concerning medications, activity levels, treatments to continue at home, and follow-up appointments are detailed in a patient's _____.
3. A nursing assistant would use a(n) _____ to measure oxygen levels in a patient's blood.

Know and Understand the Facts

4. Identify two ways a person can be admitted to a healthcare facility.
5. What are two differences between admission, transfer, and discharge?
6. Identify two examples of needed information that is collected during admission.
7. What is a discharge plan, and how is it used?

Analyze and Apply Concepts

8. Explain how to prepare a room for admission.
9. Using what you have learned so far, describe two actions you could take to help a patient adjust on admission to a healthcare facility.
10. Identify three steps a nursing assistant performs to ensure a safe and effective transfer.
11. What information does a patient need to ensure a safe and effective discharge?

Think Critically

Read the following care situation. Then answer the questions that follow.

You have just admitted a new patient, Mrs. H. Once she settles into her bed, you check her vital signs and weight. Mrs. H seems very upset, and her blood pressure is above normal. She seems to have trouble understanding what you are saying. You think she may not understand English very well. You are concerned she may not understand everything you told her during admission. In particular, you are concerned she does not understand how to call for help using the call light.

12. What could you do to ensure Mrs. H understands what you are saying?
13. Would you need to inform your charge nurse about Mrs. H's blood pressure reading?
14. What steps could you take to help Mrs. H understand the use of the call light?

Key Points

Reviewing the key points for this chapter will help you practice more safely and competently as a holistic nursing assistant and will help you prepare for the certification competency examination.

- Levels of care describe the types and amounts of care that residents require. The three levels of care are skilled care, intermediate care, and supportive care.

- The types of nursing care delivery typically seen today are functional nursing, team nursing, progressive care, and patient-centered care.

- Delegation occurs when a licensed nursing staff member asks a nursing assistant to perform specific tasks. These tasks must always be within a nursing assistant's scope of practice.

- The nursing process is a method in which licensed nursing staff members use critical thinking, analytical skills, and supporting evidence to plan for and deliver care. This process has five steps: assessing, making a nursing diagnosis, planning, implementing, and evaluating.

- Policies and procedures set boundaries, directions, and guidelines so that actions taken by healthcare staff are based on good evidence and best practice.

- There are three procedures involved in moving patients into, between, and out of healthcare facilities and units. These three procedures are admission, transfer, and discharge.

Action Steps to Holistic Care

Review the information in this chapter. Complete the following activities.

1. Select one type of nursing care delivery. Prepare a short paper or digital presentation that discusses the nursing assistant's role and responsibilities within this type of care delivery.

2. Write a short poem or limerick that expresses what nursing assistants should do when accepting a delegated task.

3. With a partner, prepare a poster that identifies and describes the top three most important practices that should be included in one of the procedures discussed in this chapter.

4. Find two pictures in a magazine, in a newspaper, or online that best demonstrate the steps in the nursing process. Describe each image and provide a rationale for why it was selected. Explain the responsibilities nursing assistants have in each step of the nursing process.

5. Admission to, transfer within, or discharge from a healthcare facility can leave a patient or resident feeling anxious or uncertain. Prepare a list of possible sources of anxiety a patient or resident might experience during each of these procedures. Then brainstorm ways you, as a holistic nursing assistant, could help ease the resident's anxiety.

 Preparing for the Certification Competency Examination

To prepare for the nursing assistant certification competency examination, you will need to know content found in this chapter. This content may be tested in the knowledge (written or oral) and skills (hands-on demonstration) portions of the exam. The following areas will be emphasized:

- professional work habits
- the importance of the delegation process
- facility policies and procedures
- admission, transfer, and discharge skills

These sample test questions are similar to ones you will find on the certification competency exam. See how well you can answer them. Be sure to select the *best* answer.

1. During which step in the nursing process might a nursing assistant provide information?
   A. making a nursing diagnosis
   B. appraising
   C. evaluating
   D. activating

2. If a resident receives 24-hour direct care in a healthcare facility, what level of care would be assigned?
   A. intermediate care
   B. skilled care
   C. long-term care
   D. supportive care

3. Which of the following best describes a policy?
   A. a set of steps
   B. a process
   C. an action
   D. a rule or guideline

4. A new nursing assistant is giving care assigned by the charge nurse. What type of nursing care delivery is being practiced on his unit?
   A. total patient care
   B. team nursing
   C. patient-focused care
   D. supplemental care

5. Which of the following is one of the five rights of delegation?
   A. right action
   B. right process
   C. right person
   D. right environment

6. Mr. L, an older gentleman, is being transferred to a long-term care facility after suffering a mild stroke. What is the first thing that must be done after the doctor's order is received and before the transfer can occur?
   A. Mr. L's permission must be obtained.
   B. Transport must be arranged.
   C. The RN must call Mr. L's destination facility.
   D. Mr. L's belongings must be packed.

7. A nursing assistant has been asked to discharge Mr. S from a rehabilitation facility. Mr. S plans to go home with his wife. Which of the following actions should the nursing assistant not take?
   A. help Mr. S gather all of his belongings
   B. make sure there is a doctor's order for Mr. S's discharge
   C. let the licensed nursing staff know Mr. S is ready for his discharge orders
   D. let Mr. S's wife help him to their car

8. The charge nurse has delegated a task to a nursing assistant who works on the day shift. The task is part of the nursing assistant's scope of practice, but she does not remember how to do it correctly. Which of the following should the nursing assistant do?
   A. take more time to do the task
   B. ask another nursing assistant to help her
   C. tell the charge nurse she needs some training before she can do the task
   D. tell the charge nurse that she doesn't think she will have time today to do the task

9. What is the first action a nursing assistant should take when admitting a patient?
   A. make sure the bed and bedside stand are ready
   B. get the admission kit and ensure it contains all necessary components
   C. check with the charge nurse and consult the admission forms
   D. tell the patient's roommate about the arrival

10. Why is a discharge plan important?
    A. It provides information about the patient's history.
    B. It provides a set of instructions for the patient.
    C. It provides data on the patient's family.
    D. It provides information about the patient's pain.

11. Which of the following explains why nursing assistants should always follow facility procedures?
    A. Procedures provide helpful information needed to provide care.
    B. Procedures are written at a level that they can be understood.
    C. Procedures ensure that all healthcare providers give consistent care.
    D. Procedures are simple and provide just a few steps to follow.

12. A new nursing assistant received a delegated assignment to prepare a room for resident admission. Which healthcare staff member on her unit delegated this assignment?
    A. the RN
    B. the HUC
    C. the doctor
    D. the social worker

13. The decision to select a particular type of nursing care delivery is usually based on which of the following?
    A. philosophy
    B. goals
    C. vision
    D. values

14. How are level-of-care assignments used?
    A. to decide on the best facility based on a person's needs
    B. to determine how to share a resident's progress with his or her family
    C. to help design facilities so they provide the best services
    D. to put standards in place so that the environment is safe

15. Before a patient can be admitted, transferred, or discharged, which of the following must occur first?
    A. The family must agree to the decision.
    B. The patient must be provided information.
    C. The RN must provide an assessment.
    D. There must be a doctor's order.

Did you have difficulty with any of the questions? If you did, review the chapter to find the correct answer(s).

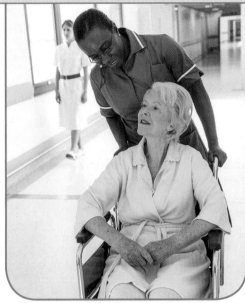

Spotmatik Ltd/Shutterstock.com

Chapter Outline

Section 6.1
Human Needs and Growth

Section 6.2
Human Behavior

Section 6.3
Body, Mind, and Spirit

Welcome to the Chapter

This chapter will help you understand what motivates people, how to recognize human needs, and how people grow. This will help you feel empathy for others, which can help you build understanding and openness. You will also learn how behavioral and generational differences can make it challenging to develop positive, productive communication and relationships. As a holistic nursing assistant, you can learn to respond to and bridge differences with the skills and knowledge in this chapter.

While reading this chapter, you will also discover the three major dimensions that affect how each of us feels and behaves: the *body*, *mind*, and *spirit*. These dimensions are key to understanding yourself, attaining a healthy lifestyle, and helping others achieve health and well-being. With this understanding, you will be able to broaden and strengthen your relationships. Forming and developing holistic relationships will directly influence the way you interact with others and the quality of care you deliver.

What you learn in this chapter will help you develop your knowledge and skills to become a holistic nursing assistant. The topics discussed in the chapter are highlighted on the Providing Holistic Care Framework.

You are now ready to start this chapter, *Human Behavior and Development*.

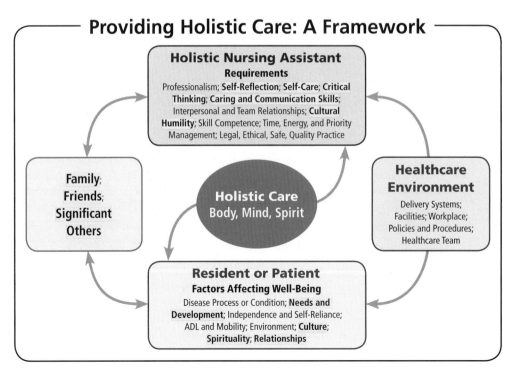

Providing Holistic Care: A Framework

Holistic Nursing Assistant
Requirements
Professionalism; **Self-Reflection; Self-Care; Critical Thinking; Caring and Communication Skills;** Interpersonal and Team Relationships; **Cultural Humility;** Skill Competence; Time, Energy, and Priority Management; Legal, Ethical, Safe, Quality Practice

**Family;
Friends;
Significant
Others**

Holistic Care
Body, Mind, Spirit

**Healthcare
Environment**
Delivery Systems;
Facilities; Workplace;
Policies and Procedures;
Healthcare Team

Resident or Patient
Factors Affecting Well-Being
Disease Process or Condition; **Needs and Development;** Independence and Self-Reliance; ADL and Mobility; Environment; **Culture; Spirituality; Relationships**

Objectives

Using a holistic approach to promote positive relationships with residents and coworkers will help you provide the best possible care. To do this, you must be aware of people's motivation, the basis of human needs, and the stages of human growth. To achieve the objectives for this section, you must successfully

- **discuss** the types, components, and theories of motivation;
- **list** the human needs that impact the attitudes, feelings, and behaviors of others;
- **explain** why human needs must be satisfied to achieve well-being; and
- **describe** the stages of human growth and development.

Key Terms

Learn these key terms to better understand the information presented in the section.

empathy
genuine
homeostasis
motivation

respect
self-actualization
self-esteem
self-respect

Questions to Consider

- Why do you do things you like or want to do? Are there actions you take that you don't want to do? Why do you think that happens?
- What needs do you have in your life? For example, you may need to live in a safe environment, get good grades to achieve your career goal, or feel appreciated by your friends.
- How important are your needs? What can you do to better meet your needs? What do you think would happen if your needs were not met? How would you feel?

How Are People Motivated?

When people have **motivation**, they are prompted to actively pursue actions or goals. For example, a person may be motivated to get something to eat (from an emotional response to a stimulus) or to go back to school and gain new knowledge or skills (from a conscious decision that directs behavior).

There are two types of motivation. The first is *extrinsic* (or external). Extrinsic motivation results from outside factors, such as receiving awards, getting a raise in salary, or avoiding punishment. Extrinsic motivation can result in the improvement of a person's performance, but is usually short term. *Intrinsic* (or internal) motivation arises from within people. It is often called *self-motivation* because actions that result from intrinsic motivation align with a person's values, beliefs, and emotions; fulfill an important desire; or result in personal satisfaction. Intrinsic factors that lead to motivation include curiosity, a challenge, a desire to help others, or recognition. The two types of motivation can work together or conflict with each other. For example, a person may be offered a new job in another city with an increased salary (extrinsic) and also see the job as a great challenge (intrinsic). Conversely, the same person can be offered that new job (extrinsic), but turn it down because it conflicts with his or her children's educational opportunities (intrinsic).

Motivation requires more than just initial action. If a person is hungry, for example, he or she will still need to initiate the action of eating. This is the first component of motivation and is called *activation*. The second component is *persistence*. If a person decides to go back to school and start a program, persistence will require that he or she continues the effort to complete the program, even through obstacles. The last component of motivation is *intensity*. Intensity refers to the concentration and effort taken when pursuing a goal or action. For example, two friends may be motivated to lose weight and set a goal for completion. One person may start the eating plan, stay with it to the end, and achieve the goal weight. The other person may not always stay on the plan and may not achieve the goal as planned.

There are several theories of motivation. Each theory takes a different perspective. In one theory, people are motivated as a result of extrinsic rewards or punishment. For a person to continue acting toward a goal, rewards must be reinforced or punished. In some situations, people choose certain actions to gain rewards. The greater the perceived rewards are, the more strongly people will be motivated to pursue actions that are reinforced. In another theory, known as the *humanistic theory of motivation*, people have strong reasons that prompt various actions. This theory is best represented by *Maslow's hierarchy of needs*, which shows that people have needs at different levels and are motivated by both extrinsic and intrinsic factors.

What Are Human Needs?

All people have needs, and needs change over a person's life span. In the 1940s, psychologist Abraham Maslow developed a hierarchy to help people understand human needs. This hierarchy, called *Maslow's hierarchy of needs*, is still regarded as an important way of explaining human needs and the impact of these needs on motivating action or behavior.

According to Maslow, human needs are ordered from low-level needs, the lowest of which are *basic needs* (requirements for food, water, sleep, and elimination), to high-level needs, the highest of which he called **self-actualization**. When people achieve self-actualization, they fulfill their potential. Maslow's hierarchy of needs is illustrated as a pyramid, with basic needs at the bottom and high-level needs at the top (Figure 6.1). Maslow believed that needs influence action or behavior and feelings. He also believed that people must satisfy needs at the bottom of the hierarchy before satisfying needs at the next level.

As you read more about Maslow's hierarchy of needs, think about your own needs. Have you met all of your basic needs? If you have, then do you find yourself experiencing needs for safety and security? According to Maslow, it will be challenging for you to feel love and a sense of belonging if you have not met your needs at the first two levels—basic needs and safety and security.

Your coworkers and those in your care also have these same needs. Keep in mind, however, that each person has his or her own experience with and perception of needs. Therefore, you cannot determine where your residents fall on the hierarchy of needs without observing and communicating with them about their needs.

Basic Needs

The first set of needs is physiological, or *basic*, needs. Physiological needs are at the lowest level and include needs for food, water, sleep, and elimination (urination and bowel movements). Meeting these basic needs helps your body achieve a state of internal balance known as **homeostasis**.

Consuming adequate amounts of water, eating a nutritious diet, and getting sufficient sleep will help your body achieve homeostasis and will meet your physiological needs. The average adult body is approximately 60 percent water, but this number may decline to 45 percent in older or obese people. Drinking water every day is an important part of meeting your physiological needs. Eating a balanced diet of fruits, grains, vegetables, and protein and getting between seven and nine hours of sleep every day are also recommended.

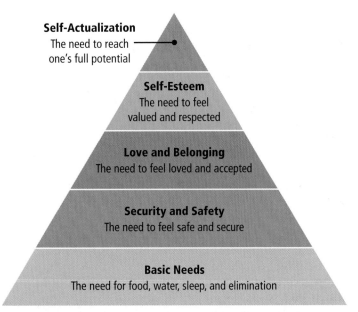

Figure 6.1 Maslow's hierarchy of needs contains five levels of needs: basic needs, security and safety, love and belonging, self-esteem, and self-actualization.

It is important to urinate and have bowel movements regularly; however, the frequency of elimination may differ between people. It is helpful to ask residents about their elimination patterns. Finally, sexual reproduction is considered a need at this level because it is essential for the survival and propagation of the human species. When basic needs at the lowest level of Maslow's hierarchy are met, needs at the next level for security and safety emerge as important.

Security and Safety

The second level of Maslow's hierarchy of needs is security and safety. These needs include the needs for

- the feeling or knowledge of living in a safe environment;
- a safe and secure place to live;
- stable finances; and
- a feeling of satisfaction with one's state of health, property, and home.

You can often see how needs influence behaviors and attitudes at this level of needs. This is especially true as a person ages and moves to the end of his or her life span. What once might have felt safe can change with the loss of mobility or the loss of a sense, such as eyesight or hearing.

Because security and safety needs are not as direct as physiological needs, you will have to listen carefully to what people are saying to understand their levels of safety or security. For example, a resident might say, "I am so worried about my daughter. Her baby is sick, and I am not there to help her care for him." This may be the resident's way of expressing her insecurities as she ages and her role changes. A helpful and holistic response might be to suggest the resident, in her new role, support her daughter by listening and by telling her daughter how strong she is, that she has confidence in her, and that she loves her. If you have permission, you can hold the resident's hand while talking to express your care and concern. These actions demonstrate **empathy** (understanding for another person's feelings and emotions), which helps you achieve a deeper connection with the resident without violating professional boundaries (Figure 6.2). All of these actions can ease the resident's concern and show that you consider her fears important.

Love and Belonging

Needs related to love and belonging can only be achieved after needs at the second level for safety and security have been met. People may express a lack of love or belonging in the things they say and do. Comments such as "I feel lost" or "I wish I could join those ladies over there" can be a clue. Body language, such as slumped shoulders, crossed arms, or time spent staring off into space, might also signal loneliness. Recognizing and responding to these behaviors and feelings in residents can help a great deal in easing residents' loneliness. You may not be able to change residents' feelings of loneliness, but you can empathize with residents and try engaging them in conversation.

Self-Esteem

The fourth level of Maslow's hierarchy of needs is **self-esteem**, which describes a person's confidence and regard for himself or herself. You can help strengthen the self-esteem of residents by exhibiting interest in what residents have done and recognizing and appreciating the experiences they have had. You can also show **respect** (admiration and appreciation)

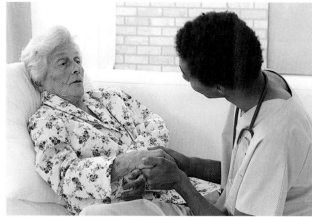

Figure 6.2 Holding a resident's hand can express empathy and caring.

and acknowledge residents' feelings, needs, and knowledge. Remind residents that they are important to their families and friends and have worth. For example, you might ask a resident if he or she has a story about helping a family member or doing something special for a friend. The more a resident recognizes his or her own value and self-worth, the more self-esteem will be strengthened, thus helping fulfill needs at this level.

Self-Actualization

The highest level of Maslow's hierarchy is *self-actualization*, in which people have become everything they hope to be. Self-actualization is more difficult to understand because its meaning is unique to each person. People have the capacity within themselves to heal and grow. This capacity in people is similar to that of the acorn, which has the potential to become *actualized* as a whole tree. Every person has the potential to become self-actualized, just as each acorn has the potential to grow into a tree. Self-actualization does not stop at a particular age and can occur as a result of changing circumstances. For example, when someone is diagnosed with a severe illness, he or she could focus energy on getting well. Because of meaningful life events, people can experience new realizations that could potentially lead to greater self-actualization.

You will always have the capacity to support, encourage, and promote self-actualization. You can do this by respecting that residents have the ability to solve their own problems and are special because of their knowledge and experiences. Your support should bring out residents' very best qualities.

Your knowledge and awareness of Maslow's hierarchy of needs can affect your relationships with coworkers and residents, as well as the care you give. Achieving self-actualization can make the difference between an impersonal, ordinary relationship and one that is **genuine** (honest, open, and sincere).

How Do People Grow and Develop?

People grow physically. They become taller and increase their weight, and their appearance and body functions also change. People also develop mentally, emotionally, and socially based on their unique characteristics. Change happens at different life stages from conception until death. Genetics (heredity), family history, and the environment in which a person lives can influence growth and development.

There are several ways growth can be discussed. Doctors often use *growth charts*, which show average growth patterns (for example, how much a toddler should weigh at two years of age). As people grow physically, they are also developing critical thinking and problem-solving skills, learning language, and building social skills.

Growth and development occur throughout a person's life span and usually happen in sequences of steps or stages. For example, children must learn to walk before they can run. Simple skills are developed first and build to more complex abilities. Each stage of development has a specific purpose, or task, that must be accomplished before the next stage can take place. Growth and development are different for every person. They can happen unevenly, or in *spurts*. For example, a person may grow faster physically than he or she develops emotionally, or vice versa.

Growth and development models, or *theories*, demonstrate how physical, mental, and emotional growth occur. These models explore the influence of growth and developmental stages for particular age groups.

Physical Development

Physical growth charts track the growth of infants, children, and adolescents by comparing physical growth with specific measurements that are expected at certain ages. These charts are available for both girls and boys. Growth charts might measure body length or height from birth to three years of age or track the weight of a child over time.

There are several different age categories for periods of physical growth, including infancy (birth–one year), toddlerhood (one–three years), the preschool years (three–five years), the school-age years (six–12 years), and adolescence (12–18 years). Figure 6.3 shows physical growth milestones for each age category.

Physical Development of Children and Adolescents	
Growth Period	**Expected Physical Growth**
Infancy (birth–one year)	• Infants typically lose about 5–10 percent of their birthweights soon after birth. • Infants should start to gain weight about two weeks after birth and should grow quickly; by four–six months, they should have doubled their birthweights. • Infants develop gross-motor skills, such as controlling the head, sitting, crawling, and may take their first few steps. • Infants develop fine-motor skills, such as holding a spoon and picking up food. • Infants' senses, including sight, hearing, taste, touch, and smell, improve. • Infants communicate using sounds and some words.
Toddlerhood (one–three years)	• Toddlers may eat less at meals, will eat frequently throughout the day, and will improve their skills in feeding themselves. • Toddlers learn to walk alone, and by two years of age, will begin to run and learn to stand on their tiptoes. • Toddlers can say several single words by 15–18 months of age; can use simple phrases by 18–24 months of age; and know nearly 1000 words by three years of age. By three years of age, they can point to objects when asked and can make simple requests based on wants. • Toddlers can follow two- or three-step directions, can sort by shape and color, and master hide and seek games. • Toddlers are aware of themselves and gradually want and enjoy the company of other children. • Toddlers want increasing independence, have mood shifts, and may begin to show defiant behavior by two years of age. • Toddlers have the cognitive development to begin toilet training around three years of age.
Preschool years (three–five years)	• Preschoolers gain 4–5 pounds and grow 2–3 inches per year. • Preschoolers have all 20 primary teeth by age three and have 20/20 vision by age four. • Preschoolers sleep 11–13 hours per night, usually without a daytime nap. • Preschoolers develop gross-motor skills, such as running, jumping, and kicking. • Around age three, preschoolers develop fine-motor skills for drawing a circle, beginning to use blunt-tip scissors, and dressing with assistance. • Around age four, preschoolers develop fine-motor skills for drawing a square and triangle, using scissors (and eventually cutting a straight line), putting on clothes properly, managing a spoon and fork, and spreading with a knife.
School-age years (six–12 years)	• Changes in height and weight vary and are influenced by genetics, nutrition, and exercise. • School-age children usually have strong motor skills and varying abilities related to eye-hand coordination, endurance, balance, and physical abilities. • Fine-motor skills, such as the ability to neatly write or make a bed, vary widely. • Some school-age children start developing secondary sexual characteristics, such as breast development for girls and the growth of the testicles and penis for boys.

(continued)

Figure 6.3 Even after childhood, people continue to develop physically as their bodies mature and change.

Physical Development of Children and Adolescents	
Growth Period	**Expected Physical Growth**
Adolescence (12–18 years)	**Girls** • Girls' growth spurts peak around age 11 and slow around age 16. • Breast buds begin to develop as early as eight years of age, and full breast growth occurs between the ages of 12 and 18. • Pubic, armpit, and leg hair begin to show around ages nine–10. • Menstrual periods (menarche) typically begin about two years after early breast and pubic hair development; in the United States, 12 is the average age for menstruation to begin. **Boys** • Boys' growth spurts peak around age 13 and slow around age 18. • The testicles and scrotum start to grow as early as age nine; genitals usually reach their adult size and shape by ages 17–18. • Nocturnal emissions of semen begin during the peak of a boy's growth spurt. • Pubic, armpit, leg, chest, and facial hair begin to show around age 12. • Boys' voices change around the same time the penis starts to grow.

Figure 6.3 *(Continued)*

Psychosocial Development

Psychosocial development refers to mental, social, and emotional changes. Psychosocial development occurs in a series of stages, sometimes called *life stages*. There are several different models and theories of psychosocial development. One model is Jean Piaget's theory of cognitive (mental) development, which was published in the early 1900s. Piaget's theory of cognitive development states that, as children develop, they become able to perform increasingly complex daily functions and activities. For example, children ages 7–11 can focus on more than one situation at a time; this is something they were not able to do when they were younger. Another widely accepted model of growth and development is Erik Erikson's theory of psychosocial development, which was developed in the 1950s. Erikson believed that certain psychological and social issues, or *conflicts*, occur at different stages of growth in a person's life. If these issues and conflicts are resolved, people grow to be successful human beings.

Erikson's model is considered one of the best ways to understand human growth and development. The model includes eight stages of growth, from infancy to old age. Erikson believed that every person passes through these stages. When each stage is successfully completed, a person reaches the potential for his or her age group. Resolving the conflicts associated with each stage creates positive outcomes as a person enters adulthood. For example, according to Erikson, when you resolve the central conflict of the adolescent stage, you will achieve **self-respect** (appreciation and acceptance of yourself). This is important because respecting one's self is the basis for respecting others, no matter what age you are.

Review the stages of psychosocial development in Figure 6.4. Can you identify any stage where you had difficulty or were unable to resolve the stage's conflict?

Erikson's Stages of Psychosocial Development

Stage	Conflict	Possible Outcomes
Infancy	Basic trust versus mistrust	Nurturing at this stage allows infants to develop optimism, trust, and confidence. If nurturing does not occur, infants will feel insecure and worthless and will lack the ability to trust.
Toddlerhood	Autonomy versus shame	At this stage, children begin to build self-esteem and autonomy by learning new skills and understanding right from wrong. If children do not learn these skills, they may have low self-esteem and feel shame as adults.
Preschool years	Initiative versus guilt	During this stage, children copy adults and take initiative by playing out or experimenting with real-life situations. If children become frustrated during this process and are not able to achieve these natural desires and goals, they may experience guilt.
School-age years	Industry versus inferiority	Children develop a sense of industry as they focus on learning, creating, and accomplishing new knowledge and skills. Children are at a social stage of development and can develop feelings of inadequacy and inferiority compared to their peers if they have problems building competence. At this stage, parents recede in importance as authorities, and peers become important.
Adolescence	Identity versus confusion	In this stage, emphasis is placed on discovering identity, working out social interactions, trying to fit in, and learning right from wrong. If unsuccessful in accomplishing the tasks of this stage, adolescents may experience role and identity confusion.
Early adulthood	Intimacy versus isolation	During this stage, young adults look for companionship and love. They seek intimacy and fulfilling relationships. If they are unsuccessful, they may experience isolation.
Adulthood	Generativity versus stagnation	In this stage, career, work, and responsibilities are important. Generativity occurs when adults attempt to produce something that makes a difference to society. Important relationships are formed within the family, workplace, and community. Due to major life changes in this stage, some people may feel challenged with finding their purpose or a new purpose. Stagnation or inactivity can then occur.
Aging years	Integrity versus despair	Reflection occurs in this stage, as successful adults look back on life with contentment and fulfillment. Other adults may reflect, view their experiences as failures, and feel a sense of despair. As a result, these adults may fear death while they struggle to find purpose.

Figure 6.4 Erikson's theory of psychosocial development identifies a central conflict for each life stage.

Using the Key Terms

Complete the following sentences using the key terms in this section.

1. _____ prompts people to act in a particular way.

2. _____ relationships are open, honest, and sincere.

3. At the highest level of Maslow's hierarchy, _____ is achieved, and the individual becomes everything he or she hoped to be.

4. Asking a resident to share a story about a time he or she did something special for a friend can help strengthen the resident's _____.

5. _____, or internal balance within the body, is achieved by meeting the body's basic needs for food, water, sleep, and elimination.

6. Appreciation for one's self, known as _____, is achieved after the central conflict of the adolescent stage is resolved.

7. Nursing assistants can achieve a deeper connection with residents by demonstrating _____, or understanding for another's feelings and emotions.

Know and Understand the Facts

8. Explain the differences between extrinsic and intrinsic motivation.

9. Describe the five levels in Maslow's hierarchy of needs.

10. Identify three conflicts in Erikson's stages of psychosocial development and the corresponding positive outcomes if these conflicts are resolved.

11. What happens during a male adolescent's physical growth?

12. Why do doctors use growth charts?

Analyze and Apply Concepts

13. Why is it helpful for holistic nursing assistants to understand Maslow's hierarchy of needs?

14. Explain how you can assist residents in meeting a particular need, such as safety and security.

15. How can recognizing the different stages of psychosocial development influence people's growth and success as adults?

Think Critically

Read the following care situation. Then answer the questions that follow.

When you enter Mrs. D's room in your community's assisted living facility, you find Mrs. D sitting in a chair. Mrs. D is still in her pajamas and is looking out the window. You ask if Mrs. D would like to go to breakfast and you offer to assist her to the dining room. Mrs. D doesn't smile, but simply shakes her head. This is not her usual behavior—Mrs. D is always ready to go for meals and seems to enjoy eating with her friends. You know that yesterday Mrs. D's daughter visited and was crying. After the visit, Mrs. D also cried and slept poorly.

16. What do you think might have caused the change in Mrs. D's behavior?

17. In your opinion, what level of Maslow's hierarchy of needs has Mrs. D achieved?

18. What can you do to respect Mrs. D's desire to avoid the dining room while still ensuring her needs are met?

Objectives

Being aware of the origins and causes of behavior is essential to understanding why people act the way they do. It is important to recognize and understand how generational differences impact behaviors. Knowledge of behavior and generational differences will help you provide quality holistic care. To achieve the objectives for this section, you must successfully

- **examine** differences in behavior;
- **explain** how differences in behavior can influence relationships and care; and
- **describe** the behaviors and attitudes of different generations.

Key Terms

Learn these key terms to better understand the information presented in the section.

behavior
covert
generation
generation gap

overt
stereotypes
taboos

Questions to Consider

- During what year were you born? Do you know the name of the generation into which you were born?
- Have you noticed generational differences between yourself and your parents or grandparents? Have you experienced conflict because of generational differences? If so, what have you done to resolve this conflict?

What Is Behavior?

When we talk about **behavior**, we are referring to actions that occur in response to a stimulus and can be seen or observed by others. Behavior differs from attitude. In chapter 1, you learned that an *attitude* is a way of feeling or thinking about a person, object, or situation. When these feelings and thoughts are acted on, they become behaviors. For example, think back to a time when you had a negative attitude about a situation. The behaviors you used to express your feelings may have included using a loud voice, making sarcastic comments, or scowling.

Most behaviors are **overt**, or open to view. Examples of overt behaviors are smiling or opening a door. Behaviors can also be **covert**, or concealed. Covert behaviors are inferred or self-reported. For example, a patient may be fearful of a procedure, and this may be signaled by his or her physiological responses.

People exhibit many different behaviors throughout their lives. Some behaviors are a result of a person's developmental stage. Behavioral differences can also arise as a result of people learning, goals changing, or generational differences. Research shows that each **generation**, or group of people who are born during the same time, has distinctive attitudes, behaviors, expectations, and habits. Each member of a generation experiences similar significant events within his or her lifetime. Specific ideas and experiences motivate the members of a generation. Because most members of a generation are around the same age, each generation's members seem to have similar ideas, problems, and attitudes.

Culture may also affect behavior. As you learned in chapter 1, *culture* is the traditions, beliefs, rituals, customs, and values that are specific to a group of people. Cultural differences that impact behavior affect how people communicate, eat, dress, and carry out their traditions. You will learn more about diverse cultures and their impact on holistic nursing care in Chapter 11, *Appreciating Diversity*.

Remember

The dynamics of the mind and relationships with others are fundamental to what it means to be human and what it means to bring healing into the world.

Daniel Siegel, MD, clinical professor of psychiatry

Culture Cues

Practicing Cultural Awareness

Being aware of cultural values, beliefs, and practices gives you the opportunity to build trusting relationships. *Cultural awareness* promotes positive interactions and helps you provide care that is culturally sensitive and acceptable. Always remember to ask if you are in doubt about a cultural belief or practice. This allows a resident to share what is acceptable and preferred.

This strategy promotes wellness, harmony, a safe environment, and good communication. Recognizing that residents may have diverse cultural backgrounds will help you develop holistic relationships and deliver holistic care.

Apply It

1. What cultural beliefs and practices do you follow that may influence your ability to develop holistic relationships and provide holistic care?
2. Think about a recent conversation you had. Did you consider your conversation partner's cultural beliefs and practices while you talked? If you did not, would considering your conversation partner's culture have changed the way you interacted with him or her?

How Do Generational Differences Affect Behavior and Attitudes?

Think About This

There are at least four different generations in today's workforce. Each generation brings its own unique experiences and perspectives.

A **generation gap** occurs when people from different generations have trouble communicating because of differences in traditions, attitudes, or beliefs. For example, older generations (such as baby boomers) may have more **taboos** (practices that are considered improper) and may communicate more formally than your generation does.

While it is helpful to know and understand the behaviors associated with different generations, do not become preoccupied with these differences. Doing so might cause you to believe **stereotypes** (simplifications or biases) about a particular generation. When you interact with members of other generations, set aside any assumptions or judgments and talk openly with people to learn about each individual. For example, you may think older residents do not know enough about modern subjects and technology to be interesting in conversation. After getting to know an older resident, however, you may find that this is untrue. Stereotypes can be a barrier. Instead of accepting stereotypes, recognize generational differences and value the qualities of each generation. The better you understand your residents' generations, the easier it will be for you to build rapport through improved communication (Figure 6.5).

As a holistic nursing assistant, you will be caring for members of various generations. Understanding the key characteristics of each generation will help you effectively have intergenerational communication and form positive relationships.

Monkey Business Images/Shutterstock.com

Figure 6.5 Positive intergenerational relationships are built on understanding and good communication.

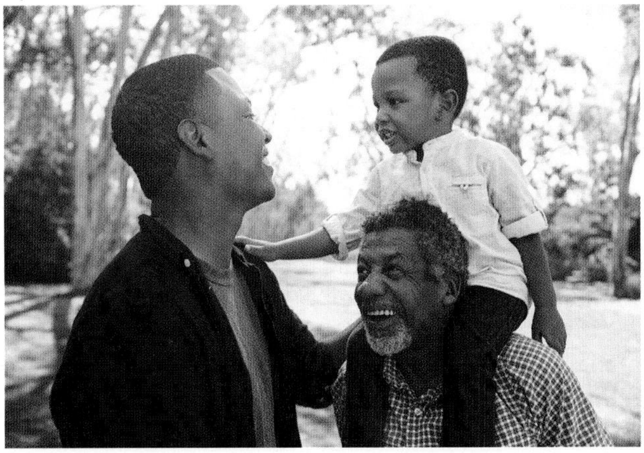

The Silent Generation (1928–1945)

Members of *the silent generation* have strong feelings of patriotism, are work oriented and quiet, are respectful of authority, and have a sense of moral obligation. People of this generation experienced economic downturn during the Great Depression and lived through World War II, and these experiences caused them to be financially conservative. People of this generation tend to save their money, maintain low debt, and pursue secure financial investments. This generation also values security, comfort, and familiar activities and environments.

The Baby Boomers (1946–1964)

Baby boomers experienced the Civil Rights Movement, the sexual revolution, several assassinations, the Korean War, and political scandals. These incidents provided a shared experience that resulted in a strong work ethic. This hardworking generation enjoyed good economic opportunities when entering the workforce and is very driven to achieve professional goals. In fact, baby boomers often define themselves by their professional accomplishments. Baby boomers are often self-reliant, independent, optimistic, confident, and patriotic. This is one of the few generations in which youth is idolized and adored.

Generation X (1965–1976)

Members of *generation X* have been called *latchkey kids* because their parents often worked, and as kids, members of this generation let themselves into the house after school. As a result, people of this generation are extremely entrepreneurial, self-sufficient, focused on financial planning, and independent. Generation X is the best-educated generation, and 29 percent of its members have obtained at least a bachelor's degree. Members of generation X started families more cautiously than their parents did and hoped to avoid raising their children the way they were raised.

Millennials (1977–1995)

Millennials make up the largest generation since the baby boomers. Sophisticated and technologically savvy, millennials may be more isolated as individuals because of the rapid expansion of technology during their youth. Millennials are immune to most traditional marketing and sales pitches because they have been exposed to these efforts since childhood. As a result, this generation is less brand loyal, more flexible, and more comfortable with changing fashion. Millennials tend to be civic minded and often volunteer or give to causes in which they believe. They also value exercise and enjoy travel.

Generation Z (1995–2004)

Because *generation Z* is still in its youth, there is not as much known about its members compared to earlier generations. This generation's environment is quite diverse and includes technology that is used in new, more significant ways than in the past. The highly sophisticated media and technology utilized daily have caused this generation to be more Internet and technologically savvy than members of previous generations. Members of generation Z tend to be very independent and use the Internet and social media as primary forms of communication.

> **Remember**
>
> *This time, like all times, is a very good one, if we but know what to do with it.*
>
> Ralph Waldo Emerson, American essayist, lecturer, and poet

Healthcare Scenario
An Intergenerational Team

Each year, the hospital in your community holds a hospital-wide Innovation Award competition. In last month's newsletter, Floor A's nursing team participated in the competition by reporting the team's innovations in staffing. Floor A's nursing team includes individuals from several generations, including baby boomers and millennials. The team reported initial challenges getting work done because of constant bickering among nursing staff and an inability to agree. Once the team members acknowledged their generational differences, however, communication improved. As a result, Floor A's nursing team developed an outstanding solution for weekend and holiday staffing. Because of the team's ability to find positive ways of communicating, hospital CEO Janet Gilford presented them with the Innovation Award.

Apply It

1. What differences do you think needed to be overcome between the baby boomers and millennials on this team?

2. How do you think acknowledging generational differences helped the team win this award?

Using the Key Terms

Complete the following sentences using the key terms in this section.

1. A young nursing assistant may struggle to communicate with an older patient because of the _____, or lack of communication, between their age groups.

2. _____, such as the use of sarcasm or scowling, are actions that occur in response to a stimulus.

3. If behaviors are inferred, they are considered _____.

4. Two people who were born during the same period of time would belong to the same _____.

5. Each generation has its own _____, or practices that are considered improper.

6. Smiling is an example of a(n) _____ behavior.

7. The assumption that an older patient would struggle to use modern technology is an example of a(n) _____.

Know and Understand the Facts

8. What is the difference between an attitude and a behavior?

9. How are overt and covert behaviors different?

10. Identify three reasons that individuals may have different behaviors.

11. Describe three similarities and three differences between two of the generations discussed in this section.

Analyze and Apply Concepts

12. What are two reasons why there are differences in people's behavior?

13. Would it be more difficult to understand an overt behavior or to understand a covert behavior? Why?

14. What can you do to avoid stereotyping residents based on the generations to which they belong?

15. Give one example of a situation in which you could bridge the gap between your generation and your residents' generation.

Think Critically

Read the following care situation. Then answer the questions that follow.

You are caring for Mr. Z, who is a member of the baby boomer generation. Mr. Z is confident, has had a very successful career, and is now in rehabilitation for a total knee replacement. Today, you are to assist Mr. Z with his ADLs because he is still having some problems with flexibility and movement. You will need to set up Mr. Z's shaving equipment and help him prepare for his morning bath. Mr. Z is in a lot of pain and is not in a very good mood. He is used to being completely independent and doesn't like having to ask for help.

16. How do the values of Mr. Z's generation shape his behavior?

17. In what ways could you help Mr. Z feel more comfortable?

18. What skills could you use to build rapport with Mr. Z and assure him that his goal to regain independence is possible?

Objectives

To provide the best possible care, you must be respectful of your own body, mind, and spirit. You must also be respectful of the bodies, minds, and spirits of patients and residents, their families, and your coworkers. Your understanding of the relationship between the body, mind, and spirit is linked to your wellness and to your ability to develop and maintain holistic relationships. To achieve the objectives for this section, you must successfully

- **explain** the body, mind, and spirit and how they relate to holistic relationships and care;
- **examine** the impact the body, mind, and spirit have on your self-image, health, and wellness; and
- **describe** care strategies that include recognition of and sensitivity to your body, mind, and spirit.

Key Terms

Learn these key terms to better understand the information presented in the section.

autonomy

conscious

parasympathetic nervous
   system (PNS)

rapport

self-image

subconscious

sympathetic nervous system (SNS)

Questions to Consider

- Were you aware that the body, mind, and spirit are all connected?
- Have you noticed this connection in your own life? For example, when you feel stressed (mind), do you also get a headache (body)? When you no longer want to do something (spirit), do you find reasons not to (mind)?

What Are Body, Mind, and Spirit?

The most positive and functional link between the body, mind, and spirit is the interaction between them. The body, mind, and spirit interact and overlap with each other, creating a connection so that people can live their lives as "whole" human beings (Figure 6.6).

Body

You already know that the body requires food and water, which are basic needs. The human *body* is a highly complex, integrative system. While each body performs the same functions, each body is also unique. How the body responds to its basic needs and how the body's needs affect a person's mind can vary. These interactions are what make each of us a special, interconnected system.

Mind

Your *mind* is constantly thinking, inquiring, and directing your behavior based on your perception of the world. Your mind becomes aware of situations through your senses of hearing, sight, taste, smell, and touch. Your thoughts can be either **conscious** (aware) or **subconscious** (unaware).

The connection between the mind and body is evident when a thought develops into a physical reaction in the body. For example, it is possible to lessen feelings of anxiety by using relaxation

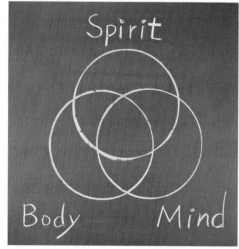

Anson0618/Shutterstock.com

Figure 6.6 The body, mind, and spirit interact and overlap, creating a connection so that people can live their lives as "whole" human beings.

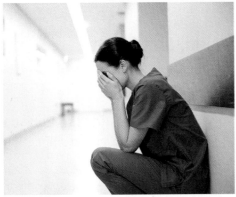
Syda Productions/Shutterstock.com

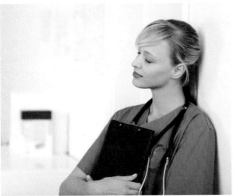
racorn/Shutterstock.com

Figure 6.7 Consider the two images in this figure. Which portion of the nervous system (sympathetic or parasympathetic) is at play in each image?

techniques, such as deep breathing, to calm yourself. When you stop thinking about the source of your anxiety and focus instead on your breathing, you immediately create a relaxation response in the body. Breathing has the ability to relax the nervous system and the entire body, especially in the abdominal region where tension and anxiety are held. Once you begin deep-breathing exercises, the **parasympathetic nervous system (PNS)** takes over and returns your body to a homeostatic state. You begin to feel calm and more open to problem solving and decision making.

The opposite occurs when the **sympathetic nervous system (SNS)** triggers the fight-or-flight response. In the *fight-or-flight response*, increased blood flow to the lungs and heart prepare a person to run or fight. At this time, the brain is not functioning optimally. It is hard for the mind to be optimistic and see possibilities and it is difficult to make decisions (Figure 6.7).

Spirit

The spirit is also connected to the body and mind. Your *spirit* is the essence of who you are inside, or your inner qualities. A sense of spirituality is present in each of us. It is said that a person's spirit is the truest part of who he or she is. When a person is said to have *spirituality*, he or she is typically seen as honest, loving, and caring and possesses wisdom, imagination, and compassion.

Sometimes, when spirit is discussed, only a person's religion is considered, but the spirit is more than this. The spirit is a person's *higher self*, or the inner qualities that help a person feel whole and achieve a sense of inner peace and harmony. Some ways to get to know your spirit are through meditation, prayer, poetry, music, and talks with friends. These activities have been proven to calm the body and mind. This feeling of calm can create a connection between the body and mind. As the body and mind influence each other, you will have a better sense of well-being and peace.

Positive connections between the body, mind, and spirit help create a healthy lifestyle. Some exercises and activities you can do to strengthen these connections include walking, participating in yoga or tai chi, weight lifting, and hiking. Eating a nutritious diet (consisting of four or five cups of fruits and vegetables a day), spending time with friends and family, writing in a journal, or doing some creative activity will also help promote positive connections between your body, mind, and spirit.

How Does the Body-Mind-Spirit Connection Influence Caregiving?

Connections between the body, mind, and spirit greatly influence the quality of care you give to others. Not only is it important to understand your own body-mind-spirit connection, but it is also essential that you, as a holistic nursing assistant, are sensitive to and aware of how connections between the body, mind, and spirit affect patients, residents, and their families.

Your Body-Mind-Spirit Connection

When your body, mind, and spirit are connected, you will begin to feel confident because your body is as healthy as it can be, your mind is clear, and your spirit is in harmony with your body and mind. This connection will help you feel strong and self-assured. It will also help you develop a positive **self-image** (view of yourself).

When you have a strong body-mind-spirit connection, your presence will be strong, but gentle and caring, when you enter a resident's room. You will be able

Remember
I am one and whole as I was created to be.
Unknown

to sense when residents are stressed and help them use calming breaths. You will understand the importance of maintaining a healthy lifestyle and will encourage residents to do the same. You will be able to focus on the unique needs and desires of those in your care and promote resident **autonomy** (personal independence). Encouraging residents to be as independent as possible will help residents maintain strong body-mind-spirit connections.

The Body-Mind-Spirit Connection and Caregiving

The body-mind-spirit connection not only affects you personally, but also impacts your caregiving. When you understand your own body-mind-spirit connection, your approach to residents will be positive, you will use supportive communication, and you will be better able to build mutual respect. Remember that the way you deliver holistic care is an extension of who you are as an individual. You, and no one else, can build a strong connection between yourself and those in your care.

Holistic care begins when you first meet a resident. This is the resident's first impression of you, and you only get one first impression. Pay close attention to the way you walk into the room, the tone of your voice, and the way you make contact. Remember that the resident's room is his or her personal space. Create trust by looking directly at the resident, being attentive, and showing appropriate concern. Be respectful and use the resident's title and last name, such as *Mr. Antar*.

It is important to always explain what care you will provide. Create **rapport** (mutual understanding in relationships) with residents by taking time to listen to them. Avoid interrupting or making judgmental statements, such as "You don't look well today." Listening helps develop positive regard, trust, and mutual respect between the nursing assistant and resident. When you listen well, your communication will be caring and sincere. In addition to listening, always try to answer any questions residents have. You may also want to use touch, if appropriate, such as a handshake or pat on the arm, when communicating (Figure 6.8).

Becoming a Holistic Nursing Assistant
Assessing Your Own Body, Mind, and Spirit

How does a person learn more about connections between the body, mind, and spirit? One important way to learn more about this is to become aware of your own body, mind, and spirit. Gaining this awareness can strengthen your body-mind-spirit connection.

The following statements represent qualities of strong connections between the body, mind, and spirit. Consider which statements apply to you. The more statements that apply to you, the stronger your connections are in that area.

Are you aware of your body? Consider which statements apply to you.

- I eat between four and five cups of fruits and vegetables daily.
- I exercise regularly.
- I sleep between seven and nine hours every night.

Are you aware of your mind? Consider which statements apply to you.

- I find time during the day to relax, even if only for a few minutes at a time.

- I communicate effectively with all types of people and am a strong listener.
- I have written goals that will help me achieve my life and career goals.

Are you aware of your spirit? Consider which statements apply to you.

- I am able to enjoy the environment on a regular basis by walking or playing outside.
- I would describe myself as a happy person.
- I have positive relationships with my family and friends.
- I like what I am presently doing—for example, going to school or a job.

Apply It

1. How many statements applied to you in each category?
2. If some statements did not apply to you, what actions can you take to change this?

Chapter 6 Human Behavior and Development

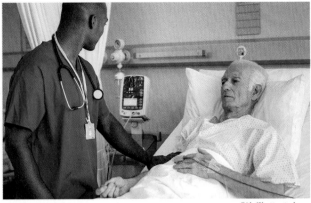

Rido/Shutterstock.com

Figure 6.8 With the patient's permission, you can use touch to communicate you are listening.

The holistic nursing assistant's role in giving care is always to build rapport, positive regard, and trust through the use of empathy, respect, genuineness, and effective communication. Relationships are built on a foundation of respect and trust. Respect and trust are choices people make. When you give respect and build trust, you will get them in return. The saying "Treat others how you want to be treated" applies to holistic nursing care.

Section 6.3 Review and Assessment

Using the Key Terms

Complete the following sentences using the key terms in this section.

1. The _____ nervous system triggers the fight-or-flight response.
2. Thoughts that you are aware of are considered _____ thoughts.
3. By listening without interruption, nursing assistants can create _____, or mutual understanding, between themselves and residents.
4. A nursing assistant who has a positive _____, or view of himself or herself, is more likely to have a strong body-mind-spirit connection.
5. After a high-anxiety situation, the _____ nervous system returns the body to a homeostatic state.
6. Encouraging residents to be as independent as possible promotes feelings of _____ and helps maintain strong body-mind-spirit connections.
7. Thoughts that occur without your active awareness are called _____ thoughts.

Know and Understand the Facts

8. In your own words, explain the connection between the body, mind, and spirit.
9. What is the difference between conscious and subconscious thoughts?
10. Describe two ways you can develop holistic relationships that consider connections between the body, mind, and spirit.

Analyze and Apply Concepts

11. Describe three actions you can take to strengthen your spirit.
12. How can understanding the body, mind, and spirit assist you in delivering care?

Think Critically

Read the following care situation. Then answer the questions that follow.

Mr. J is a retired army officer. He has been in a nursing home for the past month due to complications from an ulcer. Although Mr. J is in a lot of pain, he is very outspoken about his desire to go home. When Mr. J communicates with staff, his responses are very short and sometimes rude. This morning, Sarah, a nursing assistant, is assigned to help him wash, clean his dentures, and get dressed.

13. What can Sarah do to ensure the connection between her body, mind, and spirit is strong so she can best care for and respond to Mr. J?
14. What strategies should Sarah use to build a strong holistic relationship with Mr. J?

Key Points

Reviewing the key points for this chapter will help you practice more safely and competently as a holistic nursing assistant and will help you prepare for the certification competency examination.

- When people are motivated, they are prompted to actively pursue actions or goals.
- When delivering care, you must understand the basic human needs all people have. According to Maslow's hierarchy of needs, needs are ordered from low-level needs, the lowest of which are basic needs (requirements for food, water, sleep, and elimination), to high-level needs, the highest of which is called self-actualization.
- People develop physically, mentally, emotionally, and socially based on their unique characteristics.
- Caring for different generations is an opportunity to learn and grow. Understanding generational differences can help you connect with residents and provide quality holistic care.
- A strong body-mind-spirit connection will help you see yourself as a whole person.

Action Steps to Holistic Care

Review the information in this chapter. Complete the following activities.

1. Select one stage of physical growth. Prepare a short paper or digital presentation that discusses information about this stage.
2. With a partner, prepare a poster that illustrates two challenges people of different generations face.
3. Find pictures in a magazine, in a newspaper, or online that best demonstrate providing holistic care to a resident. Describe each image and provide a rationale for why it was selected.
4. Research one growth and development model not discussed in this chapter. Write a brief report that summarizes the theory or model.
5. With a partner, prepare a poster or digital presentation that illustrates each of the growth periods discussed in Figure 6.3. For each growth period, include an image of a child or adolescent in that stage. Also research the emotional and mental changes and developments typical during each growth period and include this information as well.

Preparing for the Certification Competency Examination

To prepare for the nursing assistant certification competency examination, you will need to know content found in this chapter. This content may be tested in the knowledge (written or oral) and skills (hands-on demonstration) portions of the exam. The following areas will be emphasized:

- basic human needs across the life span
- human growth and development
- supportive communication
- behavior that is positive and nonthreatening
- the nursing assistant's role in accommodating spiritual differences

These sample test questions are similar to ones you will find on the certification competency exam. See how well you can answer them. Be sure to select the *best* answer.

1. Which of the following is *not* an intrinsic motivational factor?
   A. a desire to help others
   B. a desire for recognition
   C. awards
   D. a challenge
2. Which type of behavior is a resident displaying when he talks with his family?
   A. covert   C. overt
   B. active   D. passive
3. A resident sometimes gets mad and yells at the nursing staff. He is very proud and does not want to be in the facility. What would be the best strategy to use when you first meet him?
   A. go inside and introduce yourself, and then sit down for a moment and listen to him
   B. tell the resident that no one wants to take care of him
   C. observe the resident in a nonjudgmental way and slowly start taking care of him
   D. go into the room smiling and begin to prepare him for his morning meal

(continued)

4. As you approach Mrs. S's room, you hear her crying. What should you do?
   A. don't go in and ask someone else to go in and check on her
   B. take a breath, knock, go in, approach Mrs. S, gently touch her shoulder, and ask if you can help
   C. go away, wait for an hour, and then come back to see Mrs. S
   D. go in and tell Mrs. S to stop crying, reminding her that things could be worse

5. Mr. C shares with you that no one cares about him anymore. You've noticed that he has not had visitors this past month. What need is Mr. C expressing?
   A. self-esteem
   B. self-actualization
   C. basic and physiological
   D. love and belonging

6. What characteristics or qualities are needed to develop a positive relationship?
   A. being in control
   B. knowing all the answers
   C. being caring and professional
   D. showing sympathy

7. Mrs. M recently had a hip fracture that required surgery. When you encourage Mrs. M to get up and use her walker to go to the restroom, she refuses. What question should you be asking yourself?
   A. Is Mrs. M experiencing pain or discomfort?
   B. Is Mrs. M angry about her hip surgery?
   C. Is Mrs. M giving you trouble because she doesn't care for you?
   D. Is Mrs. M just being difficult because she wants sympathy?

8. Which of the following is one way to create a healing environment that recognizes the body, mind, and spirit?
   A. use behaviors that communicate that patients will get better soon
   B. be present and listen to patients whenever it is appropriate and helpful
   C. talk about ways patients will be able to take care of themselves when they get home
   D. keep busy in patients' rooms and get as much done as you possibly can

9. Which of the following generations is most likely to idolize and adore youth?
   A. the baby boomers
   B. millennials
   C. the silent generation
   D. generation Z

10. Mr. J is a 23-year-old man who recently had one leg amputated. He appears very nervous. Which of the following would be the best way to approach him?
    A. feel sorry for Mr. J
    B. encourage and teach Mr. J to try a breathing exercise, if he consents
    C. tell Mr. J to try to think about happy things in his life
    D. reassure Mr. J that there are people who have it worse

11. According to Erikson, which of the following is the central conflict for adolescents?
    A. identity versus confusion
    B. industry versus inferiority
    C. intimacy versus isolation
    D. integrity versus despair

12. A nursing assistant wants to help a resident having difficulty with his physical therapy. Which of the following should she do?
    A. observe the resident and talk about what his job was in the service
    B. tell the resident he does not have a good self-image and needs to focus
    C. ask the resident if there is an exercise he used to do that could be modified to suit his current abilities
    D. get upset and tell the resident he needs to exercise to feel better

13. Which need is fulfilled when a person feels satisfied with his or her state of health, property, and home?
    A. basic needs
    B. love and belonging
    C. self-esteem
    D. safety and security

14. Which of the following is a strategy a holistic nursing assistant can use to strengthen his or her spirit?
    A. studying hard
    B. exercising daily
    C. listening to music
    D. watching family-oriented movies

15. During which stage of development do children begin running and jumping?
    A. infancy   C. adolescence
    B. school-age years D. preschool years

Did you have difficulty with any of the questions? If you did, review the chapter to find the correct answer(s).

CHAPTER 7 Health and Wellness

Welcome to the Chapter

This chapter provides information about the unique relationship between wellness and illness. *Wellness* (a feeling of good health) and *illness* (a feeling of poor health) can occur at the same time. For example, people can have chronic illnesses, but still learn to live their lives healthfully. Understanding the relationship between wellness and illness will allow you to use a variety of health and wellness strategies to promote healthful living. Some of the health and wellness strategies you will learn about are considered *integrative* or *complementary and alternative* to the healthcare typically delivered in hospitals and in other healthcare facilities.

In this chapter, you will also learn about the power of stress and ways to manage stressful situations. As part of managing stress, you will identify ways to set personal and professional priorities. Setting these priorities will allow you to better manage your time and energy and establish a positive balance between your personal and professional lives. Properly managing the stressors in your life will help you effectively care for others and for yourself.

What you learn in this chapter will help you develop your knowledge and skills to become a holistic nursing assistant. The topics discussed in the chapter are highlighted on the Providing Holistic Care Framework.

You are now ready to start this chapter, *Health and Wellness.*

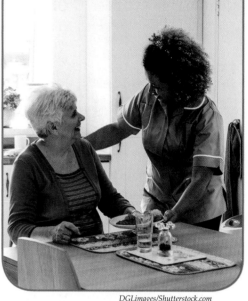
DGLimages/Shutterstock.com

Chapter Outline

Section 7.1
Wellness and Illness

Section 7.2
Work-Life Balance and Stress Management

Section 7.3
Health Promotion and Integrative Medicine

Providing Holistic Care: A Framework

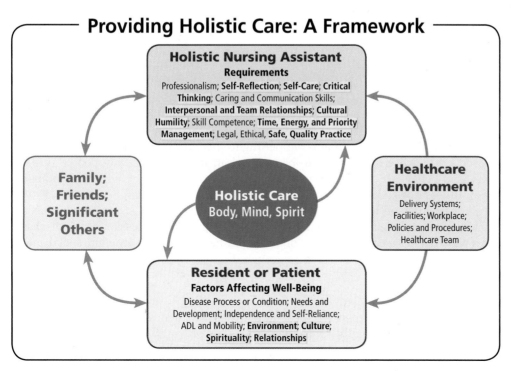

Holistic Nursing Assistant
Requirements
Professionalism; **Self-Reflection; Self-Care; Critical Thinking;** Caring and Communication Skills; **Interpersonal and Team Relationships; Cultural Humility;** Skill Competence; **Time, Energy, and Priority Management;** Legal, Ethical, **Safe, Quality Practice**

Family; Friends; Significant Others

Holistic Care
Body, Mind, Spirit

Healthcare Environment
Delivery Systems; Facilities; Workplace; Policies and Procedures; Healthcare Team

Resident or Patient
Factors Affecting Well-Being
Disease Process or Condition; Needs and Development; Independence and Self-Reliance; ADL and Mobility; **Environment; Culture; Spirituality; Relationships**

Questions to Consider

- Do you consider yourself to be *well*? Why or why not? What do you do to keep yourself well?
- When was the last time you felt ill? How did it feel to be ill? What did you have to do to feel well again?

Objectives

Understanding the unique relationship between wellness and illness is essential to providing safe, quality care. People's perceptions and understanding of wellness and illness may influence their health, and this is important to remember when you begin working as a holistic nursing assistant. To achieve the objectives for this section, you must successfully

- **describe** the relationship between wellness and illness;
- **explain** the differences between health, wellness, and illness; and
- **discuss** strategies to achieve wellness.

Key Terms

Learn these key terms to better understand the information presented in the section.

disease

health

illness

well-being

What Is the Relationship Between Wellness and Illness?

The relationship between *wellness* (a feeling of good health) and **illness** (a feeling of poor health) is not as simple as it may seem. Some healthcare providers use a straight line—with *wellness* on one end and *illness* on the other—to show the relationship between the two. This is not always an accurate picture, however. Even when people experience illness, parts of their bodies and minds can still be well. For example, when you catch a cold, you may have a cough, have a runny nose, and feel "sick." At the same time, however, your heart is beating properly, your muscles and bones enable you to walk, and you may still have a good appetite.

Illness Versus Disease

Being ill, or having an illness, is not the same as having a disease. A **disease** is caused by an incorrectly functioning organ or body system and is usually accompanied by specific symptoms that can be diagnosed by a licensed healthcare provider, such as a doctor. An *illness*, on the other hand, may be your personal interpretation of how you are feeling. You may feel dizzy even if nothing is wrong with any of your body systems. Anxiety or fear may be causing shallow, rapid breathing, which leads to you feeling dizzy.

People may interpret what is happening to them differently after they are diagnosed with a disease. These interpretations can influence the way people think, feel, and behave. If people's illnesses make sense to them, they will likely adjust. If an illness does not make sense, people may react with fear and confusion. How well or ill a person feels is not always the result of a disease. A person who has a disease, but still feels well, is more likely to manage the progression of the disease in a way that has a positive impact on his or her **health** (physical, mental, social, and spiritual condition).

Well-Being

The relationship between wellness and illness influences a person's sense of **well-being** (state of health). Every person has his or her own sense of well-being, and this sense is not necessarily affected by disease. A person may have a disease, but may still have a positive sense of well-being. This is important to remember as you care for others. Regardless of how ill a resident may be, some level of wellness is always within his or her reach (Figure 7.1).

How Can You Help Yourself and Residents Achieve Wellness?

Achieving wellness is a daily, 24-hour responsibility. Eating a healthy meal one day a week is not enough to achieve wellness. Achieving wellness requires self-awareness, commitment to wellness strategies, and ongoing change. Using wellness strategies will not only allow you to achieve your own wellness, but will also help you care for others.

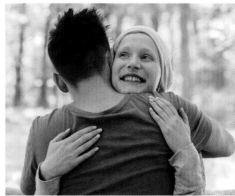

Photographee.eu/Shutterstock.com

Figure 7.1 Even if a person has a serious disease, he or she can achieve wellness.

Wellness and the Holistic Nursing Assistant

To help residents in your care achieve optimal health and well-being, you must be fully aware of your *own* health and well-being. Becoming more aware starts with determining how you see *illness*, *wellness*, and *health*. As you develop your own personal meanings for each of these terms, you will be better able to personalize your care for others. Start by being alert, present, and nonjudgmental. Committing to actions that maintain your health and well-being will help you succeed.

The following questions will help you assess your own level of health and well-being:

- What are your eating habits? Do you routinely select healthy foods? Do you snack on candy or skip meals? Do you eat in front of the television, or do you sit down at a table and eat your meal slowly?
- How often do you exercise and participate in physical activities? Do you maintain a healthy weight and exercise at least 150 minutes each week?
- Do you abstain from tobacco products and drugs, and do you keep your alcohol consumption to a minimum?
- Do you get between seven and nine hours of sleep each night?
- Do you often feel stressed? Have you found strategies to effectively manage your stress?
- Do you regularly participate in social activities? Are you part of a group that enjoys playing sports or going to the movies?
- Do you have a strong support network of family and friends?
- How happy do you feel on a daily basis? Do you wake up and look forward to your day? Do you appreciate nature and the environment around you?
- Do you consider safety in your daily habits? Do you avoid driving when you are tired? Do you never text and drive at the same time?
- Do you promote disease prevention and control? Do you wash your hands or use hand sanitizer before meals? Do you cover your mouth when you cough or sneeze?

Consider your responses to these questions. Do you feel you have achieved optimal health and well-being, or is there room for improvement?

Wellness and Residents

As a holistic nursing assistant, you can make a difference in the wellness and well-being of residents. You can also influence residents' perceptions of wellness or illness. You can do this even for residents who have acute or chronic diseases.

To help others, you must maintain your own health and wellness. For example, learning health and wellness strategies that work for you will allow you to be more helpful to others. Remember that, while you can support and promote residents' wellness and well-being, residents have the responsibility to take action and improve their own states of health, wellness, or illness. If you find that a facility or healthcare provider is more focused on residents' diseases and illnesses than on health and well-being, do not let that stop you from promoting wellness as you work with residents.

Use a positive approach and attitude when you care for residents. Your support can make a difference in residents' wellness and can help residents choose to feel better about themselves and their situations. Residents with diseases—particularly chronic diseases—may feel that they are defined by a disease, and much of these residents' time is focused on symptoms and treatment. Your support and encouragement, however, can help residents see themselves as worthwhile.

Encourage residents to be as independent and self-reliant as possible. Ask residents to play a larger role in their daily hygiene, such as bathing or oral care, whenever possible. When appropriate, encourage increased activity and ambulation. Participating in daily hygiene and enjoying activities will help residents establish a sense of normalcy and will allow residents to feel capable. Retaining some independence may be comforting to a resident, particularly if the resident is experiencing illness.

Seek to increase residents' social interactions and activities. If a resident has not been out of his or her room, and is capable, encourage the resident to visit the dining room or participate in a facility activity. Participating in social activities is a strategy for attaining wellness. Sometimes a simple invitation or suggestion can make a difference. By establishing supportive, positive relationships with residents, you can have a remarkable influence on residents' wellness.

Section 7.1 Review and Assessment

Using the Key Terms
Complete the following sentences using the key terms in this section.

1. The condition of a person's physical, mental, social, and spiritual self is known as _____.
2. A resident can have a(n) _____, or a feeling of poor health, even if other parts of his or her body and mind are still well.
3. _____ describes the state of a person's health.
4. A(n) _____ is caused by an incorrectly functioning organ or body system, is usually accompanied by specific symptoms, and can be diagnosed by a licensed healthcare provider.

Know and Understand the Facts

5. Explain the relationship between illness and wellness.
6. What is the difference between illness and disease?
7. Why is it important for nursing assistants to achieve wellness?

Analyze and Apply Concepts

8. Give one example of how perception can impact illness or wellness.
9. Describe one way that you can develop a sense of wellness or well-being.
10. Describe one way that you can help a resident develop a sense of wellness or well-being.

Think Critically
Read the following care situation. Then answer the questions that follow.

When you enter Mrs. J's room, you ask her how she is doing today. Mrs. J says she feels like she is of no use to anyone. She says she is very tired and cannot do any of the activities she used to do. She sadly says to you, "I have felt useless ever since I was diagnosed with cancer."

11. How can you demonstrate to Mrs. J that you care about her wellness?
12. What could you do to help Mrs. J improve her sense of wellness or well-being?

Objectives

To provide the best possible care, you need to understand sources of stress, the ways that stress impacts health and well-being, and techniques to manage stress. In this section, you will learn about how balancing your personal and professional responsibilities and managing your time and priorities can not only benefit you personally, but can also help you become a more effective holistic nursing assistant. To achieve the objectives for this section, you must successfully

- **identify** sources of stress;
- **list** techniques that can be used to manage stress;
- **describe** the importance of time and energy management;
- **evaluate** your own work-life balance; and
- **discuss** ways to improve your work-life balance.

Key Terms

Learn these key terms to better understand the information presented in the section.

distress

energy

energy rhythm

eustress

hormones

prioritizing

stress management

work-life balance

Questions to Consider

- Have you ever felt stressed because of a situation or person? What do you think caused the stress?
- How do you experience stress? Do you get a headache or stomachache? Does your heart beat faster, or do you feel short of breath? Do you feel that you are running out of time and can't seem to get anything done? What effect does your stress have on others in your life?
- How do you manage the stress in your life? Does the way you manage stress help you balance school, work, and other aspects of your life?

What Is Stress?

As you learned in chapter 4, *stress* is a physical or psychological response to a situation that causes worry or tension. Stress occurs as a result of physical, mental, or emotional pressures. Stress is considered normal, but it affects each person differently. Because of stress, some people get headaches, have trouble sleeping, experience sore muscles, or may even become depressed.

There are many potential sources of stress in life. Stress can come from external factors, such as your environment or different social situations. Stress can also be the result of an illness or medical procedure.

Eustress Versus Distress

Everyone experiences stress, and some stress can actually be good. **Eustress**, or *good* stress, can be beneficial and can motivate you to do new or challenging tasks. Eustress might motivate you to study hard and ace an upcoming test or to apply for a job you have been wanting. When stress remains at a high level, lasts for a long time, or gets out of control, however, it can turn into *bad* stress, or **distress**. When someone is in distress, his or her body may not function properly, and he or she may have unhealthy feelings and emotions.

When a person is stressed, his or her body releases **hormones**, which are chemical substances that regulate body processes. Hormones help protect the body and prepare the body for the challenges of stress. At this time, the *sympathetic nervous system (SNS)* also triggers the *fight-or-flight response*, which you learned about in chapter 6. During the fight-or-flight response, our hearts may beat faster, we may start to sweat, our stomachs may stop digesting food, and sometimes our immune systems are not able to keep up the body's defenses. This response helps us gear up, focus, and be alert in case we need to defend ourselves. When this response continues over time, however, it can harm physical and emotional health.

Signs and Symptoms of Stress

There are several signs and symptoms of stress. These signs and symptoms can affect mental, emotional, physical, and behavioral health:

- **Mental symptoms**: inability to concentrate, constant worry, or ability to see only the negative
- **Emotional symptoms**: moodiness, short temper, agitation, loneliness, or depression
- **Physical symptoms**: aches and pains, dizziness, nausea, rapid heartbeat, or frequent colds
- **Behavioral symptoms**: procrastination, isolation, nervous habits, or the use of alcohol or drugs to relax

It is not possible to completely eliminate all stress from your life. You can, however, determine what common sources of stress, or *stressors*, you may experience. Typically, people have their own unique reactions to stressors. For example, some people may get headaches, others may need more sleep, and some may become tense and angry. Recognizing stressors is the first step to controlling them (Figure 7.2).

Identifying the stressors in your own life can help you recognize the stressors that others experience. This can be very helpful when you care for residents. Stress can interfere with residents' abilities to achieve wellness. Be sure to report any signs or symptoms of stress in residents to the licensed nursing staff. This is very important information.

How Can Stress Be Managed?

Stress management is the process of using strategies to handle and control stress. Stress-management strategies are important not only for yourself, but also for your work as a holistic nursing assistant. Understanding how to manage stress will enhance how you work with others and how you care for patients and residents. When you manage stress, you will find your work environment more enjoyable and productive.

Identifying Stressors

The first way to manage stress is to identify stressors before they cause strong stress reactions. To do this, take a breath to relax your body and begin to identify any sources of stress. Stop for a moment and decide to focus on relaxing so you can identify any stressors that are making you tight and tense.

Identifying each stressor will help you determine if your stressors are relevant. For example, are you worrying about an event that might happen in the future, but is not happening now? Perhaps you feel stressed because you are running out of time to finish a task. Examine what is true in the moment and what is not. You may feel stressed about an event that has not happened yet, or you may feel stress from external pressures.

Practice becoming more aware of your stressors and determining if they are relevant. The goal of this practice is to stop strong stress responses before you and your body react to them. Responding proactively, rather than reacting, to stressors helps you take slower and more deliberate action. If you do this, you may not experience a fight-or-flight response.

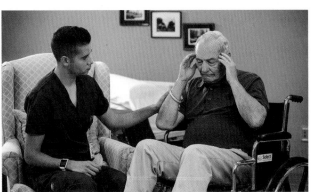

© Tori Soper Photography

Figure 7.2 Stress can come from external factors, such as illness, or internal factors, such as frustration or unmet expectations.

As a holistic nursing assistant, you should also try to identify the stressors affecting residents in your care. Residents may feel worried and stressed about not having any visitors, becoming forgetful, or losing people they love. You can help residents identify these stressors and determine if stressors are relevant. Consider a resident who is worried that he or she will not have visitors. Explore the reality of this situation with the resident by asking when he or she last had visitors and who those visitors were. Ask when these visitors said they would return. You may find that the resident is concerned only about who is visiting today, not about never having visitors.

Think About This

In a recent poll, 89 percent of people interviewed said they had experienced serious stress in their lives. According to the American Academy of Family Physicians, two-thirds of office visits to family doctors are for stress-related symptoms.

Changing Focus

Another stress-management technique is to shift focus away from a stressor and onto something that is not stressful—for example, a sport, book, candle, deep breathing, a quote or saying, or a game. Focusing on something that is not stressful will give you and your body a break. You and your body learn how it feels to be relaxed and not stressed. If you are feeling stressed, you may want to take a walk. Your body may be tense, and walking will help the body release tension. As you walk, focus on your surroundings or your breathing.

Humor is another way to relieve stress. Even just smiling creates a relaxation response in the body. Laughing is very good for the body and spirit as well. Once you experience not being stressed, you will want more of this feeling, and so will those in your care (Figure 7.3).

Using Support from Others

Relying on a strong support network of family and friends is another stress-management technique. Often, a network of family and friends can provide needed

Remember

Nature does not hurry, yet everything is accomplished.

Lao Tzu, Ancient Chinese philosopher and poet

Becoming a Holistic Nursing Assistant
Reactions to Stress

One way to track your own stress levels is to chart stressors and the effects of stress on your body, mind, emotions, and behavior. Below is an example of a chart you could use to track your stress. As you chart your stress, follow these directions:

1. Think about situations that cause you to feel stress. Identify the individual stressors in these situations and list them in the first column.
2. In the second column, describe how each stressor affects your body. List the physical symptoms you experience as you react to stress.
3. Use the third column to document what you are thinking during the stressful situation. Note any mental symptoms of stress you experience.
4. In the fourth column, explain what you are feeling during the stressful situation. List these feelings, as well as any emotional symptoms of stress.

5. Use the fifth column to list what behaviors you demonstrate in reaction to stress. Include any behavioral symptoms of stress you exhibit.

Now, each time you experience this stressful situation, you can anticipate your physical, mental, emotional, and behavioral responses. This will enable you to quickly respond to stress and eliminate negative reactions.

Apply It

1. Was it difficult to identify what stresses you in situations? What made it difficult?
2. Were you surprised by any of the symptoms of stress you identified? What was surprising?

Stressors	Physical Symptoms	Mental Symptoms	Emotional Symptoms	Behavioral Symptoms

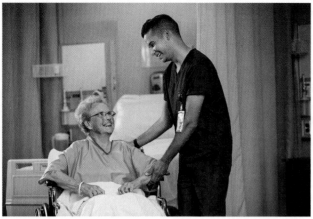

© Tori Soper Photography

Figure 7.3 Laughter and humor can help you reduce and manage stress.

assistance during difficult times and can help you feel more positive and optimistic. Studies have shown that, when people are supported by those who care for them, recovery time is reduced.

Managing Time and Energy

Using your time and **energy** (power and drive) wisely is an important and essential strategy for managing stress. Being aware of time and planning your day will allow you to more easily get your work done. The same is true for energy. If you are aware of your energy levels and understand how you can increase them, you will not only get your work done, but you will also feel good about what you are doing.

Consider that, if you live to be 77 years old, you will have 40,548,200 minutes of life available to you. It is up to you how you use these minutes. Being in control of your time, not overcommitting, and not saying *yes* to activities you really do not want to do are important time-management strategies. Adding too many commitments can rob you of your time and create stress.

One of the first steps in properly managing your time is analyzing how you spend it. One way to do this is to record what you did last week, including specific details about how each day was spent. Make sure the week you analyze is representative of a typical week in your routine schedule.

Once you have tracked exactly how you spend your time, you can decide what changes, if any, you would like to make. Perhaps you would like to spend less time watching television or playing on the computer and more time reading. Once you decide what changes you want to make, you can prioritize them. Then make the change by taking action.

Other time-management strategies you can use include the following:

- Use your time effectively. Notice if you are wasting time or checking your phone every minute (Figure 7.4).
- Break large projects up into small tasks. For example, when you work on a research paper, first create an outline of the paper's topics. Then use the outline to begin your draft.
- Say *no* or negotiate for more time when you do not have the necessary time to complete a task properly. This is a way to respect yourself and others.

Use your personal **energy rhythm** (sequence of energy peaks) to plan your work. If you are a morning person and have more energy in the morning, complete difficult or time-consuming work during the morning hours. Conversely, if you have more energy during the evening hours, use that time to complete challenging tasks.

Be aware of other people's energy levels and the effect on you. If another person's energy is low, this may lower your energy level. Knowing the type and level of energy that surrounds you is helpful, as those in your care may have low energy levels due to illness. You may have to tone down your energy level to be in sync with others.

Protect yourself against distracting or negative energy, such as a negative attitude that someone has. If you can, distance yourself from this attitude. If you cannot distance yourself, don't let the person's

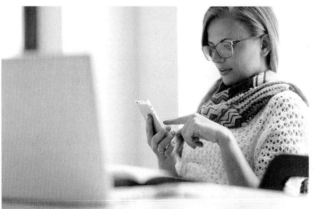

lenetstan/Shutterstock.com

Figure 7.4 In today's ever-connected world, your smartphone can be huge source of distraction, preventing you from managing your time wisely.

negative attitude affect how you interpret or handle your energy. Stressful or difficult events may leave you feeling drained. When this happens, you can restore your energy by relaxing or by refocusing on your responsibilities and the tasks required of you (Figure 7.5).

The key to effective time and energy management is to be mindful of what needs to be done and how it can be done. This ensures that what you do is satisfying and nurturing for yourself and, if possible, for others.

Establishing Priorities

All of the aforementioned stress-management strategies are very helpful in a professional setting. One technique in particular, however, helps keep work challenges under control. This technique is **prioritizing**, or organizing responsibilities or tasks so that the most important tasks are completed first. Prioritizing is also an important time-management strategy, especially when you need to complete many routine tasks for residents. When you set priorities, you determine which tasks are urgent and should come before others. Some people are comfortable using *to-do lists* to prioritize. You can even create a quick to-do list at work once you are given an assignment.

The best way to set priorities is to use either your personal to-do list or an assignment sheet. On the list or sheet, write an *A* next to tasks that are high priority and that need to be done that day. Write a *B* next to items that can wait until after A-level tasks are completed. Write a *C* next to tasks that you would like to get done, but can complete after A and B tasks are completed (Figure 7.6).

As you prioritize, think about how much time each task might take. Always allow extra time to solve any problems that may arise. Be flexible, when possible. You may finish a task early. If you do, then just move on to the next prioritized item. Be sure to figure in routine breaks, relaxation, and time for yourself. Also figure in time-outs if you are at a computer or are sitting for long periods of time.

When using a to-do list at work, be sure to review the priorities you list with the licensed nursing staff. You will need to complete all of the A-level tasks on your list. Check the list often to ensure you are on track. Feel free to reprioritize tasks if there is a change in a resident's condition or in your assignments. Remember to mark any tasks completed. This will give you a sense of accomplishment.

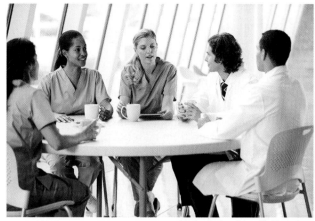
Monkey Business Images/Shutterstock.com

Figure 7.5 Relaxing can take many forms. For example, you could relax by talking with your colleagues during your break.

Priority	Mr. D	Mrs. S	Ms. D	Mr. F	Mrs. G
A	Assist with ambulation with new cane two times for 20 minutes	Measure intake and output	Apply warm compress to right foot for 20 minutes	Fall risk; remind him to ask for help to the bathroom	Turn and position every two hours
B	Assist with dressing change	Assist with shower	Frequently check pain levels during shift	Assist with eating breakfast and lunch	Give a partial bed bath and pay special attention to perineal care
C	Assist with shaving	Urinary leg bag change	Keep fresh water available to encourage fluids	Take him to afternoon facility activities	Provide snacks two times during shift

Figure 7.6 This is an example of a priority list for a nursing assistant for one shift.

Prioritizing is meant to decrease stress, not to cause it. Therefore, be sure your priorities are organized and realistic. Understanding how to set priorities can be a very valuable skill for holistic nursing assistants. Prioritizing will allow you to accomplish more than you usually would in the same time period.

What Is the Best Way to Create a Work-Life Balance?

When you are employed as a holistic nursing assistant, you will find that achieving a positive **work-life balance** is another way to manage stress. Work-life balance describes the state of a person's time and energy contributions to career, work, and family commitments (Figure 7.7). When you are stressed at work, that stress may interfere with your ability to provide quality care to others. Work-related stress can also interfere with your home life. A positive work-life balance allows you to be mentally present at home when you are home and to focus on your work responsibilities when you are at work. Doing this can help you feel more in control, which can reduce stress levels. Doing this will also make you feel much more accomplished.

The best way to determine if you have a positive work-life balance is to reflect on your answers to the following questions:

- Do you consider yourself healthy?
- Are your relationships strong, supportive, and caring?
- Are you aware and respectful of your environment?
- Are you able to rest and relax?

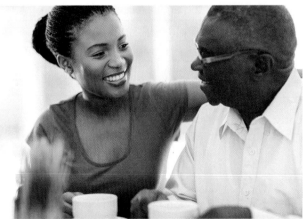

michaeljung/Shutterstock.com

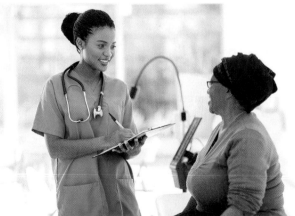

michaeljung/Shutterstock.com

Figure 7.7 Spending time with family can be a positive way to relieve stress, improving your ability to provide quality care while at work.

- Do you spend time on your own personal development?
- Do you have enough money for your current and future needs?
- Are you happy with your career? If you are not, do you have a plan to further your education and training?
- Do you have passion for what you are currently doing?

If your answer to each of these questions is *yes*, this indicates that you have the potential for an outstanding work-life balance. This is not realistic, however. Each of us will have one or more areas that need work. Identify those areas and determine how you will strengthen them. In each area that is strengthened, work and life will become more balanced. This will make each day less stressful as you work.

Section 7.2 Review and Assessment

Using the Key Terms

Complete the following sentences using the key terms in this section.

1. Your _____ is your power and drive to complete tasks.
2. _____, or organizing responsibilities so that the most important tasks are completed first, is one method of effectively managing stress.
3. Good stress, known as _____, might motivate you to do new or challenging tasks.
4. A morning person might have a(n) _____ that has more peaks in the morning than it does later in the day.
5. Chemical substances that regulate body processes are called _____.
6. _____ describes the state of a person's time and energy contributions to career, work, and family commitments.
7. Bad stress is known as _____.
8. _____ is the process of using strategies to handle and control stress.

Know and Understand the Facts

9. Name one physical and one mental effect of stress.
10. Identify two sources of stress.
11. What are three possible symptoms of stress in residents?

Analyze and Apply Concepts

12. What are two ways holistic nursing assistants can manage their stress?
13. What can holistic nursing assistants do to help reduce the stress of those in their care?
14. Describe how to prioritize work tasks and responsibilities.
15. What might cause a negative work-life balance, and what can you do to correct this balance?

Think Critically

Read the following care situation. Then answer the questions that follow.

Mrs. P, one of the residents on your unit, is sweating and appears anxious. She is trying to locate her glasses, but cannot seem to find them. Mrs. P seems to be irritated with herself for losing her glasses. She wants to be independent, so she doesn't feel she should ask for assistance. When you come into Mrs. P's room to help her with morning care, you hear her quietly repeating that she cannot find her glasses.

16. What signs do you observe that might indicate Mrs. P is stressed?
17. What can you do to help Mrs. P relieve her stress?

Questions to Consider

- What do you do to stay healthy? Do you use any particular wellness strategies?
- If you do use wellness strategies, which wellness strategies have worked the best for you? If you don't use any strategies, would you be willing to try new methods that promote health? Why or why not?

Objectives

When you work as a holistic nursing assistant, it is important to remember that health and wellness are each individual's responsibility. As a healthcare provider, however, you must recognize and use helpful strategies within your scope of practice to promote health and wellness in others. To achieve the objectives for this section, you must successfully

- **describe** the knowledge and skills holistic nursing assistants need to help promote health and wellness;
- **explain** strategies that will assist in the promotion of health and wellness in others; and
- **identify** how integrative medicine can help promote health and wellness.

Key Terms

Learn these key terms to better understand the information presented in the section.

complementary and alternative
 medicine (CAM)
contraindicate
conventional medicine

health promotion
integrative medicine (IM)
intuition
probiotic

What Is Health Promotion?

Health promotion is the process of helping people, groups, and communities improve or increase their control over health and wellness. The primary goal of health promotion is to share healthy ideas, beliefs, and experiences with the goal of motivating people to adopt healthy behaviors. One example of a health promotion goal is the cessation of smoking. Health promotion can be used in different ways. It can help one person stop smoking, provide smoking cessation classes for groups of people, or prompt people in a community to create a contest to reduce or quit smoking.

A major principle of health promotion is that you must know a person's, group's, or community's state of health and understand what helps people, including yourself, stay well and healthy. If you are not aware of your *own* health and wellness, it will be hard for you to help others achieve health and wellness. One way to become aware of your health and wellness is to become fully aware of your own body, mind, and spirit, as discussed in chapter 6. This is an ongoing process because people grow and change. A person may be healthy, catch a cold, and then have to recover. A healthy person may break a bone, which then has to heal. Regardless of one's state of health, the goal of health promotion is always to help people strive for the highest level of wellness.

Awareness is an important step in health promotion. You must be sensitive to yourself and to your environment to best understand levels of health and wellness. This sensitivity may come from observation or from **intuition** (feelings not based on facts). When you use intuition, there may not be any direct evidence of your intuitive feelings. Still, you trust those feelings to be true. Intuitive feelings may give you awareness about those in your care. For example, you may know something is different about a resident in your care, but not be sure exactly what the difference is.

Many times, your intuition can sense changes that are not yet observable, but that need to be explored. This information, even if it is based on a feeling, must always be reported to the licensed nursing staff.

Health promotion is an important part of giving care. At the national level, the *National Prevention Strategy* guides the United States in findings ways to improve health and well-being and to build the foundation for holistic care.

The National Prevention Strategy is comprised of four strategic directions that work toward promoting health, preventing disease, and ensuring safety. The goal of the National Prevention Strategy is to help Americans lead longer, healthier lives. The National Prevention Strategy also contains seven priorities, which provide evidenced-based recommendations for reducing the causes of preventable diseases and death. These priorities include

- tobacco-free living;
- the prevention of drug abuse and excessive alcohol use;
- healthy eating;
- active living;
- injury- and violence-free living;
- reproductive and sexual health; and
- mental and emotional well-being.

These priorities guide the actions of many healthcare agencies and facilities. You will find that they are equally important when you provide holistic care.

What Strategies Are Used to Promote Health?

There are many strategies used to accomplish health promotion's goal. Health policies, laws, and regulations (such as the National Prevention Strategy) can promote health. Health is also promoted through community health and disease prevention programs, such as diabetes awareness programs or blood pressure clinics. These programs and clinics provide information and resources to motivate small and large groups, families, and individuals to adopt healthy behaviors.

On a smaller scale, holistic nursing assistants promote the health of residents on a daily basis. Holistic nursing assistants can use their knowledge of residents' conditions to help residents progress. For example, a nursing assistant might help a resident maintain skin integrity or encourage as much independence as possible. Holistic nursing assistants can also promote health using strategies that focus on areas such as diet, exercise, rest and relaxation, stress management, and self-care techniques (Figure 7.8).

Educating others can be challenging, but is worthwhile. Developing a plan for educating residents is the responsibility of the licensed nursing staff. Licensed nursing staff members may encourage nursing assistants to participate in the plan developed. As a nursing assistant, you may also find other opportunities during your shift to promote health and informally provide information to residents while giving care. For example, you can show a resident the importance of exercising hands and feet when assisting with daily hygiene. You can remind residents of important safety precautions while helping them ambulate. You might also find time to provide health promotion during mealtimes (for example, by helping residents learn how to best use assistive eating devices). Paying attention to possible opportunities

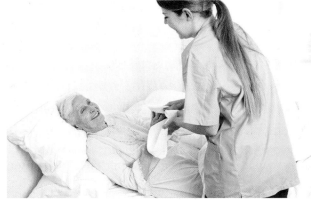

Robert Kneschke/Shutterstock.com

Figure 7.8 As they provide care, nursing assistants have the opportunity to educate residents about self-care.

can be very beneficial. The following are helpful learning principles as you encounter opportunities for health promotion:

1. Identify a readiness to learn in residents. You might recognize a readiness to learn when a resident starts asking questions about his or her care.

2. Pay attention to how residents learn best. Do residents learn best using visuals, or do they prefer hands-on experiences? Sometimes language and cultural differences influence how people learn.

3. Keep instructions simple. Don't use complicated words or medical terms. Provide printed materials if they are available and if residents are able to use them.

4. Be patient. Repetition helps residents, particularly older residents, learn. You may need to repeat the same information several times.

5. Use demonstration as an effective way to reinforce the information provided. Show residents what they need to learn and then have residents demonstrate what they learned back to you. Give residents feedback about their demonstrations.

6. If a resident is stressed or is expecting visitors, don't try to provide health promotion. Find a better time when the resident will be able to pay attention and be motivated.

7. If you do provide instruction, make sure you report what happened and document it in the resident's chart or EMR.

What Is Integrative Medicine?

Integrative medicine (IM) is a coordinated approach to the diagnosis, treatment, and prevention of diseases. In IM, healthcare providers see people as *whole individuals* and focus on the energy of the body. IM includes healthcare delivery approaches, or treatments, that are different from those usually found in hospitals and other healthcare facilities. Some IM approaches include acupuncture, hypnotherapy, meditation, therapeutic massage or touch, or even holistic nutrition. These approaches are used to treat specific conditions or diseases and are always meant to promote higher levels of health and wellness.

The use of the term *integrative medicine* is relatively new. Previously, this approach was called **complementary and alternative medicine (CAM)**. CAM focused on providing treatments either in conjunction with or in place of **conventional medicine** (treatments performed by healthcare providers who use evidence-based scientific data). IM has become more accepted because it emphasizes the importance of coordinating and integrating all treatments with the goals of disease prevention or management and health promotion.

Healthcare Scenario
The Power of Health Promotion

A large healthcare system recently received an award for its health promotion program. The system was able to show that its patients had lower rates of death as a direct result of the system's health promotion programs. The system was also commended for achieving shorter hospital stays for patients. When the system was presented with the award, the nursing, rehabilitation, and social services departments were praised for the tremendous support they gave. Support from these departments resulted in discharged patients being able to more effectively manage themselves after discharge. The system's administration credited the work and commitment of caregivers as the reason the organization was recognized.

Apply It

1. Why do you think this healthcare system won an award for health promotion?

2. What actions taken by the system and its workers do you think led to improved health?

IM has become very popular in the United States, but IM is often not covered by insurance. Those who are interested in IM must be willing to pay out-of-pocket for these services. In other countries, IM approaches are an accepted part of healthcare delivery and are often covered by healthcare insurance. As a result, more people commonly use these treatments (Figure 7.9).

In the United States, IM approaches are becoming more commonplace in healthcare facilities and among doctors and other licensed healthcare providers. IM typically includes the use of natural products, mind and body practices, Ayurvedic medicine, traditional Chinese medicine (TCM), homeopathy, and naturopathy.

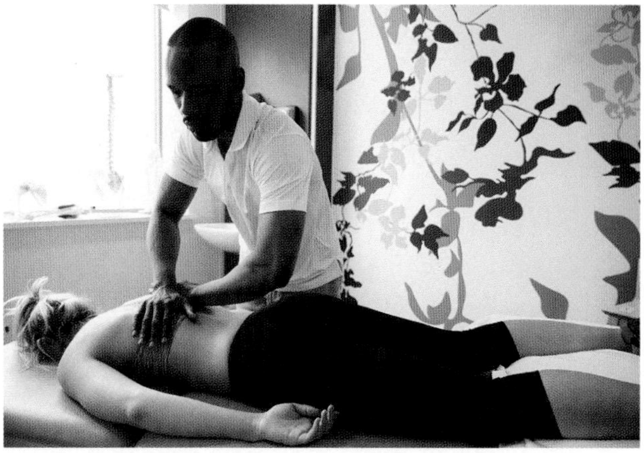

Monkey Business Images/Shutterstock.com

Figure 7.9 Massage therapy is an example of an IM approach that is sometimes covered by insurance in the United States and used in other countries.

Natural Products

Natural products include herbs or botanicals, vitamins, minerals, and **probiotics** (supplements that contain live, beneficial bacteria). Natural products are often used in IM and are easily available. They are often sold over the counter at retail pharmacies, typically as dietary supplements. Natural products are the most popular and most used IM approach among Americans.

Mind and Body Practices

Mind and body practices are performed by trained and often licensed practitioners. These practices provide a variety of ways to deliver IM. Each mind and body practice has its own origins, treatment principles, and approaches. There are several types of mind and body practices, including the following:

- **Hypnotherapy**: a procedure in which a practitioner suggests that a person experience changes in sensations, perceptions, thoughts, or behavior. Suggestions are made through a process called *being induced*. During hypnotherapy, a person is asked to concentrate on an object or point and then hears the practitioner provide helpful, calm, and focused suggestions. This technique may be effective for people who want to stop smoking or lose weight. Hypnotherapy has also been helpful for treating several health conditions, such as sleep disorders, depression, post-traumatic stress disorder (PTSD), and obesity.

- **Massage therapy**: a technique in which the soft tissues of the body are manually manipulated. Massage therapy is often used to promote relaxation or for pain management.

- **Meditation**: a technique in which a person learns to focus his or her attention inward or outward onto specific objects. Meditation can be used to help people become more mindful and manage stress.

- **Relaxation techniques**: techniques that reproduce the body's natural relaxation response. Breathing exercises and guided imagery are two examples of relaxation techniques.

- **Spinal manipulation**: a technique in which a healthcare provider applies a controlled force to a joint or the spine (Figure 7.10). Chiropractors, osteopathic and naturopathic physicians, physical therapists, and some doctors perform spinal manipulation using their hands or a device (such as a device that provides electric stimulation or traction). It is believed that misalignment and nerve pressure can cause problems in specific areas of the body, such as the neck or back. Spinal manipulation is often effective for treating muscle spasms of the back or neck and headaches.

Think About This

The most commonly used IM approaches in the United States include natural products, deep breathing, yoga, tai chi, qigong, chiropractic or osteopathic manipulation, meditation, and massage.

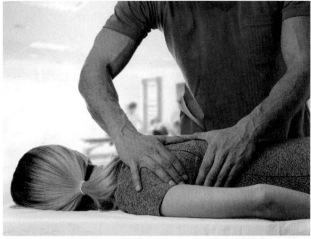

Albina Glisic/Shutterstock.com

Figure 7.10 Spinal manipulation is believed to cause temporary musculoskeletal pain relief.

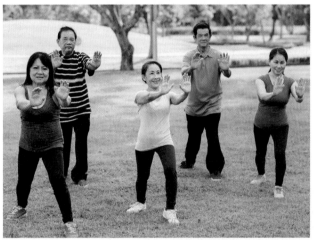

Dragon Images/Shutterstock.com

Figure 7.11 Originally developed for self-defense, tai chi is characterized by gentle, low-impact movements that many people find help reduce stress.

- **Tai chi and qigong**: the combination of specific movements or postures, coordinated breathing, and mental focus to delay aging, prolong life, increase flexibility, strengthen muscles and tendons, and aid in the treatment of health conditions (Figure 7.11). There is some evidence to support that tai chi helps people achieve balance and prevents falling.

- **Yoga**: a technique that combines physical postures or movements, focused concentration, and breathing techniques to integrate the body, mind, and spirit. There are many different forms of yoga. Yoga can be used to improve fitness, flexibility, and posture; promote stress relief; and aid in weight loss.

Ayurvedic Medicine

Ayurvedic medicine originated in India more than 3000 years ago. In Ayurvedic medicine, practitioners use herbal compounds, special diets, and lifestyle recommendations to treat arthritis and other inflammatory conditions. Practitioners believe that each person is made of five basic elements found in the universe—space, air, fire, water, and earth. These elements combine in the human body to form three life forces, which are called *doshas*.

Doshas control different body functions, and there are three doshas: vata dosha (space and air), pitta dosha (fire and water), and kapha dosha (water and earth). Each person inherits a unique mix of these three doshas; however, one dosha is usually stronger than the others and becomes that person's type. People tend to make lifestyle and diet decisions based on their doshas. The goal is to promote balance within the doshas. When people live in conflict with their natures (doshas), unhealthy patterns can lead to physical and mental imbalances. Ayurvedic medicine provides specifically tailored, individual recommendations that range from general lifestyle changes to the treatment of disease. Underlying concepts of Ayurvedic medicine include universal interconnectedness among people, their health, and the universe; the body's constitution; and the life forces.

Traditional Chinese Medicine (TCM)

Dating back more than 2500 years, *traditional Chinese medicine (TCM)* is based on the principle that *qi*, the body's core or vital energy, flows throughout the body. Qi must be balanced for optimal health and is influenced by the opposing forces of *yin* (negative energy) and *yang* (positive energy). When the flow of qi is disrupted, causing yin and yang to become imbalanced, disease results. There are many practices within TCM, including herbal and nutritional therapy, acupuncture, acupressure, restorative physical exercises, and meditation.

Acupuncture is a technique in which a licensed practitioner inserts thin needles through the skin to stimulate specific points on the body. Acupuncture is used to treat many conditions, such as headache, nausea, and fibromyalgia. It is often used for pain management (Figure 7.12).

Homeopathy

Homeopathy is based on the concept that the body has the ability to heal itself and that symptoms of an illness are the body's way of regaining health. The principle of homeopathy is that, if a substance causes certain symptoms in a healthy person, giving a person a very small amount of that substance may cure an illness with the same symptoms. Therefore, a disease is treated with minute, undetectable doses of substances that produce symptoms similar to symptoms produced by the disease. This type of treatment is similar to treatments used for allergies in conventional medicine. The substances, or remedies, come from plants, minerals, or animals. Remedies are administered using pellets placed under the tongue, ointments, gels, drops, creams, or tablets. Treatments are individualized, or specific to each person.

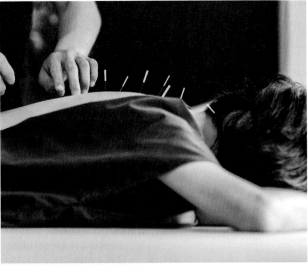

Juri Pozzi/Shutterstock.com

Figure 7.12 Acupuncture involves the insertion of thin needles into the body.

Naturopathy

Naturopathy is a system of therapy and treatments based on preventive care. It uses physical forces such as heat, water, light, air, and massage as primary treatments. Naturopathic providers provide treatments such as nutrition counseling; vitamins, minerals, and other supplements; herbal medicines; homeopathy; hydrotherapy; therapeutic massage and joint manipulation; exercise therapy; and lifestyle counseling.

Residents Using IM

The goal of IM is always to promote higher levels of health and wellness. When appropriate, IM is used in some conventional healthcare facilities. IM approaches used in conventional healthcare facilities may include tai chi, yoga, or massage therapy (Figure 7.13).

When you work as a nursing assistant, you may find that some residents used one or more IM approach prior to admission because they found these to be helpful. People do not always tell their doctors about the IM approaches they choose to use. Recently, questions regarding the use of IM have been included in admission assessments completed by licensed nursing staff. It is important that licensed nursing staff members know about the IM approaches used by residents. Some IM approaches may be **contraindicated** (advised against) for treatments residents are currently receiving and might be outside of the resident's plan of care. If a nursing assistant becomes aware of a resident using IM, he or she should report this to the licensed nursing staff. As a nursing assistant, you should never recommend or suggest an IM approach to a resident.

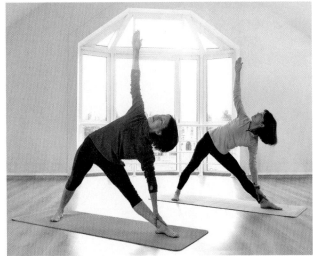

misfire_studio/Shutterstock.com

Figure 7.13 Yoga is a type of IM often used in conventional healthcare facilities. Many people find yoga to have both mental and physical health benefits.

Using the Key Terms

Complete the following sentences using the key terms in this section.

1. Feelings that are not based on facts are part of _____.
2. _____ is a type of medicine that is often used as a replacement for conventional medicine.
3. _____ contain live, beneficial bacteria.
4. _____ medicine uses evidence-based scientific data.
5. Starting a community program for smoking cessation is an example of _____.
6. Some IM approaches are _____, or advised against, for treatments residents are currently receiving.
7. In _____, healthcare providers see people as whole individuals and focus on the energy of the body.

Know and Understand the Facts

8. What is the goal of health promotion?
9. Discuss two reasons why health promotion is important when considering resident well-being.
10. Identify three strategies a holistic nursing assistant can use to promote their own health.
11. Explain three IM approaches or treatments.

Analyze and Apply Concepts

12. What specific strategies can holistic nursing assistants use to promote the health of residents?
13. In what ways does IM assist in the promotion of health?
14. Why it is important for nursing assistants to alert the licensed nursing staff if a resident is using IM approaches?

Think Critically

Read the following care situation. Then answer the questions that follow.

Mr. W is in a rehabilitation facility after having knee surgery. In addition to his knee replacement, he has rheumatoid arthritis. As Brianna, a nursing assistant at the facility, helps Mr. W with his shoes one morning, Mr. W asks her about the therapy he is receiving. He asks if she thinks he will ever be able to walk without the aid of a walker. Mr. W seems concerned about the effectiveness of his therapy and expresses this concern to Brianna. He tells her that, prior to his knee replacement, he did yoga, had acupuncture, and took supplements for his arthritis. All three treatments seemed to be effective in improving flexibility and relieving pain. Mr. W shares his concern about not continuing the IM treatments he utilized prior to his surgery.

15. How might Brianna respond to Mr. W concerning the effectiveness of his current therapy?
16. Should Brianna discuss the benefits of his previous therapies for treating arthritis? If so, what should she say?
17. What should Brianna report to the licensed nursing staff and to the physical therapist about her conversation with Mr. W?

Key Points

Reviewing the key points for this chapter will help you practice more safely and competently as a holistic nursing assistant and will help you prepare for the certification competency examination.

- The relationship between wellness and illness is not a straight line. A person can experience both wellness and illness at the same time. Even when a person is considered ill, parts of his or her body and mind can still have some level of wellness.

- Stress is something we all experience. Not all stress is bad stress (distress). We sometimes need good stress (eustress) to motivate us to do certain tasks. There are ways to manage stress, including identifying stressors, changing your focus, relying on your support network, managing time and energy appropriately, and establishing priorities.

- Health promotion is wide-ranging, and the primary goal of health promotion is to encourage healthy ideas, beliefs, and experiences and motivate people to adopt healthy behaviors.

- Integrative medicine (IM) is becoming a popular way to promote health. Recognizing different IM approaches and treatments can help you ensure safe, quality care.

Action Steps to Holistic Care

Review the information in this chapter. Complete the following activities.

1. Select one time-management strategy discussed in this chapter and research it further. Prepare a short paper or digital presentation that discusses information about this strategy.

2. With a partner, write a short song or poem that expresses the signs and symptoms of stress.

3. Create a to-do list of all the responsibilities and tasks you have to perform in the next week or two. Then practice prioritizing your responsibilities and identify the order in which the tasks must be completed. Write a brief report reflecting on this activity. Did prioritizing your tasks help you reduce stress, complete your responsibilities on time, or make it easier for you to manage your time?

4. Find two pictures in a magazine, in a newspaper, or online that best demonstrate work-life balance. Describe each image and provide a rationale for why it was selected.

5. Research one IM approach or treatment. Write a brief report that summarizes the approach or treatment and explains why it is important for holistic nursing assistants to know this information.

Preparing for the Certification Competency Examination

To prepare for the nursing assistant certification competency examination, you will need to know content found in this chapter. This content may be tested in the knowledge (written or oral) and skills (hands-on demonstration) portions of the exam. The following areas will be emphasized:

- sources of stress
- appropriate stress-relieving techniques
- signs and symptoms of stress
- time-management skills

These sample test questions are similar to ones you will find on the certification competency exam. See how well you can answer them. Be sure to select the *best* answer.

1. Which of the following statements best describes the relationship between wellness and illness?
   A. A person can be both ill and well at the same time.
   B. Illness and wellness are represented by a line, with illness on one end and wellness on the other end.
   C. Illness and wellness are the same.
   D. Illness and wellness are represented by a line separating those who are ill from those who are well.

2. A nursing assistant is having a discussion with the charge nurse about a resident. The nursing assistant reports that Mr. W is acting fidgety and is complaining of a headache. What should the nursing assistant say to the charge nurse?
   A. "It saddens me that Mr. W is being difficult."
   B. "Mr. W is different today. He seems to be showing signs of stress."
   C. "I don't think Mr. W wants to get better because he is so negative about his treatments."
   D. "Mr. W doesn't want to get better."

(continued)

3. Which of the following is an example of health promotion?

   A. going to the doctor and trusting that the care you receive will make you well
   B. exercising at the gym daily for several hours, even though it hurts
   C. paying attention to stressors and finding ways to manage them
   D. eating a diet of French fries, soft drinks, and red meat on a regular basis

4. Which of the following statements about reporting symptoms of stress to the licensed nursing staff is correct?

   A. Reporting is important, but is not necessary.
   B. Reporting is helpful for the family of the resident.
   C. Reporting is mandatory and is essential to providing safe, quality care.
   D. Reporting is useful for teaching residents.

5. Which of the following would help you achieve a positive work-life balance?

   A. achieving harmony in your life by using stress-management tools
   B. letting your work affect your emotions and home life
   C. ignoring your emotions because they won't affect your work
   D. identifying that work is stressful and realizing that is just the way it is

6. Which of the following statements about stress is true?

   A. Everyone reacts to stress in the same way.
   B. Stress management is easy to include in your life.
   C. Stress cannot be managed; instead, it manages you.
   D. Stress is different for everyone.

7. Which of the following are effective techniques for managing stress?

   A. eating, drinking, and being merry
   B. going for a walk, smiling, and laughing
   C. knowing what stress is and pushing through it
   D. ignoring stress and trusting it will eventually go away

8. Which of the following are *not* symptoms of stress?

   A. feeling alone or paranoid and being unable to do a good job at work
   B. feeling tension in the stomach and having tight shoulders
   C. eating for comfort, drinking alcohol a little more than usual, and snapping at people
   D. daydreaming, taking short naps, and eating midday snacks

9. A nursing assistant in an assisted living facility is responsible for 20 residents. He cannot find enough time to care for all of the residents. He is feeling frustrated and doesn't know what to do. Which of the following should you do to help him?

   A. tell him to complain to the charge nurse that he has too much work and that it isn't fair
   B. agree with him that it is just too much work for the time he has on the shift
   C. tell him to quit his job since this is just not the right job for him
   D. encourage him to see if he has set the right priorities for his work

10. Which of the following is a key strategy to achieving health and wellness?

    A. having good insurance
    B. knowing an acupuncturist
    C. taking responsibility for your own care
    D. taking a daily nap

11. Which type of medicine uses treatments as a replacement for conventional medicine?

    A. alternative medicine
    B. complementary medicine
    C. integrated medicine
    D. interactive medicine

12. In a to-do list, which of the following letters identifies the most important priority?

    A. B   C. F
    B. C   D. A

13. A nursing assistant finds that she is more productive in the morning than late at night. If she does her challenging work in the morning, she is considering which of the following?

    A. her homeostasis
    B. her energy rhythm
    C. her stressors
    D. her intuition

14. What is good stress called?

    A. distress   C. astress
    B. prestress   D. eustress

15. Which technique combines physical postures or movements, focused concentration, and breathing techniques to integrate the body, mind, and spirit?

    A. yoga
    B. tai chi
    C. Ayurvedic medicine
    D. spinal manipulation

Did you have difficulty with any of the questions? If you did, review the chapter to find the correct answer(s).

CHAPTER 8

The Healthy Body: Anatomy and Physiology

Welcome to the Chapter

When providing care as a holistic nursing assistant, you will need to understand the structure of the healthy human body and the way the human body functions at its optimum level. This knowledge is important because many of the procedures you will perform affect the body in different ways. This chapter covers the structure of the body, from microscopic cells; to body directions, planes, and organs; to the structure and function of the 12 body systems. You will discover not only how the body systems work, but also how they are affected by lifestyle choices and aging. You will also learn the importance of medical terminology, the structure of medical terms, and medical terms related to specific body structures and functions.

What you learn in this chapter will help you develop your knowledge and skills to become a holistic nursing assistant. The topics discussed in the chapter are highlighted on the Providing Holistic Care Framework.

You are now ready to start this chapter, *The Healthy Body: Anatomy and Physiology.*

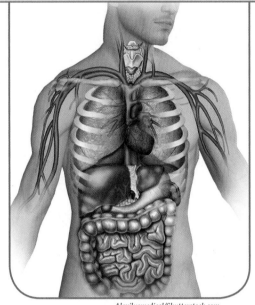

Alexilusmedical/Shutterstock.com

Chapter Outline

Section 8.1
Medical Terminology and Body Structures

Section 8.2
Body Systems

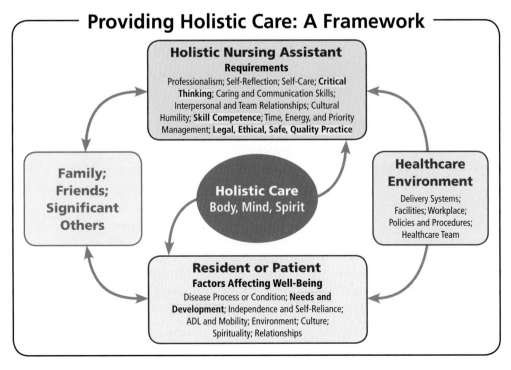

Providing Holistic Care: A Framework

Holistic Nursing Assistant
Requirements
Professionalism; Self-Reflection; Self-Care; **Critical Thinking**; Caring and Communication Skills; Interpersonal and Team Relationships; Cultural Humility; **Skill Competence**; Time, Energy, and Priority Management; **Legal, Ethical, Safe, Quality Practice**

Holistic Care
Body, Mind, Spirit

Family; Friends; Significant Others

Healthcare Environment
Delivery Systems; Facilities; Workplace; Policies and Procedures; Healthcare Team

Resident or Patient
Factors Affecting Well-Being
Disease Process or Condition; **Needs and Development**; Independence and Self-Reliance; ADL and Mobility; Environment; Culture; Spirituality; Relationships

Questions to Consider

- Think about your body and about how it looks and functions. You might want to view yourself in a mirror as you are doing this. In what ways is your body similar to the bodies of others?
- What about your body is different from others' bodies? Why do you think these similarities and differences exist?

Objectives

To achieve the objectives for this section, you must successfully

- **form** medical terms using root words, combining vowels, combining forms, prefixes, and suffixes;
- **recognize** medical abbreviations;
- **identify** the medical terminology used to describe body positions, directions, planes, cavities, and movements;
- **explain** cell structure and function; and
- **describe** the four types of body tissues, the body membranes, and the actions of these structures.

Key Terms

Learn these key terms to better understand the information presented in the section.

acronyms	nutrients
atrophy	organs
body cavities	peristalsis
cell	prone position
coronal plane	sagittal plane
Fowler's position	secretion
lateral position	supine position
medical terminology	tissue
membranes	transverse plane
neurons	tumor

What Is Medical Terminology?

Medical terminology is the language of medicine. You will use medical terminology every day as a holistic nursing assistant. Correct pronunciation and spelling are critical when providing and documenting care and when communicating with others in the healthcare facility.

Learning medical terminology requires more than simply recognizing medical terms. You must also learn to utilize medical word parts to build new terms. A strong understanding of medical word parts will allow you to deconstruct unfamiliar terms and learn their meanings.

Medical Word Parts

There are five word parts that can be used to form a medical term. Some medical terms are composed of all five word parts, while others may have just two word parts. The five word parts used in medical terminology are the root word, combining vowel, combining form (root word plus combining vowel), prefix, and suffix.

The *root word*, which is often derived from Greek or Latin, is the central part of a medical term. Root words are always part of a medical term and never stand alone. An example of a root word is *cardi*, which means "heart."

A *combining vowel* is a vowel attached to the end of a root word. Combining vowels link word parts for easier pronunciation and include *a, e, i, o,* or *u.* A combining vowel is *not* used between a root word and a suffix when the suffix begins with a vowel. The most commonly used combining vowel is *o.* The root word plus its combining vowel is known as a *combining form.* For example, the root word *cardi* and the combining vowel *o* make the combining form *cardi/o.*

A *prefix* is a part of a medical term that is attached to the beginning of a root word. Prefixes usually indicate location, time, or number. An example of a prefix is *peri-,* which means "around" or "surrounding."

The *suffix* is the part of the medical term attached to the end of a root word. Suffixes usually indicate a condition, disease, diagnosis, surgical intervention, or therapy. For example, when the suffix *-itis* (meaning "inflammation") is attached to the root word *card* (also meaning "heart"), this forms the word *carditis,* which means "inflammation of the heart." As another example, the word *cardiologist* contains the root word *cardi,* the combining vowel *o,* and the suffix *-logist* (which means "specialist"). The word *cardiologist* means "heart specialist." In this example, you must use the combining vowel *o* because the suffix does not start with a vowel.

The Structure of Medical Terms

You can form many different medical terms using just one root word and various combining forms, prefixes, and suffixes. For example, the following medical terms use the root words *cardi* and *card*:

tachy- / card / -ia = fast heart rate
  P   + RW + S

cardi / o / -pathy = heart disease
  RW + CV +   S

cardi / -ac = pertaining to the heart
  RW + S

cardi / o / -logy = study of the heart
  RW + CV +   S

peri- / card / -itis = inflammation of the lining around the heart
  P   + RW + S

P = Prefix
RW = Root Word
S = Suffix
CV = Combining Vowel

As with most English words, many medical terms can be made plural by adding an *-s* or *-es.* There are different rules for creating plural forms for terms that derive from Greek or Latin, however. For example, the singular term *bronchus* becomes *bronchi* when plural. Similarly, the term *diagnosis* becomes *diagnoses* when plural.

At the end of this chapter, you will find a glossary of common combining forms, prefixes, and suffixes. Studying these word parts will help you begin to form medical terms and start using medical terminology. This resource will also help you prepare for the certification competency exam and begin working as a holistic nursing assistant.

Medical Abbreviations

Medical terminology includes *abbreviations,* which are used to speed up communication in healthcare facilities. Abbreviations are usually short combinations of letters used to represent longer words. For example, the abbreviation *AM* stands for "morning," and the single letter *q* represents the word *every.* Medical terminology also uses **acronyms,** which are formed from the first letters or groups of letters in a phrase. An example of an acronym is *BP* for "blood pressure."

Many medical abbreviations are recognized and accepted within healthcare across the United States. Some abbreviations are used regionally, and others may be specific to particular healthcare facilities. It is important to become familiar with common medical abbreviations. You will hear, read, and use these abbreviations daily as you provide care. Figure 8.1 lists many of the common abbreviations and

Medical Abbreviations and Acronyms

Abbreviation or Acronym	Meaning	Abbreviation or Acronym	Meaning
ABC	airway, breathing, circulation	ED	emergency department
abd	abdomen	EKG; ECG	electrocardiogram
ac; a.c.	before meals	ENT	ear, nose, throat
ACLS	advanced cardiac life support	ER	emergency room
Ad Lib	as desired	FB	foreign body
ADLs	activities of daily living	FH	family history
ADM	admission	Fx	fracture
AM	in the morning	GB	gallbladder
AMA; a.m.a.	against medical advice	GI	gastrointestinal
Amb	ambulatory	GTT; gtt	drops
AMT	amount	Hgb; hgb	hemoglobin
AS	left ear	H&P	history and physical
AU	each ear	hs	hour of sleep; bedtime
BID; b.i.d.	twice a day	Hx; hx	history
BLS	basic life support	IM	intramuscular
BM	bowel movement	I&O	intake and output
BMR	basic metabolic rate	IV	intravenous
BP; B/P	blood pressure	LOC	level of consciousness
bpm	beats per minute	mg	milligrams
BRP	bathroom privileges	MRI	magnetic resonance imaging
BS	breath sounds	MRSA	methicillin-resistant *Staphylococcus aureus*
c̄	with	NEG	negative
cap	capsule	NG; ng	nasogastric
CATH	catheter	NKA	no known allergies
CBC	complete blood count	NPO; n.p.o.	nothing by mouth
CHF	congestive heart failure	N/V	nausea, vomiting
CNS	central nervous system	OD	right eye; overdose
c/o	complains of	OP	outpatient
COPD	chronic obstructive pulmonary disease	OR	operating room
CPR	cardiopulmonary resuscitation	OS	left eye
CSF	cerebrospinal fluid	OTC	over the counter
CT Scan	computerized axial tomography scan	OU	both eyes
CVA	cerebrovascular accident	P	pulse
D/C	discontinue	p.c.; pc	after meals
DNR	do not resuscitate	PO; po; p.o.	by mouth
DOA	dead on arrival	P/O; postop	postoperative
DOB	date of birth	preop	before surgery
Dx	diagnosis	PRN; p.r.n.	as needed

(continued)

Figure 8.1 Different healthcare facilities use different abbreviations. Always check a healthcare facility's policies and procedures to learn about which abbreviations are used.

Medical Abbreviations and Acronyms			
Abbreviation or Acronym	Meaning	Abbreviation or Acronym	Meaning
q	every	Sx	symptom
QID; q.i.d.	four times a day	T	temperature
R	respiration	Tab	tablet
R/O	rule out	TID; t.i.d.	three times a day
ROM	range of motion	TPR	temperature, pulse, respiration
Rx	prescribed medication; treatment	Tx	treatment
s̄	without	UA	urinalysis
SOB	shortness of breath	VS	vital signs
S/S	signs and symptoms	wt	weight
STAT	immediately		

Figure 8.1 *(Continued)*

acronyms you will encounter as a nursing assistant. Other abbreviations and acronyms are also included throughout this textbook. Abbreviations for common diseases and conditions are discussed in chapter 9.

How Is the Human Body Structured and Described?

The body has its very own *atlas*, or set of road maps, which was outlined centuries ago. Early scientists used words and pictures to organize and describe the miracle of the human body. For example, Leonardo da Vinci, a famous painter of the fifteenth century, was trained in the study of the human body. He made many sketches of the human skeleton, muscles, and organs. He sketched what is considered the first accurate illustration of the human spine.

Many terms are used to describe the body, body cavities that contain organs, and the planes of the body. There are also terms that describe body positions, directions, and movements. You will not be able to provide safe, quality care if you do not understand these terms. As a holistic nursing assistant, you will use medical terms related to the body during a variety of procedures. For instance, you may be given instructions to perform a procedure that requires placing a resident in the *supine* position. This means the resident should lie flat on his or her back.

Body Positions

As a nursing assistant, you will be asked to place residents into different body positions for a variety of reasons, including examinations, treatments, and assistance with ADLs. For example, you might place a resident into Fowler's position if the resident is eating a meal in bed or performing oral care.

To understand the different body positions, you must know the meaning of *anatomical position*. Anatomical position is the standard body position for referencing anatomical structures. In this position, the human body stands erect, the head and feet point forward, and both arms are at the sides with palms forward (Figure 8.2).

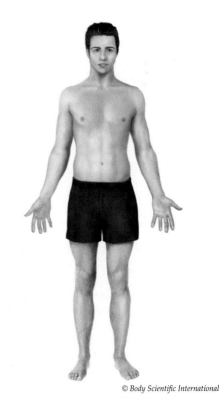

© *Body Scientific International*

Figure 8.2 In anatomical position, the left and right sides of the body are mirror images of each other.

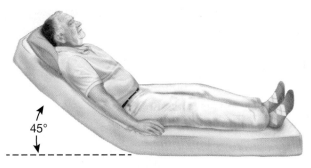

45°

Fowler's position

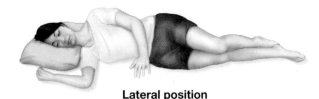

Lateral position

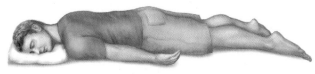

Prone position

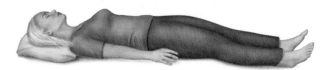

Supine position

© Body Scientific International

Figure 8.3 The four body positions shown here are used in various procedures. Pillows may be used to ensure comfort and provide support.

Both the left and right sides of the body are considered mirror images of each other, demonstrating *bilateral symmetry.*

The most common body positions you will encounter as a nursing assistant are Fowler's position, lateral position, prone position, and supine position (Figure 8.3):

- **Fowler's position:** the person is seated in bed, and the backrest of the bed is at a 45° angle; the legs are extended flat.
- **Lateral position:** the person lies on his or her side with arms free and knees slightly bent.
- **Prone position:** the person lies on his or her abdomen with arms and hands at each side, feet comfortably positioned, and head turned to the side.
- **Supine position:** the person lies flat on his or her back with the arms at each side.

Other positions will be discussed in later chapters of this textbook.

Body Planes

Body planes are imaginary lines that cut through the body and divide it into sections. These planes are used to identify and describe the body's sections (Figure 8.4). The most common planes of the body include the following:

- **Coronal plane:** divides the body into front and back halves; also known as the *frontal plane*
- **Sagittal plane:** divides the body into left and right sections; also known as the *vertical plane*
- **Transverse plane:** divides the body into upper and lower halves; also known as the *horizontal plane*

Directional Terms

Specific anatomic directional terms describe different body and body part positions and their locations (Figure 8.5). Healthcare providers, such as doctors, often write orders or give instructions using these terms. Holistic nursing assistants must also

Culture Cues
Perceptions of the Body

People have a range of unique perceptions about the body and its functions. These perceptions are influenced by people's cultures, family values about health and wellness, and experiences with health and bodily functions. For instance, if someone comes from a culture in which talking about a particular body function is not an accepted practice, that person may not communicate the relevant information to healthcare providers.

Apply It

1. What two perceptions do you have about your health and bodily functions? How have these perceptions affected your health and wellness?

2. How could you, as a holistic nursing assistant, familiarize yourself with residents' perceptions about their bodily functions?

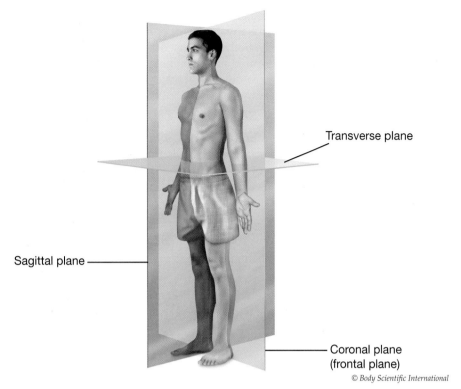

Transverse plane

Sagittal plane

Coronal plane
(frontal plane)

© Body Scientific International

Figure 8.4 The coronal plane, sagittal plane, and transverse plane divide the body into sections.

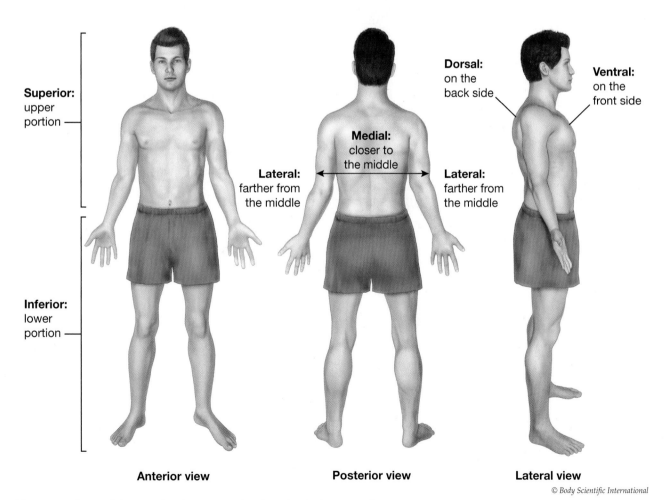

Superior:
upper
portion

Inferior:
lower
portion

Lateral:
farther from
the middle

Medial:
closer to
the middle

Lateral:
farther from
the middle

Dorsal:
on the
back side

Ventral:
on the
front side

Anterior view   **Posterior view**   **Lateral view**

© Body Scientific International

Figure 8.5 Some of the directional terms used to describe the body are illustrated here.

perform procedures following directions that use these terms. For example, a doctor's order might instruct that you place a warm compress on a resident's knee, which is on the *anterior* or ventral side of the body. A licensed nursing staff member might also direct you to look at a dressing located on a resident's back, which is on the *posterior* or dorsal side of the body.

Body Cavities

The human body is divided into **body cavities**, which are spaces in the body that contain organs. **Organs** are collections of tissues that have specific structures and functions. The two main divisions of cavities in the body are the dorsal (posterior) cavities and the ventral (anterior) cavities (Figure 8.6). The dorsal body cavity includes the cranial cavity and the spinal cavity:

- **Cranial cavity**: contains the brain (cerebrum), as well as the blood vessels and nerves that support the brain
- **Spinal cavity**: contains the spinal cord, spinal column, tailbone, and vertebrae

The ventral body cavity includes the thoracic and abdominopelvic cavities:

- **Thoracic cavity**: contains the lungs, heart, trachea, pharynx, larynx, and bronchial tubes

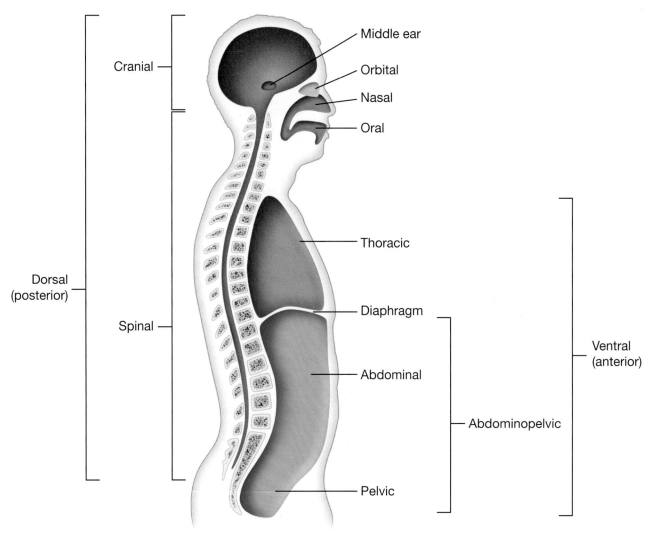

© *Body Scientific International*

Figure 8.6 The ventral cavities are those cavities near the front of the body, and the dorsal cavities are near the back of the body.

- **Abdominal cavity**: contains the liver, gallbladder, stomach, pancreas, intestines, spleen, and kidneys
- **Pelvic cavity**: contains the sigmoid colon, rectum, anus, urinary bladder, urethra, ureters, and male and female reproductive organs

Body Movements

Medical terms are also used to describe body movements (Figure 8.7). You will see terms related to movement when you provide active and passive range-of-motion (ROM) exercises for residents' joints and limbs.

What Roles Do Cells, Tissues, and Membranes Play in Body Structure?

Three essential internal structures are the foundation of life in the human body: cells, tissues, and membranes. Tissues and membranes are composed of groups of cells with similar structures and functions. *Organs* are composed of groups of tissues that work together to perform specific functions. Organs and body systems will be discussed later in this chapter.

Cells

The **cell** is the structural and functional unit of the human body. There are about 37 trillion cells in the human body and between 200 and 300 different types of cells. All cells begin as undifferentiated *stem cells*. As cells mature, they produce more stem cells and *differentiate*, or evolve, into cells that perform particular functions.

For example, some stem cells differentiate to become *white blood cells*; these cells defend the body against disease-causing microorganisms. Even though cells have different functions, most cells contain the same basic structures, which are called *organelles* (Figures 8.8 and 8.9).

Body Movements		
Movement	**Description**	**Example**
Flexion	The act of bending a joint	Bending the arm at the elbow
Extension	The act of straightening a joint	Lowering the arm back down at the elbow
Hyperextension	An exaggerated, or extreme, extension	Moving the arm from the side so that it extends behind the body
Abduction	Lateral (sideways) movement away from the midline (an invisible line running vertically through the body)	Moving the leg away from the body
Adduction	Lateral movement toward the midline of the body	Moving the leg toward the body
Rotation	Turning of a body part around an axis, or fixed point	Rotating the ankle outward so that the foot moves away from the body
Circumduction	Rotating a body part in a complete circle	Moving the pointer finger in a circular motion
Supination	Rotating a body part from the body	Rotating the forearm so that the palm faces upward
Pronation	Rotating a body part toward the body	Rotating the forearm so that the palm faces downward

Figure 8.7 Body movements are described using directional terms.

Basic Structures of the Cell

Cell Structure and Description	Location	Function
Nucleus	In the center of the cell	Directs all cell activities; found in all cells except mature red blood cells
Chromosome threadlike in shape	In the nucleus	Carries information needed for cell division; humans have 23 pairs of chromosomes
Deoxyribonucleic acid (DNA) double helix in shape	In the chromosomes	Is a chemical compound that contains instructions for developing and directing the growth and activities of living organisms
Cytoplasm a jellylike substance that is 90 percent water	Outside the nucleus	Houses the functional units (organelles) of a cell, where cell activities take place
Mitochondria relatively large structure in the cell	Suspended in the cytoplasm	Is considered the powerhouse of the cell because it maintains cell life by providing the transfer of energy
Ribosome most common structure in the cell	Suspended in the cytoplasm	Maintains the life of the cell by building specific, necessary proteins
Cell membrane	The outer layer of the cell	Selectively allows liquids and gases to pass, regulating what enters and exits the cell

Figure 8.8 Cell organelles all have specific functions in the cell.

Mature cells exist in bone, muscle, and blood. Mature cells come in a variety of different shapes—from long, thin cells to cells shaped like round discs. All cells can maintain their shape, reproduce by dividing and multiplying, use oxygen and **nutrients** (substances needed for normal body function), produce energy, and eliminate waste. Cells can also

- **atrophy**, or shrink or decrease in size;
- enlarge due to an increase in proteins in the cell membrane (called *hypertrophy*);

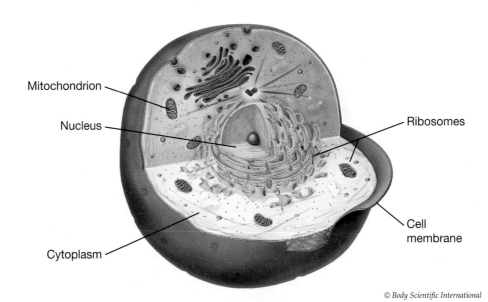

© Body Scientific International

Figure 8.9 The basic structure of the cell is illustrated here.

- increase rates of cell division, causing more cells to reproduce often to compensate for loss of cells (called *hyperplasia*);
- become abnormal in their sizes, shapes, or organization (called *dysplasia*); or
- grow into unusual shapes, called **tumors** or neoplasms. When examined, the cells in a tumor may be *benign*, or normal. The cells in a tumor may also be *malignant*, or abnormal with growth that is out of control.

Tissues

Tissues are groups of similar cells that perform a common function. The four types of tissue—connective tissue, epithelial tissue, muscle tissue, and nerve tissue—all perform unique functions.

Connective Tissue

Connective tissue connects or supports body tissues, structures, and organs. Connective tissue is composed of collagen (protein) fibers that provide strength and of elastin fibers that enable flexibility. Cartilage, bone, and blood are all types of connective tissue.

Epithelial Tissue

Epithelial tissue provides a covering for external body parts and also lines internal organs. Epithelial tissue can be found in the skin and also in the intestines. This type of tissue is classified by the arrangement of its cells (Figure 8.10). For example, *simple epithelial tissue* has a single layer of cells, which allows absorption, **secretion** (the release of chemical substances), and filtration to occur. Simple epithelial tissue is found in the intestines. *Stratified epithelial tissue* has two or more layers of cells, which provide protection in areas that experience abrasion (such as the skin).

The shape of epithelial cells is distinctive. Epithelial cells have six sides and vary in height. Epithelial cells include flat, scalelike cells; boxlike cells; and tall, column-shaped cells.

Muscle Tissue

Muscle tissue contracts, or shortens, to produce movement. There are three types of muscle tissue (Figure 8.11):

1. *Skeletal,* or *striated, muscle tissue* connects to the bones. This muscle tissue moves the skeleton by contracting and relaxing. Muscles made of this tissue are called *voluntary muscles* because they function only when a person chooses to move (for example, when a person gets up from a chair and walks).

2. *Smooth muscle tissue* moves involuntarily and is found in the walls of the intestines and other internal organs. This muscle tissue moves during normal functions of the body, such as during the ingestion of food. The involuntary movement of the intestinal muscles, called **peristalsis**, moves food through the gastrointestinal system.

Think About This

The liver can replace up to 70 percent of its cells within two weeks after an injury. Tissues that are rarely or never replaced are found in the central nervous system and in the lens of the eye.

	Simple	**Stratified**
Squamous		
Cuboidal		
Columnar		

© *Body Scientific International*

Figure 8.10 Epithelial cells come in three different shapes, and epithelial tissues can be simple or stratified.

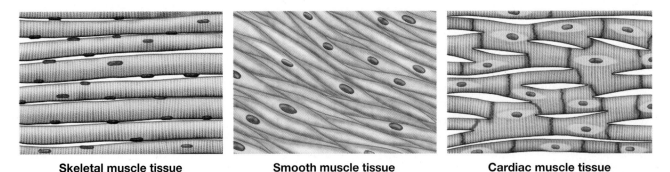

Skeletal muscle tissue   **Smooth muscle tissue**   **Cardiac muscle tissue**

© Body Scientific International

Figure 8.11 The three types of muscle tissue are skeletal muscle, smooth muscle, and cardiac muscle.

3. *Cardiac muscle tissue* makes up most of the heart wall and is also involuntary. Cardiac muscle tissue causes the heart to contract.

Nerve Tissue

Nerve tissue is composed of nerve cells, called **neurons**. Nerve tissue is found in the brain, spinal cord, and peripheral nerves. Neurons carry electrochemical messages to and from various parts of the body to produce sensation, movement, and mental activity.

Membranes

Body **membranes** are thin, soft, and flexible structures that support and protect body surfaces, organs, and joints. Some membranes separate tissues in the body and organs within body cavities. The major categories of body membranes are epithelial and connective.

Epithelial Membranes

Epithelial membranes coat and protect the surfaces of the body and internal organs. There are three types of epithelial membranes: cutaneous membranes, mucous membranes, and serous membranes.

1. *Cutaneous membranes* cover the entire body and are commonly referred to as *skin*. The skin, which is the major component of the integumentary system, will be discussed in more detail later in this chapter.

2. *Mucous membranes* line body surfaces that open directly to the outside of the body. These surfaces are found in the respiratory (nose), gastrointestinal (mouth), urinary, and reproductive systems. Mucous membranes produce a film of mucus that coats and protects underlying cells and that captures disease-causing microorganisms.

3. *Serous membranes* line the inner, closed body cavities and can be composed of several layers. The serous fluid between these layers helps prevent friction when organs move in the body cavities. Serous membranes cover the lungs and heart muscle. Serous membranes known as *mesenteries* also cover the abdominal organs.

Connective Tissue Membranes

Examples of connective tissue membranes include the *synovial membrane* and the *meninges*. Synovial membranes line joint cavities and secrete synovial fluid to prevent friction and provide lubrication to help joints move. The meninges enclose or cover the brain and spinal cord and provide protection.

Using the Key Terms

Complete the following sentences using key terms in this section.

1. Cells can _____, or shrink or decrease in size.
2. The basic structural and functional unit of the body is the _____.
3. _____ are thin, soft, and flexible structures that cover, line, or act as boundaries for cells or organs.
4. A(n) _____ is a collection of specialized cells that act together to perform specific functions.
5. Nerve tissue is composed of nerve cells, known as _____.
6. The involuntary movement of intestinal muscles, called _____, moves food through the gastrointestinal system.
7. _____ are spaces in the human body that contain organs.
8. _____ refers to the release of chemical substances.
9. A resident who lies on the bed with his legs extended and the head of the bed raised to a 45° angle is in a(n) _____.
10. _____ is a side-lying position, where the resident's arms are free and knees slightly bent.
11. Water, protein, carbohydrates, fats, minerals, and vitamins are examples of _____, which the body needs to function normally.
12. A resident lying flat on her back, with her arms at each side is in a(n) _____.
13. _____ is a body position where the resident lies on his abdomen, with arms at his sides.

Know and Understand the Facts

14. Identify the five word parts that can be used to form a medical term.
15. Describe two body positions and one body direction.
16. Where is the coronal plane of the body located?
17. List the organs in the thoracic cavity.
18. Explain two types of body movement.
19. Describe one structure and its function in a human cell.
20. What are the four types of body tissue?

Analyze and Apply Concepts

21. Form and define five medical terms that use a root word, combining vowel, and suffix.
22. Form and define five medical terms that use a prefix, root word, and suffix.
23. Working with a partner, demonstrate adduction and abduction of the leg. Evaluate your partner's performance.
24. Working with a partner, demonstrate the supine and prone positions. Evaluate your partner's performance.
25. Describe the difference between body organs and tissues.

Think Critically

Read the following care situation. Then answer the questions that follow.

Josie, a nursing assistant, has been asked to put Mr. T in Fowler's position because he has pneumonitis. Josie has also been asked to take Mr. T's B/P, P, and R. Josie finds that Mr. T has a very fast heart rate and is having trouble breathing.

26. Explain how Josie should place Mr. T in Fowler's position.
27. Deconstruct the term *pneumonitis* and examine its word elements. What does the term *pneumonitis* mean?
28. What do the medical abbreviations *B/P*, *P*, and *R* represent?
29. What are the medical terms that refer to the condition of a fast heart rate and difficulty breathing? Use the table of medical word parts at the end of this chapter to assemble the words.

Questions to Consider

- Each body system has its own specific structures and functions. The body systems interact to ensure the body is working effectively and performing essential functions. For instance, when you run (using the muscular and skeletal systems), you breathe quickly (using the respiratory system), and your heart beats fast (in the cardiovascular system). Describe two situations in which your body systems work together or perform certain functions. What were you doing?

- Consider the situations in which your body systems worked together. In these situations, which body systems were working together?

Objectives

To achieve the objectives for this section, you must successfully

- **describe** the structure of each body system;
- **explain** the primary functions of each body system;
- **identify** the medical terminology associated with each body system; and
- **discuss** the impact lifestyle choices and the aging process have on body systems.

Key Terms

Learn these key terms to better understand the information presented in the section.

alimentary canal	formed elements
anatomy	gland
antibodies	hemoglobin
appendicular skeleton	ligaments
autonomic nervous system (ANS)	pathogens
axial skeleton	peripheral nervous system (PNS)
central nervous system (CNS)	physiology
circadian rhythm	plasma
deoxyribonucleic acid (DNA)	platelets
dermis	pulse
ducts	receptors
endocrine glands	red blood cells
enzymes	somatic nervous system
epidermis	sperm
exocrine glands	sphincter
fibrous	tendons
follicles	white blood cells

What Are Anatomy and Physiology?

Human bodies are composed of systems that have particular organs, structures, and functions. These *body systems* work both independently and together to ensure the body operates effectively. In this section, you will learn about **anatomy**, or the structure of the human body, and about **physiology**, the function of the human body. You will learn about the anatomy and physiology of the following body systems:

- integumentary system
- skeletal system
- muscular system
- nervous system
- sensory system
- endocrine system

- cardiovascular system
- respiratory system
- immune and lymphatic systems
- gastrointestinal system
- urinary system
- reproductive systems

Each body system has specific medical terminology related to its anatomy and physiology. Some of these terms also apply to the anatomical structure and bodily functions of animals and plants.

There is an important relationship between human anatomy and physiology. The structure (anatomy) of the body is designed to accomplish specific functions (physiology) within each body system. As you learned in chapter 6, maintaining homeostasis requires a balance of functions. This balance is achieved using the relationship between the body's anatomy and physiology. When body systems are structured properly and function effectively, the outcome is a healthy body. Disease occurs when a structure or system in the body is injured, altered, or is malformed, impacting its function.

How Does the Integumentary System Protect the Body?

The *integumentary system* is composed of the skin; subcutaneous lipocytes (fat cells); nerves; blood vessels; and accessory organs, including sweat and sebaceous glands, hair, hair **follicles** (small sacs or cavities), nails, and nail follicles. The skin is the largest organ in the human body. As you learn about the integumentary system, it will be helpful to understand the word parts that relate to this system (Figure 8.12).

The Skin

The skin covers the body and is considered the body's greatest line of defense because it prevents disease-causing microorganisms from entering the body. The skin also shields the body from exposure to ultraviolet (UV) rays from the sun and produces vitamin D in response to sunlight. Vitamin D enables the body to develop and maintain strong bones and a healthy immune system. The elasticity of skin allows for growth and movement, as well as self-repair.

The skin contains the majority of the body's **receptors**, or sensory nerve endings, for touch, pressure, temperature, pain, and itch. The skin also plays an important role in regulating body temperature. When the body is too hot, glands in the skin produce sweat, which cools the body as it evaporates off the skin. *Capillaries* (small blood vessels) in the skin also expand to release body heat and contract to trap heat within the body. Hair follicles attached to tiny muscles cause hair on the skin to stand up and trap heat when the body is cold. Blood vessels remove waste and pass nutrients through the layers of the skin, and nerves send signals to the brain so you know how something feels.

Layers of the Skin

The skin is a *cutaneous membrane* and consists of two major layers (Figure 8.13). The outer layer is called the **epidermis**. The inner, thicker layer is called the **dermis**.

The epidermis is composed of cells containing *keratin*, a protein that makes the skin durable and waterproof. New cells are produced in the deepest layer of the epidermis, and as cells age, they move toward the surface of the skin and then shed. This process takes about four weeks. The epidermis also contains *melanin*, which determines skin's color and protects the body from the sun's UV rays.

The dermis is a **fibrous** connective tissue, meaning that it is composed of tough, thin threads. The dermis contains the proteins *collagen* and *elastin*,

Integumentary System Terminology

Combining Form	Meaning
aden/o	gland
adip/o	fat
blephar/o	eyelid
cutane/o	skin
dermat/o; derm/o	skin
hidr/o	sweat
hist/o	tissue
integument/o	covering
lip/o	fat
onych/o	nail
pil/o	hair
seb/o	oil secretion from sebaceous gland
steat/o	fat
ungu/o	nail

Figure 8.12 These combining forms relate to the integumentary system.

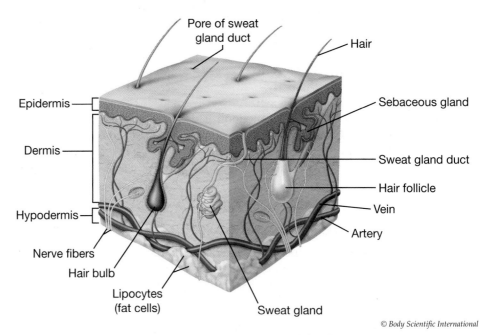

Figure 8.13 The two layers of the skin are the epidermis and dermis.

which keep skin in place and allow flexibility. Sensory nerve receptors that allow us to feel pressure, pain, and temperature are located in the dermis. Hair and nail follicles are anchored in the dermis, as are sweat and sebaceous glands.

Below the dermis lies the *hypodermis*, which is not technically part of the integumentary system. This subcutaneous layer is made up of loose connective tissue, or *adipose tissue*, that consists mainly of fat cells. This layer provides padding and insulation, keeps the body warm, and connects the skin to underlying muscles.

Sweat Glands and Sebaceous Glands

A **gland** is a group of specialized cells that secrete substances. *Sweat glands* are tiny, coiled glands that appear as pores on the surface of the skin. The palms of the hands and soles of the feet contain the most sweat glands. Sweat glands secrete *perspiration*, or sweat. Perspiration is mostly made of water and moistens the surface of the skin to cool down the body.

Sebaceous glands produce an oily substance called *sebum*. Sebum keeps the skin lubricated, which prevents infectious organisms from entering the body. It also keeps the skin smooth and soft. Sebum is released through **ducts** (tubes for conveying substances) located in hair follicles.

Hair and Fingernails

The hair and fingernails are composed of the protein keratin and epithelial cells. Hair is mostly made up of dead cells that fuse together and grow in strands from a root in the hair follicle. Hair keeps the body warm and covers the entire body, with the exceptions of the palms of the hands, soles of the feet, lips, eyelids, and scar tissue. The number of hair follicles a person has determines his or her hair color. People with blonde hair have the most hair follicles, and red-haired individuals have the fewest.

Each fingernail has a *nail plate*, a hard surface due to the presence of keratin. The *cuticle* of a nail is a band of tissue at the sides and base of the nail plate. The *nail root* anchors the nail plate. The pink color of the nail comes from blood vessels directly underneath the nail plate. The moon-shaped area on the nail is a thicker layer of cells that grows at the nail base. Nails help protect the ends of fingers and toes.

How Does the Skeletal System Support the Body?

At birth, the human body is composed of 270 bones. As an infant grows, some bones fuse together, leaving the adult skeleton with 206 bones.

The structures of the *skeletal system*

- provide structure and shape for the body
- act as levers for muscular action
- protect internal organs by shielding them with bony structure
- store calcium and phosphorus needed for regulatory functions
- form red and white blood cells and platelets in the bone marrow through *hematopoiesis*

Learning terminology related to the skeletal system will help you understand the locations and functions of bones (Figure 8.14).

Types of Bones

Bones make up the majority of the skeletal system. They come in a variety of sizes and shapes (Figure 8.15):

- **Long bones**: found in the extremities, such as the legs or arms
- **Flat bones**: found in the skull and breastbone; protect organs
- **Short bones**: found in the hands and feet
- **Irregular bones**: found in the jaw and spinal column
- **Sesamoid bones**: found in the kneecap, wrist, and feet; enable movement

Skeletal System Terminology

Combining Form	Meaning
acr/o	extremities
arthr/o	joint
brachi/o	arm
burs/o	sac of fluid near joint
carp/o	wrist
cervic/o	neck; cervix (neck of uterus)
chir/o	hand
chondr/o	cartilage
cost/o	rib
crani/o	skull
lumb/o	lumbar region
myel/o	bone marrow
oste/o	bone
pod/o	foot
rachi/o	spine; vertebrae
sacr/o	sacrum
spondyl/o	vertebra; backbone
synovi/o	lubricating fluid of the joints
tars/o	ankle
ten/o; tendin/o; tendon/o	tendon

Figure 8.14 These combining forms relate to the skeletal system.

Bone Composition

Bones are a connective tissue made of collagen, fiber, and minerals. The two types of bone tissue are compact bone and spongy bone. Compact bone tissue is dense, hard, and strong. It is located underneath the *periosteum* (outer layer of bone) and is

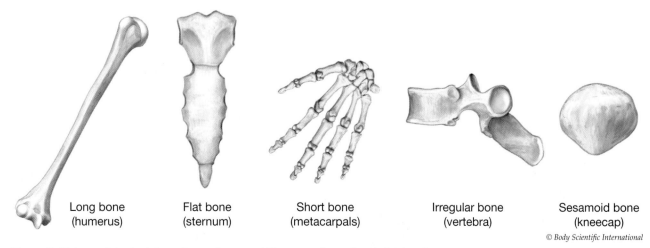

Long bone (humerus) Flat bone (sternum) Short bone (metacarpals) Irregular bone (vertebra) Sesamoid bone (kneecap)

© Body Scientific International

Figure 8.15 Long, flat, short, irregular, and sesamoid bones make up the skeletal system.

mainly found in the shaft, or *diaphysis*, of long bones. Within the diaphysis of a long bone is a hollow center containing yellow bone marrow made of fat cells. Spongy bone tissue is less dense and is usually found at the ends, or *epiphyses*, of long bones. Spaces inside spongy bone tissue contain red bone marrow. **Red blood cells, white blood cells,** and **platelets** are manufactured in red bone marrow through a process called *hematopoiesis*. Red blood cells facilitate oxygen and carbon dioxide exchange throughout the body, white blood cells fight infection, and platelets aid in clotting.

Bones have rough, exterior processes, openings, grooves, and depressions that provide structure for the attachment of muscles and tendons, for the passage of blood vessels and nerves, and for joints. A bone process found on a long bone might be a *trochanter*, or "bony bump," located at the end of a bone to accommodate a joint.

Tendons, Ligaments, and Joints

Tendons are tough, flexible bands of fibrous connective tissue that connect muscles to bones. Joints are locations where two or more bones connect. Bones are linked together by **ligaments**, which are also bands of connective tissue. Ligaments form the top layer of the *joint capsule*, which contains the junction of two bones. A *synovial membrane* lies underneath ligaments and produces synovial fluid to lubricate joints. Tendons and ligaments help stabilize joints and allow movement.

The type of joint determines the extent and direction of movement. Some joints do not allow any movement, while others enable a limb to move freely. There are three types of joints:

1. **Synarthroses:** unmovable joints, such as the sutures in the cranium
2. **Amphiarthroses:** slightly movable joints, such as the ribs
3. **Diarthroses:** freely movable joints, including gliding, hinge, pivot, condylar, saddle, and ball-and-socket joints (Figure 8.16)

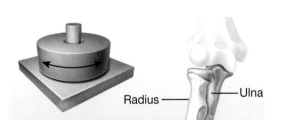

Gliding joint (intercarpal)

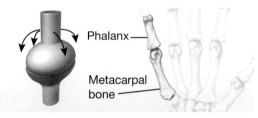

Hinge joint (humeroulnar)

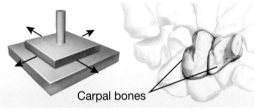

Pivot joint (radioulnar)

Condylar joint (metacarpophalangeal)

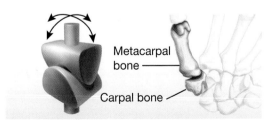

Saddle joint (trapeziometacarpal)

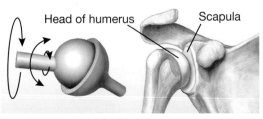

Ball-and-socket joint (humeroscapular)

© *Body Scientific International*

Figure 8.16 There are six types of freely movable joints.

The Axial Skeleton

The skeletal system has two major divisions—the **axial skeleton**, which provides stability, and the **appendicular skeleton**, which enables the body to move (Figure 8.17).

The axial skeleton includes the skull, facial bones, sternum, ribs, and spine. The skull, or *cranium*, is composed of cranial bones that are connected by *sutures*

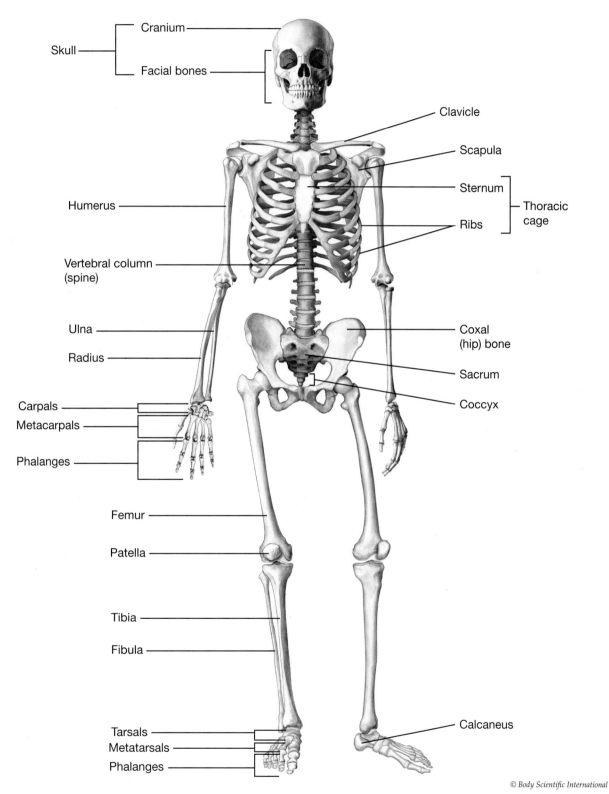

© *Body Scientific International*

Figure 8.17 The axial skeleton makes up the head and trunk of the body. The appendicular skeleton makes up the appendages (arms, shoulders, and legs).

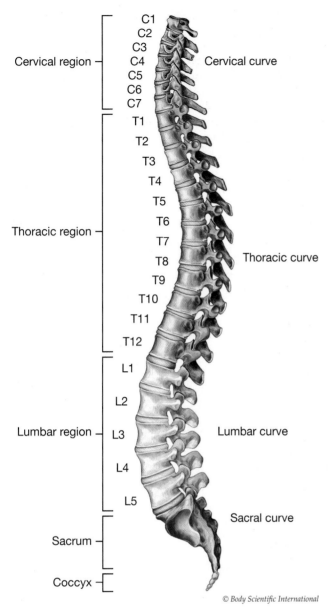

Cervical region

C1
C2
C3
C4
C5
C6
C7

Cervical curve

Thoracic region

T1
T2
T3
T4
T5
T6
T7
T8
T9
T10
T11
T12

Thoracic curve

Lumbar region

L1
L2
L3
L4
L5

Lumbar curve

Sacrum

Sacral curve

Coccyx

© Body Scientific International

Figure 8.18 The five segments of the spinal column are illustrated here.

(immovable joints) and are immobile, with the exception of the jawbone (*mandible*). The jawbone is movable and allows a person to chew and speak.

The axial skeleton also includes the sternum (*breastbone*), which protects the heart and lungs, as well as the joints attached to the sternum. These joints allow sufficient movement for breathing. There are 24 bones or 12 pairs of ribs (*costals*) attached to the sternum. The two pairs of ribs at the bottom of the ribcage are called *floating ribs* because they attach to vertebrae in the spinal column and not to the sternum.

The spinal column is made up of 26 bones, called *vertebrae*. These bones curve to protect the spinal cord. Between vertebrae are disks composed of cartilage; these disks allow movement and absorb any shocks to the body. The spinal column is divided into five segments: the cervical region, thoracic region, lumbar region, sacrum, and coccyx (Figure 8.18).

The Appendicular Skeleton

The appendicular skeleton has 126 bones; these bones can be divided into the upper and lower extremities. The upper extremities include

- the shoulder girdle (paired scapulae and clavicles, which are sometimes called collarbones);
- the arm bones (humerus, radius, and ulna);
- wrist (eight carpal bones per wrist); and
- hand bones (five metacarpals per hand and 14 phalanges that make up the fingers of each hand).

    The lower extremities include

- the pelvic girdle (coxal or hip bones, sacrum, and coccyx);
- the leg (femur, patella, tibia, and fibula);
- ankle (seven tarsal bones each); and
- foot bones (calcaneus or heel bone and five metatarsals, each with 14 phalanges or toes per foot).

How Does the Muscular System Enable Movement?

The *muscular system* is composed of more than 600 muscles and makes up 40–50 percent of the body's weight (Figure 8.19). The muscular system works with many other body systems to help the body move, respond to external stimuli, and produce heat.

    The muscular system contracts and relaxes to move the body's skeleton. Muscles have origin and insertion points. When a muscle contracts, the *insertion* of the muscle moves, while the *origin* of the muscle does not. Effective muscular function requires opposition between an agonist (which contracts) and antagonist (which relaxes). For example, if a nursing assistant lifts a resident, she will use her arm muscles. In her arm, her biceps (agonist) will contract, or flex, and her triceps (antagonist) will relax (Figure 8.20).

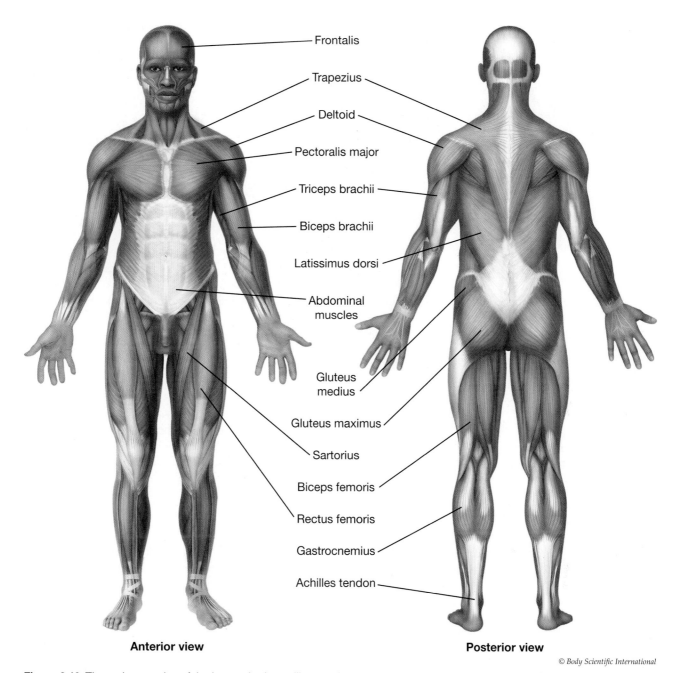

Frontalis
Trapezius
Deltoid
Pectoralis major
Triceps brachii
Biceps brachii
Latissimus dorsi
Abdominal muscles
Gluteus medius
Gluteus maximus
Sartorius
Biceps femoris
Rectus femoris
Gastrocnemius
Achilles tendon

Anterior view

Posterior view

© Body Scientific International

Figure 8.19 The major muscles of the human body are illustrated here.

In addition to movement, the muscular system has the following functions:

- provides structure using the muscles and muscle tone by holding body parts in proper position and protectively covering internal organs
- produces the majority of heat, through movement, to keep the body warm
- uses muscular action to move food through the gastrointestinal system and to move blood and fluids through the body's vessels

Familiarizing yourself with the terminology related to the muscular system will help you better understand its structure and function (Figure 8.21).

Muscle tissue has particular characteristics. This type of tissue must be able to contract, must be elastic and stretchable, and must receive and respond to neural messages.

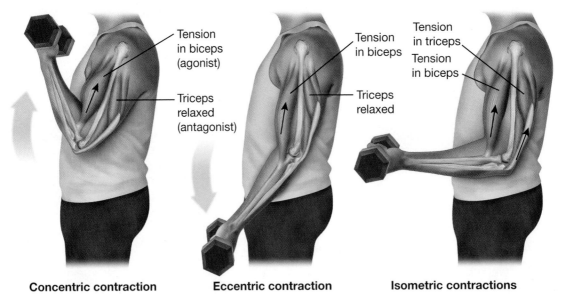

Concentric contraction   Eccentric contraction   Isometric contractions

© Body Scientific International

Figure 8.20 During concentric contraction, the biceps develop tension and shorten as your hand moves closer to your shoulder. Eccentric contraction occurs when the biceps develop tension, but lengthen, as gravity helps draw the hand and weight toward the ground. When an isometric contraction occurs in the arm, both the triceps and biceps have tension, but the length of each muscle remains the same as there is no movement.

Think About This

The muscle that lets your eye blink is the fastest muscle in your body. It allows you to blink five times per second. On average, you blink 15,000 times per day. Women blink twice as often as men.

Muscles are covered by fascia, a fibrous connective tissue that links muscles to tendons. As you have learned, tendons connect muscle to bone. Muscle is connected to bone at both ends. Within each muscle are thousands of *muscle fibers*, each with its own motor nerve ending that sends and receives signals through the nervous system. There are three types of muscle—skeletal, smooth, and cardiac.

Skeletal Muscle

Skeletal, or *striated*, *muscles* connect to bones and move the skeleton by contracting and relaxing at will. Because skeletal muscles are consciously controlled, they are considered *voluntary muscles*. These muscles are found in such areas as the scalp, face, mouth, arms, hands, abdomen, legs, and feet.

Smooth Muscle

Smooth, or *visceral*, *muscles* contract and relax without conscious control. Smooth muscles are found in the walls of organs. As they contract and relax, these muscles move the contents inside an organ. An example of smooth muscles at work is the involuntary process of *peristalsis* in the gastrointestinal tract.

Cardiac Muscle

Cardiac muscle is found only in the heart and makes up most of the heart wall. It is a striated muscle and causes the heart to contract, or *beat*. These smooth muscle contractions occur involuntarily.

How Does the Nervous System Send Signals Throughout the Body?

The *nervous system* uses billions of neurons to send electrochemical messages, also known as *neural impulses*, throughout the body. Messages are sent both consciously and unconsciously. Neurons receive information from internal and external receptors. These

Muscular System Terminology	
Combining Form	**Meaning**
articul/o	joint
fasci/o	fibrous band
fibr/o	fiber
flex/o	bend
kines/o; kinesi/o	movement
lei/o	smooth
muscul/o	muscle
my/o; myos/o	muscle
sarc/o	connective tissue
tens/o	stretched; strained
ton/o	tone; tension

Figure 8.21 These combining forms relate to the muscular system.

receptors interpret information so the body can respond either voluntarily (*consciously*) or involuntarily (*unconsciously*). Voluntary responses are controlled mostly by the brain. The two types of involuntary responses—autonomic responses and reflexes—regulate the body's internal environment (for example, blood pressure) or cause a reaction that originates in the spinal cord.

The nervous system is composed of the central and peripheral nervous systems. The **central nervous system (CNS)** consists of the brain and spinal cord. The **peripheral nervous system (PNS)** consists of 12 pairs of cranial nerves and 31 pairs of spinal nerves. Together, the CNS and PNS control many functions of the body.

Examine the table in Figure 8.22 to learn the word parts associated with the nervous system and to improve your understanding of the nervous system's structures and functions.

Neurons and Message Transmission

The basic unit of the nervous system is the *neuron*. Neurons transmit electrochemical messages throughout the body. Many neurons in a bundle are called a *nerve*.

Nervous System Terminology	
Combining Form	**Meaning**
cephal/o	head
cerebell/o	cerebellum
cerebr/o	cerebrum
crani/o	skull
dur/o	dura mater
encephal/o	brain
esthes/o; esthesi/o	nervous sensation
medull/o	medulla oblongata
mening/o; meningi/o	meninges
neur/o	nerve
phren/o	mind
psych/o	mind
synaps/o; synapt/o	point of contact
thec/o	sheath

Figure 8.22 These combining forms relate to the nervous system.

Neurons are composed of a cell body, dendrites, and axons (Figure 8.23). Both dendrites and axons extend outside of the cell body. Dendrites receive messages and stimuli and transport them into the cell body. Axons are responsible for transmitting messages from the cell body to axon terminals. The axons of some neurons are wrapped in a fatty, white substance called the *myelin sheath*. Myelin protects an axon and speeds the conduction of neural messages. Neural messages then cross the gap, or *synapse*, between the axon terminal and another neuron. This is how neural messages are transmitted throughout the body.

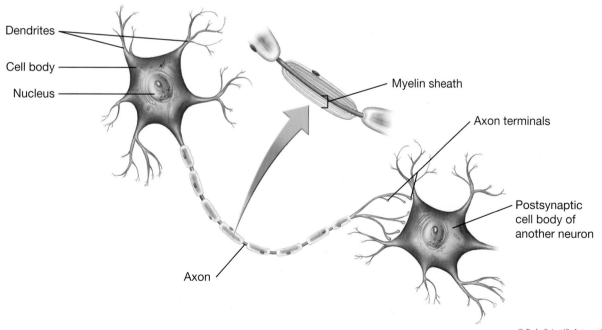

© *Body Scientific International*

Figure 8.23 Neurons are nerve cells that transmit messages throughout the body.

Central Nervous System (CNS)

The *central nervous system (CNS)* is considered the command center of the body. The structures of the CNS respond to all neural messages in the body, monitor functions throughout the body, and help maintain homeostasis. The brain is the center of *cognition*, or mental functions such as thinking, reasoning, and remembering. The spinal cord is the neural connector between the brain and the rest of the body.

The brain and spinal cord are covered with three layers of tissue known as *meninges*. The outer layer, called the *dura mater*, is a tough, protective membrane. The middle layer, the *arachnoid mater*, is a thin, transparent membrane resembling a loosely fitting sac. The arachnoid mater connects the dura mater with the innermost tissue layer, the *pia mater*. The pia mater is a thin membrane that adheres to the surface of the brain and the spinal cord. The pia mater has a rich supply of blood vessels that provide nutrients to nerve tissue. *Cerebrospinal fluid* fills the brain cavities and the central canal of the spinal column to cushion and protect these structures from injury.

Regions of the Brain

The brain is divided into four areas—the cerebrum, cerebellum, diencephalon, and brain stem (Figure 8.24). Each area plays an important role in the complex functions carried out by the brain.

- **Cerebrum**: The cerebrum is the largest region and is located in the superior and anterior parts of the brain. It is divided into left and right hemispheres, which are connected by a bundle of nerves called the *corpus callosum*. The right and left hemispheres are divided into four lobes (Figure 8.25). The cerebrum is covered by the *cerebral cortex*, which contains gray matter arranged in folds and depressions. The cerebrum controls high-level cognitive functions such as language, reasoning, memory, and sensory integration.

- **Cerebellum**: Located in the posterior part of the brain, the cerebellum controls the body's sense of balance and equilibrium. It also coordinates the voluntary movement of muscles.

- **Diencephalon**: Found beneath the cerebrum, the diencephalon houses three glands: the thalamus, pineal gland, and hypothalamus. The *thalamus* plays a role in memory and sends messages such as pain from the sensory organs to the cerebrum. The *pineal gland* helps regulate the body's **circadian rhythm**, or 24-hour sleep-wake cycle. Finally, the *hypothalamus* monitors and controls involuntary body functions such as heart rate, blood pressure, temperature, and digestion.

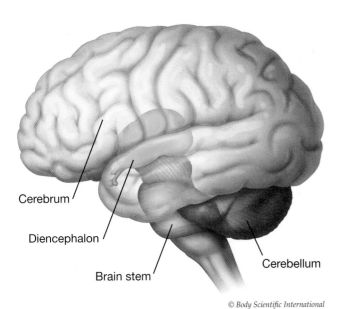

Cerebrum

Diencephalon

Brain stem

Cerebellum

© *Body Scientific International*

Figure 8.24 The structures of the brain are illustrated here.

Lobes of the Brain		
Lobe	**Location**	**Function**
Frontal	Anterior	Controls movement, reasoning, planning, problem solving, speech, and emotions
Parietal	Superior	Processes senses such as touch, pressure, temperature, and pain
Occipital	Posterior	Controls vision
Temporal	Lateral	Processes senses such as hearing and smell; factual and visual memory; and language

Figure 8.25 Each lobe of the brain specializes in different functions.

- **Brain stem**: The brain stem connects the cerebrum with the spinal cord and has three parts: the midbrain, pons, and medulla oblongata. The *midbrain* is the passageway through which neural messages travel from the brain to the spinal cord. The *pons* connects the cerebellum to the rest of the brain and plays a role in breathing. The *medulla oblongata* connects the brain to the spinal cord and regulates heart rate, breathing, and blood pressure.

Spinal Cord

The *spinal cord* extends from the base of the brain to the lower back. It is encased in the spinal column and is protected by vertebrae (Figure 8.26). The average spinal cord is 15 inches long and 1/2 inch wide. It is composed of nerve tissue, and 31 pairs of spinal nerves branch off of it and exit through either side of the spinal column. The spinal cord is divided into four regions: the cervical (C) region, thoracic (T) region, lumbar (L) region, and sacral (S) region.

Neural messages travel up and down the spinal cord and make it possible for the brain and body to communicate. Sensory neurons in the CNS transmit messages to the brain and control basic body functions. Motor neurons transmit messages away from the brain, stimulating skeletal and smooth muscle to enable voluntary and involuntary movements. For example, if you touch something hot, neurons in the spinal cord will activate the speedy reflex needed to quickly move your hand before you get burned.

Peripheral Nervous System (PNS)

The *peripheral nervous system (PNS)* connects the CNS with the rest of the body. Cranial nerves transmit neural messages to and from the brain, while spinal nerves transmit neural messages to and from the spinal cord. The PNS is divided into the autonomic and somatic nervous systems (Figure 8.27).

Autonomic Nervous System (ANS)

The **autonomic nervous system (ANS)** controls involuntary, unconscious body functions. The two divisions of the ANS are the sympathetic and parasympathetic

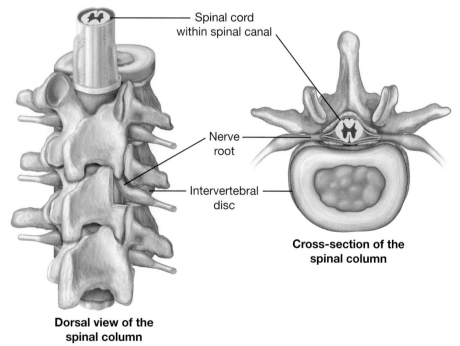

Spinal cord within spinal canal

Nerve root

Intervertebral disc

Cross-section of the spinal column

Dorsal view of the spinal column

© Body Scientific International

Figure 8.26 The spinal cord is protected by the spinal column.

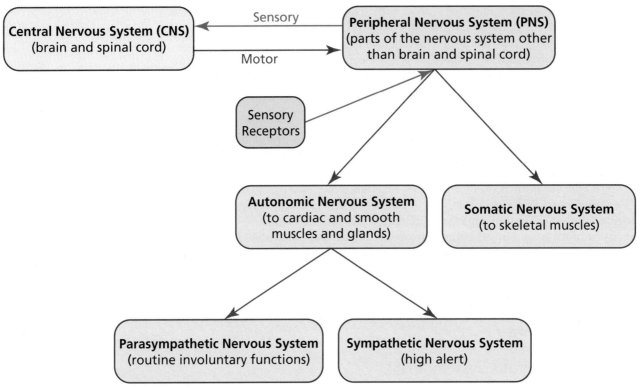

Figure 8.27 This diagram shows the divisions of the nervous system.

nervous systems, which you learned about in chapter 6. The *sympathetic nervous system* controls the body's *fight-or-flight response*, which prepares the body for an emergency. Physical reactions to the fight-or-flight response include a racing heart and rapid breathing. The *parasympathetic nervous system* controls the body's *rest-and-digest response*, which calms the body after the fight-or-flight response by decreasing heart rate and respirations.

Somatic Nervous System

The **somatic nervous system** controls voluntary body functions and stimulates skeletal muscle. This system also sends neural messages about pain.

What Is the Role of the Sensory System?

The *sensory system* is composed of sense organs, some of which are shared with other body systems. These sense organs include the eyes, ears, nose (also part of the respiratory system), tongue (also part of the gastrointestinal system), and skin (also part of the integumentary system). The structures of the sensory system transmit neural messages that enable the senses of vision, hearing, smell, taste, and touch. Important medical terminology associated with the sensory system can be found in Figure 8.28.

The Eye

The eye is the sense organ that enables vision. It has external and internal structures that receive and translate light into neural messages (Figure 8.29).

External Structures

External structures of the eye include the eyelashes and eyebrows, which help prevent foreign substances from entering the eye. Lacrimal glands located in the socket above the outer corner of the eye secrete lacrimal fluid, or *tears*. Tears moisten the eyes and keep them free from dust. The lacrimal canaliculi, or *tear ducts*, at the corners of the eyes collect, store, and drain tears. In addition, sweat glands called *ciliary glands* are located at the base of the upper and lower margins of the eyelid (where the eyelashes can be found). Ciliary glands secrete a protective lubricant onto the eyeball.

The eye is protected by the orbital socket in the skull. The orbital socket also protects the internal structures of the eye. Orbital muscles are responsible for moving the eye within the eye socket.

Internal Structures

The internal structures of the eye receive and translate light into neural messages. A clear, colorless mucous membrane, called the *conjunctiva*, lines the eyelid and covers the anterior portion of the eyeball. The fibrous sclera, commonly referred to as the *white of the eye*, protects the eye and maintains the eye's shape. The transparent, anterior portion of the sclera is the *cornea*, which protects the iris and the pupil. The iris and the pupil are located beneath the cornea. The *iris* is a colored, muscular layer of tissue. It surrounds the *pupil*, which is the small, black, circular opening at the center of the eye. The pupil lets light into the eye, and light then passes through a *lens*, which is a flexible, clear, curved structure that focuses images on the retina at the back of the eye.

The interior of the eye has two chambers. The anterior chamber is the area between the cornea and the lens. The anterior chamber contains *aqueous humor*, a clear, watery fluid that gives the eyeball shape. The posterior chamber is the area between the back of the lens and the retina. It contains a clear, gel-like substance called the *vitreous humor*, which helps keep the retina in place. The *ciliary muscle* inside the eye regulates the shape and thickness of the lens, which allows the lens to focus light on the retina.

Sensory System Terminology

Combining Form	Meaning
acous/o	hearing
acoust/o	hearing; sound
ambly/o	dull; dim
audi/o; audit/o	hearing
blephar/o	eyelid
cochle/o	cochlea
conjunctiv/o	conjunctiva
corne/o	cornea
cor/o; core/o	pupil
gustat/o	taste
ir/o; irid/o	iris
kerat/o	cornea
lacrim/o	tears
myring/o	eardrum
ocul/o	eye
olfact/o	smell
opthalm/o	eye
opt/o; optic/o	vision
ot/o	ear
papill/o	optic disc
phac/o; phak/o	lens of the eye
phot/o	light
retin/o	retina
vitre/o	glassy
vitr/o	vitreous body

Figure 8.28 These combining forms relate to the sensory system.

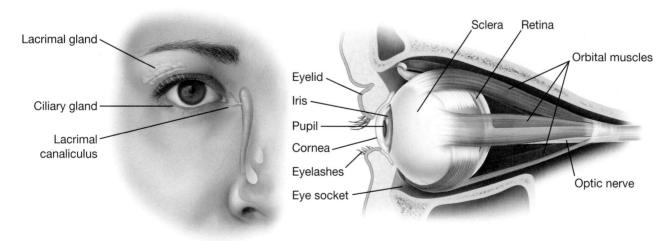

© *Body Scientific International*

Figure 8.29 The external and internal structures of the eye are important for protecting the eye and providing vision.

The *retina* consists of special, light-sensitive receptor cells known as *rods* and *cones*. Photosensitive rods and cones cast images onto the retina to enable vision. The brain then interprets what is seen on the retina. The 120 million rods in the retina are sensitive only to black and white and allow a person to see in dim light. Rods also provide peripheral (lateral) vision. The 6–7 million cones in the retina are sensitive to color and provide more acute vision.

The *optic nerve* located at the back of the eye transmits neural messages from the retina to the brain. The place where the optic nerve leaves the eyeball does not contain rods or cones. This area is called the *optic disc* or the "blind spot."

The Ear

The ear has three divisions: the outer (external) ear, the middle ear (tympanic cavity), and the inner (internal) ear (Figure 8.30). All three sections of the ear are responsible for hearing, and the inner ear also plays a role in balance and equilibrium.

Outer Ear

The structure of the outer ear consists of the auricle, or *pinna*. The auricle is composed of skin-covered cartilage that projects away from the head. Connected to the auricle is the *auditory canal*. The auditory canal is lined with hair and with *ceruminous glands* that secrete cerumen, or *earwax*. Earwax helps clean and protect the ear.

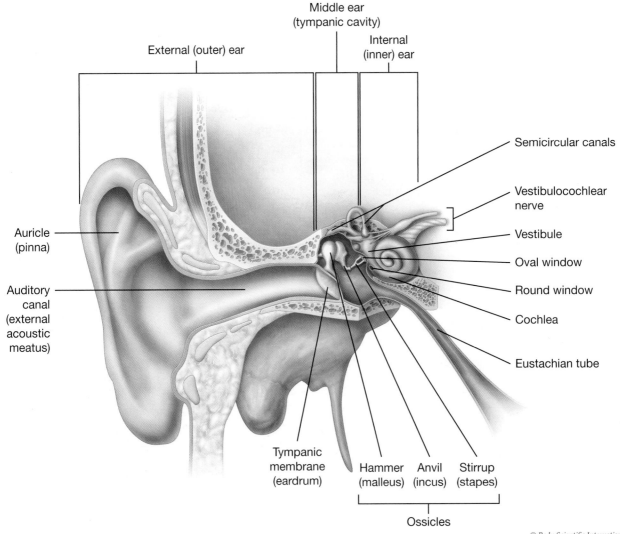

© *Body Scientific International*

Figure 8.30 The structures of the ear are illustrated here.

Middle Ear

The eardrum, also known as the *tympanic membrane*, separates the outer and the middle ear. The middle ear is also called the *tympanic cavity*. Three *ossicles*, which are the smallest bones in the body, are found in the tympanic cavity:

- **Malleus**: the hammer-shaped, outermost bone
- **Incus**: the anvil-shaped, middle bone
- **Stapes**: the stirrup-shaped, innermost bone

Sound that comes through the auditory canal is translated into sound waves, or vibrations, in the eardrum. Ossicles then transmit this vibratory motion from the eardrum to the fluid in the cochlea of the inner ear.

The tympanic cavity connects to the throat via the Eustachian tube. The Eustachian tube is closed except when a person swallows. It helps equalize pressure within the ear.

A membrane-covered opening called the *oval window* connects the middle ear to the inner ear. Beyond the oval window is the *round window*, which leads from the middle ear to the cochlea in the inner ear.

Inner Ear

The inner ear consists of three structures: the cochlea, the vestibule, and semicircular canals. The *cochlea* is a snail-shaped structure filled with fluid. Within the cochlea is the *organ of Corti*, which is the primary receptor for hearing. The organ of Corti contains four rows of hair cells that respond to sound vibrations. These cells transmit neural messages using the *cochlear nerve* and help a person determine the pitch and loudness of another person's voice. The cochlear nerve transmits neural messages to the auditory center of the brain, where sound is processed and interpreted.

The inner ear also contains structures and receptors to sense static and dynamic equilibrium. At the base of the cochlea is the *vestibule*, which connects the cochlea to fluid-filled semicircular canals. Sensory information regarding equilibrium is transmitted from the vestibule via the *vestibular nerve* to the neurons that control eye movements, to the muscles that keep the body erect, and to the brain (so that the body's position can be adjusted). Together, the cochlear nerve and vestibular nerve form a cranial nerve called the vestibulocochlear nerve.

Other Sense Organs

The nose, tongue, and skin are also considered sense organs. Inside the nose are thousands of olfactory (smell) receptor cells containing *olfactory hairs*. When these hairs are stimulated by smell, neural messages are transmitted via the *olfactory nerve* (a cranial nerve) to the brain, where smell is processed.

The average adult tongue contains about 5000 working taste buds. *Taste buds* are specialized receptors on the surface of the tongue. They sense the flavor of food, as well as temperature. Chemical receptors within tastes buds respond to sweet, salty, bitter, sour, and savory flavors, as well as fat. As you learned earlier in this chapter, the skin contains sensory receptors responsible for touch, pressure, temperature, pain, and itch.

How Do Hormones of the Endocrine System Regulate Body Functions?

The endocrine system is composed of **endocrine glands**, which are different from **exocrine glands**. *Endocrine glands* are located throughout the body (Figure 8.31) and secrete *hormones*, or chemical messengers that initiate and regulate specific body processes. Endocrine glands are ductless and secrete hormones directly into the bloodstream. *Exocrine glands* have ducts that transport substances to other organs or to the surface of the skin. Sweat glands are an example of exocrine glands because sweat is secreted through ducts in the skin. The pancreas is unique, as it has both an endocrine and exocrine function.

Think About This

According to the American Academy of Ophthalmology,

- thirty-two percent of Americans have blue or gray irises;
- fifteen percent have blue, gray, or green irises with brown or yellow flecks;
- twelve percent have green or light brown irises with minimal flecks;
- sixteen percent have brown irises with dark flecks; and
- twenty-five percent have uniformly brown irises.

Across the world, more than 50 percent of the population have brown irises.

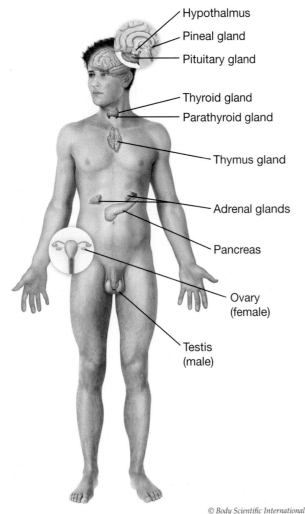

Figure 8.31 Endocrine glands throughout the body make up the endocrine system.

| Hypothalmus |
| Pineal gland |
| Pituitary gland |
| Thyroid gland |
| Parathyroid gland |
| Thymus gland |
| Adrenal glands |
| Pancreas |
| Ovary (female) |
| Testis (male) |

© Body Scientific International

Endocrine System Terminology

Combining Form	Meaning
acid/o	acid
aden/o	gland
adip/o	fat
adren/o; adrenal/o	adrenal gland
crin/o	secrete
gluc/o; glyc/o	sugar; glucose
immun/o	immune
myx/o	mucus
parathyroid/o	parathyroid gland
pituitar/o	pituitary gland
thyr/o; thryroid/o	thyroid gland

Figure 8.32 These combining forms relate to the endocrine system.

Figure 8.32 identifies combining forms related to the endocrine system. Learning this medical terminology will help you understand the forms and functions of the glands in this body system.

Hypothalamus

It is important to start the discussion of the endocrine system, hormones, and glands with the *hypothalamus*, which directly or indirectly controls all other endocrine glands. The hypothalamus is also part of the nervous system and coordinates responses and activities of these two body systems. The hypothalamus is located in the brain near the pituitary gland. Hormones secreted from the hypothalamus control such body functions as temperature regulation, thirst, hunger, sleep, mood, and sex drive. The hypothalamus also releases hormones that stimulate other glands to release specific hormones. For example, the hypothalamus releases growth-hormone-releasing factor (GRF), which stimulates the pituitary gland to release growth hormone (GH).

Pituitary Gland

The *pituitary gland* is a small gland located below the hypothalamus. It has two lobes—the anterior pituitary and the posterior pituitary.

The anterior pituitary secretes the following hormones:

- **Adrenocorticotropic hormone (ACTH):** influences the production of cortisol (which regulates blood glucose) in the kidneys.
- **Thyroid-stimulating hormone (TSH):** helps regulate the thyroid and stimulates the production of thyroid hormones, which affect the rate of metabolism in the body's tissues.
- **Follicle-stimulating hormone (FSH):** helps regulate reproductive processes and stimulates the secretion of estrogen.
- **Growth hormone (GH):** stimulates growth and development.
- **Luteinizing hormone (LH):** stimulates the production of testosterone in males and ovulation in females.
- **Melanocyte-stimulating hormone (MSH):** stimulates melanin to darken skin.
- **Prolactin (PRO):** stimulates milk production and breast development in females.

The posterior pituitary secretes *antidiuretic hormone (ADH)*, which controls water absorption in the kidneys; and *oxytocin*, which stimulates uterine contractions during childbirth and promotes the release of milk in nursing mothers.

Pineal Gland

Located in the thalamus in the brain, the *pineal gland* releases melatonin when the body is exposed to darkness. *Melatonin* is the hormone that regulates circadian rhythm, or the 24-hour sleep-wake cycle. When melatonin is released, you feel sleepy.

Thyroid Gland

The *thyroid* is a butterfly-shaped gland that wraps around the front and sides of the windpipe, or *trachea*. The thyroid gland releases triiodothyronine (T_3) and thyroxine (T_4). Together, T_3 and T_4 are known as *thyroid hormone*. Thyroid hormone controls metabolism, regulates body temperature, and increases the rate of protein production. The thyroid gland also releases *calcitonin*, which regulates the amount of calcium in the blood and helps the body maintain strong, stable bones. Calcitonin works with parathyroid hormone (PTH).

Parathyroid Glands

Two pairs of *parathyroid glands* are located on the back of the thyroid gland. Each parathyroid gland is smaller than a grain of rice. The parathyroid glands release *parathyroid hormone (PTH)*, which helps balance levels of calcium in the blood and stimulates the activation of vitamin D.

Thymus

The *thymus* is located in the chest under the sternum. This gland shrinks in size as people age and is very small by the time people reach adulthood. The thymus releases *thymosin*, a hormone that helps with the development and maturation of immune cells. As a result, the thymus is considered part of the endocrine and immune systems.

Adrenal Glands

The two *adrenal glands* sit on the tops of the kidneys. The adrenal glands have two layers. The outer layer, the *adrenal cortex*, releases cortisol and cortisone. *Cortisol* promotes the use of carbohydrates, fats, and proteins and increases the storage of blood glucose. *Cortisone* regulates blood glucose levels. The adrenal cortex also secretes *aldosterone*, which regulates blood pressure and fluid volume.

The inner layer, the *adrenal medulla*, releases *epinephrine*, which triggers the body's fight-or-flight response. The adrenal medulla also secretes *norepinephrine*, which narrows blood vessels and raises blood pressure. The adrenal glands also release some sex hormones.

Pancreas

The *pancreas* is a long, thin gland located behind and below the stomach. It serves as an exocrine gland by secreting **enzymes** (chemical agents that cause specific reactions) during digestion. The pancreas is also an endocrine gland. Within the pancreas, islets of Langerhans release the hormones insulin and glucagon. *Insulin* lowers blood sugar levels, and *glucagon* stimulates the liver to increase blood sugar levels when needed.

Ovaries

The two oval-shaped *ovaries* are located on either side of the uterus and are part of the female reproductive system. The ovaries secrete the majority of *estrogen* in the body. Estrogen regulates the female reproductive system and stimulates secondary sex characteristics. The ovaries also produce *progesterone*, which stimulates the growth of the mammary glands, regulates menstruation, and promotes the growth of the endometrium (the mucous membrane lining the inside of the uterus).

Testes

The two oval-shaped *testes* are located in the scrotal sac. The testes release *testosterone*, which regulates secondary sex characteristics and is essential for sperm maturation.

How Does the Cardiovascular System Pump Blood Through the Body?

One way to remember the anatomy of the *cardiovascular system* is to analyze the word parts in the term *cardiovascular*. The combining form *cardi/o* means "heart," and the root word *vascul* refers to the blood vessels. The suffix *-ar* means "pertaining to." Therefore, the cardiovascular system includes the heart and blood vessels.

The primary function of the cardiovascular system is to circulate oxygen-rich blood throughout the body and to remove carbon dioxide and other waste products. To accomplish this task, the cardiovascular and respiratory systems work together to complete the exchange of oxygen and carbon dioxide.

Figure 8.33 identifies combining forms related to the cardiovascular system. Learning this medical terminology will help you understand the form and function of this body system.

Cardiovascular System Terminology

Combining Form	Meaning
angi/o	vessel (blood)
aort/o	aorta
arteri/o	artery
ather/o	fatty buildup; plaque
cardi/o	heart
coagul/o	clotting
constrict/o	narrowing
coron/o	heart
cyan/o	blue
dilat/o	enlarge; expand
erythr/o	red
hem/o; hemat/o	blood
leuk/o	white
morph/o	shape
phleb/o	vein
sept/o	wall; partition
ser/o	serum
sphygm/o	pulse
systol/o	contraction
thromb/o	clot
vascul/o	blood vessel
vas/o	vessel; duct
ven/i; ven/o	vein
ventricul/o	ventricle

Figure 8.33 These combining forms relate to the cardiovascular system.

The Heart

The *heart* is located in the thoracic cavity and is composed of involuntary cardiac muscle, which contracts and relaxes in a rhythmic cycle (Figure 8.34). These contractions circulate blood through the heart to the rest of the body. The heart sits in a sac called the *pericardium* and is made up of three layers of muscle:

- **Epicardium**: serous, thin, watery layer
- **Myocardium**: located in the middle of the heart
- **Endocardium**: the innermost layer that lines the chambers of the heart

The heart is divided into right and left sides by the *septum*. Each side of the heart is further divided into an upper and lower chamber. The upper chambers are called *atria*, and the lower chambers are called *ventricles*. The lowest point of the heart is called the *apex*.

Blood Flow Through the Heart

The heart is the engine that circulates blood through the body. Blood flows in one direction, through the upper chambers of the heart to the lower chambers, and valves between the chambers prevent any backflow. Once blood leaves the heart, it circulates throughout the body via blood vessels (Figure 8.35).

Heart Rate and Blood Pressure

The heart's muscle fibers allow it to contract, relax, and pump blood through the heart. This action is regulated by the autonomic nervous system, which operates unconsciously. The heart's actions are also regulated by an electrical system consisting of sites throughout the heart muscle. The process by which the heart is electrically stimulated is *conduction*. During this process, electrical impulses in the atria and ventricles stimulate contractions needed for the heart to circulate blood. When the heart contracts, blood is forced through the arteries to the rest of the body. This is called *systole*. Between contractions, the heart relaxes (*diastole*) and fills with blood. Blood pressure measures the contraction (systolic) and then the relaxation (diastolic) of the heart. The normal range for an adult's blood pressure is 120/80 mmHg or below.

The normal **pulse**, or number of heart beats per minute, for adults is 60–100 beats per minute and depends on a person's health and physical activity. Pulse is most commonly felt and measured at the wrist, but is sometimes taken at the apex of the heart using a stethoscope. Pulse can also be taken at other points on the body. See chapter 18 for a detailed discussion about measuring and recording blood pressure and pulse.

Blood Vessels

Blood vessels provide nourishment for the heart and transport blood between the heart and the rest of the body. Many different blood vessels play a role in circulating blood throughout the body. Arteries, arterioles, and capillaries transport fully oxygenated blood from the heart to the body. Veins and venules carry oxygen-poor blood from the body back to the heart.

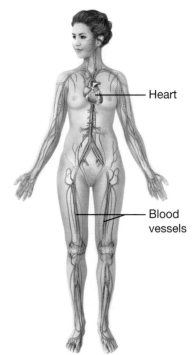

© *Body Scientific International*

Figure 8.34 The heart is located in the thoracic cavity.

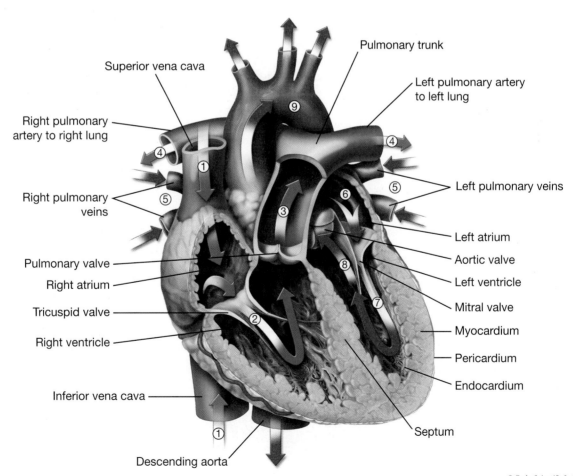

© *Body Scientific International*

Figure 8.35 Using this diagram, you can follow the flow of blood through the heart.

Think About This

There are 60,000 miles of blood vessels in a human body, enough to wrap around the Earth twice.

Blood

The average adult has between 10 and 15 pints of blood. *Blood* has two basic components: blood cells and plasma. Blood cells are referred to collectively as the **formed elements** of blood. The liquid component of blood, called **plasma**, makes up one-half of the blood's volume. Plasma is composed mostly of water, but also transports hormones, protein, sugar, and waste products to or from the body tissues.

The formed elements include three types of blood cells. Red blood cells (RBCs), or *erythrocytes*, are responsible for carrying oxygen throughout the body and removing carbon dioxide, a waste product. **Hemoglobin** molecules on red blood cells carry oxygen from the lungs to body organs and tissues and carry carbon dioxide from body organs and tissues to the lungs. This exchange of gases is vital to life. White blood cells (WBCs), or *leukocytes*, defend the body against disease-causing microorganisms called **pathogens**. Both red and white blood cells are manufactured primarily in the bone marrow. Platelets, or *thrombocytes*, help the blood clot when there is an injury.

How Does the Respiratory System Supply the Body with Oxygen?

The *respiratory system* contains organs that allow us to breathe in oxygen and get rid of carbon dioxide. Breathing, or *respiration*, is the primary function of the respiratory system. During respiration, oxygen is inhaled (inspired) and transported to the body's cells, organs, and tissues. Carbon dioxide, a waste product, is exhaled (expired) from the body. This process is carried out by several respiratory organs and by the cardio-vascular system.

The process of breathing includes two activities: ventilation and gas exchange. *Ventilation* is the movement of oxygen-rich air into the lungs and the movement of carbon dioxide out of the lungs. Ventilation is measured by counting each inspiration and expiration. The normal ventilation rate for adults is 12–20 breaths per minute.

Gas exchange occurs in the alveoli of the lungs. After oxygen is inhaled into the body, it moves to the alveoli. Here, oxygen diffuses or passes through a membrane and into capillaries so it can be circulated by blood vessels throughout the body. At this same site, carbon dioxide diffuses from the capillaries into the alveoli so it can be breathed out into the environment (Figure 8.36).

The respiratory system is divided into two parts: the upper and lower respiratory tracts. The upper respiratory tract consists of the nose and nasal cavities, mouth,

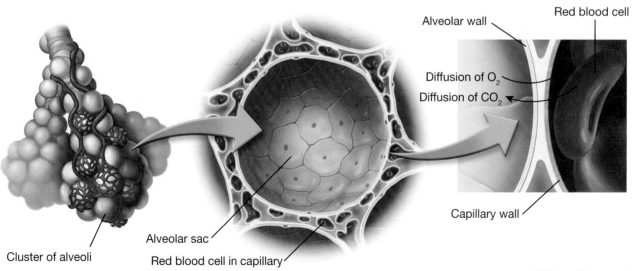

Alveolar wall

Red blood cell

Diffusion of O_2

Diffusion of CO_2

Capillary wall

Cluster of alveoli

Alveolar sac

Red blood cell in capillary

© *Body Scientific International*

Figure 8.36 Oxygen and carbon dioxide are exchanged in the alveoli of the lungs.

pharynx, and larynx. The lower respiratory tract consists of the trachea, bronchi, bronchioles, and two lungs (which contain alveoli). The upper and lower respiratory tracts work together to accomplish the respiratory system's primary function of ventilation and gas exchange.

Pair the combining forms in Figure 8.37 with the prefixes and suffixes you have learned earlier in this chapter to create medical terms related to the respiratory system.

Upper Respiratory Tract

The upper respiratory tract begins with the nose. The nose is composed of bone and cartilage and is divided by a septum (Figure 8.38). Air enters the body through the nose and flows into the *nasal cavity*, the space behind the nose. Tiny hairs called *cilia* line the nasal cavity and filter pathogens from the air. These tiny hairs also enable the senses of smell and taste and warm and moisten air. Four air-filled sinus cavities are also found behind the nose.

The pharynx, or *throat*, is the passageway into the body for air, liquid, and food. As such, it is shared with other body systems. The pharynx is divided into three sections:

1. **Nasopharynx**: serves as a passageway for air and houses the Eustachian tubes, which lead to the middle ear.
2. **Oropharynx**: houses the pharyngeal tonsil or *adenoid*.
3. **Laryngopharynx**: allows air to move into the trachea and allows liquids and food to enter the esophagus.

| Respiratory System Terminology ||
Combining Form	**Meaning**
alveol/o	air sac
aspir/o	removal
bronchi/o	bronchiole
bronch/o	bronchial tube
diaphragmat/o	diaphragm
epiglott/o	epiglottis
laryng/o	larynx; voice box
lob/o	lobe
nas/o	nose
ox/o; ox/i	oxygen
pharyng/o	pharynx; throat
pleur/o	pleura
pneum/o; pneumon/o	lung; air; gas
pulmon/o	lung
py/o	pus
rhin/o	nose
sinus/o	sinus
spir/o	breathing
thorac/o	chest
trache/o	trachea; windpipe
tub/o	tube

Figure 8.37 These combining forms relate to the respiratory system.

The final organ in the upper respiratory tract is the semirigid larynx, or *voice box*. The larynx houses the vocal folds (commonly called the *vocal cords*), movable mucous membranes that produce sound. Part of the larynx is a large plate of thyroid cartilage known as the *Adam's apple*, which is more prominent in males than in females. The epiglottis lies between the larynx and the tongue. When the epiglottis is open, it allows air to flow through the trachea into the lower respiratory tract. The epiglottis closes over the trachea when food and liquid are ingested, thus preventing these solids and liquids from passing into the trachea.

Lower Respiratory Tract

The lower respiratory tract begins with the trachea, or *windpipe*. The trachea is made of cartilage and is covered with a mucous membrane lined with cilia. The *cilia* trap foreign substances and sweep them up toward the larynx and pharynx.

Midway down the chest, the trachea divides into the right and left bronchi. The bronchi are the passageways into the lungs. Air flows into the bronchi, into smaller structures called bronchioles, and finally into the alveoli. *Alveoli* are tiny sacs in the lungs; in the alveoli, the gases oxygen and carbon dioxide are exchanged.

The lungs are the principal organs of the respiratory system (Figure 8.39). There is a right and a left lung. The right lung sits a little higher in the thoracic cavity than the left due to the location of the liver. There are three lobes in the right lung (superior, middle, and inferior) and two lobes in the left lung (superior and inferior). The area between the two lungs is called the *mediastinum*. Several organs and structures are found in the mediastinum, including the heart.

The lungs are made of porous, spongy tissue. A *pleural membrane* covers the lungs and reduces friction during breathing. Fluid fills the pleural cavity in which the lungs are located. Each lung is cone shaped and contains a network of blood, lymph vessels, and nerves. At the base of the lungs is the *diaphragm*, a muscle that contracts to help inflate the lungs.

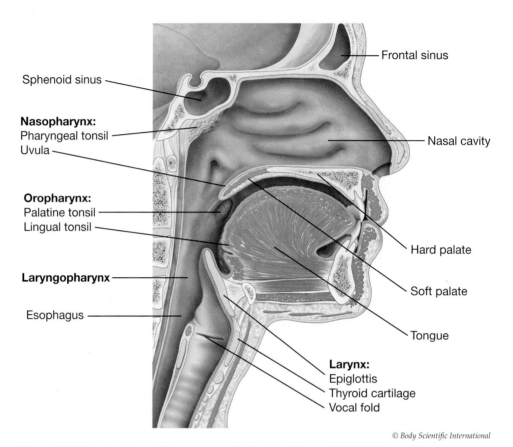

© Body Scientific International

Figure 8.38 The structures of the upper respiratory tract filter and direct air toward the lungs.

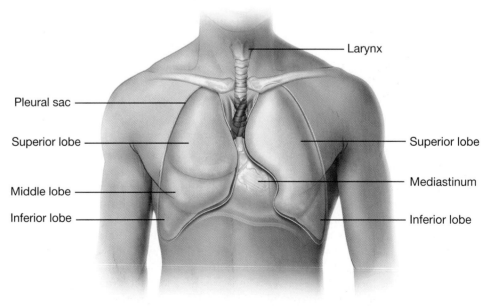

© Body Scientific International

Figure 8.39 The lower respiratory tract includes the lungs.

How Do the Immune and Lymphatic Systems Keep You Healthy?

The *immune* and *lymphatic systems* protect the body against pathogens. The immune system does not have its own set of organs or vessels. Instead, it relies on organs from other body systems to complete its vital tasks. The lymphatic system also plays a major role in immunity and protection against pathogens.

Figure 8.40 lists combining forms related to the immune and lymphatic systems. Learning these terms will help you better understand these systems.

Immune and Lymphatic System Terminology	
Combining Form	**Meaning**
adenoid/o	adenoids
immun/o	immune
lymphaden/o	lymph vessel
lymph/o; lymphat/o	lymph
phag/o	eat; engulf
tonsill/o	tonsils
vir/o	virus

Figure 8.40 These combining forms relate to the lymphatic and immune systems.

Types of Immunity

The immune and lymphatic systems aid in immunity. *Immunity*, which is a person's ability to resist infection, is an important part of protection against pathogens. There are two different types of immunity:

- **Natural immunity**: is a type of immunity humans have when they are born. Natural immunity is affected by a person's race, gender, genes, and cells (such as white blood cells).

- **Acquired immunity**: is a type of immunity that humans develop. This type of immunity can be active or passive. People develop *active immunity* through being exposed to a disease or through *immunization*. Immunization is a process in which a small or modified dose of a pathogen is injected to stimulate the production of **antibodies** (blood proteins that reduce the effects of bacteria and viruses). *Passive immunity* is short term and passes from one body to another. For example, a fetus can develop passive immunity when a mother passes antibodies through the placenta.

Immune Cells

The immune system is activated when pathogens attack the body. A variety of cells are involved in responding to this attack. *T cells* are a type of white blood cells and include *cytotoxic cells*, which destroy cells that are considered harmful. White blood cells known as *B cells* transform into plasma and secrete antibodies for protection. When these antibodies are released into blood and lymph, they target foreign substances and destroy them.

Lymph and Lymph Vessels

Lymph is a colorless fluid that originates in the capillaries of the cardiovascular system and travels through lymph vessels. As it travels, lymph replaces harmful substances in the body with healthy white blood cells and plasma before returning to the cardiovascular system. The primary cell found in lymph is the *lymphocyte*, a type of white blood cell that is specialized to defend the body against pathogens. *Lymph vessels* include ducts that propel lymph through the body.

Lymph Organs

Organs of the lymphatic system include the lymph nodes, spleen, tonsils, and thymus (Figure 8.41). *Lymph nodes* are small organs located throughout the body. Some lymph nodes can be found in the armpit (*axilla*), for example. Lymph nodes contain lymphocytes that detect and destroy cells that are foreign to the body.

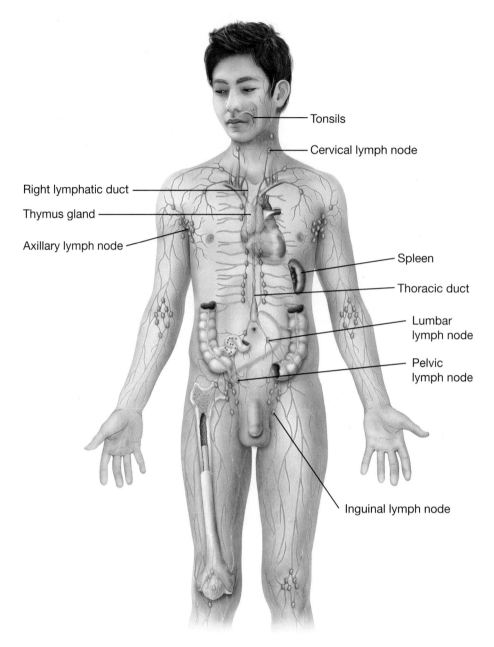

Tonsils

Cervical lymph node

Right lymphatic duct

Thymus gland

Axillary lymph node

Spleen

Thoracic duct

Lumbar lymph node

Pelvic lymph node

Inguinal lymph node

© Body Scientific International

Figure 8.41 The lymphatic organs work together to circulate and filter lymph.

The *spleen* is the largest organ in the lymphatic system. It is filled with blood vessels and a reserve of blood. The spleen is essential to destroying worn-out red blood cells, producing lymphocytes, storing platelets, and increasing blood volume in the body. Other organs that are part of the lymphatic system include the tonsils, thymus, and liver.

What Is the Gastrointestinal System's Role in Nutrition?

The *gastrointestinal system* has several essential functions related to the ingestion, breakdown, absorption, and elimination of food and liquid:

- Food and liquid enter the body through a process called *ingestion*. Liquid is swallowed, and food is chewed (masticated) during ingestion. This begins the process of digestion where food is mechanically (chewing and grinding) and chemically (saliva and its enzymes) broken down into smaller components.

- Food continues to be broken down into smaller, more manageable components during *peristalsis* (involuntary smooth muscle contractions). Peristalsis also aids in digestion by helping food mix with gastric juices. Gastric juices break down food so it is more easily absorbed by the body.

- Peristalsis continues through the small intestine to aid in further digestion. Nutrients enter the bloodstream in the small intestine and then travel to the rest of the body.

- Food that was not absorbed by the body enters the large intestine and is ultimately eliminated from the body through the anus. This is called *defecation*.

The structures and organs of the gastrointestinal system work together to absorb nutrients from the foods you eat and give you the energy you need to survive and thrive. The gastrointestinal system begins with the oral cavity, which includes the mouth, tongue, teeth, and salivary glands. The pharynx, esophagus, stomach, small and large intestines, anus, gallbladder, liver, and pancreas are also part of this body system.

Figure 8.42 provides pertinent combining forms associated with the gastrointestinal system. You can form medical terms related to the gastrointestinal system using appropriate prefixes and suffixes found earlier in this chapter.

Alimentary Canal

The gastrointestinal system includes the gastrointestinal tract (*GI tract*), which is designed to support the ingestion, digestion, absorption, and elimination of liquid and food. Another name for the gastrointestinal tract is the **alimentary canal**. The alimentary canal leads from the mouth to the anus and connects many digestive organs. Many accessory organs accompany the alimentary canal in achieving gastrointestinal functions.

The Mouth

Food and liquid enter the mouth (*oral cavity*) through the lips, or *labia* (Figure 8.43). The mouth is lined with a mucous membrane that secretes *saliva* produced by the salivary glands. This membrane provides a barrier that helps avoid injury during chewing. The membrane also helps sense hot and cold temperatures and prevents pathogens from entering the body. The lips and cheeks make up the front and the lateral walls of the mouth, and the hard and soft palates form the top, or *roof*, of the mouth. The *uvula*, a fingerlike projection anchored to the soft palate, hangs at the very back of the mouth to prevent liquid and food from entering nasal passages.

The *tongue*, which is attached to the floor of the mouth, is an accessory organ that aids in chewing (*mastication*). The tongue uses muscular action to direct and move food in the mouth toward the pharynx. On the surface of the tongue are tiny bumps called *papillae* that contain taste buds. The underside of the tongue is made up of tiny blood vessels that aid in absorption. Because of these blood vessels, medications can be administered under the tongue, or *sublingually*.

Gastrointestinal System Terminology	
Combining Form	**Meaning**
abdomin/o	abdomen
an/o	anus
append/o; appendic/o	appendix
bil/i	bile
cec/o	cecum
chol/e	gall; bile
cholecyst/o	gallbladder
cirrh/o	orange-yellow
col/o; colon/o	colon; large intestine
dent/i	tooth
duoden/o	duodenum
esophag/o	esophagus
gastr/o	stomach
gingiv/o	gums
gloss/o	tongue
hepat/o	liver
ile/o	ileum
inguin/o	groin
jaund/o	yellow
jejun/o	jejunum
labi/o	lip
ling/o	tongue
odont/o	tooth
or/o	mouth
pancreat/o	pancreas
proct/o	rectum; anus
rect/o	rectum
sigmoid/o	sigmoid colon
splen/o	spleen

Figure 8.42 These combining forms relate to the gastrointestinal system.

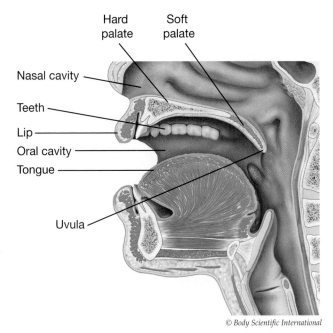

Hard palate
Soft palate
Nasal cavity
Teeth
Lip
Oral cavity
Tongue
Uvula

© Body Scientific International

Figure 8.43 The structures of the oral cavity are illustrated here.

The *teeth* are accessory organs designed to aid in the mastication and grinding of food. Each tooth is divided into two areas: the crown and the root. The outermost layer of the tooth is *enamel*. Enamel covers the tooth's second layer, known as *dentin*. At the center of the tooth is the *pulp*, which contains blood vessels and nerves. The pulp cavity extends into the root of the tooth, creating the root canal. The root of each tooth is surrounded by bone and by a layer of soft tissue called *gingiva* or *gums*.

Three *salivary glands* surround the oral cavity and play an essential role in digestion. These accessory organs produce 10,000 gallons of saliva over a person's lifetime. An enzyme called *amylase* is found in saliva and aids in the chemical breakdown of food.

Pharynx and Esophagus

The pharynx, or *throat*, is the passageway to the mucus-lined, muscular esophagus. The *epiglottis*, discussed as part of the respiratory system, allows only liquid and food to enter the esophagus. At the end of the esophagus is a **sphincter**, called the *cardiac sphincter*, that controls the flow and backflow of food and liquid traveling from the esophagus to the stomach.

Stomach

Think About This

The tongue can identify five basic tastes: sweet, sour, bitter, salt, and *umami* (meaty or savory). All parts of the tongue can detect these tastes, but the sides of the tongue are more sensitive than the middle of the tongue, and the back of the tongue is most sensitive to bitter tastes.

The *stomach*, which looks like a sac, has three major sections: the fundus, body, and antrum (Figure 8.44). The stomach also has three layers of muscle (longitudinal, circular, and oblique) that give it strength when it expands. These muscle layers also help mix food during digestion. The stomach is lined with a mucous membrane containing *rugae* (folds), which allow the stomach to expand when filled with food. This membrane also protects the lining of the stomach from harsh gastric acid. When food is mixed with gastric acid in the stomach, the mixture becomes *chyme*. Chyme enters the small intestine through a narrow passageway called the *pylorus*. The size of the pylorus is regulated by the pyloric sphincter.

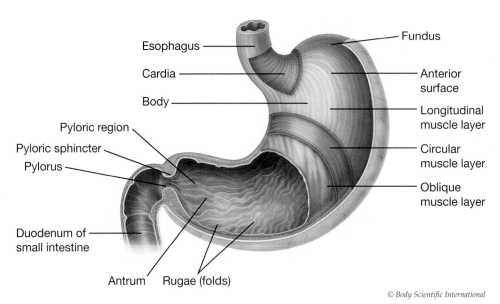

Esophagus
Cardia
Body
Pyloric region
Pyloric sphincter
Pylorus
Duodenum of small intestine
Antrum
Rugae (folds)
Fundus
Anterior surface
Longitudinal muscle layer
Circular muscle layer
Oblique muscle layer

© Body Scientific International

Figure 8.44 The stomach is made up of the fundus, body, and antrum.

Small Intestine

In the average adult, the *small intestine* is between 17 and 20 feet long. The small intestine is the longest section of the alimentary canal. The small intestine continues the process of digestion and facilitates *absorption* (the passing of nutrients, water, and electrolytes such as sodium into the blood) using small, threadlike extensions called *villi* that line the small intestine. Villi help move chyme along the twisted path of the small intestine and absorb nutrients. The small intestine consists of three sections:

1. **Duodenum**: where food is digested; digestion is aided by bile from the liver and gallbladder and by enzymes from the pancreas
2. **Jejunum**: where nutrients are absorbed into the bloodstream
3. **Ileum**: where vitamin B_{12} is absorbed into the bloodstream and where unused food and waste enter the large intestine through the ileocecal sphincter

Large Intestine

The mucus-lined large intestine gets its name because it is considerably larger in diameter than the small intestine (Figure 8.45). There are six sections in the large intestine. The first section, the *cecum*, is connected to the ileum in the small intestine and receives unused food and waste. The *appendix*, which has no known function, hangs from the lower part of the cecum. The second, third, and fourth parts of the large intestine are the ascending, transverse, and descending colons. The *ascending, transverse,* and *descending colons* surround the small intestine. The *sigmoid colon* leads into the rectum, and the *rectum* stores waste (*feces*) until waste can be eliminated in a process called *defecation*.

Anus

The *anus* is the last structure of the alimentary canal. With help from the nervous system, voluntary and involuntary sphincters within the anus help regulate and control elimination, or the evacuation of feces from the body.

Accessory Organs

Three additional accessory organs within the gastrointestinal system aid digestion. These are the pancreas, liver, and gallbladder (Figure 8.46).

Pancreas

The *pancreas* is a long, thin gland that lies behind the bottom part of the stomach. As you learned earlier in this chapter, the pancreas produces insulin and glucagon. The pancreas also produces enzymes that are secreted through the pancreatic duct into the small intestine. These enzymes assist in chemical digestion and include

- *amylase* to break down carbohydrates;
- *lipase* to break down fats; and
- *protease* to break down proteins.

Liver

The *liver* is a large organ that is divided into right and left lobes. It is located on the upper right side of the trunk of the body behind the ribcage. The liver's key function is to make *bile*, which is needed to digest food and break down fat in the small intestine. The liver also stores nutrients, filters and removes waste products from the bloodstream, and converts carbohydrates into sugar (glucose).

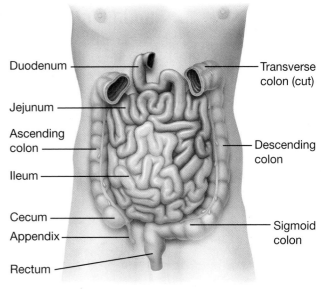

© *Body Scientific International*

Figure 8.45 The structures of the small and large intestine are illustrated here.

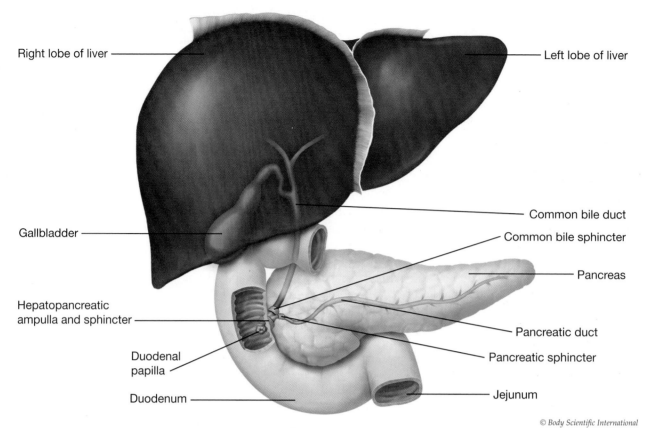

Right lobe of liver

Left lobe of liver

Gallbladder

Common bile duct

Common bile sphincter

Pancreas

Hepatopancreatic
ampulla and sphincter

Pancreatic duct

Pancreatic sphincter

Duodenal
papilla

Duodenum

Jejunum

© Body Scientific International

Figure 8.46 The liver, gallbladder, and pancreas are accessory organs to digestion. Ducts in the liver transport bile to the gallbladder and out into the body.

Gallbladder

The *gallbladder* is a small, pear-shaped pouch just beneath the liver. The gallbladder stores bile produced by the liver. When bile is needed, it travels to the duodenum in the small intestine via cystic and bile ducts. The gallbladder is not an essential organ.

How Does the Urinary System Produce, Store, and Eliminate Urine from the Body?

The *urinary system* is responsible for filtering the blood and eliminating liquid waste from the body in the form of urine. This system determines which waste products need to be filtered from the blood and which can be reabsorbed. It also maintains the body's homeostasis by monitoring fluid levels and electrolytes in the body. Fluids and electrolytes will be discussed in more detail in chapter 22.

The urinary system is composed of two kidneys, two ureters, the urinary bladder, and the urethra. The kidneys produce urine using waste products that need to be *excreted*, or expelled from the body. The urinary bladder stores urine until it is ready to be excreted through the urethra. Gravity and peristalsis move urine through the urinary system. Learning the combining forms that describe the structures and functions of the urinary system will help you better understand this body system (Figure 8.47).

Kidneys

The *kidneys* are two bean-shaped organs that weigh approximately 4–6 ounces each and are found in the abdominal cavity. Fat (*adipose*) and connective tissue line the kidneys to protect them and hold them in place. The kidney is made up of three regions: the renal cortex, renal medulla, and renal pelvis (Figure 8.48).

Renal Cortex

The outer layer of the kidney is the *renal cortex*. The renal cortex is composed of microscopic *nephrons* that filter blood and remove waste products from the body. Blood enters the kidney via the renal artery and circulates through the *Bowman's capsule*, a membrane surrounding the glomerulus of each nephron in the kidney. The *glomerulus* is a ball of capillaries with thin walls that allow only certain substances, such as water, waste products, and *urea* (waste from proteins broken down by the liver), to leave the bloodstream. A *renal tubule* attached to the Bowman's capsule accepts waste products and reabsorbs any useful substances into the bloodstream. Not all waste products are reabsorbed. Some pass to the renal medulla as *urine*, which is 95 percent water and 5 percent waste products (mostly urea).

Renal Medulla

The inner region of the kidney, the *renal medulla*, contains pyramid-shaped structures that carry urine from the renal cortex to chambers of the kidney known as *renal calyces*. Urine passes from the renal calyces into the renal pelvis.

| Urinary System Terminology ||
Combining Form	Meaning
albumin/o	albumin
calcul/o	stone
cali/o	calyx
cyst/o	cyst; fluid sac
glomerul/o	glomerulus
lith/o	stone
meat/o	meatus
nephr/o	kidney
olig/o	scanty; very small
pyel/o	renal pelvis
ren/o	kidney
ureter/o	ureter
urethr/o	urethra
urin/o	urine
ur/o	urine
vesic/o	urinary bladder

Figure 8.47 These combining forms relate to the urinary system.

Renal Pelvis

The *renal pelvis* is the lower part of the kidney and the upper part of the ureter. In the renal pelvis, urine passes to the ureters. The *hilum* is a recessed opening in the renal pelvis through which blood vessels, nerves, and the ureter pass.

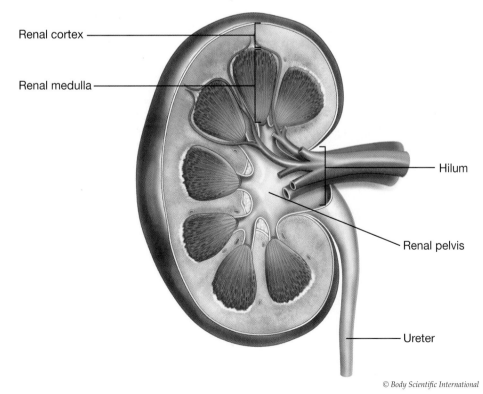

Renal cortex

Renal medulla

Hilum

Renal pelvis

Ureter

© *Body Scientific International*

Figure 8.48 The kidney's three regions play different roles in filtering the blood and storing urine.

Ureters, Urinary Bladder, and Urethra

The two *ureters* are narrow tubes that transport urine from the renal pelvis to the urinary bladder. The hollow, muscular *urinary bladder* stores urine until it is excreted from the body. The urinary bladder can store up to 16 ounces of fluid before nerves in the bladder send a message to the brain that the bladder needs to be emptied. The *urethra* is the tube that excretes urine out of the body. Two sphincters control the flow of urine out of the body. The first sphincter is the *internal urethral sphincter*, which is located at the place where the urinary bladder and the urethra meet. The internal urethral sphincter moves involuntarily. The second sphincter is the *external urethral sphincter* and is located at the end of the urethra. The external urethral sphincter is voluntary. In both males and females, urine passes out of the body through an opening called the *meatus* (Figure 8.49).

How Do the Male and Female Reproductive Systems Differ?

There are several anatomical and physiological differences between the male and female reproductive systems; however, both systems are designed to achieve the same purpose—to produce offspring. The *male reproductive system* is designed to facilitate *conception* (the union of a sperm and an ovum). To do this, the male

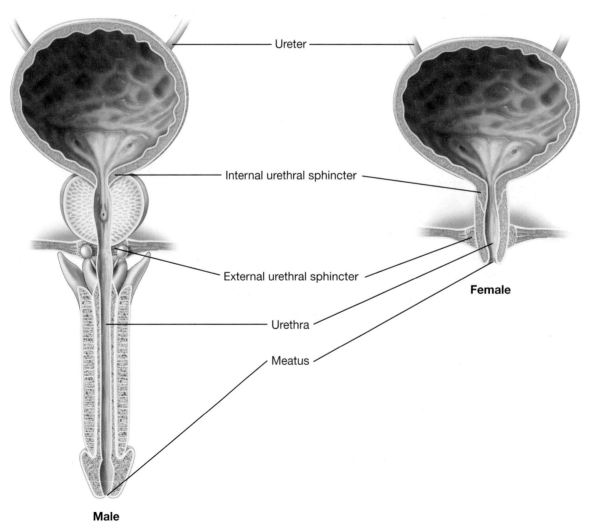

Ureter

Internal urethral sphincter

External urethral sphincter

Urethra

Meatus

Female

Male

© Body Scientific International

Figure 8.49 The ureters, urinary bladder, and urethra store urine and transport it out of the body.

reproductive system produces sufficient sperm to fertilize an ovum, or *egg*. The *female reproductive system* produces ova, supports the development of an embryo, and nourishes a baby through lactation after birth.

The male reproductive organs include the scrotum and testes, interior duct system, seminal vesicles, prostate gland, and penis. The female reproductive organs include the ovaries, fallopian tubes, uterus, vagina, vulva, and mammary glands. Learning the combining forms that describe the structures and functions of the reproductive systems will help you better understand these body systems (Figure 8.50).

Male Reproductive System

In the male reproductive system, there are external and internal organs and structures (Figure 8.51). The external organs are the scrotum and the penis. Internal organs help in the creation, storage, and transport of **sperm**. The sperm is the male reproductive cell that fertilizes a female's ovum.

External Male Reproductive Organs

The *scrotum* is a pouch covered by skin that hangs outside the body between the thighs. The scrotum contains the testes, or *testicles*, glands responsible for developing sperm.

Sperm form in small tubes, called *seminiferous tubules*, within the testes. Sperm then move to the *epididymis*, a tube located outside the testes. Sperm continue to mature, and each sperm develops a tail called a *flagellum*, which will help the sperm move up the vagina. Luteinizing hormone (LH) and testosterone are essential to the proper growth of sperm. Testosterone is also important for the development of male secondary sex characteristics, including facial, underarm, and pubic hair growth; increased muscle mass; and a deeper voice.

The penis is located above the scrotum and is composed of three layers of spongy erectile tissue and sensory receptors. The penis is responsible for excreting both urine and sperm through the *glans penis*, the portion located at the distal end. In uncircumcised men, a fold of skin, called the foreskin or *prepuce*, covers the glans penis.

Internal Male Reproductive Organs

The internal male reproductive organs include the interior duct system, seminal vesicles, and prostate gland. The interior duct system moves sperm from the epididymis to the *vas deferens*. From there, sperm are transported to the pelvic cavity and to ejaculatory ducts within the prostate gland. The prostate gland opens into the urethra.

Seminal vesicles located in the pelvic cavity produce *semen*, the fluid that transports sperm during sexual intercourse. Semen empties into the ejaculatory duct until it is released during a process called *ejaculation*. The muscular *prostate gland*, located under the urinary bladder, secretes a thick fluid that lowers the acidity of semen and also aids in the release of semen during ejaculation.

Reproductive System Terminology	
Combining Form	**Meaning**
amni/o	amnion
andr/o	male
balan/o	glans penis
cervic/o	neck; cervix (neck of uterus)
colp/o	vagina
epididym/o	epididymis
episi/o	vulva
fet/o	fetus
gon/o	seed
gynec/o	female
hyster/o	uterus
lact/o	milk
ligat/o	binding; tying
mamm/o	breast
mast/o	breast
men/o	menstruation
metr/o; metri/o	uterus
nat/i	birth
oophor/o	ovary
orch/o; orchi/o; orchid/o	testicle
ovari/o	ovary
ov/o; ovul/o	ovum; egg
prostat/o	prostate gland
salping/o	fallopian tube
semin/i	semen
sperm/o; spermat/o	sperm
test/o	testicle
uter/o	uterus
vagin/o	vagina
vener/o	sexual contact
vesicul/o	seminal vesicle
vulv/o	vulva

Figure 8.50 These combining forms relate to the male and female reproductive systems.

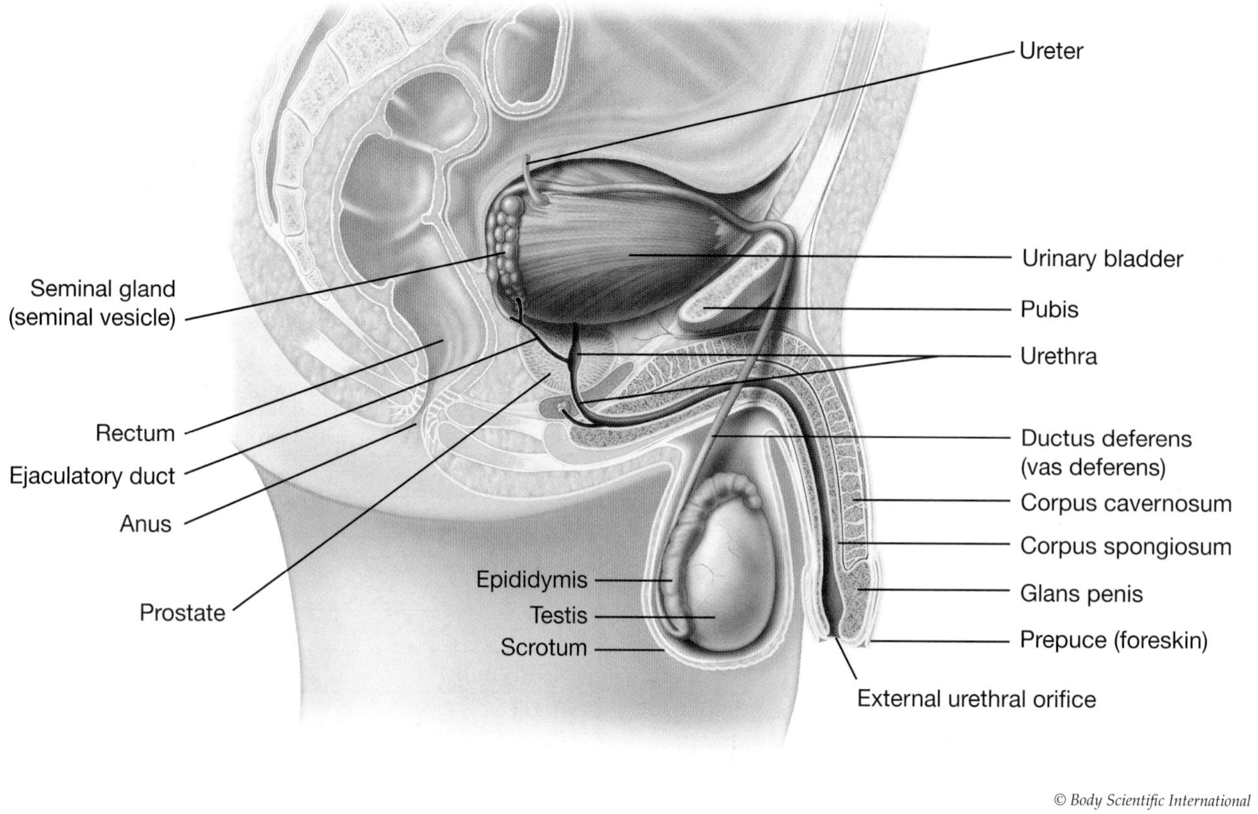
Ureter
Urinary bladder
Pubis
Urethra
Ductus deferens
(vas deferens)
Corpus cavernosum
Corpus spongiosum
Glans penis
Prepuce (foreskin)
External urethral orifice
Seminal gland
(seminal vesicle)
Rectum
Ejaculatory duct
Anus
Prostate
Epididymis
Testis
Scrotum
© Body Scientific International

Figure 8.51 The organs of the male reproductive system create and transport sperm.

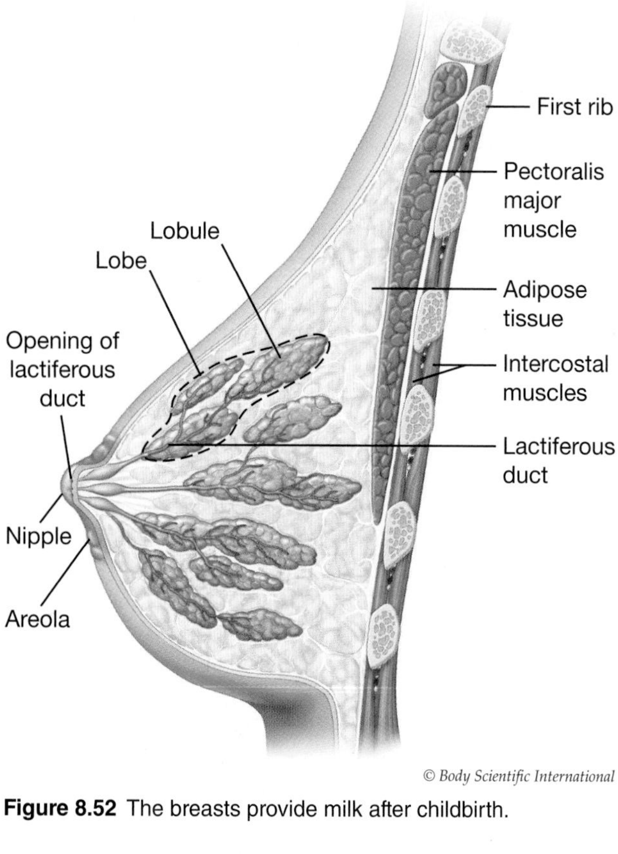
First rib
Pectoralis
major
muscle
Lobule
Lobe
Adipose
tissue
Opening of
lactiferous
duct
Intercostal
muscles
Lactiferous
duct
Nipple
Areola
© Body Scientific International

Figure 8.52 The breasts provide milk after childbirth.

Female Reproductive System

Like its male counterpart, the female reproductive system has both external and internal organs and structures. The external structures include the breasts, vulva, labia, and clitoris. Internal structures include the vagina, uterus, fallopian tubes, and ovaries.

External Female Reproductive Organs

The primary external female reproductive organs are the mammary glands, or *breasts* (Figure 8.52). Breasts change in size and function during puberty, during pregnancy, and after childbirth. On the outsides of the breasts are nipples surrounded by dark areas called *areolas*. Within the breasts are lobes, and each lobe contains lobules. Lobules produce breastmilk after childbirth. The milk produced by lobules is carried to the nipples via *lactiferous ducts*. Layers of fat (adipose) tissue surround the internal structures of the breast.

In females, the external genitalia is called the *vulva*. The vulva includes the *mons pubis*, where pubic hair grows (Figure 8.53). Two pairs of skin folds called the *labia* protect the vulva, vagina, and urethra from pathogens. Each outer fold of the labia is a *labium majus* (collectively called the *labia majora*). Each inner fold is a *labium minus* (collectively called the *labia minora*). Between the labia minora is the *vestibule*, an area that contains the openings of the urethra (meatus) and vagina. Glands on the sides of the vaginal opening

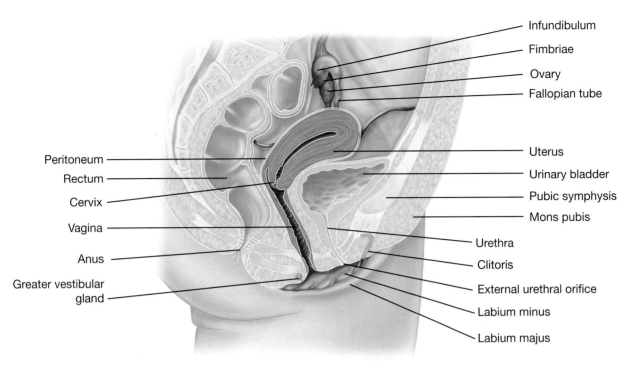

Peritoneum

Rectum

Cervix

Vagina

Anus

Greater vestibular
gland

Infundibulum

Fimbriae

Ovary

Fallopian tube

Uterus

Urinary bladder

Pubic symphysis

Mons pubis

Urethra

Clitoris

External urethral orifice

Labium minus

Labium majus

© Body Scientific International

Figure 8.53 This side view of the female reproductive system shows both the external and internal female reproductive organs.

secrete mucus for lubrication. Also located at the anterior end of the vestibule is the *clitoris*, which is composed of erectile tissue.

Internal Female Reproductive Organs

The *vagina* is a flexible, tubelike structure with a mucous lining (Figure 8.54). The vagina conducts monthly menstrual flow, receives sperm during intercourse, and serves as the birth canal. The vagina extends into the body and is attached to the uterus at the cervix. The *uterus*, a hollow, muscular organ, is sometimes called the *womb*. It is located between the urinary bladder and rectum. The uterus has a mucous lining and a rich blood supply.

The two ovaries located in the pelvic cavity are filled with ova (*eggs*), the female sex cells. The ova grow within fluid-filled sacs called *follicles*. Once a female reaches puberty, she starts ovulating, and ova are released into the fallopian tubes. This process is aided by follicle-stimulating hormone (FSH), luteinizing hormone (LH), and estrogen.

Two fallopian tubes extend from the ovaries to the top of the uterus. The fallopian tubes transport ova that have been released from the ovaries during ovulation. Small, hairlike projections in the fallopian tubes capture ova and move them toward the uterus. If an ovum is not fertilized by a sperm, it will be removed from the uterus during *menstruation*, the monthly shedding of the uterine lining. If the ovum is fertilized, it will implant in the body of the uterus. The uterus provides the "home" for a *fetus*, or unborn child. The uterus has enough elasticity to manage the growth of a fetus for an average of 40 weeks.

DNA and Reproduction

Deoxyribonucleic acid (DNA) plays an important role in reproduction. DNA molecules are found within the nucleus of every human cell. The complete set of DNA is known as the *genome*. The genome contains the instructions needed for an organism to reproduce, develop, and survive. It also contains the biological instructions that make each of us unique. Each DNA sequence that contains these instructions is called a *gene*.

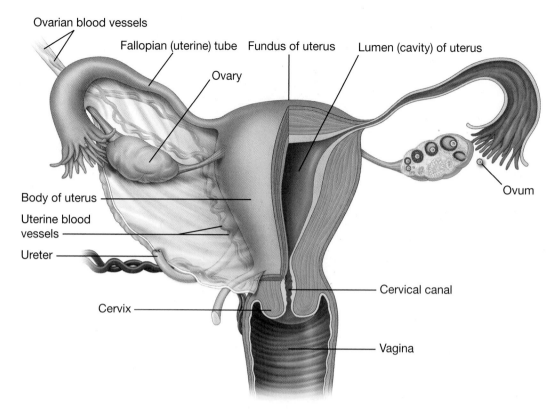

Figure 8.54 The internal organs of the female reproductive system create and transport ova and can house a developing fetus.

Ovarian blood vessels
Fallopian (uterine) tube
Fundus of uterus
Lumen (cavity) of uterus
Ovary
Ovum
Body of uterus
Uterine blood vessels
Ureter
Cervical canal
Cervix
Vagina

© Body Scientific International

DNA molecules are tightly packaged and only unwind when DNA replication occurs. When DNA molecules are packaged, they are called *chromosomes*. The complete DNA genome has approximately 20,000 genes on 23 pairs of chromosomes. When reproduction occurs, humans inherit half of their DNA from their fathers and half from their mothers.

How Do Lifestyle Choices and Aging Affect Body Systems?

Not only are people responsible for forming opinions about their health and levels of wellness or illness, but they also make lifestyle choices that ultimately affect the body's health as they age. For instance, maintaining a healthy weight during adulthood and exercising regularly will help prevent certain diseases and conditions,

Healthcare Scenario
Pharmacogenomics

John recently read a report online about a local company that was offering people the opportunity to learn about their DNA. The company was offering to analyze an individual's genome using a sample of saliva. The program, called "Getting to Know Your Genome," claimed it could help individuals be more aware of their genetic risks. It also claimed that individuals would learn how to choose the best medications and doses as part of a new science called pharmacogenomics.

Apply It

1. Identify the possible advantages of John and his family participating in this program.

2. What possible disadvantages might John and his family experience if they decide to participate in this program?

such as diabetes, that often come with age. Exercise also increases mobility and balance, which help people avoid the risk of falling. As another example, smoking as a young adult may create a compromised respiratory system later in life and lead to breathing problems, such as chronic obstructive pulmonary disease (COPD).

Even if people follow the best health practices and make the best lifestyle choices, the body will change with age. These changes include alterations in the structures and functions of individual cells and major body systems.

Changes to Cells, Tissues, and Organs

When cells age, they begin to function poorly or even abnormally. Cells also die as a part of normal bodily processes, usually to make room for new cells. Cells also die because they can only divide and multiply a limited number of times over a lifetime. If a cell cannot divide, it will grow larger and then die. Cells will also die if they are damaged by harmful substances such as sunlight, radiation, or certain medications.

Body tissues also change with age. For example, connective tissue becomes stiff. This causes organs and airways to become more rigid, which makes it more difficult for the body to breathe and receive adequate nutrition. Tissue can also shrink (*atrophy*) or develop lumps called *nodules*.

Because of cell and tissue changes, organs also change and begin to function less effectively. Most bodily functions peak shortly before age 30 and then begin to gradually decline. As we age, our organs do not have the same capacity to function as they once did. Overworking a weak organ can result in damage to the organ or even organ failure.

Over time, the most significant organ changes occur in the heart, lungs, and kidneys. Not all organs lose a large number of cells or lose capacity, however. For example, healthy individuals do not lose as many brain cells as unhealthy individuals. Losses in brain cells may occur due to damage, such as a stroke, Alzheimer's disease, or Parkinson's disease. Often, the aging of one organ also affects the functions of other organs. A person with rigid or narrow blood vessels may also experience breathing problems because the cardiovascular and respiratory systems share the responsibility of oxygen transport.

Becoming a Holistic Nursing Assistant
The Effects of Aging

Aging has many consequences on the human body. A resident's physical dexterity and movement can be greatly affected. A resident's appearance may also change, and personal hygiene and eating may be less of a concern. As people age, reading and oral communication may slow down, and people may become frustrated with their slowness and memory changes. Attention to detail and the ability to organize information may lessen or deteriorate, leading to changes in daily habits, personal interests, and even the desire to drive. Some people may avoid older adults and believe they are less interesting. Older adults may also lose their interests in interacting with others.

Changes that residents experience due to aging can have a significant impact and can greatly influence residents' lifestyles, needs, and desires.

As a holistic nursing assistant, you must be sensitive to residents' responses to aging. You should also look out for opportunities to promote residents' well-being and support their physical, emotional, and spiritual needs.

Apply It

1. Have you had experiences with older adults? If you have, what have you noticed about how older adults deal with their physical and mental changes?

2. If you were asked to care for an older adult, what could you do to help the adult improve his or her physical activity or lifestyle?

3. Now that you know the effects of aging, what efforts can you make to slow down your aging process?

The Aging Body

Remember

*It's not how old you are,
it's how you are old.*

Jules Renard, French author

All people age differently; however, the first signs of aging usually involve the skeletal and muscular systems. As people age, they begin to lose bone density, lose balance, and have problems with mobility. These signs may be followed by changes in the eyes and ears. If people invest in maintaining and actively using their bodies when they are younger, the aging process may be delayed. Figure 8.55 outlines common changes associated with age in each body system.

Body System Changes with Age	
Body System	**Signs of Aging**
Integumentary system	• Skin tears, bruises, and takes longer to heal. • The ability to tolerate cold decreases. • Old-age spots appear on the skin. • Blood flow to the skin decreases. • Skin becomes dry. • Nerve endings become less sensitive to sensations such as pain. • Skin has a harder time converting sunlight to vitamin D. • Hair thins and becomes gray or white. • Fingernails become rigid and may yellow or split. • Toenails change shape and thicken.
Skeletal system	• Bone loss occurs (called *osteoporosis*). • The face may sag, and eyes appear to shrink into the head. • Vertebral degeneration at the top of the spine causes the head to tip forward. • Cartilage lining the joints thins, loosens, and becomes less flexible. • Lubricating fluid in the joints depletes, causing ligaments to harden.
Muscular system	• Muscle tissue and strength starts decreasing at age 30. • Fast-contracting muscle fibers lessen in activity. • The number and size of muscle fibers permanently decrease. • Muscle is replaced by fatty or fibrous tissue, making muscles stiff. • Muscle is replaced by body fat. This changes the shape of the body its in.
Nervous system	• Changes in the myelin sheath cause chemical messages in the brain to slow down. • Sensation and strength may decrease. • Blood flow to the brain decreases. • The cerebellum may deteriorate, causing loss of balance. • By age 70, short-term memory, the learning of new material, and recall may be more difficult.
Sensory system	• The lens of the eye stiffens, making it harder to focus on close objects. • The lens becomes denser, and it is more difficult to see in dim light. • The lens yellows, changing the way colors are perceived. • Sensitivity to glare increases. • The eyes produce less fluid and tears, making them feel dry. • Tiny black specks (floaters) move across the field of vision. • Changes in ear structure and nerve cells cause age-related hearing loss. • Inner ear structures stiffen and deteriorate slightly, making a person unsteady. • Hearing worsens, making it harder to hear high- and low-pitched sounds.

(continued)

Figure 8.55 Aging affects all of the body systems.

Body System Changes with Age

Body System	Signs of Aging
Endocrine system	• The thyroid may shrink and function less effectively with age. • Metabolism of sugar and carbohydrates is less effective. • Levels and activity of growth hormones decrease. • Metabolism of fat, cholesterol, calcium, and vitamin D may be altered.
Cardiovascular system	• Heart muscles reduce in size, and blood vessels become stiff and less elastic. • Plaque accumulates on the insides of the arteries (*atherosclerosis*). • Arteries harden and lose their elasticity (*arteriosclerosis*). • The amount of bone marrow decreases. • Blood cell production slows.
Immune and lymphatic systems	• The thymus slows down. • Cells are less able to destroy pathogens and other foreign substances.
Respiratory system	• Alveoli, airways, and tissues lose elasticity and become more rigid. • The diaphragm weakens. • Pathogen-fighting cells fail, making it harder for the lungs to fight infection. • A person's cough weakens, making it harder to clear the lungs.
Gastrointestinal system	• Muscles in the esophagus weaken, sometimes causing problems with swallowing. • The stomach is less elastic and holds a smaller amount of food. • Less lactase (an enzyme needed to digest milk) is produced. • Food moves more slowly through the large intestine. • Liver enzymes function less effectively. • Taste buds lose sensitivity. • The sense of smell lessens. • Mouth dryness increases because less saliva is produced. • Dry mouth and loss of taste and smell reduce the ability to taste food. • Teeth weaken and become brittle, and tooth enamel tends to erode. • Gums may start to recede, causing the gumline to become exposed.
Urinary system	• The number of kidney cells decreases, causing the kidneys to shrink in size. • Fewer nephrons filter the removal of waste products. • Bladder volume can shrink by one-half, causing more frequent urination. • Overactive bladder muscles may cause a feeling of needing to urinate, and muscles can weaken so the bladder is not completely emptied. • Weakened urinary sphincter muscles may cause leakage. • The prostate gland may enlarge, interfering with the passage of urine. • Older men may experience a longer start to their urine streams, have less force when urinating, and dribble at the end of urination.
Reproductive systems	• Estrogen levels decrease, causing the ovaries and uterus to become smaller and the vagina to become thinner, drier, and less flexible. • Breasts may become less firm and more fibrous and often will sag. • Male sex drive decreases. • Less sperm are produced. • Erectile dysfunction may occur due to changes in aging blood vessel circulation.

Figure 8.55 (*Continued*)

Using the Key Terms

Complete the following sentences using key terms in this section.

1. B cells secrete _____, which reduce the effects of bacteria and viruses.
2. Disease-causing microorganisms are known as _____.
3. Hormones secreted by exocrine glands are transported through _____ to other organs in the body.
4. Circular muscles known as _____ help regulate the flow of urine out of the body.
5. The pancreas secretes _____, or chemical agents, that aid digestion.
6. Hair _____ are small sacs or cavities that contain hair.
7. A(n) _____ is a group of specialized cells that secrete substances.
8. The liquid component of blood is known as _____.
9. _____ are the components of the blood responsible for oxygen and carbon dioxide exchange.
10. The _____ is the outermost layer of the skin.
11. The components of the blood that fight infection and provide protection are _____.
12. _____ enable the blood to clot.
13. When taking a(n) _____, you are measuring the beat of the heart through the walls of a peripheral artery.

Know and Understand the Facts

14. Which organ is primarily responsible for breathing?
15. Which body systems are responsible for body movement?
16. Describe how the urinary system excretes waste.
17. List one lifestyle habit that can be changed to delay the aging of a body system.
18. Identify two organs that are affected by aging and explain how they change.
19. Identify the five word parts used to form medical terms.
20. Describe the difference between Fowler's, lateral, prone, and supine positions.

Analyze and Apply Concepts

21. Select one body system and describe the locations and functions of its organs.
22. Form and define three medical terms for each of the 12 body systems.
23. Identify two body systems whose organs work together to achieve a particular function and describe that function.
24. Explain how the hormones of the endocrine system regulate body functions.

Think Critically

Read the following care situation. Then answer the questions that follow.

Sixteen-year-old Lawrence was hospitalized last night after a very bad car accident. His right humerus, wrist, ankle, and two ribs are fractured. He has many bruises and cuts on his face and neck, and there is R/O concussion. Prior to the accident, Lawrence was being treated for hypothyroidism. His VS show that he has tachypnea, and he is complaining of dysuria.

25. Identify and define each of the medical terms and abbreviations used in this care situation.
26. Which body systems will be affected by Lawrence's accident?
27. List three body functions that will be affected by Lawrence's injuries.

Word Parts

Combining Forms

Combining Form (Root Word Plus Combining Vowel)	Meaning	Combining Form (Root Word Plus Combining Vowel)	Meaning
anter/o	front	infer/o	below
arthr/o	joint	later/o	side
bi/o	life	lip/o	fat
cardi/o; card/o	heart	log/o	study
caud/o	tail	medi/o	middle
cephal/o	head	my/o	muscle
cervic/o	neck; cervix (neck of uterus)	neur/o	nerve
col/o; colon/o	colon; large intestine	path/o	disease
cost/o	rib	pneum/o	lung; air; gas
cyt/o	cell	poster/o	back; behind
dist/o	away from the point of origin	proxim/o	near the point of origin; close
dors/o	back of the body	sarc/o	connective tissue
enter/o	intestine (small)	super/o	above
gastr/o	stomach	thorac/o	chest
glyc/o	sugar	ventr/o	front side of the body
hepat/o	liver	viscer/o	internal organ
hist/o	tissue		

Combining Forms

Prefix	Meaning	Prefix	Meaning
a-; an-	not; without	eu-	good
ab-	away from	exo-	outward
ad-	toward	hemi-	half
ante-	before	hetero-	different
anti-	against	homo-	same
auto-	self	hyper-	above normal; excessive
bi-	two; both	hypo-	below normal; less than
brady-	slow	in-	into
circum-	around	infra-	beneath; below; under
con-	together	inter-	between
dia-	through; complete	intra-	within; into
dis-	apart; abnormal	macro-	large
dorsi-	back	mega-	big
dys-	bad; difficult; painful	meta-	change; after
ec-	outside	micro-	small
echo-	reflected sound	mono-	one
en-; em-	in; within	neo-	new
endo-	in; within	non-	not
epi-	on; over; upon	pan-	all
eso-	inward	para-	near; beside

(continued)

Combining Forms

Prefix	Meaning	Prefix	Meaning
per-	through	supra-	above; over
peri-	around; surrounding	syn-	together; with
poly-	many	tachy-	fast
post-	after; behind	trans-	across
pro-	forward; in front of	tri-	three
quadri-	four	ultra-	beyond; excess
sub-	below; under		

Combining Forms

Suffix	Meaning	Suffix	Meaning
-ac; -al; -ar; -ary; -atic; -iac; -ial; -ic; -ical; -ior; -ory; -ous; -tic	pertaining to	-ectomy	surgical removal
-algesia	pain; sensitivity	-edema	swelling
-algia	pain	-ema	condition
-ant	substance that promotes	-emesis	vomiting
-arche	beginning	-emia	blood condition
-ase	enzyme	-emic	pertaining to blood condition
-assay	analyze	-esthesia	condition of feeling or sensation
-asthenia	weakness	-fusion	to pour
-ation	process	-gen	substance that produces
-blast	developing cell	-genesis	formation
-capnia	carbon dioxide	-genic	produced by; in
-cele	swelling; protrusion	-gram	record; image
-centesis	procedure to remove fluid	-graphy	process of recording
-chezia	defecation	-gravida	pregnant
-clysis	irrigation; washing	-ia; -ism	condition
-crit	to separate	-in; -ine	chemical
-cusis	hearing	-ion	process
-cyte	cell	-ist	specialist
-dipsia	thirst	-itis	inflammation
-dynia	pain	-lepsy	seizure or sudden attack
-ectasis	dilation; expansion	-logist	one who specializes in the study

(continued)

Combining Forms

Suffix	Meaning	Suffix	Meaning
-logy	study of	**-poiesis**	formation
-lysis	breaking down	**-porosis**	condition of small holes
-lytic	pertaining to breakdown or destruction	**-prandial**	meal
-malacia	softening	**-ptosis**	droop; sag
-megaly	enlargement	**-rrhage**	rupture
-meter	measure	**-rrhaphy**	suture
-metry	process of measuring	**-rrhea**	flow
-oid	like; resembling	**-salpinx**	fallopian tube
-oma	tumor	**-sclerosis**	hardening
-opia	vision condition	**-scope**	instrument used to view
-opsy	view of	**-scopy**	visual examination with a scope
-orexia	appetite	**-sis**	state; condition
-osis	abnormal condition	**-spasm**	muscle contraction
-osmia	smell	**-stalsis**	contraction
-otia	ear condition	**-stasis**	stoppage of flow
-paresis	weakness	**-stenosis**	narrowing
-partum	childbirth	**-stitial**	standing; positioned
-pathy	disease	**-stomy**	new opening
-penia	decrease; deficiency	**-taxia**	muscle coordination
-pepsia	digestion	**-tension**	pressure
-pexy	surgical fixation	**-therapy**	treatment
-phagia	eating; swallowing	**-thorax**	chest
-phasia	speech	**-tomy**	incision
-pheresis	removal	**-trophy**	condition of growth
-phoresis	transmission	**-tropic**	turning
-plasia	development; formation	**-tropin**	hormone
-plasm	formation; structure	**-tripsy**	process of crushing
-plasty	surgical repair	**-um; -us**	structure; thing; membrane
-plegia	paralysis	**-uria**	condition of urine
-plegic	pertaining to paralysis	**-version**	to turn
-pnea	breathing	**-y**	process of

Key Points

Reviewing the key points for this chapter will help you practice more safely and competently as a holistic nursing assistant and will help you prepare for the certification competency examination.

- Holistic nursing assistants use medical terminology daily to make observations, understand and provide descriptions, and receive and give instructions about care.

- Specific terms refer to body cavities, body positions, and planes of the body. There are also terms that refer to body directions and movements. Cells, membranes, and tissues are the foundation of life and have unique and specific functions.

- The body systems include the integumentary, skeletal, muscular, nervous, sensory, endocrine, cardiovascular, lymphatic and immune, gastrointestinal, respiratory, urinary, and reproductive systems. These body systems work independently and as a whole.

- People make lifestyle choices that ultimately affect their health as they grow older. While following best health practices helps the aging process, the body will change regardless. Changes will occur in the structures and functions of individual cells and major body systems.

Action Steps to Holistic Care

Review the information in this chapter. Complete the following activities.

1. As a nursing assistant, you will be expected to know many medical abbreviations and acronyms. Using Figure 6.1 as a guide, create flashcards by writing the abbreviation or acronym on one side and the definition on the other. Then review these with a partner.

2. Research one body system and describe two facts about the system that were not discussed in this chapter.

3. With a partner, prepare a poster about the structure or function of a body system or organ. List the information that is most important to know when providing care.

4. Find two pictures in a magazine, in a newspaper, or online that best demonstrate the aging process. Explain why you selected these images.

5. Body systems often work together to achieve homeostasis. Identify two body systems that work together, explain their relationship, the contributions of each system, and the shared goal. Then prepare a report outlining your findings.

Preparing for the Certification Competency Examination

To prepare for the nursing assistant certification competency examination, you will need to know content found in this chapter. This content may be tested in the knowledge (written or oral) and skills (hands-on demonstration) portions of the exam. The following areas will be emphasized:

- medical terminology and abbreviations
- the structure of the body and body systems, including cells, tissues, and organs
- the functions and normal aging of the following body systems: integumentary, muscular, skeletal, respiratory, cardiovascular, nervous, sensory, lymphatic and immune, gastrointestinal, endocrine, urinary, and reproductive systems

These sample test questions are similar to ones you will find on the certification competency exam. See how well you can answer them. Be sure to select the *best* answer.

1. Which of the following is the smallest structural and functional unit of the human body?
   - A. tissue
   - B. membrane
   - C. cell
   - D. organ

2. What is the medical abbreviation for *activities of daily living*?
   - A. ACLs
   - B. ACDLs
   - C. ADALs
   - D. ADLs

3. A nursing assistant is asked to write the medical term meaning "disease of the nerves." Which of the following terms should he or she use?

   A. neuralgia
   B. neuropathy
   C. arthroscopy
   D. arthritis

4. What is a ligament?

   A. a fibrous cord of tissue that attaches bone to bone
   B. a fibrous cord of tissue that attaches muscle to bone
   C. a fibrous cord of tissue that attaches muscles to vessels
   D. a fibrous cord of tissue that attaches bone to nerves

5. You are taking care of Mr. M, an 85-year-old resident. He shares that his eyes feel very dry and itchy. Why might this be happening?

   A. aging of his skin and eyes
   B. playing cards too much
   C. being out in the sun
   D. not using glasses for reading

6. The medical term *arthritis* is composed of a(n)

   A. root word and prefix
   B. prefix and suffix
   C. root word and suffix
   D. root word and combining vowel

7. A nursing assistant strained a muscle in his arm when helping move a resident. Which type of muscle did he injure?

   A. synovial muscle
   B. involuntary muscle
   C. smooth muscle
   D. skeletal muscle

8. A new nursing assistant is asked to turn Mrs. A. She will be using the muscles in her arms and legs. For her muscles to contract, which of the following must occur?

   A. opposition between an agonist and antagonist
   B. alignment with her striated and smooth muscles
   C. opposition between abduction and adduction actions
   D. alignment with the tendons and ligaments

9. Which of the following is a change associated with the aging process?

   A. Skin becomes thick and calloused.
   B. Skin becomes less sensitive to pain.
   C. Skin becomes very hairy.
   D. Skin becomes very flexible.

10. Which of the following directs all of a cell's activities?

    A. mitochondria
    B. ribosome
    C. nucleus
    D. chromosome

11. Which of the following cells helps blood clot?

    A. fibrinogen
    B. red blood cell
    C. white blood cell
    D. platelet

12. Which of the following terms describes the front part of the body?

    A. ventral
    B. dorsal
    C. coronal
    D. proximal

13. Which word part is the central part of a medical term?

    A. suffix
    B. prefix
    C. acronym
    D. root word

14. Mrs. M has arthritis and cannot ambulate well. As a result, she has trouble having bowel movements. Which part of her gastrointestinal tract is affected?

    A. large intestine
    B. gallbladder
    C. esophagus
    D. small intestine

15. Which of the following terms is used to describe the structure of the human body?

    A. chemistry
    B. physiology
    C. biology
    D. anatomy

Did you have difficulty with any of the questions? If you did, review the chapter to find the correct answer(s).

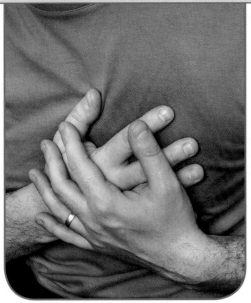

andriano.cz/Shutterstock.com

Welcome to the Chapter

As a holistic nursing assistant, you will provide safe, quality care for patients and residents who are experiencing various diseases and conditions. This presents both challenges and rewards. In this chapter, you will learn the signs, symptoms, treatments, and care considerations for the diseases and conditions you will most often encounter when providing care. The body systems discussed in chapter 8 provide the framework for this discussion. You will also learn relevant medical terminology and abbreviations.

Diseases and conditions often cause pain. Understanding the nature of pain and knowing the best ways to observe and report it will provide you with the knowledge and skills you will need to promote comfort.

What you learn in this chapter will help you develop your knowledge and skills to become a holistic nursing assistant. The topics discussed in the chapter are highlighted on the Providing Holistic Care Framework.

You are now ready to start this chapter, *Diseases, Conditions, and Pain*.

Chapter Outline

Section 9.1
Common Diseases and Conditions

Section 9.2
Pain Relief

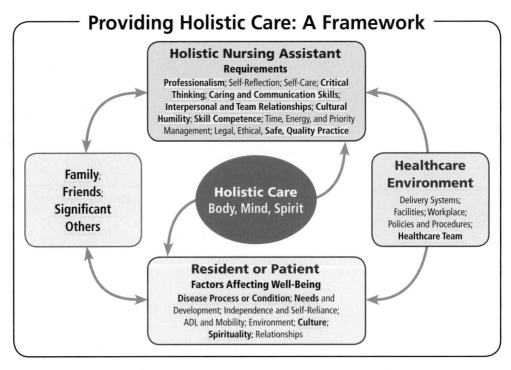

Providing Holistic Care: A Framework

Holistic Nursing Assistant
Requirements
Professionalism; Self-Reflection; Self-Care; **Critical Thinking**; **Caring and Communication Skills**; **Interpersonal and Team Relationships**; **Cultural Humility**; **Skill Competence**; Time, Energy, and Priority Management; Legal, Ethical, **Safe, Quality Practice**

Family; Friends; Significant Others

Holistic Care
Body, Mind, Spirit

Healthcare Environment
Delivery Systems; Facilities; Workplace; Policies and Procedures; **Healthcare Team**

Resident or Patient
Factors Affecting Well-Being
Disease Process or Condition; **Needs** and Development; Independence and Self-Reliance; ADL and Mobility; Environment; **Culture**; **Spirituality**; Relationships

Objectives

To achieve the objectives for this section, you must successfully

- **explain** the difference between acute and chronic diseases and conditions;
- **identify** the signs and symptoms of common diseases and conditions for each body system;
- **describe** the treatments and care considerations for common diseases and conditions; and
- **use** medical abbreviations and terminology associated with the diseases and conditions discussed in this section.

Key Terms

Learn these key terms to better understand the information presented in the section.

abrasion	hypertension
abscess	immobility
acute disease	incontinence
analgesic	inflammation
anesthetic	ischemia
aneurysm	lesions
aphasia	malignant
arrhythmias	metastasis
arteriosclerosis	monotone
atherosclerosis	morbidity
benign	mortality
biopsy	necrosis
catheter	nodules
chronic disease	pathology
coma	plaques
condition	predisposition
decubitus ulcer	sclerosis
dialysis	sign
edema	symptom
fistula	topical
flares	ultrasound
hemiplegia	

Questions to Consider

- Living with a disease or medical condition can be very challenging and difficult. Do you know someone who is living with a serious or chronic disease or condition? If so, what has this person told you about the experience?
- What changes has the person made to accommodate the disease or condition? Have these changes been helpful?

How Do Diseases and Conditions Differ?

In the United States today, the average life expectancy at birth is 78.8 years—81.2 years for women and 76.4 years for men. Rates of **mortality** (the numbers of deaths) show that the top 10 causes of death are heart disease, cancer, chronic lower respiratory disease, accidents (unintentional injuries), cerebrovascular accidents (strokes), Alzheimer's disease, diabetes, influenza and pneumonia, nephritis and nephrosis, and suicide.

Rates of **morbidity** (the number of people who have a disease) show that the most common diseases and conditions in the United States include heart disease, stroke, cancer, type 2 diabetes, obesity, and arthritis.

Defining Diseases and Conditions

Think About This

According to recent reports, heart disease is the leading cause of death for Caucasian, African-American, American Indian, and Alaska Native populations. Heart disease is the second leading cause of death for Asian populations or Pacific Islanders. Cancer is the leading cause of death for Asian or Pacific Islander populations and the second leading cause for Caucasians, African-Americans, American Indians, and Alaska Natives. For Hispanic populations, cancer is the leading cause of death, and heart disease is the second leading cause of death.

As you learned in chapter 7, a *disease* is a deviation from a normal, healthy state. Disease occurs when an organ or body system incorrectly functions and exhibits particular signs and symptoms. In contrast, the term **condition** refers to a particular physical or mental state of health or illness. For example, a person might say, "I have a heart condition," which means the person's heart may not be functioning properly. The person may have coronary artery disease due to a buildup of plaque in the arteries.

Classifying Diseases and Conditions

Diseases may be classified in a variety of ways. The purpose of classification is to examine commonalities and differences among diseases. Diseases are also classified as a way to study the trends, causes, and effects of certain diseases and conditions in particular populations. The following classifications discuss the causes of diseases:

- **Genetic or congenital disorder**: caused by a person's genes or by a birth event. Examples of genetic or congenital disorders include Down syndrome, sickle cell anemia, and cerebral palsy (Figure 9.1).
- **Infectious disease**: also called *pathogenic disease* and caused by microorganisms such as bacteria or viruses. Pathogenic microorganisms can be passed from person to person, transferred by an insect bite, or ingested from contaminated food or water. Examples of infectious diseases include hepatitis (caused by a virus) or tuberculosis (caused by bacteria).
- **Degenerative disease**: a result of cell breakdown over time, which causes changes in tissues and organs. Examples of degenerative diseases include arthritis and Parkinson's disease.
- **Nutritional disease**: a deficiency or excess in a person's diet. An example of a nutritional disease is rickets, which is caused by vitamin deficiency.
- **Cancer**: caused by the production of abnormal or excess body cells. Examples of cancers include melanoma, breast cancer, and leukemia.

Conditions are categorized using the body system or organ that is affected. For example, a person may have a skin or lung condition.

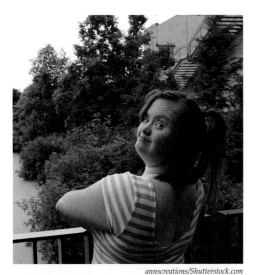

annscreations/Shutterstock.com

Figure 9.1 Down syndrome is an example of a genetic or congenital disorder.

What Are Acute and Chronic Diseases or Conditions?

Diseases or conditions can be acute or chronic. An **acute disease** is short-term and usually has an abrupt onset. A **chronic disease** is long-term or recurring.

Acute Diseases and Conditions

An acute disease or condition has a sudden onset and lasts a short amount of time. Examples of acute diseases or conditions include a cold or pneumonia, a bone fracture, or a skin rash. These diseases or conditions last only a few days or weeks. With treatment, they will go away or will not recur for a long time.

Chronic Diseases and Conditions

For a disease or condition to be classified as chronic, it must last for at least three months. Most chronic diseases and conditions, however, become lifetime challenges. Consider, for example, a person with arthritis. A person with arthritis has joint damage and lives with ongoing **inflammation** (swelling and redness) and pain. As another example, a person who has eczema (a skin condition) may have skin **lesions** (areas of damaged tissue) that worsen, stay the same, or improve for a period of time. Regardless, the person's condition will never go away. Recent statistics indicate that about one-half of all adults have one or more chronic diseases or conditions. One in four adults have two or more chronic diseases or conditions.

Living with any chronic disease or condition can be frightening and frustrating. A chronic disease will often last a lifetime and will require constant attention. Many people with chronic diseases or conditions go through periods of sadness, discouragement, hopelessness, anger, and depression.

When working with people who have chronic diseases or conditions, holistic nursing assistants must always try to be understanding. Nursing assistants should help these residents achieve the best possible quality of life and assist with minimizing daily challenges. Some strategies you may use as a holistic nursing assistant include

- being knowledgeable about a resident's disease or condition;
- observing and reporting changes in the resident's disease or condition to the licensed nursing staff;
- having a positive attitude and approach when providing care;
- encouraging healthful habits, such as good nutrition and exercise;
- suggesting healthy activities, such as reading, journal writing, listening to music, deep breathing, and meditation;
- promoting the resident's quality time with family and friends; and
- identifying useful sources of information and local support groups.

Care for Acute and Chronic Diseases or Conditions

The types of care, treatment, and healthcare facilities needed will differ between acute and chronic diseases or conditions. For example, care for acute diseases and conditions is typically short-term, and recovery is quick. The same is not true for people with chronic diseases or conditions. Chronic diseases or conditions require continuous care over a long period of time, and people may never recover. In fact, the disease or condition may get worse. For some people, a disease or condition may become *terminal*. Terminal illnesses cannot be cured and will result in death within a short period of time.

Acute and chronic diseases or conditions also require different types of health-care facilities. A person with an acute disease may enter a hospital through the emergency room due to the severity of the disease and the need for immediate care. A person with a chronic disease or condition will regularly see a doctor unless an

---

Becoming a Holistic Nursing Assistant
Helping Residents with Diseases or Conditions

Residents who have diseases or conditions, whether acute or chronic, may sometimes feel they are defined by their diseases or conditions. A resident may have been labeled or referred to as "Mrs. J, the resident who had a stroke" or "Mr. D, the resident with terrible skin lesions." Holistic nursing assistants must never define residents by their diseases or conditions. It is true that, as a holistic nursing assistant, you must be knowledgeable about a resident's disease, treatment plan, and care requirements. In the end,

however, residents are human beings who have feelings and emotions just like you.

Apply It
1. As a holistic nursing assistant, what can you do to be sure residents are not labeled?
2. Describe how you might demonstrate your care and support for residents who have diseases or conditions.

Abbreviations and Acronyms Related to Diseases and Conditions

Abbreviation or Acronym	Meaning
A-FIB	atrial fibrillation
ALS	amyotrophic lateral sclerosis
AIDS	acquired immunodeficiency syndrome
AMD	age-related macular degeneration
BPH	benign prostatic hypertrophy
CA	cancer
CABG	coronary artery bypass graft
CAD	coronary artery disease
CHF	congestive heart failure
COPD	chronic obstructive pulmonary disease
CP	chest pain
CSF	cerebrospinal fluid
CVA	cerebrovascular accident
EKG; ECG	electrocardiogram
GERD	gastroesophageal reflux disease
HBV	hepatitis B virus
HDL	high-density lipoprotein cholesterol
HIV	human immunodeficiency virus
HTN	hypertension
IBS	irritable bowel syndrome
LDL	low-density lipoprotein cholesterol
MI	myocardial infarction
MRI	magnetic resonance imaging
MS	multiple sclerosis
PE	pulmonary embolus
PVC	premature ventricular contraction
PVD	peripheral vascular disease
SLE	systemic lupus erythematosus
STD	sexually transmitted disease
STI	sexually transmitted infection
TB	tuberculosis
TIA	transient ischemic attack
URI	upper respiratory infection
UTI	urinary tract infection
VD	venereal disease
VF	ventricular fibrillation

Figure 9.2 Always reference your healthcare facility's policies to learn which abbreviations and acronyms are used in the facility.

acute episode occurs. If this happens, the person may need care in an emergency room. A chronic disease or condition may also become more severe and cause increasing loss of mobility. If this occurs, the person with the chronic disease may not be able to take care of himself or herself at home and may need to enter an assisted living or long-term care facility.

How Are Medical Terms, Abbreviations, and Acronyms Used to Describe Diseases and Conditions?

In chapter 8, you learned how to build medical terms using root words, prefixes, suffixes, and combining vowels. Suffixes are often used to form medical terms that describe diseases and conditions. For example, the suffix -itis means "inflammation," and the suffix -sclerosis means "hardening." Medical abbreviations and acronyms are also commonly used to describe various diseases and conditions (Figure 9.2).

How Are Diseases and Conditions Classified by Body System?

As you learned earlier in this chapter, diseases and conditions are often classified by cause. Another method for classifying diseases and conditions is by the affected body system. Each disease is associated with a particular **pathology**, or changes that occur in the body's tissues and organs as a result of the disease. Pathology includes a disease's signs and symptoms. A **sign** is a piece of objective, or factual, information about a disease or condition. A **symptom** is a piece of subjective information about a disease or condition based on a person's feelings or opinions. Each disease has unique signs, symptoms, treatments, and care considerations.

In this chapter, you will learn about the diseases and conditions you will most often encounter when you begin working as a nursing assistant. These diseases and conditions are classified by body system, signs, and symptoms. Care considerations are emphasized.

For many of these diseases and conditions, treatments include prescribed medications. If a resident is taking prescribed medications, be sure to observe the resident closely. If the resident deviates from his or her normal patterns—physically, mentally, or emotionally—he or she may be experiencing a side or adverse effect from the medication or an allergy or sensitivity to its chemical or natural ingredients. These observations need to be reported to the licensed nursing staff immediately so that action can be taken.

Which Diseases and Conditions Affect the Integumentary System?

Common diseases and conditions that affect the integumentary system (skin, hair, and nails) include keratosis, psoriasis, shingles, and decubitus ulcers. If a person has a skin disease or condition, a *dermatologist* (doctor who specializes in treating diseases, disorders, and injuries of the skin, hair, and nails) will likely be a key care provider. The licensed nursing staff and nursing assistants are usually responsible for carrying out a doctor's or dermatologist's instructions.

Keratosis

Keratosis is a condition in which there is too much *keratin* (a skin protein) in the skin. The two forms of keratosis discussed are keratosis pilaris and seborrheic keratosis.

Keratosis pilaris is a skin condition that cannot be prevented or cured. It is characterized by patches of thickened, dry skin; painless rough patches; and tiny bumps. Treatment usually consists of moisturizers, and in some cases, prescription creams to improve the skin's appearance.

As people age, they may also develop a noncancerous condition known as *seborrheic keratosis*. In seborrheic keratosis, round or oval-shaped growths appear on the body. These growths start as small, rough patches that develop into thick, wart-like growths. The growths look waxy and slightly raised (Figure 9.3). They are usually brown in color, but can also be yellow, white, or black.

Seborrheic keratosis runs in families, and increased exposure to the sun also increases risk. A growth should be surgically removed if it looks suspicious or is causing physical discomfort or emotional distress.

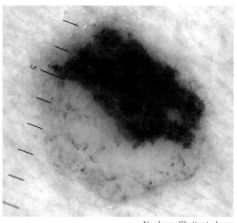

Nasekomoe/Shutterstock.com

A

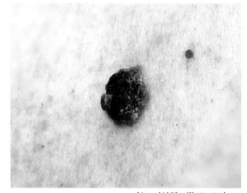

Lipowski Milan/Shutterstock.com

B

Figure 9.3 Unlike melanoma, or skin cancer, (A), seborrheic keratosis (B) causes raised, wart-like growths.

Psoriasis

Psoriasis is a condition characterized by the excessive growth of new skin cells on the top layer of the skin. This condition typically affects the knees, elbows, and scalp, but may also be found on the torso, palms, soles of the feet, and finger and toenails. In psoriasis, thick, red patches called **plaques** develop due to swollen blood vessels below the skin. Plaques are often covered with loose, silver-colored scales; may be accompanied by severe itchiness, called *pruritus*; and may be painful, crack, or bleed (Figure 9.4). Plaques can grow so large that they merge into one another, covering large areas of the body.

The direct cause of psoriasis is unknown. It may be an inherited defect of the immune system. **Flares**, or intensifications of the disease, are usually associated with a stressful situation or emotional trauma that triggers the immune response.

Treatments for psoriasis are primarily **topical**, or applied to the surface of the skin. These treatments include over-the-counter and prescription ointments, creams, and shampoos. Other treatments include oral and injectable medications and light therapies. Sunlight is also helpful for treating psoriasis, although sunscreen should be worn and sun exposure should be limited to 20 minutes daily, three days a week.

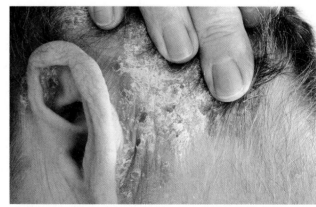

Lipowski Milan/Shutterstock.com

Figure 9.4 Psoriasis causes plaques, which are often covered with silver-colored scales.

The following are care considerations for residents with psoriasis. Always confirm with the licensed nursing staff that care considerations are consistent with facility policy, the doctor's orders, and the plan of care:

- Keep the skin moist and avoid itchiness by applying lotions or creams to the affected area. Use lotion less frequently in warm weather, as the combination of sweat and lotion can make psoriasis worse.
- Bathe the resident every other day or every third day using lukewarm water to avoid dry skin. Adding salts, oil, or finely ground oatmeal to the water will soothe the skin. After bathing, pat and do not rub the skin with a dry towel.
- Wrap the affected skin in bandage or plastic wrap and wash gently in the morning to reduce scaling.

Shingles

Shingles, or *herpes zoster*, is a painful skin rash caused by the varicella-zoster virus. The varicella-zoster virus also causes chickenpox. Everyone is at risk for shingles; however, shingles is more common among people who are over 50 years of age or who have weakened immune systems (due to stress or taking certain medications, for example).

Shingles itself is not contagious, although exposure to shingles blisters can cause chickenpox in people who have never had chickenpox or received its vaccine. Some people who get shingles get it only once, recover, and never have it again. Others may experience repeated episodes. There is now a vaccine for shingles. This vaccine lowers the chance that a person will have an episode of shingles. If a vaccinated person gets shingles anyway, the person will experience less pain and have a rash that clears more quickly.

Shingles symptoms typically develop in stages. The first stage is characterized by a headache and may be accompanied by light sensitivity and flu-like symptoms. The next stage includes tingling, itching, or pain in the area where a rash may appear. For some people, no rash appears; others have a mild rash; and yet others have a pronounced rash with fluid-filled blisters that crust over in two to four weeks and may leave scars (Figure 9.5). Shingles is treated with antiviral medications and **analgesics** (pain medications).

Following are general care considerations for residents with shingles:

- Keep any skin sores clean.
- Check the resident's pain levels and alert the licensed nursing staff if pain relief is needed.
- Remind the resident to take medications as prescribed.

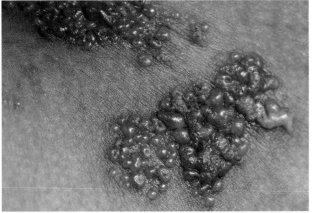

santol/Shutterstock.com

Figure 9.5 Shingles rashes often contain fluid-filled blisters.

Decubitus Ulcers

A **decubitus ulcer** is sometimes called a *bedsore*, *pressure ulcer*, or *pressure injury*. It is a skin condition caused by continuous pressure on the skin and on bony areas (or *projections*) that restricts blood circulation. Continuous pressure can result from resident **immobility** (inability to move) or from rubbing on the skin. Items that rub the skin may include bed covers, clothing, wrinkled or wadded-up sheets, tubing on or around the body, and even food crumbs in the bedding. Fragile skin is particularly susceptible to decubitus ulcers. Other risk factors for this condition are inability to feel pain, muscle spasms, poor nutrition, extreme weight loss, and **incontinence** (lack of bowel or bladder control).

Stages of Decubitus Ulcers

The appearance of a decubitus ulcer can range from a very mild, pink or red coloration of the skin to a severe wound that extends to bone and sometimes into internal organs. The severity of decubitus ulcers is identified using four stages (Figure 9.6):

- **Stage 1**: the skin is not open, but appears red on people with light complexions and blue or purple on people who have darker complexions.

- **Stage 2**: the decubitus ulcer is still considered superficial, or *shallow*, but the skin is now open. A blister filled with fluid, an **abrasion** (scraping of the outer layer of skin), or a shallow sore that looks like a crater can be seen, and the surrounding area may be irritated and red in color. As soon as the skin is broken, there is risk for *cellulitis*, or infection of the skin and connective tissue.

- **Stage 3**: the ulcer is much deeper than in stage 2 and may extend into underlying connective tissue. The sore looks more like a crater and may ooze, bleed, or contain pus.

- **Stage 4**: the damage is deep and may reach muscles, tendons, ligaments, joints, and bone. The ulcer will bleed, and skin and tissue **necrosis** (death) may occur. At this stage, there is risk not only of bone and joint infections, but also of system-wide infection leading to *sepsis* (a life-threatening infection in the bloodstream) and organ failure.

Stages of Decubitus Ulcers

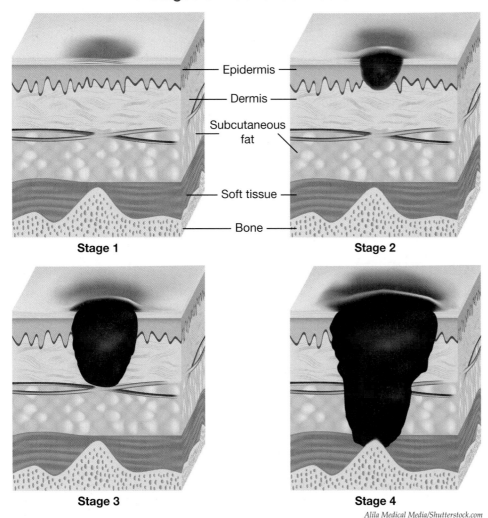

Alila Medical Media/Shutterstock.com

Figure 9.6 The stages of a decubitus ulcer are illustrated here.

Sometimes a decubitus ulcer is considered *unstageable*. This happens when the ulcer is covered by a mass of dead tissue or contains dry scabs. In these situations, it is difficult to see the depth of the ulcer, and therefore, its stage cannot be identified.

Pressure Points

Certain areas of the body are more likely to develop decubitus ulcers than others. These susceptible areas are known as *pressure points*. Pressure points can be found where skin covers the bony areas of the body (Figure 9.7).

Prevention, Treatment, and Care Considerations for Decubitus Ulcers

As a holistic nursing assistant, you should focus on preventing the formation of decubitus ulcers. To do this, provide good skin care each time a resident's position is changed. You will learn more about skin care in chapter 20, but basic guidelines follow:

- Keep pressure points dry and clean.
- Ulcers must be kept clean, and dressings should be applied when needed.
- Wet or creased dressings and bandages should be changed regularly.

When possible, and as directed by a doctor's order, help residents ambulate and perform range-of-motion exercises regularly. See chapter 17 for ambulation, range-of-motion (ROM) exercises, and positioning procedures. If a resident is immobile, the resident's position in bed or in a chair should be changed at least every two hours on a schedule, and support devices for positioning should be used. Bed linens should be smooth and free from crumbs.

In the event that a resident develops a decubitus ulcer, apply these guidelines:

- Help ensure good nutrition to promote wound healing.
- Assist with pain relief.
- Observe and report on the resident's condition, as needed. Note any existing ulcers upon admission. Immediately report any new redness or ulcers. Residents who have a healed decubitus ulcer are at higher risk of developing the same ulcer again.

How Do Diseases and Conditions Influence Skeletal System Function?

Diseases of the skeletal system may affect a resident's mobility, cause joint pain, and increase the risk for broken bones. Common skeletal diseases and conditions include osteoporosis, arthritis, and fractures.

Osteoporosis

Think About This

Bone is so strong that 1 cubic inch of bone can withstand 19,000 pounds or more, roughly the weight of five standard pickup trucks.

The term *osteoporosis* means "porous bones." Thus, osteoporosis is a condition in which the bones are *porous*, or full of holes (Figure 9.8). Osteoporosis occurs when the body makes too little bone or starts losing bone density, or *mass*. Bone cells are constantly regenerating; however, as people age, bone mass does not renew itself as quickly. This results in less bone density. Approximately 54 million people in the United States have osteoporosis and low bone mass. Other risk factors for osteoporosis include

- race;
- sex (women are more likely to develop osteoporosis due to hormonal changes);
- family history;
- lifestyle choices (sedentary activities, excessive alcohol consumption, and tobacco use increase the risk of developing osteoporosis);
- medical conditions, such as kidney or liver disease, arthritis, and cancer; and
- certain medications, such as steroids.

Pressure Points for Decubitus Ulcers

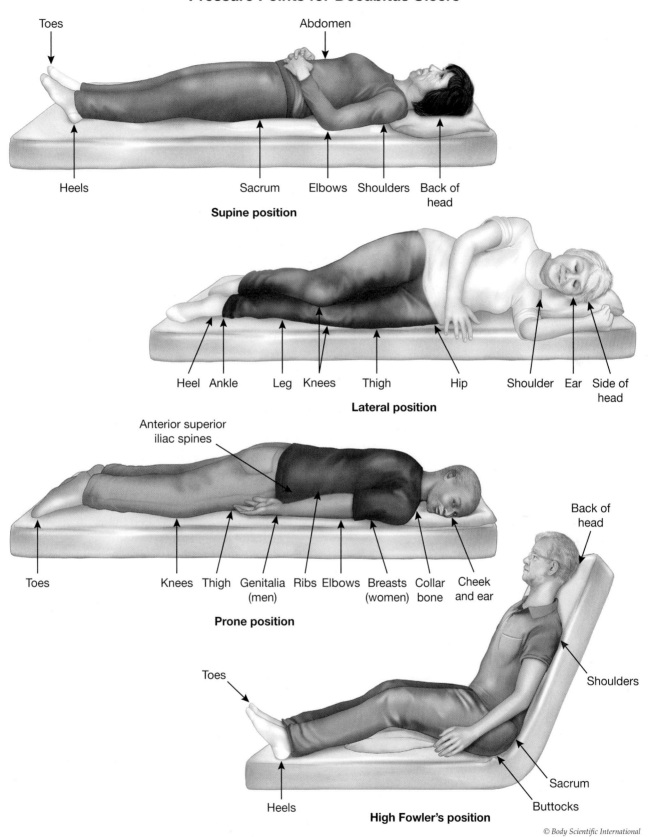

Supine position

Toes

Abdomen

Heels

Sacrum

Elbows

Shoulders

Back of head

Lateral position

Heel   Ankle   Leg   Knees   Thigh   Hip   Shoulder   Ear   Side of head

Prone position

Anterior superior iliac spines

Toes

Knees   Thigh   Genitalia (men)   Ribs   Elbows   Breasts (women)   Collar bone   Cheek and ear

High Fowler's position

Back of head

Shoulders

Toes

Heels

Sacrum

Buttocks

© *Body Scientific International*

Figure 9.7 Decubitus ulcers are more likely to develop at pressure points. Bed linens may create pressure points on the toes or abdomen if the resident is lying in supine position, for example.

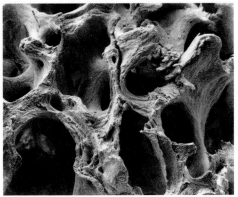

Dee Breger/Science Source

Figure 9.8 Osteoporotic bone is full of holes, as shown here.

Osteoporosis Symptoms

Osteoporosis is a silent disease. Symptoms usually do not occur until the bones begin to weaken, and then symptoms may include back pain and the loss of height if osteoporosis affects the vertebrae. As a result, some people with osteoporosis become stooped or hunched (Figure 9.9). Osteoporosis leads to a high risk of bone fractures, typically in the hip, spine, or wrist. A *bone density test* is performed to determine the presence of osteoporosis and also monitors the effectiveness of treatment.

Care Considerations for Osteoporosis

Lifestyle changes are usually recommended to treat osteoporosis. These lifestyle changes may include smoking cessation, increased physical activity, and a balanced diet. Some people who are at high risk for or who have osteoporosis are on prescription medications to both prevent and treat the disease. The plan of care for those with osteoporosis usually focuses on supporting a healthy lifestyle. People who have osteoporosis should eat a diet rich in calcium and vitamin D. A weight-bearing exercise plan is also recommended to prevent further bone loss and fractures. If a resident has osteoporosis, extra attention should be paid to how the resident is moved, positioned, and assisted with ambulation. The resident may need gentle assistance. In addition, fall-prevention strategies must be in place (see chapter 16).

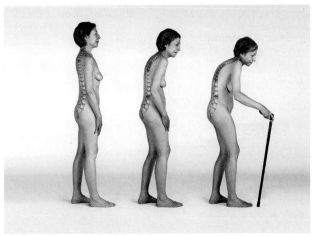

Gustoimages/Science Source

Figure 9.9 A person with osteoporosis can appear stooped or hunched.

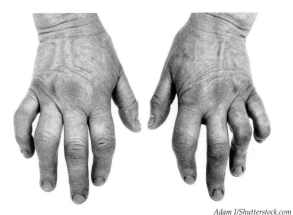

Adam J/Shutterstock.com

Figure 9.10 One effect of arthritis is inflammation of the joints.

Arthritis

Arthritis describes a variety of chronic diseases and conditions characterized by joint inflammation. Inflamed joints are usually swollen, tender, and red. Approximately one out of every five adults in the United States has been diagnosed with arthritis. This condition is a common cause of chronic pain, can lead to permanent joint changes, and is the leading cause of disability. Arthritis is often the result of lifelong joint use and repeated injury. While the risk of arthritis does increase with age, about two-thirds of people with arthritis are younger than 65. Arthritis is more common among women than men and affects all racial and ethnic groups.

Types of Arthritis

Some of the most common types of arthritis are osteoarthritis, rheumatoid arthritis, systemic lupus erythematosus (SLE or lupus), fibromyalgia, and gout. Common symptoms include pain, aching, stiffness, and swelling in or around joints, leading to decreased range of motion (Figure 9.10). The joints most commonly affected by arthritis are in the hands, lower back, hips, knees, and feet. Rheumatoid arthritis and lupus also affect multiple organs. Symptoms may appear suddenly or develop gradually.

Care Considerations for Arthritis

Treatment for arthritis centers on good lifestyle habits. For example, a healthy diet and exercise help maintain a normal weight, ensuring extra weight does not press on inflamed, sore joints. While exercise can be painful and tiring, it is very important for maintaining range of motion. Rest periods can help with endurance, and mobility aids can assist with stability, balance, and gait.

You can help residents who have arthritis become more comfortable by using positioning, giving a warm bath, and maintaining a restful environment. These actions will lead to better and more restful sleep and will help the resident conserve energy.

Pain is another consideration in treating arthritis. As a nursing assistant, you can assist the licensed nursing staff by providing routine information about pain levels. Support residents by combining prescribed pain-relief medications with nonmedical pain-relief techniques, as ordered by the doctor.

One method of nonmedical pain relief, which must be ordered by a doctor, is the use of warm and cold applications on affected joints. Dry or wet heat relaxes muscles and increases blood flow, or *circulation*. Some examples of applications are hot compresses, heating pads, heated pools, and warm baths and showers. Cold compresses or ice packs reduce swelling and numb the nerves to relieve pain. Both warm and cold applications should be used for no more than 20 minutes, so the skin can return to its normal temperature between applications. Observe whether warm or cold applications work best for a resident and report that information to the licensed nursing staff and document it in the resident's EMR. More information about warm and cold applications can be found in chapter 21.

Fractures

Both osteoporosis and arthritis can increase the risk of broken bones, or *fractures*. Fractures are common skeletal system conditions that can occur throughout life, but are more frequent for children and older adults, due to falls. Although the entire healthcare team will provide care in the case of a fracture, an orthopedist or orthopedic surgeon will likely be key care providers.

Fractures occur when an outside force is stronger than the bone on which it is exerting pressure, causing the bone to crack. Certain medications, lack of proper nutrition or activity, and osteoporosis can also lead to fractures, particularly in the hip. Women over 65 years of age have the highest risk of hip fractures. Some hip fractures are repaired surgically; in other cases, the hip is replaced with a prosthesis.

Types of Fractures

There are different types of fractures (Figure 9.11). In a *displaced fracture*, the bone snaps into two or more parts and moves so the bone itself is no longer in place. In a *nondisplaced fracture*, the bone does not move; rather, the fracture runs part or all of the way through the bone. In an *open fracture*, the bone breaks through the skin, which increases risk for infection. In a *closed fracture*, there is no puncture or open wound. Some fractures are considered *pathologic* because they are caused by the weakening of bones due to disease. A *stress fracture* is a hairline crack in a bone.

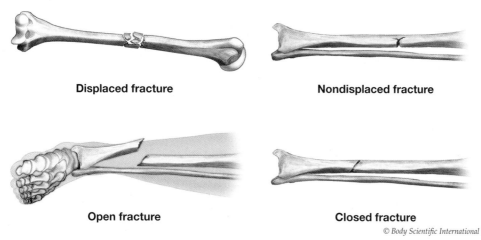

Displaced fracture   Nondisplaced fracture

Open fracture   Closed fracture

© Body Scientific International

Figure 9.11 Four types of fractures are illustrated here.

Care Considerations for Fractures

After a fracture occurs, a bone needs to be set, or positioned into its proper place, using a process called *reduction*. No surgery is required for a closed reduction; in a closed reduction, a plaster or fiberglass cast is used to immobilize the fractured bone. Sometimes bones need to be pinned together, which requires surgery through open reduction. In open reduction, rods, screws, or plates are used to properly position the bone before a cast is applied.

When a cast is applied, it needs to be kept dry to prevent a bad smell and skin irritation. Skin care will be needed at the edges of the cast. When caring for a resident with a cast, cover the cast with plastic and do not let water get under the cast during bathing. Keep the cast from becoming soiled if the resident uses a bedpan or urinal. Sometimes sprinkling baking soda or rubbing a fabric softener wipe on the outside of the cast can help reduce any odor. Remind residents to never push items such as hangers or pencils under the cast if the skin is itching. This can damage the skin and dislocate the cast.

Casts must never restrict circulation. Observation of a resident with a cast is extremely important. When caring for a resident, ask if there is numbness and tingling, which are signs of restricted circulation. Feel the exposed area outside of the cast to determine if it is cold; this may also indicate restricted circulation. Another sign of restricted circulation is a pale or bluish tinge (called *cyanosis*) to the skin.

Infection may occur under a cast. When observing a resident, note if the skin around the cast is unusually warm or if there is odor or drainage coming from under the cast. A resident with an infection may also experience chills or a fever. Immediately report any of these signs to the licensed nursing staff.

Supportive devices such as pillows, trochanter rolls, and footboards can be used to provide proper positioning and comfort for a resident in a cast. See chapter 17 for more information on the use of such devices.

Which Common Diseases Are Associated with the Muscular System?

There are several common muscular system diseases. Two will be discussed in this section: muscular dystrophy (MD) and amyotrophic lateral sclerosis (ALS).

Muscular Dystrophy (MD)

Muscular dystrophy (MD) is a group of diseases that cause progressive weakness and loss of muscle mass due to atrophy. In MD, abnormal genes interfere with the production of proteins needed to maintain healthy muscle tissue.

There are different types of MD. Each type is caused by a unique genetic mutation, which is usually inherited. There is no cure for MD. Some people with MD will lose the ability to walk and have trouble breathing and swallowing.

The main sign of MD is progressive muscle weakness. Other symptoms begin at different ages and in different muscle groups, depending on the type of MD. About one-half of MD cases are *Duchenne MD*, which typically affects young boys. Early signs of Duchenne MD include difficulty getting up from a lying or sitting position, frequent falls, walking on the toes, and muscle pain and stiffness. Other types of MD are milder, progress more slowly, and occur in adulthood. In these types, muscles often cannot relax following contraction, and facial and neck muscles are the first to be affected. The progressive weakness associated with MD can affect breathing, and residents with MD may need breathing assistance, such as a *ventilator* (a machine that forces air in and out of the lungs). MD can reduce the efficiency of the heart muscle and also cause difficulty swallowing (*dysphagia*).

Amyotrophic Lateral Sclerosis (ALS)

Amyotrophic lateral sclerosis (ALS) is characterized by the gradual decline and deterioration of motor neurons in the brain and spinal cord. In ALS, motor neurons in the spinal cord degenerate, which leads to scarring or **sclerosis** (hardening) of the muscles they control. As a result, muscles will waste away, or *atrophy*. When motor neurons die, the brain's ability to initiate and control muscle movement is lost. Because voluntary muscle action is affected, a person with ALS may lose the ability to speak, eat, move, and breathe.

The onset of ALS is gradual and often occurs between the ages of 40 and 70. On average, people with ALS survive 5–10 years after diagnosis. Initial symptoms may vary; one person may experience trouble speaking, and another may have a hard time picking something up. Because ALS affects only motor neurons, the senses of sight, touch, hearing, taste, and smell, as well as the muscles of the eyes and bladder, are generally not affected.

There are a variety of ways a holistic nursing assistant can provide care for those with progressive muscular diseases or conditions. Each of these should be guided by the resident's plan of care (Figure 9.12). Any observed changes in a resident's status should be reported to the licensed nursing staff immediately.

Care Considerations for Muscular Diseases	
Area	**Care Considerations**
Mobility	• Encourage the continuation of daily routines and low-impact aerobic exercise, such as walking and swimming • Assist with physical activity, ADLs, strengthening strategies for unaffected muscle groups, and stretches • Encourage the use of canes, walkers, orthopedic appliances, and wheelchairs to help maintain mobility and independence • Provide range-of-motion (ROM) exercises, as ordered • Practice fall-prevention strategies to prevent injury
Positioning	• Provide proper positioning, change positions every two hours, and always check for redness over bony prominences • Use assistive devices, such as slings, for weak extremities
Skin	• Provide care that prevents skin breakdown
Respiration	• Elevate the head of the bed to ease shortness of breath and provide comfort • Assist with deep breathing and coughing exercises, use of incentive spirometer, and postural drainage, as ordered
Nutrition	• Promote a low-calorie, high-protein, and high-fiber diet with adequate fluids to prevent constipation • Suggest smaller, more frequent meals and easy-to-eat foods • Explain the importance of weight control • Suggest eating techniques such as sitting up straight, putting the chin on the chest when swallowing, and concentrating while eating
Hydration	• Monitor daily fluid intake—2500 ccs, unless contraindicated because of difficulty swallowing

(continued)

Figure 9.12 Holistic nursing assistants can provide care to help residents with mobility, positioning, skin, respiration, nutrition, hydration, elimination, speech, and emotional support.

Care Considerations for Muscular Diseases	
Area	**Care Considerations**
Elimination	• Observe for signs and symptoms of a possible urinary tract infection (for example, frequency, urgency, painful urination, and fever) • Be aware of bowel patterns, such as constipation, diarrhea, or an impaction
Speech	• Encourage slowing of speech and pausing between breaths
Emotional support	• Be sensitive to potential emotional issues, such as alterations in body image, mood changes, and depression • Be patient and supportive • Provide information about resources and support groups for residents and their families • Provide comfort and alert the licensed nursing staff if the resident expresses feelings of pain

Figure 9.12 *(Continued)*

How Is the Nervous System Affected by Disease?

Think About This
The brain does not have any pain receptors, and consequently, cannot feel pain.

Common nervous system diseases include multiple sclerosis (MS), Parkinson's disease, and peripheral neuropathy. Injuries to the spinal cord, discussed in chapter 21, also affect the function of this body system. If a resident has a nervous system disease, a neurologist is likely a key care provider.

Multiple Sclerosis (MS)

Multiple sclerosis (MS) is a condition in which the immune system attacks *myelin*, the protective material that surrounds nerve fibers in the brain and spinal cord. Eventually, nerves themselves may become damaged, and nerve signals to the body may slow or be blocked (Figure 9.13). There are treatments for this disease, but there is no cure.

The first symptoms of MS usually appear between the ages of 20 and 50. Women are more likely to be diagnosed with MS than men. There are four major types of MS.

- **Relapsing-remitting MS:** is the most common type. In this type of MS, a person experiences relapses (*attacks*) following by recovery (*remissions*).

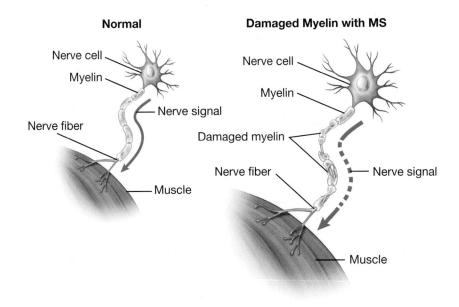

© Body Scientific International

Figure 9.13 Damage to myelin slows and interrupts the transmission of neural messages.

- **Secondary progressive MS**: develops from relapsing-remitting MS after 10–20 years. This type of MS does not have relapses or remissions.
- **Primary progressive MS**: is the third type. People with this type of MS experience gradual worsening of their symptoms over time, no well-defined attacks of symptoms, and little or no recovery. People with primary progressive MS are usually diagnosed when they are older and experience disability sooner.
- **Progressive relapsing MS**: is the least common. In this type of MS, relapses happen occasionally, and symptoms worsen between relapses.

While symptoms vary depending on the type of MS, there are some common signs and symptoms. Early MS signs and symptoms include fatigue; muscle stiffness, weakness, or spasms; tingling; numbness in the face, body, arms, or legs; trouble walking; blurred vision; difficulty processing thoughts; pain; and depression. MS is hard to diagnose, and several tests are performed to rule out other diseases with similar signs and symptoms. These tests usually include physical examinations to assess balance and coordination and magnetic resonance imaging (MRI) to examine the body's structure in detail using a magnetic field and pulses of radio wave energy.

The type of MS determines the severity of the disease and the effectiveness of treatment. Treatment may consist of medications to ease symptoms and manage stress. Rehabilitation may be used to promote strength and balance and reduce fatigue. People who have difficulty speaking or swallowing may also receive occupational therapy.

Parkinson's Disease

Parkinson's disease progresses gradually and causes neurons in the brain to gradually break down or die. Neurons in the brain are responsible for producing *dopamine*, a vital chemical messenger. Decreased dopamine levels cause abnormal brain activity that leads to the signs and symptoms of Parkinson's disease.

Risk factors for Parkinson's disease include

- gender (men are more likely than women to get Parkinson's disease);
- age (Parkinson's disease often begins toward the middle or end of a person's life);
- heredity;
- the environment, such as exposure to certain toxins; and
- changes in the brain, including the presence of Lewy bodies, which are markers for Parkinson's disease.

Symptoms of Parkinson's disease usually begin on one side of the body. This side will always exhibit the worst symptoms, even if symptoms eventually appear on the other side of the body. Typical signs and symptoms include a characteristic movement called *pill rolling* (rubbing the tip of the thumb and the forefinger back and forth); tremors in the head, hands, and fingers (when relaxed), which make writing difficult; slow movement (*bradykinesia*); shorter steps than usual; stooped posture; balance problems; and stiff muscles (Figure 9.14). Vocal changes also occur and make speech soft, quick, slurred, and **monotone** (flatsounding). Difficulty processing thoughts, frequent

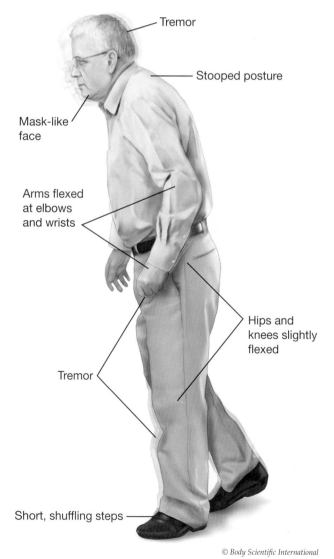

Tremor

Stooped posture

Mask-like face

Arms flexed at elbows and wrists

Hips and knees slightly flexed

Tremor

Short, shuffling steps

© *Body Scientific International*

Figure 9.14 The symptoms of Parkinson's disease are illustrated here.

waking during the night, fatigue, difficulty swallowing, accumulation of saliva in the mouth (causing drooling), depression, anxiety, constipation, and bladder control issues may also occur.

There are no specific tests for diagnosing Parkinson's disease. Typically, a medical history is reviewed for signs and symptoms. A physical and neurological exam is conducted, along with an MRI and **ultrasound** (use of ultrasonic waves to view internal structures) of the brain.

A treatment plan of care for Parkinson's disease may include different types of prescription medications to help improve movement and walking, reduce tremors, and treat depression. Physical therapy, speech-language therapy, and attention to lifestyle issues (such as exercise and diet) may be helpful. Integrative medicine (IM) approaches are often considered and include acupuncture; massage; tai chi; yoga; meditation; and music, art, or pet therapy. Surgery may also be performed to regulate certain parts of the brain and improve symptoms, but is only advised for certain residents.

Neuropathy

A *neuropathy* is a disease that can affect three types of nerves—sensory, motor, or autonomic.

- If neuropathy affects sensory nerves, the signs and symptoms include tingling, pain, and numbness.
- If neuropathy affects motor nerves, there is weakness in the feet and hands.
- If neuropathy affects autonomic nerves, there may be problems with internal organs, which can increase heart rate and lower blood pressure.

Neuropathy can involve a single nerve (*mononeuropathy*) or many nerves (*polyneuropathy*). About one-third of all neuropathies are *idiopathic*, which means the cause is unknown.

Peripheral neuropathy is a type of neuropathy in which nerves carrying messages to the body are damaged or diseased. Peripheral neuropathy is one of the most common neuropathies and can be a side effect of many medications. Diabetes, vitamin deficiencies, some cancers, chronic kidney disease, and inflammatory conditions can also cause peripheral neuropathy. Injury, infection, or pressure from a tumor or broken bone lying next to or on a nerve can trigger neuropathy.

Treating neuropathy may include over-the-counter and prescription pain medications, as well as topical medications such as **anesthetic** (a medication that produces a loss of sensation). Mechanical aids, including braces or specially fitted shoes, help with muscle weakness to better support walking and reduce pain. IM approaches such as acupuncture, massage, and herbal medications may also helpful for some residents.

Care Considerations for Residents with Neurological Diseases

There are several ways a holistic nursing assistant can assist in providing care for residents with neurological diseases:

- Help promote regular activity, stretching, and range-of-motion (ROM) exercises.
- Support residents who use assistive ambulatory devices, such as canes and walkers.
- Pay attention to the resident's balance and ensure fall-prevention measures are in place.
- Observe for and ask about pain; inform the licensed nursing staff of any pain. Use nonpharmacological strategies per the plan of care to help relieve pain.
- Assist with eating, when required, and encourage the resident to drink plenty of fluids to prevent constipation.
- Provide appropriate protection and assistance for residents with bladder control issues.

- Be aware that residents may have cognitive or thinking challenges. Communicate clearly, slowly, and in simple terms, when necessary.
- Be sensitive to changes in body image and mood, as well as depression.
- Be patient and supportive. Report any emotional or behavioral changes to the licensed nursing staff.
- Assist in providing information about resources and support groups for residents and their families.

How Does Disease Alter Sense Organ Function?

Common sensory system diseases and conditions are cataracts, glaucoma, macular degeneration, otitis media, and Ménière's disease. Care considerations for vision and hearing impairment or loss are discussed in detail in chapter 24. Diseases and conditions of the sense organs are usually treated by healthcare providers such as ophthalmologists, optometrists, or otolaryngologists. Holistic nursing assistants provide care according to the plan of care and directions from the licensed nursing staff.

Cataracts

A *cataract* is a condition in which a slow buildup of protein on the lens of the eye causes clouding (Figure 9.15). The lens must be clear to let light through to the retina. The buildup of protein on the lens causes light to scatter and makes it harder for light to pass through the lens. This affects sight. When there is too much protein on the lens, a person is not able to see clearly. Cataracts can occur in one or both eyes. They are not harmful to the eye, are not contagious, and do not spread from eye to eye. Cataracts may form in the center of the lens, at the edge of the lens, or at the back of the lens.

Most cataracts form due to aging, but cataracts can also develop as a result of other diseases, such as diabetes or long-term use of steroid medications. Injury to the eye and congenital disorders can also cause cataracts. Risk factors for cataracts include smoking and alcohol use, family history, and prolonged exposure to the sun. More than one-half of people over age 80 in the United States have a cataract or have had cataract surgery.

The most common sign of cataracts is blurry vision as the cataract grows. The lens may become yellow or brown and make reading difficult, make images less sharp, and make colors dull. Some people with cataracts are more sensitive to light and glare and see halos (rings) around lights. Eyeglass or contact lens prescriptions may change frequently for people with cataracts. Tests used to identify cataracts include a visual acuity test (eye chart), light and magnification of the eye to see eye structures using an ophthalmoscope, and dilation of the eyes to see the retina.

People with cataracts may benefit from changing eyeglass or contact lens prescriptions, using anti-glare sunglasses and magnifying lenses, using brighter lamps, and limiting night driving. Surgery to replace the eye's lens with an artificial lens is recommended only when vision loss interferes with normal living activities, such as driving or reading. Cataract surgery is performed on one eye at a time and is usually done in an outpatient facility. It is a common operation in the United States and is considered safe, relatively painless, and very effective (although there are some risks, such as retinal detachment).

Glaucoma

Glaucoma is a condition in which the optic nerve is damaged, possibly resulting in vision loss and blindness. There is no cure for glaucoma, and lost vision cannot be restored. *Open-angle glaucoma* is the most

Think About This
The eyes heal very quickly. It takes only 48 hours for a scratch on the cornea to mend.

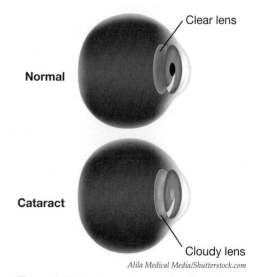

Normal

Clear lens

Cataract

Cloudy lens

Alila Medical Media/Shutterstock.com

Figure 9.15 A cataract causes clouding of the lens.

common type of glaucoma and occurs when fluid builds up at the open angle of the eye (where the cornea and iris meet). Fluid buildup creates pressure in the eye, which can damage the optic nerve. The amount of intraocular pressure (pressure within the eye) that the optic nerve can tolerate is unique to each person.

Other types of glaucoma include low-tension or normal-tension glaucoma and angle-closure glaucoma. In *angle-closure glaucoma*, fluid at the front of the eye cannot drain through the angle and is blocked, creating very severe pressure. This is considered a medical emergency. People over the age of 60, African-Americans over the age of 40, people with a family history of glaucoma, and those with high blood pressure are at risk.

Glaucoma can occur in one or both eyes. Initially, open-angle glaucoma has no symptoms; however, without treatment, side vision (*peripheral* vision) is lost. If allowed to progress, glaucoma can cause tunnel vision and ultimately blindness. Glaucoma can be treated using prescription oral medications and eye drops that lower eye pressure or cause the eye to make less fluid. Other treatments may include surgery to promote better fluid drainage.

Tests that determine if a person has glaucoma include a visual acuity test (eye chart), a visual field test to determine peripheral vision, and a measurement of the pressure inside the eye. Early diagnosis is important to prevent vision loss.

Macular Degeneration

Macular degeneration is an incurable eye disease caused by the deterioration of the *macula*, the central portion of the retina (Figure 9.16). When the macula is damaged, the eye does not receive images correctly, and a person's ability to read, drive a car, see details, and recognize faces or colors is compromised.

There are two types of macular degeneration—wet and dry. *Dry macular degeneration* is significantly more common and is characterized by yellow deposits called *drusen*. Drusen are composed of *lipids*, or fatty proteins that form when the eye fails to dispose of waste products. When drusen are small and scattered, they may not affect vision. When they become large and grow close together, *wet macular degeneration* can develop and cause more severe vision loss. Wet macular degeneration is caused by the growth of abnormal blood vessels underneath the macula.

The biggest risk factor for macular degeneration is age. *Age-related macular degeneration (AMD)* refers to macular degeneration that develops over the age of 60. Other risk factors are genetics, race (as Caucasians are more likely to develop the disease than other races), smoking, and cardiovascular disease.

The early stages of macular degeneration will have no noticeable symptoms. As macular degeneration progresses, people will experience wavy or blurred vision. Central vision may be completely lost over time and may leave people legally blind (Figure 9.17). In AMD, peripheral vision is not affected because the retina still functions properly.

Nutrition is an important element for preventing macular degeneration. A diet high in antioxidants (found in foods with vitamins K and C) is important because antioxidants slow down chemical reactions that can lead to cell damage. Exercising regularly, avoiding smoking, and protecting the eyes from sunlight are also essential prevention strategies. Wet AMD may be treated with the use of a laser to lower intraocular pressure, with chemical injections, and with prescription medications.

Otitis Media

Otitis media, commonly called an *ear infection*, is the most common cause of earaches. Although otitis media usually affects infants and children, it can also affect adults. Otitis media has a sudden onset,

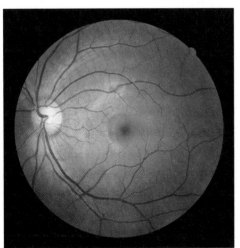

Figure 9.16 The macula is the lighter portion of the retina shown here.

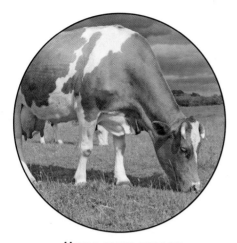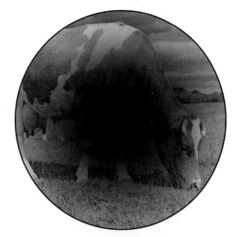

How a scene appears with normal vision

How a scene appears with vision affected by macular degeneration

Smereka/Shutterstock.com; concept adapted from Lighthouse International

Figure 9.17 In macular degeneration, central vision deteriorates most quickly.

and the common signs and symptoms in adults include ear pain or an earache, drainage of fluid from the ear, and diminished hearing.

In otitis media, infection is located in the middle ear. Infection is usually associated with a cold, influenza, or other respiratory infection. Infection can also be caused by allergies, smoke, fumes, and other environmental toxins. In otitis media, the eardrum will be red and will appear to be bulging.

Ménière's Disease

Ménière's disease affects the inner ear. This condition causes spontaneous episodes of spinning (called *vertigo*); hearing loss; ringing, buzzing, roaring, whistling, or hissing in the ear (called *tinnitus*); and a feeling of fullness or pressure in the ear. Ménière's disease usually begins between the ages of 20 and 50. A combination of factors may contribute to Ménière's disease, including allergies, viral infection, improper fluid drainage or blockage in the inner ear, migraines, or a genetic **predisposition** (tendency to suffer from a condition).

Ménière's disease is chronic and does not have a cure; however, medications, rehabilitation to improve balance, hearing aids, and sometimes surgery can help reduce the severity and frequency of vertigo episodes. Vertigo episodes can occur weeks or years apart, and symptoms may improve or disappear entirely between episodes. In most cases, Ménière's disease affects only one ear.

Vertigo may cause people to lose their balance easily, resulting in a high risk of falling. Sudden movements and bright lights should be avoided during an episode, and people should rest after an episode before returning to normal activities.

How Do Diabetes and Thyroid Disease Affect the Endocrine System?

Diabetes mellitus and thyroid disease (hyperthyroidism and hypothyroidism) are common diseases of the endocrine system. Although these diseases originate in the endocrine system, they impact the whole body. People with diabetes or thyroid disease will be cared for by a variety of healthcare providers, but an endocrinologist (doctor specializing in the endocrine system) and a diabetes educator will likely be key care providers.

Diabetes Mellitus

Diabetes mellitus, commonly referred to as *diabetes*, is a disease in which the body's ability to produce or respond to insulin is damaged. This causes abnormal *metabolism* (chemical reactions in the body that maintain cells and the organism) of carbohydrates and elevates glucose (*sugar*) levels in the blood and urine.

There are four types of diabetes: type 1 diabetes, type 2 diabetes, prediabetes, and gestational diabetes. *Gestational diabetes* occurs during pregnancy and often goes away after the baby is born. In some cases, gestational diabetes can develop into type 2 diabetes if the woman had risk factors prior to pregnancy. This section focuses on type 1 and type 2 diabetes.

According to recent statistics, diabetes affects 8 percent of the US population and is one of the most common diseases. While type 1 diabetes can develop at any age, it typically begins during childhood or adolescence. Type 2 diabetes more commonly appears after age 40.

Type 1 Diabetes Mellitus

In *type 1 diabetes*, the immune system destroys insulin-producing cells in the pancreas, leaving little or no insulin that can be transported throughout the body. As a result, instead of moving into cells, glucose builds up in the bloodstream and causes *hyperglycemia* (high blood glucose levels). Symptoms of type 1 diabetes include increased thirst or hunger, frequent urination, mood changes, blurred vision, fatigue, and weakness.

Risk factors for type 1 diabetes include family history; environmental factors, such as exposure to viral illness; the presence of damaging immune cells called *autoantibodies*; and possibly the kinds of foods eaten. The specific cause of type 1 diabetes is unknown.

Type 2 Diabetes Mellitus

As with type 1 diabetes, the specific cause of *type 2 diabetes* is unknown. Type 2 diabetes develops when cells become resistant to insulin and when the pancreas is unable to make enough insulin to overcome this resistance. Instead of moving into cells, glucose builds up in the bloodstream.

Type 2 diabetes has the following risk factors:

- age (type 2 diabetes more commonly occurs in people who are older)
- overweight (the more fatty tissue there is, the more resistant cells are to insulin)
- lack of exercise
- family history
- race (African-Americans, Hispanics, American Indians, and Asians are at higher risk than people of other races)
- high blood pressure
- abnormal cholesterol and triglyceride levels

Signs and Symptoms of Diabetes Mellitus

The signs and symptoms are the same for both type 1 and type 2 diabetes:

- increased thirst
- frequent urination
- extreme hunger
- unexplained weight loss, even though a person is eating more
- tingling pain or numbness in the hands and feet (usually in type 2 diabetes)
- ketones in the urine (ketones are by-products of muscle and fat breakdown and develop when there is a lack of available insulin)
- fatigue and irritability

- blurred vision
- slow-healing sores and frequent infections (specifically related to the gums, skin, and vagina)

Some people with type 2 diabetes have symptoms so mild they go unnoticed for a time.

Tests for Diagnosing Diabetes Mellitus

Diabetes is often diagnosed using a blood test called *glycated hemoglobin (A1C)*, which measures the percentage of blood glucose attached to *hemoglobin* (oxygen-carrying molecules in red blood cells). When glucose levels are high, more glucose attaches to hemoglobin. Other tests determine the amount of glucose in the blood under different conditions; the normal range of blood sugar is 70–100 mg/dl:

- **Random blood sugar**: a blood sample is taken at a random time to determine the level of blood glucose.
- **Fasting blood sugar**: a blood sample is taken after a person has not eaten overnight.
- **Oral glucose tolerance test**: after fasting, a person drinks a sugary liquid, and blood glucose levels are tested over a two- or four-hour period.

If type 1 diabetes is suspected, a urine test may be performed to detect the presence of ketones. A doctor may also order a test to check for autoantibodies (damaging immune cells) in the blood. This is done to distinguish between type 1 and type 2 diabetes.

Those who have diabetes may experience long-term complications if they fail to manage their blood glucose levels. People's abilities to manage their levels may be compromised by inactivity, obesity, or poor nutrition. Resulting complications can include dry skin conditions, hearing loss, heart disease, cerebrovascular accidents (strokes), kidney damage, retinopathy (eye damage), peripheral neuropathy, and severely limited blood circulation (gangrene) to the lower limbs (Figure 9.18). Gangrene can lead to amputation of the toes and feet.

Care Considerations for Diabetes Mellitus

Diabetes cannot be cured, but symptoms can be managed when blood glucose levels are carefully monitored. Using glucometers or continuous glucose monitors, people with diabetes can check and record their blood glucose levels to ensure they stay within the target (Figure 9.19). This is the only reliable way to monitor

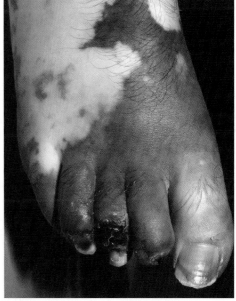

Biophoto Associates/Science Source

Figure 9.18 Gangrene is a result of severely limited circulation.

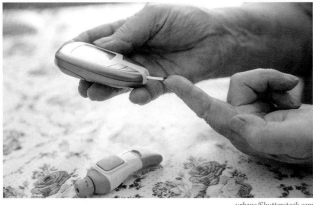

urbans/Shutterstock.com

A

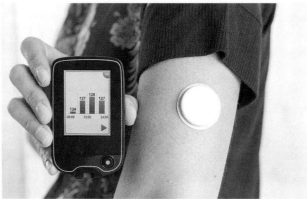

Click and Photo/Shutterstock.com

B

Figure 9.19 Glucometers (A) and continuous glucose monitors (B) help people check their glucose levels.

glucose levels on a continuous basis. Monitoring is particularly important for those who use insulin replacement. Glucose levels may be checked between four and eight times a day or several times a week.

Type 1 diabetes requires that insulin be replaced, either by injection or via an insulin pump. An insulin pump is attached to the body by a **catheter**, which is a tube inserted into the body. The insulin pump is programmed to dispense prescribed amounts of insulin. There are three different types of insulin: rapid-acting, intermediate, and long-acting insulin. Insulin may be prescribed for type 2 diabetes; however, oral medications are used more often to stimulate insulin production and slow the production and release of glucose by the liver.

Diet and exercise are particularly important for managing diabetes. A dietitian may help people with diabetes design meal plans that align with their lifestyles and prescribed medications.

It is important that people with diabetes follow their prescribed diets and exercise plans to help manage blood glucose levels. People with diabetes should limit alcohol consumption and can maintain a healthy weight by eating designed meal plans filled with fruits, vegetables, and whole grains. Meals should be eaten on a regular schedule, and people with diabetes should not skip meals or eat partial meals.

As a holistic nursing assistant, you may care for residents with diabetes. It is important to carefully document what a resident has eaten during a meal and to report this to the licensed nursing staff. When caring for residents with diabetes, assist with the regimen of exercise and activities prescribed by the doctor (for example, walking, aerobic exercise, resistance training, or physical therapy). Exercise lowers blood glucose levels and increases sensitivity to insulin.

Even if residents with diabetes carefully manage their blood glucose levels, they must be observed closely for three possible conditions:

- **Hyperglycemia**: high blood sugar. Blood glucose levels can become too high if residents overeat, have an illness, or do not take sufficient prescribed medications. Signs and symptoms of hyperglycemia include excessive thirst, a dry mouth, fatigue, nausea, and blurred vision. Hyperglycemia is commonly treated by adjusting a resident's meal plan, prescribed medications, physical activity, or exercise.

- **Diabetic ketoacidosis**: buildup of ketones in the urine. When the body lacks adequate insulin, it breaks down fat for energy, causing ketones to build up in the blood. Diabetic ketoacidosis most commonly occurs in type 1 diabetes and may occur due to illness or missed doses of insulin. Signs and symptoms include loss of appetite, weakness, confusion, vomiting, fever, stomach pain, and fruity-smelling breath. Checking for excess ketones in the urine can detect diabetic ketoacidosis (Figure 9.20). Diabetic ketoacidosis can lead to coma and death and is a serious condition that may require emergency care.

- **Hypoglycemia**: low blood sugar. Blood glucose levels sometimes drop too low if a person does not have enough calories at a meal, skips a meal, significantly increases physical activity, drinks large amounts of alcohol, or takes too much of a prescribed medication. Signs and symptoms of hypoglycemia include sweating, shakiness, weakness, hunger, dizziness, headache, blurred vision, heart palpitations, irritability, slurred speech, drowsiness, confusion, fainting, and seizures. Hypoglycemia can be remedied if a person consumes a quick source of sugar, such as fruit juice, regular soda, or glucose tablets. Some people with diabetes keep a prescribed glucagon emergency injection kit consisting of a syringe and glucagon that can be injected into the arm, thigh, or buttocks. There is no danger of overdose with glucagon. This kit is helpful if a quick source of energy is not available or if hypoglycemia is severe.

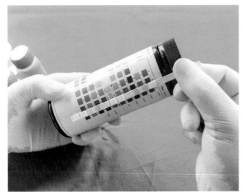

Figure 9.20 Ketone test strips help detect ketones in the urine.

Signs of hyperglycemia, diabetic ketoacidosis, or hypoglycemia must be reported immediately to the licensed nursing staff.

Foot care is essential for residents who have diabetes. Feet should be washed daily in lukewarm water, dried gently (particularly between the toes), and moisturized. Do not cut the toenails of residents with diabetes, unless permitted. These residents will usually need professional foot care. Do, however, look for any blisters, cuts, sores, redness, or swelling that may lead to gangrene. Dental and gum care are also important, so observe the resident for red or swollen gums. Help promote smoking cessation, as smoking may lead to cardiovascular disease. Stress management is also an important part of caring for people with diabetes, as stress can prevent insulin from working properly and cause blood glucose levels to rise.

Thyroid Disease

There are many different kinds of thyroid disease, and thyroid diseases range from problems with thyroid hormone production to cancer. *Hyperthyroidism* and *hypothyroidism* are the two types of thyroid disease you will most commonly encounter when working as a holistic nursing assistant.

The risk factors for thyroid disease include gender (since women are more likely to experience thyroid disease than men), age (over 50), family history (especially with autoimmune disease), smoking, radioactive iodine treatments, iodine deficiency, some medications and treatments, and stress. Thyroid disease is diagnosed through physical examinations, laboratory tests, and ultrasounds; these tests help doctors detect nodules and determine how well the thyroid is functioning. Radioactive iodine uptake tests also allow doctors to measure how much thyroid hormone is being produced.

Hyperthyroidism

Hyperthyroidism refers to excess production of the thyroid hormone. Hyperthyroidism can be caused by Graves' disease, in which the immune system attacks the thyroid gland and the thyroid reacts by making too much thyroid hormone. Other common causes of hyperthyroidism include **nodules** (knotlike collections of body tissue), which develop in the thyroid gland and increase the secretion of thyroid hormone, and cancerous growths, which are rare.

Although signs and symptoms may vary, people with hyperthyroidism often experience nervousness, tremors, agitation, *tachycardia* (rapid heartbeat), heart palpitations, heat intolerance, mental fogginess and poor concentration, and menstrual changes (reduced flow). Signs and symptoms of Graves' disease include protruding eyeballs, red or swollen eyes, tearing or discomfort in one or both eyes, light sensitivity, and blurry or double vision.

Goiter

When the thyroid gland enlarges, it may create a growth called a *goiter*. For example, when a person has Graves' disease, the entire thyroid gland can become enlarged, forming a goiter. A goiter can also form when nodules in the thyroid develop and cause increased production of thyroid hormone.

Hypothyroidism

Hypothyroidism occurs when the thyroid gland does not produce enough thyroid hormone. The most common cause of hypothyroidism is an autoimmune disorder called *Hashimoto's thyroiditis*. In Hashimoto's thyroiditis, the body produces antibodies that attack and destroy the thyroid gland, and the thyroid gland becomes inflamed.

Symptoms commonly associated with hypothyroidism include feeling cold, sluggishness, depression, menstrual changes (excessive flow or prolonged cycle), mental fogginess and poor concentration, a bloated feeling, weight gain, and high cholesterol levels.

Care Considerations for Thyroid Disease

Hyperthyroidism is treated by slowing down or stopping excess thyroid hormone production. Some common treatments prescribed are radioactive iodine treatments, a year of antithyroid medications, or sometimes surgery.

Hypothyroidism is treated with lifelong thyroid hormone replacement using prescription medications. Side effects of these medications might include nervousness or even chest pain. Some medications, such as antidepressants, can interfere with thyroid hormone replacement.

When caring for a resident with thyroid disease, observe the resident for any signs or symptoms of changes or side effects from medications. Report any signs or symptoms to the licensed nursing staff. Also be sensitive to and watch for any emotional issues, such as mood changes or depression, and report them to the licensed nursing staff. Assist in providing information about resources for residents and their families.

How Does Disease Affect the Cardiovascular System?

Common cardiovascular system diseases include coronary artery disease, angina (*chest pain*), myocardial infarction (*heart attack*), and congestive heart failure. Cerebrovascular accidents (CVAs), or *strokes*, and peripheral vascular disease are also common. A *cardiologist* (a doctor who specializes in heart diseases and conditions) and cardiac surgeon will likely be key care providers for people with cardiovascular diseases. Neurologists may be involved because of damage to the central nervous system due to hemorrhaging after a stroke.

Coronary Artery Disease

Coronary artery disease occurs when there is damage, injury, or disease in the inner layers of coronary arteries. These layers supply the heart with blood, oxygen, and nutrients. When these layers are damaged, plaque and other waste products form at the site, resulting in a condition called **atherosclerosis** (Figure 9.21). Plaque hardens and narrows the arteries, allowing less blood to flow to the heart. As the surfaces of arteries become more clogged with plaque, a person will experience chest pain (*angina*) and shortness of breath. If the arteries become completely blocked, this causes a myocardial infarction (*heart attack*). If the surface of the plaque ruptures, platelets that clump at that site to repair it may block the artery in the process and cause a heart attack.

Many people with coronary artery disease may not realize that plaque is building up because they do not experience symptoms until they have a significant blockage. Risk factors for coronary artery disease include aging; gender (as men are more likely to develop the disease); family history; smoking; high blood pressure; high LDL (low-density lipoprotein, or bad cholesterol) levels; overweight or obese; lack of physical activity; and excessive, unrelieved stress. Recent research has found that certain conditions may lead to coronary artery disease, including

- sleep apnea (repeatedly stopping and starting breathing during sleep);
- greater levels of high-sensitivity, C-reactive protein (a substance produced by the liver that increases when there is inflammation in the body); and
- higher levels of triglycerides (fat in the blood).

Angina

Angina is caused by reduced blood flow to the heart. This type of chest pain has been described as a sensation of squeezing, pressure, heaviness, and tightness in the center of the chest. The pain can be a one-time occurrence or can recur and can make normal daily activities very difficult and uncomfortable. Shortness of breath; sweating; and pain in the arms, neck, jaw, or shoulder may accompany chest pain.

Think About This

On Earth, blood pools in the feet because of gravity. When you are standing, the pressure from gravity is 200 mmHg at your feet and 60–80 mmHg in the brain. In space, blood pools in the chest and head (called a *fluid shift*) rather than only in the feet, and this causes the pressure to equalize due to the lack of gravity. As a result, astronauts have stuffy noses, headaches, puffy faces, and thin legs.

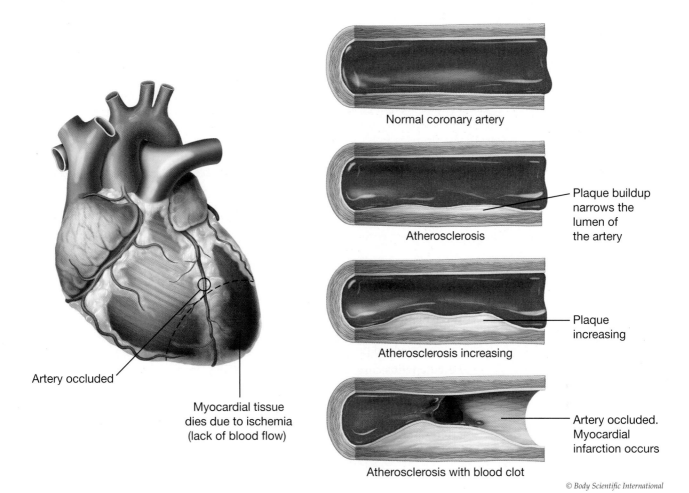

Normal coronary artery

Atherosclerosis

Plaque buildup narrows the lumen of the artery

Atherosclerosis increasing

Plaque increasing

Atherosclerosis with blood clot

Artery occluded. Myocardial infarction occurs

Artery occluded

Myocardial tissue dies due to ischemia (lack of blood flow)

© *Body Scientific International*

Figure 9.21 Atherosclerosis narrows the arteries, restricting blood flow.

Stable angina is caused by physical activity that makes the heart work harder and that demands more blood than what is available due to narrowed arteries. Stable angina usually lasts for a few minutes and will disappear with rest or prescribed medications. *Unstable angina*, which is more serious, can occur even at rest and is unexpected. Unstable angina may occur due to a rupture of plaque, causing blockage in the artery. Unstable angina will last longer and may not disappear with prescribed medications. Unstable angina is a medical emergency.

Myocardial Infarction

Myocardial infarction, or *heart attack*, occurs when a completely blocked coronary artery causes **ischemia**, or lack of blood flow to the heart (Figure 9.21). This lack of blood flow damages the heart muscle. The amount of damage that occurs typically depends on how quickly a person receives treatment. Classic signs and symptoms of a heart attack include crushing or squeezing pain in the center of the chest; pain in the shoulder, arm, back, teeth, and jaw; shortness of breath; sweating; prolonged pain in the upper abdomen; and nausea and vomiting. In some cases, a person who is having a heart attack will not experience any signs or symptoms. Women tend to experience less classic signs and symptoms and may not experience neck or jaw pain.

Congestive Heart Failure

Congestive heart failure occurs when the heart does not have the oxygen and nutrients it needs to pump blood effectively. This weakens the heart's pumping power. Congestive heart failure often results from reduced blood flow or damage from a heart attack. When congestive heart failure occurs, blood moves through the heart at a slower-than-normal pace, and pressure in the heart increases. Congestive heart failure can affect the kidneys and cause **edema**, or retention of fluid in the body. Fluid also builds up in the arms, legs, ankles, feet, and lungs.

The signs and symptoms of congestive heart failure include fluid buildup in the lungs, which causes shortness of breath and sometimes a dry, hacking cough or wheezing. Fluid buildup can also cause swelling in the ankles and legs, bloating in the abdomen, and weight gain. Dizziness, fatigue, rapid heartbeats, and **arrhythmias** (abnormal heart rhythms) may also occur due to interference with the heart's electrical impulses.

Coronary artery disease is diagnosed by a doctor who collects medical history, performs a physical examination, and orders special blood tests to check for enzymes that signal damage to the heart. A chest X-ray will help a doctor see if the heart is enlarged due to damage to the heart muscle and thinning and stretching of the heart walls. Other diagnostic tests include an electrocardiogram (EKG or ECG), echocardiogram, stress test, coronary angiography, or computerized tomography (CT) scan.

Care Considerations for Coronary Artery Disease

Prescribed medications such as aspirin are often used to reduce blood clotting and decrease arterial obstructions in people who have coronary artery disease. Various other prescription medications may be used to widen blood vessels, relax blood vessels to improve blood flow, slow heart rate, decrease blood pressure, or lower blood cholesterol. The following medical procedures may also be appropriate for some people:

- **Percutaneous coronary intervention (PCI)**: Coronary artery stenosis (narrowing) often requires percutaneous coronary intervention (PCI). During this procedure, a catheter with a tiny balloon at the tip is inserted into the narrowed artery. The balloon inflates, widening the blocked artery, and a small wire mesh coil called a *stent* is inserted to keep the artery open (Figure 9.22).

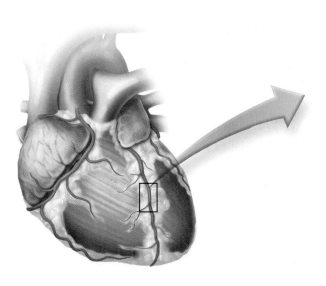

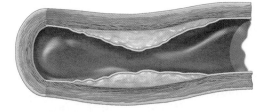

A Cholesterol buildup partially blocking blood flow through the artery.

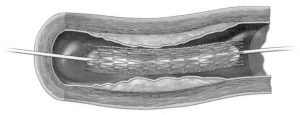

B A stent with a balloon is inserted into the partially blocked artery.

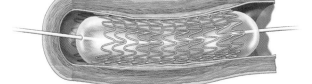

C The balloon is inflated to expand the stent.

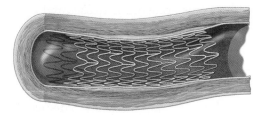

D The balloon is then removed from the expanded stent.

Figure 9.22 Stents are inserted to keep arteries open.

- **Coronary artery bypass surgery**: When an artery is very narrow or is blocked, a surgeon may use a vein or artery from another part of the body as a *graft* (a healthy tissue that replaces diseased tissue). During this surgery, (also called *coronary artery bypass grafting* or *CABG*) the graft is used to bypass the blocked or narrow coronary artery, allowing blood to flow around it. This surgery is most appropriate for people who have multiple narrowed arteries.

Lifestyle changes are typically part of the plan of care for people with coronary artery disease. These lifestyle changes may include smoking cessation, healthful eating, weight loss, regular exercise, and stress reduction. Promoting and supporting needed changes in the following ways is essential to delivering holistic care:

- Help residents eat their healthful special diets, including whole grains, fruits and vegetables, and limited amounts of saturated fat. Have residents avoid large meals that will make them feel too full and that will require their already damaged hearts to overwork.

- If residents are overweight, support changes in caloric and food intake and remind residents why healthy weights help their hearts work more effectively.

- Assist in residents' prescribed exercise plans. Be sure residents pace themselves and take rest breaks.

- If residents smoke, assist with smoking cessation plans. Remind residents to avoid exposure to secondhand smoke.

- Find ways to help residents relax and avoid stress. Pay attention to any fears or anxieties residents share about their disease and report these to the licensed nursing staff.

- Check to see if residents have taken all of their prescribed medications.

- Observe and immediately report any changes in residents, including blood pressure, pulse, respiration, and mental or emotional behaviors or attitudes.

- Current research has shown that some dietary supplements may be helpful for those with coronary artery disease. Helpful dietary supplements include fish and fish oil, flax and flaxseed oil, and oat bran and oatmeal. These supplements should only be used if they are ordered as part of the plan of care.

Cerebrovascular Accident (CVA)

A *cerebrovascular accident* (*CVA*) or *stroke* occurs when a blood vessel in the brain becomes blocked due to atherosclerosis or **arteriosclerosis** (hardening of the arteries) or bleeds due to a ruptured **aneurysm** (distended or weak area in a blood vessel, as illustrated in Figure 9.23).

Types of Strokes

There are three types of strokes: ischemic stroke, hemorrhagic stroke, and transient ischemic attack (TIA). *Ischemic strokes* are the most common and account for approximately 85 percent of all strokes. Ischemic strokes occur due to blocked arteries, which keep blood from nourishing the brain (Figure 9.24).

Hemorrhagic stroke occurs when an artery in the brain leaks blood or ruptures due to an aneurysm. The bleeding places damaging pressure on brain cells. The two types of hemorrhagic strokes are *intracerebral* and

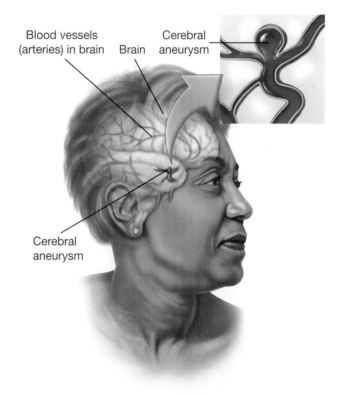

Blood vessels (arteries) in brain   Brain   Cerebral aneurysm

Cerebral aneurysm

© *Body Scientific International*

Figure 9.23 An aneurysm is a weakened area of an artery.

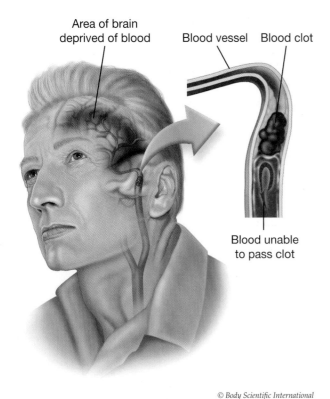

Area of brain deprived of blood

Blood vessel   Blood clot

Blood unable to pass clot

© Body Scientific International

Figure 9.24 Ischemic strokes result from blocked arteries in the brain.

subarachnoid. Intracerebral hemorrhagic strokes are the most common and occur when an artery bursts and bleeds into surrounding brain tissue. In a subarachnoid hemorrhagic stroke, bleeding occurs between the brain and its tissue covering. Risk factors for hemorrhagic stroke include smoking, diabetes, high cholesterol, and **hypertension** (high blood pressure).

A *transient ischemic attack (TIA)* is also called a *ministroke* because it lasts for only a short amount of time. Like an ischemic stroke, a TIA is caused by a blocked artery in the brain. It is not uncommon for a person to have a TIA and not know it. Approximately one-third of all people who have TIAs will likely have major strokes within one year if they do not receive treatment.

Symptoms of Stroke

The signs and symptoms of a stroke include a sudden, severe headache that feels different from other headaches experienced. A person who is having a stroke may also experience numbness; tingling; weakness (causing drooping of the face and mouth); loss of movement in the face, arm, or leg; or **hemiplegia** (loss of movement on one whole side of the body). These symptoms may make it difficult for a person to walk. Trouble seeing, slurred speech, **aphasia** (inability to understand and use words), confusion, dizziness, and difficulty understanding simple statements may also occur.

Time is critical for treating strokes. The longer a person goes without treatment, the greater the damage from the stroke will be. Strokes can be diagnosed using blood tests, EKGs or ECGs, X-rays that can visualize bleeding in the brain and the type of stroke, and an MRI. Other tests may be used if a person has a history of coronary artery disease.

Care Considerations After a Stroke

The prescribed treatment for a stroke depends on the type of stroke experienced. If a person has a hemorrhagic stroke, treatment will focus on quickly controlling bleeding, reducing pressure in the brain, and stabilizing blood pressure.

One of the most important care considerations after a stroke is the damage the stroke may leave. Damage from a stroke can significantly affect people physically, mentally, and emotionally. After people have strokes, they want to regain control over their lives and recover the abilities they had prior to the stroke. Ways to support residents who have suffered from a stroke include the following:

- Assist with ambulation. Many residents will need a cane or walker. Ensure that fall-prevention and protection strategies are in place.

- Assist with dressing. Mobility lost because of the stroke may make dressing difficult. Devices such as reachers and buttonhooks can be very helpful.

- Assist residents with eating if the stroke has affected their mouths and arms. Help residents eat and drink slowly to prevent choking and the spitting up of food.

- Assist with potential bladder problems. Some residents will experience a loss of bladder control. Change these residents quickly to prevent skin irritation.

- Assist if there are any vision problems. Residents with right-side paralysis may also have difficulty seeing on the right. Be sure residents are oriented to the room and do not try to get up on their own.

If a resident has paralysis or problems with speech or eating, physical or occupational therapy will usually be ordered. It is important to be patient and respectful with residents who have had a stroke. Residents will be very frustrated if they can no longer do what they were able to do prior to the stroke. This is especially true if residents have aphasia. When caring for these residents, speak slowly and listen carefully. Also encourage residents' families to provide support during recovery. Show residents' families proper and supportive ways they can help.

Generally, the goal of treatment after a stroke is to manage the effects of the stroke and prevent another stroke. Medications may be prescribed to dissolve and prevent blood clots and lower cholesterol and blood pressure. Lifestyle changes related to smoking cessation, healthy eating, and physical activity are important.

Peripheral Vascular Disease (PVD)

Peripheral vascular disease (PVD), or *peripheral artery disease*, occurs when there is damage to the blood vessels that supply blood to areas of the body other than the brain and heart. Damage usually occurs due to atherosclerosis and arteriosclerosis. The buildup of plaque and hardening of the blood vessels can progress over time until arteries become narrow or blocked. Other causes of PVD include the presence of a blood clot, inflammation of the arteries (*arteritis*), infection, or injury. Blood vessels in the legs are most often affected, but blood vessels in the arms and kidneys may also experience narrowing and blockage.

Risk Factors for PVD

Men over age 60 are more likely to have PVD than women and will often find the disease disabling. PVD is more common among people who have diabetes, smoke, are overweight, are not active, have high blood pressure, have high cholesterol, and have a family history of PVD. The risks of heart attack and stroke are greater for people with PVD and vice versa. If a person has coronary artery disease or has had a heart attack or stroke, he or she is at risk for PVD.

PVD Symptoms

The first signs of PVD begin slowly. A person may feel discomfort, such as fatigue or cramping, in the legs due to inadequate blood supply to the leg muscles. Intermittent, dull pain and cramping may occur in one or both calves, thighs, or hips. During walking, this pain is more evident and goes away when a person is at rest. Other signs and symptoms are numbness, tingling, or weakness in the legs; burning or aching pain in the feet or toes, even at rest; cold feet; loss of hair on the legs; and change of skin color (to a pale and bluish color). When symptoms are more severe, pain is present even during rest at night. If PVD is left untreated, gangrene can develop in the affected limb, and tissues may die and decay. This can lead to amputation.

PVD is diagnosed through medical evaluation by a doctor. This evaluation may include tests that assess pain and changes in blood pressure in the limbs; a treadmill test that determines a person's ability to walk and blood pressure; an angiography (X-ray of blood vessels that uses dye for visualization) to determine blockage; an ultrasound; and an MRI.

Care Considerations for PVD

Treatment for PVD depends on the underlying cause of the disease. One of the greatest risk factors for PVD is smoking, particularly if a person also has diabetes. Helpful strategies for the treatment of PVD include smoking cessation, a healthful diet, physical activity, and efforts to lower blood pressure and cholesterol. A holistic nursing assistant can provide care by helping residents find comfortable positions and observing for any changes in the skin (sores that do not heal) or complaints of new sensations or pain in the legs. If these changes and complaints occur, they need to be reported to the licensed nursing staff immediately.

Care may also include prescription medications that dilate (open) the blood vessels, prevent blood clots, relieve pain, and lower blood pressure and cholesterol. Surgical interventions may include an *angioplasty* (procedure used to widen narrow or obstructed arteries or veins), stenting, an *atherectomy* (surgical removal of plaque), or coronary artery bypass grafting (CABG). Surgery may be helpful but is usually only performed if medication has not treated PVD successfully.

How Does Disease Affect Respiratory System Structures?

The *common cold* is a viral infection of the respiratory system and affects the nose and throat. Because most people have experienced a cold in their lifetimes, this section will focus on two other common respiratory diseases: asthma and chronic obstructive pulmonary disease (COPD). Chronic bronchitis and emphysema are two conditions related to COPD. Influenza, pneumonia, and tuberculosis (TB) are discussed in chapter 14. Although respiratory diseases are treated by all members of the healthcare team, a *pulmonologist* specializes in this area and will be a key care provider.

Think About This

The medical term for sneezing is *sternutation*. One sneeze will spray about 100,000 germs about 3–5 feet.

Asthma

Asthma is a chronic lung disease in which the airways become inflamed, swell, and narrow. Inflammation causes mucus to develop, which narrows the airways even more and reduces airflow to the lungs.

Approximately 25 million people in the United States have asthma. For many people, asthma starts during childhood. No one is quite sure what exactly causes asthma. Some possible causes include genetics, family history, respiratory infections, environmental irritants such as secondhand smoke, and airborne allergens.

Signs and Symptoms of Asthma

Asthma may cause periods of wheezing, which is characterized by a high-pitched, whistling sound during expiration. Other symptoms may include a tight chest; shortness of breath; and coughing, usually at night or early in the morning. For some people, symptoms are mild and go away with or without treatment. For others, symptoms get worse, and attacks or *flares* may occur.

Asthma attacks are usually triggered by particular substances or circumstances. Triggers are typically specific to the individual. A trigger can be dust, animal fur, mold, pollen, cigarette smoke, a new chemical used in the home, a certain food, exercise, a newly prescribed medication, or an upper respiratory infection.

Tests for Diagnosing Asthma

Along with medical history and a physical examination, *spirometry* (a lung function test) is used for diagnosis. Using a spirometer, doctors measure how much air is inhaled, how fast air is inhaled, and how much air and how fast it is exhaled (Figure 9.25). Sometimes an inhaled medication is used to open airways.

A *peak flow meter* may be used to determine how well air moves in and out of the lungs (Figure 9.26). The peak flow meter provides a score, or *peak expiration flow rate (PEFR)*, to indicate how well a person's lungs are functioning. Before using the peak flow meter, a baseline measurement for lung function should be established when no asthma symptoms are present. This baseline measurement represents the highest peak flow rate a person can achieve and establishes

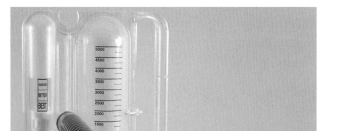

glenda/Shutterstock.com

Figure 9.25 A spirometer measures the amount of air inhaled and exhaled.

the person's normal range. Thereafter, the reading should be between 80 and 100 percent of the usual peak flow rate. Any reading below the person's normal range is a sign that the airway is narrowed. Keeping track of lung function daily can help a person know when his or her breathing is getting worse. It can also help a doctor know if medications are effective.

Other lung function tests include the *lung volume test*, which measures the amount of air left in the lungs after taking a deep breath and exhaling fully. *Pulse oximetry* measures how much oxygen is in the blood (and is further discussed in chapter 18). Analyzing arterial blood gases is another way of measuring oxygen levels.

Care Considerations for Asthma

There is no cure for asthma. Treatment focuses on controlling asthma symptoms. When symptoms are under control, they appear no more than two days a week, sleep is uninterrupted, and quick-relief medications are only needed two days a week.

Prescription oral medications and medications taken though an inhaler or nebulizer are used to manage asthma symptoms. When a handheld *inhaler* is used, medication goes directly to the lungs as the person breathes in the dry medication. A *nebulizer* is a machine that delivers a fine mist of liquid medicine that goes directly into the lungs. These are long-term medications that are taken daily and are not considered quick relief for asthma symptoms (Figure 9.27).

Quick-relief or rescue inhaler medications relax tight muscles in the airways during a flare. These medications cause the airways to open so air can flow to the lungs. They do not reduce inflammation. Sometimes rescue inhalers do not provide relief, and a person may become out of breath and have trouble talking and walking. This is an emergency, and 9-1-1 should be called.

Asthma triggers and conditions that can make asthma harder to manage should be avoided. Some of these conditions include a runny nose, sinus infections, reflux disease, and stress. Efforts to reduce triggers should not interfere with physical activity, which is important to maintain. When caring for residents who use inhalers and nebulizers, be sure you understand the purpose of the inhaler or nebulizer and check with the licensed nursing staff to ensure a quick-relief inhaler is nearby.

Residents who use an inhaler are at risk for developing *thrush*, a fungus that builds up on the lining of the mouth. Thrush causes the formation of creamy, white lesions on the tongue, inner cheeks, and sometimes the roof of the mouth and the back of the throat (Figure 9.28). To reduce the risk of thrush, a spacer is placed in the holding chamber of an inhaler to prevent medications from reaching the mouth or back of the throat. Oral hygiene is critical for residents using inhalers. Rinsing the mouth with water after using an inhaler can lower the risk of thrush.

Chronic Obstructive Pulmonary Disease (COPD)

Chronic obstructive pulmonary disease (COPD) is also known as *chronic obstructive airway disease* or *chronic obstructive lung disease*. In COPD, thick, inflamed airways filled with mucus reduce the amount of airflow into the body. When people have COPD, they usually have two conditions—chronic bronchitis and emphysema (Figure 9.29). The severity of these conditions will vary for each person.

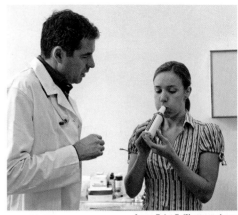

Image Point Fr/Shutterstock.com

Figure 9.26 A peak flow meter provides a PEFR, or lung function score.

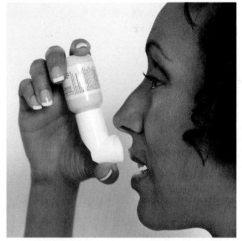

sirtravelalot/Shutterstock.com

A

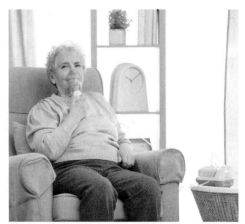

Africa Studio/Shutterstock.com

B

Figure 9.27 People with asthma use inhalers (A) and nebulizers (B) for relief.

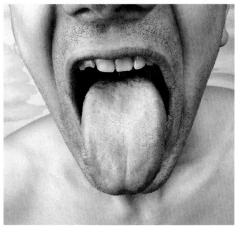

Adam J/Shutterstock.com

Figure 9.28 One area thrush can form is on the back of the tongue.

Chronic Bronchitis

Bronchitis is a condition in which the bronchial passages become inflamed. Irritated membranes in the bronchial passages swell and narrow the airways to the lungs. Bronchitis can be acute (lasting one to three weeks) or chronic (lasting three months or longer). When people have acute bronchitis, they experience a persistent, hacking cough; mucus in their airways; and a feeling of breathlessness. These people may also have an upper respiratory infection (URI), as acute bronchitis is most often the result of a viral infection. Once the acute phase of bronchitis passes, membranes in the bronchial passages usually return to normal. Treatments for acute bronchitis usually include cough suppressants, over-the-counter medications to relieve fever and body aches, rest, and fluids.

Chronic bronchitis is long-term, is progressive, and requires ongoing medical treatment. Repeated episodes of acute bronchitis, which weaken the airways, may result in chronic bronchitis. Other causes of chronic bronchitis are smoking and the inhalation of secondhand smoke. Over time, damage to the cilia in the lungs can result in improper functioning.

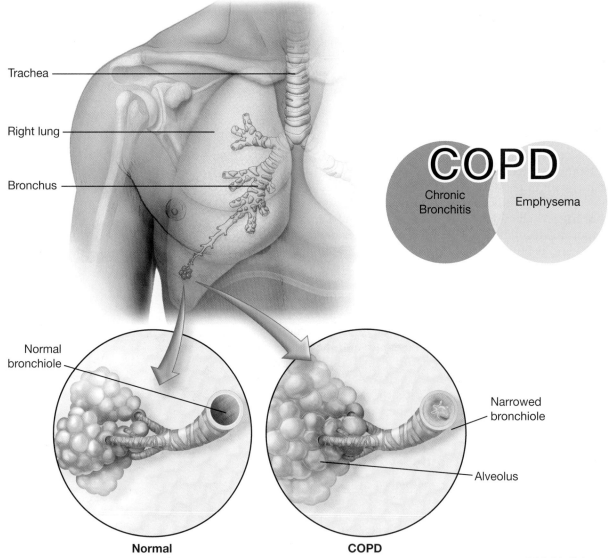

© Body Scientific International

Figure 9.29 COPD includes chronic bronchitis and emphysema.

Emphysema

Emphysema causes damage to the walls of air sacs (*alveoli*) in the lungs, which reduces the amount of gas exchange that can occur. Because the alveoli do not work properly, carbon dioxide becomes trapped during exhalation, leaving no room for fresh oxygen during inhalation. People with emphysema experience a gradual increase in shortness of breath, even at rest. Heart problems may also result from this disease.

Signs and Symptoms of COPD

COPD is the third-leading cause of death in the United States. Symptoms of COPD appear slowly and worsen over time, limiting activities of daily living. Symptoms of COPD include a persistent cough that produces large amounts of mucus, a tight-feeling chest, shortness of breath (usually with physical activity), and wheezing. Severe symptoms—such as difficulty catching one's breath, tachycardia (rapid heart rate), edema, mental confusion, and weight loss—can reflect the amount of lung damage. There is no cure for COPD; lung damage is irreversible.

COPD is most often seen in middle-age and older adults. To diagnose COPD, doctors take a medical and family history and perform spirometry and other lung function and blood tests. A chest X-ray or chest CT scan may also help determine the amount of damage.

Care Considerations for COPD

The goals for treating COPD are to relieve symptoms, slow disease progression, improve tolerance to activity, and prevent complications. *Bronchodilators*, inhaled medications that relax muscles around the airways, help improve breathing. Long-acting bronchodilators are used daily, while short-acting bronchodilators are used only when needed. Other medications may help reduce inflammation when COPD is severe. Residents who have severe COPD may also need oxygen therapy delivered by nasal cannulas (Figure 9.30). Residents with COPD should receive an annual flu shot and pneumonia vaccine to prevent complications. Surgery may benefit those with severe COPD or emphysema.

Living with COPD can be frustrating, be scary, and cause stress and depression. Lifestyle modifications for those with COPD include smoking cessation, avoidance of secondhand smoke, and removal of environmental irritants. Holistic nursing assistants can assist by listening and providing support and resources, as directed.

As a holistic nursing assistant, you can help residents with daily activities and ensure activities are done slowly to conserve breathing. Residents also need to have personal items within easy reach, have assistive devices, and receive help eating due to shortness of breath. If residents are on oxygen therapy, good hygiene around the nose and mouth is essential. Maintaining good hygiene is also important, as there may be large amounts of coughed-up mucus. Always observe residents for worsening symptoms, such as trouble breathing, gasping, or changes in attitude or emotions. Notify the licensed nursing staff immediately if these occur.

How Are the Immune and Lymphatic Systems Affected by Disease?

The primary function of the immune system is to defend the body against infection. As you learned in chapter 8, there are two different types of immunity. *Natural immunity* is the immunity with which people are born. *Acquired immunity* is immunity to specific bacteria or viruses and gives the body the ability to protect itself. There are several ways the immune system can malfunction and result in particular diseases and conditions (Figure 9.31).

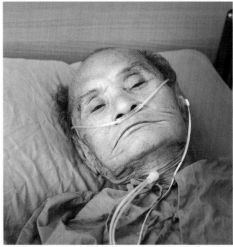

iidea studio/Shutterstock.com

Figure 9.30 A nasal cannula can help a resident with COPD breathe.

Diseases and Conditions of the Immune System		
Disease or Condition	**Cause**	**Example**
Primary immune deficiency	Being born with a weak immune system	*Severe combined immunodeficiency (SCID)*: a person is born with a lack of vital white blood cells.
Acquired immune deficiency	A disease that weakens the immune system	*HIV/AIDS*: important white blood cells are destroyed, leaving a person at risk for contracting opportunistic infections (which are difficult to overcome).
Allergic reaction	An overly active immune system	*Eczema*: an allergen causes an itchy rash.
Autoimmune disorder	Immune system attacks itself	*Systemic lupus erythematosus (SLE or lupus)*: the body develops autoimmune antibodies that attack and damage its own tissue; most commonly affects the joints, lungs, blood cells, nerves, and kidneys.

Figure 9.31 Some common types of immune system diseases are described here.

Autoimmune Disorders

When a person has an *autoimmune disorder*, the body produces antibodies that attack the body's own tissues instead of fighting infection. There is no known cause of autoimmune disorders, although a person's genes, in combination with infection and other environmental factors, play a role. There are more than 80 autoimmune disorders, and these disorders tend to run in families. Women (particularly African-American, Hispanic, and Native American women) are at higher risk for some autoimmune disorders.

Treatments for autoimmune disorders generally focus on using medications and other approaches to reduce immune system activity. No cure has been discovered.

Several diseases and conditions, including rheumatoid arthritis and multiple sclerosis (MS), are thought to be affected by the autoimmune response. Another autoimmune disorder is *systemic lupus erythematosus* (commonly called *lupus* or *SLE*). People who have lupus develop autoimmune antibodies that attack multiple body tissues. While lupus is different for each person, it typically affects the joints, lungs, blood cells, nerves, kidneys, and skin. *Ulcerative colitis* and *Crohn's disease* are autoimmune inflammatory bowel diseases (IBD). These diseases cause antibodies to attack the lining of the intestines, resulting in abdominal pain, diarrhea, rectal bleeding, fever, and weight loss. Another autoimmune disorder called *vasculitis* results in the immune system attacking and damaging blood vessels.

HIV/AIDS

Human immunodeficiency virus (HIV) weakens the immune system and causes people to become sick with infections that would not normally affect them. *Acquired immunodeficiency syndrome (AIDS)* is considered the most advanced stage of HIV.

HIV is transmitted through blood, semen, vaginal fluid, and breast milk. It is not transmitted by simple casual contact, such as kissing or sharing drinking glasses. HIV is most commonly spread by

- vaginal or anal intercourse without a condom with someone who has HIV/AIDS;
- the sharing of needles or syringes with someone who has HIV/AIDS;
- deep puncture with a needle or surgical instrument contaminated with HIV;
- HIV-infected blood, semen, or vaginal secretions that get into open wounds or sores; and
- birth or breast-feeding when the mother is infected with HIV/AIDS.

Recent US statistics show that 1.1 million people are living with HIV. Since the early 1980s, over 1 million people have been diagnosed with AIDS.

HIV/AIDS Signs, Symptoms, and Diagnosis

HIV symptoms vary depending on the stage of the virus. In the first stage of HIV infection, people may experience a fever, headache, diarrhea, sore throat, swollen lymph glands (in the neck), muscle aches and joint pain, and red rashes that do not itch. These symptoms will usually last for a few weeks. At this time, the virus is highly infectious.

The second stage of HIV is called *clinical latent infection* (or *chronic HIV*). There are no specific signs or symptoms of this stage; however, some people continue to have swollen lymph glands. At this stage, untreated HIV will continue to attack and destroy the immune system, leaving a person susceptible to other serious infections. This stage can last for a very long time and will usually not progress if the person is taking medication.

HIV may progress to the third and final stage, which is AIDS. The signs and symptoms of AIDS are

- constant tiredness;
- headaches and dizziness;
- swollen lymph glands in the neck or groin;
- a fever that lasts more than 10 days;
- night sweats;
- unexplained weight loss of 10 or more pounds;
- purplish spots on the skin or mouth;
- shortness of breath;
- a persistent, deep, dry cough;
- severe, chronic diarrhea;
- yeast infection in the mouth (thrush), throat, or vagina;
- unexplained bruises or bleeding from a body opening;
- frequent or unusual skin rashes;
- severe numbness or pain in the hands or feet, loss of muscle control and reflexes, paralysis, or loss of muscular strength; and
- confusion, personality changes, or decreased mental abilities.

People with AIDS who do not take medications will only survive about three years, less if they get a serious infection.

Only testing confirms the presence of HIV. Testing is usually a two-step process. The first test detects HIV-specific antibodies in the blood or saliva. If this test is positive, a second test is done to confirm the first result. If a person does get HIV/AIDS, he or she should seek immediate treatment. There is currently no cure for HIV/AIDS, but there are treatments.

Care Considerations for HIV/AIDS

People who are at high risk of getting HIV may take a medication called *pre-exposure prophylaxis (PreP)*. PreP helps reduce a person's risk of getting HIV. *Post-exposure prophylaxis (PEP)* medications may be prescribed for people who have been infected as a result of sexual assault, unprotected sex, or the sharing of needles with someone who is HIV-positive. PEP must be taken within 72 hours of exposure and can have unpleasant side effects. There is no guarantee it will prevent the transmission of HIV.

The current treatment for HIV/AIDS is a combination of medications (called a *cocktail*) that helps control the growth of the virus. These cocktails also keep HIV from progressing into AIDS, improve the function of the immune system, and slow or stop symptoms. Cocktails for AIDS may not be available to everyone, can be expensive, and may have serious and uncomfortable side effects. They may only work for some people and only for limited periods of time. IM approaches such as vitamins, minerals, herbs, yoga, massage therapy, meditation, and acupuncture may be used alongside medications.

Protection against HIV/AIDS is very important. The surest way to prevent HIV/AIDS is to abstain from sexual intercourse and from sharing needles. If people choose to have sex, they should practice safe or safer sex (for example, using condoms for protection) to reduce the risk of exchanging blood, semen, or vaginal fluids.

Holistic nursing assistants are involved in several care considerations for residents with HIV/AIDS. As a holistic nursing assistant, you should use consistent hand hygiene and put on gloves if touching infected fluids or waste. It is also important to prevent skin puncture; pay attention to any potential sharp instruments that have been exposed to bodily fluids and left in the linens. If present, these instruments must be removed carefully.

As a holistic nursing assistant, encourage mobility if the resident is weak and frail and maintain skin integrity through frequent positioning and by keeping the skin clean and dry. Mobility can also be improved through range-of-motion (ROM) exercises and gentle massage, if ordered.

Be aware of potential side effects from medications and observe and report to the licensed nursing staff any physical, behavioral, or emotional changes. Good nutrition, fluids, exercise, rest, and stress management are important for helping residents maintain a healthy lifestyle.

How Does Disease Influence Gastrointestinal System Function?

The gastrointestinal (GI) system uses its essential functions of ingestion, digestion, absorption, and elimination to transform foods eaten into energy that is needed to survive and thrive. Any change or disruption in this process may result in a gastrointestinal disease or condition. Common gastrointestinal system diseases and conditions are gastroesophageal reflux disease (GERD), peptic ulcers, gallbladder disease, and diverticulitis. While the entire healthcare team will provide care, a *gastroenterologist* will likely be a key care provider.

Gastroesophageal Reflux Disease (GERD)

Gastroesophageal reflux disease (GERD) is commonly called *acid reflux* and is characterized by the flow of acidic stomach contents back into the esophagus. This backflow occurs when the lower esophageal sphincter between the esophagus and the stomach is either weak or relaxes when it should not. The severity of GERD depends on the severity of the sphincter's dysfunction. The cause of GERD is sometimes a *hiatal hernia* (the bulging of the stomach into the chest through the diaphragmatic hiatus). Severe coughing, vomiting, or straining are possible causes of a hiatal hernia.

Signs and Symptoms of GERD

The key symptom of GERD is *heartburn*, which is also called *indigestion*. In the United States, nearly 15 million people suffer from heartburn daily, and 60 million have heartburn at least once a month. Heartburn feels like a burning pain in the middle of the chest. This is different from chest pain that is felt during a heart attack and that gets worse with exercise. The burning sensation during heartburn is sometimes accompanied by an acidic taste. Food may also move up the throat and into the mouth. Heartburn can last as long as two hours and is usually worse after eating, lying down, or bending over.

Other symptoms of GERD include a chronic cough, laryngitis, and nausea. A serious complication is *esophagitis*, or damaging inflammation in the esophagus that may be accompanied by esophageal bleeding and ulcers.

Care Considerations for GERD

Easing the symptoms of heartburn is an important step in treating GERD. Simply standing erect may reduce heartburn, and taking over-the-counter antacids will neutralize acid in the stomach. Adopting a diet that excludes chocolate, peppermint, coffee, fried or fatty foods, citrus fruits and juices, tomato products, pepper, and alcohol will also help residents find relief. If an appropriate diet does not ease heartburn, or if heartburn becomes chronic, a doctor will order special diagnostic procedures. One procedure might be an *upper GI series*, in which the esophagus, stomach, and upper part of the small intestine are viewed using a special X-ray procedure.

Changes in diet can reduce reflux and damage to the lining of the esophagus and can usually relieve GERD. Dietary changes can be challenging, particularly if excluded foods are favorites or are an important part of the resident's culture. Controlling portions and eating at least two to three hours before going to bed can also decrease GERD. Elevating the head of the bed or sleeping on wedges will minimize reflux. Do not use pillows for these positions, as they may increase pressure on the stomach. If feeding a resident, position the head of the bed at 75–90 degrees and leave the head of the bed elevated for one to two hours after eating. Encouraging weight loss for overweight residents can provide relief.

Smoking cessation is also known to relax the sphincter responsible for GERD. Some residents use prescription medications to reduce the secretion and amount of acid in the stomach. Surgery may be necessary to treat very severe GERD.

Peptic Ulcers

Peptic ulcers are sores or sometimes holes in the lining of the GI tract. A *gastric ulcer* forms in the stomach, and the more common *duodenal ulcer* forms in the small intestine. *Esophageal ulcers* (in the lower part of the esophagus) are rare and usually form due to the use of medications or alcohol (Figure 9.32).

One in 10 people experience an ulcer sometime in life. Risk factors for developing a peptic ulcer include a family history of ulcers, stress, diet, long-term use or abuse of over-the-counter pain medications, and smoking (which increases stomach acid). A bacterial infection caused by *Helicobacter pylori* (*H. pylori*) is present in most people who have duodenal and gastric ulcers and may be the primary cause of ulcers. Ulcers are more likely to develop in older adults, as older adults may take medications that irritate the GI tract.

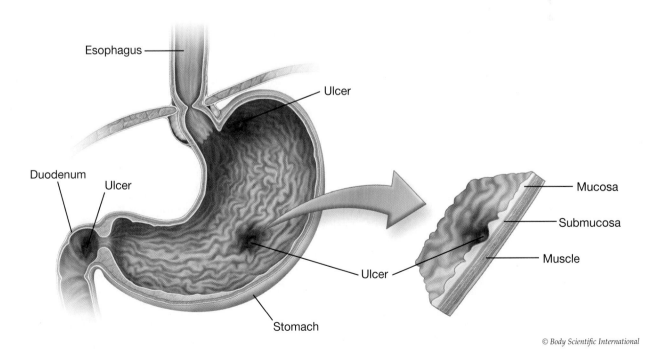

© *Body Scientific International*

Figure 9.32 The three types of peptic ulcers are illustrated here.

Signs and Symptoms of Peptic Ulcers

Peptic ulcers cause a dull abdominal pain that becomes more intense when the stomach is empty. Bloating, burping, acid reflux, weight loss (because it hurts to eat), and nausea or vomiting are other symptoms. Symptoms that require immediate treatment are continuing, sudden sharp pain in the abdominal area; black or bloody stools; and bloody vomit that looks like coffee grounds. These signs suggest that the ulcer has worn through the stomach lining or that a blood vessel has broken.

Doctors identify peptic ulcers by examining medical history and current symptoms. A blood, stool, or breath test will determine the presence of *H. pylori*. Other tests might include an endoscopy or barium X-ray. In a barium X-ray, barium (a thick, white fluid) is swallowed and coats the stomach and small intestine. This fluid makes it easier to see an ulcer on the X-ray.

Care Considerations for Peptic Ulcers

There are various treatment options for peptic ulcers, and treatment should start early to prevent further damage and possible hemorrhage. If *H. pylori* is present, antibiotics are given to kill the bacteria. Antacids and prescription medications may be used to decrease stomach acids. Ulcers must be monitored to ensure they do not worsen. If an ulcer does not heal, if there is bleeding, or if there is a tear in the GI lining, the next step may be blood transfusions or surgery.

While ulcer-related symptoms may subside quickly with treatment, prescribed medications must be taken, and smoking, alcohol, and foods that trigger symptoms must be avoided. Managing stress also helps alleviate symptoms. As a holistic nursing assistant, observe and report any side effects that may accompany treatment. These side effects include headaches, dizziness, and diarrhea.

Gallbladder Disease

Gallbladder disease occurs when *gallstones* (hardened composites of cholesterol and other substances found in bile) form in the gallbladder. Gallstones range from very small (the size of gravel) to the size of a golf ball (Figure 9.33). Gallstones only cause problems when they block the bile duct. Gallstones can form if the gallbladder does not empty normally. People who are overweight are at greater risk for gallstone formation.

Signs and Symptoms of Gallbladder Disease

Gallbladder disease sometimes causes mild pain in the upper right part of the abdomen, and pain may spread to the right upper back or shoulder blade. The pain can be steady or come and go and may get worse when a person eats. Most people who have gallstones do not have symptoms until a bile duct is blocked. Then people may experience pain, as well as fever and chills. In gallbladder disease, the skin and the whites of the eyes can become yellow, or *jaundiced*. This symptom could mean that gallstones are in the bile duct or that there is an infection in the gallbladder. This is an emergency.

To determine if there is gallbladder disease, a doctor will ask about a resident's pain, the time that the pain started, and the pain's location and duration. An ultrasound can reveal the presence of gallstones.

Care Considerations for Gallbladder Disease

To prevent or reduce the risk of gallstones, residents should not skip meals, should maintain a healthy weight, and should lose weight slowly if needed. Prescription medications may be used to dissolve gallstones. More commonly, surgical removal of the gallbladder (called a *cholecystectomy*) is required if gallstones become large and if attacks recur frequently. The gallbladder is not a crucial organ, so its removal does not affect vital body function.

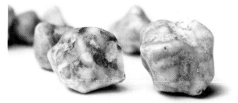

Roblan/Shutterstock.com

Figure 9.33 Gallstones form in various shapes and sizes.

If caring for residents who have had a cholecystectomy, be aware that they may experience diarrhea for a short period while their bodies become accustomed to changes in digestion.

Diverticulitis

Diverticulitis occurs when pouches in the wall of the colon, called *diverticula*, become inflamed or infected. Low fiber in the intestine can create pressure, which causes diverticula to form in weak spots in the intestinal wall. Risk factors for diverticulitis include aging, a diet high in animal fat and low in fiber, lack of exercise, obesity, smoking, and certain medications.

Signs and Symptoms of Diverticulitis

Signs and symptoms of diverticulitis include intense pain in the lower left abdomen that worsens during activity, fever and chills, bloating and gas, nausea and vomiting, and diarrhea or constipation. The presence of diverticula is determined through examining a medical history and conducting a physical examination, blood test, and X-ray or CT scan.

Care Considerations for Diverticulitis

Treatment for diverticulitis varies based on the severity of symptoms. Prevention is important to ensure that diverticula do not become inflamed or infected. As a holistic nursing assistant, you should follow the resident's plan of care. Residents should be encouraged to maintain a high-fiber diet with whole grains and fresh fruit and vegetables. These foods will help digested food pass through the intestines quickly, thus reducing pressure. Encourage residents to consume fluids to ensure that fiber is not constipating. Exercise also helps promote normal bowel function. During a mild diverticulitis attack, low heat on the abdomen, if prescribed, can be comforting. Guiding a resident through relaxation techniques, such as deep breathing and the use of pain medications (as ordered), may also be helpful. Prescription medications, including antibiotics, are given if there is an infection. At first, solid food should be replaced with liquids to allow the intestine to heal. Severe attacks may require intravenous (IV) antibiotics. If complications such as a perforation (hole), **abscess** (collection of pus that causes swelling), or **fistula** (an abnormal opening) occur, a bowel resection surgery may be the next step.

During a *bowel resection surgery*, diseased parts of the intestine are removed, and healthy portions of the intestine are reconnected. In addition to bowel resection, a colostomy (surgical opening in the abdomen for passing waste into an external bag) may be necessary. A colostomy allows the intestine to rest and inflammation to subside. Once healed, the colostomy can be reversed and the intestine reconnected. For information about ostomy care, see chapter 22. For post-surgical care, see chapter 24.

How Is the Urinary System Affected by Disease?

Urinary tract infections (UTIs), kidney stones, and acute kidney failure are common urinary system diseases and conditions. You will learn about a urinary condition called *incontinence* in chapter 23. *Urologists* are doctors who specialize in diagnosing and treating diseases and conditions of the urinary system.

Think About This
When the urinary system is healthy, urine can stay in the bladder for up to five hours before being excreted.

Urinary Tract Infection (UTI)

A *urinary tract infection (UTI)* is an infection in any part of the urinary system. UTIs typically develop when pathogens enter the body through the urethra and begin to grow. The body usually defends effectively against these bacterial invasions, but sometimes the body fails, resulting in an infection. UTIs can occur in the kidneys (*pyelonephritis*), urinary bladder (*cystitis*), or urethra (*urethritis*).

Common causes of UTIs include the transfer of bacteria from the anus, sexual activity, certain types of birth control, menopause, kidney stones, an enlarged prostate, the presence of a urinary catheter, or a surgical procedure. Women are at greater risk for UTIs due to their anatomy, as the female urethra is located very close to the anus. UTIs that women get are usually cystitis or urethritis.

Signs and Symptoms of UTIs

Signs and symptoms of UTIs are specific to the infection's location. In general, UTIs are accompanied by a strong and persistent urge to urinate and a burning sensation when urinating. When a person has a UTI, very small amounts of urine may be excreted, and urine may appear cloudy and have a strong smell. Blood may also be present in the urine, causing urine to look red, bright pink, or cocoa colored. People who have UTIs may experience confusion and disorientation, and women may experience pain in the pelvic area. UTIs in the kidneys may cause upper back and side pain, fever, and chills. In urethritis, there may be discharge from the urethra. If left untreated, UTIs may lead to serious complications, such as multiple and more serious infections, urethral narrowing (called a *stricture*), and kidney damage.

Tests for diagnosing a UTI usually include a urine sample for laboratory analysis (to determine the types of cells present in the urine). Another test that helps diagnose a UTI is a *urine culture*, in which a small amount of urine is tested to identify the specific bacteria present. See chapter 19 for more detailed information about collecting urine samples. When diagnosing a UTI, a doctor may also want to look at the structure of the urinary system using a CT scan or an MRI. When people have recurring infections, a doctor may also perform a *cystoscopy*, which involves the insertion of a long, thin catheter with a lens into the urethra and urinary bladder to view the organs' linings.

Care Considerations for UTIs

Antibiotics are typically used to treat UTIs, and several different antibiotics may be used. The results of a urine culture help in selecting the right antibiotic. The duration of antibiotic treatment depends on the infection and on medical history.

UTIs are usually painful; therefore, an analgesic may be prescribed. As a holistic nursing assistant, you can care for residents with UTIs by paying attention to residents' levels of pain and reporting that information to the licensed nursing staff. Sometimes it is helpful to apply heat to the resident's abdomen using a warm, dry compress or a heating pad, if ordered. Keep residents hydrated and avoid irritating fluids such as coffee, soft drinks, and citrus juices. Irritating fluids can aggravate tissue linings in the urinary system and increase the frequency and urgency of urination. If a resident has a urinary catheter, provide thorough catheter care to prevent UTIs (see chapter 23). Provide excellent hygiene for residents by giving daily perineal care (see chapter 22); ensuring cleanliness after elimination; and keeping dressings, briefs, and other linens near the urethra dry and clean.

Kidney Stones

Kidney stones (*renal lithiasis*) are small, hard deposits that form in the kidneys. They are composed of minerals and acid salts. Kidney stones can form when the urine becomes concentrated and contains more crystal-forming substances than urine is able to dilute. Urine may also lack the necessary substances to prevent crystals from sticking together. While there is no single cause for kidney stones, dehydration; diets high in protein, salt, and sugar; obesity; gout; family or personal history; gastrointestinal diseases; and side effects of some medications are possible causes.

The type of kidney stone can help determine the cause. Some kidney stones are composed of calcium, and other kidney stones may be caused by a UTI. These kidney stones grow quickly and are large (Figure 9.34).

Signs and Symptoms of Kidney Stones

A person can have a kidney stone and not be aware of it. This is because symptoms may not occur until the stone starts to move. Signs and symptoms of moving kidney stones include

- pain that comes in waves, changes in intensity, is located in the side and back below the ribs, and spreads to the lower abdomen and groin;
- pink, red, or brown urine that is foul smelling;
- a persistent need to urinate, urination of small amounts, and pain during urination;
- fever and chills, if an infection is present; and
- nausea and vomiting.

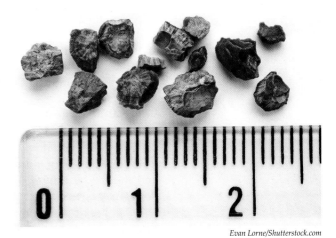

Evan Lorne/Shutterstock.com

Figure 9.34 Kidney stones vary in size and shape.

Care Considerations for Kidney Stones

Treatment for kidney stones varies depending on the type of kidney stone and the cause. The focus of treatment is on passing the kidney stone, which can be very painful. Strategies for helping people pass small kidney stones include drinking a great deal of water (between 2 and 3 quarts) until urine is clear, using pain medications, and sometimes using prescribed medications that relax the muscles in the ureter. Larger kidney stones may require the use of sound waves to break up the kidney stones, the use of a scope to remove kidney stones, or surgery. Prescription medications will control the amount of minerals and acid found in the urine and prevent the formation of kidney stones.

As a holistic nursing assistant, encourage residents who have a history of kidney stones to drink plenty of fluids. Be aware of any foods that promote the forming of kidney stones. Some of these include foods with a lot of salt; animal protein; and foods with oxalate (a compound found in food that is excreted in the urine) such as beets, spinach, sweet potatoes, nuts, chocolate, and soy products. If you are caring for a resident who is passing a kidney stone, follow the instructions given by the licensed nursing staff.

Renal Failure

When the kidneys become unable to filter waste products from the blood, a condition called *renal failure* or *kidney failure* occurs. Renal failure causes an accumulation of dangerous levels of waste products and creates an imbalance in the body's chemical composition.

Renal failure can develop over a long period of time or in a few hours, depending on the cause. Failure that develops quickly, or *acute renal failure*, is an emergency. If not treated, it can be irreversible and fatal. A person can also have chronic kidney disease, or *chronic renal failure*, in which there is a gradual loss of kidney function.

Usually, renal failure is the result of some other disease such as hypertension, diabetes mellitus, or PVD. Other causes are urinary blockage, infections, allergic reactions, medications, blood loss, severe burns, or cancer.

Signs and Symptoms of Renal Failure

Signs and symptoms of renal failure are decreased urine output, edema, shortness of breath, chest pain, muscle weakness, drowsiness and fatigue, confusion, and nausea. Advanced stages of renal failure or end-stage renal disease (ESRD) can lead to seizures or a **coma** (a state of deep and prolonged unconsciousness). Complete loss of kidney function leads to death.

Tests for diagnosing renal failure include the measurement of urinary output to determine if it is within normal limits (between 800 and 2000 milliliters daily). A *urinalysis* examines the chemical composition of the urine. A doctor may also use blood tests to determine the level of kidney function, an ultrasound, a CT scan, and a **biopsy** (the removal of a small piece of tissue for testing) to test kidney tissue.

Care Considerations for Renal Failure

Renal failure may require hospitalization. Treatment goals will be established to balance fluids, and prescription medications may be used to control high potassium levels due to lack of kidney filtering. High potassium levels can cause arrhythmias and muscle weakness. Temporary **dialysis** (removal of waste products from the body) may be needed to get rid of wastes, toxins, and excess fluids from the blood.

Diet is extremely important for treating renal failure, and low-potassium foods are an essential component. Low-potassium foods include apples, cabbage, green beans, and strawberries. A diet that limits salt and phosphorus is also a requirement to reverse renal failure. Phosphorus is a mineral found in milk, cheese, and nuts. Limiting protein and calcium intake may also be recommended.

When kidneys are so damaged they cannot function and have nearly or completely failed, a resident has *end-stage renal disease (ESRD)*. Dialysis is necessary in this case. The resident may receive *hemodialysis* (through a machine that filters the blood) or *peritoneal dialysis* (through a catheter inserted into the abdominal cavity that delivers a solution that absorbs waste and excess fluids). When the kidneys are no longer able to remove waste products, a kidney transplant may be appropriate.

Which Diseases Are Associated with the Reproductive Systems?

A common reproductive system disease for males is benign prostatic hypertrophy (BPH). Reproductive system diseases for females include vaginitis and uterine prolapse. A discussion of sexually transmitted infections (STI) is included in Appendix B. While the entire healthcare team provides care, a *urologist* and *gynecologist* will likely be key care providers.

Benign Prostatic Hypertrophy (BPH)

Benign prostatic hypertrophy (BPH), also called *benign prostatic hyperplasia*, is an enlarged prostate gland. Due to hormonal changes and cell growth, this is a common occurrence for men as they age. When the prostate gets bigger than normal, it can partially block the urethra (Figure 9.35). This can cause problems with urination.

Signs and Symptoms of BPH

The signs and symptoms of BPH include

- trouble starting the urine stream and difficulty stopping it, which causes "dribbling";
- a weak urine stream;
- the feeling that the bladder is not completely empty after urination; and
- extreme difficulty urinating when the bladder is nearly blocked, which can cause a backup of urine (called *urinary retention*), infections, and kidney damage.

BPH is noncancerous and does not interfere with the ability to achieve an erection. It is diagnosed by taking a medical history and conducting a physical examination. A urinalysis may be done, and a *digital* (using the fingers) *rectal exam* by a doctor can determine the size of the prostate. Some doctors also perform a special blood test (called a *prostate-specific antigen* or *PSA* test) to help rule out prostate cancer.

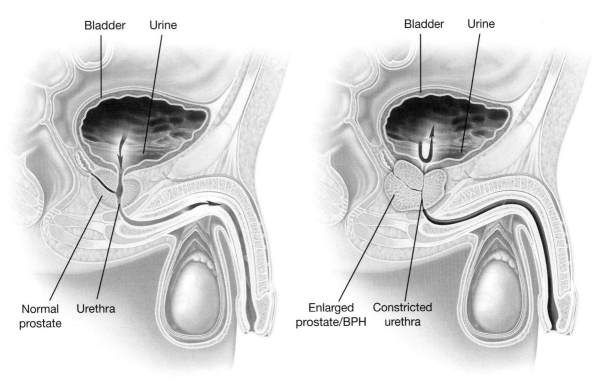

Bladder   Urine

Bladder   Urine

Normal   Urethra
prostate

Enlarged   Constricted
prostate/BPH   urethra

© *Body Scientific International*

Figure 9.35 BPH can block the male urethra if the prostate grows too large.

Care Considerations for BPH

The focus of BPH treatment is on reducing or controlling any symptoms. Medications may be prescribed, and lifestyle and physical strategies may be recommended to control symptoms. If symptoms are severe, surgery may be performed to remove part of the prostate gland.

When it is difficult to urinate, a resident may become anxious and fearful. This anxiety may cause the resident to be tense, making it even more difficult to urinate. Encourage residents to relax and stay calm. You can also help residents *double urinate*, or urinate as much as possible, relax for a moment, and then urinate again. Avoiding caffeine and alcohol will help lessen the need to urinate. As a holistic nursing assistant, you can help residents maintain good body hygiene and skin care and provide special briefs if there is dribbling. Be respectful and do not call these briefs diapers.

Vaginitis

Vaginitis is an infection or inflammation of the vagina. The source of the infection might be bacteria, a virus, or yeast. Some cases of vaginitis are considered noninfectious. Each type of vaginitis causes different symptoms; however, more than one source can cause infection. As a result, telling the types of vaginitis apart is challenging.

Common causes of vaginitis relate to normal organisms found in the vagina. A healthy vagina may have a clear or slightly cloudy discharge. Vaginitis can be caused by a *yeast infection*, or an overgrowth of the yeast normally found in the vagina. The same is true of bacterial infection; vaginitis may result when there are more bacteria than usual in the vagina. Vaginitis may result from sexual contact; poor hygiene; lower levels of hormones, which make the vagina dry; or allergic reactions to detergents, fabric softeners, soaps, or vaginal sprays.

Signs and Symptoms of Vaginitis

The signs and symptoms of vaginitis include changes in the color, smell, and texture of vaginal discharge. For example, a yeast infection may cause vaginal discharge to look like cottage cheese. Vaginal discharge may also have a fishy smell if the infection is bacterial. Irritation, itching, or burning during urination may also occur. Determining which type of vaginitis is present is important to ensure the cause of vaginitis is identified and treated correctly.

Care Considerations for Vaginitis

Medications and topical creams may be prescribed to treat vaginitis, and people with vaginitis should avoid irritants, use cold compresses, and abstain from sex until the infection is completely gone. To prevent vaginitis, encourage residents to maintain good hygiene and avoid using sprays or perfumed soaps. For immobile residents, providing daily perineal care is essential. (See chapter 21 for the perineal care procedure.) Vaginal irrigation (*douching*) is not recommended, as it can disrupt the normal organisms in the vagina and increase the risk of another infection. Clothes such as nylon or tight pants that hold in heat and moisture will further the problem of vaginitis. Yogurt with active cultures may help reduce infection.

Uterine Prolapse

Uterine prolapse occurs when the muscles and ligaments of the pelvic floor stretch, weaken, and provide inadequate support for the uterus. The uterus can then slip down into the vagina or even protrude out of the vagina (Figure 9.36).

Uterine prolapse can vary in its severity and can happen to women of any age. It can be caused by damage to tissues during pregnancy and childbirth, large babies, loss of muscle tone, loss of estrogen during menopause, or continuous straining during elimination. Additional risk factors include age, obesity, heavy lifting, excessive coughing, and genetic predisposition.

Signs and Symptoms of Uterine Prolapse

Mild uterine prolapse usually goes unnoticed. The signs and symptoms of moderate-to-severe prolapse include

- tissue protruding from the vagina or the feeling that something is falling out of the vagina;

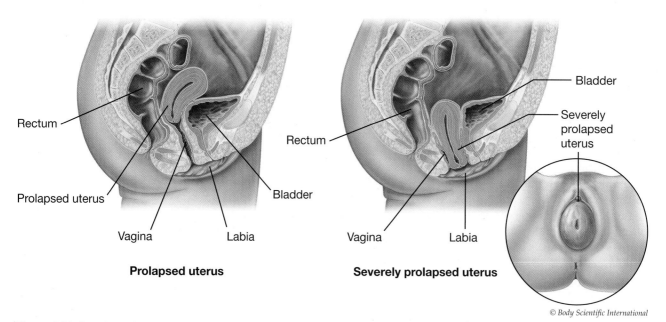

Prolapsed uterus

Severely prolapsed uterus

© *Body Scientific International*

Figure 9.36 A prolapsed uterus can slip into or protrude from the vagina.

- urine leakage or retention;
- trouble having a bowel movement;
- a feeling of pulling in the pelvis; and
- low back pain.

Symptoms of moderate-to-severe uterine prolapse can worsen at the end of the day. Possible complications of uterine prolapse include ulcers (due to rubbing on underwear) and possible prolapse of other pelvic organs, such as the urinary bladder or bowel. Diagnosis is made through physical examination.

Care Considerations for Uterine Prolapse

As a holistic nursing assistant, you can encourage residents with uterine prolapse to drink plenty of fluids, eat high-fiber foods (if appropriate), avoid straining during elimination, and suppress coughing. You can also assist by reminding residents to use good body mechanics when lifting and maintain a proper weight (if needed) to decrease pressure. Sometimes a *vaginal pessary*, a device that fits inside the vagina and holds the uterus in place, may be ordered. A vaginal pessary is not helpful if the prolapse is severe. The vaginal pessary can also be irritating to surrounding tissue. Surgery is usually required to repair a severe prolapse.

How Does Cancer Affect the Body?

The final disease this section will discuss is *cancer*. The effects of cancer provide a good representation of the holistic interconnectedness of body systems. Cancer can begin at an original site in one body system and then spread to other systems. If it spreads, it will not only affect the structure and function of the system where it started, but will also affect other systems.

Cancer occurs when cells grow abnormally and out of control, crowding out normal cells. Some cancers grow quickly, while others are slow growing. There are many types of cancer, and cancer cell growth can start in any location of the body.

Cancer cells spread to other locations in the body through a process called **metastasis**. When metastasis occurs, cells from the original site of cancer (for example, the intestine) spread to other parts of the body (for example, the bones). Once cancer metastasizes, it is much harder to treat. The most common cancers are breast, lung, prostate, intestine and rectum, urinary bladder, skin, thyroid, and pancreatic cancer.

In many cancers, a lump called a *tumor* forms; ais **malignant**, it is cancerous (Figure 9.37). If a tumor is **benign**, it does not contain cancer cells. A tumor might also be a *lipoma*, which consists of fat cells. Some cancers, such as blood cancer, do not form tumors. Blood cancer occurs within blood cells.

Stages of Cancer

The classification system for cancer uses stages and progresses from stages 1 to 4. The stages describe how far the cancer has spread. Stage 1 indicates that cancer has not likely spread from its original site. As the stage numbers increase, cancer has spread farther from the original site. Stage 4 is the most advanced stage of cancer. The stage of cancer helps determine treatment. For example, at stage 1, treatment might be surgery because of the limited spread. Later stages, however, may require a combination of surgery, chemotherapy, or radiation.

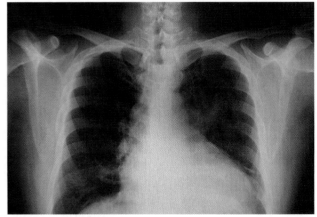

create jobs 51/Shutterstock.com

Figure 9.37 A lung tumor is visible on this chest X-ray.

Cancer Risk Factors, Signs and Symptoms, and Diagnosis

Factors that reduce the risk of developing cancer include living a healthy lifestyle; not smoking; and avoiding toxic substances such as secondhand smoke. Risk factors for cancer include age, family history of cancer, and exposure to sunlight without protection.

The signs and symptoms of cancer are different depending on the type and location of the cancer. For example, breast cancer often causes a lump to form in the breast, while a lesion on the skin may signal melanoma. Some general signs and symptoms of cancer include

- weight loss of 10 or more pounds with no reason;
- consistent fatigue and fever;
- pain that does not go away;
- changes in the color or texture of the skin;
- sores that do not heal;
- changes in elimination;
- unusual bleeding or discharge;
- lumps;
- trouble swallowing; and
- ongoing hoarseness and coughing.

X-rays, blood tests, or a biopsy are usually performed to diagnose cancer.

Cancer Treatments

Common treatment approaches for cancer usually include some combination of surgery, chemotherapy agents (toxic drugs), or radiation. The treatment method used depends on the type of cancer, its stage, and individual response.

Surgery

If surgery is required, one option is prophylactic surgery. In *prophylactic surgery*, an organ is removed before its cells become cancerous because the person has a known high risk for cancer in that particular organ. If a malignant tumor is present, the goal of surgery is to remove the entire tumor and its edges and be sure no cancerous cells remain. During surgery, sometimes the surgeon also removes surrounding tissue to prevent possible spread. Sometimes a person has a course of chemotherapy prior to surgery to shrink a tumor.

Chemotherapy

Surgery is not the only treatment option available. *Chemotherapy* (sometimes called *chemo*) is another choice. Chemotherapy consists of a group of drugs (chemotherapy agents) that target cancer cells. There are many different chemotherapy agents. Some destroy cancer cells, some keep cancer from spreading, or others shrink tumors before surgery or radiation therapy.

Chemotherapy drugs may be administered using a variety of methods, including injection, an intravenous (IV) catheter, injection into the peritoneal cavity, topical administration, and oral administration. Chemotherapy is usually administered in timed cycles, allowing the body to build new, healthy cells between treatments. For example, one week of chemotherapy may be followed by two weeks of rest.

Common side effects of chemotherapy include fatigue, dry mouth, sores in the mouth, easy bruising, appetite and weight changes, nausea and vomiting, constipation or diarrhea, hair loss, and changes in mood and concentration. Side effects can subside quickly after treatment, though some may take much longer to go away or last a lifetime.

Radiation

Radiation is used to kill or slow the growth of cancer cells. A radiation treatment consists of high-energy waves directed at cancer cells. Side effects of radiation are different for each person, are associated with the location of radiation therapy, and can be mild or severe. Early side effects generally include nausea, fatigue, and skin problems. If radiation is administered to the scalp, hair loss may be a side effect. Eating problems may result if treatment is administered to the head, face, or throat. Resulting eating problems usually do not last long.

Cancer Survival Rates

Some people will completely recover from cancer, some will live with cancer for many years in remission, and others will die of cancer. Nearly 40 percent of men and women receive a diagnosis of cancer during their lifetimes. Mortality from cancer accounts for 185 deaths per 100,000 men and women every year. Mortality is higher for men than for women, is highest among African-American men, and is lowest among Asian and Pacific Islander women. Approximately 64 percent of cancer survivors have lived more than five years after diagnosis. Only 15 percent of survivors have lived for 20 or more years after diagnosis. Nearly one-half of cancer survivors are age 70 or older.

While many people survive cancer today, every person is different. Some people have different stages of cancer and respond to treatment better than others do. It is hard to estimate the survival rate for cancer, particularly if a person has other illnesses.

Care Considerations for Cancer

When people receive a diagnosis of cancer, their lives may no longer be the same. People will experience many changes in their self and body images, work schedules, family lives, and daily routines. Many people become frightened and anxious, worrying about what will happen next and how long they will live. This can be overwhelming. After a cancer diagnosis, there are many decisions to make and much to think about—not only for the present, but also for the future.

Providing Emotional Support

Each person will react uniquely and respond to treatment differently. Some people become discouraged, some experience denial, and others feel like they can overcome the diagnosis and anything else that comes their way. It is important for a holistic nursing assistant to be sensitive to and aware of a resident's feelings about and approaches to cancer diagnosis and treatment. Supportive care and attention to residents' needs are fundamental. Being positive and adding humor, when appropriate, can be helpful.

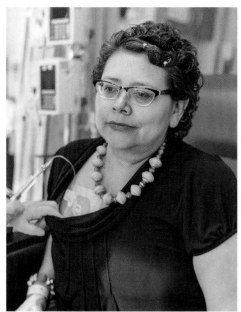

Emerald Raindrops/Shutterstock.com

Figure 9.38 Chemotherapy is delivered via a catheter and port.

Responding to Treatment Side Effects

If a resident has had surgery, he or she will need post-surgical care, which can include dressing changes, proper positioning, and careful monitoring of blood pressure. If a resident is having chemotherapy, he or she may have a catheter, port, and attached pump to control the delivery of medications (Figure 9.38). Skin care and observation for possible infection are critical.

Chemotherapy

Attention to a resident's response to chemotherapy and its side effects requires good observation and reporting.

- If a resident feels fatigued, be sure he or she rests after treatment and takes short naps during the day. If ordered and appropriate, mild exercise, such as a short walk, can boost energy. Practice fall-prevention strategies.

- If a resident feels nauseous, small, frequent meals can help, as can apples, juice, tea, and flat ginger ale. Sometimes drinking fluids slowly before and after, but not during, meals can also help. Avoid strong-smelling foods, sweets, and fried fatty foods. Food may taste metallic and plastic utensils may help.

- If a resident is experiencing hair loss, use a soft-bristle brush during hair care and mild, moisturizing shampoo and conditioners. Shorter hair may make hair appear fuller. The resident should only wear a wig if the scalp is clean and free from irritation or sores. Be sure the wig is clean.

- If a resident seems to have mental fog after treatment (sometimes called *chemo brain*), provide daily activities, talk with the resident, and focus on one thing or task at a time.

- Sun sensitivity is another side effect of chemotherapy. Residents should go outside when the sun is the weakest (before 10 a.m. and after 4 p.m.). Sunscreen with an SPF of 30 or higher should be used. In addition, skin should be covered, and a wide-brimmed hat should be worn to keep the face shaded.

Be aware of and immediately report any unusual side effects. Side effects may include a very high fever, shortness of breath or trouble breathing, bleeding, a rash or allergic reaction, difficulty swallowing, chills, or long-lasting diarrhea.

Some people try IM approaches to relieve nausea and vomiting. Deep breathing and meditation are two relaxation techniques that may also help.

Radiation

If a resident's treatment plan includes radiation, there will likely be side effects. Skin may look sunburned; get swollen or blistered; or become dry, flaky, and itchy. When caring for residents, be gentle during skin care and use mild soap and luke-warm water. Check to see what ointment or lotion is ordered and be sure not to use hot or cold compresses, tape, or bandages unless instructed.

As you would for residents undergoing chemotherapy, use sun precautions even after the radiation has ended. Radiation therapy to certain parts of the body can have side effects that influence eating and cause nausea. Follow the same care considerations discussed for residents experiencing nausea after chemotherapy. If radiation is administered to the head and neck, residents may experience mouth sores, lack of or thick saliva, and trouble swallowing. Take special care during oral hygiene (see chapter 20). Diarrhea is another side effect. A doctor may prescribe medications and change the diet to ensure there is adequate nutrition. Be sure to keep the resident's skin and bed linens clean and dry. If you are caring for patients in their childbearing years, note that radiation therapy can lower a person's sex drive and sperm count. Pregnancy is not advised during treatment.

End-of-Life Care

For some, poor quality of life and the spread of cancer lead to a decision to end treatment. Holistic care is most essential when this happens. Some people choose to receive end-of-life care at home, others stay in long-term care settings, and others who are close to death may choose to use hospice services. Prescription medications are often used to relieve pain and other symptoms, including shortness of breath, nausea, or constipation. Excellent hygiene and skin care are most important to ensure other issues, such as decubitus ulcers, do not arise.

As you will learn in chapter 27, the end-of-life experience is different for each person. Some residents desire alone time, others are worried and fearful, and others prefer to communicate with family members and those around them. Be sure to provide whatever is needed, including a back massage, assistance with eating and elimination, listening, or helpful resources. Alert the licensed nursing staff if pain relief is needed.

Section 9.1 Review and Assessment

Using the Key Terms

Complete the following sentences using key terms in this section.

1. A weak area in an artery in the brain is a(n) _____.
2. One possible effect of a stroke is _____, or the inability to use or understand words.
3. Abnormal heart rhythms are called _____.
4. The condition in which the arteries harden is called _____.
5. The buildup of plaque in the arteries, restricting blood flow, is _____.
6. If a tumor is not cancerous, it is _____.
7. The term _____ refers to the retention of fluid in the body.
8. If a person is paralyzed on one whole side of the body, he or she has _____.

Know and Understand the Facts

9. What is the difference between an acute and chronic disease?
10. List two risk factors for one of the diseases discussed in this chapter.
11. What is hypertension, and how does it affect the body?
12. Explain the difference between atherosclerosis and arteriosclerosis.
13. Describe what happens when a person has a hemorrhagic stroke.

Analyze and Apply Concepts

14. Discuss the typical treatment for a resident with diabetes mellitus.
15. Identify the care considerations you would follow for a resident who has cancer.

Think Critically

Read the following care situation. Then answer the questions that follow.

Mrs. M was diagnosed with type 2 diabetes 15 years ago. She is 25 pounds overweight and has maintained her diabetic management plan for several years. Last month, she had a stroke. Mrs. M is now in a skilled nursing facility because she has left-sided weakness and is having trouble with her speech. The doctor feels that her diabetes is not stable enough, so he has prescribed insulin injections.

16. Which signs and symptoms should you watch for to determine if Mrs. M becomes hypoglycemic or hyperglycemic?
17. How are hypoglycemia and hyperglycemia treated?
18. Describe three considerations that will be important when caring for Mrs. M.

Pain Relief

Questions to Consider

- We have all experienced pain in our lives. Think about the last time you felt physical pain. Did you hurt yourself, or was the pain from an illness?
- What was your initial reaction to pain? How long did the pain last? What did you do to lessen the pain?

Objectives

When a person has a disease or condition or experiences trauma, there is usually pain. Pain is the body's alert or alarm system. It lets people know they need to stop doing something, such as touching a hot surface. It can also alert people that the body is experiencing internal distress, such as a GI upset or trauma from a fall. In this section, you will learn about the types of pain, the way pain is felt, people's reactions to pain, pain levels and intensity, and pain-relief techniques. To achieve the objectives for this section, you must successfully

- **describe** types of pain and the pain cycle;
- **explain** reactions to pain and pain's impact on people's lives;
- **use** scales and measures to determine pain levels; and
- **discuss** different ways to relieve pain and provide comfort.

Key Terms

Learn these key terms to better understand the information presented in the section.

acute pain   pain scales

chronic pain   stoic

nonpharmacological

What Is Pain?

Pain is something everyone experiences. It is an uncomfortable feeling or sensation recognized by each of us. Sometimes pain occurs suddenly and goes away quickly. Pain may also start slowly and last for a long time. There are many types of pain and ways to describe the feeling.

Pain can be mild, moderate, or severe. When asked, people often describe their pain in different ways. Some might say pain is sharp, dull, aching, throbbing, stabbing, crushing, or stinging. Pain can start as a sharp feeling and become achy, or it can begin as a dull pain and become crushing.

Many factors influence the development and severity of pain. Pain's origin, such as arthritis, a cut, or an abrasion, influences its sensation and severity. Other factors, such as the individual's experience, cultural and ethnic influences, and the length of time pain is experienced, must also be considered when understanding pain.

Pain is felt, or *perceived*, when pain receptors in the nervous system are stimulated. Pain receptors send a signal that travels through nerves to the spinal cord (Figure 9.39). The spinal cord responds to pain by causing a reflex action and signaling motor nerves to act on the sensation of pain. The spinal cord also carries the pain message to the brain, where the message is received by the thalamus and interpreted in the cerebral cortex. Sometimes the pain message is also sent to other parts of the brain, and these parts of the brain cause particular reactions, such as increased heart rate or sweating. This process happens very swiftly so your body can take immediate action.

Remember

Never underestimate the pain of a person, because in all honesty, everyone is struggling. Some people are just better at hiding it than others.

Will Smith, American actor

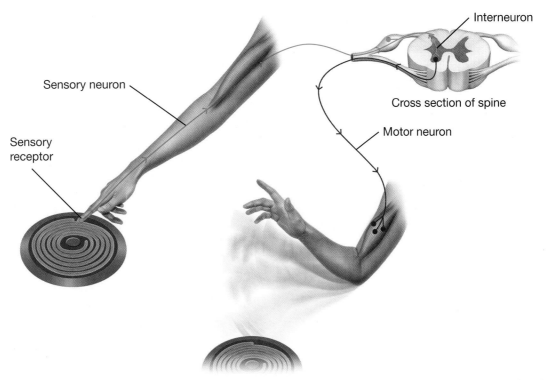

Interneuron

Sensory neuron

Cross section of spine

Sensory
receptor

Motor neuron

Figure 9.39 Sensory receptors in the finger transmit pain messages to the spinal cord and brain to alert the person to remove his finger from the hot stove.

Acute and Chronic Pain

When pain is sudden and goes away relatively quickly with treatment (within six months), it is acute. **Acute pain** may be the result of an injury, such as a broken bone, surgery, or even childbirth. When pain persists over time, it is chronic. **Chronic pain** may be the result of a past injury, disease, or condition. Some examples of chronic pain are low back pain, recurrent headaches, or joint pain from arthritis.

Acute pain is felt (often intensely), begins to subside, and typically goes away quickly with or without treatment. Because chronic pain is usually associated with a disease, a person may experience continuing pain from degenerative diseases, such as arthritis. People with chronic pain tend to interpret messages differently, as their nervous systems react in altered ways to long-standing pain. For those with chronic pain, even the slightest touch can feel severe. Often, chronic pain becomes an endless cycle, and people may feel there is no way out.

Cycle of Chronic Pain

Chronic pain occurs over and over again and feels endless to those experiencing it. This is why people with chronic pain experience the *cycle of chronic pain*. A repeating cycle of pain can lead to decreased activity, low interest in daily living, and diminished feelings of happiness and joy. Both physical reactions and psychological (emotional) responses are part of the cycle of chronic pain.

For example, consider a resident who has chronic, painful muscle spasms in his lower back. Physically, the resident feels pain when he moves because movement causes immediate muscle tension or spasms. Muscle spasms lead to less circulation, inflamed muscles, reduced mobility, muscle weakness, and decreased activity. When the resident moves and feels severe pain, he guards against or avoids further activity to reduce his pain.

The psychological or emotional dimension of the cycle of chronic pain includes fear, anxiety, and a stress response to pain. The resident who has muscle spasms may become depressed due to his physical pain. Depression may lead to even more

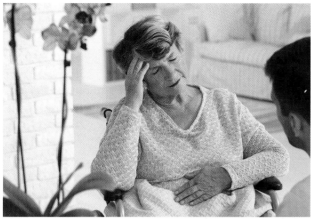
Photographee.eu/Shutterstock.com

Figure 9.40 Chronic pain can have a significant impact on residents' lives.

inactivity, as the resident may have little desire to do anything. If the resident uses pain medications for a long time, he may experience a deadening and disorienting effect and desire to move even less (Figure 9.40).

It is easy to imagine how the cycle of chronic pain affects people's lives. Endless time is spent focusing on the pain, and less attention is spent on living life. Limited mobility leads to muscle tightening and atrophy, which cause little motivation for activity that is now very painful. There is little joy, happiness, and desire. These experiences lead to frustration, sadness, depression, grief, and anger about a life that feels lost. It is not surprising that people who are in chronic pain have very little interest in activities of daily living and resist requests to exercise, be active, or socialize. While this is the cycle of chronic pain, not all people who have chronic pain experience it in this way. A great deal depends on how a person perceives pain. This is an individual response.

The Pain Experience

Each individual is the best judge of his or her own pain. One's experience and interpretation of pain can either strengthen or weaken the ability and willingness to withstand pain. A person who has a weakened capacity for pain may describe even the smallest pain as severe. We all have different pain thresholds, or limits. For some, the threshold is high; these people are not particularly sensitive to pain. Others have a low threshold for pain; these people feel pain to a greater degree and feel stressed and emotionally spent.

The experience of pain also influences how people respond to pain medications. For some people, the need for medications to relieve pain is great. These people expect that, if medication is taken, the pain will go away. This may not always happen, however. A medication may not relieve the pain or may not be the right strength.

If medications are taken too often or for too long a period, they may become less effective, and the body may require larger amounts to reach the same relief. Some people are **stoic** (detached from feeling) and feel that they can withstand pain without the help of medication. This is based on the person's pain threshold.

Culture Cues
Expressions of Pain

In some cases, a person's background may influence their response to, and expressions of, pain. Some people are very expressive about pain, while stoic residents may feel they should bear pain silently, perhaps even smiling through the pain.

A resident's willingness to report pain may be influenced by his or her cultural background. Bearing pain means suffering pain well, a quality valued by some. Not everyone in every culture conforms to a set of expected behaviors or beliefs; however, being mindful and sensitive to how others respond to and express pain is important when giving care.

Apply It

1. What assumptions or values do you have about pain based on your culture and family values?

2. How have your assumptions or values affected your response to pain?

3. In your opinion, what two actions can you take as a holistic nursing assistant to demonstrate you are aware of a resident's pain?

It is always hard to judge others when it comes to perceived pain. The balance is a person's desire to control pain, the relief felt from pain medication, and efforts to avoid developing resistance to pain medication.

Cultural and ethnic differences also influence a person's response to pain. A person's feelings about disease, pain, and the use of pain medications are often learned through tradition and family values. For example, a person may have learned growing up that pain should be ignored and that it is just part of life. As a result of their experiences, people will be affected by pain differently. Some people may need a great deal of pain relief, and others will not ask for or even require it.

What Is the Best Way to Observe and Report Pain?

When working as a holistic nursing assistant, you will need to determine the level and intensity of a resident's pain so you can report it properly. This is important because it helps licensed nursing staff members be knowledgeable about the pain and ensure that the most appropriate and effective pain medication is provided. This knowledge can also help holistic nursing assistants take **nonpharmacological** (not medication-based) actions, based on the plan of care, to help comfort and ease pain.

Awareness of Pain

The first step in determining others' pain is to be self-aware about your beliefs, attitudes, and feelings about pain. For example, if you have a high threshold for pain and come from a culture that is stoic, you might not be as sensitive to and aware of others' pain.

The next step is to understand how people express their pain. Many residents can describe their pain in detail. Others may just say, "I hurt." Many times, a resident's facial expressions and gestures are key indicators of pain. For example, a resident who keeps her eyes closed and tenses the muscles in her jaw may be in pain. Other gestures that indicate pain include keeping the hands closed around the body or rubbing the part of the body that hurts.

Pain Scales

When providing holistic care, you must always be objective in how you observe and report the resident's subjective perceptions and feelings. **Pain scales**, or devices used to measure the perception of the severity of pain, can help you do this (Figure 9.41).

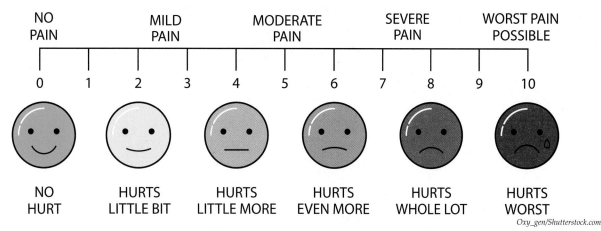

Oxy_gen/Shutterstock.com

Figure 9.41 Pain scales may use numbers and faces to help residents identify their levels of pain.

Check to see which scales your healthcare facility uses. Pain scales can help you ask residents to verbally describe the intensity of pain using numbers from 0 (no pain) to 10 (severe pain).

A pain scale that uses expressive cartoon faces to illustrate different levels of pain can be helpful when working with young patients or with residents who do not speak English well. The patient or resident selects the face that best describes the intensity of pain on a range from *does not hurt* to *hurts a whole lot*.

Pain scales also exist for residents who cannot communicate verbally. These pain scales require that you observe residents for certain expressions and gestures classified as pain indicators. For example, these pain scales will ask you to look at a resident's face and determine, based on expressions, where the resident falls and how much pain the resident is experiencing. These scales may also assess the resident's level of activity—from lying quietly to thrashing about in the bed—and whether the resident is crying, moaning, or whimpering. Careful listening and observation enable a holistic nursing assistant to find out the real story behind a resident's pain.

Pain Relief

Depending on the pain and its severity, pain may be relieved using over-the-counter medications or prescribed pain medications. Physical therapy and pain-relief therapy can also help.

As you learned in chapter 7, IM approaches can be used to relieve pain. Some IM approaches used for pain relief include

- acupuncture or acupressure;
- relaxation techniques, such as deep breathing;
- meditation;
- massage therapy;
- biofeedback (the use of a device to practice relaxation techniques);
- hypnotherapy;
- yoga; and
- tai chi or qigong.

IM approaches must be reviewed by a doctor before they are used to ensure they do not interfere with pain-relief goals or the disease process.

Some IM approaches are more effective when combined with other methods. For example, prescribed medications are more effective when combined with massage or meditation. Residents might need to try various methods to maintain maximum pain relief. A pain-relief action plan or a consultation with a pain-relief specialist can be helpful. To assist in pain relief, a holistic nursing assistant can

- be sensitive to and aware of a resident's pain during care;
- help residents relax before, during, and after procedures by encouraging them to use deep breathing during times of pain;
- provide comfortable positioning;
- encourage residents to listen to favorite music before, during, and after procedures as a means of staying calm;
- talk with residents about their memories of peaceful and calm experiences;
- use distraction by providing reading materials, favorite television shows, or opportunities to talk with family and friends;
- provide a gentle massage, which is particularly helpful during bathing;
- apply warm and cold packs and compresses, if ordered; and
- use pleasing aromas in the room, if acceptable.

If you have residents who have difficulty talking about pain, you might ask them to write about their pain and discuss their thoughts with family members, a doctor, or the licensed nursing staff.

Using the Key Terms

Complete the following sentences using key terms in this section.

1. _____ is pain that goes away relatively quickly with treatment.
2. Pain that persists over time is _____.
3. _____ are devices used to measure the perception of the severity of pain.
4. Approaches to pain that are not related to medication are _____.
5. If a person is detached from feeling, he or she is _____.

Know and Understand the Facts

6. Describe the two types of pain.
7. What is the difference between acute and chronic pain?
8. Identify two nonpharmacological or IM approaches to pain relief.
9. Descirbe the cycle of chronic pain.

Analyze and Apply Concepts

10. Describe three ways pain can impact people's lives.
11. How might the chronic pain cycle affect a resident's pain experience?
12. Explain two reasons why people might react to pain differently.
13. Describe why and how pain scales are used.
14. A nursing assistant is providing morning care for a resident. The resident states that she has pain in her right wrist and arm. What three actions can the nursing assistant take to assist with pain relief?

Think Critically

Read the following care situation. Then answer the questions that follow.

You are caring for Mrs. G in an assisted living center. Mrs. G has advanced rheumatoid arthritis that affects many of her joints. She also has COPD. Your assignment is to help Mrs. G with bathing and ambulation. Mrs. G is 82 years old and has been at the center for six months. She is quite thin and frail. She uses a walker for ambulation and seems very independent. When you walk into Mrs. G's room, she tells you that today she has quite a bit of pain in her hips and would rather stay in bed and not bathe.

15. How should you respond to Mrs. G using what you know about arthritis and COPD?
16. How can you best determine Mrs. G's pain intensity and level so you can inform the licensed nursing staff?
17. What do you need to know about Mrs. G's diseases to help with pain relief?
18. What nonpharmacological approaches might you use with Mrs. G?
19. Identify two care considerations that will enable you to provide safe, quality, holistic nursing care.

Key Points

Reviewing the key points for this chapter will help you practice more safely and competently as a holistic nursing assistant and will help you prepare for the certification competency examination.

- Diseases and conditions can be acute or chronic. An acute disease or condition lasts a short amount of time and has a rapid onset. Chronic diseases or conditions last for at least three months and are often lifetime challenges.

- A holistic nursing assistant must be knowledgeable about common diseases and conditions and their causes, signs and symptoms, general treatments, and care considerations.

- Pain is an uncomfortable feeling or sensation. Pain that is sudden and goes away relatively quickly with treatment is acute. When pain does not go away over time, it is chronic.

- Pain can be severe, moderate, or mild, and the interpretation of pain is unique to each person. Diseases or conditions, individual and familial experiences with pain, cultural and ethnic influences, and how long pain is experienced all influence a person's interpretation.

- Pain scales help determine levels of pain and intensity and provide important information for the licensed nursing staff.

- Nonpharmacological actions such as deep breathing and massage can help comfort and ease pain.

Action Steps to Holistic Care

Review the information in this chapter. Complete the following activities.

1. Prepare a poster or digital presentation that outlines the differences between acute and chronic diseases or conditions. Identify three diseases or conditions that fall under each category. Be sure to explain how each type of disease affects the care that is needed and which type of healthcare facility is most appropriate. Finally, consider whether you would prefer caring for patients with acute diseases or conditions or residents with chronic diseases or conditions and explain your choice.

1. Select a disease or condition not discussed in this chapter. Conduct research and prepare a short paper or digital presentation that summarizes the causes, signs and symptoms, and three care considerations.

2. With a partner, prepare a poster that illustrates five facts about a disease or condition discussed in this chapter.

3. Find two pictures in a magazine, in a newspaper, or online that best demonstrate various levels and intensities of pain. Describe each image and discuss how it represents pain.

4. Select one cultural, ethnic, or religious group and research values or traditions they might have surrounding pain. Describe these values or traditions and identify two special considerations for providing care.

Preparing for the Certification Competency Examination

To prepare for the nursing assistant certification competency examination, you will need to know content found in this chapter. This content may be tested in the knowledge (written or oral) and skills (hands-on demonstration) portions of the exam. The following areas will be emphasized:

- common health problems involving the body systems
- signs and symptoms of common health problems, types of pain, and factors that lead to discomfort and pain
- expressions and gestures that indicate discomfort and pain
- scales and measures for determining level of pain
- nonpharmacological measures that nursing assistants can use to enhance comfort

The sample test questions are similar to ones you will find on the certification competency exam. See how well you can answer them. Be sure to select the *best* answer.

1. Which of the following describes pain that goes away rather quickly?
   - A. chronic
   - B. mild
   - C. acute
   - D. sharp

2. Mrs. M has had psoriasis for several years. How would you expect her skin to look?
   - A. very dry, thick, or scaly and itchy
   - B. with rough patches and thick, wartlike growths
   - C. dry with rough patches and tiny bumps
   - D. thick with red patches or plaques

3. Mr. J is admitted to the emergency department with severely low blood sugar. What is this condition called?

   A. hypotension
   B. hypoglycemia
   C. hyperglycemia
   D. hypertension

4. When a resident is diagnosed with arthritis, this is considered a(n)

   A. degenerative disease
   B. infectious disease
   C. nutritional disease
   D. environmental disease

5. Mr. D has coronary artery disease. He is complaining of pain in his chest. This is called

   A. angina
   B. lupus
   C. vaginitis
   D. BPH

6. A nursing assistant wants to help Mrs. M be more comfortable and get some relief from her back and hip pain. Which of the following actions would *not* be helpful?

   A. using the pain scale to report the level of pain
   B. making Mrs. M walk around the room to exercise her back and hip
   C. helping Mrs. M deep-breathe and think about a pleasant experience
   D. using distraction by suggesting a favorite TV program to watch

7. A nursing assistant is caring for a resident who has had a stroke. The resident is having trouble speaking. What is this symptom called?

   A. GERD
   B. hemiplegia
   C. metastasis
   D. aphasia

8. Today, Dr. Smith told Mr. O that the cancer in his right lung is in only one lobe and has not spread. Which stage of cancer does this represent?

   A. stage 2
   B. stage 1
   C. stage 3
   D. stage 4

9. Mrs. D has a superficial decubitus ulcer on her hip. The ulcer has only one blister filled with fluid, and the surrounding area is irritated and red. What stage is the decubitus ulcer?

   A. stage 4
   B. stage 2
   C. stage 1
   D. stage 3

10. Ms. A has COPD. Her primary symptoms are most likely

    A. mental confusion
    B. nausea and vomiting
    C. coughing and mucus
    D. chest pain

11. Research has indicated that bacterial infection causes

    A. GERD
    B. gastritis
    C. diverticulitis
    D. peptic ulcer

12. Which of the following is another name for myocardial infarction?

    A. heartburn
    B. angina
    C. stroke
    D. heart attack

13. What is one way to prevent a resident from contracting a UTI?

    A. provide good catheter and perineal care
    B. make sure you use warm compresses on the urethra
    C. be sure the resident takes daily medications
    D. keep the linens free from crumbs and wrinkles

14. Mr. A has glaucoma. Which part of the eye does this disease damage?

    A. the retina
    B. the lens
    C. the iris
    D. the optic nerve

15. Your best friend has asthma. She usually is able to control her flares, but today she is short of breath and is having trouble breathing. What should she do first?

    A. use her quick-relief inhaler
    B. call 9-1-1
    C. call her doctor
    D. use her nebulizer

Did you have difficulty with any of the questions? If you did, review the chapter to find the correct answer(s).

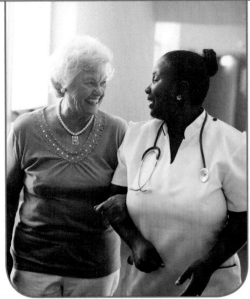

Jacob Lund/Shutterstock.com

Welcome to the Chapter

In this chapter, you will learn how to use verbal and nonverbal communication to positively influence your interpersonal relationships with others. You will also develop listening skills and learn to overcome communication barriers. As a holistic nursing assistant, you will help licensed nursing staff members communicate important information about residents' health. Learning to communicate holistically will help you establish positive, caring relationships with residents. In this chapter, you will also learn to recognize how anxiety, fear, anger, and conflict affect communication and interpersonal relationships and how you can respond effectively to these emotions and situations.

What you learn in this chapter will help you develop your knowledge and skills to become a holistic nursing assistant. The topics discussed in the chapter are highlighted on the Providing Holistic Care Framework.

You are now ready to start this chapter, *Communication and Caring*.

Chapter Outline

Section 10.1
Holistic Communication and Health Literacy

Section 10.2
Caring Skills and Interpersonal Relationships

Section 10.3
Anxiety, Fear, Anger, and Conflict

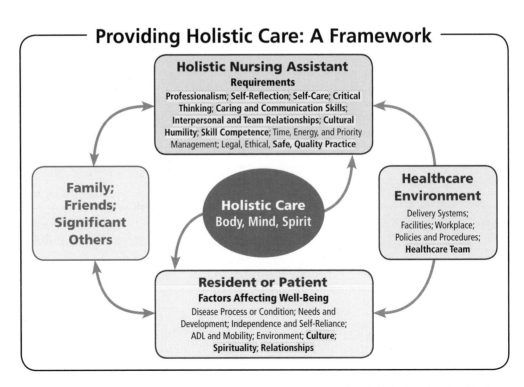

Providing Holistic Care: A Framework

Holistic Nursing Assistant
Requirements
Professionalism; Self-Reflection; Self-Care; Critical Thinking; **Caring and Communication Skills; Interpersonal and Team Relationships;** Cultural Humility; **Skill Competence;** Time, Energy, and Priority Management; Legal, Ethical, **Safe, Quality Practice**

Holistic Care
Body, Mind, Spirit

Family; Friends; Significant Others

Healthcare Environment
Delivery Systems; Facilities; Workplace; Policies and Procedures; **Healthcare Team**

Resident or Patient
Factors Affecting Well-Being
Disease Process or Condition; Needs and Development; Independence and Self-Reliance; ADL and Mobility; Environment; **Culture; Spirituality; Relationships**

Objectives

To provide the best possible care, you must understand the fundamentals of communication, including verbal and nonverbal communication, communication barriers, questioning, and listening. You must also know how to interact with others holistically. Doing so will empower residents in your care to be health literate. People who are health literate fully comprehend and use information about their diseases or conditions, treatments, and medications. To achieve the objectives for this section, you must successfully

- **explain** the basic principles of holistic communication;
- **describe** the role holistic nursing assistants play in increasing health literacy;
- **describe** verbal and nonverbal communication and active listening;
- **identify** the barriers to holistic communication; and
- **demonstrate** holistic communication strategies.

Key Terms

Learn these key terms to better understand the information presented in the section.

active listening	defense mechanisms
body language	health literacy
clarification	interpreter
closed-ended question	jargon
communication barriers	labeling
congruent communication	open-ended question

Questions to Consider

- Do you enjoy talking with others?
- Do you think you are an effective communicator? What special qualities and characteristics do you possess that allow you to communicate effectively with others?
- What can you do to improve your communication skills?

Humans have been communicating with one another since the beginning of time. Even before people began to speak and write, they used cave paintings, rock carvings (*petroglyphs*), and rock paintings (*pictographs*) to communicate. We have come a long way since those very early days.

Today, people communicate with one another in many ways. In addition to face-to-face communication and chatting on the telephone, technological advancements have made digital communication increasingly popular. Smartphones, tablets, and laptops give people the ability to communicate electronically using e-mail, text messaging, video chatting, and social media. Healthcare facilities also use digital communication, including e-mail, video conferencing, and social media, to communicate with staff, advertise services, and provide education.

What Is Holistic Communication?

A large part of your responsibility as a nursing assistant will be communicating effectively. *Communication* is the way people exchange information with one another. We send and receive messages—both verbal and nonverbal—with the goal of communicating thoughts, needs, and feelings.

When communication is holistic, it considers all aspects of a resident's body, mind, and spirit. *Holistic communication* is more than just talking. It is being fully present and fully focused on an exchange with another person. Holistic communication promotes healing and well-being and keeps lines of communication open to achieve a caring environment. Successful holistic communicators are accurate, honest, timely, and nonjudgmental. Holistic communication helps nursing assistants and residents develop trusting, respectful relationships, which are critical to delivering safe, quality care.

Components of Communication

As a holistic nursing assistant, you will communicate verbally with residents, residents' families, and members of the healthcare team. You will give residents instructions, converse with residents and their families, share information about resident care with the healthcare team, and discuss procedures with the licensed nursing staff. These are only a few examples of how you will communicate verbally during your shift. The ability to communicate effectively, ensuring your message is heard and understood, is necessary for delivering safe, quality care. To communicate a message effectively, you must understand the four basic components of communication (Figure 10.1):

1. the sender
2. mode of communication
3. recipient
4. feedback

Sender

The *sender* initiates communication, determines the content of his or her message, and evaluates the best way to deliver the message clearly. The sender also chooses the *mode of communication*, or the way in which the message will be sent.

Modes of Communication

There are four modes of communication for sending a message: speaking, listening, using gestures or body language, and writing. The mode of communication chosen should always fit the situation. For example, facility policies are usually written first and then shared verbally with staff, who can refer to the written document for further clarification. Clarity is important for ensuring the intended message is received. To communicate clearly, senders should make sure their words and facial expressions or body language match. When verbal and nonverbal communication match, this is called **congruent communication**.

Recipient

Once a message is sent, the *recipient* receives the message by carefully listening to the spoken words and by observing the tone and pitch of the sender's voice and the sender's body language. When communication is digital, nursing assistants should

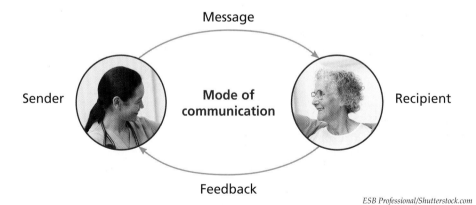

Message

Sender   Mode of communication   Recipient

Feedback

Figure 10.1 The four components of communication are the sender, mode of communication, recipient, and feedback.

pay attention to the words that are sent for the best understanding. The recipient is as important as the sender, and this approach gives the recipient the best chance to fully understand the intended message.

Feedback

Feedback is a response from the recipient that confirms the sender and the recipient have the same, or a similar, perception of the message. Examples of giving feedback include answering a question, confirming that you understand what is being asked of you, or saying, "I understand how you are feeling." Feedback should be brief, timely, and relevant.

Verbal and Nonverbal Communication

Verbal communication occurs when people use spoken words to express themselves. Only about 10 percent of communication is verbal. The remaining 90 percent of communication is nonverbal and does not use words. Examples of *nonverbal communication* include pointing your finger, shaking your head, making facial expressions, or using body gestures. Body posture also reflects your feelings. For example, standing with your back straight indicates confidence, while slumped shoulders can convey a lack of confidence or indifference.

Body language is a type of nonverbal communication that uses gestures and body movements. Messages sent using body language can be indirect or straightforward. For example, giving a thumbs-up reflects a positive feeling, while giving a thumbs-down reflects a negative feeling. When you shake hands with someone, you are welcoming him or her. Tapping your fingers on a desk or fidgeting can communicate boredom or impatience.

Body language can be a powerful communication tool. Unfortunately, people are not always aware of their body language. A person might communicate an opinion verbally, but communicate a differing opinion with his or her body language. Even when body language accurately communicates thoughts or feelings, others may not interpret the body language in the way it was intended.

Other types of nonverbal communication include making eye contact, moving the eyebrows and forehead, using touch, and navigating zones of personal space. In the United States, comfortable zones of personal space are expressed in the following ways:

- *Intimate space* (1.5 feet or less) might be shared with family, very close friends, and pets.
- *Personal space* (1.5–4 feet) is reserved for friends and acquaintances.
- *Social space* (4–12 feet) is often observed in business settings or when meeting new people.
- *Public space* (12 feet or more) is observed when speaking in front of a group of strangers.

In your role as a nursing assistant, you will routinely "invade" the personal space of residents. You will be a stranger to residents, but you still must enter residents' intimate space to deliver care. When entering a resident's intimate space, remember to be courteous and respectful. Ask permission to touch the resident prior to each procedure. If doing a procedure that involves an intimate body part, move slowly and explain what you are doing. If you stand over a resident, he or she may become uncomfortable, so avoid standing over residents if you can. When possible, remain at the resident's eye level when you are working or talking (Figure 10.2). If you use your hands to deliver care, ensure that your hands are warm. If you need to use gloves, explain why.

Remember

The most important thing in communication is to hear what isn't being said.

Peter Drucker, management consultant, educator, and author

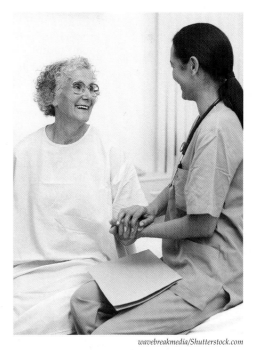

wavebreakmedia/Shutterstock.com

Figure 10.2 Talking with residents at eye level will help residents feel more comfortable.

Observation

To communicate holistically, you must use your senses of sight, smell, touch, and hearing. Using your senses will improve your observations, improve the care you give, and make your interactions more meaningful. One way to use your senses is to observe changes in residents. For example, observing a resident's facial expressions can let you know if the resident is in pain. You may use your sense of smell to identify a foul odor, which can alert you to a possible new condition. Your sense of touch can help others feel cared about and also allow you to detect changes in skin temperature.

Your senses are extremely important during observation. As a holistic nursing assistant, you will use your senses to report any resident observations you make. *Objective observations* are observations that provide measurable facts without your personal interpretation. For example, when you measure a resident's blood pressure, you report only the readings you take.

You might also use *subjective observations*. Subjective observations are based on opinions and personal interpretation. A subjective observation could be a resident's account of his or her experience or level of pain. It could also be an interpretation based on an objective observation, such as a resident seeming more confused today than yesterday. You will learn more about this way of observing and reporting in chapter 12.

What Are Barriers to Effective Holistic Communication?

Communication barriers are actions, behaviors, or situations that interfere with or block effective holistic communication. For example, language can be a communication barrier. You can avoid this barrier by using words that others will understand. You may need to adjust these words if a resident speaks another language or does not have a good understanding of English. If a resident speaks a different language, be sure to ask for an **interpreter** who can translate for you. If there are no interpreters available, use pictures to convey your message.

Jargon and Slang

Jargon and slang are words, phrases, and language used by a specific group of people or culture. The use of jargon or slang is another barrier to effective holistic communication. The words in jargon and slang may be unfamiliar to residents and can complicate a conversation or cause misunderstanding. People from different generations, cultures, or geographical areas may have their own unique jargon or slang. Examples of slang include the word *selfie* and *lol* (short for laugh out loud).

Some jargon is specific to healthcare and is acceptable to use with other healthcare staff members. Examples of healthcare jargon include medical abbreviations, such as *BP* for "blood pressure"; *NPO*, which means "nothing by mouth"; or *vitals*, which is short for "vital signs." Do not use healthcare jargon with patients or residents. Instead, use words that everyone you work with and care for will understand. If you must use a word that may cause confusion, provide an explanation of the word.

Stereotypes and Labels

Another barrier to communication is *stereotyping*. In chapter 6, you learned that a *stereotype* is a simplification or bias about a group that shapes the treatment of all group members. Some people use stereotypes to justify negative and discriminatory behaviors against others. To avoid this communication barrier, always be aware of any biases you have against groups or types of people. It is important to treat everyone with respect.

Labeling, or negatively describing someone in one word or a phrase, is also a barrier to communication. Labeling can cause *prejudice*, and prejudice can prevent people from examining whether there is truth to a label. Labeling is also hurtful to the person who is labeled. For example, saying that someone who talks a lot has a "big mouth" may make that person hesitant to share an important opinion. If you call someone lazy and laugh, the other person may feel hurt.

Words can hurt others. Think about the words you use and eliminate any labels that are part of your day-to-day communication. The role of the nursing assistant is to assist others in their daily lives, not to hinder them.

Advice

Giving advice is another important barrier to effective communication. It is not the nursing assistant's role or responsibility to give advice or opinions to residents, family members of residents, or healthcare staff. If nursing assistants give advice instead of listening, they may ignore what a resident really wants to communicate, and this will result in a poor quality of care. Giving personal advice crosses professional boundaries. Giving medical advice about a resident's disease, condition, or treatment plan is outside the scope of practice for a nursing assistant and can be dangerous or harmful. Instead of giving medical advice, refer any medical questions to the licensed nursing staff. If you are asked a question you cannot answer, be polite and explain that you will let the licensed nursing staff know about the concern.

Cultural Barriers

Cultural differences may be another barrier to communication. As you have learned, *culture* is the traditions, beliefs, rituals, values, and customs shared by a particular group of people. It is important for caregivers to be aware of other people's cultures. If you do not know a resident's culture or beliefs, you may unintentionally offend the resident.

As much as possible, take time to learn about residents' cultural beliefs. Where are residents from? Do they speak English? Do they have cultural beliefs that influence how they communicate (for example, not making eye contact with others)? As a holistic nursing assistant, always look for any special attention or changes in care that residents may require as a result of cultural beliefs.

Hearing Impairments

The tone of your voice and the rate at which you speak may present a challenge when you communicate with residents who have hearing impairments. When caring for a resident who has a hearing impairment, always approach the resident from the front. When talking, always face the resident, use good eye contact, and avoid mumbling (Figure 10.3). You may need to speak slower or louder for those who

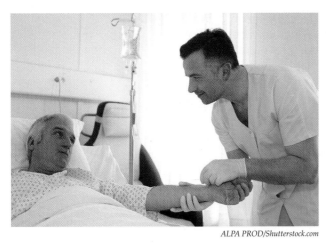
ALPA PROD/Shutterstock.com

Figure 10.3 Always make eye contact when communicating with a resident who has a hearing impairment.

cannot hear well, but you do not need to yell. Use short sentences and simple words. Remember that high-pitched tones may be difficult to hear, even if a resident uses a hearing aid. Always make sure that residents' hearing aids are turned on and that hearing aids' batteries are working.

Some residents and their families may rely on *sign language* to communicate. In these situations, an American Sign Language (ASL) interpreter may be needed. An ASL interpreter may be particularly helpful when very important instructions or information need to be communicated. Check with the licensed nursing staff to learn how you can access this resource.

Vision Impairments

Eyesight tends to worsen as people age, so many residents will have vision impairments, and some may wear eyeglasses. The holistic nursing assistant's responsibility is to make sure that eyeglasses are clean and fit well. If eyeglasses are not clean, use a soft cloth to clean them. If there are any problems with the eyeglasses or if a resident refuses to wear his or her eyeglasses, tell the licensed nursing staff.

To avoid startling residents, knock on the door before entering a resident's room and always announce who you are. This is very important for all residents, but is even more critical for those with vision impairments who may have difficulty seeing you without eyeglasses. When entering a resident's room, you could say, "Good morning, Mrs. J. I'm Tammy, your nursing assistant. I'm here to help you get dressed."

Speech Impairments

Speech impairments may make it harder for residents to communicate with you. For example, *aphasia* is one speech impairment you may experience when caring for residents. Aphasia may be caused by a stroke, brain tumor, brain injury, infection, or dementia.

There are different types of aphasia. In one type, residents know what they want to say, but have difficulty communicating. In another type, residents struggle to find the right words to speak or write. At its most severe, aphasia causes difficulty speaking and understanding words.

When working with residents who have speech impairments, check for comprehension. Speak slowly and calmly in simple sentences. Give residents the time they need to talk, and do not finish residents' sentences or correct errors. Gesturing or pointing to objects can also help with explanations.

Cognitive Disorders

People with cognitive disorders experience thinking challenges and may forget events, have trouble learning, be unable to process and understand information, and exhibit inappropriate behavior. These challenges are the result of organic changes in the brain. Progressive, permanent cognitive disorders are called *dementia* and have a range of symptoms that begin slowly and gradually get worse. The two most common dementias are Alzheimer's disease (AD) and vascular dementia.

Dementia causes *cognitive changes* that affect communication. These changes include memory loss, confusion about time and dates, disorientation, and trouble finding appropriate words or participating in a conversation. Holistic nursing assistants should approach residents with dementia in a calm, professional manner and should use proper body language to show respect and interest. As a nursing assistant, you may smile and gently touch or hug a resident, when appropriate. Always keep an even tone of voice, as loud noises can cause an aggressive response. Maintain eye contact and calmly explain why you are there and what is needed. Keep instructions simple and break them down into steps and wait between questions for answers. When needed, use closed-ended questions, such as, "Would you like to wear this sweater today?" Use simple words, such as "Roll to the right" or "Stand up," followed with praise.

Defense Mechanisms

Some of the most serious barriers to communication are **defense mechanisms**. Defense mechanisms are unconscious behaviors that enable people to ignore or forget situations or thoughts that cause fear, anxiety, and stress. Defense mechanisms are a form of stress management. For example, a person may deny that he or she has an illness such as diabetes to decrease feelings of fear or anxiety.

Defense mechanisms can prevent people from being honest about and sharing their feelings. There are many defense mechanisms, and only some of them interfere with communication. Common defense mechanisms that may create communication barriers include the following:

1. **Denial**: rejecting the truth about one's feelings, experiences, or facts. An example of denial is a resident insisting he feels fine when he does not. The resident is using the defense mechanism to convince himself and others that he is fine.

2. **Repression**: refusing to remember a traumatic or painful situation. An example might be forgetting a terrifying childhood event.

3. **Regression**: reverting back to childlike behaviors when fearful, anxious, or angry. A resident who has a temper tantrum may be exhibiting signs of regression.

4. **Displacement**: transferring a bad or negative feeling, such as anger, away from the source and onto someone or something else. For example, you might be angry with your friend, but hold the anger in until you get home and snap at a family member.

5. **Projection**: believing that others feel a certain way when, in fact, the feelings are yours. For example, you might say, "I know my teacher dislikes me," when the real truth is that you dislike your teacher.

6. **Reaction formation**: feeling one way inside, but outwardly expressing the feeling in an opposite way. For example, you may not like a person, but still go out of your way to be nice to her.

7. **Intellectualizing**: focusing on facts, logic, and reasoning instead of a stressful feeling or uncomfortable emotion. For example, a resident recently diagnosed with a terminal illness may focus on learning everything about the disease and possible treatments instead of dealing with his or her feelings about the diagnosis.

8. **Rationalization**: using logic to excuse unacceptable behaviors and feelings. Often, people use this defense mechanism after they have done something they regret. An example would be stealing money from a friend and then making it sound acceptable by saying, "She owed me money anyway."

We all use defense mechanisms. When defense mechanisms are overused, however, they are no longer protective and can become harmful. It is important to recognize when defense mechanisms are being used, either by yourself or by others. Recognizing defense mechanisms is a good first step in making sure defense mechanisms do not become barriers to communication.

How Can Communication Be Improved?

What should you do if people have difficulty understanding what is being communicated? When you encounter difficult communication situations, be patient, listen carefully, and try to clarify and reflect what is being communicated. You can use a communication strategy called *active listening,* which uses clarification and reflection. Proper questioning will also help improve communication.

Active Listening

Active listening promotes understanding and successful communication. Active listening involves showing interest in the person speaking, showing interest in what is being said by paying attention, and providing good eye contact. As you listen, look directly at the speaker, but do not stare. Eye contact helps the speaker feel that what he or she is saying is important and that the message has been received. Eye contact also shows you are willing to take the time to pay attention. Sitting down, leaning toward the speaker, and nodding your head also show you are actively listening (Figure 10.4).

Clarification involves restating what you believe was said to make sure you heard the message correctly. To ask for clarification, you might say to the speaker, "I want to be sure I understand. What I heard you say was...." You could also ask another person to clarify a message you have communicated by saying, "I want to be sure you understood what I said. Would you repeat back what you heard?"

Reflection is a technique in which you listen, identify feelings a resident is expressing nonverbally, and ask a question to bring forward those feelings. For example, you might ask, "Are you feeling frustrated about not being able to walk as independently as you did yesterday?" The goal of reflection is to identify a resident's feelings so they can be expressed and discussed. Often, just acknowledging a feeling will relieve a resident's tension and frustration and lead to increased comfort and well-being.

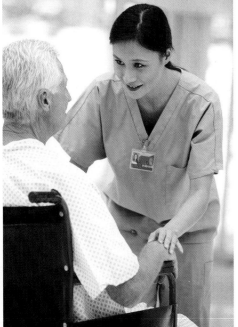

Figure 10.4 This nursing assistant is demonstrating that she is actively listening.

Questioning

Questions are an effective communication tool. The most effective questions are **open-ended questions** that lead to more than a one-word answer. Open-ended questions help you get the information you need to provide safe, quality holistic care.

An example of an open-ended question is "Can you tell me how well you slept last night?" This question requires a resident to answer with more than one word. As the resident considers the answer to this question, he or she may also think of other details to share and tell you that he or she had a good, quality sleep.

Some people share more freely when answering an open-ended question than when answering a more specific or **closed-ended question**. A closed-ended question, such as "Did you sleep well last night?", may result in a one-word answer of "yes" or "no." If an open-ended question had been asked, the answer might have been more detailed. For example, a resident might have answered, "Although I slept for about seven hours, I had a hard time falling asleep and had some strange dreams." This answer begins a conversation with the nursing assistant. The nursing assistant can explore the length and quality of the resident's sleep by asking more open-ended questions.

When using questioning, avoid "why" questions since these types of questions may be difficult to answer. "Why" questions can make people feel defensive, and this can create a communication barrier. An example of a "why" question that might make a resident feel defensive could be "Why did you ring your call light? I was just in your room 10 minutes ago."

What Can Nursing Assistants Do to Help Improve Health Literacy?

Health literacy is the degree to which people fully understand and use information about their health, diseases, conditions, or treatments. Having health literacy leads to people's ability to manage their health, make effective and appropriate health decisions, find necessary healthcare resources, share personal information, adopt healthy behaviors, and engage in self-care.

At the core of health literacy is the effectiveness of communication between residents and healthcare providers. The extent of a person's health literacy can be influenced greatly by common misunderstandings or communication problems. Poor health literacy can result when people ignore what they are told, misinterpret messages, or lack the information or understanding to follow instructions or report abnormal symptoms. Several factors may influence a person's level of health literacy. These may include a person's

- English reading and writing skills;
- ability to understand and calculate simple math;
- beliefs about wellness and illness; and
- depth of knowledge about healthcare topics and systems.

People who are more likely to have below-average health literacy include older adults, people from specific cultures, nonnative English speakers, and people with low incomes and educational levels. The extent of a person's health literacy is also influenced by culture, knowledge and skills, situation, and ability to communicate.

The Patient Protection and Affordable Care Act includes a National Action Plan to Improve Health Literacy. This plan seeks to help individuals make informed decisions about their healthcare. Healthcare providers are encouraged to deliver care in a way that is easy to understand and that is beneficial to patients' long-term health. The Joint Commission (TJC) has also set guidelines on health literacy.

The responsibility for improving health literacy lies with all caregivers. One primary way to ensure people are health literate is to focus on good communication skills. Following are some guidelines that nursing assistants can follow when communicating with residents about health:

- Use all forms of communication to get your message across.
- Choose words and examples that make the information understandable.
- Offer simple instructions for better understanding.
- Speak plainly. When necessary, request an interpreter so the resident's primary language is used.

- Speak slowly and actively listen.
- Ask questions in different ways.
- Check if the message was understood by asking the resident to repeat back what he or she heard.
- Always report questions and concerns to the licensed nursing staff.

Remember, every day is an opportunity to communicate.

Using the Key Terms

Complete the following sentences using key terms in this section.

1. _____ involves showing interest in the person speaking and using clarification and reflection.
2. Gestures and movements are examples of _____.
3. When you use _____, you restate what you believe was said to make sure you heard the message correctly.
4. An example of a(n) _____ is "Do you want to wear this sweater?"
5. _____ is a person's ability to fully understand and use information about health, diseases, conditions, or treatments.
6. _____ is the words, phrases, and language used by a specific group of people.
7. _____, or negatively describing someone in one word or a phrase, is also a barrier to communication.
8. An example of a(n) _____ is "Which sweater would you like to wear?"

Know and Understand the Facts

9. What is holistic communication?
10. Explain the four basic components of communication.
11. Describe the difference between verbal and nonverbal communication.
12. List three barriers to communication.
13. What is health literacy?

Analyze and Apply Concepts

14. Provide two examples of defense mechanisms and explain the influence of the two defense mechanisms on holistic communication.
15. Explain how active listening and questioning can promote holistic communication.
16. Imagine you are a nursing assistant working in a long-term care facility. Write a care situation in which holistic communication is used effectively between yourself and a resident. Identify the communication strategies used and how they affect the conversation.
17. Describe two appropriate actions that can be used to improve health literacy.

Think Critically

Read the following care situation. Then answer the questions that follow.

Harry has just started his job as a nursing assistant and is caring for Mrs. D. Mrs. D had a stroke three months ago, which paralyzed the left side of her face. As a result, she is unable to speak clearly. Mrs. D also has a hearing impairment. Harry brings lunch to Mrs. D, puts it on the overbed table, and quietly tells Mrs. D that lunch is ready. He then walks out of her room.

When Harry returns later to pick up Mrs. D's tray, he notices that nothing has been eaten. He says to Mrs. D, "Why didn't you eat anything? Well, if you don't want to eat, you don't have to." While Harry is talking, Mrs. D mumbles and points to her bathroom.

18. What are the communication barriers in this situation?
19. How could Harry make sure he is aware of Mrs. D's hearing and speaking problems?
20. What should Harry do differently in this situation?

Objectives

Understanding the process and strategies that build and maintain effective interpersonal relationships is an important part of becoming a successful nursing assistant. In this section, you will learn about the behaviors, attitudes, and skills necessary to effectively care for others. Strong interpersonal relationships and caring skills are the foundation of holistic care. To achieve the objectives for this section, you must successfully

- **explain** the four types of interpersonal relationships;
- **describe** behaviors and attitudes that demonstrate caring; and
- **discuss** how caring relationships are established.

Key Terms

Learn these key terms to better understand the information presented in the section.

caring

giving of self

interpersonal relationships

intimate relationships

Questions to Consider

- Have you ever met someone for the first time and immediately felt like that person's friend? In contrast, have you ever immediately disliked a person you just met? Why do you think you responded to these people in this way?
- Many times, our first impressions of people help us determine the nature of the relationships we build. Building relationships is even more important when we are asked to care for someone. Think of a time you were asked to care for a person or a pet. How did you feel? Was giving care a burden, or did you enjoy it? Why?

What Are Interpersonal Relationships?

Interpersonal relationships develop between two or more people who have similar interests or goals. These relationships are built and maintained when people's needs and desires are met. Strong interpersonal relationships can be found among family members or friends. Interpersonal relationships can also form between coworkers, but these relationships may not be as strong (Figure 10.5).

An interpersonal relationship outside the family may begin when you work closely with someone over a long period of time. You may want to spend time with that person and enjoy his or her company. An interpersonal relationship may also develop when you work with a person you get along with and respect. All interpersonal relationships require attention and effective communication. There are four types of interpersonal relationships: family relationships, friendships, intimate relationships, and professional relationships.

Family Relationships

Family relationships are based on interactions between parents, siblings, and extended family members. Families form their own patterns of communication, which are typically based on culture, habit, and familiarity.

Friendships

The second type of interpersonal relationship is *friendship*. Friendships are usually built on similar likes and dislikes. Future plans, goals, and desires are typically discussed at the beginning of a friendship. As time passes, more personal information is shared, and trust develops. The relationship continues to build as each

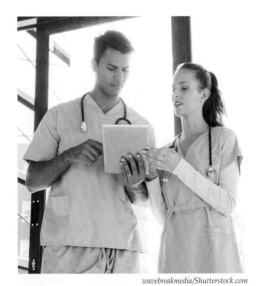

wavebreakmedia/Shutterstock.com

Figure 10.5 Interpersonal relationships may develop when you work with a person you get along with and respect.

person lets down his or her walls of defense and protection. Often, private information and secrets are exchanged. Both friendships and family relationships usually offer protection, support, and acceptance for those involved.

Intimate Relationships

The third type of interpersonal relationship is the intimate relationship. **Intimate relationships** develop from romantic feelings and love. Some intimate relationships develop over time, while others begin when there is "love at first sight." These relationships are close, romantic, and sometimes sexual. If this type of relationship is to thrive, those in the relationship must pay attention to each other's emotions and feelings.

Professional Relationships

Professional relationships are developed and maintained in professional, or work, settings. As a nursing assistant, you will develop professional relationships with coworkers, residents, and residents' family members (Figure 10.6). Interpersonal relationships in professional settings do not have the same strength as family relationships and friendships and do not always extend outside the workplace. Intimate relationships are not appropriate at all in professional settings.

Although professional relationships may not be as deep or long-lasting as other relationships, they require the same level of attention and effective communication. Developing professional relationships can improve care and health outcomes. For example, the way you approach, communicate, listen, and respond can impact a resident's desire to comply with your requests. It can also influence a resident's compliance with his or her treatment program. Residents may even feel better about themselves as a result of your relationships with them.

How Are Professional Relationships Built and Maintained?

You can use several important approaches and skills to build and maintain professional relationships. Professional relationships are at their strongest when you follow these strategies:

- Be present. Be responsive and focus on others.
- Respect others' views and opinions. Actively listen, ask open-ended questions, and show interest in what others have to say.
- Be helpful. Take the time to ensure residents and staff have the assistance they need, even when you are busy.
- Be fair. Avoid stereotypes and labels.
- Be trustworthy and reliable. Others should be able to count on you at all times.
- Be appreciative, positive, and optimistic. Offer positive feedback and comments when appropriate.
- Be a team player. Provide support and pitch in when needed, even if you are busy or tired.
- Manage anger and conflict in an appropriate manner.

The feelings you have as you give care are an important aspect of building a professional relationship. Perhaps you are caring for a resident whose

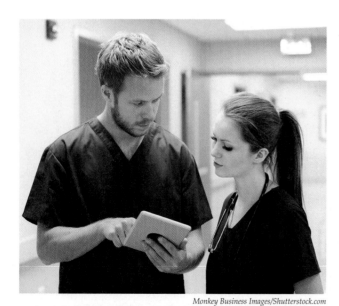

Figure 10.6 One example of a professional relationship is the relationships you have with your coworkers.

comments or behaviors remind you of someone you do not like. It is possible that, as you give care, you will transfer that feeling onto the resident. This can negatively affect your relationship with that resident and your ability to provide holistic care. The reverse may also be true if a resident unconsciously transfers feelings about another person onto you.

Feelings that are transferred because of association can be good or bad. For example, a resident may become angry with a nursing assistant for seemingly no apparent reason. The anger, however, may result from the nursing assistant reminding the resident of a disliked person from his or her past. A resident may also like a nursing assistant because he or she reminds the resident of a close friend or family member.

Feelings that are transferred are often unconscious. If you find yourself being short or angry with a resident without cause, stop and reflect on your feelings. Conversely, if you find yourself being too friendly, ask yourself why. If you experience a resident being too friendly or directing anger toward you, do not take these feelings personally. Rather, recognize and be aware of what is happening. Then focus on effective communication skills and the way you can best deliver care.

If residents exhibit strong feelings about you, do not react or respond to their feelings inappropriately and never take their feelings personally. Instead, use your active listening and questioning skills to help divert residents' feelings to their recovery, treatment, and family members. If you are unable or have difficulty diverting either your own feelings, or the feelings of a resident, let the charge nurse know. Sometimes a change of assignment helps.

What Are Caring Skills?

As a holistic nursing assistant, you will be asked to care for people who are ill. How do you feel about having this responsibility? Maybe you have already had this experience with a family member or friend.

When people hear the word *caring*, they may already have an idea of what the word means. In healthcare, the term **caring** means providing assistance and comfort to positively affect the health and well-being of a patient or resident. Caring also means going beyond the words written in your position requirements; it may involve giving of yourself, showing empathy and patience, being reliable and resourceful, and seeking information.

Giving of Self

To care for others, you must be **giving of self**. A person who is giving of self makes himself or herself available and open to others. To be giving of self, nursing assistants must understand that residents' needs come first. Nursing assistants who are giving of self, impact both the physical and emotional well-being of residents. These caregivers are positive and earn the trust and respect of others. This quality is important. Residents who do not trust or respect their caregivers may not cooperate, making it harder to provide care.

Empathy

Caring and being giving of self also require *empathy*, or understanding for another person's feelings and emotions. An example of empathy might be telling a resident, "I understand you may be frightened about your upcoming procedure." If appropriate, you could even hold a sad-looking resident's hand as an expression of caring and empathy. A good way to hold a resident's hand is to rest the resident's hand on top of yours. This allows the resident to easily remove his or her hand, if desired (Figure 10.7).

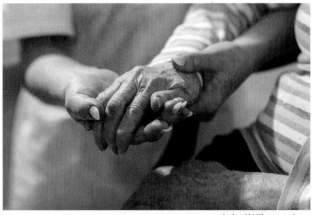
thodonal88/Shutterstock.com

Figure 10.7 It is best to hold a resident's hand in such a way that the resident can remove his or her hand if desired.

Patience and Reliability

Holistic nursing assistants who exhibit caring behaviors are *patient* and are willing to understand. They are *reliable*, never take shortcuts, and know their responsibilities. These behaviors not only characterize caring, but also demonstrate competence. They show that nursing assistants understand their roles, take the time to ensure accuracy, and are consistent in their practice.

Information Seeking

Another way to show that you care is to take the time to learn more about residents. You can use the information you learn to help residents experience their past joys and present desires (Figure 10.8). Suppose a resident has shared with you that she once enjoyed running with her dog, but can't now because she is in a wheelchair. She is depressed because she misses the companionship of her dog. By connecting with a volunteer animal therapy program, you might be able to help this resident. Animal therapy organizations bring therapy dogs into healthcare facilities and allow residents to spend time with the animals. Just seeing a dog could improve this resident's spirits and well-being.

Resourcefulness

Remember

Too often we underestimate the power of a touch, a smile, a kind word, a listening ear, an honest compliment, or the smallest act of caring, all of which have the potential to turn a life around.

Leo F. Buscaglia,
American author, motivational
speaker, and professor

People who are *resourceful* think and act quickly to overcome challenges or solve problems. Caring can be demonstrated with simple, resourceful actions.

Consider a resident with Alzheimer's disease who always sits quietly in the activity room of a long-term care facility. When nursing staff members try to talk with the resident and ask questions, the resident never responds with more than one

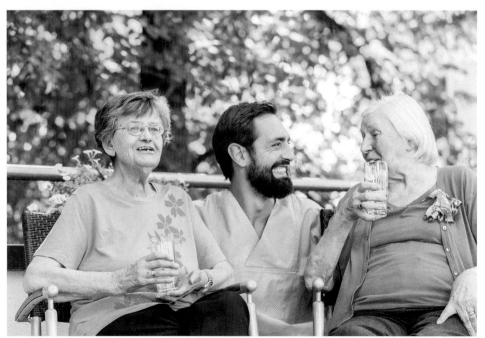
Kzenon/Shutterstock.com

Figure 10.8 Learning more about residents will help you form good relationships and deliver care.

word. A nursing assistant speaks with the resident's daughter, who says that her father loves big band music. The next day, the nursing assistant gives the resident a pair of headphones and plays big band music for him. The resident sits up in his wheelchair, sings, taps his feet, and moves his hands in a rhythmic way. As a result, the resident is more open to answering questions. More importantly, the resident and those around him experience joy. Something as simple as music and a nursing assistant's care can make a profound difference in a resident's life.

Using the Key Terms

Complete the following sentences using key terms in this section.

1. When you are _____, you put a resident's health and wellness needs before your own needs as a caregiver.
2. _____ is providing assistance and comfort to positively affect the health and well-being of a resident.
3. A relationship between two people with the same goal is a(n) _____.
4. A(n) _____ develops from romantic feelings.

Know and Understand the Facts

5. Identify and define the four types of interpersonal relationships.
6. List five strategies for building and maintaining strong professional relationships.
7. What does it mean to be *giving of self*?
8. Describe two skills that demonstrate caring.

Analyze and Apply Concepts

9. Explain how to handle a situation in which a resident tells you he or she does not like the nursing assistant who gave care yesterday.
10. Identify two qualities or behaviors you can demonstrate to help establish effective professional relationships.
11. Give two examples of situations in which a nursing assistant can demonstrate caring behaviors or actions.

Think Critically

Read the following care situation. Then answer the questions that follow.

Jennifer, a nursing assistant, has been caring for Mr. H, a war veteran, for several weeks. Both of Mr. H's legs were amputated at the knee as a result of an explosion during his tour of duty. Mr. H has always been pleasant and cooperative, and he and Jennifer have developed a good relationship. Today, Mr. H received bad news, but Jennifer was not aware of the news. When Jennifer entered Mr. H's room to help him with morning care, Mr. H threw an object from his nightstand at her. Jennifer was shocked at his behavior. She asked him what was wrong. Mr. H was crying and was embarrassed to have anyone see him cry, so he yelled, "Leave me alone!"

12. What feeling is Mr. H displaying, and is it directed toward Jennifer?
13. What should Jennifer do next to maintain her strong interpersonal relationship with Mr. H?
14. What attitudes and behaviors can Jennifer demonstrate to show she cares about Mr. H?

Questions to Consider

- Think about a time you felt anxious, fearful, or angry. What caused these feelings, and what did you do about them? If you acted on these feelings, did you feel better or worse as a result?
- Now think about a time you experienced conflict with a friend or family member. What caused the conflict? How did you and your friend or family member feel? Were you able to resolve the conflict? If you were, how was the conflict resolved?

Objectives

To provide the best possible care, you must understand, recognize, and respond appropriately to the anxiety, fear, anger, and conflict of patients and residents. Learning how to manage feelings requires skill and is important for maintaining positive relationships. To achieve the objectives for this section, you must successfully

- **identify** the causes of anxiety, fear, anger, and conflict;
- **describe** the behaviors and feelings associated with anxiety, fear, anger, and conflict; and
- **explain** strategies a holistic nursing assistant can use to ease anxiety, fear, anger, and conflict.

Key Terms

Learn these key terms to better understand the information presented in the section.

anger	conflict
assertive	fear
collaboration	phobias
compromise	

What Is Anxiety, and How Can It Be Managed?

As you learned in chapter 4, *anxiety* is a feeling of worry, uneasiness, or nervousness. Anxiety is common. Mild, brief anxiety may occur in anticipation of an event that has not yet happened. For example, a student may experience anxiety before taking an important test. Anxious feelings may produce physical reactions. Before the test, a student might feel his heart pounding, notice his foot shaking, or start chewing on his lips or fingernails. People handle anxiety differently. Some people deal with it by crying, expressing anger, or shutting down emotionally. Others do not know why they are feeling anxious and may recognize the cause of anxiety only after it has passed.

Anxiety disorders are different from experiencing mild or brief anxiety caused by a stressful event. Anxiety disorders include **phobias** (unsupported, exaggerated fears), panic, post-traumatic stress disorder (PTSD), and obsessive-compulsive disorder (OCD) and affect 40 million adults in the United States ages 18 and older. These 40 million adults make up about 18 percent of the US population. Anxiety disorders usually last at least six months and can continue for a lifetime. They get worse if left untreated.

Anxious Residents

Anxiety is something you may observe in residents. To recognize anxiety, watch for heavy, short breaths and complaints about heart palpitations or chest pain. If the chest pain is described as severe, notify the licensed nursing staff immediately.

You might also observe

- unusual shakiness;
- dizziness;

- sweating;
- muscle aches;
- dry mouth; and
- fluctuations in behavior and mood.

Some residents will tell you they feel anxious. Others might experience the physical symptoms of anxiety, but be unaware of the cause.

If a resident shows physical symptoms of anxiety, alert licensed nursing staff members so they can follow up. If a resident is experiencing anxiety, encourage the resident to talk with you about his or her feelings. Use good eye contact and be present during the conversation. You might ask if a resident would like some water, since dry mouth is often a result of anxiety. If a resident is not sure what is causing his or her feelings, know that just your calm, positive presence can help (Figure 10.9).

You can tell anxiety is subsiding, or *lessening,* when physical symptoms start to disappear. If you observe that the resident's anxiety is intense or prolonged, alert the licensed nursing staff. Some residents may need medication to relieve their symptoms. The goal of your care is to ease anxious feelings and to keep these feelings from spiraling out of control.

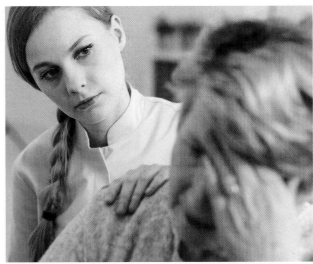

Photographee.eu/Shutterstock.com

Figure 10.9 One way to help ease resident anxiety is to just be present. Sometimes a caring touch can help residents be calm.

Anxiety as a Caregiver

Working in healthcare may expose you to many situations that can cause anxiety. For example, thinking about performing a procedure for the first time or working with a new resident may cause anxiety. As a nursing assistant, you will need to handle your feelings appropriately.

If you do feel anxious while giving care, the following suggestions may help you overcome those feelings:

- Know what causes you to feel anxious and what physical symptoms are typical for you. Recognizing your own patterns of anxiety will help you become aware of and manage them.
- If you start to feel anxious, take slow, deep breaths. This will have a calming effect.
- If you feel your anxiety is getting in the way of providing safe care, take a brief break.
- Talk about your feelings and anxiety with a coworker.
- Never feel embarrassed about your anxiety. Everyone has experienced anxiety at one time or another.

Think About This

According to the National Institutes of Mental Health, women are more than twice as likely as men to experience anxiety disorders in their lifetimes.

What Is Fear, and How Can It Be Overcome?

Some people describe **fear** as a paralyzing feeling. You may describe fear as feeling scared, feeling emotionally out of control, or being overwhelmed. Fear is different from anxiety. While anxiety occurs in response to an *anticipated* event, fear is an unpleasant emotion or feeling that occurs in response to an *identified* threat or the presence of danger.

Fear is a personal experience. Some fears may develop from terrifying and real experiences, while other fears may develop from the possibility or threat of a frightening experience. Because fear is a personal experience, reactions to fear may range from a low level of fear to debilitating fear. There are many types of fears. Common fears include fears of flying, public speaking, heights, the dark, failure, or rejection.

Fearful Residents

Depending on your point of view and experience, you can view fear as either positive or negative. Positive fear can serve as a healthy warning sign and motivate you to do or be better. Fear can also be immobilizing. Some people react to fear in an aggressive manner. They may scream, yell, or lash out physically (Figure 10.10). Others may shut down emotionally in the face of fear.

Fear has physical effects due to the actions of the *sympathetic nervous system (SNS)*, which you learned about in chapter 6. Fear can cause the *fight-or-flight response*. When people are fearful, they can become short of breath and sometimes sweat. People's hearts may race, and people may become shaky or nervous. Depending on their levels of fear and the threats they are facing, people may run and scream or stand strong and physically fight.

Fear cannot be overcome unless a person commits to reducing or eliminating his or her fear. As a nursing assistant, you may find that some residents ignore their fear. Residents may bottle the fear up inside, and all you see may be anger, self-pity, or sadness, which are feelings that often accompany fear. Holistic communication and caring, even in the form of an empathetic response of understanding, can help identify and relieve a resident's fear.

Fear as a Caregiver

Fear can sometimes be hard to recognize in ourselves. You can practice identifying your fears in writing or out loud. Once you have identified your fears, you must learn ways to manage them. Taking deep breaths when you feel fearful may help. You might also ask yourself why you are feeling afraid. This will help you understand how the fear started. You may set goals to begin overcoming your fears. For example, you might set a goal to find someone with whom to share your feelings. Some people find that professional help can assist in overcoming fears. If we do not deal with our fears, they may inhibit our ability to help others.

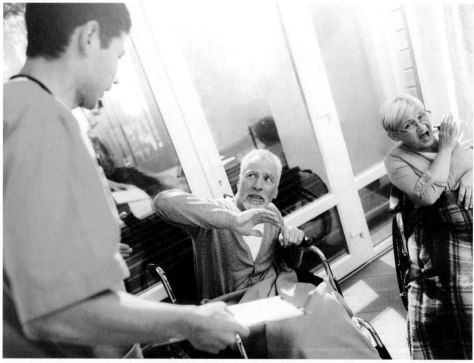

VGstockstudio/Shutterstock.com

Figure 10.10 Fear may cause residents to become angry. When this happens, it is important to remain calm, try to identify the cause of the fear or anger, and do not take their reactions personally.

What Strategies Can Be Used to Manage Anger?

Anger is a powerful feeling that develops from frustration, displeasure, or a threat (Figure 10.11). Anger can be very damaging to one's self and others. We have all experienced anger and its many degrees of intensity. *Frustration* is a mild form of anger; *rage* is an extreme form. Many situations or experiences can cause anger. Some people have personal issues that are ignited by certain situations. For example, if you are unhappy about being short and if someone calls you "shorty," you may get angry and say something hurtful in response.

Anger causes physical reactions. Some people say that anger feels like a tornado whirling inside them over which they have no control. Others have a lesser reaction to anger. Typically, when you are angry, your heart rate increases, you may frown, your eyes narrow, your body heats up, your breathing may be altered, and your feelings turn into behaviors. Some people erupt in anger and yell, scream, or pound on something. Others experience the same physical reactions, but instead of demonstrating anger outwardly, turn anger inward. This can cause serious physical symptoms and depression.

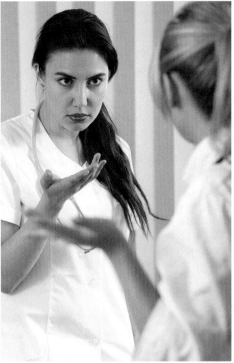

Edw/Shutterstock.com

Figure 10.11 Anger can be a powerful emotion, but it is important not to let anger keep you from acting professionally.

Angry Residents

Some residents believe they have lost control over their own lives, and this causes them to feel frustrated or helpless. Residents may not know how to talk about their feelings and instead keep them inside. As their feelings intensify, residents may become angry. The following are strategies you can use to help calm angry residents:

- Use active listening.
- Do not personally respond to the anger.
- Ask questions to clarify why the resident is angry.
- Speak in a soft tone at a low volume level. This will help defuse the anger.
- Never raise your voice or yell. Some residents just need to vent their anger.

Calming residents is critical, particularly if anger is getting out of hand or if residents are at risk of hurting themselves or others. If residents ask you to leave them alone, do that, but inform residents you will return in a certain amount of time. Always respect residents' wishes and be sure to keep residents safe. If residents do ask you to leave them alone, alert the licensed nursing staff to the situation.

Anger as a Caregiver

Managing anger is not always easy. As a nursing assistant, you will need to recognize what situations can and will make you angry. You will need to learn to control your anger. It is unprofessional to exhibit anger or to gossip about people with whom you are angry.

As a nursing assistant, you must rise above your anger and deal with it appropriately. If you feel yourself getting angry, try to remove yourself from the situation that is causing your anger. Walk away, take a break, and do some deep breathing to calm down.

As a nursing assistant, you may also need to speak up and share if someone is making you angry. If you can remain calm, you can respond to situations that cause anger. For example, if someone calls you a name that makes you angry, politely tell the person that the name hurts your feelings and that you would appreciate not being called by that name again.

Conflict Management

In last night's news broadcast, a local broadcast journalist reported on a conflict between the local community hospital and a group of citizens in the community. The citizens requested that the hospital provide community outreach services for the large population of older adults in the community. In particular, the citizens sought special resources for people with Alzheimer's and dementia and for family caregivers.

The reporter stated that, early that morning, citizens from the community were outside the hospital distributing informational leaflets. Hospital officials responded to the citizens' request with a public letter. The officials stated that they did not see how or why they should take responsibility for providing these services. The officials also said they did not have the financial resources to support such a center.

Apply It

1. What is the source of the conflict described in this scenario?

2. Did either side take any actions that increased the conflict? Explain.

3. What action could the hospital take next?

4. How would you suggest that the hospital and community members resolve this conflict?

How Can Conflict Be Resolved?

Conflict is any disagreement between two or more people. It can be as simple as a difference of opinion or as complex as a war. Conflict is not always bad. Many times, conflict helps solve problems or creates new ways of completing tasks. A conflict may be centered on facts, values, beliefs, expectations, feelings, or behaviors. Conflicts may be *external*, or exist between people or groups. Conflicts may also be *internal*. For example, a person may struggle to make an important decision. Conflict *must* be addressed and should never be ignored. If conflict is not resolved, it will continue and grow in intensity (Figure 10.12).

There are always feelings that arise during a conflict. These feelings typically include anxiety, fear, and some level of anger. These feelings must be acknowledged and responded to before any problem solving can occur to resolve the conflict. Each of us has a different style when dealing with and resolving conflict. Styles are mostly learned and are based on past experiences, approaches to problems, and communication skills. Conflict-management styles range from avoiding conflict altogether to directly dealing with conflict. Many times, *compromise* (in which both people make concessions) can help reduce a conflict situation. *Collaboration* (in which people work together to resolve conflict in a way that satisfies everyone) is considered the most inclusive and positive approach to managing conflict.

Conflict resolution is important, and it is always possible to resolve disagreements in a productive manner. The bottom line is that conflicts *must* be responded to. Otherwise, situations can get out of control. Conflict management has two components that happen in a sequence. The first component involves managing feelings, and the second component is problem solving.

The first component of conflict management is managing feelings. To manage feelings, follow these steps:

1. Cool down any angry feelings.

2. Stay in the present and focus on the situation.

3. Avoid assigning any blame.

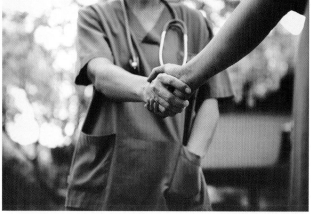

ESUN7756/Shutterstock.com

Figure 10.12 Conflict resolution is important, and it is always possible to resolve disagreements in a productive manner.

The second component of conflict management is problem solving and includes the following steps:

4. Attack the problem and not the person with whom you have the conflict.
5. Focus on the issue.
6. Don't jump to conclusions.
7. Be **assertive** (bold and clear) when expressing your feelings and requests.
8. Use active listening.
9. Seek a solution by finding common interests and agreement.

Remember that there are several styles of managing conflict, but the two conflict-management styles that work best are **compromise** or **collaboration**. When compromise occurs, both sides of a conflict experience wins and losses until the best resolution is reached. Collaboration takes place when everyone works together and agrees with the final solution.

> **Remember**
>
> *One can be the master of what one does, but never of what one feels.*
>
> Gustave Flaubert, author

Section 10.3 Review and Assessment

Using the Key Terms
Complete the following sentences using key terms in this section.

1. _____ is the process by which two sides of a conflict make concessions to find the best resolution.
2. A(n) _____ is any disagreement between two or more people.
3. The emotion of _____ results from the threat or presence of danger.
4. _____ is an emotion that develops from frustration, displeasure, or a threat.
5. Communication that is _____ is bold and clear.
6. _____ is the process by which people work together to resolve conflict in a way that satisfies everyone.
7. Unsupported, exaggerated fears are _____.

Know and Understand the Facts

8. What is the difference between fear and anxiety?
9. Identify one way a holistic nursing assistant can help relieve a resident's fear.
10. Describe three physical responses to anger.
11. Identify three strategies to calm angry residents.
12. What is the difference between compromise and collaboration?

Analyze and Apply Concepts

13. Explain two ways to deal with anxiety.
14. A resident is yelling at another resident and pounding his fists on his wheelchair. What can a nursing assistant to do help calm this resident?
15. Describe three strategies a holistic nursing assistant can use to resolve conflict.

Think Critically
Read the following care situation. Then answer the questions that follow.

Janet is a nursing assistant caring for Mrs. G, an 88-year-old woman, today. Mrs. G was admitted to a local long-term care facility yesterday afternoon. In the morning, Janet knocks on Mrs. G's door and introduces herself. Mrs. G looks frightened and pulls the bed covers up to her eyes. Janet asks if Mrs. G would like to get ready for breakfast. Mrs. G shakes her head. Janet asks her again about eating breakfast and says, "Would you like to eat in your room today?" Mrs. G continues to shake her head and keeps her covers pulled up to her neck.

16. What feelings might Mrs. G be expressing?
17. What might be the reason for Mrs. G's feelings?
18. What would you advise Janet do or say to help Mrs. G feel more comfortable?

Key Points

Reviewing the key points for this chapter will help you practice more safely and competently as a holistic nursing assistant and will help you prepare for the certification competency exam.

- Holistic communication is essential to giving safe, quality care.
- Cultural differences, labeling, jargon, and stereotyping may cause communication barriers. Defense mechanisms are unconscious ways of diminishing stress and anxiety.
- Health literacy is the degree to which people fully understand and use information about their health, diseases, conditions, and treatments.
- To build and maintain strong interpersonal relationships, you must be self-aware, respectful, helpful, fair, trustworthy, appreciative, a team player, and able to manage anger and conflict.
- Caring means providing assistance and comfort to positively affect the health and well-being of residents.
- You will encounter anxiety, fear, anger, and conflict during your work as a holistic nursing assistant. Allowing residents to share their feelings and emotions is one way to respond.

Action Steps to Holistic Care

Review the information in this chapter. Complete the following activities.

1. Working with a partner, select one barrier to holistic communication discussed in the chapter. Create a skit that shows the communication barrier in action, with one of you acting as a resident and the other as a holistic nursing assistant. Be sure to include a resolution to this barrier, using holistic communication.

2. Select one defense mechanism you learned about in this chapter. Prepare a short paper or digital presentation that describes the defense mechanism, how it is demonstrated, why a person would use this defense mechanism, and how to best respond to the defense mechanism.

3. With a partner, select one of the following: anxiety, fear, anger, or conflict. Prepare a poster that illustrates your selection. Include a definition of your selection and two action steps to decrease it.

4. Find pictures in a magazine, in a newspaper, or online that best demonstrate three types of nonverbal communication you use.

 Preparing for the Certification Competency Examination

To prepare for the nursing assistant certification competency examination, you will need to know content found in this chapter. This content may be tested in the knowledge (written or oral) and skills (hands-on demonstration) portions of the exam. The following areas will be emphasized:

- verbal and nonverbal communication
- barriers to communication
- care that supports communication and behavior in a positive, nonthreatening way
- effective communication with residents, patients, families, and the healthcare team
- dynamics of interpersonal relationships
- caring skills

These sample test questions are similar to ones you will find on the certification competency exam. See how well you can answer them. Be sure to select the *best* answer.

1. Which of the following is the most common way people communicate?
   A. verbally
   B. using slang or jargon
   C. nonverbally
   D. using active listening

2. Which of the following is the best way to communicate with someone who is hearing impaired?
   A. yell loudly until the person responds
   B. use short sentences and simple words
   C. stand behind the person while you talk
   D. increase the tone of your voice

3. Which of the following is the most effective way to be sure a resident understands your explanation of a new treatment?

   A. have the resident write it down
   B. have the resident read it from a pamphlet
   C. have the resident repeat back what he or she heard
   D. have the resident ask you questions

4. A nursing assistant wants to be sure she is expressing herself in a caring way. Which of the following qualities would best show this skill?

   A. projection   C. privacy
   B. gossip   D. respect

5. Mrs. L shares with her nursing assistant that she is afraid of dying. How should the nursing assistant best respond?

   A. He should say, "If you pray, you will not be so afraid."
   B. He should ask Mrs. L open-ended questions and listen quietly.
   C. He should tell Mrs. L that she is not going anywhere soon.
   D. He should tell Mrs. L that he will ask for medications to help calm her down.

6. When the same message is sent using both verbal and nonverbal communication, the message is considered which of the following?

   A. congruent   C. caring
   B. assertive   D. empathetic

7. How do nursing assistants show they are actively listening?

   A. by interrupting as much as possible
   B. by starting to make the bed
   C. by using good eye contact and responding appropriately
   D. by using laughter

8. What are the four components of communication?

   A. listener, receiver, communicator, and observer
   B. sender, mode of communication, recipient, and feedback
   C. observer, method of communication, receiver, and participant
   D. sender, observer, strategy, and feedback

9. Which of the following describes a health literate person?

   A. someone who is able to read books and information pamphlets about health conditions and diseases
   B. someone who is able to make informative decisions about his or her disease or condition
   C. someone who is able to search the Internet for information about specific diseases
   D. someone who is able to tell his or her friends all about what is wrong with them

10. Mr. D is angry about how ill he feels today. What would be the best way to communicate with him?

    A. yell at him and tell him to settle down immediately
    B. call his daughter and tell her that she needs to visit him
    C. ignore Mr. D and get him water to help him calm down
    D. help him share his feelings and give him time to calm down

11. Two nursing assistants have worked well together for several years. They like each other and believe they have an excellent professional relationship. Which of the following bests describe why they have this relationship?

    A. They are respectful and appreciative of each other.
    B. They have created an intimate way of talking to each other.
    C. They have formed an excellent friendship.
    D. They both like their nurse supervisor.

12. This morning, Mrs. W told you that she feels so much better today and is sure she will be going home by the end of the week. You both know she has terminal cancer and is in her final days. What defense mechanism is she using?

    A. repression   C. regression
    B. denial   D. displacement

13. A new nursing assistant is not yet comfortable in her position. She walks with a stooped posture and keeps her arms crossed over her chest when talking with staff. What mechanism is she using to express her discomfort?

    A. tone of voice   C. body language
    B. slang   D. stereotyping

14. The first action someone should take to resolve a conflict between two people is which of the following?

    A. give the two people a resource on conflict
    B. focus on the issues that are causing the conflict
    C. collaborate with all the people involved
    D. manage the feelings the people have

15. What communication barrier is present when a nursing assistant says to a resident, "I need your vitals, stat"?

    A. jargon   C. stereotyping
    B. labeling   D. empathy

Did you have difficulty with any of the questions? If you did, review the chapter to find the correct answer(s).

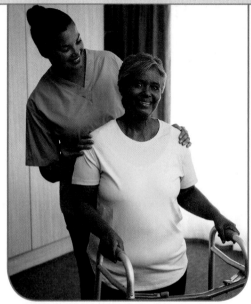

wavebreakmedia/Shutterstock.com

Welcome to the Chapter

Nursing assistants provide care to diverse patients and residents who come from all races, ethnicities, and cultures. Practicing cultural humility and respect is an important part of providing holistic care. When you practice cultural humility, you are aware of and sensitive to other cultures, including your own culture. This sensitivity leads to a deeper appreciation and understanding between people. It also helps build an open-minded relationship and stronger partnership with others. Having cultural humility and respect for diversity allows for successful cross-cultural communication with people from diverse groups and populations. This is vital to delivering safe, quality care.

What you learn in this chapter will help you develop your knowledge and skills to become a holistic nursing assistant. The topics discussed in the chapter are highlighted on the Providing Holistic Care Framework.

You are now ready to start this chapter, *Appreciating Diversity*.

Chapter Outline

Section 11.1
Diverse Cultures

Section 11.2
Cultural Humility and Cross-Cultural Communication

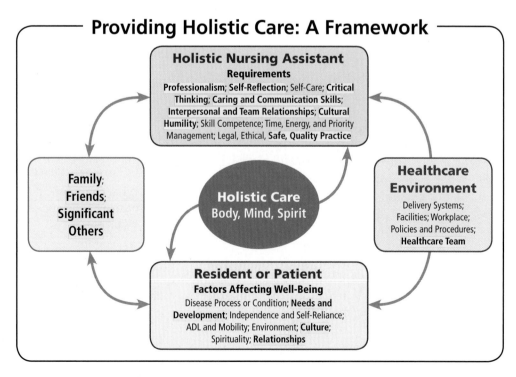

Providing Holistic Care: A Framework

Holistic Nursing Assistant
Requirements
Professionalism; Self-Reflection; Self-Care; **Critical Thinking; Caring and Communication Skills; Interpersonal and Team Relationships; Cultural Humility;** Skill Competence; Time, Energy, and Priority Management; Legal, Ethical, **Safe, Quality Practice**

Family; Friends; Significant Others

Holistic Care
Body, Mind, Spirit

Healthcare Environment
Delivery Systems; Facilities; Workplace; Policies and Procedures; **Healthcare Team**

Resident or Patient
Factors Affecting Well-Being
Disease Process or Condition; **Needs and Development;** Independence and Self-Reliance; ADL and Mobility; Environment; **Culture;** Spirituality; **Relationships**

Objectives

Caring for people from diverse cultures, groups, and populations is an important part of a holistic nursing assistant's responsibility. As a holistic nursing assistant, you need to become acquainted with the dynamics of and the differences between race, ethnicity, and culture. You also need to know about challenges that can become barriers to appreciating diversity. To achieve the objectives for this section, you must successfully

- **describe** the difference between race, ethnicity, and culture; and
- **identify** the challenges to appreciating and working within diverse cultures, groups, and populations.

Key Terms

Learn these key terms to better understand the information presented in the section.

beliefs	race
customs	racism
diversity	rituals
ethnicity	traditions
ethnocentrism	trait
prejudice	

Questions to Consider

- Have you ever communicated or worked with people who have different beliefs or who come from cultural groups different from your own? These people may have dressed differently or spoken a language other than yours.
- What did you do when you interacted with these people who were different? How did you react?
- When you interacted with these people, did you ever not know what to say or do? What feelings did that cause? How did you deal with your feelings?

What Is Diversity?

In healthcare, you will become acquainted with, care for, and work with many different people. While we all have the same basic needs, we all also come from a variety of family backgrounds, geographic locations, ethnic groups, generations, religions, orientations, and belief systems. This is **diversity**, or the presence of differences among people (Figure 11.1). There are many types of diversity, including racial and ethnic diversity, family diversity, religious diversity, geographic diversity, generational diversity, and sexual diversity, among others.

Remember

Our goal should be to understand our differences.

James D. Watson,
American scientist

Racial and Ethnic Diversity

To be comfortable with diversity, you must understand the terms related to this topic. Two terms you will hear often that relate to diversity are *race* and *ethnicity*. **Race** is linked to a person's genetic makeup and cannot be changed. Race can be identified using a person's distinctive physical characteristics, or **traits**. People of the same race may share certain aspects of their appearances, including skin, hair, or eye color.

Ethnicity describes the ethnic group a person belongs to and is different from race. Ethnicity is a group's identification with shared social, cultural, and traditional practices. For example, an Italian family that follows traditional Italian practices would be ethnically Italian. Conversely, a person who has the racial characteristics of a Hispanic may not identify with his or her Hispanic ethnicity, or social, cultural, and traditional practices.

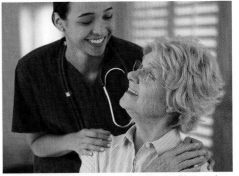

Rocketclips, Inc./Shutterstock.com

Figure 11.1 Diversity refers to the many differences among people. In healthcare, communicating and giving care require knowledge of diversity and respect for others' differences.

As you have learned, *culture* is a set of learned behaviors and is passed down through generations. People of the same culture have shared **traditions** (behaviors that have special meanings), **beliefs** (ideas accepted to be true), and languages. They also have shared **rituals** (actions always done in the same way), eating habits, dress, and **customs** (established practices and beliefs). For example, Hispanic or Latino cultures usually value family, both immediate and extended. In many Asian cultures, older adults play major roles in making decisions that can affect the entire family.

The US Census Bureau recognizes the following races in the United States: Caucasian, African-American, American Indian or Alaska Native, Asian, Native Hawaiian or other Pacific Islander, and Hispanic or Latino. Today, most of the US population is comprised of Caucasians, although the African-American and Hispanic populations are growing quickly.

Family Diversity

Diversity exists among families. Some families are considered *traditional* and include a mother, a father, and a child or children. Other families are made up of a single parent, who is either male or female, and a child or children. In *blended families*, divorced parents marry other people and may have children from both marriages. Some families have two parents of the same sex. Additionally, some families adopt or foster children. An *intergenerational family* is one in which several generations live in the same house. Interracial families have family members from different races.

Religious Diversity

Successful holistic nursing assistants should have a general familiarity with diverse religions. A *religion* is defined by a specific set of spiritual beliefs about supreme beings, a particular philosophy of life, a code of ethics, and a set of rituals. In some religions, a supreme being is seen as responsible for all healing. The religion most commonly represented in the United States is Christianity, which a little over 70 percent of people follow and which primarily includes Protestantism and Catholicism. Nearly 6 percent of people in the United States follow other religions, such as Judaism, Buddhism, and Islam. The final 23 percent of people in the United States are unaffiliated with a religion. These people may consider themselves atheists (people who deny or disbelieve the existence of a supreme being), consider themselves agnostics (people who believe they cannot know if any supreme being exists), or simply not have a formal relationship with a religion.

Geographic Diversity

The places where people live, or people's geographic locations, must also be considered when discussing diversity. Various regions of the United States may have diverse cultural practices. For example, people who grow up on the East Coast of the United States have a different experience from those who grow up in the South (Figure 11.2). Regional accents may vary, people may have familiarity with different types of food, and people may call items such as clothing or furniture by different names (for example, a *sofa, couch,* or *divan*). People may even be accustomed to different types of transportation because of their geographic locations. People who live in the city may utilize public transportation, while people in more rural areas may rely exclusively on personal vehicles.

Generational Diversity

You learned about the different generations in chapter 6. In today's society, there are five diverse generations: the silent generation, baby boomers, generation X, millennials, and generation Z. Remember that it is important not to believe stereotypes about particular generations. Rather, you should recognize generational diversity and value the qualities of each generation. The better you understand the differences between generations, the easier it will be for you to understand the members of these generations and build rapport through improved communication.

Think About This

According to the US Census Bureau, the Caucasian population will remain the largest single group of people in the United States until 2060. At that time, minorities—which now comprise 37 percent of the population—will grow to approximately 57 percent of the population. By 2060, nearly one in three US residents will be Hispanic or Latino.

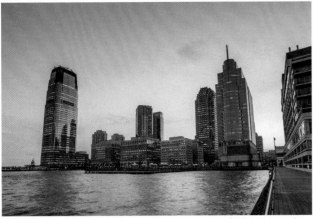

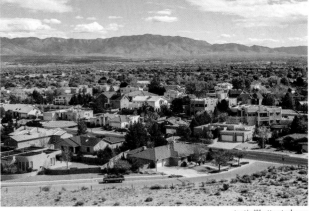

f11photo/Shutterstock.com

turtix/Shutterstock.com

A

B

Figure 11.2 Even within the United States, there is much regional diversity. Someone who grew up on the East Coast (A) would have a vastly different experience from someone who grew up in New Mexico (B).

Sexual Diversity

As a holistic nursing assistant, you will encounter people with different sexual orientations and gender identities. *Sexual orientation* describes a person's emotional, romantic, and sexual attraction to males or females. A person's sexual orientation may be

- heterosexual (attracted to members of the opposite sex);
- homosexual (attracted to members of the same sex);
- bisexual (attracted to members of both sexes); or
- asexual (lacking sexual attraction for other people).

Gender identity refers to a person's sense of being a man or a woman and the expression of that sense. For example, a person may feel that his or her assigned

Culture Cues
Valuing Diversity

The following guidelines will help you recognize and appreciate diversity as a holistic nursing assistant:

- Treat people the way *they* wish to be treated, not the way *you* wish them to be treated.
- Question your own assumptions and the assumptions of others. This will help you avoid limiting your opportunities to understand another person.
- Offer to assist others whose backgrounds and experiences are different from your own.
- When asking someone to explain a point of view or an opinion different from your own, let the person know that you are asking because you want to understand, not because you want the person to justify the opinion.
- Watch for any tendencies you might have to joke about or make fun of people's differences. When you see another person joking this way, be direct and ask him or her to stop.

- Welcome ideas that are different from your own.
- Look at issues from another person's point of view before making decisions.
- Continually monitor your thoughts and language for any assumptions or stereotypes you might have.
- Always use facility policies and procedures. Healthcare facilities often have resources, including staff members who have expertise in diversity.

Apply It

1. Which of these guidelines do you follow as part of your typical interactions with others?
2. Which of these guidelines do you not often follow? Which guidelines would you like to incorporate into your interactions with others? Explain.
3. How can you incorporate the guidelines you do not often follow into your interactions with others?

sex (male or female) is the same as his or her gender identity. Another person may feel that his or her assigned sex is incorrect and instead identify with the opposite gender. This person's assigned sex may be male, but she may have a female gender identity. People with this type of gender identity consider themselves *transgender*. Transgender people may identify with different sexual orientations.

Some people have *differences of sexual development (DSDs)*, also called *intersex*. People with DSDs are born with variations in their biological structures—that is, their sexual anatomy is not in alignment with the female or male sex. For example, a female may be born without a vaginal opening. A male may be born with a scrotum that looks like labia. A person may have male anatomy on the outside, but have typical internal female anatomy, or have a mix of XX and XY chromosomes. In some cases, a DSD is recognized at birth. In other cases, it is not identified until puberty or not identified at all.

Other types of diversity you will encounter as a holistic nursing assistant include diversity in people's mental and physical abilities, differences in levels of education, and varied political beliefs. As a holistic nursing assistant, you will likely care for many, if not all, of the diverse cultures, groups, and populations discussed. Each patient or resident, no matter his or her background, always deserves safe, quality care.

What Are Challenges to Appreciating Diversity?

Appreciating diverse cultures requires you to first develop an awareness about your *own* cultural values and beliefs. Learning about your cultural values and beliefs provides you with the information you will need to determine how your cultural perspectives differ from those you work with and those in your care. When you know your own perspectives, you will be able to recognize when your values and beliefs are different from those belonging to your patients, residents, and coworkers (Figure 11.3). This realization can help you overcome challenges related to establishing relationships and providing care. Making the conscious choice to accept and appreciate diversity will also help you avoid potential challenges and communication barriers.

Challenges to appreciating diversity include ethnocentrism, biases, prejudices, racism, and stereotypes.

- **Ethnocentrism**: involves judging another culture based on the beliefs and standards of one's own culture.

- **Bias**: is an unfair belief that some people, objects, or situations are better than others. Ethnocentrism can create a bias.

  - **Prejudice**: is an opinion or feeling that is formed without facts. Prejudice develops when a person is biased and often leads to unfair feelings of dislike for a person or group based on race, sex, or religion. For example, a family member may have had an experience with a person from another culture that caused him to form a negative opinion about that culture as a whole. This may also cause you to form prejudices against people from that culture.

  - **Racism**: is a form of prejudice. It is the belief that one's own race is superior.

  - **Stereotyping**: is also a form of prejudice. It is an oversimplified, generalized, usually unfavorable opinion about a group of people. A stereotype, for example, might be that all old people are cranky or that all people who are overweight are sloppy.

Challenges to appreciating diversity can interfere with your ability to be culturally aware, sensitive, and respectful. Overcoming these challenges, should they occur, is essential to delivering safe, quality care.

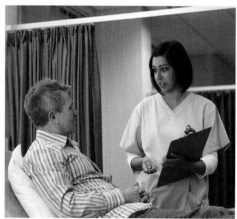
Cultura Motion/Shutterstock.com

Figure 11.3 Once you understand your own background and culture, you will be more able to communicate with people from different backgrounds and cultures.

Using the Key Terms

Complete the following sentences using key terms in this section.

1. _____ refers to a group's identification with common social, cultural, and traditional practices.
2. People of the same _____ have similar inherited characteristics, including skin, eye, and hair color.
3. _____ are ideas that a person or group of people accept to be true.
4. _____ judges another culture based on the beliefs and standards of one's own culture.
5. _____ is not based on facts and leads to unfair feelings of dislike for a person or group because of race, sex, or religion.
6. _____ refers to intolerance, discrimination, or prejudice based on race.
7. Behaviors or practices that have special meanings or symbolism are _____.
8. _____ are actions that are always done in the same way.

Know and Understand the Facts

9. In your own words, explain the meaning of diversity.
10. Explain the difference between *race, ethnicity,* and *culture*.
11. Identify and describe two types of diversity.
12. What is the difference between ethnocentrism and prejudice?
13. What is the difference between racism and stereotyping?

Analyze and Apply Concepts

14. How might the family, religious, or generational diversity among residents impact the way you give care?
15. Discuss two challenges that can interfere with a person's ability to appreciate diversity.
16. A nursing assistant has been asked to care for a resident who comes from a different generation than she, has lived in a different geographic area, and has a different cultural background. What three guidelines can she incorporate into her care to value diversity?

Think Critically

Read the following care situation. Then answer the questions that follow.

Mrs. P is a 75-year-old woman whose admission documents indicate that she is Jewish and follows Judaism's religious traditions and customs. Mrs. P had a broken hip and now needs therapy after hip-replacement surgery. After talking with her second husband and his children, Mrs. P has decided that her rehabilitation will be most successful if she spends a few weeks in a specialized facility that offers daily therapy. She will stay in the specialized facility until she is able to safely walk at home. When Aamir, a nursing assistant, meets Mrs. P and her husband, he realizes they both have heavy accents and are difficult to understand. Aamir has worked with a similar resident in the past, and it was not a good experience. Aamir found that resident demanding and stubborn.

17. Which types of diversity are present in this situation?
18. What religious traditions and customs might Mrs. P practice?
19. What challenges to appreciating diversity might arise in this situation?
20. What actions could Aamir take to prevent any challenges to appreciating diversity?

Questions to Consider

- To which races or ethnic groups do you belong? What are your family's values, traditions, and customs?
- Have people ever seen you as *different*? How did that make you feel?
- Have others understood your differences? If so, how did they show that they understood? What have you done in the past to show that you understand others' differences?

Objectives

People have cultural humility when they have awareness and respect for their own cultures as well as the cultures of others. Having cultural humility will enhance your ability to respond to residents' holistic needs and to use cross-cultural communication. To achieve the objectives for this section, you must successfully

- **identify** your own cultural beliefs, values, and traditions;
- **recognize** that routines and procedures may need to be altered due to cultural and religious traditions and customs;
- **integrate** cultural humility routinely into practice; and
- **demonstrate** cross-cultural communication when giving holistic care.

Key Terms

Learn these key terms to better understand the information presented in the section.

cross-cultural communication kinship
cultural humility

What Is Cultural Humility?

It is important to understand that people interpret their own cultures and beliefs uniquely. No two people or families are exactly the same, even if they share a common religion or cultural heritage. People within a culture or religion may interpret, practice, or feel comfortable following traditions in different ways. Therefore, it is never fully possible to understand another culture and all of the people in it.

Because of this, it is important that holistic nursing assistants practice cultural humility. **Cultural humility** has a positive effect on care. This approach acknowledges that it is impossible to learn and know everything about another person's culture. Instead, cultural humility recognizes that there are differences among all people and focuses on the importance of assessing one's own culture to understand its limitations, barriers, and gaps in knowledge. Cultural humility attempts to achieve a sense of equality by encouraging people to be respectful of one another, be open to new ideas, and understand that each person should be treated as an individual.

A person who practices cultural humility is positively curious about how other people see the world and live. This positive and respectful curiosity leads a person to be open-minded and present when observing and asking questions of others.

Respecting the beliefs and traditions of those in your care is a critical and important part of your role and responsibility as a holistic nursing assistant. As you provide care with cultural humility, you may discover differences in the ways your residents approach their health, the procedures they will follow, and the medications they are willing to take. Individuals may have particular family dynamics, communication styles, dietary preferences and restrictions, religious customs, and levels of modesty that impact the care you give.

Family Dynamics

As a holistic nursing assistant, you will come in close contact with residents' family members. In some cultures, a particularly strong emphasis is placed on family, and

Remember

Our cultural strength has always been derived from our diversity of understanding and experience.

Yo-Yo Ma, cellist and United Nations Messenger of Peace

older adults serve as decision makers for younger family members. In such cases, family members may be heavily involved in caregiving. Parents and grandparents may be respected because of their wisdom or knowledge and may be consulted during decision making. In some cultures, the father is important for decision making, while other cultures place the role of primary caregiver with the mother or grandmother. There is often **kinship** (feelings of closeness) between members of an extended family or community. A resident may be close with a support group or with people in his or her neighborhood. Sometimes these relationships are as important as relationships with family and friends. Because these relationships are so important, they should be acknowledged and respected.

Communication Styles

A nursing assistant's ability to communicate effectively with residents may be influenced by residents' cultural and communication practices. In some cultures, self-control is valued to the extent that people are unwilling to acknowledge strong emotions or pain. This may make it difficult for residents to share how they are feeling with the nursing staff. Other cultures have great respect for authority figures, such as doctors. As a result, residents may smile and nod out of respect, even if they are feeling confused or embarrassed. This reaction may be misleading. It may lead to the assumption that everything is all right with the resident, when everything is not.

Dietary Preferences and Restrictions

People's diets are often influenced by their cultural or religious practices. For example, many Buddhists abstain from consuming alcohol and are often vegetarians. Jewish individuals may follow a *kosher* diet and eat only foods that meet the requirements of Jewish dietary laws. Muslim residents may not eat pork or any foods prepared with any form of alcohol. Some religions dictate the consumption of particular foods during ceremonial times (Figure 11.4). Other religions prohibit alcohol, tobacco, tea, or coffee from being consumed. As a holistic nursing assistant, you must be aware of any medical and religious dietary restrictions your residents have and assist with accommodating any special requests, as appropriate.

Religious Customs

Residents' religions may affect the care they require even in ways beyond dietary restrictions. For example, residents' religious beliefs may prevent them from taking certain medications, receiving blood transfusions, donating or receiving organs, or allowing life support. Residents may also require specific arrangements to practice their religious beliefs. Religious beliefs may impact a resident's daily schedule as the resident integrates prayer, meditation, or other religious practices into the day.

As a holistic nursing assistant, you may be asked to ensure that residents have what they need to follow their religious traditions. For example, Muslims may require supplies and equipment for washing prior to prayer, a clean sheet to place on the floor, and assistance kneeling to get into prayer position facing the city of Mecca. Jewish residents may observe the *Sabbath*, which begins on Friday at sundown and lasts until sundown on Saturday. During the Sabbath, a Jewish person who abides by religious traditions may not write, bathe, or use electricity (for example, turn on or off lights). You may need to assist these residents with any activities they are not able to do. For example, you may need to turn lights in the resident's room on or off during Sabbath.

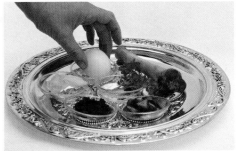

Figure 11.4 One example of a religious ceremony involving food is the Jewish Passover. This arrangement of food, known as the Seder plate, has symbolic meaning.

Levels of Modesty

Nursing assistants see residents in their most vulnerable moments. As a holistic nursing assistant, you should provide extra care and

On last night's news report, it was announced that a local residential community center received an award for demonstrating outstanding care of their diverse residents. The center was recognized for creating a feeling of respect and dignity. In particular, the nursing staff was commended for showing excellence in cultural and religious awareness. The residents, when interviewed, said they appreciated how staff members went out of their way to learn about residents' practices. Staff members also organized celebrations for all of the different holidays.

Apply It

1. What might the nursing staff be doing to show excellence in cultural and religious awareness?

2. How do you think the nursing staff might be demonstrating cultural humility?

3. What cross-cultural communication skills do staff members need to continue using to demonstrate respect and dignity?

consideration for residents whose cultural practices or religious beliefs dictate *modesty* (regard for decency of behavior, dress, and exposure of body parts to others). In an effort to maintain their modesty, some residents prefer to receive treatment from someone of the same gender. Some women may also keep their hair covered.

How Can a Nursing Assistant Integrate Cross-Cultural Communication into Care?

When holistic nursing assistants integrate cultural humility into practice, they have the ability to use **cross-cultural communication**. Cross-cultural communication uses practices and approaches that promote and improve relationships with people from different cultures. This type of communication is based on being aware and sensitive; building knowledge about another culture's values, traditions, and customs; and understanding how members of a culture communicate both verbally and nonverbally. The following guidelines are part of cross-cultural communication:

- Be present, make eye contact, and use active listening skills.
- Pay attention to your body language. Be mindful of your gestures and avoid using your arms and hands when talking, as this may seem intimidating.
- Smile and be open to hearing what is said.
- Avoid intruding on a resident's personal space.
- Use plain language when speaking. Avoid words that have dual meanings or similar sounding words (such as *pair* and *pear*).
- Avoid slang, jargon, and humor. Residents are not likely to understand them.
- Use short, simple sentences. Keep questions and answers brief.
- Speak slowly to give people time to interpret what you are saying.
- Ask the resident to repeat back what he or she heard.
- If the resident does not repeat back what you said, ask the resident if he or she has any questions.
- Ask questions so you can respect traditional practices.
- Summarize what you have said, if you can. Repeat the same message, with patience, so the resident has more time to understand what was said.
- Use other forms of communication to support oral communication.
- Attempt to learn key words in other languages.
- Provide written resources in a resident's native language.
- Ask the licensed nursing staff for an interpreter, when appropriate and necessary.

Becoming a Holistic Nursing Assistant
Cultural Humility and Cross-Cultural Communication

The following list includes qualities of holistic nursing assistants who practice cultural humility and use cross-cultural communication skills. Read through this list and consider whether you possess each quality.

- I have a good understanding of my own cultural and ethnic identity.
- I use self-reflection and avoid making assumptions or believing stereotypes.
- I respect others and do not impose my own values and beliefs on them.
- I work hard at understanding differing perspectives.
- I know that a person's skill in the English language has nothing to do with his or her level of intelligence or literacy.

- I pursue needed resources by asking questions and seeking training when I am uncertain about a cultural group or religion.
- I always use cross-cultural communication skills when working with people or groups from different cultures or religions.

Apply It

1. Which of the qualities in this list do you already possess?
2. Consider which qualities you do not possess and brainstorm ways you could develop your knowledge and skills to possess them in the future.

Section 11.2 Review and Assessment

Using the Key Terms

Complete the following sentences using key terms in this section.

1. Practices and approaches that promote and improve relationships with people from different cultures are part of _____.
2. _____ is awareness and understanding of one's own culture, as well as the cultures of others.
3. A feeling of being close is described as _____.

Know and Understand the Facts

4. Identify two ways a nursing assistant can demonstrate cultural humility.
5. Give two examples of specific religious customs holistic nursing assistants must be aware of when providing care.
6. Describe two examples of family dynamics that represent cultural diversity.
7. What is cross-cultural communication?

Analyze and Apply Concepts

8. Identify one area in which you can improve your practice of cultural humility.
9. How can cultural dietary preferences and restrictions affect care?
10. Name four cross-cultural communication skills.

Think Critically

Read the following care situation. Then answer the questions that follow.

Tiana, a nursing assistant, has been asked to care for Elena, a 16-year-old girl who has been hospitalized for an acute asthma episode. Elena spends the majority of her time with her grandparents, who immigrated to the United States from South America. As a result, Elena speaks little English. Tiana has been assigned to perform Elena's morning care. As Tiana enters the room, Elena's grandmother is feeding Elena something she brought from home.

11. What is the first action Tiana should take when she enters the room to show cultural humility?
12. What cultural knowledge will be important for Tiana to know to provide safe, quality care?
13. Which cross-cultural communication skills could help Tiana care for Elena?

Key Points

Reviewing the key points for this chapter will help you practice more safely and competently as a holistic nursing assistant and will help you prepare for the certification competency examination.

- The United States is comprised of people from a variety of races and ethnicities. Learning to appreciate others' differences, or diversity, will enable you to provide high-quality care.
- Nursing assistants will encounter residents from diverse family structures, religious beliefs, geographic locations, and generations.
- Ethnocentrism, bias, prejudice, stereotypes, and racism will prevent a nursing assistant from appreciating diversity.
- Cultural humility recognizes that there are differences among all people and focuses on the assessment of one's own culture to understand its limitations, barriers, and gaps in knowledge.
- Cross-cultural communication is based on being aware and sensitive; building knowledge about another culture's values, traditions, customs; and understanding how members of a culture communicate both verbally and nonverbally.

Action Steps to Holistic Care

Review the information in this chapter. Complete the following activities.

1. Select one challenge to appreciating diversity. Prepare a short paper or digital presentation that provides more detail than what is found in this chapter.
2. Write a short paper that explains the concept of cultural humility. Discuss why cultural humility is an important quality for holistic nursing assistants to possess. Also identify the qualities a person who practices cultural humility must have. Finally, explore an area such as family dynamics, modesty, or religious customs, that might impact the care you will give as a holistic nursing assistant and explain how you could use cultural humility to address any challenges or differences.
3. With a partner, prepare a poster that illustrates three cross-cultural communication skills. Show how these skills will lead to more effective resident interaction.
4. Research one cultural or religious group in the United States. Write a brief report describing three traditions or customs that would be important for a holistic nursing assistant to know.

Preparing for the Certification Competency Examination

To prepare for the nursing assistant certification competency examination, you will need to know content found in this chapter. This content may be tested in the knowledge (written or oral) and skills (hands-on demonstration) portions of the exam. The following areas will be emphasized:

- influence of cultural attitudes
- the nursing assistant's role in respecting and accommodating cultural differences
- recognition of cultural and religious beliefs leading to variations in diet

These sample test questions are similar to ones you will find on the certification competency exam. See how well you can answer them. Be sure to select the *best* answer.

1. When a person evaluates another culture based on the beliefs and standards of his or her own culture, this is called
   A. bias
   B. prejudice
   C. stereotyping
   D. ethnocentrism

2. A nursing assistant is caring for an older woman who practices her culture's traditions. Which of the following would *not* be a cultural or religious consideration?
   A. The woman may have cultural dietary restrictions to consider.
   B. The woman may be very modest and want to be covered.
   C. The woman may want the nursing assistant to assist her with meals.
   D. The woman may have many family members visiting at the same time.

3. Which of the following best describes the difference between race and racism?

   A. Race is a group of people who share many physical characteristics. Racism is the belief that one's race is superior.
   B. Race is intolerance or discrimination. Racism is the belief that one's race is inferior.
   C. Race is a group of people linked by family traditions. Racism is the belief that one's race is built on values.
   D. Race is related to geographic area. Racism is the belief that one's race is superior.

4. The difference between a ritual and a tradition is that a tradition is

   A. a religious ceremony
   B. a practice that requires dietary restrictions
   C. handed down from one generation to another
   D. a practice that involves only current family members

5. A new nursing assistant is caring for a Muslim resident. What should the nursing assistant know about using cultural humility in her practice?

   A. In Islam, food is used to honor the dying.
   B. She should treat each resident as an individual.
   C. She does not need to worry about any dietary customs.
   D. All Muslim people usually act the same way.

6. Which of the following is true of ethnicity?

   A. It is based on the racial roots, customs, and rituals as a group sees them and practices them.
   B. It is based on a group's decision about how they will practice their rituals and traditions.
   C. It is based on a group's identification with common social, cultural, and traditional practices.
   D. It is based on a cultural group's perception of their likes and dislikes and how they are practiced.

7. Nursing assistants who demonstrate cultural humility always

   A. use journaling to describe their experiences
   B. use team meetings to discuss conflicts
   C. use meditation to deal with stress
   D. use self-assessment to understand their own culture

8. Which of the following actions demonstrates cross-cultural communication skills?

   A. being present and using active listening skills
   B. providing clean linen during morning care
   C. providing comfortable chairs
   D. keeping the curtains closed during a procedure

9. What is a blended family?

   A. a family that consists of several generations
   B. a family of members from difference races
   C. a family that consists of remarried parents and their children
   D. a family that consists of two single people

10. What is a stereotype?

    A. an opinion that is not based on facts
    B. an oversimplified, generalized, usually unfavorable opinion about a group of people
    C. a judgment about another culture based on the beliefs and standards of one's own culture
    D. an unfair belief that some people, objects, or situations are better than others

11. If a nursing assistant is being prejudiced, she is

    A. being rude and mean to another person
    B. paying special attention to another person
    C. forming an opinion before getting the facts
    D. creating rumors and spreading them

12. Mrs. H, a 45-year-old woman, is Jewish and observes her religion's traditions and customs. What is the most important thing to know about her dietary needs?

    A. She will likely not have a midday snack.
    B. She will likely need a diet free from fats and carbohydrates.
    C. She will likely ask for a meal that has no spices or salts.
    D. She will likely need a meal that is kosher.

13. A nursing assistant is taking care of Mrs. J, an older Asian woman. Mrs. J doesn't ask for much, and the nursing assistant provides her limited care because she always seems so happy. Is this nursing assistant practicing cultural humility?

    A. yes, because he likes taking care of her
    B. no, because he provides only limited care
    C. yes, because he doesn't bother her with a lot of daily care
    D. no, because he may not really know what she needs

14. A nursing assistant who asks questions to build knowledge about a resident's cultural values, traditions, and customs is using

    A. cultural sensitivity
    B. cross-cultural communication
    C. transpersonal communication
    D. cultural awareness

15. What is sexual orientation?

    A. one's attraction to males or females
    B. one's personal identity of being male or female
    C. one's romantic engagement
    D. one's personal expression

Did you have difficulty with any of the questions? If you did, review the chapter to find the correct answer(s).

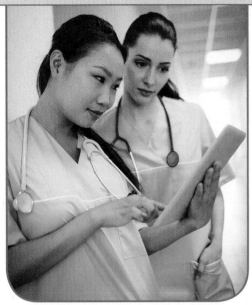

wavebreakmedia/Shutterstock.com

Welcome to the Chapter

This chapter provides information about the holistic nursing assistant's role in planning and organizing care. Some tools used to organize care include plans of care and care conferences. In this chapter, you will also learn how to use objective and subjective observation to report important information about the care you give. Reading and completing assignment sheets, participating in rounds, and filling out change-of-shift reports are other skills you will gain.

What you learn in this chapter will help you develop your knowledge and skills to become a holistic nursing assistant. The topics discussed in the chapter are highlighted on the Providing Holistic Care Framework.

You are now ready to start this chapter, *Planning, Observing, and Reporting Care.*

Chapter Outline

Section 12.1
Planning and Organizing Care

Section 12.2
Observing and Reporting Care

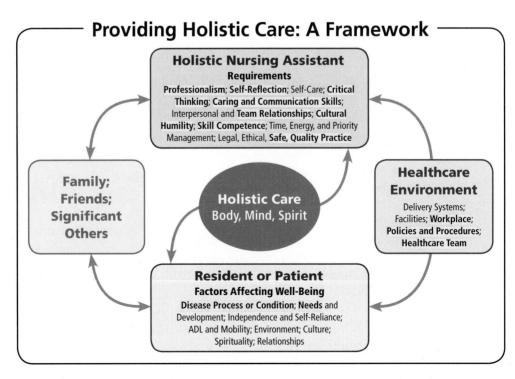

Providing Holistic Care: A Framework

Holistic Nursing Assistant
Requirements
Professionalism; Self-Reflection; Self-Care; Critical Thinking; Caring and Communication Skills; Interpersonal and **Team Relationships; Cultural Humility; Skill Competence;** Time, Energy, and Priority Management; Legal, Ethical, **Safe, Quality Practice**

Family; Friends; Significant Others

Holistic Care
Body, Mind, Spirit

Healthcare Environment
Delivery Systems; Facilities; **Workplace; Policies and Procedures; Healthcare Team**

Resident or Patient
Factors Affecting Well-Being
Disease Process or Condition; Needs and Development; Independence and Self-Reliance; ADL and Mobility; Environment; Culture; Spirituality; Relationships

Objectives

To provide effective holistic care, you must understand the holistic nursing assistant's role in care planning, care conferences, rounds, and reporting. This information will guide the care you give. Knowing how to use assignment sheets to organize and deliver care is also important for becoming a nursing assistant. To achieve the objectives for this section, you must successfully

- **identify** the purposes and key components of plans of care, care conferences, rounds, and change-of-shift reports;
- **explain** how nursing assistants participate in care planning, care conferences, rounds, and change-of-shift reports; and
- **describe** how to read and use assignment sheets to organize and deliver care.

Key Terms

Learn these key terms to better understand the information presented in the section.

care conferences   rationale

change-of-shift report   rounds

nursing orders

Questions to Consider

- Have you ever planned or organized an activity and had others count on you for the activity to be successful? The activity might have been a party, event, or pickup.
- When planning the activity, what did you do to make sure you accomplished your responsibilities?
- What type of planning was involved for the activity? Did you have to rely on the help of others? What did you learn from this experience?

What Is a Plan of Care?

As you learned in chapter 5, a *plan of care* is a written document that licensed nursing staff members develop for each resident. RNs write the plan of care, and LPNs/LVNs assist in this process. The plan of care is based on a comprehensive assessment and provides guidance for delivering individualized, consistent care. In some facilities, plans of care are called *service plans.*

Plans of care are evaluated and updated both routinely and when any changes occur. Any updates or changes in care are documented by the licensed nursing staff and then communicated to staff members across all shifts. This communication helps establish continuity of care across shifts and among members of the nursing staff. Another way that facilities provide continuity and consistency in care is using whiteboards in residents' rooms. These white boards list each resident's nurse, nursing assistant, goals for the day, and any special procedures or treatments. The information listed is changed for each shift.

Plans of care are also useful for determining what care is covered by insurance. This is because plans of care detail the types of treatments needed, schedules for observing and reporting, and the amount and type of assistance staff will be required to provide.

Plan of Care Organization

Plans of care vary by healthcare facility; however, they are generally organized using the steps of the nursing process and other important components of delivering care (for example, doctors' orders). Plans of care are usually composed of pertinent medical information, including medical diagnoses, ordered medications and treatments, nursing diagnoses, nursing goals, and **nursing orders** (instructions for achieving care goals). All of the information in a plan of care is important (Figure 12.1).

Remember

A goal without a plan is just a wish.

Antoine de Saint-Exupéry,
French writer

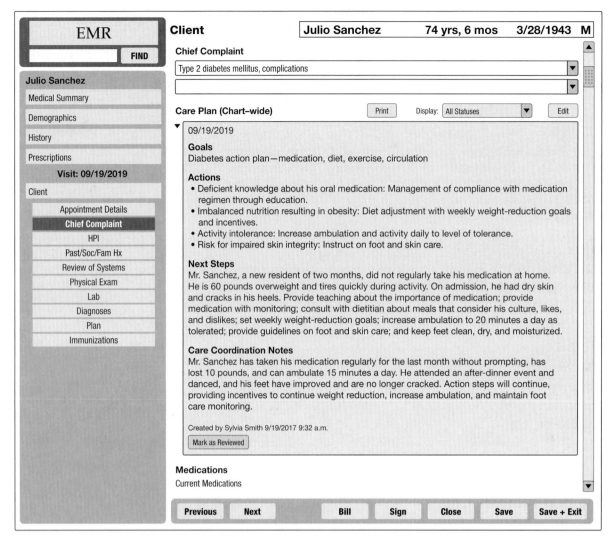

EMR

FIND

Julio Sanchez

Medical Summary

Demographics

History

Prescriptions

Visit: 09/19/2019

Client

Appointment Details

Chief Complaint

HPI

Past/Soc/Fam Hx

Review of Systems

Physical Exam

Lab

Diagnoses

Plan

Immunizations

Client | **Julio Sanchez** | **74 yrs, 6 mos** | **3/28/1943** | **M**

Chief Complaint

Type 2 diabetes mellitus, complications

Care Plan (Chart–wide) | Print | Display: All Statuses | Edit

09/19/2019

Goals
Diabetes action plan—medication, diet, exercise, circulation

Actions
- Deficient knowledge about his oral medication: Management of compliance with medication regimen through education.
- Imbalanced nutrition resulting in obesity: Diet adjustment with weekly weight-reduction goals and incentives.
- Activity intolerance: Increase ambulation and activity daily to level of tolerance.
- Risk for impaired skin integrity: Instruct on foot and skin care.

Next Steps
Mr. Sanchez, a new resident of two months, did not regularly take his medication at home. He is 60 pounds overweight and tires quickly during activity. On admission, he had dry skin and cracks in his heels. Provide teaching about the importance of medication; provide medication with monitoring; consult with dietitian about meals that consider his culture, likes, and dislikes; set weekly weight-reduction goals; increase ambulation to 20 minutes a day as tolerated; provide guidelines on foot and skin care; and keep feet clean, dry, and moisturized.

Care Coordination Notes
Mr. Sanchez has taken his medication regularly for the last month without prompting, has lost 10 pounds, and can ambulate 15 minutes a day. He attended an after-dinner event and danced, and his feet have improved and are no longer cracked. Action steps will continue, providing incentives to continue weight reduction, increase ambulation, and maintain foot care monitoring.

Created by Sylvia Smith 9/19/2017 9:32 a.m.
Mark as Reviewed

Medications
Current Medications

Previous | Next | Bill | Sign | Close | Save | Save + Exit

Figure 12.1 A sample electronic plan of care is shown here.

Nursing Diagnosis

As you learned in chapter 5, a *nursing diagnosis* is different from a medical diagnosis. A medical diagnosis identifies a disease or medical condition. In contrast, a nursing diagnosis identifies a potential or actual health problem that can be improved through nursing care. Examples of these health problems include poor nutrition, breathing difficulties, and difficulty ambulating. RNs make nursing diagnoses using clinical judgment, doctors' directions and orders, documentation about resident progress, ongoing assessment and observation, reports from healthcare staff, and evidence-based research and literature.

Nursing Goal

The *nursing goal* is the desired change or outcome in a resident's condition. For example, a nursing goal might be to promote ambulation or more independence when eating. In some facilities, nursing goals might be called *critical* or *clinical pathways*.

Nursing Orders

Nursing orders are instructions that outline the actions nursing staff members must take to help residents achieve desired goals. For example, a nursing order might state that a nursing assistant should help a resident ambulate at least twice per shift or provide an adaptive device to help with self-feeding.

Nursing orders usually contain very specific information, such as

- the date of the order;
- the action to be taken;
- the **rationale** (reasoning) for the action;
- the duration of the action; and
- the signature of the licensed nursing staff member who wrote the order.

Plan of Care Evaluation

Evaluation is ongoing and is used to track and update the progress that is made toward achieving a goal. The information provided by nursing assistants helps licensed nursing staff members determine if nursing actions should be stopped, continued, or adjusted. Evaluation is also used to assess the overall effectiveness of the nursing plan of care.

An updated, written plan of care is usually available for nursing staff to reference during a shift. This plan of care may be in the form of a *Kardex* or part of an EMR, depending on the facility's use of electronic documentation. The plan of care may be provided in total or in summary. A summary would identify the most important actions, such as treatments, medications, allergies, and special diets.

Plans of Care and the Nursing Assistant

Although nursing assistants do not create plans of care, they play an important role in the care planning process. Because nursing assistants work closely with residents, they share important observations and information that affect the plan of care. When you are a nursing assistant, your charge nurse may ask you for specific information that you have collected and may use that information to write a realistic plan of care. For example, you may have heard that a resident does not like to sleep with covers. You should share this during initial care planning, as it affects a resident's comfort and warmth.

What Is the Purpose of a Care Conference?

Care conferences, or *plan of care conferences*, are conducted on a routine basis. These conferences bring together all members of the healthcare team who deliver care to a particular resident. Nursing staff members, social workers, dietitians, and rehabilitation and therapy staff members all participate in care conferences and discuss the plan of care. The resident and a family representative may also attend. It is a resident's right to participate in care planning and care conferences.

During care conferences, plans for continuing care, progress being made, problems or challenges in providing care, and plans for discharge are discussed. Care conferences may occur weekly or monthly, depending on the need, and may last from a few minutes to one or more hours. The conference agenda may include both medical and nonmedical concerns, such as

- levels of nursing care;
- adjustments to nursing diagnoses or goals;
- changes in therapies, nutritional needs, and other services;
- any emotional needs; and
- personal concerns.

The intent of the conference is to review progress and make adjustments to the plan of care, if necessary.

During a care conference, questions may arise regarding how well a resident is eating and drinking, if a resident's weight has changed, whether or not the resident participates in activities, or if the resident needs personal items. These are questions the nursing assistant, who most often provides direct care, can typically answer. If a nursing assistant has been caring for a resident regularly, he or she may also comment on the resident's progress.

What Are Rounds?

Rounds or *rounding* are opportunities to physically monitor and discuss the status of a resident's condition or disease. Rounds are conducted in the resident's room or in the hallway right outside it.

There are different types of rounds. *Medical grand rounds* usually occur in hospitals and are led by doctors. The primary purpose of these rounds is to teach medical students, not just to monitor and discuss a particular patient's disease or condition. Medical grand rounds may be held at the patient's bedside, in a hallway near the patient's room, or in a conference room.

Nursing rounds are conducted by the licensed nursing staff. These rounds typically occur in a resident's room, either at the beginning or end of a shift, and check on the resident's condition and any special needs. Rounds are used to provide staff members with information about their assigned residents. When nursing rounds are performed at the end of a shift, they can take the place of change-of-shift reporting.

Hourly Rounds

Recently, hourly or more regular rounding has become a best practice. Hourly rounds have been shown to improve safety, encourage more effective delivery of care, and improve satisfaction. Hourly rounding involves checking on patients or residents at regular intervals during a shift to determine levels of comfort, safety, and environmental needs. Frequent and consistent monitoring helps prevent harmful events, such as possible falls or the formation of decubitus ulcers due to immobility. Rounds also allow licensed nursing staff members to monitor pain medication needs. Patient and resident satisfaction is often higher in this type of rounding, as patients and residents know their needs will be more frequently met. This also prevents patients and residents from having to always use call lights to make requests (Figure 12.2).

Regular, hourly rounding helps work organization and flow. Hourly rounds allow nursing staff members to anticipate needs and respond quickly and effectively. Rounding information may be written on a tracking document that may later be input into the electronic medical record (EMR). Some facilities provide computers directly outside each room or laptops or tablets that can be moved from room to room. In these cases, pertinent rounding information is input directly into the EMR.

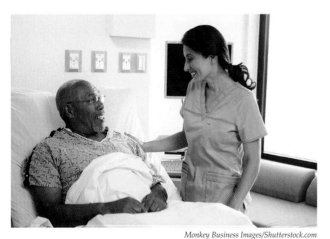

Monkey Business Images/Shutterstock.com

Figure 12.2 During rounds, nursing staff members visit patients and monitor them to anticipate their needs. This gives patients the chance to communicate their needs without using the call light.

The Role of the Nursing Assistant in Rounds

When you work as a nursing assistant, you may be included in rounds or delegated to perform rounds on assigned residents during your shift. During rounding, you may be asked to observe a resident's condition, check on the effectiveness or outcome of treatment, or ask a resident about his or her pain levels after taking medication. If you are included in rounds, provide specific, factual information about those in your care. You must conduct rounds as you are directed by the licensed nursing staff. If any follow-up care is needed, you are responsible for providing that care as directed. Follow-up care may include informing the licensed nursing staff that pain medication is needed or changing the position of a resident to prevent a decubitus ulcer.

How Is a Change-of-Shift Report Used?

The **change-of-shift report** is a verbal report that transfers essential information about patients or residents from one shift to the next. Change-of-shift reports are completed approximately 15–30 minutes prior to the end of a shift. These reports may be communicated from the outgoing charge nurse to the incoming charge nurse. In some healthcare facilities, the entire incoming nursing staff attends and listens to the outgoing charge nurse's report. Outgoing nursing assistants may also provide reports to incoming nursing assistants. The change-of-shift report is often shared in a conference or staff room on the nursing unit. Some facilities conduct change-of-shift reports during rounds. When these reports are shared during rounds, they may be called *huddles*.

Content of the Change-of-Shift Report

The content of the change-of-shift report is crucial for care delivery. When a change-of-shift report is being conducted, nursing staff members share accurate information about resident statuses. Detailed plans for future care are discussed based on reports from the outgoing nursing staff. It is critical that nursing staff members share any safety concerns (such as fall risks) and information about changes in a resident's condition or disease (such as changes in vital signs). Nursing staff members should also discuss future plans, including any tests that may affect care during the next shift and restrictions in eating or ambulation (Figure 12.3).

The Nursing Assistant's Role in the Change-of-Shift Report

Nursing assistants play an important role during the change-of-shift report. Nursing assistants may be present when the report is shared and may provide the charge nurse with information about residents in their care. Providing detailed, accurate information about a resident's status is essential to care. It can be helpful to keep notes about the care you give during a shift so you do not

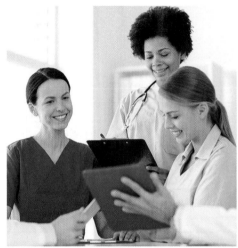
Syda Productions/Shutterstock.com

Figure 12.3 The information shared during a change-of-shift report is important. Nursing staff members should be alert and listen carefully during the report.

Culture Cues
Cultural Beliefs About Healthcare

Cultural traditions and practices help form a person's beliefs regarding healthcare, health, illness, and disease. These beliefs influence when a person seeks care and treatment and who a person is willing to see for healthcare needs. Beliefs about healthcare also affect healthcare choices, responses to specific treatments, and willingness to make necessary changes to achieve health and well-being.

For example, if a resident has been diagnosed with cardiovascular disease, she will likely need to change her dietary habits, take medications, and exercise regularly. If these requirements interfere with her healthcare beliefs and cultural traditions and practices, she will not likely adhere to the plan of care. The resident may refuse to change her diet because it does not include traditional foods she eats.

Another resident may believe that only herbal remedies work and refuse to take medications

prescribed by his doctor. If the resident does this, his disease or condition may be greatly affected, causing grave consequences. As a nursing assistant, you must pay attention to cultural practices and help, as appropriate, to balance residents' cultures with their treatment needs. This is an essential part of planning and organizing effective care delivery.

Apply It

1. Select one disease or condition and describe how cultural traditions or practices might influence treatment or care. Also explain why you selected the disease or condition.

2. Identify three specific cultural traditions or practices that could impact disease progression or treatment. Explain how these cultural traditions or practices might be accommodated.

forget important items. Some facilities provide assignment sheets to help you keep track of relevant information during your shift.

During the change-of-shift report, listen carefully and take notes, particularly about information related to your assignments and the residents in your care. Ask questions if the previous shift's change-of-shift report is unclear.

Remember ————

For every minute spent in organizing, an hour is earned.

Anonymous

What Is an Assignment Sheet?

Assignment sheets are used in healthcare facilities to identify which residents a holistic nursing assistant will be caring for and what specific care is required. These sheets provide detailed information about specific residents and will help you plan and organize your shift (Figure 12.4). Assignment sheets will also help you identify any routine or special care needed. During your shift, you may add information to the assignment sheet. For example, you may record a resident's response to treatment so you remember to report it to the licensed nursing staff.

Some facilities use single assignment sheets that include all of the important information for an assigned resident. Other facilities hand out two assignment sheets—one with the nursing assistant's specific assignments and another that details

RM	RESIDENT	BATH	ACTIVITY	TRTMT	FLUIDS	ADDED INSTR
2	John S	☑ Bed ☐ Tub ☐ Shower ☐ Shampoo ☑ Shave ☐ Nails	☑ Bed ☐ Brp/Help ☐ Amb/Help ☐ Amb ☐ Walker ☐ Whlchr ☐ Crutches	☐ Enema ☐ BM ☐ Void ☐ Incont. ☑ Bed Sore ☐ Eggcrate ☐ Handrolls	☐ Encourage ☐ Limit to ____ ☐ Sips/W ☐ I & O ☐ Dist/W ☑ Catheter	*Catheter and Skin Care*
3	Don L	☐ Bed ☐ Tub ☑ Shower ☐ Shampoo ☐ Shave ☐ Nails	☐ Bed ☐ Brp/Help ☐ Amb/Help ☑ Amb ☐ Walker ☐ Whlchr ☐ Crutches	☐ Enema ☐ BM ☐ Void ☐ Incont. ☐ Bed Sore ☐ Eggcrate ☐ Handrolls	☐ Encourage ☐ Limit to ____ ☐ Sips/W ☐ I & O ☐ Dist/W ☐ Catheter	*Warm Compress*
4	Ruth Z	☐ Bed ☐ Tub ☑ Shower ☑ Shampoo ☐ Shave ☐ Nails	☐ Bed ☐ Brp/Help ☐ Amb/Help ☐ Amb ☑ Walker ☐ Whlchr ☐ Crutches	☐ Enema ☐ BM ☐ Void ☐ Incont. ☐ Bed Sore ☐ Eggcrate ☐ Handrolls	☐ Encourage ☐ Limit to ____ ☐ Sips/W ☑ I & O ☐ Dist/W ☐ Catheter	
5A	Lillian B	☐ Bed ☐ Tub ☑ Shower ☐ Shampoo ☐ Shave ☐ Nails	☐ Bed ☑ Brp/Help ☐ Amb/Help ☐ Amb ☐ Walker ☐ Whlchr ☐ Crutches	☑ Enema ☐ BM ☐ Void ☐ Incont. ☐ Bed Sore ☐ Eggcrate ☐ Handrolls	☐ Encourage ☐ Limit to ____ ☐ Sips/W ☑ I & O ☐ Dist/W ☐ Catheter	*Foot Care*
5B	Jane D	☐ Bed ☑ Tub ☐ Shower ☐ Shampoo ☐ Shave ☐ Nails	☐ Bed ☐ Brp/Help ☐ Amb/Help ☐ Amb ☐ Walker ☑ Whlchr ☐ Crutches	☐ Enema ☐ BM ☐ Void ☐ Incont. ☐ Bed Sore ☑ Eggcrate ☐ Handrolls	☑ Encourage ☐ Limit to ____ ☐ Sips/W ☐ I & O ☐ Dist/W ☐ Catheter	

Figure 12.4 A sample assignment sheet is shown here.

each resident's care needs. Assignment sheets may include noncare assignments, such as cleaning the supply room or checking inventory. Scheduled breaks and meal times may also be listed.

When receiving an assignment sheet, take time to review it with the charge nurse. This review is especially important if you are caring for unfamiliar residents or if there have been changes in a resident's condition or progress. Also review any treatments you have not done recently.

Use assignment sheets to plan your shift and prioritize tasks. For example, if you have to give two complete bed baths and a shower, you may give the shower first since bed baths take much longer. You might also take care of urgent needs first before performing any treatments or procedures that take longer. Assignment sheets are more than words; they are planning tools for your shift. You can use them to your best advantage if you see them as organizational tools to help you be efficient and effective.

Section 12.1 Review and Assessment

Using the Key Terms

Complete the following sentences using key terms in this section.

1. _____ are opportunities to monitor and discuss the status of a resident's condition or disease.
2. A resident's plan of care is discussed by all caregivers during a(n) _____.
3. _____ outline the actions that should be taken to achieve stated goals of care.
4. A(n) _____ transfers essential information about residents from one shift to the next.
5. The research- and science-based reasoning behind a specific nursing action is the _____.

Know and Understand the Facts

6. Describe the purpose of a plan of care.
7. What is the purpose of a care conference?
8. Why are change-of-shift reports important?
9. Explain the process used to share critical information during rounds.

Analyze and Apply Concepts

10. Discuss the role nursing assistants play in providing information during care conferences.
11. What contributions can a nursing assistant make during change-of-shift reports?
12. What might a nursing assistant be asked or delegated to observe during rounds?
13. Describe how nursing assistants use assignment sheets to plan, prioritize, and organize care.

Think Critically

Read the following care situation. Then answer the questions that follow.

Sima has been caring for Mrs. F for the past week. She has enjoyed this assignment and is very comfortable with the care she is providing. Sima has become so accustomed to caring for Mrs. F that she no longer spends any time observing, asking Mrs. F questions about how she feels, or making notes on her assignment sheet. When the charge nurse asks for change-of-shift report information today, Sima says that nothing has changed.

14. Do you think Sima is properly caring for Mrs. F? Explain your answer.
15. Is Sima's answer to the charge nurse appropriate? Why or why not?
16. When you are caring for someone for a long period of time, how can you ensure you are keeping track of important and necessary information?

Questions to Consider

- How observant do you think you are?
- How well can you describe an event or situation after it has happened? Are you able to use specific details, or do you remember only generalities?
- What might you do to be more observant?

Objectives

Possessing subjective and objective observation skills is essential to providing safe, quality care. Equally essential are accurate, complete, and timely reports. To achieve the objectives for this section, you must successfully

- **explain** the difference between objective and subjective observation; and
- **describe** the process used to provide accurate, complete, and timely reports.

Key Terms

Learn these key terms to better understand the information presented in the section.

critical observation
deformity
memory
numbness

objective observations
subjective observations
tingling

Remember

Never trust to general impressions, my boy, but concentrate yourself upon details.

Sir Arthur Conan Doyle, British physician and author of the Sherlock Holmes novels

Holistic nursing assistants must be sensitive to and aware of changes in a resident's daily routine, behavior, communication, appearance, general mood, and physical health. Always expect that changes in a resident's condition will occur as the resident's condition may improve or worsen. Regularly observe residents to help identify changes. A good time to do this is during routine care. It is particularly important to practice observation when you have been asked to observe a resident for specific changes (for example, a change in breathing patterns or wound drainage).

What Are Objective and Subjective Observations?

Observation is one of the most important responsibilities of a holistic nursing assistant. A holistic nursing assistant who is observing a resident looks for physical changes, expressions of emotion, responses to treatment, and progression of the resident's disease or condition. This information, which is observed while providing care, may be either objective or subjective. **Objective observations** are based on facts. **Subjective observations** are based on feelings or opinions.

Objective Observations

The primary purpose of objective observation is to eliminate bias and personal opinions and focus instead on factual information. Objective observations are based on the senses of sight, hearing, touch, and smell. For example, the measurement of a resident's oxygen status is an objective observation (Figure 12.5). If a resident tells you about a rash she has, an objective observation would state that the resident has a red, bumpy irritation on the upper arm. You would describe only what you saw by observing the rash objectively. You would not say "the resident has a rash."

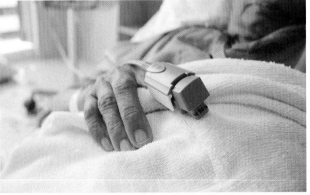

Piyada Jaiaree/Shutterstock.com

Figure 12.5 Specific measurements (for example, using a pulse oximeter) are examples of objective observations.

As another example, a resident may tell you he has a bump on his right leg near the outside of his ankle. You touch the bump and discover it is very hot and is protruding enough to stretch the skin. It is oval-shaped and about 2 inches around. The details of what you see will formulate your objective observation. You should not simply describe a "bump on the leg." You should report to the licensed nursing staff that the resident has an oval-shaped bump that is 2 inches around on his lower-right leg near the outside of his ankle. You should report that the bump is hot to the touch and is protruding enough to stretch the skin.

Subjective Observations

Subjective observations are ideas, thoughts, or opinions. While subjective observations are helpful and important observations, they are not facts. If residents provide subjective observations, the residents' exact words must be relayed to the licensed nursing staff.

As an example of subjective observation, a resident may complain of pain. To make an objective observation, you would need to see physical evidence of pain. This physical evidence might include the holding or rubbing of the painful body part, discoloration on the body part that hurts, or movement of the resident away from you when you touch that body part. Without physical evidence, there is no way to know if pain is an objective fact or not. To report the pain subjectively, you might say, "The resident states that his pain feels like a dull ache and never lets up. In the morning, it feels worse than in the evening."

Observation Challenges

Observations—both objective and subjective—present many challenges. When an observation is not reported or recorded soon after it occurs, gaps in **memory** (the storage and remembrance of past experiences) may make it difficult to recall details in the future. Another challenge to making accurate observations is *reconstructive memory*. In reconstructive memories, people recreate what they *think* they saw. Reconstructive memories are usually faulty because people add inaccurate information to fill in the specifics they do not remember. Therefore, always report or record your observations as soon as possible. If you do not remember specific events or details and if you did not record a particular observation, always tell the licensed nursing staff that you cannot recall the specifics.

Think About This

Formal statements of proof surrounding criminal actions have shown that people tend to be poor observers. Over time, what people see and remember becomes increasingly unreliable. People may not be paying full attention, particularly when a memory involves strangers. Many people think that eyewitness testimony is powerful; however, what the mind takes in and processes is highly suspicious because it is influenced by personal perceptions and attitudes. When people think back about what they have seen, they often become more certain about their observations, even if the event they observed did not happen the way they saw it.

Becoming a Holistic Nursing Assistant
Developing Observation Skills

The following guidelines will help you develop your observation skills as a holistic nursing assistant:
1. Always be mindful, or aware of what is happening, and concentrate on collecting helpful objective and subjective information.
2. Listen very carefully to what residents share with you.
3. Never judge others, no matter what they say or do.
4. When observing, always consider how residents' behaviors and feelings will affect their diseases and conditions.
5. Always carry something you can use to write notes about your observations.
6. Be timely, clear, and detailed when you communicate your observations.

Apply It
1. Which of these six guidelines do you believe you are already using effectively when observing others?
2. Which guidelines refer to skills you need to develop? Explain your answer.
3. What actions can you take to become a better observer?

To be successful and provide safe, quality care, holistic nursing assistants need to develop strong observational skills. **Critical observation** occurs when both objective and subjective observation are used appropriately. Part of critical observation is knowing when you should share your observation with the charge nurse. Some observations, such as those related to routine care or treatments, can wait until the change-of-shift report. Other critical observations, such as complaints of pain or changes in vital signs, must be reported to the charge nurse immediately.

How Does Accurate Reporting Make a Difference in Care?

The healthcare team communicates observations and other important information by accurately reporting care. Accurate reporting ensures that residents' conditions are always being effectively monitored so nursing staff members can promptly respond to any issues or concerns. Although you may need to provide a report over the telephone, reporting is best accomplished through face-to-face communication (Figure 12.6).

Always use your notes to give a specific, accurate report. Report only those details you saw or actions you did yourself. To give your report in a timely manner, communicate with the charge nurse at the change of shift. If the observation is cause for concern, share it with the charge nurse as soon as possible. Always tell the charge nurse immediately if there is a change in a resident's condition. You should particularly report any changes related to

- the resident's ability to respond;
- mobility;
- complaints of sudden, severe pain;
- a sore or reddened area on the skin or swelling;
- complaints of a sudden change in vision;
- complaints of pain or difficulty breathing;
- abnormal respirations;
- complaints or signs of difficulty swallowing;
- vomiting;
- bleeding;
- vital signs outside the normal ranges;
- joint pain, tenderness, or **deformity** (distortion);
- complaints of **numbness** (lack of feeling) or **tingling** (a sensation like sharp points digging into the skin); or
- lightheadedness or dizziness.

Healthcare Scenario
Objective and Subjective Observations

Yesterday, the local news reported that a teacher came to the rescue of a 10-year-old boy who fell off the swings at the neighborhood park. The teacher was passing by on her way home from work and saw the boy fall from the swing. It looked like the boy had let go of the chains, and he was high in the air. After the boy fell, the teacher ran over and observed that his arm was twisted. The boy was complaining of pain in his neck and head. The teacher immediately called 9-1-1.

Apply It

1. What is the teacher's objective observation in this scenario?
2. What is the teacher's subjective observation in this scenario?
3. What specifically should the teacher report to the 9-1-1 operator?

Always give a report to your charge nurse and to the person who is covering for you before you leave the unit for any reason. Whenever you are reporting, use the following steps:

1. Give the resident's name, room number, and bed number.
2. Include the time you made your observation or gave specific care.
3. Provide objective observations, such as what you saw, heard, smelled, or felt.
4. Provide only subjective observations that were communicated to you by the resident (for example, any reported feelings of pain).
5. Identify any anticipated or requested resident needs.

Finally, always be prepared to give a report during the change of shift, when there are immediate issues, and whenever the charge nurse requests you do so.

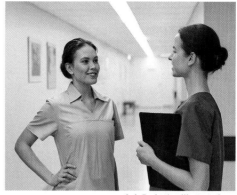

Syda Productions/Shutterstock.com

Figure 12.6 Reports are best given verbally in person.

Using the Key Terms

Complete the following sentences using key terms in this section.

1. The sensation of _____ feels like sharp points digging into the skin.
2. _____ refers to the storage and remembrance of past experiences.
3. In _____, both objective and subjective observation are used appropriately.
4. The distortion of a body part is a(n) _____.
5. _____ are observations based on facts.
6. _____ is a sensation characterized by lack of feeling.
7. Observations based on feelings or opinions are _____.

Know and Understand the Facts

8. What is an objective observation?
9. What is a subjective observation?
10. When is it appropriate to give an immediate report to the licensed nursing staff?

Analyze and Apply Concepts

11. Identify two challenges to observation and how each challenge can be overcome.
12. List three guidelines you can use to improve your observation skills as a holistic nursing assistant.
13. A nursing assistant is leaving the unit on break. List the five steps he should take when reporting to the charge nurse.

Think Critically

Read the following care situation. Then answer the questions that follow.

Jim, the charge nurse, asked nursing assistant Jaylene to check on Mr. L and see if his pain had eased. Jim gave Mr. L medication about a half hour ago for leg pain. When Jaylene got to Mr. L's room, she asked him how he was doing, but Mr. L was holding his leg and crying quietly.

14. How should Jaylene describe what she sees? What type of observation is this?
15. What should Jaylene do next? Explain your answer.
16. What type of report should Jaylene give Jim, the charge nurse, and when?

Key Points

Reviewing the key points for this chapter will help you practice more safely and competently as a holistic nursing assistant and will help you prepare for the certification competency examination.

- A written plan of care provides the necessary direction and guidance for delivering individualized, holistic care.

- Care conferences include the healthcare staff members delivering care to a particular resident. The intent of the conference is to review progress and make adjustments to the plan of care, if necessary.

- Rounds are regularly performed to monitor residents' conditions or diseases.

- Change-of-shift reports share essential information between shifts.

- Assignment sheets identify which residents each nursing assistant will be caring for during a shift.

- It is important that nursing assistants regularly observe residents for changes in daily routine, behavior, communication, appearance, general mood, and physical health.

- The healthcare team communicates observations and other important information by reporting the care given. When reporting, always use your notes to give specific information, report only what you saw or did yourself, and give your report in a timely manner.

Action Steps to Holistic Care

Review the information in this chapter. Complete the following activities.

1. Create a poster or digital presentation that explains what a plan of care is and why it is important. Discuss how and why they are created, who uses them, the information that is typically included, and how they are organized and evaluated. Then consider how a nursing assistant might utilize a plan of care or contribute to its development.

2. With a partner, write a song or a limerick about objective and subjective observation. Include an example of each.

3. With a partner, prepare a poster with information about the use of assignment sheets. Illustrate what is important about using the sheet and how the sheet can help organize care and manage time.

4. Find one picture in a magazine, in a newspaper, or online that best represents a nursing assistant providing a report to the charge nurse that a resident's condition has changed. Describe what the nursing assistant should include in the report.

5. Research current scientific information about rounding and resident care. Provide a brief report that describes three current facts about rounding not covered in this chapter.

 Preparing for the Certification Competency Examination

To prepare for the nursing assistant certification competency examination, you will need to know content found in this chapter. This content may be tested in the knowledge (written or oral) and skills (hands-on demonstration) portions of the exam. The following areas will be emphasized:

- observation and reporting of condition changes
- objective and subjective observations

These sample test questions are similar to ones you will find on the certification competency exam. See how well you can answer them. Be sure to select the *best* answer.

1. The purpose of a plan of care is to
   A. provide doctors with an opportunity to review care
   B. provide the healthcare team with a plan so they can adjust to different orders
   C. provide the necessary directions for delivering individualized, holistic care
   D. provide the resident and family with a set of teaching instructions

2. A charge nurse has written a new plan of care for Mrs. D. Which of the following should be included?
   A. nursing diagnosis
   B. nursing research
   C. nursing theories
   D. nursing steps

3. What is the purpose of a care conference?

    A. to discuss daily assignments
    B. to discuss admissions
    C. to discuss transfers
    D. to plan and change care as needed

4. A nursing assistant was asked by his charge nurse to perform rounds. The charge nurse is specifically asking the nursing assistant to

    A. monitor residents' conditions or diseases
    B. clean residents' rooms to ensure a safe and secure environment
    C. provide proper nutritional snacks when requested
    D. offer residents the opportunity to be involved in activities

5. Why are change-of-shift reports important?

    A. They give staff a chance to talk with each other about shift issues and problems.
    B. They are a time to relax and get to know staff from other shifts.
    C. They are a time to transfer essential resident information from one shift to the next.
    D. They provide time for nursing staff to document and talk with doctors.

6. A nursing assistant is struggling with her assignment. She seems confused about what she should be doing. What should she use to get organized?

    A. a care plan
    B. nursing orders
    C. nursing diagnosis
    D. her assignment sheet

7. Objective observation uses

    A. only facts
    B. opinions and beliefs
    C. opinions and facts
    D. your own beliefs

8. A nursing assistant used both objective and subjective observation to report on Mr. J's care. Which of the following is a subjective observation?

    A. Mr. J's urine appeared cloudy.
    B. Mr. J said he felt very nauseous.
    C. Mr. J felt warm to the touch.
    D. Mr. J's face was red and splotchy.

9. Which of the following should a nursing assistant immediately report to the charge nurse?

    A. the number of family members visiting
    B. preferred snacks
    C. changes in responsiveness
    D. changes in therapy schedule

10. What positive outcome can be achieved by rounding?

    A. seeing family members more often
    B. taking a few minutes to rest
    C. monitoring the number of visitors
    D. monitoring possible fall risks

11. A charge nurse wants the nursing assistants on her unit to practice holistic observation. Which skill or approach should she teach them?

    A. to improve listening
    B. to laugh more
    C. to increase relaxation
    D. to pay more attention to feelings

12. When a new nursing assistant transferred to your unit, he needed training on giving a change-of-shift report. Which skill or step is the most important?

    A. being sure to provide as much information as possible
    B. reporting only those things he saw or did himself
    C. waiting to report until he has all the information
    D. providing a report that includes the family and roommate

13. When a nursing assistant uses critical observation, she

    A. includes both logical and factual observations
    B. includes subjective observations and opinions
    C. includes objective and subjective observations
    D. includes sensitive and timely observations

14. A nursing goal is used to

    A. plan activities that ensure residents get adequate exercise and ambulation
    B. identify actions and provide instructions to achieve a desired goal for residents
    C. provide enough information to transfer a resident to another room
    D. describe a resident's condition so others know how to provide care

15. Which of the following helps ensure continuity of care?

    A. plan of care
    B. assignment sheet
    C. timely reporting
    D. subjective reporting

Did you have difficulty with any of the questions? If you did, review the chapter to find the correct answer(s).

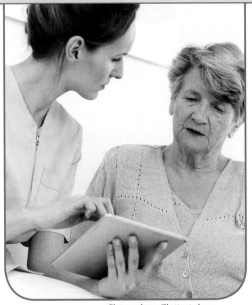

Photographee.eu/Shutterstock.com

Welcome to the Chapter

When you work as a nursing assistant, you will need to understand how to use specific types of records, technology, and digital communication devices. You will also need to know how to properly and accurately document care in an electronic health record (EHR), electronic medical record (EMR), or paper record, and how to effectively handle telephone communications. These knowledge and skills are essential to providing safe, quality holistic care.

What you learn in this chapter will help you develop your knowledge and skills to become a holistic nursing assistant. The topics discussed in the chapter are highlighted on the Providing Holistic Care Framework.

You are now ready to start this chapter, *Records and Documentation*.

Chapter Outline

Section 13.1
Health Records
and Technology

Section 13.2
Documentation

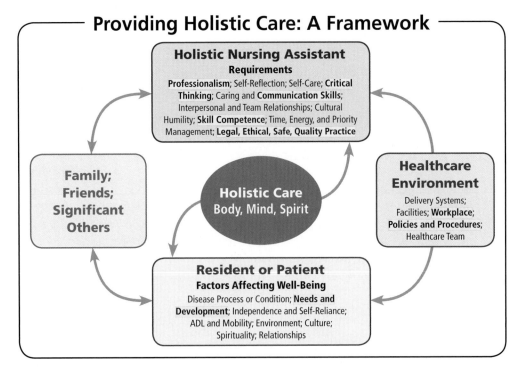

Providing Holistic Care: A Framework

Holistic Nursing Assistant
Requirements
Professionalism; Self-Reflection; Self-Care; **Critical Thinking**; Caring and **Communication Skills**; Interpersonal and Team Relationships; Cultural Humility; **Skill Competence**; Time, Energy, and Priority Management; **Legal, Ethical, Safe, Quality Practice**

Family; Friends; Significant Others

Holistic Care
Body, Mind, Spirit

Healthcare Environment
Delivery Systems; Facilities; **Workplace; Policies and Procedures**; Healthcare Team

Resident or Patient
Factors Affecting Well-Being
Disease Process or Condition; **Needs and Development**; Independence and Self-Reliance; ADL and Mobility; Environment; Culture; Spirituality; Relationships

Objectives

To provide the best possible care, you must understand the types of records, technology, digital communication, and devices used in healthcare facilities. This knowledge will help you feel more comfortable using records, documenting with technology, and operating digital communication devices. To achieve the objectives for this section, you must successfully

- **describe** the different types of records and their purposes;
- **identify** records that nursing assistants are responsible for maintaining; and
- **discuss** the types and uses of technology, digital communication, and devices typically found in healthcare facilities.

Key Terms

Learn these key terms to better understand the information presented in the section.

consultations
electronic health record (EHR)
electronic medical record (EMR)

manually
payroll
software applications

Questions to Consider

- What experiences do you have using technology for word processing, keeping electronic records, or playing games? Where do you use technology?
- What experiences do you have with digital communication and devices? Do you use smartphones, e-mail, the Internet, instant messaging, social media, or a blog? What types of digital communication do you use, and where do you use them?
- Have your experiences with technology been positive? If not, what challenges have you faced? What might make your experiences better?

What Types of Records Are Used in Healthcare?

Many types of records are used in healthcare, and each type of record has a different purpose. Some records relate directly to care, while others aid the organization and daily function of the healthcare facility. When you begin working in healthcare, using and maintaining records will be an important responsibility.

Some records are digital; others are physical forms and must be filled in **manually**, or by hand. For example, nursing assistants in some facilities record vital signs on a form; in other facilities, they enter this information into the resident's EMR (Figure 13.1). The types of records or documents used depend on the facility.

There are two primary types of records used in healthcare facilities:

1. records that support and document care
2. records that ensure all functions in a facility are organized and operate smoothly and efficiently

Records That Support and Document Care

Information related to resident health and care is documented and stored in specific types of records. These records are often digital, but manual recordkeeping may still document vital signs and fluid intake or output at the bedside. Information about residents is kept on the unit in which residents reside and is readily available. When residents are discharged or expire, their records are sent to a department that stores and maintains the facility's health records.

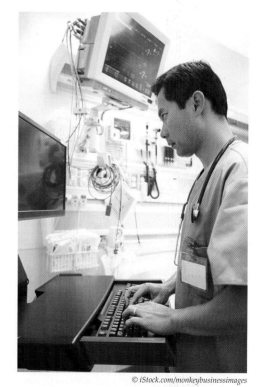

© iStock.com/monkeybusinessimages

Figure 13.1 Nursing assistants can enter information into a resident's EMR using digital devices.

As a holistic nursing assistant, you will be responsible for viewing, using, and adding to these health records. Careful, accurate documentation is essential to providing effective holistic care. Records that support and document care include EHRs; EMRs; paper records; admission, transfer, and discharge records; medication administration records (MARs); and plans of care.

Electronic Health Record (EHR)

An **electronic health record (EHR)** is a digital record that contains all of a person's health information, including medical history and healthcare experiences. An EHR can include doctors' visits, hospital stays, surgical or medical procedures, annual physical examinations, referrals, and **consultations** (meetings) with other doctors, social workers, or therapists. If you are employed in a healthcare facility that uses electronic records, you will receive special training about how to use these records properly.

EHRs make information available instantly and display all medical and healthcare information from every provider who has given care. One benefit of the EHR is that the information it contains can be shared across healthcare providers and facilities. The information in an EHR can literally travel with the patient. Another benefit is that EHRs are environmentally friendly and eliminate the vast amount of paper used with manual recordkeeping.

EHRs store specific healthcare data, demographics, medical history, diagnoses, medications, allergies, progress notes, immunization dates, laboratory test results, X-ray images, and insurance and billing data. This information can come from a variety of healthcare facilities, such as hospitals, pharmacies, or community clinics. The goal of the EHR is to contain, in one place (such as with the person's primary care provider), all medical and health records. The universal availability of the EHR enables more coordinated, patient-centered care; eliminates duplication; and allows a smooth transition from one healthcare facility to another.

For example, when a pharmacist enters medication details into a patient's record, this information becomes available to all healthcare providers. As a result, healthcare providers can see all drugs and dosages ordered throughout a patient's medical history. When an EHR system is fully functional, a patient can go to his or her own EHR to view personal information, laboratory and X-ray results, special screening outcomes (for example, from a mammogram), and summaries of notes made by specialists.

Electronic Medical Record (EMR)

An **electronic medical record (EMR)** is a component of an EHR. An EMR typically uses the same technology as an EHR; however, instead of housing the entire health record, it includes information about a patient's single stay in a facility (such as a hospital or an individual trip to the doctor's office).

The EMR contains administrative and clinical information about the patient. Administrative information includes age, gender, insurance coverage, and other data

Healthcare Scenario
Electronic Health Records

Last week, a large long-term care center in the city began installing an electronic health record system. The system is going to cost several million dollars and will not be in place for at least a year. The goal of installation is to have the system handle the new expansion of the facility and keep information about residents secure. The system being installed has been used by hospitals in this city, but has never been implemented in this type of healthcare facility.

Apply It

1. What are two benefits of installing an EHR system?

2. What challenges do you think a facility would face installing this kind of system after using paper charts for a long time?

3. What actions can a holistic nursing assistant take to ensure all electronic information collected is kept confidential?

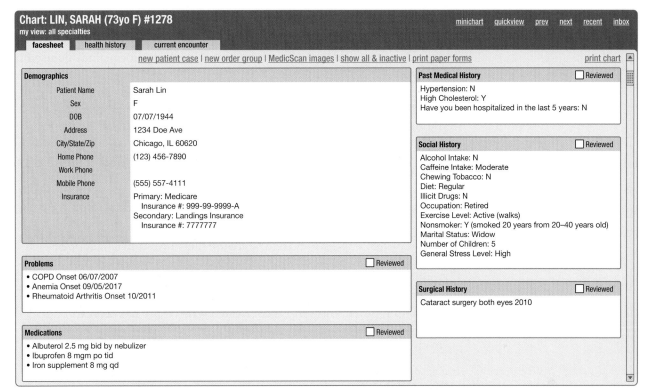

Figure 13.2 This is an example of an EMR.

such as religious preference. Clinical information includes all medical and health information, such as history, diagnosis, progress, laboratory test results, and consultations with specialists. EMRs track information over time, identify due dates for screenings or checkups, and provide trends in treatment progress and response (Figure 13.2). They can also help monitor the quality of care given.

Paper Record

A *paper record*, sometimes called a *paper chart*, is a physical document that includes administrative and clinical information about a patient or resident. This information is categorized into different sections (Figure 13.3). The paper record is stored in one facility and is more challenging to share with other healthcare providers because it is not electronic.

Admission, Transfer, and Discharge Records

Admission, transfer, and discharge records provide information needed during admission to, transfer within, and discharge from a healthcare facility. These forms are discussed in chapter 5.

Medication Administration Record (MAR)

A medication administration record (MAR) is a record of the drugs or medications administered by the licensed nursing staff during a stay at a healthcare facility. The MAR is often part of the EMR or patient chart.

Plan of Care

As you learned in chapter 12, a *plan of care* is a written document developed for each resident by the licensed nursing staff. The plan of care is based on a comprehensive assessment of the resident and provides guidance for delivering individualized and consistent care. In some facilities, plans of care are called *service plans*. Plans of care may be recorded in an EMR.

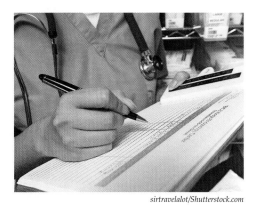

sirtravelalot/Shutterstock.com

Figure 13.3 Paper records are still used in many healthcare facilities.

Records Related to Facility Operations

Some records used in healthcare facilities are not related to patient or resident care. These records ensure the facility operates smoothly. Some forms may be used by many healthcare staff members, while others may be specific to particular healthcare functions.

- **Employment forms**: These records are completed during the process of hiring. They are usually kept in the Human Resources department and include records concerning employment, **payroll** (the amount of money paid to employees), and required health information (such as drug screenings and immunizations).
- **Policies and procedures**: These records provide guidance and instructions for delivering care and working in a healthcare facility. These are discussed in chapter 5.
- **Order forms**: This form is used to ensure there are sufficient supplies available in a healthcare facility at all times. An order form is completed routinely according to the necessary and required inventory of supplies and is submitted to the appropriate department.
- **Incident reports**: This form is completed when there has been an error or accident in a healthcare facility. Incident reports are discussed in chapter 16.

Record Life Span

The life span of records in a healthcare facility includes creation, maintenance, retention, and destruction. Because records are legal documents, their life spans are regulated by accreditation agency recommendations, federal and state retention laws and regulations, legal requirements, and in some facilities, the needs of ongoing medical research and education. All healthcare facilities have policies and procedures regarding the maintenance, retention, and destruction of records and documents.

Advantages of Using Electronic Records

There are many advantages to using electronic records. For example, researchers have found that using electronic medical records reduces medical errors. Handwritten instructions may be difficult to read, potentially causing errors, and electronic records reduce this possibility. Electronic recordkeeping has become so important that the Centers for Medicare & Medicaid Services (CMS) has instituted an EHR incentive program. The program gives healthcare providers and facilities a financial incentive to adopt, implement, upgrade, or demonstrate certified EHR technology. This technology helps facilities achieve health and efficiency goals, such as proper electronic data capture and information sharing. As a holistic nursing assistant, you must be aware of and carefully follow EHR policies, including requirements from national, state, and local entities.

How Should Health Records Be Handled?

Information documented in an EHR should concern only the patient or resident receiving care, and confidentiality must be maintained. As you learned in chapter 3, *confidentiality* requires that healthcare providers consider any information communicated by a patient or resident to be private. For example, a patient's paper record may not be read by outsiders or copied without permission. The use of electronic records has made confidentiality even more vulnerable, so extreme caution is needed.

As you learned in chapter 3, the Health Insurance Portability and Accountability Act (HIPAA) protects the rights of patients and residents regarding the confidentiality of health records. According to HIPAA, patients and residents can expect that their diagnoses, test results, and private information will be recorded accurately and kept confidential when they visit a healthcare facility. Healthcare facilities often have extensive security measures in place to protect this health information, and *health information* is considered any paper, oral, or electronic record shared with a healthcare provider, insurer, or similar entity that can be used to identify a patient. If healthcare providers share information inappropriately, this can be considered an *invasion of privacy* and have legal consequences.

When reading, using, or documenting in health records, follow these guidelines to ensure personal information is kept private and confidential:

- Maintain privacy and confidentiality at all times.
- Never take a photo or video of patients or residents or their families using a personal device.
- Do not identify patients or residents by name outside the unit and facility.
- Do not post or publish information online that may lead to patient or resident identification.
- Do not access records out of curiosity.
- Log off a computer once you are done using it (Figure 13.4).
- Choose a strong password and do not share it with others.
- Promptly report any identified breaches of confidentiality or privacy.
- Abide by the facility's policies regarding the use of employer-owned electronic devices and the use of personal devices in the workplace.
- Remember that any violation of confidentiality and privacy is grounds for discipline.

In addition to ensuring confidentiality, HIPAA also provides the right (with a few exceptions) for people to inspect, review, and receive copies of their health records. Patients and residents must complete a formal request to review these records and receive them physically or electronically. Patients and residents can also designate personal representatives, such as family members, to access their records. They may also, with permission, let other caregivers receive copies. Sometimes healthcare facilities use secure, online health portals to allow patients to access their health information. Copies of health records cannot be denied, even if a person has not yet paid for healthcare services. If mailing records, some facilities may request that their patients pay fees.

How Is Technology Used to Record and Share Health Information?

EHRs and EMRs are not the only ways information is recorded and shared in healthcare facilities. Holistic nursing assistants must be comfortable using various technologies appropriately and effectively. Although available technologies vary among healthcare facilities, nursing assistants should be able to identify and understand the uses of available devices and apps.

Digital Communication and Devices

As a nursing assistant, you may use many different types of digital devices and communication technologies, including cell phones, landline telephones, pagers and paging systems, voice mail, fax machines, e-mail, desktop computers, laptop computers, and wireless devices such as tablets. In some healthcare facilities, technology is fully integrated into daily caregiving. Other healthcare facilities still utilize more traditional communication methods, such as paper records and documentation.

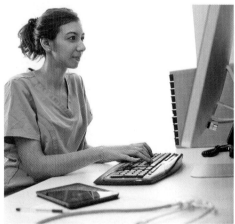

Monkey Business Images/Shutterstock.com

Figure 13.4 When using a computer to access electronic records, always log off the computer once you are done.

When you work in a healthcare facility, you may encounter *computers on wheels* or *COWs*, which are computers mounted on carts. COWs are wheeled into a patient's or resident's room and are used to input or complete necessary documentation. Nursing assistants may also carry wireless devices, such as laptops and tablets, throughout a shift. These devices are used to document care or record vital signs immediately. In some facilities, wall-mounted, touchscreen computers are located in each patient's or resident's room for this purpose.

In healthcare facilities, urgent needs and information are often communicated using a pager or paging system, landline telephone, or cell phone provided by the facility. E-mail is also used, but only for information unrelated to the patient or resident and care. For example, e-mail might be used to communicate announcements, scheduling, or meeting invitations and reminders.

Devices and digital communication methods are used not only in healthcare facilities, but also in doctors' offices and pharmacies. For example, using a wireless device such as a tablet, a doctor could review patient information and enter his notes directly into an EMR. This would both save a great deal of time and ensure accuracy. Similarly, a pharmacist could use a tablet to access information about a particular medication and to verify proper dosage by sending a message to the prescribing doctor.

Software Applications

Healthcare staff members, patients, and residents often find **software applications** (*apps*) to be extremely beneficial as references and resources. Apps are commonly found on wireless devices, such as tablets and smartphones, and can be categorized based on their use:

- disease information and diagnostic aids
- drug and nutrition references
- medical and drug conversions and calculators
- ranges of clinical laboratory values
- clinical research
- medical and healthcare training

Apps can also focus on the information needed to identify correct medical coding required for insurance, order prescription refills, and organize and simplify work assignments. Some healthcare facilities use apps to share secure, protected messages and information between healthcare providers. Apps that store or share protected health information must be HIPAA-compliant for information security.

Sometimes information saved in EHRs can be accessed through secure, HIPAA-compliant apps or through password-protected websites established by healthcare providers (called *online portals*). These online portals allow patients, residents, and their families (if the patient is a child or has a legal guardian) to view lab results, request prescription refills, schedule appointments, and access other EHR information. Patients, residents, and their families may also access health-related apps to keep track of diets, track daily exercise, and monitor blood pressure or heart rate.

Telephones

Telephones in healthcare facilities are more than just devices; they provide a way to share and gather information. Typically, landline telephones are located at a nurse's station, and answering the telephone is an important part of a holistic nursing assistant's daily responsibilities. Appropriately receiving and sharing information over the telephone helps contribute to the delivery of safe, quality care.

The same legal requirements and confidentiality that impact face-to-face and written communication also affect information shared over the telephone. If important information about a resident is shared over the telephone, you should write this information down and verify by restating the information back to the caller. If you believe taking the information is outside your legal scope of practice, let the caller know and seek a member of the licensed nursing staff. You may ask the caller to wait, but if that is not possible, take the caller's number so the appropriate person can follow up on the call. Examples of calls that are outside the scope of practice involve conveying doctors' orders, receiving or giving test results, or releasing any resident information. Treat each telephone call as a vital part of care.

The following principles and steps will help you ensure proper telephone communication. Remember to always follow facility guidelines.

1. Answer the telephone promptly. Greet callers in a friendly, professional manner. Smile when answering the call, as this improves the quality of your voice and helps you sound like you are interested in taking the call. Identify yourself and your unit. For example, you could say, "Good morning, this is Debbie Smith, certified nursing assistant, on Unit 4A. How may I help you?"

2. If you are making a call, state your name and title when your call is answered. Let the person know immediately why you are calling (Figure 13.5).

3. Speak clearly with confidence and use a low tone of voice and moderate volume and speed. Listen to the message and ask questions, if needed. When taking notes about information, ask the caller to spell his or her name and any unfamiliar words. If you are taking a message, include the date and time of the message and the name of the caller.

4. If a doctor calls to communicate medical orders, let the doctor know receiving this information is outside your scope of practice. You may ask the doctor to hold while you get a licensed nursing staff member or ask if the doctor would like his or her call returned.

5. If you need to place a caller on hold, ask for the caller's permission before doing so. For example, you might say, "May I please place you on a brief hold?" Always wait for an answer before placing the person on hold.

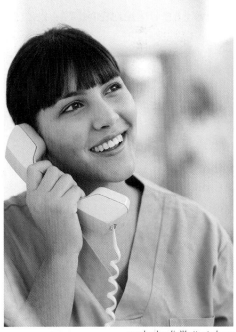

wavebreakmedia/Shutterstock.com

Figure 13.5 When calling, immediately identify yourself and the reason for the call.

6. Never use jargon or medical abbreviations, as the other person might not understand medical terminology.

7. Listen to the other person attentively to determine the best way to assist him or her.

8. Take notes while listening, wait for the other person to finish speaking, repeat key points, and ask questions to clarify the person's statements.

9. Finish the call in a friendly, professional way. For example, you could say, "Thank you. Is there anything else I can help you with?" or "Thank you for calling and have a nice day."

In many healthcare facilities, telephones are located in patient or resident rooms for convenience. Facilities may also provide secure cell phones that nursing assistants and licensed nursing staff members can use during their shifts. These phones are sometimes connected to the call lights in patient or resident rooms, allowing the nursing assistant to answer a call light using the phone.

Section 13.1 Review and Assessment

Using the Key Terms
Complete the following sentences using key terms in this section.

1. _____ are software programs that can have many health-related uses.
2. A(n) _____ contains information about a patient's single stay in a healthcare facility.
3. Meetings with healthcare experts are called _____.
4. A(n) _____ includes information about a resident's entire medical history and all healthcare experiences.
5. _____ refers to the amount of money an organization pays its staff.

Know and Understand the Facts

6. What are the two primary types of records used in a healthcare facility? Identify a record in each category.
7. Describe the difference between an EHR and EMR.
8. Identify two types of records that support and document care.

Analyze and Apply Concepts

9. List three actions a holistic nursing assistant can take to ensure confidentiality and privacy when using electronic records.
10. List two digital communication devices you might be asked to use in a healthcare facility.
11. How can apps be useful to holistic nursing assistants?
12. What are three guidelines to remember when using a telephone as a holistic nursing assistant?

Think Critically
Read the following care situation. Then answer the questions that follow.

Lucia has been a nursing assistant in a local community hospital for a few months. She enjoys working with the patients and likes using the hospital's electronic medical records. Lucia is caring for Mrs. O, who was admitted after she fainted and broke her left hip. Mrs. O had surgery to repair her hip and also has type 2 diabetes and COPD. In the afternoon, Mrs. O's son came to visit. Mrs. O could not remember what the doctor told her about her surgery, illness, and the progress she's making. Mrs. O's son asked Lucia if he could see his mother's health record to better understand her condition.

13. Can Mrs. O's son access her health record? If he can, what guidelines should be followed?
14. What digital resources could Lucia use to understand Mrs. O's condition and illnesses? Research one app she might use.

Objectives

As a nursing assistant, you must know how to properly and accurately document (or chart) in a patient's or resident's records within your scope of practice. To achieve the objectives for this section, you must successfully

- **describe** why documentation is essential when providing care;
- **explain** the documentation scope of practice for nursing assistants;
- **discuss** the sources of information used for documentation; and
- **apply** guidelines for accurate and timely documentation.

Key Terms

Learn these key terms to better understand the information presented in the section.

12-hour clock   addendum
24-hour clock   amendments

Questions to Consider

- Think about the last time you wrote something. Maybe you were writing for a school assignment or for a job. Did you plan ahead what you wanted to write, or did you just start writing?
- When you write, what steps do you take to ensure you express your thoughts effectively?

Why Is Documentation Essential to Care?

All care that is given to a patient or resident needs to be documented (or *charted*). The primary purpose of documentation is to provide a timely, ongoing record of care that includes accurate, concise information about the care that is provided. Doctors, licensed nursing staff members, and other healthcare providers use this essential information to make determinations regarding a resident's status and progress, necessary changes in treatment, medications, and care. The primary responsibility of nursing assistants is to enter information into patient or resident records and complete forms with specific information (such as vital signs or fluid intake and output measurements) within scope of practice. Nursing assistants may also fill out other facility forms, such as order forms or incident reports, as needed or requested.

When working as a nursing assistant, you must follow documentation guidelines and remember that the health record is a legal document. Never document something if it was not done. You should not wait until the end of a shift to document care, but you should also never record any care or task before it is completed. Never document for someone else, even if members of the licensed nursing staff ask you to document for them. If this situation occurs, report it to the charge nurse or the nurse manager. Documentation is always a description of what *you* have done.

What Sources of Information Are Used to Document Care?

In chapter 12, you learned that observation is a way to determine the status of and changes in a resident's condition. When observing, you should look for physical changes, expressions of emotions, responses to treatment, or the progression of a resident's disease or condition. Information observed may be either objective or subjective. As you learned in chapter 12, *objective observations* are based on facts, and *subjective observations* are based on feelings or opinions.

When documenting care, you can use the notes on your assignment sheet as a source of information. Using these notes, you can document the completion of the care provided. If care was not provided as assigned, you should document this and explain why these changes were made. Care that was not completed should also be reported to the licensed nursing staff. Another source of information for documentation is completed forms that indicate vital signs, food eaten, or the intake and output of fluids.

What Guidelines Should Be Followed When Documenting Care?

Many healthcare facilities use electronic records, but some still use manual documentation in paper records. If you work in a facility that uses paper records, you must use blue or black ink to document care per facility policy. Write legibly, so that others can easily read what you have written. Write on every line and do not skip lines. Draw a line through any blank spaces so that additional information cannot be written on the record. When you have finished documenting care, sign your full name and include your title.

If you are using electronic records, you will be given special training and a username for the electronic record system. After completing an entry in an electronic record, you should sign your full name using a digital signature and include your title.

Whether you are using electronic or paper records, follow these guidelines when documenting care:

1. Check that you are documenting in the correct resident's record.

2. Read the prior notes before you write your own to ensure continuity.

3. Identify the date and time that you are making the entry. Depending on the facility's preference, you may use a 12- or 24-hour clock (Figure 13.6). The **12-hour clock** splits each day into two 12-hour periods: the 12 hours from midnight to noon (called *a.m. hours*) and the 12 hours from noon to midnight (called *p.m. hours*). The **24-hour clock** divides the day into 24 hours, from midnight to midnight and numbered from 0 to 24. If you are using a 12-hour clock, note if the time is a.m. or p.m. If you use a 24-hour clock, you will only need to identify the time. In the 24-hour clock, noon would be 1200, and midnight would be 2400.

Becoming a Holistic Nursing Assistant
Documentation

Documentation is essential to providing safe, quality holistic care. Documentation provides ongoing information about the progress, changes, and statuses of patients and residents. It also ensures continuity of care between shifts and provides information that may be needed or required by other healthcare staff and insurance companies. When documenting care, remember that documentation must always:

- be specific to a patient or resident;
- be kept private and confidential;
- be yours (not someone else's);
- be timely (not done at the end of the shift);
- be accurate (if you are not sure how to spell a word, look it up);
- be written in sequence of care;

- contain only what was observed or performed;
- contain simple, descriptive terms and accepted abbreviations;
- be corrected immediately and according to procedure if an error occurs (by the person who made the error); and
- have a signature, title, date, and time of entry.

Remember that, if you do not document something, it is not considered done.

Apply It

1. Do you think any of these guidelines might be a challenge for you to implement? Why or why not?

2. Describe how you can overcome any challenges you may encounter documenting care.

4. Think and document in the sequence that you delivered care. If you gave a bed bath before you helped a resident walk, for example, document in that order.

5. Document only what you observed, heard, and did and how the patient or resident responded. Include objective and subjective observations. Use quotation marks when documenting subjective information (for example, if a patient tells you, "I feel so depressed today"). Do not give any of your own opinions or interpretations.

6. Always document any response or behavior that is not typical for a patient or resident.

7. Use simple, descriptive terms, but avoid words such as *normal*, *good*, or *adequate*.

8. Use commonly accepted abbreviations used by the facility in which you work.

9. Never remove pages from a paper record or delete an entry or section from an electronic record.

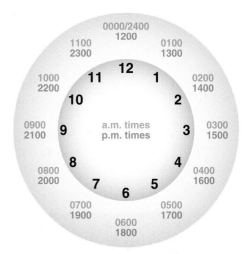

Figure 13.6 The 12- and 24-hour clocks are illustrated here.

How Are Documenting Errors Corrected?

If an error has been made during documentation, it must be corrected quickly. The only person who can change, or *amend*, a record is the person who wrote the original entry. Documentation corrections are legally called **amendments**. The following guidelines can guide you in correcting errors for both paper and electronic records. Always check your facility's guidelines for amending a health record.

1. Make sure there really is an error before you continue. If the error is not your error, consult the person who entered the incorrect information and encourage him or her to amend the problem. If the error is yours, take steps to correct it.

2. If correcting a paper record, do not erase or use any correction liquid or tape. Instead, draw a single line through the incorrect information and make sure the original entry remains legible. The new entry should be placed above or next to the error. Initial or sign and date the correction. The original and corrected entry should always be readable (Figure 13.7).

3. If correcting an electronic record, add an **addendum** to the original electronic document that provides the corrected information. *Do not* delete the original information or rewrite it. Make sure the new entry is clearly identified as an addendum on the document.

4. If you failed to enter information during documentation, add a late entry with the missing information and details.

Did not want to ambulate after morning care. Stated, "I have a terrible headache and want to take a nap." VS taken. T—100.2, P—82, R—18, BP—116/86. When asked, pain level was a 5. Observed a red rash on her
9/17/20XX SCR
~~left upper arm.~~ left lower arm. Reported VS, headache, pain level, and rash to the charge nurse.

Figure 13.7 To correct a manual record, draw a line through the incorrect information, then initial and date. Add the correct information on top of or beside the incorrect entry.

5. Once you correct an error or enter missing information, you must *authenticate* the information, or prove that it is real. To do this, digitally or manually sign the entry with your full name and title. Also include the date.

6. Ensure that the original document is retrievable. Remember that health records are legal documents that must be stored and accessible at all times.

Each healthcare facility has unique policies and procedures regarding how to handle errors. Ask questions if you are uncertain about how to amend a record.

Section 13.2 Review and Assessment

Using the Key Terms

Complete the following sentences using key terms in this section.

1. An item added to a health record is a(n) _____.
2. The _____ uses a.m. and p.m. designations.
3. The _____ divides the day into 24 hours numbered from 0 to 24.
4. _____ are corrections to a health record.

Know and Understand the Facts

5. Explain why documentation is essential.
6. Identify two sources of information used when documenting care.
7. Describe two ways to ensure accurate documentation.

Analyze and Apply Concepts

8. Why is it important to never document for another nursing assistant or healthcare provider?
9. Describe how you would correct an error in a paper record.
10. Describe how you would correct an error in an electronic record.
11. List the five guidelines that should be followed when documenting care.
12. How would you document 10 in the evening using a 12-hour clock and a 24-hour clock?

Think Critically

Read the following care situation. Then answer the questions that follow.

Mrs. J was admitted to a healthcare facility yesterday. Jack, a nursing assistant, is responsible for her care today. Mrs. J will need a complete bed bath, will need her vital signs taken every three hours, and will need to be turned and positioned every two hours. During Jack's shift, Mrs. J complains of nausea, and the charge nurse gives her medication. Jack stops providing care because Mrs. J wants to take a nap after her medication. After about an hour, Mrs. J says she feels much better, so Jack resumes care and finishes the bed bath. He turns her every two hours and measures her vital signs as requested.

13. What specific information should Jack be documenting during his shift? Where should he be documenting this information?

14. If Jack makes an error documenting his care in Mrs. J's EMR, what should he do to correct the error? What should he do if he makes an error in a paper record?

Key Points

Reviewing the key points for this chapter will help you practice more safely and competently as a holistic nursing assistant and will help you prepare for the certification competency examination.

- When working in healthcare facilities, you may use both electronic and paper health records. An electronic health record (EHR) details a patient's or resident's entire health history. An electronic medical record (EMR) provides information related to a single visit in a healthcare facility.

- Health records fall into two categories: those that support and document care and those that help a facility be organized and operate smoothly and efficiently. All healthcare facilities have policies and procedures for maintaining, retaining, and destroying records.

- Documentation must be timely, accurate, and concise. Nursing assistants are responsible for documenting in patient or resident records and recording information on forms.

- A health record is a legal document and must be accurate and maintained properly. If care is not documented, it is not considered done.

- Any documentation errors must be corrected quickly. The only person who can correct, or amend, a record is the person who made the original entry.

Action Steps to Holistic Care

Review the information in this chapter. Complete the following activities.

1. Prepare a short paper or digital presentation describing three types of records holistic nursing assistants use. Discuss how completing these records accurately promotes quality and ensures a safe environment.

2. Imagine that you are a salesperson for a company that develops electronic health record (EHR) software. What would you say to convince a potential customer to switch from using paper charts to electronic records? Include the benefits of using EHRs and the disadvantages of using paper charts. Also brainstorm potential arguments the customer might have for continuing to use paper charts.

3. With a partner, write a song or a poem about documentation guidelines. Include five guidelines in this chapter.

4. With a partner, prepare a poster outlining how to correct errors in paper and electronic health records. Include all the required guidelines.

5. Research and describe two apps holistic nursing assistants might use when providing care.

✓ Preparing for the Certification Competency Examination

To prepare for the nursing assistant certification competency examination, you will need to know content found in this chapter. This content may be tested in the knowledge (written or oral) and skills (hands-on demonstration) portions of the exam. The following areas will be emphasized:

- documentation
- confidentiality
- communication guidelines

These sample test questions are similar to ones you will find on the certification competency exam. See how well you can answer them. Be sure to select the *best* answer.

1. The phone rings at the nurse's station. What is the first thing a nursing assistant should say when answering?
   A. "Hello, this is Unit 5, Sarah. How can I help you?"
   B. "Hello, this is Unit 5, Sarah, nursing assistant. How can I help you?"
   C. "Hello, this is Sarah Jones, nursing assistant. How can I help you?"
   D. "Hello, this is Unit 5, Sarah Jones, nursing assistant. How can I help you?"

2. An electronic medical record (EMR) is an electronic document that
   A. is left at the bedside for ease of reading
   B. has health information from multiple providers
   C. has information about a specific patient's single stay
   D. is left in the medical records department so it is safe and secure

(continued)

3. A nursing assistant realizes he has made an error in an EMR. What should he do to correct the error?

   A. ask his supervisor to fix it before the shift ends
   B. check facility policy for the correct procedure
   C. cross the information out digitally and enter new information
   D. wait until the next shift

4. What is an app?

   A. a piece of computer hardware that records information
   B. a software program that develops forms
   C. a piece of computer hardware that has different uses
   D. a software program that has different uses

5. A nursing assistant is asked by her busy charge nurse to document the care given by the charge nurse. What should the nursing assistant tell her charge nurse?

   A. "I will do that after I complete Mr. D's bed bath."
   B. "I understand you are busy, but I can only document what I have done."
   C. "I will include that in my change-of-shift documentation."
   D. "I will check to see if I can document that."

6. Which of the following is an example of maintaining confidentiality?

   A. sharing someone's name, but not age or gender
   B. asking someone to keep a secret
   C. keeping something private
   D. making something available to the public

7. When a nursing assistant answers the phone, the caller is a doctor requesting a resident's laboratory results. What should the nursing assistant say to the doctor?

   A. "I am performing Mrs. K's bath right now. May I call you back?"
   B. "Sure, if you can hold, I will check the record."
   C. "I don't think those results are in yet, but I will check."
   D. "I will ask the nurse in charge to call you right back with the results."

8. If your facility uses a 24-hour clock, and you are performing care at 1:15 p.m., what time should you write on the documentation?

   A. 1315
   B. 0115
   C. 1115
   D. 1305

9. Ms. C, a new patient, shares with you that her heart is beating fast. What should you document about what she said?

   A. The patient is having a lot of pain.
   B. The patient stated that "her heart is beating fast."
   C. The patient seems to be uncomfortable.
   D. The patient feels like her heart is beating fast.

10. In which of the following records do nursing assistants do the majority of documentation?

    A. progress notes
    B. the plan of care
    C. the health record
    D. the assignment sheet

11. When documenting a telephone call, nursing assistants should always

    A. take notes after the call
    B. take notes during the call without interrupting the caller
    C. take notes at the end of the call
    D. takes notes during the call and confirm accuracy with the caller

12. What is the nursing assistant's primary purpose and responsibility when documenting?

    A. to keep track of a resident's visitors
    B. to record the different treatments given during a shift and the resident's responses
    C. to record the progress made
    D. to provide timely, accurate, and concise information about care given

13. Which of the following is the best example of an objective observation?

    A. The resident was complaining of a lot of pain.
    B. The resident's blood pressure was 165/110, and her hands were shaking.
    C. The resident stated that "she had a lot of pain."
    D. The resident seemed anxious.

14. A family member asks the nursing assistant for a copy of Mrs. P's health record. How should the nursing assistant respond?

    A. "I would be happy to get that for you."
    B. "Only the doctor can provide that information."
    C. "I can ask the nurse to check who is designated to view Mrs. P's health records."
    D. "Family members are never able to see someone else's records."

15. The proper way to sign documentation is with your

    A. first name, last name, and title
    B. last name and title
    C. first name and title
    D. first name and last name

Did you have difficulty with any of the questions? If you did, review the chapter to find the correct answer(s).

Welcome to the Chapter

You learned in chapter 8 that the immune system works to prevent disease and destroy pathogens that enter the body. This chapter explores the body's natural defenses in greater detail, particularly as they relate to infection. Immunity, or resistance to disease, develops in response to various factors. Understanding these factors and the risks that can lead to infection will help you provide safe, quality care as a holistic nursing assistant. You will also learn about how microorganisms become disease-causing pathogens.

What you learn in this chapter will help you develop your knowledge and skills to become a holistic nursing assistant. The topics discussed in the chapter are highlighted on the Providing Holistic Care Framework.

You are now ready to start this chapter, *Body Defenses and Infection.*

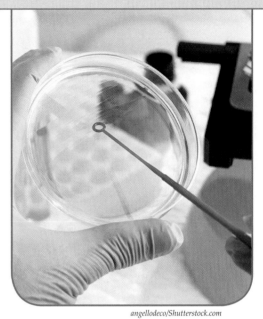

angellodeco/Shutterstock.com

Chapter Outline

Section 14.1
Body Defenses, Immunity, and Risk

Section 14.2
Pathogens and Infection

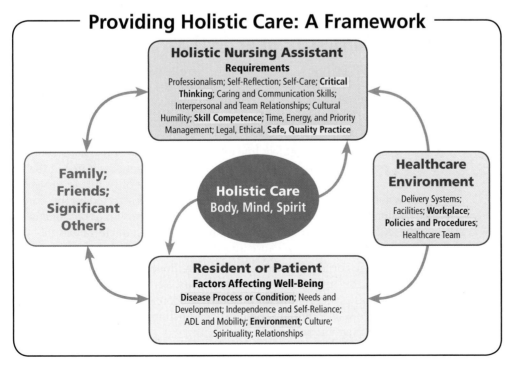

Providing Holistic Care: A Framework

Holistic Nursing Assistant
Requirements
Professionalism; Self-Reflection; Self-Care; **Critical Thinking**; Caring and Communication Skills; Interpersonal and Team Relationships; Cultural Humility; **Skill Competence**; Time, Energy, and Priority Management; Legal, Ethical, **Safe, Quality Practice**

Family; Friends; Significant Others

Holistic Care
Body, Mind, Spirit

Healthcare Environment
Delivery Systems; Facilities; **Workplace; Policies and Procedures**; Healthcare Team

Resident or Patient
Factors Affecting Well-Being
Disease Process or Condition; Needs and Development; Independence and Self-Reliance; ADL and Mobility; **Environment**; Culture; Spirituality; Relationships

Questions to Consider

- Do you remember receiving vaccinations when you were a child? Did anyone object to the vaccinations you received?
- Have you ever had a childhood disease, such as the measles or chickenpox? What was this experience like?
- Have you recently received any adult vaccinations? Did you experience any side effects from a vaccination?

Objectives

To provide the best possible care, you must understand risks for infection and the body's defenses against infection. It is important to familiarize yourself with the concept of immunity, or a person's ability to resist disease. To achieve the objectives for this section, you must successfully

- **describe** the natural lines of defense against disease in the human body; and
- **explain** the immune response, immunity, and risk for infection and disease.

Key Terms

Learn these key terms to better understand the information presented in the section.

antigens

bacteria

infection

lubricants

microorganisms

mucus

phagocytosis

saliva

toxins

The human body constantly faces possible attack from both internal and external factors. As a result, the body has its own biological armor that protects it from **infection** (invasion by harmful, microscopic organisms) and disease. The body's armor is composed of physical and chemical barriers that prevent disease-causing **microorganisms** (microscopic organisms) from entering the body. These barriers form the body's first line of defense. The body is also protected by a second, cellular line of defense called the *immune response*. The immune response describes the body's internal reaction to *pathogens* (disease-causing microorganisms). Inflammation, coughing, and sneezing also help rid the body of infection or disease.

What Are the Barriers to Infection?

Remember

Our body is a machine for living. It is organized for that, it is its nature. Let life go on in it unhindered and let it defend itself.

Leo Tolstoy, Russian author

The body's first line of defense against infection includes physical and chemical barriers in different parts of the human body. Structures and substances in the human body utilize their unique anatomy and physiology to protect the body and prevent the entry of pathogens. The physical and chemical barriers include the following structures and substances:

- The skin (*epidermis*) is the greatest line of defense because of its vast surface area. The skin creates a physical barrier between the inner structures of the human body and the outside world; however, the skin is only able to protect the body when it is healthy and intact. Natural **lubricants** secreted by the skin reduce friction and contain substances that prevent the growth of pathogens. When the skin is cut or torn, enzymes are released to kill **bacteria** (single-celled microorganisms that can cause infection) that may try to enter the body.

- The nasal passages of the respiratory system are lined with mucous membranes. Mucous membranes contain **mucus**, a thick, slippery fluid that moistens and protects parts of the body. Mucous membranes in the nasal passages contain tiny hairs called *cilia*, which trap microorganisms that may cause infection or disease.

- The eyes produce cleansing tears that protect the eye, continuously lubricate it, and keep it from becoming dry. Tears contain water, salt, antibodies, and enzymes that stop bacterial growth on the eye's surface.
- The eyelashes form a physical barrier that keeps foreign particles, such as dust and dirt, away from the eye.
- The mouth secretes **saliva**, a watery fluid that blocks the growth of pathogens.
- The gastrointestinal (GI) tract is lined with mucous membranes that trap microorganisms. The GI tract contains good bacteria called *normal flora*. Normal flora change the chemical composition of the GI environment to prevent the growth of and kill harmful bacteria. Gastric acid inside the stomach also destroys microorganisms that may be found in ingested food.
- The vagina is lined with mucous membranes and has an acidic environment that helps prevent the growth of pathogens.
- The urethra rinses pathogens out of the urinary tract and has mucous membranes for protection.

What Is the Immune Response?

The body's second line of defense, the immune response, is a cellular and chemical response that helps fight against infection. In the immune response, the body distinguishes between its own tissues and cells and outside or foreign substances. Foreign substances are known as **antigens** and may include **toxins** (poisons).

As part of the immune response, cells with foreign antigens and toxins are identified by antibodies. As you learned in chapter 8, *antibodies* are blood proteins that attach themselves to antigens and mark them for destruction by the immune system. As a result, white blood cells engulf and destroy antigens through a process called **phagocytosis** (Figure 14.1). The immune system remembers antigens after encountering them once, and if antigens appear again, the body is prepared to mount a better, faster response. Each time a new antigen enters the body, the body must develop a new set of antibodies unique to that antigen. The human body can develop around 100 million types of antibodies.

Often, once the body develops antibodies for an antigen, it is permanently immune to a disease. For example, people who get mumps build enough antibodies that they are unlikely to get the disease again. If these people do get mumps again, they will usually get a milder case. As you learned in chapter 8, immunity that develops when the body builds antibodies is called *acquired immunity*.

How Does Vaccination Create Immunity?

Immunity can also be acquired through *vaccination*, or the injection of a vaccine. As you learned in chapter 2, a *vaccine* is a mixture that contains a very mild form of a disease so the body builds antibodies against that disease. An example of a common vaccine is the annual flu shot. People who receive a flu vaccine are injected with a biological mixture containing a flu antigen that has been weakened or killed. Introducing this weakened or killed antigen prompts the body to develop antibodies specific to that antigen. As a result, the body will attack and destroy that antigen if exposed to it again. If exposed to that flu antigen, the vaccinated person will usually not get sick or will have a milder case if he or she does get sick.

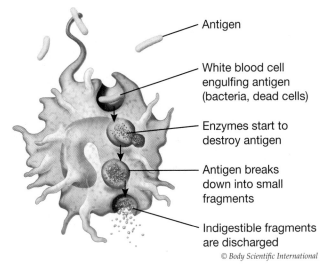

Antigen

White blood cell engulfing antigen (bacteria, dead cells)

Enzymes start to destroy antigen

Antigen breaks down into small fragments

Indigestible fragments are discharged

© *Body Scientific International*

Figure 14.1 During phagocytosis, white blood cells engulf antigens and destroy them. Antibodies mark antigens for destruction.

Vaccines are created to prevent or reduce the severity of diseases. In some cases, vaccines are developed in response to disease epidemics that can be fatal or cause disabilities (for example, smallpox or polio). Vaccines have also been developed for measles and whooping cough (*pertussis*). Vaccines continue to be developed, usually in response to outbreaks of communicable diseases such as the Ebola virus.

Sometimes vaccinations are given once, such as the vaccine for shingles (herpes zoster). Other vaccines require subsequent doses, called *boosters*, after the initial injection. Specific vaccinations are often recommended or even required when a person is traveling to another country. When a person visits another country, he or she has not been exposed to the common diseases of the area and built immunity. Examples of vaccinations required for some international travel include those for typhoid or yellow fever. Annual vaccinations are also offered for diseases such as influenza (the flu shot) or pneumonia. Most vaccinations are given by injection, though some are given orally (such as those for polio or rotavirus) or through the nose.

In the United States, the Centers for Disease Control and Prevention (CDC) provides an immunization schedule for children ages 0–18. This schedule includes vaccinations for varicella (*chicken pox*); inactivated poliovirus; and measles, mumps, and rubella (*MMR*). The CDC also provides a schedule for adult vaccinations. This schedule includes similar recommendations with additional vaccines for diseases such as human papillomavirus (HPV). Vaccinating a large majority of the population against a disease helps control the spread of the disease because most of the population is immune. When the majority of a population is immune, this is called *community immunity* or *herd immunity*.

In the United States, vaccinations are typically required for children of school age, though some states make exceptions for parents who object for religious or other reasons. Vaccinations are also required for people who work in certain professions, such as healthcare. The goal of vaccination is protection for yourself and others.

What Other Body Responses Defend Against Infection?

Other body responses also defend against infection. These responses include the inflammatory response, coughing, and sneezing. The *inflammatory response* causes *inflammation*, which is characterized by redness and swelling. Inflammation is the body's response to irritation, injury, or infection. It is caused by body tissues secreting chemicals that cause blood vessels around the damaged area to swell. Inflammation can make the affected area warm to the touch. It may also cause a person to run a fever (increased body heat), which destroys antigens or toxins. The inflammatory response signals white blood cells and other cells to travel to the injured area of the body and attack toxins. Sometimes *pus*, the aftermath of an immune response, can be found at the site of injury. Pus contains tissue, dead antigens, and white blood cells (Figure 14.2).

As a holistic nursing assistant, you will observe and report inflammation. If you observe inflammation, you might document that "the area around the wound on the upper arm was red, swollen, and warm to the touch." Often, pressure from swelling and the increased body heat associated with inflammation cause pain.

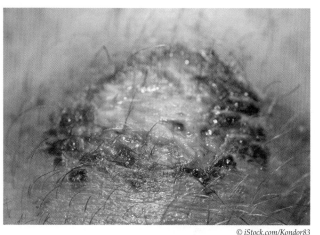

© iStock.com/Kondor83

Figure 14.2 Inflammation and pus indicate the presence of an infection.

Coughing and sneezing are additional forms of body defense. These automatic reflexes rid the body of antigens or toxins. Be aware that coughing and sneezing spray antigens and toxins into the air or onto someone else's clothing and can cause others to get sick. To reduce this risk, cover your nose and mouth with the inner part of your arm before coughing or sneezing. Do not cough or sneeze onto your hands, as this increases your chances of spreading germs to other people and surfaces.

What Increases the Risk for Infection?

Risks for infection and disease are everywhere, though some people are more vulnerable to these risks than others. People who are very old or very young have more difficulty avoiding infection, particularly during flu season or during extremely hot or cold weather. Infants and young children may have underdeveloped immune systems due to their ages. Older adults often have less resistance to infection due to increased likelihood for acute or chronic illness and a slower metabolism.

People in poor health (for example, people with respiratory or cardiovascular conditions) have limited resistance to colds and flus. These people often experience more severe symptoms than the general public. People with autoimmune disorders or human immunodeficiency virus (HIV) may experience chronic conditions that lower immunity. Also at increased risk are people who have been hospitalized or in a healthcare facility for a long time, have an artificial joint, or are on kidney dialysis.

Patients in hospitals and residents in long-term care facilities are susceptible to infection, particularly if they have urinary catheters or continuous central line intravenous (IV) catheters. Urinary catheters and IV catheters increase risk for infection because they are foreign objects placed inside the body. Increased susceptibility to infection has become a major problem in healthcare facilities; infections acquired within healthcare facilities are called *healthcare-associated infections (HAIs)*. You will learn more about HAIs later in this chapter and in chapter 15.

Using the Key Terms

Complete the following sentences using key terms in this section.

1. As part of the body's first line of defense, the mouth secretes _____, a watery mixture that blocks the growth of pathogens.
2. _____ are substances foreign to the body that are identified and destroyed by antibodies.
3. _____ are secreted by the skin to reduce friction and prevent the growth of pathogens.
4. Pathogens are disease-causing _____ that can only be seen through a microscope.
5. Single-celled, microscopic organisms that can cause infection are called _____.
6. _____ refers to the invasion and growth of harmful, microscopic organisms in the body.
7. The body's immune system distinguishes between natural cells and _____, which are also called poisons.
8. _____ is a thick, slippery fluid that moistens and protects parts of the body.
9. During the process of _____, a white blood cell engulfs and destroys foreign antigens.

Know and Understand the Facts

10. What physical barriers form the body's first line of defense?
11. What chemical barriers form the body's first line of defense?
12. Describe the immune response.
13. What is a vaccine?
14. What does community or herd immunity accomplish?

Analyze and Apply Concepts

15. What is acquired immunity?
16. What happens when inflammation occurs?
17. How do vaccines build the body's immunity against a disease?
18. Explain why age might play a role in increasing a person's risk for infection.
19. What should a person do to avoid spreading antigens or toxins when coughing or sneezing?

Think Critically

Read the following care situation. Then answer the questions that follow.

You have been asked to care for Mr. S today. He is a 75-year-old man who has a lung infection and COPD due to many years of smoking. Mr. S's wife said that he got sick two weeks ago and could not catch his breath. Mr. S was admitted to the hospital, and after two days, transferred to your facility. Mr. S also has a bandage on his arm covering an open wound. The skin around the wound looks red and has pus.

20. How do you think Mr. S's COPD affects his lung infection?
21. Why was Mr. S at risk for lung infection?
22. Explain why Mr. S's wound looks the way it does.
23. Describe how you would report and document Mr. S's wound.

Objectives

Understanding how microorganisms cause infection and disease will prepare you to provide safe, quality care. It is also important to learn about the chain of infection, signs and symptoms of infection, modes of transmission, bloodborne pathogens, and healthcare-associated infections. To achieve the objectives for this section, you must successfully

- **identify** the four types of microorganisms;
- **describe** the six links of the chain of infection;
- **explain** modes and methods of transmission, signs and symptoms of infection, and general treatment; and
- **recognize** issues related to bloodborne pathogens and healthcare-associated infections (HAIs).

Questions to Consider

- When was the last time you had an infection? How did you get the infection?
- Could the infection you got have been prevented? If so, what could you have done?
- When you had the infection, how did you feel? What did you have to do to make the infection go away?

Key Terms

Learn these key terms to better understand the information presented in the section.

aerobic	culture
anaerobic	disinfectants
antiseptics	dormant
autopsies	noncommunicable diseases
bloodborne pathogens	phenol
chlorophyll	photosynthesis
communicable diseases	

What Are Microorganisms and Pathogens?

No matter where you are, very small organisms live around and with you. These organisms are so small that they are only visible through a microscope. As a result, they are called *microorganisms,* or *microbes.*

Microorganisms can be found in many places—in the air, water, and soil and on plants, animals, and people. Some microorganisms are useful and do not cause disease. These are called *normal flora.* As you learned in the previous section, some normal flora live in the gastrointestinal tract and help with digestion.

Normal flora do not cause problems if they do not travel to new locations. Normal flora can, however, cause disease if they move away from their places of origin. When this occurs, normal flora become *pathogens.*

Prior to the 1800s, parts of the world had vastly different views of infection and disease. Some people believed disease was a punishment for evil or resulted from an imbalance of internal forces in the body. This view changed during the 1800s when several notable doctors and scientists began to understand how pathogens, or *germs,* are spread. These doctors and scientists also discovered that hand washing impacts the spread of infection.

During the 1800s, a French pharmacist found that solutions containing chlorides of lime or soda could eliminate offensive odors from human corpses and be used as **disinfectants** (chemicals used to destroy or slow the growth of microorganisms) and **antiseptics** (fluids or substances that prevent the growth of microorganisms). Hungarian doctor Ignaz Semmelweis noticed a high mortality rate among women

Remember

The body is a community made up of innumerable cells or inhabitants.

Thomas Edison, American inventor and businessman

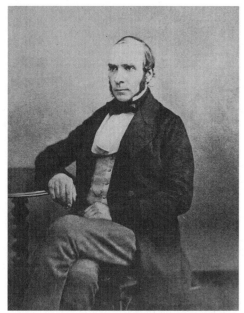
The National Library of Medicine

Figure 14.3 John Snow's discovery of the source of London's cholera outbreak in 1854 led to improvements in water and waste management.

following childbirth in a hospital. Often, women who gave birth in a hospital were treated by doctors and students who had just completed **autopsies** (examinations conducted to determine cause of death). Semmelweis hypothesized that these students and doctors were still carrying pathogens on their hands and suggested that they wash their hands in a solution of chlorinated lime water before touching pregnant patients. Semmelweis's suggestion resulted in a drastic decrease of women dying of childbirth fever. Several years after Semmelweis's discovery, an English doctor named John Snow traced a cholera epidemic in London to contaminated water. He ordered the water supply closed, and the epidemic diminished (Figure 14.3).

Even with mounting evidence, many doctors still doubted that microorganisms caused disease. Discoveries by Louis Pasteur, Robert Koch, and Joseph Lister in the latter half of the nineteenth century, however, helped people understand the connection between germs and disease. In the mid-1800s, French chemist and microbiologist Louis Pasteur discovered that heating beer and wine to a certain temperature killed bacteria that caused these liquids to spoil or change into vinegar (Figure 14.4). This heating process became known as *pasteurization* and is still used to purify foods and liquids today.

During the late 1800s, German doctor Robert Koch proved that bacteria caused disease. He showed that the bacterium *Bacillus anthracis* caused anthrax in cattle and sheep and demonstrated that an infectious agent can be isolated from an infected animal, cultivated in a **culture** (grown in a favorable substance), and then injected into a healthy animal to cause the same infection. Because of Koch's discovery, German microbiologists were able to isolate *Staphylococcus, Streptococcus,* and the microorganisms that caused cholera, typhoid fever, diphtheria, pneumonia, tetanus, meningitis, and gonorrhea.

Joseph Lister, an English doctor, applied discoveries about microorganisms and the spread of disease to his work in surgery. He soaked surgical bandages in **phenol** (an acid that can be used as a disinfectant in dilute form) to prevent postoperative infections.

These groundbreaking discoveries led to the *germ theory,* which holds that many diseases are caused by microorganisms. The discovery of the germ theory was made possible by the development of the microscope (to see tiny microorganisms), actions that prevent contamination, and *epidemiology* (the study of the patterns, causes, and effects of health and disease in specific populations).

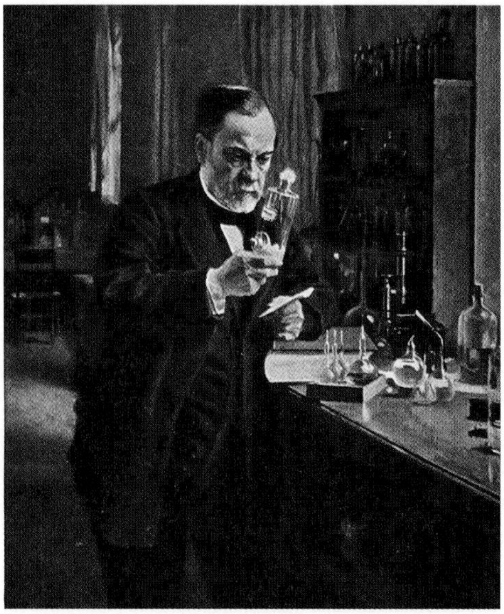

What Are the Types of Microorganisms?

There are four types of microorganisms—bacteria, viruses, fungi, and parasites. In this section, you will learn about each type of microorganism, the way the microorganism is spread and detected, common treatments, and examples of infections and diseases caused by each microorganism.

Bacteria

Bacteria are single-celled microorganisms that are often harmless, but can also cause infections in any part of the body. If bacterial infections are not treated, they may spread. Bacteria may be **aerobic** (needing oxygen) or **anaerobic** (not needing oxygen) and can only be seen under a microscope. These microorganisms are classified and named according to their sizes and shapes (Figure 14.5). There

The National Library of Medicine

Figure 14.4 Louis Pasteur's experiments confirmed that microorganisms caused the spoiling of beer and wine.

are three basic shapes of a bacterium: a spherical bacterium (*coccus*), a rod-shaped bacterium (*bacillus*), and spiral bacteria. A spiral bacterium may be shaped like a comma (*vibrio*); shaped like a rigid corkscrew (*spirillum*); or long, thin, and flexible (*spirochet*).

Bacteria group together and form colonies. Most bacteria that cause disease grow in a warm, dark, and moist environment and require nutrients (such as oxygen, if they are aerobic). Bacteria can enter the body through the skin, nose, mouth, eyes, ears, lungs, urethra, and vagina, among other places. Once bacteria gain entry, they multiply quickly, causing infection. Bacterial infection can destroy tissues and cells; bacteria may also overwhelm the body and prevent it from functioning properly.

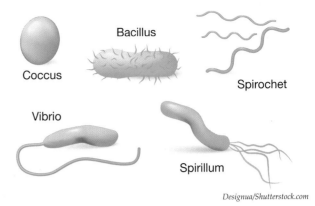

Designua/Shutterstock.com

Figure 14.5 A spherical bacterium is called a *coccus*, and a rod-shaped bacterium is called a *bacillus*. Spiral bacteria come in three shapes: *vibrio*, *spirillum*, and *spirochet*.

Bacterial Infections

Bacteria are the most common cause of infection in the body, and bacterial infections are treated with antibiotics. The type of bacterial infection depends on the type of bacteria and location in the body. Two examples of bacterial infections are tuberculosis (TB) and bacterial pneumonia.

Tuberculosis (TB) is caused by the bacterium *Mycobacterium tuberculosis*. It is not a current or major threat in the United States, but is still a concern, and is spread through droplets in the air (from coughing and sneezing). TB primarily attacks the lungs, but can also damage the kidneys, spine, and brain. Risk factors include a weakened immune system and travel to areas where TB is prevalent. In latent TB, noncontagious bacteria are in the body, but no symptoms are present. Latent TB can become active TB, the symptoms of which are painful coughing that lasts more than three weeks, coughing up blood, fatigue, fever, night sweats and chills, loss of appetite, unintentional weight loss, back pain, and blood in the urine. Patients with TB take antibiotics for at least six to nine months and must take all of the medication prescribed. Active TB can spread; therefore, infection control precautions (such as covering the mouth with a tissue and putting dirty tissue in a sealed bag) are necessary.

Bacterial pneumonia is usually caused by *Streptococcus pneumoniae* and is an infection of the lungs that causes inflammation and fluid buildup. Risk factors for bacterial pneumonia include an age over 65, asthma, diabetes, heart disease, smoking, surgery, poor nutrition, and alcohol consumption. Common signs and symptoms are high fevers; chills and sweating; greenish, yellow, or bloody mucus; dyspnea (difficulty breathing); sharp, stabbing pain in the lungs; fatigue; little appetite; cyanosis in the lips and fingernails; and confusion. Prevention strategies are regular hand hygiene, good nutrition and exercise, sufficient sleep, isolation from those who are sick, and vaccines. Effective treatments include antibiotics (until the bacteria are destroyed), medications for fever and pain, rest, plenty of fluids, a humidifier to loosen mucus, smoking cessation, oxygen therapy, and IV fluids.

Other examples of bacterial infections are acute appendicitis, diphtheria, conjunctivitis (*pink eye*), tetanus, rheumatic fever, syphilis, pertussis (*whooping cough*), and Lyme disease.

Antibiotics

Antibiotics are the most common treatment for bacterial infections and may be taken by mouth, applied to the skin, or injected intramuscularly or intravenously.

Penicillin, one of the first antibiotics, became available in the early 1940s and was used heavily during World War II. Since World War II, pharmaceutical companies have manufactured many different types of antibiotics, which have become a widespread and commonly accepted way to treat bacterial infections. The array of antibiotics available has made it easier to prescribe the correct antibiotic for a specific bacterium and eliminate the infection. One challenge of the widespread use of antibiotics is antibiotic resistance.

Antibiotic resistance develops when bacteria change to resist the effects of an antibiotic. Bacteria that survive an antibiotic treatment multiply into bacteria that are resistant to that antibiotic. Bacteria that are resistant to more than one antibiotic are called *multidrug-resistant organisms (MDROs)*. Examples of MDROs are methicillin-resistant *Staphylococcus aureus* (MRSA) and vancomycin-intermediate or vancomycin-resistant *Enterococcus* (VRE). Antibiotic resistance has consequences for those who have infections. For example, when a person has an infection that is antibiotic resistant, recovery time can be very slow. In some cases, death can occur if the infection cannot be treated. Good hygiene, cleanliness, and the cautious use of antibiotics can help prevent antibiotic resistance. Some facilities have antibiotic policies and guidelines regarding the use of antibiotics and ways to manage antibiotic resistance.

Viruses

Viruses are the smallest microorganisms. They are 100 times smaller than bacteria. Viruses are small bundles of protein that cannot grow or multiply by themselves and instead take over host cells (usually plant or animal cells). After taking over a host cell, a virus injects genetic material into the host and takes possession of its functions. The host cell, now infected with the virus, reproduces the viral protein and genetic material, causing the virus to spread. Some viruses spread through saliva, coughing, sneezing, or sexual contact. Others are contracted through the *fecal-oral route* (through water or food contaminated with feces).

Viral infections cannot be treated with antibiotics, but are instead treated with antiviral prescription medications. Like antibiotics, antiviral medications are specific to particular viruses, but rather than destroying a virus, they slow virus development. Antiviral medications exist for AIDS and the flu, for example. Vaccinations can also prevent or slow the development of a virus, even if the virus has been recently contracted. Vaccinations exist for viral pneumonia, the flu, polio, measles, mumps, rubella, and smallpox (Figure 14.6).

The common cold and influenza (commonly called the *flu*) are both viral infections. Both infections affect the respiratory system and are contagious, but are caused by different viruses. Compared to the common cold, the flu has a sudden onset, more intense symptoms, and more serious health issues and complications (such as pneumonia, bronchitis, and in some cases, death).

People over the age of 65, people with chronic medical conditions, pregnant women, and young children are at greatest risk for contracting the flu. Flu symptoms include fever, chills, cough, sore throat, runny or stuffy nose, muscle or body aches, headache, and fatigue. Antiviral medications can lessen symptoms, shorten the time a person is sick by one or two days, and prevent serious flu complications. These medications are best taken within two days of getting the flu. Infection control precautions (such as practicing good hand hygiene and disinfecting contaminated surfaces), rest, and increased fluids are important for recovery.

Other examples of viral infections are chickenpox, measles, hepatitis, mononucleosis (*mono*), polio, rabies, shingles, HIV, and Ebola.

Fungi

A *fungus* is an organism that lacks **chlorophyll** (a substance found in plants that absorbs and transfers light). Fungi reproduce through *spores*, which are single-celled units capable of reproducing on their own. Fungi must digest food to live, since they are incapable of **photosynthesis** (the process of converting energy from the sun into chemical energy). Types of fungi include mushrooms, molds, yeasts, and parasitic fungi.

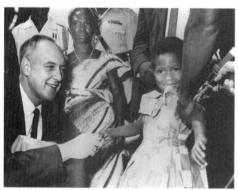

National Library of Medicine

Figure 14.6 Between 1966 and 1980, the World Health Organization eradicated smallpox through global mass vaccination and containment measures. Smallpox was declared eradicated in 1980. Today, the smallpox vaccine is only given to people who work with the virus in labs.

Fungi are common. In fact, people breathe in or come into contact with fungal spores daily without getting sick. The human body naturally contains some fungi, including yeasts and parasitic fungi. Yeast infection can occur when the amount of yeast in the body becomes imbalanced. This can result when people take antibiotics over a long period of time or when bacteria that naturally keep yeast from growing become too suppressed, causing more yeast to grow than normal. Opportunistic fungi can also cause infection. Opportunistic fungi take advantage of opportunities to cause infection (for example, a weak immune system caused by HIV/AIDS).

Fungal infections are typically treated using over-the-counter or prescription antifungal creams, ointments, or medications. Examples of fungal infections include thrush, athlete's foot, vaginal yeast infections, ringworm, fungal eye infections, and pneumocystis pneumonia.

Parasites

Parasites are organisms that live on or in other organisms, or *hosts*. Parasites feed from and sometimes at the expense of the host. Some parasites do not affect the host, while other parasites make the host organism sick. Parasitic infections can be caused by three types of organisms (Figure 14.7):

1. **Protozoa**: live in drinking water; one example is the *Plasmodium* parasite, which causes malaria
2. **Helminths**: commonly live in the intestines; include tapeworms, ringworms, and hookworms
3. **Ectoparasites**: live in or feed off human skin; include fleas and ticks

Parasites can be spread through contaminated water, waste, fecal matter, blood, sexual contact, and mishandled or undercooked food. Some parasitic infections are spread by insects, which carry the disease and transmit it while feeding off the host. One example is malaria, which is spread by mosquitos.

Parasites thrive in warm, moist climates, such as those found in tropical or subtropical regions of the world. People who travel to these regions are at increased risk for contracting parasitic infections. A compromised immune system also increases the chance of developing a parasitic infection. One parasitic infection that is common with preschool and school-age children is head lice. Lice are spread through personal contact, combs, brushes, hats, and other clothing.

Not all parasitic infections can be treated, though antibiotics and other medications (such as lotions or creams) can be helpful for treating particular infections. Treatment should also include removal of the infestation (for example, bedbugs or lice). Other examples of parasitic infections include bedbug bites, pinworm, foodborne diseases, head and body lice, malaria, and trichinosis (caused by eating raw or undercooked pork or wild game infected with roundworm eggs).

How Are Infections Categorized?

Infections are categorized as either local, systemic, or opportunistic. Some infections result from specific situations, such as a patient's stay in a hospital.

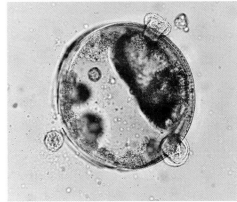

Rattiya Thongdumhyu/Shutterstock.com

A

Rattiya Thongdumhyu/Shutterstock.com

B

Choksawatdikorn/Shutterstock.com

C

Figure 14.7 Protozoa (such as the *Vorticella* parasite shown in A) are microscopic. Helminths include various types of worms, including the tapeworm shown in B. An ectoparasite might be a flea (C) or a tick.

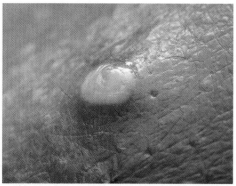

khlungcenter/Shutterstock.com

Figure 14.8 A skin boil is an example of a local infection.

Local Infections

Local infections are confined to one area of the body. For example, a local infection might be a *boil* (a reddened bump filled with pus surrounded by tender, swollen skin) or a wound on the skin (Figure 14.8). Signs and symptoms of a local infection include fever; redness, heat, pain, and swelling at the site; and pus or discharge that may be foul smelling.

Systemic Infections

A *systemic infection* is widespread and travels throughout the body via the bloodstream. The flu is an example of a systemic infection. The signs and symptoms of a systemic infection include aches, sometimes chills and fever, nausea and vomiting, and general overall weakness.

Opportunistic Infections (OIs)

Opportunistic infections (OIs) develop only under certain circumstances as a result of a weakened immune system. An opportunistic infection develops when a person's immune system has been weakened by another infection. The opportunistic infection takes advantage of the weakened immune system and creates a second infection. For example, pneumocystis pneumonia is a common opportunistic infection in people who have HIV/AIDS.

Healthcare-Associated Infections (HAIs)

A *healthcare-associated infection (HAI)*, also known as a *nosocomial infection*, is an infection that is acquired in a hospital or other healthcare facility. Examples of these infections include central line-associated bloodstream infections (CLABSIs) from a central intravenous catheter, catheter-associated urinary tract infections (CAUTIs), and ventilator-associated pneumonia (VAP). Infections that occur at surgery sites are known as surgical site infections (SSTs). *Clostridium difficile* or *C. difficile* is another HAI. Older adults and people with diseases or conditions that require the prolonged use of antibiotics are at greater risk of acquiring this infection. *C. difficile* bacteria are transmitted by surfaces or instruments contaminated with infected feces (for example, commodes, bathtubs, and rectal thermometers).

Healthcare facilities have regulations and standards that must be followed to prevent HAIs. These regulations, along with care considerations, prevention, and control strategies for nursing assistants, are discussed in detail in chapter 15.

Healthcare Scenario
HAIs in Long-Term Care

Yesterday, it was reported that a long-term care center downtown has seen a significant increase in HAIs among its residents in the last month. The center is owned by a large healthcare corporation and has numerous residents who are over 85 years old, have catheters, and have difficulty ambulating. The center has also experienced staffing changes. The nursing director was replaced two months ago, and as a result, some staff members left.

Apply It

1. Why do you think the HAI rate increased in this center?

2. What can the facility, licensed nursing staff, and nursing assistants do to lower the rate of HAIs?

What Is the Chain of Infection?

For an infection to develop, a particular sequence of events must occur. The sequence of events that leads to infection is known collectively as the *chain of infection*. There are six links in the chain of infection (Figure 14.9):

1. **Infectious agent**: An infectious agent, or *pathogen*, must be present to cause infection. The pathogen might be a bacterium, virus, fungus, or parasite. It must have the capacity to cause disease, multiply and grow, and enter the body.

2. **Reservoirs**: The pathogen needs a *reservoir* where it can live and reproduce. Reservoirs can be environmental or human. A potential reservoir for infection might be a toilet seat or feces.

3. **Portal of exit**: Pathogens need a *portal of exit*, or a way to leave the reservoir. A portal of exit can be through a sneeze, a cough, blood, or feces.

4. **Means of transmission**: There must be a means of transmission, or a *carrier*, for the pathogen to move from one place to another. Pathogens can be transmitted directly (between two people, such as through a sneeze or cough) or indirectly (from a contaminated piece of equipment). Sometimes human carriers can incubate a disease and be harmful to others, even if they are not sick themselves.

5. **Portal of entry**: A *portal of entry* must exist for the pathogen to enter a person. The portal of entry could be the respiratory system (through breathing in), the gastrointestinal system (through eating contaminated food), or an open wound.

6. **Susceptible host**: A susceptible host that cannot resist the pathogen will become ill. The potential for infection depends on several risk factors, including the host's age, existing diseases and conditions, and the amount of infectious agent.

The purpose of infection control is to break the links in the chain of infection. Infection control will be discussed in more detail in chapter 16.

Think About This

Approximately 1 out of every 25 hospitalized patients has an HAI at any given time. This means that nearly 650,000 patients develop an HAI annually. Recent statistics show that about 75,000 people die as a result of an HAI acquired during hospitalization, and more than one-half of these fatal HAIs are acquired on a patient care unit.

In long-term care, infections are one of the most common reasons residents are admitted to hospitals. Each year, between one and three million residents contract a serious infection, such as a urinary tract infection (UTIs), diarrheal disease, or antibiotic-resistant *Staphylococcus* (staph) infection. As many as 380,000 residents die each year as a result of infection.

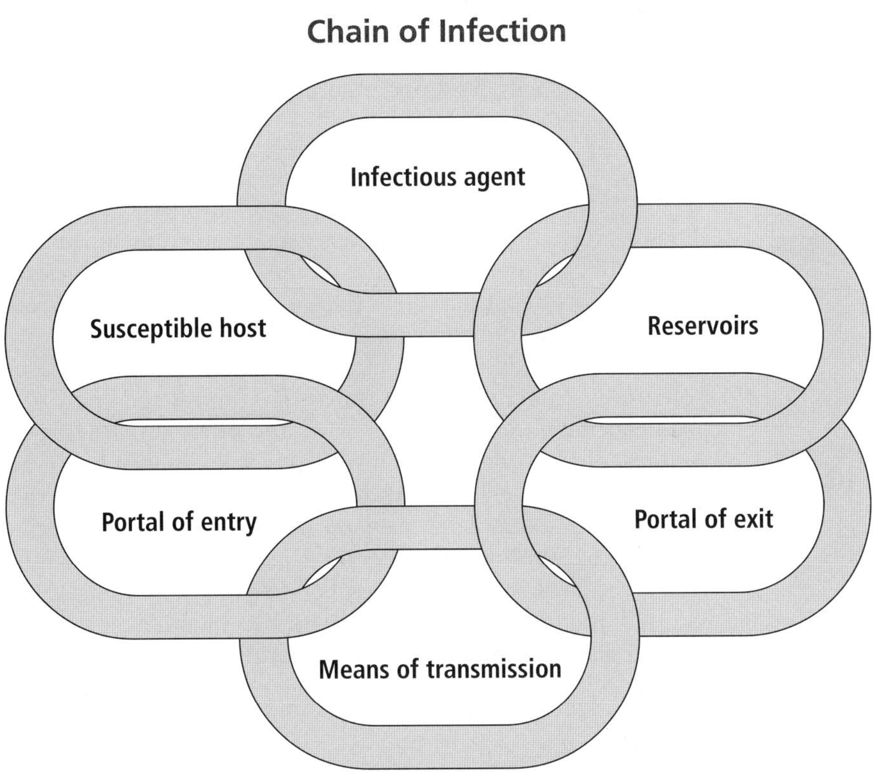

Chain of Infection

Figure 14.9 The chain of infection consists of six links: the infectious agent, reservoirs, portal of exit, means of transmission, portal of entry, and susceptible host.

How Are Communicable Diseases Transmitted?

Diseases and infections can be categorized by how they are transmitted. Diseases that cannot be transmitted between people, objects, and animals are *noncommunicable*, or not contagious. Examples of **noncommunicable diseases** include genetic diseases, cancers, mental disorders, autoimmune diseases, and heart disease.

Communicable diseases are contagious and can be transmitted between people, objects, and animals. Communicable diseases can spread through airborne transmission, contact transmission, vehicle or vector transmission, and bloodborne pathogens. These diseases can also develop opportunistically or due to the reactivation of a **dormant**, or *latent*, organism (an organism with slowed or stopped functions).

Airborne Transmission

Airborne or *droplet transmission* occurs when microscopic pathogens become suspended and move in the air or become trapped in dust. If these pathogens are inhaled by a susceptible host, they can cause illness. Airborne transmission can occur when someone who is ill coughs, sneezes, talks, laughs, sings, or spits.

Contact Transmission

Contact transmission occurs when an infectious agent or reservoir housing a pathogen comes into contact with a host. Contact can be direct—through touch; sexual contact; blood; or body fluids such as drainage, urine, feces, mucus, saliva, or vomit. Contact can also be indirect—through contaminated items such as soiled linen, clothing, a dressing soaked with drainage, or used specimen containers.

Vehicle and Vector Transmission

Another mode of transmission is *vehicle transmission*. Vehicle transmission occurs when an infectious agent is ingested via contaminated food or water. An example of a disease spread by vehicle transmission is *dysentery*. *Vector transmission* occurs when an infection is introduced into the skin or mucous membranes through an animal or insect bite. The mosquito is a common vector and can cause diseases such as malaria, Zika virus, and West Nile virus (Figure 14.10). Ticks, fleas, and other insects can also serve as vectors for disease.

Bloodborne Pathogens

Bloodborne pathogens are disease-causing microorganisms found in an infected person's blood. Some examples of bloodborne pathogens are hepatitis B virus (HBV), hepatitis C virus (HCV), and human immunodeficiency virus (HIV). Bloodborne pathogens can be transmitted through exposure to human blood and other potentially infectious body fluids, sharps-related injuries and needlesticks (punctures of the skin), and other injuries that break the skin. Bloodborne pathogens are especially dangerous in healthcare settings, where healthcare staff members may be exposed to blood. For example, a licensed nursing staff member may be exposed to bloodborne pathogens if he accidentally sticks himself with a needle after giving an injection to a person with HBV. OSHA safety standard requirements related to bloodborne pathogens and needlestick prevention can be found in chapters 15 and 16.

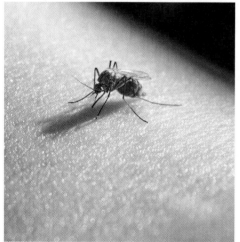

Alexander Penyushkin/Shutterstock.com

Figure 14.10 Mosquitoes are common vectors of many diseases.

How Are Infections Identified?

A person who suspects he or she has an infection should seek medical attention from a doctor. Observing related signs and symptoms can lead to the identification of an infection. An infection can also be detected using various laboratory tests and X-rays.

Typically, the first tests taken are blood tests. A common blood test to identify infection is a white blood cell count. The body releases increased numbers of white blood cells into the bloodstream when an infection is present. White blood cells fight infection. As a result, an elevated white blood cell count can indicate the presence of an infection.

Blood or fungi cultures may be used to determine the type of microorganism causing the infection. These cultures also help determine what type of treatment is needed. A patient may be put into an isolation room until the results of a blood culture are available. This is for the patient's protection and for the protection of others, as it will help prevent the spread of infection.

Specific infections may require additional tests. A urinary tract infection (UTI), for example, is tested using urine samples and a urine culture. To diagnose pneumonia, a doctor may order an X-ray of the lungs and a sputum test. Skin tests can also be used to identify specific infections. For example, the Mantoux tuberculin skin test (TST) is used to identify TB. During this test, a small amount of TB antigens is injected under the top layer of skin on the inner forearm. If a person has TB, his or her skin will react to these antigens. Some of these tests will be discussed in chapter 19.

Becoming a Holistic Nursing Assistant
Caring for Residents with Infections

When caring for residents with infections, holistic nursing assistants must remember several important considerations. Often, the focus of care is stopping the infection process as quickly as possible. It is also important, however, to consider the psychosocial aspects of care.

When providing holistic care, be aware of and sensitive to the resident's fear or guilt surrounding an infection. Perhaps the resident knew someone who died from an infection; perhaps the resident did not keep a wound clean enough. It is important to recognize pain associated with an infection. Being sensitive to, observing, and reporting levels of pain will help relieve pain and promote healing.

Some people may be embarrassed by the odor associated with seepage from wounds or rashes. As a holistic nursing assistant, maintain the resident's good hygiene and keep any dressings clean and fresh. This will help eliminate the smell and any embarrassment.

Finally, realize that personal protective equipment (PPE) and the processes used in infection control may be frightening to residents. The sight of a mask and gown can be upsetting, especially to children or older adults. Provide advance notice about the use of PPE and explain why PPE is necessary.

Apply It

1. Think back to a time when you were sick. Did you find your symptoms embarrassing or painful? What made you feel more at ease?

2. Some people find caring for a resident with an infection difficult or unpleasant. What actions might a holistic nursing assistant take to ensure he or she feels competent providing such care?

Using the Key Terms

Complete the following sentences using key terms in this section.

1. _____ are examinations conducted to determine cause of death.
2. Infectious microorganisms that are found in the blood are called _____.
3. Diseases can develop due to the reactivation of a(n) _____ organism, or an organism that has slowed or stopped functions.
4. Bacteria that are _____ need oxygen to live.
5. _____ bacteria do not need oxygen to live.
6. Diseases that can be transmitted from one person, object, or animal to another are called _____.
7. _____ are not contagious and cannot be transmitted by contact.
8. The acid _____ can be used as a disinfectant in dilute form.
9. Performing a(n) _____ involves cultivating living tissue cells in a substance favorable to their growth.
10. _____ are chemicals used to destroy or slow the growth of microorganisms to prevent them from spreading.

Know and Understand the Facts

11. Describe the four types of microorganisms.
12. List the six links in the chain of infection.
13. Identify and describe one method of infection transmission.
14. What are bloodborne pathogens?
15. What is an OI and what does it do?
16. What does the acronym HAI mean?

Analyze and Apply Concepts

17. Describe the signs and symptoms of a local wound infection.
18. Describe the sequence of events that must occur to create a chain of infection.
19. Explain the difference between communicable and noncommunicable diseases. Give one example of each.
20. Explain the uses and challenges of antibiotic treatment.

Think Critically

Read the following care situation. Then answer the questions that follow.

Ten-year-old Jake was hospitalized yesterday due to a serious bacterial infection on his lower leg. He fell while riding his bicycle last week and suffered a deep gash. His mother stopped the bleeding, cleaned the wound, and put on a large bandage, but several days later, Jake told his mother that his leg really hurt and that "icky" stuff was coming out of the wound. Jake's mother cleaned the wound again and told him to be careful. The next day, Jake had a high fever, and the wound was very swollen with seeping, watery discharge and pus.

21. What signs and symptoms indicate the presence of an infection?
22. What tests might be done to determine the type of bacterial infection?
23. What type of care might you be asked to provide as a nursing assistant?
24. What holistic care considerations should you be aware of when caring for Jake?

Key Points

Reviewing the key points for this chapter will help you practice more safely and competently as a holistic nursing assistant and will help you prepare for the certification competency examination.

- Antibodies fight infection by identifying and destroying foreign substances (antigens and toxins) through phagocytosis.

- Microorganisms that can cause disease are called pathogens. There are four types of pathogens: bacteria, viruses, fungi, and parasites.

- Infections can be local, systemic, or opportunistic. Healthcare-associated infections (HAIs) arise as a consequence of a person's stay in a healthcare facility.

- The chain of infection includes six links: an infectious agent, reservoir, portal of exit, means of transmission, portal of entry, and susceptible host.

- Communicable diseases can be transmitted between people, objects, and animals; noncommunicable diseases cannot.

- Infection can be transmitted through airborne transmission, contact transmission, vehicle or vector transmission, and bloodborne pathogens.

Action Steps to Holistic Care

Review the information in this chapter. Complete the following activities.

1. Select one of the following: central line-associated bloodstream infection (CLABSI), catheter-associated urinary tract infection (CAUTI), or ventilator-associated pneumonia (VAP). Prepare a short paper or digital presentation describing how nursing assistants can prevent this infection. Be sure actions promote safe, quality care.

2. With a partner, write a song or a poem about the four different types of microorganisms. Include the characteristics of each and give an example of a disease caused by each, including the appropriate treatment.

3. With a partner, prepare a poster discussing one category of infection, including a specific example and its location. Also include the signs and symptoms and possible treatment.

4. Research current scientific information about vaccinations. Write a brief report describing three current facts about vaccinations not covered in this chapter.

 Preparing for the Certification Competency Examination

To prepare for the nursing assistant certification competency examination, you will need to know content found in this chapter. This content may be tested in the knowledge (written or oral) and skills (hands-on demonstration) portions of the exam. The following areas will be emphasized:

- types of microorganisms
- the immune response, immunity, and vaccination
- people at risk for infection
- the infectious process and chain of infection
- modes and methods of transmission
- signs and symptoms of infection
- bloodborne pathogens and healthcare-associated and nosocomial infections

These sample test questions are similar to ones you will find on the certification competency exam. See how well you can answer them. Be sure to select the *best* answer.

1. Which of the following is a microorganism that causes infection?

   A. culture
   B. phenol
   C. pus
   D. pathogen

2. Which of the following are links in the chain of infection?

   A. host and parasite
   B. reservoir and source
   C. portal of exit and portal of entry
   D. transmission and virus

(continued)

3. A nursing assistant is working with an older man who has pneumonia. She should be aware that pneumonia can be transmitted by
   A. droplets
   B. white blood cells
   C. serum
   D. bile

4. Which of the following patients is most at risk for getting an infection?
   A. Janie, 16 years old
   B. Mrs. F, 85 years old
   C. Lester, 8 years old
   D. Ms. J, 45 years old

5. A new nursing assistant is caring for an older woman who has an intravenous catheter. Which HAI might the woman be at risk for contracting?
   A. trichinosis
   B. pneumocystis pneumonia
   C. central line-associated infection
   D. hepatitis B

6. Which of the following is the body's first line of defense?
   A. blood
   B. skin
   C. stomach
   D. ligaments

7. When a body part is warm to the touch, red, and swollen and has pus, these are signs of a(n)
   A. systemic infection
   B. regional infection
   C. local infection
   D. area infection

8. Which microorganism most commonly causes infection?
   A. fungus
   B. microbe
   C. virus
   D. bacterium

9. A nursing assistant is helping care for a patient when she observes that a blood-soaked dressing has fallen onto the bed linens. This patient has hepatitis. The nursing assistant informs the licensed nursing staff member about the fallen item. She has just prevented a possible infection from
   A. viral pathogens
   B. bloodborne pathogens
   C. normal flora
   D. protozoan pathogens

10. During vaccination, people are injected with a(n)
    A. biological preparation of an antigen that has been weakened or killed
    B. antibiotic that will kill antigens in the body
    C. antiviral medication that will decrease the toxicity of the host
    D. microscopic preparation of an antibody that is ready to kill an antigen

11. Which of the following indicates the presence of inflammation?
    A. There are visible sores and swelling.
    B. There is pus, the area is cool to the touch, and the patient is feverish.
    C. The area is swollen, cool to the touch, and red.
    D. The area is swollen, warm to the touch, and red.

12. What are antibodies?
    A. blood proteins that mark antigens for destruction
    B. blood proteins that help antigens grow
    C. blood proteins that help white blood cells develop
    D. blood proteins that attack and destroy red blood cells

13. Ms. C has acquired an infection. In the chain of infection, she is which link?
    A. reservoir
    B. susceptible host
    C. portal of exit
    D. portal of entry

14. When residents cough or sneeze without covering their mouths, they are transmitting possible infection via
    A. a vehicle
    B. contact
    C. droplets
    D. environment

15. For a virus to cause an infection, it must have a(n)
    A. fungus
    B. pathogen
    C. antigen
    D. host

Did you have difficulty with any of the questions? If you did, review the chapter to find the correct answer(s).

Welcome to the Chapter

In chapter 14, you learned about the chain of infection. As a holistic nursing assistant, you must also know how to break the chain of infection and thereby prevent and control infections. Following standard and transmission-based precautions can help prevent and control infections in healthcare facilities. In this chapter, you will learn important skills related to infection prevention and control. These skills include following proper hand hygiene practices, using personal protective equipment (PPE), double-bagging biohazardous waste, transporting patients to and from isolation, following exposure control plans, and cleaning rooms after discharge. You will also learn about the types of wounds and wound care, including ways to maintain a sterile field and the nursing assistant's responsibilities during dressing changes.

The information and procedures presented in this chapter will help you build the knowledge and skills needed to become a holistic nursing assistant. Check with your instructor to ensure these procedures are within your state's regulations for nursing assistant practice. The topics discussed in the chapter are highlighted on the Providing Holistic Care Framework.

You are now ready to start this chapter, *Infection Prevention and Control*.

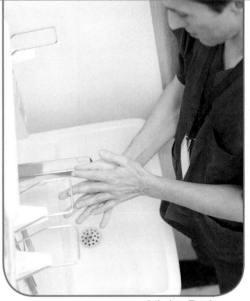
© iStock.com/TommL

Chapter Outline

Section 15.1
Standard and Transmission-Based Precautions

Section 15.2
Wound Care

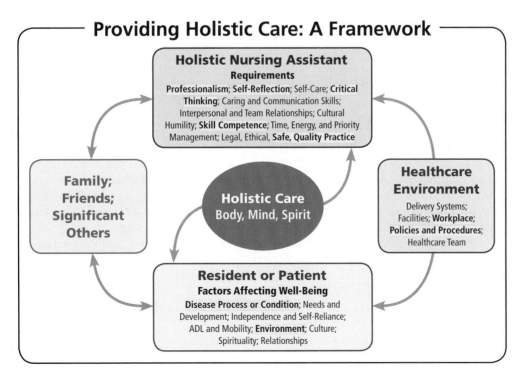

Providing Holistic Care: A Framework

Holistic Nursing Assistant
Requirements
Professionalism; **Self-Reflection**; Self-Care; **Critical Thinking**; Caring and Communication Skills; Interpersonal and Team Relationships; Cultural Humility; **Skill Competence**; Time, Energy, and Priority Management; Legal, Ethical, **Safe, Quality Practice**

Family; Friends; Significant Others

Holistic Care
Body, Mind, Spirit

Healthcare Environment
Delivery Systems; Facilities; **Workplace; Policies and Procedures**; Healthcare Team

Resident or Patient
Factors Affecting Well-Being
Disease Process or Condition; Needs and Development; Independence and Self-Reliance; ADL and Mobility; **Environment**; Culture; Spirituality; Relationships

Standard and Transmission-Based Precautions

Questions to Consider

- How many times per day do you wash your hands? Do you wash your hands only in certain situations, such as before eating, after you have coughed or sneezed, or after going to the bathroom?
- Think about why you wash your hands. Do you wash your hands for cleanliness, out of habit, or because someone said you should? When you wash your hands, do you think about your own cleanliness or the health of others?

Objectives

As a nursing assistant, you must have a working knowledge of infection prevention and control. Standard and transmission-based precautions are used in healthcare facilities to prevent the spread of infection and protect healthcare staff, patients, residents, and visitors. You will need to follow standard procedures regarding hand hygiene and the use of personal protective equipment. Additional precautions may be needed to prevent the spread of pathogens through contact or droplets in the air. If contact with infectious bodily fluids or blood does occur, healthcare staff members follow the facility's exposure control plan to protect themselves and others. Measures such as double-bagging biohazardous materials, following proper procedures for transporting patients to and from isolation, and cleaning a room after discharge are also discussed. To achieve the objectives for this section, you must successfully

- **explain** the principles and procedures required in standard and transmission-based precautions;
- **describe** the parts of an exposure control plan;
- **explain** how to perform proper hand hygiene;
- **identify** the steps needed to correctly put on and remove personal protective equipment (PPE); and
- **describe** double-bagging, proper transport to and from isolation, and procedures for cleaning a room after discharge.

Key Terms

Learn these key terms to better understand the information presented in the section.

alcohol-based hand sanitizer

asepsis

dressing

excretions

friction

isolation

personal protective equipment (PPE)

secretions

sharps

sterile

World Health Organization (WHO)

What Is Asepsis?

As a holistic nursing assistant, you will be responsible for helping prevent the spread of infection in a healthcare facility. One way nursing assistants prevent infection is by helping ensure **asepsis** (the absence of infections or infectious material). In healthcare, the terms *clean* and *dirty* are used when discussing asepsis. Items that have come in contact with potential pathogens are considered *dirty*, and items that have not been exposed to potential pathogens are considered *clean*.

When giving care, work with clean surfaces and then move to dirty surfaces. For example, always touch clean body parts or surfaces before touching those that are dirty or contaminated. Do not touch your own face, nose, or eyeglasses prior to touching a resident. Following these guidelines will help prevent *touch contamination* (the transfer of potential pathogens from a dirty to a clean surface or object).

There are two types of asepsis. *Medical asepsis* is a clean technique used to reduce the number and spread of microorganisms and prevent and control infection. Medical asepsis procedures include hand hygiene, the use of **personal protective equipment (PPE)**, and isolation. PPE includes specialized clothing and accessories (such as gloves, gowns, masks, and goggles) that protect against infection or injury. *Surgical asepsis* is a sterile technique used to completely eliminate microorganisms from the surface of an object. Surgical asepsis will be discussed in more detail in chapter 25.

What Are Standard Precautions?

To achieve medical asepsis, healthcare staff members follow standard and transmission-based precautions. *Standard precautions* are basic infection prevention and control practices used to prevent the spread of disease. Transmission-based precautions supplement standard precautions to prevent the spread of disease via direct contact with pathogens, droplets of infected respiratory secretions, and airborne pathogens. You will learn more about transmission-based precautions later in this section.

Standard precautions are infection prevention and control measures used to deliver safe, quality care. In the United States, these measures are guided by the Centers for Disease Control and Prevention (CDC) and are supported by evidence-based research. Standard precautions protect staff, patients, residents, family members, and visitors from diseases that can be spread through contact with blood, bodily fluids, breaks in the skin (including rashes), and mucous membranes. Standard precautions include hand hygiene, the use of PPE, respiratory hygiene, cough etiquette, safe injection practices, safe handling of **sharps** (objects, such as needles, that can penetrate the skin) to prevent injuries, and careful management of potentially contaminated equipment and surfaces. You will learn about the safe handling of sharps in chapter 16. Standard precautions should be used appropriately and consistently with every patient or resident.

Hand Hygiene

The role of hand washing for preventing the spread of infection was discovered in the nineteenth century and continues to be a critical infection control practice today. If all people routinely washed their hands, one million deaths each year could be prevented. According to the CDC, proper hand washing with soap and water could reduce diarrheal-associated deaths by 50 percent, reduce respiratory infections by 16 percent, and eliminate the majority of foodborne illnesses such as norovirus (viral gastroenteritis) and salmonella (bacterial infection causing diarrhea, fever, and abdominal cramps).

Hand hygiene includes both hand washing with soap (sometimes antimicrobial) and water and the use of an **alcohol-based hand sanitizer**, which is a liquid, gel, or foam preparation that kills most bacteria and fungi and stops some viruses found on the skin (Figure 15.1). The CDC and the **World Health Organization (WHO)** are leaders in setting hand hygiene guidelines. The WHO is an agency of the United Nations that focuses on international public health.

The epidermis, or outer surface, of the skin on the hands is tough and is composed of 10–20 layers of cells. These cells are constantly being renewed. They and many microorganisms picked up during routine daily activities can remain on the hands (Figure 15.2). Unless microorganisms are removed, they can survive 30–180 minutes on the hands. Therefore, hand hygiene (hand washing or using hand sanitizer) is critical. When working in a

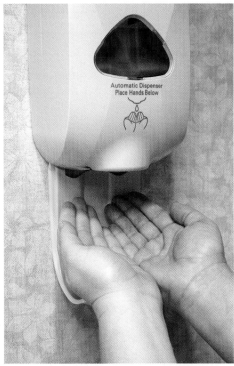

Paul Velgos/Shutterstock.com

Figure 15.1 In a healthcare facility, alcohol-based hand sanitizer can often be found in hand sanitizer dispensers.

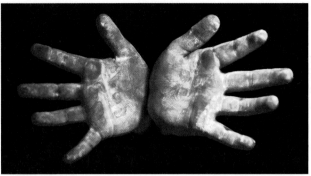

James King-Holmes/Science Source

Figure 15.2 The hands in this image have been lit with a UV light to show the areas (in light blue) that have not been adequately washed and that still contain microorganisms.

healthcare facility, nursing assistants should follow facility policy regarding when hand hygiene should be practiced. Generally, hand hygiene should be practiced

- when first entering a healthcare facility;
- before going on break or eating a meal;
- before leaving a shift;
- after using the restroom;
- before entering and upon leaving a resident's room;
- after touching a resident;
- before putting on and taking off gloves;
- before handling a meal tray;
- before getting clean linens;
- after exposure to bodily fluids;
- before and after procedures;
- after picking up an object from the floor or a dirty surface; and
- whenever hands are visibly soiled (in this case, always hand wash).

Alcohol-based hand sanitizers can be easily purchased and are often found in dispensers (for example, in healthcare facilities, grocery stores, and other public places). Effective hand sanitizers usually contain at least 60–95 percent alcohol.

During hand washing and using hand sanitizer, **friction** (resistance produced by rubbing two surfaces) helps remove microorganisms. Remember that wearing gloves is not a substitute for proper hand hygiene. Knowing how to effectively perform hand hygiene procedures is essential to infection prevention and control.

Procedure Hand Washing

Rationale
Standard precautions require routine and proper hand washing to remove and prevent the spread of microorganisms.

Preparation

1. Locate a sink near the place you will give care. There must be
   - a sufficient supply of antimicrobial soap;
   - a sink with warm, running water;
   - clean paper towels in a dispenser; and
   - an appropriate waste container nearby.
2. If your sleeves are long, use a clean, dry paper towel to push them up your arms until they are close to your elbows.
3. Remove any watches or rings. If you cannot remove a watch, use a clean, dry paper towel to push it up your arm away from your hand. If you cannot remove your rings, you will have to lather soap underneath them.

Best Practice
Always consider the sink to be contaminated. Stand far enough away from the sink that your clothing does not touch it (Figure 15.3). Do not touch the inside of the sink at any time. Always rewash your hands if they touch the sink at any time.

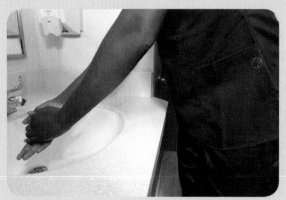

Figure 15.3

The Procedure

4. Using a clean, dry paper towel, turn on the faucet. Do not turn on the faucet with your bare hands. Adjust the water temperature until the water is warm. Be sure the water does not splash on your scrubs.

5. Thoroughly wet your hands, wrists, and the skin 1–2 inches above your wrists.

6. Remove your hands from the water stream. Apply enough soap and work it into a thick lather over your hands, wrists, and the skin at least 1–2 inches above your wrists (Figure 15.4). If you have not removed your rings, lather soap underneath them.

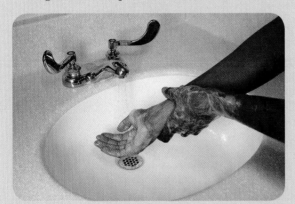

Figure 15.4

> **Best Practice**
> When washing your hands, keep your hands and forearms below your elbows. Water should flow down off your fingertips and should never flow up your arms.

7. Rub your palms together in a circular, counterclockwise motion.

8. Push the fingers of the right hand between the fingers of the left hand and rub up and down.

9. Push the fingers of the left hand between the fingers of the right hand and rub up and down.

10. With fingers interlaced, rub the palms together from side to side.

11. Bend your fingers and interlock them. The backs of your fingers should touch the opposite palm. Rub from side to side (Figure 15.5). Clean under your fingernails by rubbing them against the other palm and forcing soap underneath them. Continue rubbing to clean around the tops of your nails. Reverse hands and repeat this step.

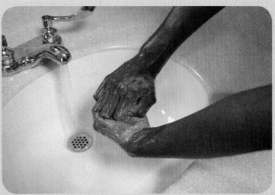

Figure 15.5

12. Hold the left thumb in the palm of the right hand. Rub in a circular, counterclockwise motion.

13. Hold the right thumb in the palm of the left hand. Rub in a circular, counterclockwise motion.

14. Hold the fingers of the right hand together and place them in the middle of the left palm. Rub in a circular, counterclockwise motion.

15. Hold the fingers of the left hand together and place them in the middle of the right palm. Rub in a circular, counterclockwise motion.

> **Best Practice**
> Work up a good foam as you wash over every part of your hands and wrists.

16. Wash your hands for a minimum of 20 seconds. You can use different methods to ensure you reach the 20-second minimum. For example, you could sing the "Happy Birthday" song twice from beginning to end.

17. Hold your hands under the running water with your fingers pointing downward (Figure 15.6). Rinse your wrists and hands thoroughly.

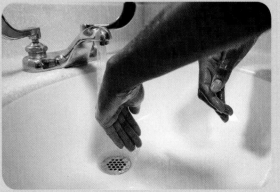

Figure 15.6

(continued)

18. Using a clean, dry paper towel, dry your hands and then your wrists, moving from your clean hand up toward the dirty forearm. Grab only one paper towel from the dispenser. Do not touch the dispenser and do not shake water from your hands.

19. Drop the used paper towel into the waste container. If another paper towel is needed, use the same procedure. Never touch the waste container.

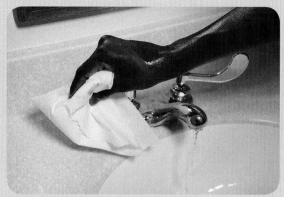

Figure 15.7

Follow-Up

20. Use a clean, dry paper towel to turn off the sink faucet (Figure 15.7). Your bare hand should not touch the sink faucet. The faucet is always considered contaminated.

21. Discard the paper towel into the waste container. Never touch the waste container.

Reporting and Documentation

This is an accepted, standard procedure. It does not need to be reported or documented.

Images courtesy of Wards Forest Media, LLC

Procedure | Using Hand Sanitizer

Rationale

Standard precautions require routine and proper hand hygiene. Using an alcohol-based hand sanitizer can help remove and prevent the spread of microorganisms.

Preparation

1. Locate the nearest hand sanitizer dispenser.

2. If your sleeves are long, use a clean, dry paper towel to push them up your arms until they are close to your elbows.

3. Remove any watches or rings. If you cannot remove a watch, use a clean, dry paper towel to push it up your arm away from your hand. If you cannot remove your rings, you will have to cover the rings with hand sanitizer.

The Procedure

4. Squeeze hand sanitizer from the dispenser into the cupped palm of one hand. Use enough hand sanitizer, usually one full pump, to cover the surfaces of the palms and fingers and perform the entire procedure.

Best Practice
This procedure should take at least 20 seconds. Add more hand sanitizer to your hands, if needed.

5. Rub your palms together in a circular, counterclockwise motion (Figure 15.8).

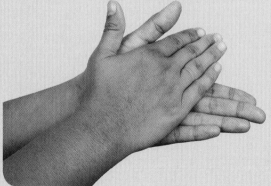

Figure 15.8

6. Push the fingers of the right hand between the fingers of the left hand and rub up and down (Figure 15.9).

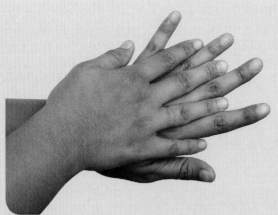

Figure 15.9

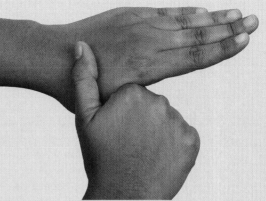

Figure 15.12

7. Push the fingers of the left hand between the fingers of the right hand and rub up and down.

8. With fingers interlaced, rub the palms together from side to side (Figure 15.10).

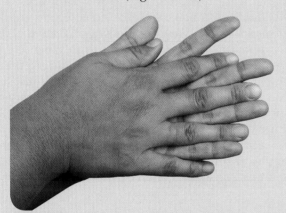

Figure 15.10

9. Bend your fingers and interlock them. The backs of your fingers should touch the opposite palm (Figure 15.11). Rub from side to side. Reverse hands and repeat this step.

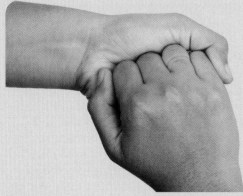

Figure 15.11

10. Hold the left thumb in the palm of the right hand. Rub in a circular, counterclockwise motion (Figure 15.12).

11. Hold the right thumb in the palm of the left hand. Rub in a circular, counterclockwise motion.

12. Hold the fingers of the right hand together and place them in the middle of the left palm. Rub in a circular, counterclockwise motion (Figure 15.13).

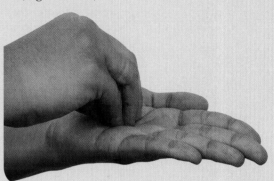

Figure 15.13

13. Hold the fingers of the left hand together and place them in the middle of the right palm. Rub in a circular, counterclockwise motion.

14. Continue to rub your hands for the full 20 seconds.

> **Best Practice**
> Creating friction is just as important when using hand sanitizer as it is when washing the hands.

Follow-Up

15. When the hands feel dry, the procedure is complete.

Reporting and Documentation

This is an accepted, standard procedure. It does not need to be reported or documented.

Images courtesy of Gratsias Adhi Hermawan/Shutterstock.com

Personal Protective Equipment (PPE)

Personal protective equipment (PPE) is specialized clothing and accessories that protect the wearer from exposure to infectious materials. PPE creates barriers that prevent microorganisms from making contact with the wearer's skin or mucous membranes. PPE also protects patients with compromised immune systems from caregivers. To be effective, PPE must be put on (*donned*) and taken off according to procedure.

PPE includes gloves, gowns, masks, respirators, goggles, face shields, and in some cases, head covers and protective gear for the feet (such as booties). Gloves *must* be worn when touching blood, bodily fluids, mucous membranes, **secretions** (substances produced by cells or organs), **excretions** (waste products expelled from the body), breaks in the skin, and contaminated items. You should also wear gloves if the resident's disease or condition requires them; if the resident has open or seeping sores or rashes; if you are handling soiled linens; and if you have scrapes, scratches, or chapped skin. For example, if a nonsterile **dressing** (protective material placed on a wound) needs to be changed, you will need to wear nonsterile, disposable gloves. You will need to use **sterile** gloves that are completely free of living microorganisms if a sterile dressing is changed or a sterile procedure is being performed. Hypoallergenic gloves and other types of nonallergenic gloves should also be available, if needed.

Gowns are required for completing certain procedures, particularly those that involve contact with blood, bodily fluids, secretions, and excretions. Gowns are also required for care given in an isolation room. Wearing a gown protects the skin and clothing from contamination. Some gowns are disposable, while others can be laundered and reused. A gown should be selected based on its resistance to fluids. For example, if fluid is likely to penetrate the gown during care, a fluid-resistant gown should be used. Clean and sterile gowns also exist. Clean gowns are used when caring for residents in isolation. A sterile gown is usually necessary during an invasive procedure (a procedure that enters the body) such as surgery.

Face protection is necessary for certain procedures and types of care. For example, face protection is required if splashes or sprays of blood, bodily fluids, or secretions are anticipated or if the resident is in an isolation room. There are different types of face protection (Figure 15.14):

- **Goggles**: the most reliable and practical eye protection against splashes, sprays, and respiratory droplets. Goggles protect the eyes effectively, but do not protect other parts of the face from splashes or sprays. Personal or safety eyeglasses are not substitutes for goggles.

- **Face shield**: protects the face, mouth, nose, and eyes. A face shield protects the face from the chin to the forehead and sometimes over the top of the head; it should wrap around the face to the ear. This reduces the possibility of a splash going around the edge of the shield and reaching the eyes.

- **Mask**: worn to protect the nose and mouth from splashes or sprays of blood or bodily fluids, to prevent droplets from being transmitted by close contact, and to prevent the contamination of a patient's wounds by a caregiver's mucus and saliva. Masks do not fit snugly on the face or provide a tight seal, so they are not reliable protection against airborne transmission. Masks may also be given to patients to limit the spread of their infectious respiratory secretions.

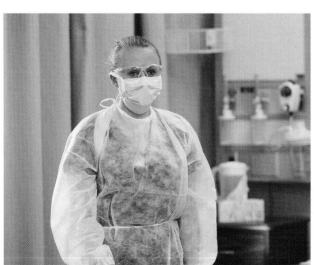

© Tori Soper Photography

Figure 15.14 This nursing assistant is wearing goggles and a mask for face protection.

- **Respirator**: protects the nose and mouth and filters the air to prevent the inhalation of airborne microorganisms. A respirator must fit the wearer's face and provide a tight seal to be effective. Types of respirators include disposable respirators; powered, air-purifying respirators (PAPRs), and self-contained breathing apparatus (SCBA) respirators.

Procedure | Putting On and Removing Disposable Gloves

Rationale

Standard and transmission-based precautions require the use of disposable, nonsterile gloves for a variety of procedures. Putting on and removing gloves properly helps ensure infection prevention and control.

Preparation

Best Practice
The following procedure is performed only when putting on or removing disposable gloves in a resident's room.

1. Bring two pairs of disposable gloves in the correct size into the resident's room and place them on a clean surface. A box of disposable gloves may already be in the room. If a box is available, be sure the gloves are the correct size.
2. Before putting on the gloves, inspect them for cracks, holes, tears, or any discoloration. Gloves may become punctured by rings and fingernails; avoid these to protect yourself and the resident. Discard damaged gloves.
3. If a gown is required, put on the gown before putting on the gloves.

The Procedure: Putting On Disposable Gloves

4. Wash your hands or use hand sanitizer to ensure infection control.
5. Your hands should be dry. Gloves are easier to put on dry hands.
6. Pick up one glove by its cuff (Figure 15.15). The outside of a nonsterile glove is always considered contaminated, so keep your gloved hands away from your clothing and other areas.

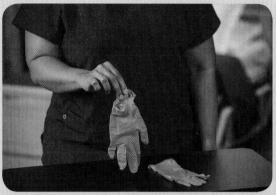
Figure 15.15

7. Pull the glove onto your hand (Figure 15.16).

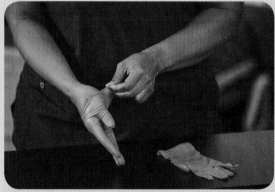
Figure 15.16

8. Repeat steps 6 and 7 with the glove for your other hand.
9. Interlace your fingers to adjust the gloves on your hands.
10. If you are wearing a gown, pull the cuffs of the gloves up over the sleeves of the gown (Figure 15.17).

(continued)

Putting On and Removing Disposable Gloves *(continued)*

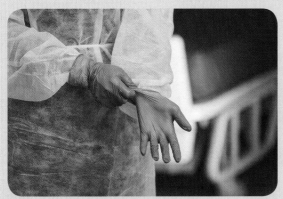
Figure 15.17

> **Best Practice**
> Always remove gloves if they become torn or soiled during a procedure. Then wash your hands or use hand sanitizer to ensure infection control and put on another pair of gloves using the same procedure.

The Procedure: Removing Disposable Gloves

11. To remove your gloves, use the gloved fingers of one hand to grasp the other, gloved hand. Grasp the gloved hand just below the cuff of the glove.

12. Pull the cuff of the glove down, drawing it over your hand and turning it inside out (Figure 15.18).

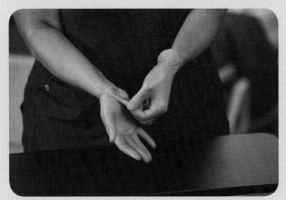
Figure 15.18

13. Pull the glove off your hand and hold it in the palm of the other, gloved hand (Figure 15.19).

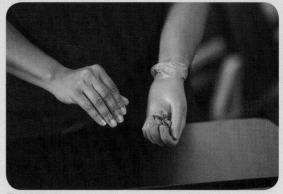
Figure 15.19

14. Insert the fingers of the ungloved hand under the cuff of the remaining glove on the other hand.

15. Slowly pull the glove off, turning it inside out and drawing it over the first glove.

16. Drop both gloves into the appropriate waste container.

> **Best Practice**
> Never wash or reuse gloves.

Follow-Up

17. Wash your hands to ensure infection control.

Reporting and Documentation

This is an accepted, standard procedure. It does not need to be reported or documented.

Images courtesy of © Tori Soper Photography

Rationale

Standard and transmission-based precautions require that healthcare staff members wear gowns during procedures in which they might be exposed to or transmit microorganisms. Gowns create barriers that protect healthcare staff. In some situations, such as caring for residents in isolation, gowning must occur prior to entering the room.

Preparation

1. Select the appropriate gown.
2. Remove any watches or jewelry.
3. If wearing long sleeves, roll them up above your elbows.

> **Best Practice**
> As often as possible, carry out all procedures that require a gown at one time. This avoids regowning for multiple entries into and exits from the same room.

The Procedure: Putting On a Gown

4. Wash your hands or use hand sanitizer to ensure infection control.
5. Hold the gown by the shoulders out in front of you. The back of the gown should face you.
6. Unfold the gown carefully. Do not shake it open.
7. Slide your hands and arms into each of the sleeves of the gown (Figure 15.20).

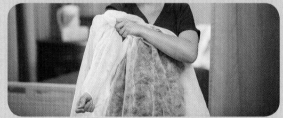

Figure 15.20

8. Pull the top of the gown around your neck to cover your scrubs.
9. Reach behind the gown and tie the neck ties using a simple shoelace bow.
10. Reach behind the gown again. Grab the open edges of the gown and pull them together so they overlap. Your clothing should be covered completely.

11. Tie the waist ties in the back using a simple shoelace bow (Figure 15.21).

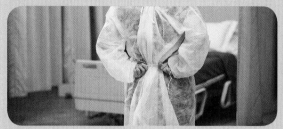

Figure 15.21

12. Put on disposable gloves. Always put on gloves after putting on a gown. Pull the gloves up over the cuffs of the gown sleeves.

The Procedure: Removing a Gown

13. Before removing your gown, first remove and discard your gloves. Be careful not to contaminate yourself.

> **Best Practice**
> Do not touch the outside of the gown as you remove it.

14. Reach behind the gown and untie both the neck and waist ties.
15. Slide your hands back into the sleeves of the gown. Using one hand (still inside the sleeve), hold the cuff of the opposite sleeve and begin pulling your arm out of that sleeve (Figure 15.22). Be careful not to touch the outside of the gown.

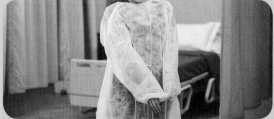

Figure 15.22

16. Repeat step 15 to begin pulling the other arm out of its sleeve (Figure 15.23). Do not touch the outside of the gown with your hands as you pull the gown down off your shoulders and arms.

(continued)

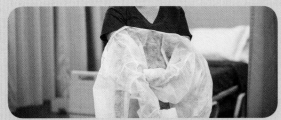

Figure 15.23

17. Turn the gown inside out as you remove it.

18. Hold the gown, turned inside out, away from your clothing.

19. Roll the gown so the contaminated outside faces inward toward the gown (Figure 15.24).

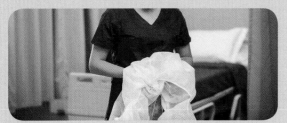

Figure 15.24

20. The gown is now considered infectious waste. Dispose of the gown in the appropriate waste container before leaving the room. Do not wear the gown again. If the gown is a reusable cloth gown, it should be worn only once and should be handled as contaminated linen according to facility policy.

Follow-Up

21. Wash your hands to ensure infection control.

Reporting and Documentation

This is an accepted, standard procedure. It does not need to be reported or documented.

Images courtesy of © Tori Soper Photography

Procedure   Wearing Face Protection

Rationale

The proper application of a mask, respirator, goggles, or face shield provides a barrier that protects those who are giving and receiving care. In some situations, such as working with residents in isolation, this PPE must be put on outside the room.

Preparation

1. Assemble the necessary equipment (the mask, respirator, goggles, or face shield).

2. Wash your hands or use hand sanitizer to ensure infection control.

The Procedure: Putting On a Mask or Respirator

3. Pick up the mask or respirator by its ties or elastic band. Place the mask or respirator over your nose, face, and chin. Secure the ties or elastic band of the mask or respirator behind your head and neck (Figure 15.25).

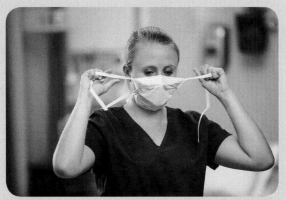

Figure 15.25

4. Do not touch the portion of the mask or respirator that will cover your face. Only handle the ties or elastic band.

5. Adjust the mask or respirator over your nose, mouth, and chin by pinching the flexible portion over the bridge of the nose. The mask or respirator should fit snugly over the nose and under the chin. If you wear eyeglasses, the mask must also fit snugly under the bottom of your eyeglasses.

6. Check that the mask or respirator fits properly and seals tightly on your face.

7. Try to avoid coughing, sneezing, and unnecessary talking while wearing the mask or respirator to prevent contamination. If the mask or respirator becomes moist, contaminated, or damaged, replace it.

8. Do not let the mask or respirator hang around your neck when not in use.

The Procedure: Removing a Mask or Respirator

9. If you are wearing gloves, remove and discard them. Be careful not to contaminate yourself.

10. Before removing the mask or respirator, wash your hands or use hand sanitizer to ensure infection control.

11. Untie the ties or remove the elastic band of the mask or respirator. Start with the ties or elastic band at the bottom of the mask or respirator and then untie or remove the ties or elastic band at the top.

12. Grasp the mask or respirator by its ties or elastic band. Use both hands to pull the mask or respirator away from the face. Dispose of the contaminated mask or respirator according to facility policy.

The Procedure: Putting On Goggles or a Face Shield

13. Place the goggles or face shield on your face and eyes and adjust them so they protect the face and eyes.

> **Best Practice**
> Personal eyeglasses or contact lenses are not considered adequate eye protection.

14. Try to avoid coughing, sneezing, and unnecessary talking while wearing a face shield to prevent contamination. If the goggles or face shield become moist, contaminated, or damaged, replace them.

15. Do not let the goggles or face shield hang around your neck when not in use.

The Procedure: Removing Goggles or a Face Shield

16. If you are wearing gloves, remove and discard them. The outside of the goggles or face shield is contaminated, so do not touch it with your bare hands.

17. Wash your hands or use hand sanitizer to ensure infection control.

18. With ungloved, clean hands, remove your goggles or face shield by grasping the clean earpiece with both hands and lifting the goggles or face shield away from your face.

19. Discard the goggles or face shield in the designated receptacle according to facility policy.

Follow-Up

20. Do not reuse any disposable face protection.

21. Wash your hands to ensure infection control.

Reporting and Documentation

This is an accepted, standard procedure. It does not need to be reported or documented.

Image courtesy of © Tori Soper Photography

Respiratory Hygiene and Cough Etiquette

In addition to hand hygiene and the use of PPE, respiratory hygiene and cough etiquette are also standard precautions that protect others from the spread of infection. Actions related to respiratory hygiene and cough etiquette prevent transmission and contain the respiratory secretions of residents who exhibit the signs and symptoms of a respiratory infection. These actions include

- covering one's mouth and nose with a tissue when coughing or sneezing;
- coughing or sneezing into one's upper sleeve or elbow (not into the hands) if a tissue is not available (Figure 15.26);
- using the nearest waste container to dispose of a tissue after its use;
- washing the hands or using hand sanitizer after contact with respiratory secretions and contaminated objects or materials;
- placing a napkin over a resident's mouth if he or she coughs during mealtime to prevent droplet contamination of other residents' food;

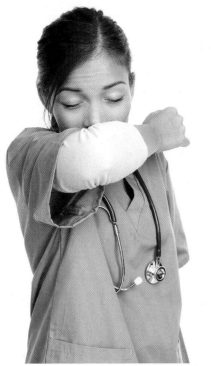
Maridav/Shutterstock.com

Figure 15.26 Coughing into the arm prevents droplets with pathogens from spraying into the environment and contaminating the hands.

- providing tissues and no-touch waste containers for tissue disposal;
- placing hand sanitizer dispensers, tissues, and waste containers in convenient, public areas;
- providing soap dispensers and clean paper towels next to sinks; and
- offering masks to people who have signs or symptoms of a respiratory infection.

One way to encourage respiratory hygiene and cough etiquette is to hang informational posters where they can be seen by visitors, family members, patients, and residents. Posters should be written in languages appropriate to the geographic area.

Potentially Contaminated Equipment or Surfaces

In healthcare, the risk of spreading pathogens through contact always exists. All equipment and surfaces have the potential to become contaminated. For example, hands and gloves can easily pick up microorganisms after contact with contaminated surfaces and equipment and can transfer microorganisms to residents and other surfaces. As a result, all equipment and working surfaces must be cleaned and decontaminated (to reduce the number of pathogens and prevent transmission) after contact with blood or other potentially infectious materials.

The first step in eliminating microorganisms from contaminated surfaces and equipment is cleaning. During *cleaning*, foreign materials are removed from surfaces and equipment. Cleaning must always precede disinfection and sterilization procedures. Healthcare facilities usually have schedules and procedures for cleaning and specific methods for decontamination. Cleaning is usually done with water, scrubbing, and detergents. Sometimes products containing natural enzymes are more effective than detergents on stubborn stains or waste. During *disinfection*, germicides known as *disinfectants* prevent microorganisms from spreading and destroy many microorganisms depending on their strength. Disinfectants are available in wipes or sprays. *Sterilization* completely eliminates all forms of microorganisms using extreme physical or chemical processes, such as steam under pressure or liquid chemicals.

Gloves must always be worn during cleaning, disinfection, and sterilization procedures. All disposable equipment can be used only once and then must be thrown away. Contaminated equipment, clothing, and supplies are double-bagged in biohazard waste bags for proper handling and disposal.

Procedure | Double-Bagging

Rationale
The proper removal and disposal of infectious waste from an isolation room protects healthcare staff and prevents contamination of the environment.

Preparation
1. This procedure requires two healthcare staff members. One staff member should stand inside the isolation room, and the other should stand outside the room. The procedure will require
   - disposable gloves; and
   - 2 leak proof, plastic biohazard waste bags (Figure 15.27).

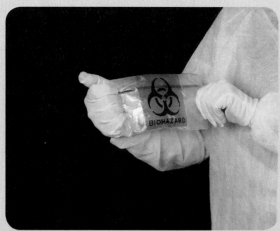

Figure 15.27

The Procedure: Inside the Isolation Room

2. Wearing disposable gloves and other appropriate PPE, stand in the room by the doorway with the full bag of waste. Be sure the contaminated biohazard waste bag is closed tightly.

3. Wait until the staff member outside the room folds the top of a clean biohazard waste bag into a cuff.

4. Place the contaminated biohazard waste bag inside the clean biohazard waste bag (Figure 15.28).

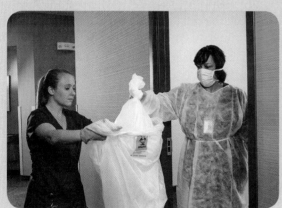

Figure 15.28

The Procedure: Outside the Isolation Room

5. Wearing disposable gloves, stand outside the doorway with a clean biohazard waste bag.

6. Fold the top of the clean biohazard waste bag into a cuff. The cuff protects your hands from contamination.

7. Hold the clean biohazard waste bag wide open.

8. Remain standing outside the doorway while the staff member inside the room places the contaminated biohazard waste bag inside the clean biohazard waste bag.

9. Tie the clean biohazard waste bag with the biohazard waste and take it to the appropriate department for disposal, disinfection, or sterilization.

Follow-Up: Inside the Isolation Room

10. Remove your PPE before leaving the room.

11. Wash your hands to ensure infection control.

Follow-Up: Outside the Isolation Room

12. Remove and discard your gloves.

13. Wash your hands to ensure infection control.

Reporting and Documentation

This is an accepted, standard procedure. It does not need to be reported or documented.

In addition to handling potentially contaminated equipment or surfaces, holistic nursing assistants also ensure that rooms are cleaned after discharge (sometimes called *terminal cleaning*). This type of cleaning ensures that rooms are prepared for the next resident and are free from soil and microorganisms. Depending on facility policy, this procedure may be carried out by a nursing assistant, shared with the housekeeping department, or completed only by housekeeping staff.

Procedure | Cleaning a Room After Discharge

Rationale

Cleaning a room properly after discharge removes soil and microorganisms and readies the room for the next admission.

Preparation

1. Bring the necessary equipment into the room. Place the following items in an accessible location:
   - a basin of warm water
   - cleaning cloths
   - a disinfectant solution
   - a container for soiled linen
   - plastic bags
   - disposable gloves
   - PPE, as needed
   - label and pen

The Procedure

2. Put on disposable gloves.
3. Remove and place all disposable materials in plastic bags to be discarded.
4. Separately bag and label any personal items that may have been left behind and might be claimed later. Make a list that contains each item. When finished with the cleaning procedure, you will take the personal items and the list to the licensed nursing staff.
5. Remove all items from the bedside stand. Clean, disinfect, or sterilize items according to facility policy.
6. Remove linen from the bed and all other linen from the room.

> **Best Practice**
> All linen in the room, even clean linen, is considered soiled and must not be reused.

7. Place the linen in the appropriate laundry container.
8. Wash any special equipment with disinfectant solution and return the equipment to its proper storage location.
9. Wash the following items with a disinfectant solution:
   - plastic covers on mattress and pillows
   - bed frame
   - bedside table and stand
   - bedside chair
10. Clean the light fixture, call light, telephone, and windows with the appropriate disinfectant solution.
11. Remove and discard your gloves.
12. Wash your hands or use hand sanitizer to ensure infection control.
13. Restock the room with any necessary supplies and make the bed according to facility policy.
14. Check the call light, light fixture, and telephone to ensure they are in working order.
15. Place a new bag liner in the waste container.
16. Check the bed's side rails, if used, to make sure they are securely attached and in the down position.

Follow-Up

17. Return cleaning supplies to their proper storage location.
18. Wash your hands to ensure infection control.

Reporting and Documentation

19. Alert the appropriate staff that the room has been cleaned and is ready for admission.

What Are Transmission-Based Precautions?

Transmission-based precautions supplement standard precautions. They are used for patients who are known or suspected to be infected with specific pathogens. Transmission-based precautions include contact precautions, droplet precautions, and airborne precautions. One example of a transmission-based precaution is wearing goggles or face shields during contact, not just when splashes or sprays are anticipated.

Contact Precautions

Contact precautions are used when microorganisms may be spread by direct or indirect contact (for example, contact with draining wounds, feces, vomit, head lice, or other bodily fluids). Contact precautions require that gloves and a gown be worn upon entering a room and when coming into contact with residents, surfaces, or objects in the room (Figure 15.29). Contact precautions also require that reusable items be cleaned or disinfected and that nonreusable items be discarded immediately after use.

Droplet Precautions

Droplet precautions are used when an infection can be spread by respiratory droplets or by contact with mucous membranes. Two examples of these infections are influenza and pertussis (*whooping cough*). Respiratory droplets do not usually travel more than 3–6 feet. When following droplet precautions, wear a face mask upon entering the room and within 3 feet of anyone who is known or suspected to have a droplet-spread disease. These precautions are very important if the resident also has a fever.

Airborne Precautions

Airborne precautions are required when a disease can be spread by microorganisms circulated in air currents. Two examples of these diseases are the measles and tuberculosis. You should follow airborne precautions when entering the room of a resident suspected or known to have such a disease.

Airborne precautions usually require the use of a respirator certified by the National Institute of Occupational Safety and Health (NIOSH). In some cases, a high-efficiency particulate air (HEPA) filtration unit may also be used to filter out airborne pathogens in the room.

Enteric, Wound, and Skin Precautions

In healthcare, you may also encounter other specific precautions. *Enteric precautions* help control diseases that can spread through direct or indirect oral contact with infected feces or contaminated articles. *Wound* and *skin precautions* help prevent the spread of microorganisms found in infected wounds and heavy secretions.

Bloodborne Pathogen Precautions

Special Occupational Safety and Health Administration (OSHA) safety standards apply to bloodborne pathogens such as HIV, hepatitis B and C, the *Plasmodium*

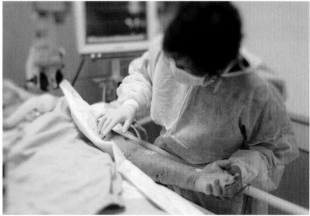
© iStock.com/PongMoji

Figure 15.29 Contact precautions prevent direct contact with contaminated objects. These precautions include wearing a gown and gloves. This nursing assistant is also wearing a mask to prevent the spread of infection via respiratory droplets.

parasite (which causes malaria), *Treponema pallidum* bacteria (which cause syphilis), and the Ebola virus. Bloodborne pathogen precautions protect healthcare staff and others who come into contact with blood and other potentially infectious materials (OPIM), such as semen and vaginal secretions. Contact may occur through needle-sticks; cuts from procedures; or direct contact between infected blood or secretions and broken skin, mucous membranes, or the eyes. The use of OSHA safety standards prevents exposure to bloodborne pathogens and reduces the chances of infection if contact occurs accidentally. These standards also require that facilities develop and implement an *exposure control plan*, which includes specialized requirements, procedures, and training for staff members who are exposed to blood and OPIM.

Isolation

When transmission-based precautions are in place, a resident may be placed in **isolation**, which uses specific preventive measures to limit or eliminate the spread of microorganisms from an infected person to others. Isolation protects both residents and healthcare staff, and isolation rooms are labeled with a sign on the door (Figure 15.30). Staff members entering an isolation room must wear masks, gowns, gloves, and any other PPE required. Isolation includes additional guidelines for cleaning and disinfecting equipment and disposing of trash in proper waste containers. There are several categories of isolation, which depend on the disease's mode of transmission and isolation requirements:

1. **Strict isolation**: used to prevent the transmission of all highly communicable diseases spread by contact or airborne routes

2. **Respiratory isolation**: used to prevent the transmission of microorganisms spread by droplets that may be sneezed out or breathed in; may use special ventilation and filtration systems

3. **Protective isolation**: used to protect those vulnerable to pathogenic microorganisms due to lowered immunity (for example, residents with leukemia and those receiving treatments that decrease resistance to disease)

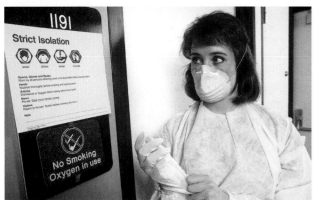

Doug Martin/Science Source

Figure 15.30 Signs should mark isolation rooms and the type of isolation.

Procedure — Transporting to and from Isolation

Rationale

When patients in isolation need to be transported to or from the room for diagnostic tests or procedures, contact precautions should be followed during transport. Use of PPE will be determined by facility policy, the type of isolation, and precautions.

Preparation

1. Ask the licensed nursing staff how this procedure fits into the plan of care, if there are doctor's orders for the procedure, if there are any special instructions or precautions, and if the resident can be moved into the positions required for this procedure.

2. Notify the department that will receive the patient from isolation.

3. Wash your hands or use hand sanitizer to ensure infection control.

4. Put on PPE as required by the type of precautions in place.

5. Knock before entering the room.

6. Introduce yourself using your full name and title. Explain that you work with the licensed nursing staff and will be providing care.

7. Greet the patient and ask the patient to state his or her full name, if able. Then check the patient's identification bracelet.

8. Use Mr., Mrs., or Ms. and the last name when conversing.

9. Explain the procedure in simple terms, even if the patient is not able to communicate or is disoriented. Ask permission to perform the procedure.

10. Bring the necessary equipment into the room. Place the following items in an accessible location:
    - transport vehicle, such as a wheelchair or stretcher
    - clean sheet(s)
    - bath blanket
    - mask for the patient, if needed

11. Maintain safety by asking for assistance. If using a stretcher, ask another staff member to assist you.

12. Cover the stretcher or wheelchair with a clean sheet. Do not let the sheet touch the floor.

The Procedure

13. Provide privacy by closing the curtains, using a screen, or closing the door to the room.

14. Raise or lower the bed to the appropriate position for the transport vehicle. The bed should be in the low position for the wheelchair or should be raised to the height needed for a stretcher.

15. Lock the wheels on both the bed and the transport vehicle.

16. Ensure safety during the procedure. If there are side rails, raise and secure the rails on the opposite side of the bed from where you will be working. Lower the rail on the side you are working.

17. Put a mask on the patient, if instructed and according to facility policy.

18. Help the patient into the wheelchair or onto the stretcher. Allow the patient to do as much as possible.

19. If using a wheelchair, wrap a sheet or bath blanket around the patient and then cover the patient with another sheet or bath blanket. Make sure the sheet or bath blanket does not touch the floor. If using a stretcher, cover the patient with a sheet or bath blanket.

20. If appropriate to facility policy, the type of isolation, and precautions, remove your PPE and wash your hands or use hand sanitizer to ensure infection control.

21. Open the door and move the patient out of the isolation unit (Figure 15.31).

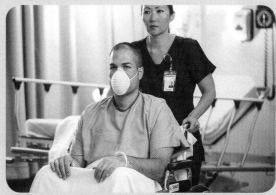

Figure 15.31

22. To return the patient to isolation, place the wheelchair or stretcher holding the patient near the door of the room. Put on PPE before entering the isolation room.

23. Enter the isolation room and unwrap the patient. Remove the patient's mask, if used.

24. Discard the mask in the biohazard waste container located in the room.

25. Assist the patient from the wheelchair or stretcher back to bed.

26. Check to be sure the bed wheels are locked, then reposition the patient and lower the bed.

27. Follow the plan of care to determine if the side rails should be raised or lowered.

28. Remove, clean, and store equipment in the proper location. Remove soiled linens and discard disposable equipment.

Follow-Up

29. Make sure the resident is comfortable and place the call light and personal items within reach.

30. Conduct a safety check before leaving the room. The room should be clean and free from clutter or spills.

31. Remove your PPE before leaving the room.

32. Wash your hands or use hand sanitizer before leaving the room.

33. Remove the transport vehicle from the isolation room. Clean and store the transport vehicle according to facility policy.

Reporting and Documentation

34. Communicate any specific observations, complications, or unusual responses to the licensed nursing staff. Record this information, along with the care provided, in the chart or EMR.

Image courtesy of © Tori Soper Photography

Becoming a Holistic Nursing Assistant
Providing Care in Isolation

Isolation in a healthcare facility can be very frightening and lonely. Healthcare staff members, family members, and friends have to wear gowns, gloves, and masks to protect themselves and the resident when they enter the isolation room. Family members and friends may be scared to enter the isolation room, which can cause the resident in isolation to feel alone and rejected. Residents may also worry about giving a disease to a family member or loved one. These feelings of fear and loneliness can create communication barriers and make it difficult for the resident to express feelings and emotions. The supplies and waste containers in an isolation room may make personal items less readily available. If personal items are inaccessible, the isolation room can feel even more unpleasant and distressing.

The following care considerations will help you provide holistic care to those in isolation:

- Be sure the resident and the resident's family members understand why isolation and precautions are necessary.
- Ensure that the resident's rights are maintained even during isolation.
- Remind the resident that the protection offered by isolation is beneficial to well-being.
- Let the resident know when you are entering the room. The door will be closed, so be sure to knock first.

- When talking with the resident, smile behind your mask and continue to smile whenever you can. Even if your mask covers your mouth, your smile will be expressed in your eyes. It will go a long way to help the resident feel comfortable and accepted.
- Spend time with the resident and talk with him or her during and after procedures and care.
- Check with the resident before leaving the room to determine if there is more you can do for him or her. This reduces the number of times you will have to reenter the room. Reentering the room requires masking, gowning, and gloving and increases the risk for cross-contamination.
- Keep the room clean and free from clutter. This maintains safety and helps the resident better see his or her own belongings.

Apply It

1. Have you ever been alone and isolated from others? If you have, how did it feel? What would have helped you feel less isolated?
2. Review the care considerations for residents in isolation. Which ones do you think will be most helpful to residents in isolation? Explain your answer.

What Is an Exposure Control Plan?

OSHA guarantees the right to a safe workplace to all staff, and particularly to staff who may be exposed to contaminated blood or bodily fluids. Healthcare facilities must provide annual, cost-free training during work hours about the hazards, risks, and measures of protection related to exposure. Healthcare facilities must also provide all necessary equipment and a system for reporting exposure. If a healthcare staff member is exposed to blood or bodily fluids, he or she should follow the facility's *exposure control plan*. In addition, healthcare facilities must provide free hepatitis B vaccines and immediate, confidential medical evaluation and follow-up for anyone exposed to blood or bodily fluids.

Healthcare staff members also have responsibilities in preventing exposure. They must always follow standard precautions, be immunized against hepatitis B, report all exposures immediately, and comply with recommended post-exposure treatment. Healthcare staff members should also support others who have been exposed and maintain their confidentiality.

A written exposure control plan should include

- a list of all job positions at risk for exposure;
- requirements for hepatitis B vaccination;
- policies related to standard precautions, including hand hygiene practices and the use of PPE;
- safe management and disposal of sharps;
- procedures for isolation and the management of isolation care;

Remember

In life, be careful in each of your actions and use your efforts, and time carefully.

Anurag Prakash Ray,
inspirational author

- hazard communication, including common and clear classifications of any chemicals used, hazard information on labels, and training;
- procedures for transferring patients with suspected or confirmed infections to isolation rooms and;
- specific precautions to be taken before and during transfer to and from isolation;
- procedures for cleaning and disinfecting contaminated equipment and surfaces;
- waste-management procedures;
- postexposure follow-up; and
- work practices that reduce or eliminate exposure to blood and OPIM (for example, not eating or drinking in potentially contaminated areas).

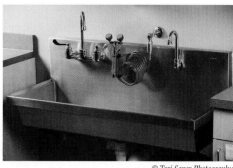

© Tori Soper Photography

Figure 15.32 An exposure control plan must include procedures for using emergency eye-washing equipment shown in this photo.

If exposure does occur, healthcare facility procedures must be followed. These procedures may include washing needlesticks or cuts with soap and water; flushing any splashes to the nose, mouth, or skin with water; washing the eyes with clean water, saline, or sterile solutions (Figure 15.32); and immediately reporting the exposure incident so that instructions for treatment (along with any possible risks) can be provided and started as soon as possible.

Section 15.1 Review and Assessment

Using the Key Terms

Complete the following sentences using key terms in this section.

1. A(n) _____ instrument is one that is free from living microorganisms.
2. _____ includes specific preventive measures that limit or eliminate the spread of microorganisms from an infected person to others.
3. The absence of infection or infectious material is known as _____.
4. Waste products expelled from the body are called _____.
5. _____ are substances produced by cells and organs.

Know and Understand the Facts

6. Discuss three standard precautions.
7. Identify three transmission-based precautions.
8. Identify three actions associated with proper respiratory hygiene and cough etiquette.
9. List four parts of an exposure control plan.

Analyze and Apply Concepts

10. Discuss three ways to provide holistic care for patients in isolation.
11. Explain the procedure for hand washing.
12. Describe the proper procedure for putting on and taking off a gown.

Think Critically

Read the following care situation. Then answer the questions that follow.

Keiko, a new nursing assistant, was asked to take care of Mr. D, an older patient who is in isolation with hepatitis B. Mr. D has several decubitus ulcers that are draining. This is the first time Keiko is taking care of Mr. D.

13. What specific precautions are necessary when caring for Mr. D?
14. What PPE should Keiko wear?
15. To provide holistic care, what approach should Keiko take when she enters Mr. D's room?

Questions to Consider

- What types of wounds have you, a friend, or a family member had? Was the wound a result of an accident at home, in a car, or because of surgery?
- Did the wound bleed a lot or require stitches? How quickly did it heal?
- Did you get an infection with the wound? If so, how was the infection treated?

Objectives

When you begin working as a nursing assistant, you will care for residents with various types of wounds. Being familiar with different types of wounds and their care will enable you to provide safe, quality care. In this section, you will learn how to maintain a sterile field, put on and remove sterile gloves, and assist with nonsterile dressing changes.
To achieve the objectives for this section, you must successfully

- **describe** the characteristics of penetrating and nonpenetrating wounds;
- **explain** the steps in assisting with the changing of a nonsterile dressing;
- **identify** the requirements to maintain a sterile field; and
- **list** the steps for putting on and removing sterile gloves.

Key Terms

Learn these key terms to better understand the information presented in the section.

contusions	nonpenetrating wounds
exudate	penetrating wounds
frostbite	sterile field
lacerations	wound

How Are Wounds Categorized?

A **wound** is an injury to body tissue that can be caused by a cut, blow, or other force. There are two major categories of wounds: penetrating wounds and nonpenetrating wounds. **Penetrating wounds** are characterized by a break in the skin. **Nonpenetrating wounds** do not break through the skin.

Penetrating Wounds

Penetrating wounds break through the skin and are often deep enough to cut through body tissues and organs. Some examples of penetrating wounds include

- simple cuts that cause an opening in the skin and bleeding;
- decubitus ulcers that wear through the skin's surface;
- stab wounds from a sharp object, such as a knife or a needle (Figure 15.33);
- gunshot wounds; and
- surgical wounds from a surgical procedure.

Nonpenetrating Wounds

Nonpenetrating wounds are caused by rubbing or friction on the surface of the skin. They do not break through the skin. These wounds include

- abrasions that result from being hit by or falling against a blunt object;
- decubitus ulcers that do not penetrate the skin;
- **lacerations**, or tear-like wounds that have ragged edges and may be caused by falling against a rough surface;

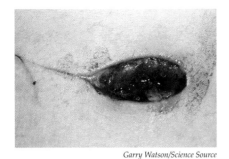

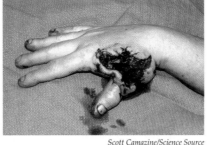

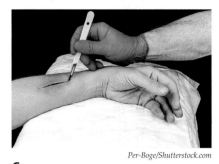

A

B

C

Figure 15.33 Illustrated here are a stab wound (A), gunshot wound (B), and surgical wound (C).

- **contusions**, or swollen bruises that are caused by broken blood vessels and may result from falling or being hit by a blunt object (Figure 15.34); and
- concussions, which cause no visible external wounds to the skin, but do cause internal damage to the brain and brain tissue.

Other Types of Wounds

Nursing assistants will also encounter other types of wounds while giving care. For example, another type of wound might be a bite or a sting from an insect or animal. *Thermal wounds* may result from exposure to extreme temperatures. Examples of thermal wounds include sunburn, burns from a fire, and **frostbite** (a condition in which extreme cold temperatures cause freezing and damage to body tissues). *Chemical wounds* result from the inhalation of or contact with chemical substances, and can cause skin or lung damage (Figure 15.35). In *electrical wounds*, high-voltage electrical currents enter the body and cause serious internal damage, even if the skin only has a minor burn.

What Should Be Observed and Reported About Wounds?

As a nursing assistant, you should be able to observe, report, and document the condition of a wound. For example, if the edges of the wound are red and swollen, this may indicate a possible infection. Also report and document the color, amount, and smell of drainage from a wound. Drainage that is thin, watery, and slightly yellow or colorless is called *clear* or *serous drainage*. Other types of drainage may be thin, watery, and slightly pink from blood (serosanguinous). These types are usually considered normal early in the healing process.

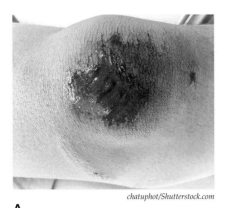

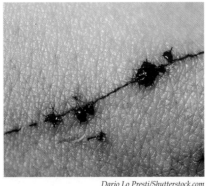

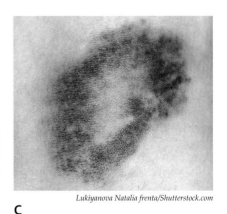

A

B

C

Figure 15.34 Illustrated here are an abrasion (A), laceration (B), and contusion (C).

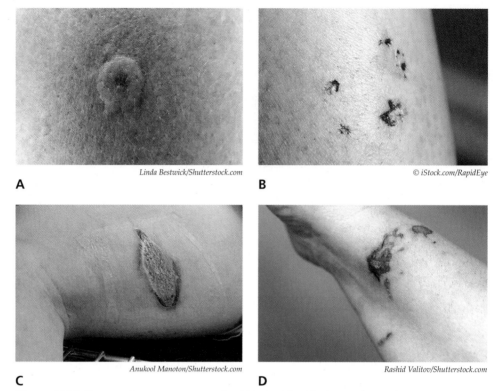

Linda Bestwick/Shutterstock.com

© iStock.com/RapidEye

Anukool Manoton/Shutterstock.com

Rashid Valitov/Shutterstock.com

A   B   C   D

Figure 15.35 Illustrated here are a wasp sting (A), dog bite (B), thermal burn (C), and chemical burn (D).

Drainage of an abnormal color might be tinged with large amounts of blood (sanguinous) or be mostly blood. Another abnormal type of drainage is *purulent drainage*, which is filled with pus. Purulent drainage is typically gray, green, or yellow and is often thick in consistency. This type of drainage usually signals an infection.

Some drainage is always expected during wound healing, and minimal to moderate drainage is usually normal. If drainage soaks a dressing, however, this needs to be reported immediately. The odor of a wound is usually not as important as the color and amount of drainage, though a very strong or foul odor might suggest an infection. Some wounds, particularly surgical wounds, will have a drain, or small tube, surgically inserted within or underneath the wound (Figure 15.36). The drain ensures fluid is easily drained.

Culture Cues
Cultural Responses to Wounds

Different cultures view the process of healing in many different ways. These varying perceptions may also extend to wounds, scarring, treatment, and the pain associated with wounds. For example, a resident may tolerate wound pain in a dignified manner and not tell you about its severity, which may lead to poor pain relief. Poor pain relief can affect the healing process; therefore, it is important to understand how cultural issues can pose potential barriers to healing.

Apply It

1. Think about how people react to their wounds and their treatment. What reactions are unfamiliar to you?

2. What actions could you take as a holistic nursing assistant to be sensitive to and aware of potential cultural differences affecting wound care?

What Types of Dressings Are Commonly Used?

Many patients and residents will have wounds that are covered with dressings. Dressings are used to protect wounds, absorb drainage, and promote comfort and healing. Several factors help or hinder the wound healing process. These include the health and age of the person, nutritional and respiratory status, medications, cultural and socioeconomic factors, and other diseases. For example, people with diabetes often have slower healing processes due to poor blood circulation.

There are many types of dressing materials. Gauze dressings are used most often, but dressings may also be made of other materials such as transparent adhesive film. The dressing material is selected based on what is needed for effective wound healing. For example, an absorptive dressing might be used for a wound that has a lot of drainage and needs minimal dressing adherence. Gauze dressings may be made of cotton, polyester, or rayon and are available in sterile or nonsterile packaging. Gauze dressings come in different sizes, such as 2 × 2 (2 inches by 2 inches) or 4 × 4. A dressing changing kit consisting of a covered tray with gloves, a waterproof drape, a mask, dressings, bandages, and tape may also be available. Some kits also include small scissors and measuring tape (for determining the size of the wound) and a cleaning solution such as saline.

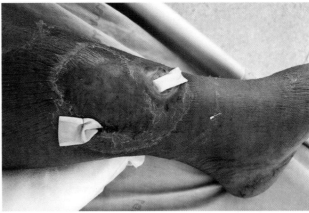

Tewan Banditrukkanka/Shutterstock.com

Figure 15.36 Drainage tubes help wounds drain and heal.

Some dressings are held in place by bandages. Bandages range in sizes and types of material. For example, Montgomery ties or straps are often paired with adhesive tapes applied to either side of a wound (usually an abdominal wound). Montgomery ties or straps have perforated edges, which eliminate the need to remove and reapply tape during every dressing change.

There are many types of dressings. Dry dressings are applied in several layers to absorb drainage. Wet dressings are saturated with a prescribed solution to promote healing. They are usually covered with dry dressings. Dressings may be nonsterile or sterile.

Nonsterile Dressings

Nonsterile dressings protect open wounds from contamination and absorb **exudate**, or drainage. Nonsterile dressings are routinely changed and are changed more often if there are large amounts of drainage. Licensed nursing staff members may ask nursing assistants to assist with these dressing changes. This is an important responsibility. During dressing changes, hand hygiene and careful observation of the wound and drainage are critical.

Procedure   Assisting with Nonsterile Dressing Changes

Rationale

Using the correct procedure to assist with changing a nonsterile dressing will help prevent infection and promote healing.

Preparation

1. Ask the licensed nursing staff how this procedure fits into the plan of care, if there are doctor's orders for the procedure, if there are any special instructions or precautions, and if the patient can be moved into the positions required for this procedure.

(continued)

Assisting with Nonsterile Dressing Changes *(continued)*

2. Wash your hands or use hand sanitizer before entering the room.

3. Knock before entering the room.

4. Introduce yourself using your full name and title. Explain that you work with the licensed nursing staff and will be providing care.

5. Greet the patient and ask the patient to state his or her full name, if able. Then check the patient's identification bracelet.

6. Use Mr., Mrs., or Ms. and the last name when conversing.

7. Explain the procedure in simple terms, even if the patient is not able to communicate or is disoriented. Ask permission to perform the procedure.

8. Bring the necessary equipment into the room. Place the following items in an accessible location:
   - at least four pairs of disposable gloves
   - PPE, as needed
   - tape or Montgomery straps
   - dressing supplies or a dressing changing kit, as directed by the licensed nursing staff (Figure 15.37)

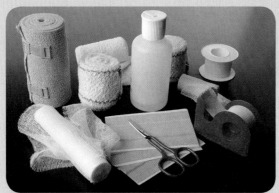

Figure 15.37

   - saline solution or cleaning solution, as directed by the licensed nursing staff
   - tape-adhesive remover
   - plastic bag or a biohazard waste bag, if needed
   - bath blanket
   - disposable protective pad
   - waterproof drape

Best Practice
Arrange your equipment on the overbed table so you do not have to reach over or turn your back on your work area.

The Procedure

9. Provide privacy by closing the curtains, using a screen, or closing the door to the room.

10. Lock the bed wheels and then raise the bed to hip level.

11. Ensure safety during the procedure. If there are side rails, raise and secure the rails on the opposite side of the bed from where you will be working. Lower the rail on the side you are working.

12. Assist the patient into a comfortable position.

13. Place a bath blanket over the top linens. Then fanfold the linens (fold them back on themselves) underneath to prevent exposing the patient.

14. Expose only the affected body part and place the waterproof drape (if available) around it. If a waterproof drape is not available, use a disposable protective pad.

15. Make a cuff at the top of the plastic bag and place it within reach.

16. Wash your hands or use hand sanitizer to ensure infection control.

17. Put on disposable gloves and PPE, as required.

18. Remove tape or Montgomery straps to expose the existing dressing.

19. If needed, wet a 4×4 dressing with tape-adhesive remover and clean around the tape for easier removal. Always wipe away from the dressing.

20. Remove each layer of the existing dressing, starting with the top dressing. A licensed nursing staff member may also perform this task. Place the used dressings in the plastic bag.

Best Practice
Avoid allowing the patient to see the soiled side of the dressing, as this may make the patient feel uncomfortable.

21. Very gently remove the dressing that covers the wound. A licensed nursing staff member may also perform this task. If the dressing sticks to the wound or to the drain site, moisten the dressing with saline before removing it. Place the used dressing in the plastic bag.

22. Observe the wound, wound drainage, and the drain site. A licensed nursing staff member will likely inspect the wound.

23. Remove your gloves and place them in the plastic bag.

24. Wash your hands or use hand sanitizer to ensure infection control.

25. Put on a new pair of disposable gloves.

26. Open new dressings and cut the length of tape needed.

27. Clean the wound with saline or another solution, as directed by the licensed nursing staff. Start cleaning at the top of the wound and work your way down to the bottom. Clean by stroking out and away from the wound toward the surrounding skin. Use a new piece of gauze for each stroke. Place soiled gauze in the plastic bag.

28. Apply clean dressings as directed by the licensed nursing staff. Do not touch the side of the dressing that will cover the wound.

29. Secure the dressings in place using tape or Montgomery straps. Nonallergenic tape is available if the resident has an allergy.

30. Remove your gloves and place them in the plastic bag.

31. Wash your hands or use hand sanitizer to ensure infection control.

32. Put on a new pair of disposable gloves.

33. Cover the patient with the top linens and remove the bath blanket by rolling it up, with the patient side facing inward, underneath the top linens.

34. Discard used supplies in the plastic bag. Ask the licensed nursing staff member if he or she would like to see the soiled dressing. Tie the plastic bag and discard it according to facility policy.

35. Remove and discard your gloves.

36. Wash your hands or use hand sanitizer to ensure infection control.

37. Put on a new pair of disposable gloves.

38. Check to be sure the bed wheels are locked, then reposition the patient and lower the bed.

39. Follow the plan of care to determine if the side rails should be raised or lowered.

40. Remove, clean, and store equipment in the proper location. Remove soiled linens and discard disposable equipment.

Follow-Up

41. Remove and discard your gloves.

42. Wash your hands to ensure infection control.

43. Make sure the patient is comfortable and place the call light and personal items within reach.

44. Conduct a safety check before leaving the room. The room should be clean and free from clutter or spills.

45. Wash your hands or use hand sanitizer before leaving the room.

Reporting and Documentation

46. Communicate any specific observations, complications, or unusual responses to the licensed nursing staff. Record this information, along with the care provided, in the chart or EMR.

Image courtesy thodonal88/Shutterstock.com

Sterile Dressings

Sterile dressings are applied in a sterile field. A **sterile field** is an area that is free from living microorganisms. A sterile field may be required for changing the dressing of a wound with microorganisms or for performing specific procedures. Only equipment and supplies that have been sterilized can be placed or used in a sterile field. Specific guidelines help maintain a sterile field:

- Sterile gloves and drapes are used to secure and maintain the sterile field.
- The 1-inch margin, or space, around the sterile field is considered sterile. Any area beyond that margin is considered contaminated.
- Nonsterile items should never be used. Sterile gloves or sterile forceps are used to touch other sterile items in the sterile field.
- You should never turn your back on the sterile field or leave the sterile field unattended, as the sterile field may become contaminated without your knowing.

- You should check the expiration dates on all sterile items before using them. A sterile package that is open, torn, punctured, moist, or wet is contaminated. Note that some sterile items do not expire and remain sterile as long as the packaging is intact and stored properly.
- The sterile field must remain dry. Anything in the sterile field that becomes wet by a nonsterile item is contaminated.
- Airborne microorganisms can contaminate sterile items or the sterile field. To avoid this, prevent drafts and do not cough, sneeze, talk, or laugh. If you need to talk during a procedure, wear a mask.
- Any time an item or the sterile field has been contaminated, remove the contaminated item and correct the procedure. If necessary, start over with sterile supplies.

As a nursing assistant, you may be asked to wear sterile gloves to help maintain a sterile field or assist with sterile procedures or dressing changes.

Procedure | Putting On and Removing Sterile Gloves

Rationale

Only sterile items can touch other sterile items. Therefore, sterile gloves must be worn when performing any sterile procedure.

Preparation

1. Locate a package of sterile gloves in the correct size. Sterile gloves should have both an outer and inner package. Check that the gloves have not expired. Inspect the package to ensure it is dry and free from tears, holes, punctures, or watermarks.

2. Arrange the area in which you will be putting on the sterile gloves. Ensure that you have enough room to maintain a sterile field.

3. Prepare the work surface so it is at waist level and within your sight.

4. Clean and dry the work surface.

> **Best Practice**
> Do not turn your back on the sterile field or leave the sterile field unattended.

5. Wash your hands or use hand sanitizer to ensure infection control.

6. If a gown is required, put the gown on before putting on the gloves.

The Procedure: Putting On Sterile Gloves

7. Open the outer package of the gloves by grasping and gently peeling back the flaps.

8. Remove the inner package. Place it on the work surface.

9. Read the manufacturer's instructions on the inner package. The package should be labeled with directional terms such as *right*, *left*, *up*, and *down*.

10. Arrange the inner package on the work surface so that the right glove lies near your right hand and the left glove lies near your left hand. The cuffs of the gloves should lie near you, and the fingers of the gloves should point away from you.

11. Using the thumb and index finger of each hand, grasp the folded edges of the inner package.

12. Fold back the inner package to expose the gloves (Figure 15.38).

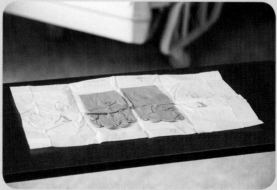

Figure 15.38

> **Best Practice**
> The inside of the sterile package is a sterile field. Do not touch or otherwise contaminate the inside of the package or the gloves.

13. Each glove will have a cuff about 2–3 inches wide. The cuffs and insides of the gloves are *not* considered sterile.

14. Pick up one glove at the cuff with your thumb, index finger, and middle finger. If you are right-handed, put on the right glove first. If you are left-handed, put on the left glove first. Always pick up a glove with the opposite hand.

15. Turn your hand so that the palm side of the glove faces up. Lift the cuff up and slide your fingers and hand into the glove (Figure 15.39).

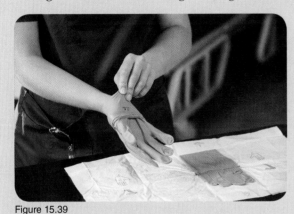

Figure 15.39

16. Pull the glove up over your hand. If some of your fingers get stuck, leave them that way until you put on the other glove. Do not use your ungloved hand to straighten the glove.

> **Best Practice**
> Do not let the outside of the glove touch any nonsterile surface.

17. Leave the cuff turned down on the second glove.

18. Reach under the cuff of the second glove using the four fingers of your gloved hand (Figure 15.40). Be careful not to contaminate your thumb.

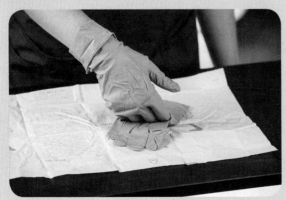

Figure 15.40

19. With your fingers under the cuff, put on the second glove. Your gloved hand should not touch the cuff itself or any surface.

20. Adjust each glove for comfort with the opposite hand.

21. Slide your fingers under the cuffs to pull them up.

22. Touch only sterile items while wearing sterile gloves.

> **Best Practice**
> Keep your gloved hands and the sterile field above your waist. To avoid possible contamination, interlace your fingers away from your scrubs while waiting for the procedure.

The Procedure: Removing Sterile Gloves

23. Grasp one gloved hand just below the cuff with the gloved fingers of your other hand.

24. Pull the cuff of the glove down, drawing it over your hand and turning it inside out.

25. Pull the glove off your hand and hold it in the palm of your other, gloved hand.

26. Insert your ungloved fingers under the cuff of the remaining glove.

27. Slowly pull the glove off, turning it inside out and drawing it over the first glove.

28. Drop both gloves into the appropriate waste container.

> **Best Practice**
> Never reuse sterile gloves.

Follow-Up

29. Wash your hands to ensure infection control.

Reporting and Documentation

This is an accepted, standard procedure. It does not need to be reported or documented.

Image courtesy of © Tori Soper Photography

Using the Key Terms

Complete the following sentences using key terms in this section.

1. _____ are wounds caused by rubbing or friction on the surface of the skin.
2. Wounds that break the skin are called _____.
3. A(n) _____ is an area that is aseptic.
4. _____ are swollen wounds caused by broken or damaged blood vessels.
5. Wounds that tear body tissue, resulting in ragged edges, are _____.
6. A(n) _____ is any injury to body tissue.
7. Tissue damage causes _____, or liquid that drains from a wound.
8. In _____, extreme cold temperatures cause freezing and damage to body tissues.

Know and Understand the Facts

9. What is the difference between a penetrating and nonpenetrating wound? Give two examples of each.
10. Describe two types of wounds that are neither penetrating or nonpentrating.
11. What three properties should be observed, reported, and documented about wound drainage?
12. List three guidelines for maintaining a sterile field.

Analyze and Apply Concepts

13. List the steps for changing a nonsterile dressing.
14. Describe the type of wound drainage that may indicate the presence of an infection.
15. What should be done if a sterile field becomes contaminated?
16. Explain the correct procedure for putting on and removing sterile gloves.

Think Critically

Read the following care situation. Then answer the questions that follow.

Mr. Y was admitted to a skilled care facility with a large wound on his left arm. He is Asian-American, 78 years old, and frail. He has had this wound intermittently for the past year, and his doctor feels that regular, supervised dressing changes will improve healing. Amelia, a nursing assistant, is assigned to Mr. Y's care. When Amelia enters Mr. Y's room, she observes that Mr. Y is holding his arm close and breathing quickly. When Amelia asks if Mr. Y is in pain, he smiles and says, "No." Amelia is assigned to change Mr. Y's first nonsterile dressing.

17. What should Amelia do to follow up on her observations prior to the dressing change? Should Amelia change the dressing even if she believes Mr. Y is in pain? Explain your answer.
18. What questions regarding Mr. Y's wound should Amelia ask the charge nurse before changing Mr. Y's dressing?
19. Describe how Amelia should clean the wound during the dressing change.

Key Points

Reviewing the key points for this chapter will help you practice more safely and competently as a holistic nursing assistant and will help you prepare for the certification competency examination.

- Asepsis, or the absence of microorganisms, is important for preventing the spread of infection.

- Standard precautions (hand hygiene, PPE, respiratory hygiene, cough etiquette, safe injection practices and handling of sharps, and careful management of potentially contaminated equipment or surfaces) and transmission-based precautions (contact precautions; droplet precautions; airborne precautions; enteric, wound, and skin precautions; bloodborne pathogen precautions; and isolation) prevent and control infection.

- Exposure control plans establish procedures to prevent exposure to contaminated blood or bodily fluids.

- Dressings may be wet or dry, sterile or nonsterile. Sterile dressings require sterile gloves and a sterile field. Nonsterile dressings help prevent contamination and absorb drainage.

Action Steps to Holistic Care

Review the information in this chapter. Complete the following activities.

1. With a partner, practice the procedures for donning and doffing personal protective equipment (PPE). Use disposable gloves, a gown, and face mask. Take turns practicing the procedures and evaluating each other's performance. Note any steps in the procedures that your partner performed incorrectly or forgot. Afterwards, review the procedures to reacquaint yourself with any steps you may have performed inaccurately or forgotten.

2. With a partner, prepare a poster about taking care of a resident in isolation. Include infection control, transmission-based precautions, and supportive approaches and actions.

3. Find two pictures in a magazine, in a newspaper, or online that best represent the two categories of wounds. Explain why you selected each picture.

4. Research sterile and nonsterile dressings. Write a brief report describing three current facts not covered in this chapter.

 Preparing for the Certification Competency Examination

To prepare for the nursing assistant certification competency examination, you will need to know content found in this chapter. This content may be tested in the knowledge (written or oral) and skills (hands-on demonstration) portions of the exam. The following areas will be emphasized:

- infection control procedures, including hand hygiene and PPE
- standard and transmission-based precautions
- bloodborne pathogen standards
- respiratory hygiene and cough etiquette
- sterile dressings
- maintenance of sterile fields
- procedure for putting on and removing sterile gloves
- exposure control plan and reporting

These sample test questions are similar to ones you will find on the certification competency exam. See how well you can answer them. Be sure to select the *best* answer.

1. Standard precautions include which of the following?
   A. isolation techniques
   B. the use of sterile gloves
   C. cleansing draining wounds
   D. proper hand washing

2. What is the most important guideline for caring for a resident in isolation?
   A. being very careful when touching the resident
   B. not giving some care because the resident is in isolation
   C. wearing PPE when caring for the resident
   D. ensuring all supplies and equipment are sterile

(continued)

3. When nursing assistants are exposed to a blood spill or splash, what is the first thing they should do?

   A. put on a pair of new gloves and a mask
   B. follow the healthcare facility's exposure control plan
   C. keep working until finished and then alert the charge nurse
   D. wipe off the blood with a sterile dressing

4. Transmission-based precautions include

   A. infection precautions
   B. pathogen precautions
   C. contact precautions
   D. respiratory precautions

5. A resident has a wound that is swollen and bruised. What is this called?

   A. laceration
   B. contusion
   C. concussion
   D. abrasion

6. What type of isolation is used when a patient's resistance and immunity to microorganisms are low?

   A. respiratory isolation
   B. strict isolation
   C. protective isolation
   D. pathogenic isolation

7. Which of the following is an example of a penetrating wound?

   A. abrasion
   B. rash
   C. frostbite
   D. cut

8. Which of the following is a guideline for ensuring proper hand hygiene?

   A. use a hand sanitizer for at least 20 seconds
   B. dry your hands thoroughly after turning off the faucet
   C. wash your hands for at least 10 seconds
   D. use only very hot water and alcohol-based soap

9. Mr. J requires a procedure in a sterile field. Which guideline should be followed?

   A. keep all items at least 1 inch outside the field
   B. only use sterile items in the sterile field
   C. wear clean, disposable gloves
   D. check with the charge nurse to see what equipment will be needed

10. When removing a gown, a nursing assistant should

    A. remove gloves last
    B. pull the gown off and leave on gloves
    C. remove gloves first
    D. be sure the gown is folded carefully after use

11. Mrs. G has just been discharged, and the nursing assistant has been asked to clean the room. What is the most important thing the nursing assistant should do?

    A. leave items left in the room to be picked up later by the family
    B. return all clean linen to the linen closet
    C. keep all unused, disposable items for later use
    D. wash the bed, bedside table, and chair with disinfectant solution

12. The inside of a sterile package of gloves is considered

    A. clean
    B. dirty
    C. contaminated
    D. sterile

13. Which of the following is an important factor in helping a wound heal?

    A. vigorous exercise
    B. proper nutrition
    C. walking often
    D. massaging the wound

14. A patient has just been put into isolation and is very depressed. What could a nursing assistant do to provide holistic care?

    A. tell the patient not to worry, as this is only a temporary measure
    B. talk with the family and ask them to bring something the patient likes
    C. explain why being in isolation is important right now
    D. avoid going into the room, as not to disturb the patient

15. Hand hygiene must be used

    A. before handling a meal tray
    B. after charting
    C. before going to a meeting
    D. after eating a meal

Did you have difficulty with any of the questions? If you did, review the chapter to find the correct answer(s).

Welcome to the Chapter

This chapter provides information you will need to understand to maintain a safe culture and environment for yourself and those in your care. This chapter will focus on identifying potential hazards, preventing common accidents and injuries, properly reporting safety issues, and keeping residents free from harm. You will also learn about quality measures for maintaining a safe culture, the need for safety plans, safety awareness, and the importance of safety checks.

What you learn in this chapter will help you develop your knowledge and skills to become a holistic nursing assistant. The topics discussed in the chapter are highlighted on the Providing Holistic Care Framework.

You are now ready to start this chapter, *Maintaining a Safe Environment and Practice.*

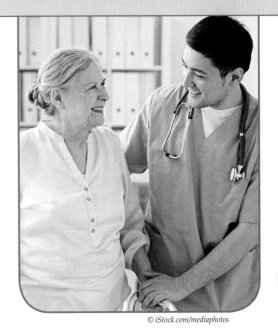

© iStock.com/mediaphotos

Chapter Outline

Section 16.1
A Culture and Environment of Safety

Section 16.2
Fall Prevention

Section 16.3
Restraint-Free Care

Section 16.4
Fire, Electrical, Chemical, and Oxygen Safety

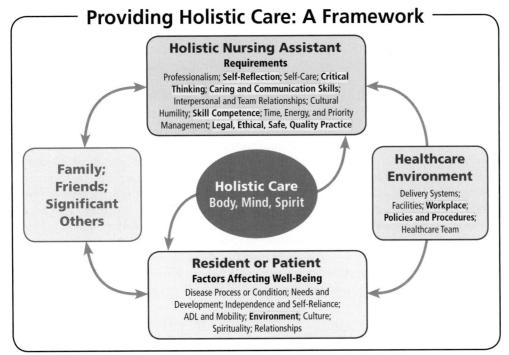

Providing Holistic Care: A Framework

Holistic Nursing Assistant
Requirements
Professionalism; **Self-Reflection**; Self-Care; **Critical Thinking**; **Caring and Communication Skills**; Interpersonal and Team Relationships; Cultural Humility; **Skill Competence**; Time, Energy, and Priority Management; **Legal, Ethical, Safe, Quality Practice**

Family; Friends; Significant Others

Holistic Care
Body, Mind, Spirit

Healthcare Environment
Delivery Systems; Facilities; **Workplace**; **Policies and Procedures**; Healthcare Team

Resident or Patient
Factors Affecting Well-Being
Disease Process or Condition; Needs and Development; Independence and Self-Reliance; ADL and Mobility; **Environment**; Culture; Spirituality; Relationships

Questions to Consider

- Safety is an essential need that all people share. How would you define *safety*?
- How do you ensure that you and those important in your life remain safe?
- When you become a nursing assistant, what safety practices do you think will become most important?

Objectives

To safely provide care as a holistic nursing assistant, you must make safety and the removal of potential hazards a part of your everyday awareness, attitudes, and behaviors. To achieve the objectives for this section, you must successfully

- **describe** the importance of a culture of safety, safety checks, and compliance with the healthcare facility's safety plans;
- **identify** potential hazards, common accidents and injuries, and ways to prevent and properly report these issues; and
- **include** safety awareness and risk prevention as essential parts of daily nursing assistant practice.

Key Terms

Learn these key terms to better understand the information presented in the section.

always events
clinically adverse events
culture of safety
entrapment
harm

near misses
needlesticks
never events
transparency

Safety has always been an essential and desired outcome in healthcare, and it is more important today than ever. In 1999, the Institute of Medicine (IOM) published the landmark report *To Err Is Human*, which shocked healthcare providers and the public by finding that 98,000 deaths per year were due to medical errors. Many of these deaths were preventable. *To Err Is Human* was the first of many IOM reports that continue to raise awareness about the hazards and potential harm that can occur during healthcare delivery.

Along with the IOM and other reports, both government and private agencies determined that quality and safety were extremely important and that specific measures of quality and safety should be regularly monitored and reported by and about hospitals and long-term care facilities. As a result, the performance of healthcare facilities in reporting and meeting set standards is now tied to financial reimbursement. If care given in a facility does not meet safety and quality standards, Medicare and some insurance companies may not reimburse the facility for the cost of care.

The Centers for Medicare & Medicaid Services (CMS) monitors quality measures such as clinical care, patient outcomes, and recent hospital experiences. Quality measures also exist for other types of facilities. Long-term care facilities are required to perform initial assessments on admission, to conduct periodic assessments over the course of a resident's stay, and to develop *minimum data sets (MDSs)* that set a foundation for the assessment of all residents. Assessment information is used to help develop, review, and revise the resident's plan of care with the goal of coordinating care and services to enable the highest possible physical, mental, and psychosocial well-being. A *resident assessment instrument (RAI)* must be used to gather specific information and ensure residents are provided a level of care that promotes quality of life.

Remember

Safety isn't just a slogan; it's a way of life.

Anonymous

What Does Safety Mean in Healthcare?

Quality of care and safety are interconnected. A healthcare facility must use safe practices to attain expected and required quality standards and measures. Safety encompasses many dimensions. For example, both the environment and the equipment used must be safe. Healthcare staff members must maintain safety standards and follow facility safety plans to ensure their safety and the safety of patients, residents, family members, and other visitors (Figure 16.1).

Being safe and promoting safety are important responsibilities of holistic nursing assistants. Several definitions of safety are commonly used in healthcare. Familiarizing yourself with these definitions is important, as facilities may use one or more to direct their facility safety plans.

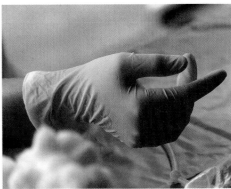

Pornprasit/Shutterstock.com

Figure 16.1 Safety standards, such as the use of PPE, ensure the safety of both healthcare staff and residents.

The World Health Organization (WHO) defines patient safety as the prevention of errors and harmful effects to patients. *Unsafe events* are processes or acts of omission (not doing the right thing) or commission (doing the wrong thing) that result in hazardous healthcare conditions or **harm** (unintended injury). The Agency for Healthcare Research and Quality (AHRQ) defines patient safety as freedom from accidental or preventable injuries resulting from medical care. Care that improves patient safety reduces the occurrence of preventable, harmful outcomes.

The IOM holds that people should not be harmed by care intended to help them. Care should be based on sound scientific knowledge and should respond to individual preferences, needs, and values. Unnecessary waits and harmful delays should be reduced, and care should not be wasteful or vary in quality due to patient diversity. Safety is an important requirement for patient care delivery, and healthcare facilities must demonstrate **transparency** (honesty) in reporting safety issues.

Finally, the National Quality Forum (NQF) states that safety practices are processes that provide evidence-based care, reduce the likelihood of harm, and maximize the likelihood of avoiding errors with effective systems and processes.

Definitions of safety should guide your practice as a holistic nursing assistant. Following are important guidelines drawn from the main points of these commonly accepted safety definitions and standards:

- Be aware and mindful of safety at all times.
- Always work to prevent errors or harm.
- Learn from errors that do occur.
- Work to assure a culture of safety that includes all healthcare staff members, facilities, patients, and residents.

How Can You Recognize a Culture of Safety?

The Centers for Disease Control and Prevention (CDC) defines a **culture of safety** as the shared commitment of a healthcare facility's leadership and staff to ensure a safe work environment. A healthcare facility with a culture of safety has the necessary systems, procedures, and teamwork to achieve safe, high-quality performance from the nursing and healthcare staff. Healthcare facilities that enjoy a culture of safety promote the occurrence of **always events**. Always events are routine activities and processes that are so important they must be performed reliably and consistently; always events result in effective admissions, transfers, discharges, and handoffs (change-of-shift reporting, for example).

It is impossible to eliminate all errors in a healthcare facility. When errors occur in a culture of safety, the focus is on *what happened*, not on *who did it*. The goal of this approach is to bring failures and issues out into the open immediately and deal with them in a blame-free, nonbiased, and nonthreatening way. As a result, in a culture of safety, **clinically adverse events** (medical errors) and **near misses** (unplanned health outcomes that do not cause harm) can be reported without fear of punishment. A culture of safety is always willing to address and resolve all safety concerns.

Sometimes nursing and healthcare staff members may not think or act safely due to lack of time, inexperience, or shortcuts. This type of behavior does not support a culture of safety. To create a culture of safety, holistic nursing assistants must

- abide by all safety principles, policies, and procedures;
- be aware of safety issues;
- pay attention to how personal, cultural, and ethnic differences impact safety;
- voice opinions and concerns to the charge nurse;
- suggest solutions to problems;
- report errors both informally to the charge nurse and formally through documentation; and
- report errors in a timely and specific way using the facility's policy, procedure, and forms.

Using a safety-oriented approach demonstrates that you value and are committed to your own personal safety and the safety of others.

How Do Nursing Assistants Ensure Safety?

Hazards and accident risks for residents in long-term care facilities include falls; burns; decubitus ulcers; blood clots; medication errors; healthcare-associated infections (HAIs), such as *Staphylococcus* (staph) or urinary tract infections and pneumonia; and entrapment. The majority of these complications are temporary and treatable; however, some of them may cause life-threatening injuries or even contribute to death. Holistic nursing assistants are responsible for ensuring resident safety by avoiding never events, preventing accidents, conducting safety checks, preventing sharps-related injuries, and following facility safety plans.

Avoiding Never Events

Never events are actions or errors that lead to serious resident harm, disability, or death. Never events are serious, reportable events and are grouped into seven categories: surgical events, product or device events, resident protection events, care management events, environmental events, radiologic events, and criminal events. Some examples of never events are

- a fall while a resident is receiving care;
- an infection or decubitus ulcer due to improper or lack of care; or
- a burn (from any source) from a procedure.

As a holistic nursing assistant, you must avoid never events by always following facility policy and practicing safely.

Preventing Accidents

Preventing accidents requires personal awareness of safety hazards, safety promotion, safety policies and the facility's safety plan, risks, safety equipment, and infection prevention and control. For example, as a nursing assistant, you can prevent falls by understanding and reducing their risks. Following these general guidelines will help you ensure resident safety by reducing the risk of an accident:

- Before providing care, always check the resident's identification to be sure you are providing care to the correct resident. You will need two identifiers to verify the resident, such as name, a facility-assigned identification number or bar code, date of birth, phone number, social security number, address, or photo. In most instances, you would say the resident's name, ask the resident to give you his or her name, and compare the name with

Think About This

Cultures use colors differently to signal warnings or danger. In the United States, the color red is often used as a warning to signal danger. Healthcare facilities use red or sometimes orange to identify hazards. Other cultures may use different colors to communicate warnings. Chinese culture, for example, uses the color yellow for this purpose.

the identification bracelet (Figure 16.2). In some healthcare facilities, such as in assisted living, residents prefer not to wear identification bracelets as they do not want to be seen as ill or feel as if they are in a hospital setting, where ID bracelets are common. Rather, these residents may be identified by at least one identifier verification and their photo, which can be found in the EMR (Figure 16.2). You may need to verify the identification of residents who are unable to communicate. Follow facility policy for identification verification.

- Make sure there is adequate lighting when you work around and with residents.

- When transferring residents between beds, stretchers, or wheelchairs, always lock the equipment wheels before moving the resident.

- Make sure all equipment is in good repair and functions properly.

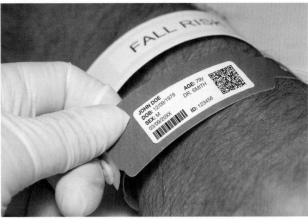

Sherry Yates Young/Shutterstock.com

Figure 16.2 Checking the identification bracelet can ensure you are delivering care to the correct resident.

Conducting a Safety Check

Safety checks play an important role in reducing risks and preventing accidents. A safety check should be performed as you give care in a resident's room and always before you leave the resident's room. During a safety check, make sure the resident is safe and comfortable in bed, in a chair, or in a wheelchair. The bed or wheelchair must be in the locked position so that it does not roll when the resident moves into or out of the bed or wheelchair. If side rails are used on the bed, the resident must be situated to prevent **entrapment**, a harmful event in which the resident falls between the bed and side rails. Entrapment can cause injury or death. If side rails are not used, the bed must be placed in its lowest position so the resident does not fall.

After positioning a resident properly, check that any tubing (from an IV or Foley catheter, for example) is attached properly and is not kinked. Place the call light in an accessible place for the resident. Pick up any debris or items on the floor, clean up any spills on the floor, and position any furniture or obstacles so they will not get in the way if the resident moves around the room.

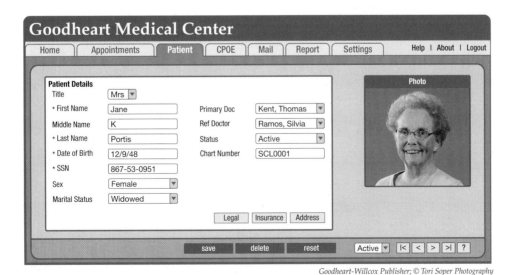

Goodheart-Willcox Publisher; © Tori Soper Photography

Figure 16.3 Upon admission, a resident's photograph is normally taken and saved in the EMR to be used for identification purposes.

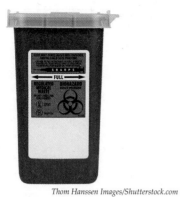

Thom Hanssen Images/Shutterstock.com

Figure 16.4 Used sharps and needles should be disposed of in sharps containers.

Preventing Sharps-Related Injuries and Needlesticks

Sharps-related injuries are caused by sharp objects (such as razors, broken glass, or rough edges) that break the skin. **Needlesticks** are punctures of the skin by needles (for example, from an IV catheter or medication). These pose another safety risk, as puncture wounds from used needles can transmit pathogens. When handling exposed sharps or needles, pay attention to the safety of the resident and other staff. Visually inspect trays and other surfaces (including the bed) that may contain waste materials from a procedure. Make sure no sharps or needles are left behind after procedures.

Sharps and needles must be disposed of in designated *sharps containers* (Figure 16.4). When disposing of sharps and needles, do not bring your hands close to the opening of the sharps container and never place your hands or fingers into the container. Visually inspect the sharps container for hazards, such as overfilling, which can cause injuries from exposed sharps.

Following Facility Safety Plans

The *facility safety plan* outlines policies and procedures that need to be followed by all healthcare staff. These plans comply with federal, state, and local laws and regulations related to health and safety. They also comply with facility-specific requirements. Facilities often have departments or staff responsible for maintaining and updating the plan, investigating and reducing or removing hazards or risks, and conducting research to achieve compliance. Facility safety plans usually include regulations and guidelines related to the following workplace safety concerns:

- fire safety
- biosafety (related to the treatment of human blood, bodily fluids, body tissues, or pathogenic organisms)
- radiation and chemical safety
- hazardous waste and materials (HAZMAT) management and emergency response
- accident investigation and mitigation (to reduce or remove accident risks)

What Work Hazards Affect Nursing Assistants?

The Occupational Safety and Health Administration (OSHA) estimates that 5.6 million nursing and healthcare staff members are at risk for occupational exposure to bloodborne pathogens such as HIV, the hepatitis B virus (HBV), and the hepatitis C virus (HVC). To reduce these risks, nursing assistants should follow the bloodborne pathogen precautions outlined in chapter 15. Other safety hazards include needlesticks, sharps-related injuries, and musculoskeletal disorders (MSDs).

Nursing staff members have reported high rates of MSDs, such as back and shoulder injuries (Figure 16.5). The most common cause of MSDs is moving and repositioning residents. Other risk factors for developing MSDs include

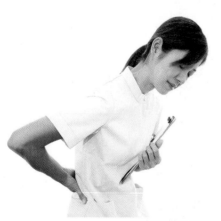

sunabesyou/Shutterstock.com

Figure 16.5 MSDs and back pain are common among nursing staff.

- overexerting;
- performing multiple lifts;
- lifting a resident alone;
- lifting uncooperative or confused residents;
- lifting residents who cannot support their weight or who are heavy;
- performing work beyond one's physical capabilities;

- moving an object or resident improperly;
- moving a resident in a confined space or awkward position; and
- not being adequately trained in body mechanics (see chapter 17).

As a nursing assistant, you will be responsible for following safety principles and practices at all times, both during work and in your everyday life. Being aware and taking extra steps to prevent hazards and harm can make a difference in your life and in the lives of others.

Section 16.1 Review and Assessment

Using the Key Terms

Complete the following sentences using key terms in this section.

1. When an error occurs in a(n) _____, the focus is on what happened, not who did it.
2. In _____, residents experience harm when they fall between the bed and side rails.
3. Unintended physical injury is known as _____.
4. _____ are unplanned health outcomes that do not cause harm.
5. A(n) _____ is a puncture wound from a needle.
6. Serious events that result in harm, death, or significant disability are called _____.
7. A culture of safety is characterized by _____, or honesty.
8. _____ are routine activities and processes that are so important they must be performed reliably and consistently.
9. Medical errors are also known as _____.

Know and Understand the Facts

10. List three common hazards or risks for residents in healthcare facilities.
11. What is the difference between an always event and a never event?
12. In a culture of safety, what is the goal of dealing with errors?
13. Why are safety checks important?
14. What is a safety plan, and what does it usually include?

Analyze and Apply Concepts

15. What are the characteristics of a culture of safety?
16. How can a nursing assistant help maintain a culture of safety?
17. List three actions a holistic nursing assistant should perform when conducting a safety check.

Think Critically

Read the following care scenario. Then answer the questions that follow.

Veronica has cared for older adults at her facility for the past five years and prides herself in the care she provides. She feels that all healthcare staff members should have the same level of commitment. Yesterday, Veronica saw Daniel, another nursing assistant, taking care of Mrs. G, who is 85 years old and has Alzheimer's disease. Mrs. G had a cold, and Daniel did not wash his hands when he entered the room. Daniel also did not make sure Mrs. G was safe in her bed when he briefly left the room. This is not the first time Veronica has noticed Daniel's lack of safety awareness.

18. What risks or safety hazards did Veronica observe?
19. Should Veronica mind her own business or should she report Daniel's actions? Explain your answer.
20. If Veronica does report Daniel's actions, what should she say, and whom should she tell?

Questions to Consider

- Falls are more common among older adults; however, OSHA reports that slips, trips, and falls cause 15 percent of all accidental deaths, second only to traffic fatalities. Have you experienced a fall? What was its cause?
- Could the fall you experienced have been prevented? If so, explain what you could have done.

Objectives

To help prevent residents from falling, you must be aware of fall risks and ways to avoid them. To achieve the objectives for this section, you must successfully

- **identify** the causes of falls and those who are at risk for falling;
- **describe** ways to prevent falls; and
- **explain** what a nursing assistant should do if a resident falls.

Key Terms

Learn these key terms to better understand the information presented in the section.

commode   hypothermia

gait   incident report

gait belt   osteoporosis

Falls can cause serious injury, especially for older adults. One out of every three adults age 65 or older falls each year. More falls occur as a person ages. Those who fall once are likely to fall again.

Falls cause 25 percent of all hospital admissions and 40 percent of admissions to long-term care facilities. Most falls occur in a resident's room between 10:00 p.m. and 6:30 a.m. This window of time poses more risks because there are usually fewer staff members and less activity in a resident's room at night. Residents are more likely to leave their beds to go to the bathroom without asking for assistance and may fall.

Twenty to thirty percent of people who fall suffer moderate-to-severe injuries such as dislocations, bruising, cuts to the skin, muscle tears, hip fractures, or head traumas. Injuries are more likely to affect residents who have **osteoporosis** (a condition of porous bones). Bones weakened by osteoporosis increase a person's risk of falling, and if a person with osteoporosis does fall, the injury is usually more severe.

What Causes Falls?

Falls happen for a variety of reasons. Inadequate handrails, a slippery tub, an icy sidewalk, or even a pet can cause a person to fall. Falls can also occur because of poor or unstable footwear and insufficient lighting. Health issues may also increase a person's risk of falling. For example, low blood pressure, sensory loss, stroke, dementia, medications, and nervous system disorders such as Parkinson's disease can cause a person to fall. A person's ability to get up after a fall can also affect the outcome. Immobility after a fall can cause complications such as dehydration, decubitus ulcers, **hypothermia** (a condition of low body temperature), and pneumonia.

Older adults need to be particularly cautious about falls, as age alone is a significant risk factor. Many older adults rely on assistive devices such as walkers and canes; however, these devices can increase the risk of falling if they fit poorly or are defective. An older adult is also more likely to fall if he or she has difficulty with balance, strength, perception, vision, range of motion, or coordination. Twenty to thirty percent of older adults fear falling.

When caring for a resident who may be at risk for falling, you should always pay attention to his or her

- balance and strength;
- potential loss of sensation or sensory impairment;
- level of vision and hearing; and
- joint range of motion and **gait** (manner of walking).

Balance, gait, muscle, or range-of-motion exercises can be very helpful for preventing falls in some residents. Building strength and balance also promotes self-confidence, which decreases a resident's likelihood of falling.

How Can Falls Be Prevented?

Holistic nursing assistants play a vital role in preventing residents from falling. The first step in preventing falls is identifying residents who are at risk for falls. Usually, a doctor, licensed nursing staff member, or physical therapist will conduct an assessment of a resident. This assessment will review a resident's medications, any fall risk factors, and strategies to overcome risks. This assessment forms the basis of the *fall risk program*, which is developed as part of the resident's plan of care.

Identification of Residents with Increased Fall Risk

Healthcare facilities often use a visual alert, such as a sign, picture, or wristband, to indicate that a resident has an increased risk for falling. Fall risk images are located either within a resident's room or in the hall near the doorway (Figure 16.6). Some facilities may use resident seat monitors, bed and chair exit alarms, and wrist or room motion monitors to alert nursing staff that an at-risk resident is mobile without assistance. A resident's independence must always be balanced with safety needs.

Observation and Prevention Strategies

There are many fall-prevention strategies that holistic nursing assistants can use to prevent resident harm. First, work slowly and steadily when you provide assistance with ADLs and ambulation. Do not rush residents. Follow the acronym *ACT*:

- be **A**ware.
- **C**orrect risks.
- **T**ake precautions.

Strong observation skills can help prevent resident falls. Holistic nursing assistants should frequently monitor and observe residents and listen for calls for help, banging, or falling objects. In facilities that use bed and chair alarms, nursing assistants can listen for alarms that signal a resident's weight has been removed.

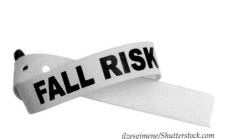

ilzesgimene/Shutterstock.com

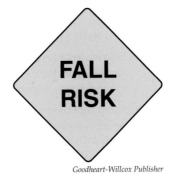

FALL RISK

Goodheart-Willcox Publisher

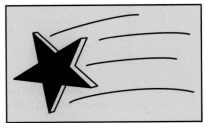

Goodheart-Willcox Publisher

Figure 16.6 Fall risk bracelets, signs, and falling stars signal that a resident has an increased risk for falling.

The following guidelines will also help holistic nursing assistants practice safely and prevent falls:

- Ensure a working call light is always within each resident's reach. Instruct residents to call for assistance instead of trying to get up themselves. Answer call lights promptly.
- Keep the resident's bed at the lowest possible level and place mats around the bed, if necessary. If side rails are used, keep them in the down position for mobile residents.
- Make sure the resident's room is well lit and does not have glare (especially important for residents with poor eyesight).

  - Keep the room clean, dry, and uncluttered. Place the resident's personal items within his or her reach. Clean up small, nonhazardous spills immediately or block off the area if you must wait for someone to clean up the spill.
  - Check to be sure there are no wires, cords, or other tripping hazards in the room.
  - Encourage residents to use handrails and grab bars, especially in bathrooms and ambulating areas (for example, hallways). Provide shower chairs, if needed.
  - Be sure chairs are stable and sturdy, are at a good height, and have armrests to assist residents who want to stand.
  - Be aware of any changes in a resident's medications and understand how changes may affect the resident. Observe for dizziness, sleepiness, and blood pressure changes.
  - Keep a bedside **commode** (chair containing a chamber pot) nearby, so it can be used safely (Figure 16.7). If needed, install high toilet seats so residents do not have to bend down too far when using the toilet.

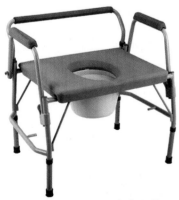

focal point/Shutterstock.com

Figure 16.7 A bedside commode can help residents eliminate without walking to the bathroom.

- Check with the licensed nursing staff before applying creams, bath oils, or powders to a resident's skin, as these substances can make surfaces slippery.
- If a resident wears eyeglasses, ensure that the eyeglasses fit properly and are nearby so the resident can reach them easily.
- Discourage residents from wearing long gowns or robes.
- Be sure that ambulatory residents have sturdy, nonskid shoes or footwear (Figure 16.8). Also ensure that canes, walkers, and chair legs have nonskid tips. Lock the wheels on beds and wheelchairs whenever a resident is moving into or out of the bed or wheelchair.
- Provide assistive devices, such as a **gait belt** (a safety device that fits around the waist), when a resident ambulates (Figure 16.9).
- If a resident begins to fall while ambulating, ease him or her down using guidelines provided in chapter 17.

Remember to always report resident falls immediately and to report any changes in a resident's condition. Document and report your observations and any actions taken. Resident safety and fall prevention should be top priorities for all nursing assistants.

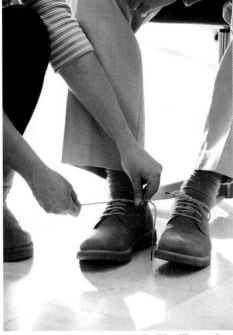

SpeedKingz/Shutterstock.com

Figure 16.8 Make sure the resident's nonskid footwear fits properly and is securely fastened, if necessary.

What Should Be Done If a Resident Falls?

If a resident falls, you must act quickly. Stay with the resident and do not move him or her, as the fall may have caused an injury, and moving the resident can make injuries worse. Alert the charge nurse immediately and then stay with the charge nurse as he or she assesses the resident. The charge nurse's assessment will determine the next action. Once the assessment is completed, the resident's vital signs may need to be taken frequently. You will need to observe the resident for unusual changes, such as headache, fever, drowsiness, dizziness, vomiting, or double vision. Be sure to notify the charge nurse if these occur.

A resident's recovery from a fall depends on the extent of injury and the resident's medical condition prior to the fall. Regaining mobility is always the goal, especially for older adults, who can rapidly lose strength and function if immobile.

An **incident report**, or *occurrence* or *accident report*, will likely be required if a resident falls. Incident reports record information about unusual events, such as resident injuries. The purpose of an incident report is to document the exact details of an incident and provide factual information for reviewing and responding to the event. Incident reports record the details of any injuries, such as falls, needlesticks, or burns; errors in care; resident complaints; faulty equipment; and incidents that put patients, residents, or staff members at risk.

An incident report must be written as soon as possible after the event. This ensures that details are not forgotten or remembered incorrectly. Incident reports are completed according to facility policy and procedure, and the appropriate facility form is used.

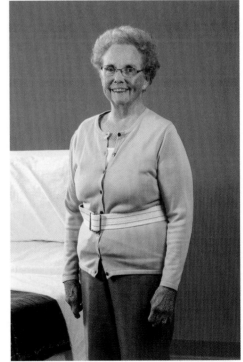

© Tori Soper Photography

Figure 16.9 When worn around the resident's waist, a gait belt allows the nursing assistant to assist the resident in standing, transferring, and ambulating.

Details should be recorded in sequence, should be complete, and should be accurate and include objective (factual) information. If subjective information is recorded, it should be directly quoted. Write only what was observed and do not make assumptions or place blame. Usually, the following information is requested:

- where and when the incident occurred
- the events surrounding the incident
- whether injury was a direct result of the incident

Reporting incidents is critical to maintaining a safe environment. Never try to cover up or hide an injury or mistake.

Remember

Safety first is safety always.

Charles M. Hayes

Section 16.2 Review and Assessment

Using the Key Terms

Complete the following sentences using key terms in this section.

1. A(n) _____ is a safety device used when a resident stands or ambulates.
2. The condition _____ is characterized by low body temperature.
3. A bedside _____ is a chair containing a chamber pot.
4. When assessing fall risk, you should pay attention to a resident's _____, or manner of walking.
5. Porous bones are a sign of _____.
6. A(n) _____ records information about an unusual event.

Know and Understand the Facts

7. What are three common causes of falls among older adults?
8. List four actions that can help prevent resident falls.
9. Describe the purpose of an incident report.
10. In which three ways can facilities alert staff that a resident is a fall risk?

Analyze and Apply Concepts

11. What does the acronym *ACT* stand for?
12. Describe the first two actions a nursing assistant should take when a resident falls.
13. Identify three important guidelines to follow when completing an incident report.
14. What might a nursing assistant be asked to observe after a resident has fallen?

Think Critically

Read the following care situation. Then answer the questions that follow.

Mr. T has been at a skilled nursing facility for only one week, and Luis, a new nursing assistant, has been assigned to take care of him. Mr. T is 73 years old, has COPD, and is very thin. He was admitted to the facility after falling several times at home and has several bruises on his arms and legs. Mr. T is very independent and does not like to use his walker. Luis has been assigned to help Mr. T with his morning shower and ensure he ambulates several times a day.

15. What are two reasons Mr. T may be considered a fall risk?
16. What actions should Luis take to prevent Mr. T from falling?
17. What should Luis do if Mr. T does fall?

Objectives

To safely provide care as a nursing assistant, you must work to achieve a restraint-free environment for residents. If the use of restraints is ordered by a resident's doctor, careful application and observation will be required. To achieve the objectives for this section, you must successfully

- **identify** different types of restraints;
- **discuss** alternative strategies to restraints;
- **identify** situations in which a restraint may be ordered; and
- **explain** how to observe, monitor, and care for residents in restraints.

Key Terms

Learn these key terms to better understand the information presented in the section.

Alzheimer's disease (AD)   restraint

range of motion (ROM)

Questions to Consider
- Have you ever been confined somewhere or held back physically from doing something?
- If so, what was it like to be restrained? How did you feel?

As a holistic nursing assistant, you will care for some residents whose physical activity requires monitoring due to disease or medications. For example, residents may be disoriented, confused, or very aggressive or may tend to wander due to dementia or **Alzheimer's disease (AD)**. AD is a degenerative brain disease that leads to memory loss, impaired thinking, disorientation, and changes in personality and mood. When residents exhibit these behaviors, doctors may order restraints to keep residents from falling or harming themselves or others. The decision to use a **restraint** (a device or substance that inhibits movement) is very difficult, and healthcare facility policies and federal and state regulations regarding the use of restraints must be followed. Preventive or alternative measures must be tried before restraints can be applied. If restraints are used, they must be ordered by a doctor and accompanied by training, careful observation, monitoring, and care.

What Is a Restraint?

A restraint is anything that prevents a resident from moving freely. Restraints can be physical or chemical. A *physical restraint* is a device, material, or equipment that is placed on or near a resident and restricts his or her freedom of movement. A *chemical restraint* is a medication that makes a resident drowsy or sleepy and unable to move freely. Restraints can only be used to treat medical conditions or prevent residents from causing physical harm to themselves or others.

If restraints are necessary, they must be used in ways that do not cause injury or emotional harm. Observation and monitoring of a restrained resident's physical and psychological status are essential and required.

Types of Physical Restraints

Only the least restrictive restraints may be applied in healthcare facilities. The type of restraint is determined by the doctor, who will choose a restraint that keeps the resident safe and also provides the greatest amount of freedom.

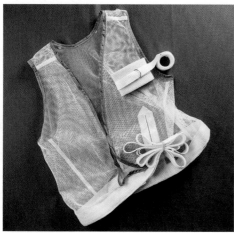

© Tori Soper Photography

Figure 16.10 A vest restraint secures a resident's trunk to a bed or chair.

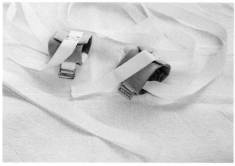

Kim M Smith/Shutterstock.com

Figure 16.11 Wrist restraints secure a resident's arms and hands to a bed or chair.

Physical restraints used in healthcare facilities should never be makeshift (like a sheet, for example). Restraints should always be designed and purchased for a particular use and should be the correct size. Some physical restraints include

- a vest or trunk restraint (Figure 16.10);
- a belt;
- soft-padded wrist or ankle restraints (Figure 16.11);
- a lap tray to keep a resident from falling forward or out of a chair; or
- a mitten used to stop a resident from pulling on a urinary catheter.

Tucking a resident into bed too tightly is considered a restraint. The side rails on a resident's bed are also considered restraints. Side rails are often used to assist with and enhance the mobility of residents, enabling residents to move in bed and get in and out of bed. When side rails prevent residents from leaving their beds or become dangerous, however, they are considered physical restraints.

Risks Associated with Restraint Use

Several risks are associated with the use of restraints. Bruises, choking, loss of muscle tone, decubitus ulcers, falls, and loss of dignity are just a few examples. Residents can become depressed, withdrawn, or agitated when their movements are restricted. The use of side rails as restraints has also led to severe injury and death, as struggling residents become trapped between the side rails and the bed mattress while trying to leave the bed. This is called *entrapment*. There are seven entrapment zones (Figure 16.12). Each entrapment zone has great potential for causing injury or death.

As a result of possible entrapment, many long-term care facilities avoid using side rails. Instead, beds are lowered close to the floor, and wheel locks are engaged for safety. If a resident is at risk for falling out of bed, mats are placed next to the lowered bed. Some beds that do have rails have *mobility rails*, which are smaller than side rails and provide handholds for residents who need help getting in and out of bed.

In long-term care centers that use side rails, licensed nursing staff members must perform ongoing assessments of the resident's physical and mental status to authorize side rail use. If used, side rails must be in proper working order. The bed used should have a proper-sized mattress or a mattress with raised foam edges. There should never be a gap wide enough to entrap a resident's head or body between the mattress and the bed or side rail. Close monitoring is required to ensure safety and determine if a resident's status has changed.

How Is a Restraint-Free Environment Promoted and Maintained?

The use of restraints is regulated by state and federal laws. For example, Medicare- and Medicaid-certified nursing homes cannot use restraints except to treat medical symptoms. Certified nursing homes must provide care that maintains or enhances residents' quality of life. As a result, the goal of care is always to keep residents free from harm using restraint alternatives.

One key action that helps avoid the use of restraints is answering call lights immediately. Answering call lights immediately prevents residents from wandering, becoming confused, or getting out of bed. Responding quickly to resident needs and

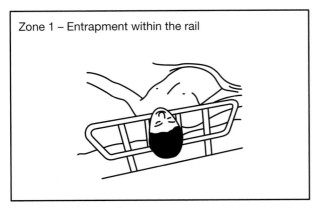

Zone 1 – Entrapment within the rail

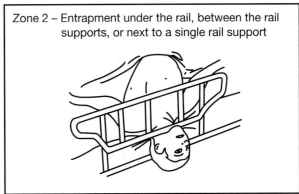

Zone 2 – Entrapment under the rail, between the rail supports, or next to a single rail support

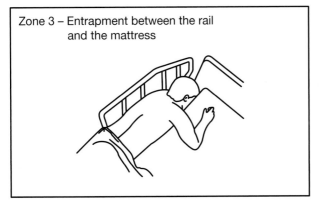

Zone 3 – Entrapment between the rail and the mattress

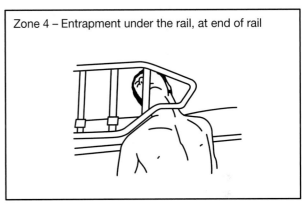

Zone 4 – Entrapment under the rail, at end of rail

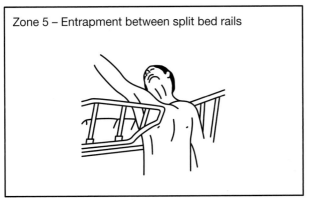

Zone 5 – Entrapment between split bed rails

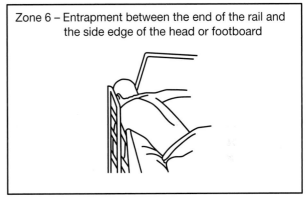

Zone 6 – Entrapment between the end of the rail and the side edge of the head or footboard

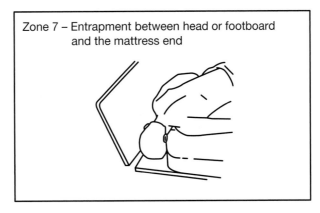

Zone 7 – Entrapment between head or footboard and the mattress end

US Food and Drug Administration

Figure 16.12 The seven entrapment zones describe the seven areas a resident can become entrapped.

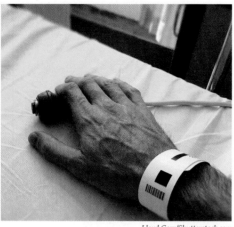

Lloyd Carr/Shutterstock.com

Figure 16.13 Easy access to a call light and a prompt response from nursing staff will reassure residents their needs will be tended to quickly, discouraging them from attempting to get out of bed when it is unsafe to do so.

offering physical, behavioral, or emotional support can be used as alternatives to restraints. Following are some other guidelines, usually directed by the plan of care, for providing alternatives to restraints:

- Place the call light close to the resident or attach the call light to the resident's gown or clothing (Figure 16.13). Remind the resident to use the call light.

- Suggest that the resident be moved to a room or bed more visible to the nursing or healthcare staff.

- Always keep the resident's bed in the lowest position possible. This reduces the risk of injury if the resident falls.

- Check on residents who are at risk for harm more often. Increase the frequency of rounds from every hour to every 15 minutes.

- Use alternative restraint devices, such as door, bed, and chair alarms or recliners that can be adjusted to upright or fully extended, reclined positions.

- Remind family members or special private sitters hired by the family to monitor the resident, particularly during the night hours.

- Place a dim night-light in the room so the resident can safely walk to the bathroom at night without tripping or falling. For residents who are not a fall risk, you might also place a bedside commode or urinal close to the bed within the resident's reach.

- Remind the resident to use grab rails in the hallways and bathrooms (Figure 16.14).

- Redirect the resident from trying to pull on a catheter, tube, or line. A long-sleeve gown or robe over an IV catheter may prevent a resident from pulling it out.

- Encourage the resident to use his or her eyeglasses, hearing aids, cane, or walker. Explain that these devices will help the resident better respond to the environment and socialize with others.

- Decrease resident confusion by providing links to reality. For example, you could turn on the television or radio or place a calendar and clock in the room.

- Provide distraction for residents by visiting, holding hands, providing enjoyable activities, encouraging residents to hold on to a favorite item, offering a snack or something to drink, and promoting socialization with other residents.

- Be aware of actions that may trigger aggressive or combative behaviors and learn what actions may be calming.

- Provide restorative care, such as walking; scheduled toileting; and independent eating, dressing, and bathing programs.

- Tell residents when their behavior is unsafe. Provide safety reminders. Reward residents with praise when they act safely.

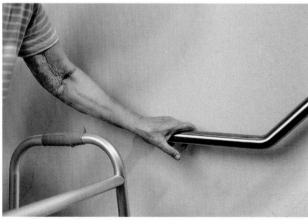

Toa55/Shutterstock.com

Figure 16.14 Using grab rails in the hallways and bathrooms will help residents ambulate safely.

The goal of care is to provide as much independence as possible while still keeping the resident safe. There is convincing evidence that a safe environment can be provided without physical restraints, which restrict freedom and can create other serious risks. Safe care can use alternative safety measures tailored to meet individual needs and assure the best possible quality of life. While all healthcare facilities work toward providing restraint-free care, restraint-free care is not always possible. Sometimes restraints are needed to keep a resident safe and free from harm. Holistic nursing assistants can help prevent any issues or challenges related to restraints by

- applying restraints in the correct manner, when directed by the licensed nursing staff, using proper procedure;
- providing excellent care;
- monitoring and observing residents; and
- reporting any problems to the licensed nursing staff immediately.

When Should Restraints Be Used?

Restraints should only be used to protect residents from harming themselves or others when preventive actions or alternative measures have failed. Restraints should *never* be used for the convenience of the nursing and healthcare staff or to punish the resident.

The use of a restraint requires a doctor's order. In a restraint order, the doctor must give the medical reason for the restraint, the circumstances under which the restraint can be used, and the length of use. Before a restraint can be used, a resident's family member or guardian is consulted, and the family member or guardian must sign an informed consent document if the resident is unable. Because residents have the right to make decisions about their care and treatment, restraints cannot be used without the consent of residents, their family members, or guardians. The resident and his or her family member or guardian are always informed about the potential risks of using the restraint.

Restraint use must be monitored, and its effectiveness must be continuously observed and evaluated. Nursing assistants must be aware of healthcare facility policy regarding the use of restraints.

How Are Restraints Safely Applied and Monitored?

Once the doctor has ordered a restraint and the informed consent document has been reviewed and signed, licensed nursing staff members have full responsibility for applying, monitoring, and removing restraints. Licensed nursing staff members assess the resident's condition and then plan for and provide preventive actions for restraint safety. Only in emergency situations can licensed nursing staff members apply short-term restraints without a doctor's order.

Nursing assistants provide direct care to residents with restraints; may apply and remove restraints, if assigned by the licensed nursing staff; and observe and report residents' conditions and responses to restraints. Nursing assistants must always follow the healthcare facility's procedure for applying a restraint and must not make any changes to the approved procedure.

Applying a Restraint

The procedure for applying a restraint will vary depending on the type of restraint and the facility. The following general guidelines ensure the resident's comfort and the safe, proper application of the restraint:

- Tell the resident (and family members, if present) what you are doing and why. For example, you could say, "Mrs. J, I am going to put this padded, soft restraint on your right wrist because you are trying to pull out the IV on your left arm. You need the IV to receive your medication."

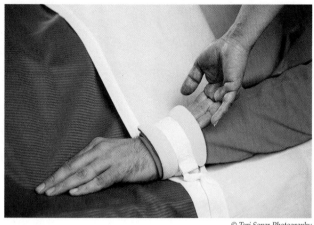

© Tori Soper Photography

Figure 16.15 You should be able to fit three fingers between the resident's body and the restraint used.

- Check that you have the right restraint type and size. The restraint should not be frayed or torn. Check the restraint's fit by making sure three fingers will fit between the restraint and the resident's body (Figure 16.15).

- Always apply the restraint over clothing, not on bare skin. Padding should be used for any bony projections.

- Be sure the resident is properly positioned in bed while wearing the restraint.

- Never tie a restraint to a movable part of the bed or to a movable chair. For example, a vest restraint should never be tied to a side rail.

- Ensure the restraint does not interfere with the resident's breathing or circulation.

- Do not put a restraint on an arm with an IV catheter; on skin that is burned, sore, or injured; or on a broken arm or leg.

- Make sure the resident cannot reach the ties of the restraint.

- Tie the restraint using a slipknot for quick release (Figure 16.16).

- Put the call light in a place the resident can easily use it.

- Assure the resident or family members that you and other healthcare staff members will regularly observe and check on the resident.

- Report to the licensed nursing staff immediately if the resident or a family member does not want the restraint. If the resident is stable, you can leave the room to give the report. If the resident is not stable, use the call light or ask someone to get a licensed nursing staff member so you can stay in the room.

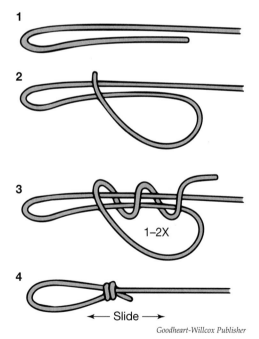

← Slide →

Goodheart-Willcox Publisher

Figure 16.16 To tie a slipknot, follow the four steps in this illustration.

Observing a Restrained Resident

Restrained residents must be observed or checked on regularly. Observing residents means monitoring their physical and emotional reactions and responses to the restraint. Depending on the resident's condition, you may need to observe the resident every 5, 10, or 15 minutes. Stable and safe residents may be observed hourly, but licensed nursing staff members make this determination. When observing a resident, carefully consider the following:

- **The resident's physical state**: Is the resident safe from injury? Is the resident's skin pink, blue, or gray? Is the skin warm or cool to the touch? What is the color of the resident's lips or nails? Is the restraint comfortable—not too tight or loose? Does the resident feel tingling in any restrained body part? Does the resident have a diminished or absent pulse? Is the resident breathing normally? Does he or she appear weaker than usual? Is the resident complaining about pain on or near the restraint? Are nutrition, elimination, and hygiene needs being met?

- **The resident's emotional state**: Is the resident afraid or nervous? What is the resident saying about the restraint? Does the resident appear confused? Is he or she upset, angry, or agitated?

- **The resident's response to the restraint**: Is the restraint keeping the resident from harm? Has the resident improved enough that he or she no longer needs the restraint? Have the behaviors that prompted the use of the restraint disappeared?

If you notice that something is not normal or correct during observation, report it to the licensed nursing staff immediately. Fix any problems you are qualified and able to fix (for example, readjusting the restraint). If you cannot fix the problem, call for help, but do not leave the resident alone.

Residents in restraints need more frequent care than residents without restraints. Care for residents with restraints should be given at least every two hours and more often when needed. Restraints should be released for at least 10 minutes during care. Care for residents with restraints should include a plan for

- sufficient movement and toileting;
- **range of motion (ROM)**, or the amount of voluntary motion, for the restrained body parts (unless the resident is sleeping);
- turning and positioning, if the resident is not able to turn and position himself or herself;
- skin care, as needed;
- cleaning, bathing, and drying; and
- nourishment and fluids.

Observations about restraints should always be documented. Be sure you are familiar with the documentation procedures and forms required by your health-care facility. Some facilities use *restraint flow sheets*, which track the care given (such as monitoring every two hours, turning, or positioning). Other facilities require progress notes that include the same information and also comment on how well residents are adjusting to restraints. It is important to know which form is required by your healthcare facility.

How Is Restraint Use Discontinued?

The use of restraints can be discontinued only when there is a doctor's order. The discontinuation of a restraint is ordered when a resident's behavior has improved to the point that the restraint is no longer needed. Restraints are usually removed gradually according to a plan that includes the use of alternative safety measures. Restraints should never be removed abruptly, as they can bruise and damage the skin and strain joints. Licensed nursing staff members may ask nursing assistants to continue closely observing a resident for a short period of time after a restraint has been discontinued. This ensures the resident stays safe and free from harm.

Section 16.3 Review and Assessment

Using the Key Terms

Complete the following sentences using key terms in this section.

1. A(n) _____ is any physical equipment or chemical substance that prevents a resident from moving freely.

2. _____ is a degenerative brain disease that leads to memory loss, impaired thinking, disorientation, and changes in personality and mood.

3. The amount that a person can move a joint voluntarily is _____.

Know and Understand the Facts

4. What are physical restraints?
5. What are three types of physical restraints?
6. What are chemical restraints?
7. What is entrapment, and how can it be prevented?
8. Identify two risks associated with the use of restraints.

Analyze and Apply Concepts

9. What are four alternative safety measures to using restraints?
10. What is one reason the use of restraints might be ordered by a doctor?
11. Describe three observations that nursing assistants must make when residents are in restraints.
12. What three actions should nursing assistants take when caring for a resident in a restraint?

Think Critically

Read the following care situation. Then answer the questions that follow.

Tom is a nursing assistant at a small community hospital. Today, he is providing care for a newly admitted patient—Mr. C, a 65-year-old Hispanic gentleman. Mr. C was transferred from the emergency department about two hours ago and was admitted after a serious car accident. Mr. C is very agitated and does not speak English well. He seems to be trying to remove his IV and get out of bed. He is moaning and appears to be in a lot of pain. Tom has been asked by the charge nurse to check on Mr. C to see how he is doing.

13. What should Tom immediately do to make sure Mr. C is safe?

14. What should Tom say to the charge nurse about his observations regarding Mr. C's present condition?

15. Do you think Mr. C should be put in restraints? If not, how should the situation be handled? If you think he should be in restraints, what would be the next steps?

Objectives

To help promote a safe environment as a nursing assistant, you must be aware of fire, chemical, and electrical risk and prevention strategies. You must also be able to maintain an appropriate and safe environment for residents using oxygen. To achieve the objectives for this section, you must successfully

- **describe** ways to prevent fires and eliminate chemical and electrical risks;
- **identify** what to do in case of a fire; and
- **explain** the actions required to safely care for residents using oxygen.

Key Terms

Learn these key terms to better understand the information presented in the section.

fire triangle   RACE
flow meter   safety data sheet (SDS)
nasal cannula

Questions to Consider

- Have you ever experienced a fire—either small or large?
- If you have experienced a fire, what was your immediate reaction? Were you unable to move, or did you get a burst of energy and immediately spring into action?
- Did you use some form of fire suppression like a fire extinguisher? If so, what was that experience like?

Healthcare facilities face considerable risks because of their large populations of non-ambulatory residents and the difficulty of evacuation. As a result, nursing and healthcare staff members must know how fires can start and how to prevent them. They must be knowledgeable about fire safety rules, plans, and procedures. They must also know how to prevent fires and what to do if a fire starts.

How Do Fires Start?

For a fire to start, three elements must be present—fuel, oxygen, and heat. These three elements form the **fire triangle** (Figure 16.17). Fuel is any flammable solid, liquid, or gas. If any one part of the fire triangle is missing, a fire will not start.

You can help prevent fires by keeping heat away from flammable items. For example, you should keep resident clothes away from potentially hot items, such as a frayed electrical wire.

How Should a Nursing Assistant Respond to a Fire?

When you begin working as a nursing assistant, you may hear a facility fire alarm or an overhead announcement, even if you do not see a fire. If the facility fire alarm sounds or if you are alerted by an overhead announcement, abide by the facility guidelines and

- listen for the facility code announcement to identify the location of the fire;
- close the nearest resident, office, laboratory, and utility room doors;
- clear the corridors and elevator lobbies on the floor of the fire alarm and on other floors, if instructed;

Think About This

According to the CDC, someone in the United States dies in a fire approximately every 169 minutes. Fires injure someone every 30 minutes. Most people who encounter fire will die from smoke inhalation or toxic gases, not from burns. Those most at risk for fire-related injuries are older adults, who may have difficulty escaping from a fire due to disabilities.

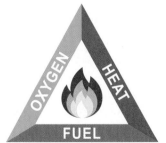

BALRedaan/Shutterstock.com

Figure 16.17 The fire triangle consists of fuel, oxygen, and heat—the three elements needed to start a fire.

- remain alert and await further instructions on the announcement system;
- do not evacuate unless specifically instructed to do so; and
- resume normal activities when the facility code indicates all is clear.

If a fire starts in your facility, you must act very fast. The first few minutes can be a matter of life and death. Use the **RACE** system and always follow your healthcare facility's specific fire plan (Figure 16.18).

Classes of Fire and Types of Fire Extinguishers

You should only attempt to extinguish a fire using a fire extinguisher after the rescue, activate the alarm, and confine the fire steps are accomplished and the fire department is on the way. Do *not* use fire extinguishers unless you are trained and confident about using them. There are several fire extinguishers; each type is designed to extinguish a particular class of fire:

- **Class A fire**: ordinary, solid materials such as wood, paper, cloth, or trash; a water or multipurpose dry chemical extinguisher is used.
- **Class B fire**: gasoline, oil, paint, or other flammable liquids; a carbon dioxide or multipurpose dry chemical extinguisher is used.
- **Class C fire**: wiring, fuse boxes, computers, or other electrical sources; a dry chemical or multipurpose dry chemical extinguisher is used.
- **Class D fire**: powders, flakes, or shavings from metals; a class D extinguisher is used.
- **Class K fire**: combustible fluids, such as oils and fats; a dry or wet chemical extinguisher is used.

The facility fire plan should indicate when fire extinguishers must be checked. Fire extinguisher checks should be performed on a regular basis by a designated person and should make sure extinguishers are fully charged and ready for use in case of an emergency.

Understanding the RACE Acronym	
R—Rescue	Remove residents from danger by helping them to a safe place (usually designated by the facility fire plan). Move residents outdoors only if there is no safe indoor option. Unlock bed wheels to move residents quickly. All personal items should be left behind.
A—Activate alarm	Follow the facility fire plan procedure and begin the alarm or alert. This may involve telling a fellow staff member to call the fire department, activating a manual pull station, or sending out the prescribed code over the announcement system. Early fire department notification is essential.
C—Confine the fire	Fire doors should freely close when there is a fire or smoke. These doors confine fires to small areas. Close fire doors behind the last person leaving an area. Confining the fire limits the spread of heat and smoke, as residents are moved elsewhere on the floor or out of the building.
E—Extinguish	Extinguish the fire if you can do so safely without causing danger to anyone. If the fire is very small and can quickly and safely be extinguished using water or a fire extinguisher, extinguish it. If the fire is large, begin evacuating residents when directed. Only a staff member who is competent to use a fire extinguisher and who has a clear, unobstructed exit should use the extinguisher. In all other cases, qualified, professional firefighters should extinguish the fire.

Figure 16.18 The RACE system consists of four steps: rescue, activate the alarm, confine the fire, and extinguish.

Using a Fire Extinguisher

Once you have obtained the proper fire extinguisher for the type of fire present, you must use the extinguisher in accordance with your training. When using a fire extinguisher, remember the acronym *PASS* (Figure 16.19):

- **P—Pull** the lock pin.
- **A—Aim** the nozzle low at the base or bottom of the fire or flames.
- **S—Squeeze** the handles together while holding the extinguisher straight.
- **S—Sweep** the nozzle from side to side at the base of the flames until the fire is extinguished.

A slight kickback may accompany the activation of the extinguisher. Carbon dioxide extinguishers may make a noise as the extinguishing agent rushes out of the extinguisher. Before using an extinguisher, identify an exit behind you in case the fire extinguisher fails to operate properly or you cannot completely extinguish the fire.

How Can a Fire Be Prevented?

Preventing fires is a critically important part of a nursing assistant's responsibilities. Taking specific actions to prevent fires will help keep residents free from harm:

- Familiarize yourself with the locations of smoke detectors and fire alarms in your facility (Figure 16.20). Smoke detectors should never be disabled. A periodic beep or chirp from a smoke detector means the battery is low and must be changed immediately. If you hear this, report it to the licensed nursing staff.
- Know the facility fire plan, the locations of fire extinguishers, and the proper methods of using fire extinguishers. Become familiar with the facility's escape routes and actively participate in facility fire drills.
- Check that sprinklers are in working order and are not obstructed by any objects. Do not store items near sprinkler heads, as items may prevent water from spraying on the fire.

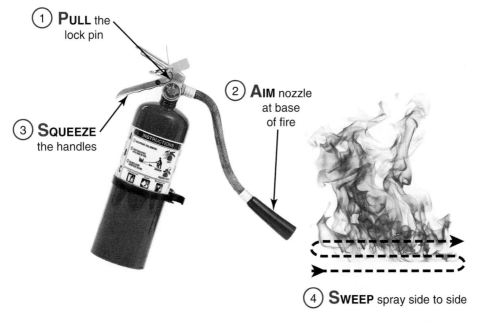

① **PULL** the lock pin

② **AIM** nozzle at base of fire

③ **SQUEEZE** the handles

④ **SWEEP** spray side to side

Thomas M Perkins/Shutterstock.com, Valeev/Shutterstock.com

Figure 16.19 The four steps in extinguishing a fire are pulling the lock pin, aiming the nozzle, squeezing the handles, and sweeping from side to side.

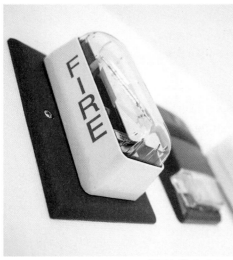

B Calkins/Shutterstock.com

Figure 16.20 In many healthcare facilities, fire alarms will sound an alarm and flash when there is a fire.

- Keep hallways and exit doors clear.
- Store flammable materials properly.
- Enforce no-smoking rules.
- Teach mobile residents about fire safety. Educating residents about responding in the event of a fire is an important method for ensuring safety.
- Show residents the proper escape routes from their rooms. Remind mobile residents to use the stairs and not the elevator if there is a fire. Let those who use wheelchairs, canes, or walkers know that assistance will be provided.
- Tell residents to shut the door if a fire is blocking the doorway, as this will keep the fire out. Residents or nursing assistants should also put towels or blankets along the bottom of the door to keep smoke out of the room (Figure 16.21). If they are able, residents should yell for help or call 9-1-1 from their room phones.
- Instruct residents to feel the door before opening it if they hear a fire alarm. The door should not be opened if it feels hot. If the door is hot, a fire is just on the other side. Opening the door will spread the flames and smoke into the room. If the door is hot, the resident should put a towel or blanket along the bottom of the door to keep the smoke out and signal or call for help.

What Are Electrical and Chemical Hazards?

Nursing assistants must also be aware of electrical and chemical hazards. Understanding these hazards helps nursing assistants maintain the safety of residents, family members, and facility staff.

Electrical Safety

Electrical hazards can result in bodily shock, electrical fires, and explosions. There are four main types of electrical injuries: electrocution, electrical shock, burns, and falls caused by contact with electricity. Hazards include electrical cords that are damaged or aging, faulty electrical equipment, and damaged electrical wall receptacles. The facility safety plan should provide directions regarding electrical safety, as many OSHA standards must be met. General guidelines must also be observed to maintain electrical safety:

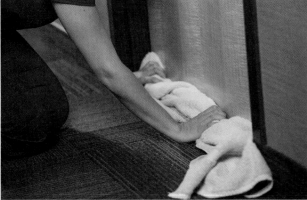

© Tori Soper Photography

Figure 16.21 A towel or blanket will help prevent smoke from entering the room.

- Never overload electrical outlets or use an item with a damaged electrical cord. Do not use extension cords and do not turn on an electrical razor while oxygen is in use.
- Check that all equipment used for residents has been inspected and is safe. Many facilities use stickers or tags to identify electrical equipment as safe.
- Ensure there is sufficient working space around all electrical equipment to permit the safe operation and maintenance of equipment.
- Check that all outlets near sources of water are properly grounded with a three-pronged outlet to prevent shocks or electrocution.
- Do not plug in or unplug electrical equipment when your hands are wet.

- Keep all electrical appliances at least 3–4 feet from any sink, tub, shower, or stove.
- If you are concerned about an electrical outlet or piece of equipment, do not use it. Report it to the licensed nursing staff.

Chemical Safety

Many hazardous chemicals are present in healthcare facilities and pose the threat of toxic exposure for patients, residents, and healthcare staff. Toxic exposure to hazardous chemicals can result from topical and spray medications; anesthetic gases; and chemicals used to clean, disinfect, and sterilize work surfaces and equipment.

OSHA hazard standards and facility-specific guidelines for chemical safety are often outlined in the facility safety plan. General guidelines for maintaining chemical safety include the following:

- Familiarize yourself with the information provided in the **safety data sheet (SDS)**, or *material safety data sheet (MSDS)*, for each hazardous chemical. The SDS (provided by the facility and typically found in the safety plan) contains information about potential hazards; the safe use, storage, and handling of chemical products; and emergency procedures.
- Check that all hazardous chemicals are clearly labeled.
- Use appropriate PPE (such as gloves, goggles, and gowns) when handling hazardous detergents and chemicals.
- If the eyes or body are exposed to hazardous chemicals, quickly flush the body or eyes using facility equipment according to procedure (Figure 16.22).

What Is Oxygen Therapy?

Oxygen therapy is a lifeline for many people. Without oxygen therapy, some people might not survive a respiratory illness or might not be able to perform simple ADLs. Oxygen is safe to use under the right conditions and can be used at home or in healthcare facilities. Oxygen will not explode or burn, but can cause things that are already burning to burn hotter and faster.

The need for oxygen therapy is determined by a doctor. The doctor also identifies the *rate*, or amount, of oxygen to be delivered based on what the resident needs. In healthcare facilities, licensed nursing staff members are responsible for setting up oxygen equipment and tubing and adjusting the rate of oxygen given to a resident. The nursing assistant observes that the amount of oxygen delivered is accurate and that equipment and tubing are properly placed. Any changes or problems are reported to the licensed nursing staff.

The following supplies are typically used for administering oxygen:

- **Flow meter**: ensures a resident gets the prescribed amount of oxygen (1–6 liters per minute, if delivered through a nasal cannula); also called a *regulator*
- **Pressure gauge**: shows the amount of oxygen being delivered (Figure 16.23)

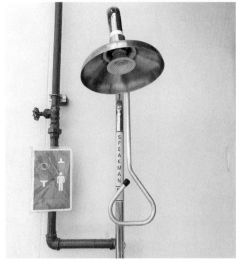

Niwat panket/Shutterstock.com

A

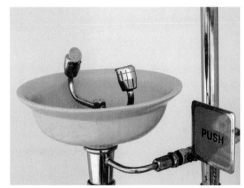

Niwat panket/Shutterstock.com

B

Figure 16.22 Healthcare facilities may have emergency showers (A) and eyewash stations (B) to flush the body and eyes if they are exposed to hazardous chemicals.

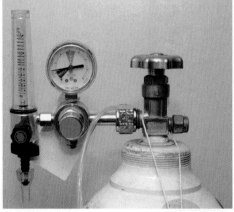

WeStudio/Shutterstock.com

Figure 16.23 Flow meters, or regulators, ensure the correct amount of oxygen is delivered. Pressure gauges show the amount of oxygen being delivered.

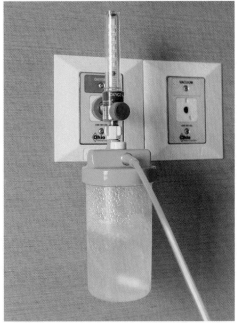

Nednapa Sopasuntorn/Shutterstock.com

Figure 16.24 Oxygen tubing connects the oxygen mask or nasal cannula to the source of oxygen (in this case, an oxygen wall unit).

- **Oxygen tubing**: used to move oxygen from the tank, cylinder, or wall unit to the resident (Figure 16.24)
- **Nasal cannula**: most commonly used to deliver oxygen; has two small prongs that deliver oxygen into the nose; is placed about 1/2 inch into the nostrils (Figure 16.25)
- **Masks**: used if a resident has difficulty breathing through the nose or needs a large amount of oxygen; covers the nose and mouth
- **Humidifier**: adds moisture to oxygen and prevents the resident's nasal passages from drying

Oxygen tanks and cylinders are labeled with a United States Pharmacopeia (USP) code and are marked with a colored diamond that reads *Oxygen* (Figure 16.26). The USP code indicates that the oxygen is being used for medical purposes. Oxygen tanks and cylinders contain gas under high pressure. If they are not handled correctly, their high pressure can cause serious damage, injury, or death.

All supplies and equipment involved in oxygen therapy must be kept clean and in good, working order. Any connections should be in good condition. As a holistic nursing assistant, report any needed repairs to the licensed nursing staff. Keep equipment clean and safe by wiping down the outsides of the equipment with a damp, soapy cloth on a regular basis. If the resident is using a humidifier, empty the water from the reservoir and wash the reservoir in hot, soapy water every day. Nasal cannulas and masks are usually changed at least every two to four weeks. The tubing should be changed at least once a month. Change the tubing and mask often if the resident has a cold or the flu; however, always check facility policy regarding changing equipment, nasal cannulas, tubing, and masks.

Promoting Oxygen Safety

Oxygen must always be used safely. Follow these important safety rules both in healthcare facilities and at home:

- Ensure precautions for oxygen safety are posted outside any room or building in which oxygen is used or stored.
- When oxygen is in use, prevent static electricity (for example, from skin rubbing on sheets or blankets and the use of hand sanitizer).
  - Prevent fires by never using oil-based face creams, hair dryers, or electrical razors while oxygen is in use. Instead, use water-based cosmetics or creams.
  - Maintain oxygen therapy precautions (such as keeping a resident away from flammable items or static electricity) and follow facility procedures when transporting residents receiving oxygen.
  - Place no-smoking signs throughout the facility and the room in which oxygen is being used.
  - Keep tanks and cylinders, if used, at least 10 feet from open flames, space heaters, large windows, or any other source of heat. Make sure that stored oxygen tanks and cylinders will not tip over or fall. Keep liquid oxygen upright so that it does not spill. Liquid oxygen may cause skin damage.

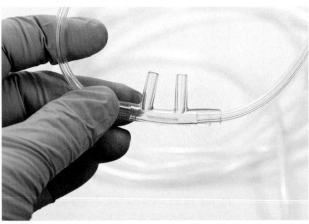

Sherry Yates Young/Shutterstock.com

Figure 16.25 A nasal cannula is most often used when a low to medium flow of oxygen is required.

- Do not use cleaning solutions, paint thinners, or aerosol spray cans near oxygen, as these can ignite a fire.
- Never use grease or oil near oxygen, as these are flammable materials. Grease and oil can be found in hand lotions, hair lubricants, and petroleum jelly. Aerosol sprays, such as hairsprays, are also flammable and should not be used near oxygen equipment.
- If the person receiving oxygen therapy is cooking, ensure that the cannula is secured over the ears and behind the head, not under the chin.
- Secure tubing to the side of clothing with a large safety pin (though be sure not to puncture the tubing). This will keep the tubing away from any heat source.

Caring for Residents on Oxygen Therapy

Residents receiving oxygen therapy need safe, quality care. As a holistic nursing assistant, you should observe and report skin irritation, changes in breathing, changes in vital signs, or changes in the operation of equipment to the licensed nursing staff. You should also do the following:

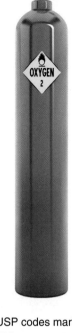

cigdem/Shutterstock.com

Figure 16.26 USP codes mark oxygen used for medical purposes.

- Make sure an *Oxygen in Use* sign is posted on the door to the room and on the wall over the bed.
- Regularly check oxygen flow, as directed by the licensed nursing staff, and remove possible tubing kinks that can minimize or prevent the flow of oxygen.
- Keep any tubing off the floor.
- Be sure the cannula or mask and tubing are placed correctly, as they can be easily displaced when a resident moves or sleeps.
- Observe the skin around the nasal cannula or mask for irritation. Give frequent skin care to the face or nose. Use water-soluble lubricants on these sensitive skin areas and do not use any oil-based products.
- Tuck some gauze under the nasal cannula tubing to prevent the cheeks or skin behind the ears from becoming sore (Figure 16.27).

Healthcare Scenario
Oxygen Safety

Joy, a nursing assistant in a long-term care center, found Mr. A, a 75-year-old resident, on the floor near his bed. Oxygen tubing and an electrical cord were wrapped around Mr. A's neck, and the electrical cord was tied to the call light cord hanging over his bed. Joy immediately called the charge nurse for help. The charge nurse removed Mr. A's restraints and administered CPR. Unfortunately, Mr. A was pronounced dead at 12:15 a.m. The coroner stated that it appeared as though Mr. A was trying to get out of bed and got tangled in the cords and tubing.

Apply It
1. Why did Mr. A get tangled in the tubing and cords?
2. Could Joy have done any more than she did? Explain your answer.

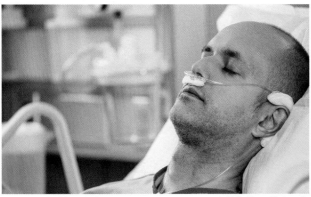
© Tori Soper Photography

Figure 16.27 Placing gauze beneath the nasal cannula and its tubing can reduce soreness around the nose and ears.

- Promote breathing comfort for residents in bed by keeping the head of the bed raised. Use pillows to support residents who are seated.
- Observe changes in skin color. Gray or blue skin could indicate that the resident is not getting sufficient oxygen. Alert the licensed nursing staff immediately if this occurs.
- Remove items that may cause a fire (for example, electrical equipment that may cause sparks or flammable fluids).

Section 16.4 Review and Assessment

Using the Key Terms

Complete the following sentences using key terms in this section.

1. _____ stands for *rescue, activate alarm, confine the fire,* and *extinguish.*
2. A(n) _____ has two small prongs that deliver oxygen into the nose.
3. Fuel, heat, and oxygen make up the _____.
4. During oxygen therapy, the _____ makes sure a resident gets the prescribed amount of oxygen.
5. A(n) _____ contains information about the potential hazards of a chemical product.

Know and Understand the Facts

6. What are the three elements needed to start a fire?
7. What does the acronym *RACE* stand for?
8. What does the acronym *PASS* stand for?
9. Identify two pieces of equipment used in oxygen therapy. Explain how each piece is used.

Analyze and Apply Concepts

10. What should a nursing assistant do if a fire alarm is activated in the facility?
11. Describe five guidelines a nursing assistant should follow to prevent a fire.
12. Explain two actions a nursing assistant can take to maintain electrical safety.
13. Identify five guidelines that must be followed to ensure oxygen safety.

Think Critically

Read the following care situation. Then answer the questions that follow.

Mary is a nursing assistant at a skilled nursing facility and is caring for Ms. J, who was transferred from the hospital with moderate respiratory distress caused by serious pneumonia. Ms. J is 75 years old and very independent. She is mobile, but will need oxygen therapy while she recovers. Ms. J is not happy about being in the skilled nursing facility and complains about the nasal cannula. Her nose is sore, and she does not like the sign that shows she is on oxygen.

14. What can Mary do to help Ms. J with her nasal cannula and sore nose?
15. If you were Mary, how would you explain the importance of the sign to Ms. J?
16. Identify three oxygen safety guidelines Mary should follow when caring for Ms. J.

Key Points

Reviewing the key points for this chapter will help you practice more safely and competently as a holistic nursing assistant and will help you prepare for the certification competency examination.

- Preventing risks and accidents requires personal awareness about safety hazards, safety promotion, safety policies, infection control, risk management, and the use of safety equipment.

- To prevent falls, always work slowly and steadily and *ACT* (be aware, correct risks, and take precautions).

- A restraint-free environment must be promoted and maintained whenever possible. A doctor's order is required to use a restraint and all federal, state, and facility policies must be followed to ensure residents have a good quality of life.

- Nursing assistants should always use and teach residents fire-prevention skills and be familiar with the facility's fire safety plan.

- When caring for residents on oxygen therapy, observe and report signs of skin irritation, changes in breathing and vital signs, or changes in the operation of equipment to the licensed nursing staff.

Action Steps to Holistic Care

Review the information in this chapter. Complete the following activities.

1. Prepare a short paper or digital presentation that describes how nursing assistants contribute to a culture of safety. Discuss how a culture of safety supports quality and ensures a safe environment.

2. With a partner, write a song or a poem about fire safety. Include how fires can start and how to prevent them.

3. With a partner, prepare a poster about fall prevention. Include risks for falls and prevention measures nursing assistants can take.

4. Research current scientific information about electrical and chemical safety in healthcare facilities. Write a brief report describing three current facts not covered in this chapter.

5. Create a poster or digital presentation that outlines five work-related safety hazards that affect nursing assistants. Include strategies for avoiding each hazard.

✓ Preparing for the Certification Competency Examination

To prepare for the nursing assistant certification competency examination, you will need to know content found in this chapter. This content may be tested in the knowledge (written or oral) and skills (hands-on demonstration) portions of the exam. The following areas will be emphasized:

- general resident safety
- safety hazards
- accident prevention and reporting
- fall prevention
- use of restraints
- fire prevention and oxygen safety

These sample test questions are similar to ones you will find on the certification competency exam. See how well you can answer them. Be sure to select the *best* answer.

1. A doctor has ordered restraints for Mr. S. Which of the following is true?
   A. Mr. S will be at a lower risk for developing respiratory problems.
   B. Mr. S will be at a greater risk for developing decubitus ulcers.
   C. Mr. S will become more hungry and thirsty.
   D. Mr. S will be at a greater risk for falling out of bed.

2. A fire starts in Mr. G's room. The first thing a nursing assistant should do is
   A. try to put out the fire
   B. get Mr. G out of the room safely
   C. pull the fire alarm
   D. inform the charge nurse

(continued)

3. Mr. D has been identified as a fall risk. The first thing a nursing assistant should do is
   A. put a restraint on Mr. D
   B. tell Mr. D to be careful getting out of bed
   C. advise Mr. D's family that he is a fall risk
   D. put a fall risk sign on Mr. D's bed or outside his door

4. A nursing assistant sees that Mrs. C, who is in restraints, is half out of bed. What should the nursing assistant do?
   A. put the restraint back on tightly so Mrs. C cannot move
   B. leave the restraint off and report to the charge nurse
   C. call for help to get Mrs. C back to bed and reapply the restraints
   D. put a different type of restraint on Mrs. C

5. A nursing assistant sees that Mr. J is not getting enough oxygen through his tubing. What should the nursing assistant do?
   A. turn up the oxygen
   B. turn off the oxygen
   C. check the oxygen tubing for kinks
   D. ask Mr. J to take deeper breaths

6. To prevent back strains and injuries, nursing assistants should
   A. wear sturdy shoes
   B. not try to lift very heavy residents without help
   C. ask for help on all of their activities
   D. use correct-size bed sheets when making beds

7. To ensure electrical safety, a nursing assistant should do all of the following except
   A. use extension cords to keep equipment away from a water source
   B. not unplug equipment with wet hands
   C. not switch on an electrical razor while oxygen is in use
   D. leave sufficient working space around all electrical equipment to permit safe operation

8. When using a fire extinguisher, be sure to
   A. use it only after the rescue, activate the alarm, and confine the fire steps
   B. use it only at the start of a fire
   C. use it only for small fires
   D. use it only for midsize or large fires

9. Which of the following is not an important safety guideline?
   A. be aware and mindful of safety at all times
   B. always work to prevent errors or harm
   C. learn from errors if they occur
   D. never report an error because you can get in trouble

10. What are the three elements needed to start a fire?
    A. oxygen, fuel, and water
    B. oxygen, heat, and nitrogen
    C. fuel, oxygen, and heat
    D. heat, nitrogen, and fuel

11. During a safety check, a nursing assistant should
    A. turn off the television
    B. make sure the call light is accessible
    C. close the bathroom door
    D. straighten the bed linens

12. A nursing assistant must complete an incident report about a fall. What should be included in the incident report?
    A. the person the nursing assistant thinks is to blame
    B. detailed facts about what the nursing assistant witnessed
    C. the resident's actions prior to the fall
    D. the resident's attire during the fall

13. A nursing assistant's left eye was exposed to a chemical spray during cleaning. What should the nursing assistant do?
    A. quickly report the exposure to the charge nurse
    B. see the doctor after getting home
    C. quickly flush the eye per facility procedure
    D. wipe the eye with a clean, wet dressing

14. To prevent falls, a nursing assistant should
    A. provide comfortable chairs for residents
    B. move potential obstacles in common areas and resident rooms
    C. place extra blankets on the resident in bed
    D. assist residents in dressing and wearing loose-fitting clothing

15. When an error occurs in a culture of safety, the focus is on
    A. what happened, not who did it
    B. who made the error and the result
    C. how many times the error was made
    D. what will happen to the person who made the error

Did you have difficulty with any of the questions? If you did, review the chapter to find the correct answer(s).

Welcome to the Chapter

As a nursing assistant, you will be responsible for promoting, supporting, and assisting with mobility. Maintaining mobility is essential for resident well-being. When positioning, turning, transferring, and lifting residents, nursing assistants must use proper body mechanics and appropriate techniques and procedures that ensure the safety of residents and nursing assistants. In this chapter, you will learn about the importance of ambulation and about ways to aid residents who use assistive ambulatory devices such as canes, walkers, and wheelchairs. You will also learn the importance of rehabilitation and restorative care, ways to assist residents with range of motion, and guidelines for helping residents maintain as much independence and self-reliance as possible.

The information and procedures presented in this chapter will help you build the knowledge and skills needed to become a holistic nursing assistant. Check with your instructor to ensure these procedures are within your state's regulations for nursing assistant practice. The topics discussed in the chapter are highlighted on the Providing Holistic Care Framework.

You are now ready to start this chapter, *Promoting Mobility*.

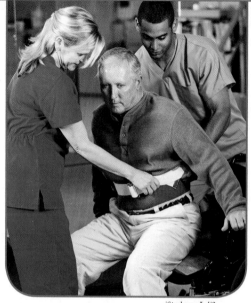

iStock.com/kali9

Chapter Outline

Section 17.1
Body Mechanics

Section 17.2
Positioning, Turning, Transferring, and Lifting

Section 17.3
Ambulation and Assistive Ambulatory Devices

Section 17.4
Rehabilitation and Restorative Care

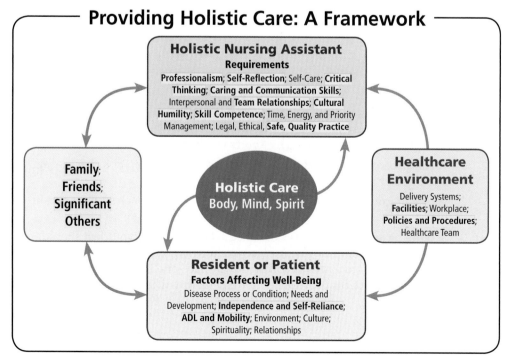

Providing Holistic Care: A Framework

Holistic Nursing Assistant
Requirements
Professionalism; Self-Reflection; Self-Care; Critical Thinking; Caring and Communication Skills; Interpersonal and Team Relationships; Cultural Humility; Skill Competence; Time, Energy, and Priority Management; Legal, Ethical, Safe, Quality Practice

Family; Friends; Significant Others

Holistic Care
Body, Mind, Spirit

Healthcare Environment
Delivery Systems; Facilities; Workplace; Policies and Procedures; Healthcare Team

Resident or Patient
Factors Affecting Well-Being
Disease Process or Condition; Needs and Development; Independence and Self-Reliance; ADL and Mobility; Environment; Culture; Spirituality; Relationships

Questions to Consider

- On a scale of 1–10, with 10 being the best, how would you rate your posture? Do you stand up straight or do you hunch your back?
- If you gave yourself a low rating, what do you think causes you to have poor posture? What might you do to improve your posture?
- How might poor posture affect a person's health and well-being?

Objectives

To promote and support resident mobility, you must first understand the principles of body mechanics. Once you are familiar with these principles, you can put them to use.
To achieve the objectives for this section, you must successfully

- **describe** the four main principles of body mechanics; and
- **demonstrate** proper body mechanics when working with residents.

Key Terms

Learn these key terms to better understand the information presented in the section.

body mechanics   joints
connective tissue   posture

What Are Body Mechanics?

You learned in chapter 16 that moving and positioning residents puts nursing assistants and other healthcare staff at greater risk for developing *musculoskeletal disorders (MSDs)*. Nursing staff members frequently report high rates of back and shoulder injuries. Most of these injuries can be prevented by using proper body mechanics. **Body mechanics** are actions that promote safe, efficient movement by using the correct muscles and movements to avoid straining muscles or joints. Proper body mechanics allow nursing assistants to safely and efficiently complete tasks such as positioning residents.

Mobility, or the ability to move, enables you to walk, climb stairs, or drive a car. Mobility only occurs through the contraction of muscles. When muscles contract, they move bones with the help of **connective tissue** (which joins muscles and bones together). For example, two muscle groups contract to move your upper arm: the biceps located on the front of your upper arm and the triceps located on the back of your upper arm. The contraction of these muscles is aided by connective tissue. Mobility is essential for your well-being and the well-being of residents.

Remember ────

Movement is a medicine for creating change in a person's physical, emotional, and mental states.

Carol Welch-Baril,
educational director
of BioSomatics

Principles of Body Mechanics

Proper body mechanics prevent muscle and joint strain and promote good posture. **Posture** refers to the way in which a person holds his or her body. There are four main principles that characterize proper body mechanics:

1. **A stable center of gravity**: is established when you keep your back straight and bend only at the knees and hips.

2. **A line of gravity**: is established when you keep your back straight and lift objects close to your body.

3. **A wide base of support**: is established when you keep your feet shoulder-width apart (about 12 inches), place one foot slightly in front of the other, slightly bend your knees to absorb any impact, and turn with your feet first. These practices provide maximum stability while lifting.

Why Do Some Healthcare Staff Members Wear Back Belts?

Some healthcare facilities ask that healthcare staff members wear specially designed *back belts* to protect against back injuries during care (Figure 17.4). Unless it is required, wearing a back belt is usually a matter of choice, as research has not shown that back belts actually prevent back injuries. If a back belt is used, it should be worn properly. Wearing a back belt should never be a substitute for proper body mechanics and good lifting skills.

There are several types of back belts. Back belts typically worn in healthcare facilities are lightweight, are elastic, and are worn around the lower back. Some back belts have suspenders that hold them in place.

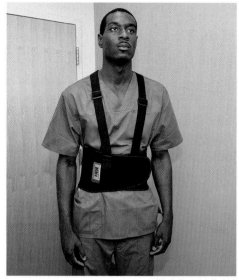

Wards Forest Media, LLC

Figure 17.4 Back belts can help reduce a nursing assistant's chance of back injury.

Section 17.1 Review and Assessment

Using the Key Terms

Complete the following sentences using key terms from this section.

1. Proper body mechanics can reduce strain on _____, or locations where two bones meet.
2. The way in which a person holds his or her body is called _____.
3. _____ is a type of tissue that joins muscles and bones.
4. Actions that promote safe, efficient, strain-free movement are _____.

Know and Understand the Facts

5. Identify the four main principles of body mechanics.
6. What are three benefits of using proper body mechanics?
7. What actions should be taken to achieve proper posture when standing?

Analyze and Apply Concepts

8. Describe the proper body mechanics for lifting objects.
9. Describe proper body mechanics for sitting in a chair.
10. List two guidelines for incorporating proper body mechanics into your daily life.

Think Critically

Read the following care situation. Then answer the questions that follow.

Priya, a nursing assistant, was helping Mrs. G with her bath when several bath towels on the bedside table dropped to the floor. Priya did not want to leave the bath towels because she was concerned she might trip on them. Priya quickly stooped over, picked up the towels, and placed them off to the side with the other dirty linens.

11. Did Priya do the right thing by picking up the linens right away? Should she have left them there? Explain.
12. Was Priya using proper body mechanics when she picked up the linens? Explain your answer and what, if anything, Priya should have done differently.

Questions to Consider

- Have you ever stayed in one position for too long? Maybe you had to lie in bed for a lengthy period of time due to illness or sat for hours working on a computer.
- How did you feel after staying in one position for too long? Did you experience aches and pains in particular body parts? If so, what did you do to relieve these aches and pains?

Objectives

As a holistic nursing assistant, you will use your knowledge of body mechanics to promote and support resident mobility, safety, and skin integrity. Using proper body mechanics will ensure that you and residents are properly aligned at all times, even when residents are being positioned, turned, transferred, or lifted. Proper alignment reduces the stress on fragile bones and joints; allows residents to remain mobile, even if they are bedridden; and maintains safety. Proper alignment also helps ensure skin integrity by preventing rubbing, chafing, or pressure on the skin. To achieve the objectives for this section, you must successfully

- **explain** the importance of proper body alignment, positioning, and safe handling techniques;
- **identify** different body positions; and
- **demonstrate** the procedures for positioning, turning, transferring, and lifting residents.

Key Terms

Learn these key terms to better understand the information presented in the section.

ankylosis

body alignment

contracture

foot drop

orthostatic hypotension

syncope

trochanter rolls

Nursing assistants are responsible for monitoring and changing resident positions to prevent the effects of immobility. Immobility may develop due to surgery, partial paralysis, or weakness from diseases or conditions. The nursing assistant's responsibility may include positioning a resident in bed, moving a resident up in bed, turning a resident, helping (transferring) a resident into a wheelchair, or lifting a resident. It is critical that residents maintain proper body alignment during these procedures.

Why Is Body Alignment Important?

Body alignment is the optimal placement of all body parts such that bones and muscles are used efficiently. It is essential for correct posture. Proper body alignment describes how the head, shoulders, spine, hips, knees, and ankles relate to and line up with each other. For example, when you are standing with good body alignment, your shoulder blades should be back, your chest should be forward, the top of your head should align with the ceiling, and your knees should be straight. When a resident is lying in bed, the spine should not be crooked or twisted, and the arms and legs should be comfortably positioned.

The goal of proper body alignment is to reduce the amount of stress on joints and skin. If body parts are in correct alignment, they will remain functional, healthy, and stress free.

How Should Residents Be Positioned, Turned, Transferred, and Lifted?

As a nursing assistant, you will be responsible for positioning, turning, transferring, and lifting residents to prevent the effects of immobility. The benefits to residents include the following:

- **Increases comfort and helps residents relax**: being in any position, even one that feels comfortable, can become unbearable after a long period of time. Repositioning residents may relieve restlessness and help residents who have trouble sleeping.

- **Restores body function**: changing positions and maintaining the natural curves of the body can help improve respiratory and gastrointestinal function. These actions can also stimulate circulation, which prevents the buildup of fluid in the lungs and the possible formation of blood clots in the legs.

- **Prevents deformities**: when they are not actively moving, muscles can atrophy (waste away) and develop **contracture** (shortening) and **ankylosis** (stiffening). Residents with **foot drop** (a condition in which the feet and toes drag) will be unable to lift the front part of one or both feet due to muscle weakness or paralysis. Proper positioning and support in bed are especially important for this condition.

- **Relieves pressure and strain on the skin**: relieving pressure prevents the formation of a decubitus ulcer.

Using Equipment and Devices

Different types of equipment and devices are used for positioning. If you are uncertain about using a type of positioning equipment or device, check with the licensed nursing staff, as some equipment and devices may be contraindicated. Be aware that some equipment and devices can be used or interpreted as restraints, which can violate resident rights and cause harm (for example, smothering from a pillow or possible entrapment). Examples of positioning equipment and supportive and friction-reducing devices include

- pillows of various sizes to help protect the skin; prop up a limb; or support the head, a limb, or the back for comfort;

- folded or rolled towels and blankets to prop up and support the resident and maintain proper body alignment;

- **trochanter rolls**, made from rolled towels or blankets, that span from the top of the pelvic bone to the mid thigh to prevent external rotation of the hips (Figure 17.5);

- a *draw sheet* (also called a *pull sheet*, *turning sheet*, or *lift sheet*) that is folded in half, placed on the middle of the bed, and used by the nursing assistant to turn the resident;

- cotton padding to protect the skin and bony areas;

- a *footboard*, which is a flat panel placed at the end of the bed to prevent foot drop (Figure 17.6);

- a *hip abduction wedge*, which is usually made of stiff foam rubber material cut into a wedge and is used to prop up the hip (Figure 17.7); and

- a *bed board*, which is a wide board placed under the mattress that provides additional support.

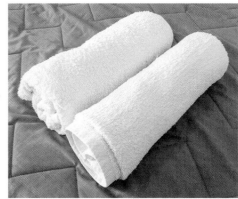
Wanlika Thongthup/Shutterstock.com

Figure 17.5 Trochanter rolls are made of rolled towels or blankets and are placed outside the legs to prevent external hip rotation.

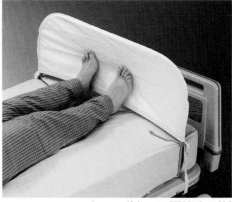
Image provided courtesy TIDI Products, LLC

Figure 17.6 The footboard helps prevent foot drop.

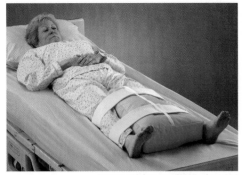

Image provided courtesy TIDI Products, LLC

Figure 17.7 The hip abduction wedge props up the hip.

Understanding Body Positions

Repositioning residents includes moving them into different body positions on a regular basis. Doctors will usually prescribe a specific schedule for placing residents, particularly bedridden residents, into different positions, sometimes every hour. Even if there is no doctor's order, residents should be moved or repositioned every two hours. There are several different types of positions. At a minimum, residents should be rotated through at least four body positions during a shift, unless a particular position is *contraindicated*, or harmful, due to a resident's disease or condition. Supportive devices such as pillows, towels, blankets, padding, trochanter rolls, and footboards may be used to maintain alignment. Position changes and the types of positions used should be recorded to make sure a correct schedule is maintained.

Fowler's Position

- The resident is seated in bed, and the head of the bed is raised to a 45° angle (Figure 17.8). In *high Fowler's position*, the bed is raised to a 60–90° angle.
- The resident's knees may be elevated with a pillow under the knees and a pillow may also be used to support the resident's head.

Semi-Fowler's Position

- The resident is seated in bed, and the head of the bed is raised to a 30° angle (Figure 17.9).
- Support the resident's head with a pillow.
- The resident's knees may be elevated with a pillow under the knees.
- You may need to use a foot support (such as a footboard) to prevent foot drop, if ordered by the appropriate healthcare provider.

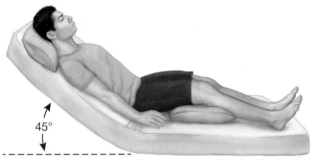

© Body Scientific International

Figure 17.8 In Fowler's position, the head of the bed is elevated to 45°.

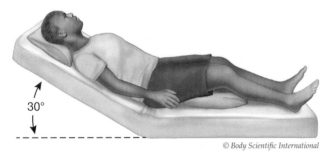

© Body Scientific International

Figure 17.9 In semi-Fowler's position, the head of the bed is elevated to 30°.

Supine Position

- The resident is lying faceup, flat on the back (Figure 17.10).
- The bed is flat, and both of the resident's arms and legs are extended.
- Support the resident's head with a pillow.
- If necessary, support the resident's arms and hands with pillows.
- You may need to support the small of the resident's back with a small, rolled towel or blanket and place a small, folded towel under the knees to relieve strain on the back.
- Use a footboard, if ordered by the appropriate healthcare provider, to prevent foot drop.
- You may need to place a trochanter roll to prevent the resident's hips from rotating outward.
- If needed, use padding to protect pressure points on the resident's elbows, knees, and tailbone.

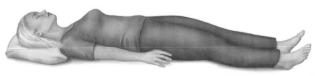

© Body Scientific International

Figure 17.10 In supine position, the resident or patient lies flat on his or her back.

Trendelenburg Position

- Trendelenburg position is a special supine position often used for residents who need certain medical or surgical procedures. The resident's legs are raised above the head (Figure 17.11).
- The resident's legs may be extended or bent.

Prone Position

- The resident is lying facedown, flat on the abdomen (Figure 17.12).
- The resident's legs are extended, and the head is turned to one side.
- The resident's arms are extended down at the sides. The arms may also be bent upward at the elbows.
- You may need to support the resident's head and abdomen with pillows.
- If needed, place a pillow under the resident's lower legs to reduce pressure on the toes. The resident's feet may hang off the bed to relieve pressure on the toes.

Lateral Position

- The resident is lying on the left side (called *left lateral*) or the right side (called *right lateral*), as shown in Figure 17.13.
- Support the resident's head with a pillow.
- The resident's lower arm should be flexed.
- The resident's upper leg and hip should be bent at the knee to relieve pressure on the back.
- You may need to place a pillow against the resident's back to maintain the position.
- If needed, place a small pillow under the arm.
- If needed, place a pillow between the resident's knees for protection and alignment.

Sims' Position

- Sims' position is a partly left lateral and partly prone position (Figure 17.14).
- Support the resident's head and shoulder with a pillow.
- The resident's left leg and arm should be extended, and the right leg and arm should be flexed.
- The resident's left arm should rest behind him or her.
- The flexed right leg should be supported with a pillow.
- The flexed right hand and arm should be supported with a pillow.

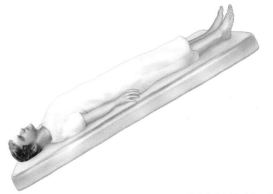

© *Body Scientific International*

Figure 17.11 In Trendelenburg position, the resident or patient lies on his or her back. The legs are raised above the head.

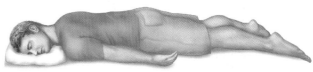

© *Body Scientific International*

Figure 17.12 In prone position, the resident or patient lies facedown.

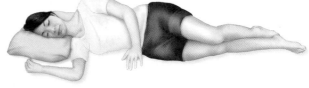

© *Body Scientific International*

Figure 17.13 In lateral position, the resident or patient lies on one side.

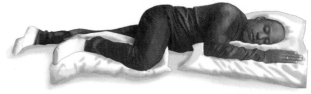

© *Body Scientific International*

Figure 17.14 In Sims' position, the resident or patient lies partly prone and partly lateral.

Following Positioning Guidelines

Properly positioning and repositioning residents requires a working knowledge of the different body positions, familiarity with needed equipment, and attention to the condition of the resident and the resident's skin. Always practice safety by using proper body mechanics and by asking for assistance if the resident is frail, is overweight, or has drainage tubes or an IV catheter.

Safe Handling

Maintaining safe resident-handling techniques at all times is vital when positioning or repositioning residents. General safety guidelines include the following:

- Maintain a wide, stable base with your feet.
- Position the bed at the correct height (waist level when providing care, hip level when moving a resident).
- Try to keep your work directly in front of you and avoid rotating your spine.
- Keep the resident close to your body to minimize reaching.
- Always observe the skin before and after changing a resident's position. Give skin care to pressure points. Protect the resident from tubing that may rub the skin.
- Provide the most support to the heaviest part of the resident's body. Avoid placing one body part directly on top of another.
- Move the resident carefully and smoothly. Avoid *shearing*, or abrasion, of the skin.
- Always check that the bed linens are clean, dry, and smooth. Ensure that folds in the linens or food crumbs do not rub the skin and increase the risk of decubitus ulcers.
- Pay attention to any complaints of dizziness, shortness of breath, rapid heartbeat, chest or head pain, changes in ability or strength, or pain when bearing weight during positioning. If the resident makes one of these complaints, stop the procedure, maintain resident safety, and alert the licensed nursing staff immediately.

Preparation

Resident-handling procedures such as positioning, turning, transferring, and lifting require safe preparation. When preparing for any resident-handling activity, you should follow specific guidelines:

1. Observe the resident and determine what supplies or equipment may be needed to ensure safety. Examples of equipment include mechanical, full-body lifts (either mobile or ceiling-mounted); mobile, sit-to-stand lifts; and gait (transfer) belts. These types of equipment help reduce the resident load on the nursing assistant.
2. Know how positioning equipment works and understand the procedure for using it.
3. Gather the appropriate supplies and equipment and other staff members, if needed.
4. Organize the physical environment and equipment to ensure safe completion of the procedure. Lock the wheels of the bed or wheelchair, raise or lower the bed or stretcher to the correct height, remove clutter, and check if any equipment needs to be charged.
5. If other staff members are needed for the procedure, make sure they know what to do.
6. Position yourself using the principles of body mechanics.

Understanding Directions

As a holistic nursing assistant, you should always explain what you are doing when positioning or moving residents. Residents who do not speak your language, however, may have a hard time understanding what is expected of them. You may need to ask for an interpreter or a family member to help explain the procedure. Understanding may be difficult even when an interpreter is used or when English is the resident's second language. Thus, move and speak slowly. Ask questions along the way to be sure you are understood. Showing residents what you want them to do can be helpful.

Language proficiency and cultural differences may interfere with communication as you ask residents to turn, sit up, or move from the bed to a chair. Be observant and watch residents' nonverbal communication and body reactions, as many cultures believe that people should be polite and show respect to those perceived as authority figures (such as healthcare providers). Residents may follow your directions even if they do not understand, are uncomfortable, or do not really want to participate. Residents may frown as they are moved, and their bodies may become stiff due to pain. If this occurs, stop changing the resident's position. There may be other ways to change the position (for example, by finding a more comfortable position or supporting the body with additional pillows, towels, blankets, or padding to relieve pressure). Always work to maintain safety and prevent incorrect twisting or turning, which can increase risk for skin rubs, irritation, bruising, or falls.

Apply It

1. What two actions can a holistic nursing assistant take to ensure residents understand what is expected of them?

2. What precautions can be taken to prevent possible bodily harm or pain, maintain skin integrity, and reduce safety risks during a position change?

---

7. Tell residents what actions you expect from them. Show residents what to do and then help them during the procedure. Ask residents to assist as much as they safely can and to the extent of their ability. Be sure to ask if residents are in pain. If a resident is in pain, let the licensed nursing staff know before changing a position.

8. Some residents (for example, residents who are paralyzed) may not be able to tell you if they are uncomfortable. You must pay special attention to these residents to prevent possible problems due to poor body alignment.

Procedure | Positioning in Bed

Rationale

Proper positioning in a bed provides good body alignment, helps maintain skin integrity, prevents decubitus ulcer formation, and promotes comfort and relaxation.

Preparation

1. Ask the licensed nursing staff how this procedure fits into the plan of care, if there are doctor's orders for the procedure, if there are any special instructions or precautions, and if the resident can be moved into the positions required for this procedure.

2. Practice safety by asking for assistance from a coworker.

3. Wash your hands or use hand sanitizer before entering the room.

4. Knock before entering the room.

5. Introduce yourself using your full name and title. Explain that you work with the licensed nursing staff and will be providing care.

6. Greet the resident and ask the resident to state his full name, if able. Then check the resident's identification bracelet.

7. Use Mr., Mrs., or Ms. and the last name when conversing.

8. Explain the procedure in simple terms, even if the resident is not able to communicate or is disoriented. Ask permission to perform the procedure.

(continued)

9. Bring the necessary equipment into the room. Place the following items in an accessible location:

- pillows of various sizes, if available and needed
- folded or rolled towels and blankets
- trochanter rolls
- draw sheet
- padding for skin and possible pressure points
- bed board
- footboard, if used to prevent foot drop
- hip abduction wedge

If you are unsure how to use a positioning device, check with the licensed nursing staff.

> **Best Practice**
> An immobile resident, whether in bed or seated in a chair, should be repositioned at least every two hours. Some residents may need to be repositioned more often. Follow the plan of care.

The Procedure

10. Provide privacy by closing the curtains, using a screen, or closing the door to the room.

11. Lock the bed wheels and then raise the bed to hip level.

> **Best Practice**
> Disposable gloves are worn only if required for infection prevention and control.

12. Ensure safety during the procedure. If there are side rails, raise and secure the rails on the opposite side of the bed from where you will be working. Lower the rail on the side you are working.

13. While the position may be prescribed by the plan of care, there may be times when residents can be asked about their personal comfort preferences. Be sure any tubing, such as IV catheters or urinary drainage bags, are not dislodged or kinked during or after positioning.

14. If moving an immobile resident up in bed, place pillows under the head and against the headboard for safety. The resident should be in a supine position. Ask another nursing assistant to help you with this procedure and stand on the opposite side of the bed from the other nursing assistant. Grasp each side of the draw sheet, and in unison (on the count of three), gently slide the resident up in the bed. Use proper body mechanics by standing straight and facing the bed with your knees slightly bent and your feet pivoted toward the head of the bed.

15. If moving a resident with some mobility up in bed, place pillows under the head and against the headboard for safety. Put one arm under the resident's shoulders and the other arm under the resident's hips. The resident should be in a sitting position in bed. Ask the resident to bend his knees, brace his feet firmly against the mattress, and place both hands on the mattress alongside his legs. On the count of three, ask the resident to push toward the head of the bed with his hands and feet. At the same time, slide the resident while still supporting his shoulders and hips. Use proper body mechanics by bending your knees, bending your body from the hips, pivoting toward the head of the bed, and shifting your weight from foot to foot as the resident moves.

16. Place pillows; soft, rolled towels; trochanter rolls; or blankets under the appropriate body areas, such as the head, shoulders, and small of the back; arms and elbows; thighs (tucking under to prevent external hip rotation); and ankles, calves, and knees (to raise the heels off the bed).

17. Do not raise the resident's ankles without first supporting the knees and calves.

18. If the knees are flexed, support them with a small pillow or blanket roll.

19. If appropriate, place a small pillow or blanket roll at the feet to prevent foot drop. (Use a footboard only if approved.)

20. Position the resident so the body is properly aligned. Then straighten the bed linens.

> **Best Practice**
> Pay attention to all possible pressure points on the resident's body. Provide support and padding for these areas, as needed.

21. Raise the head of the bed to a level appropriate for the position.

22. Check to be sure the bed wheels are locked and lower the bed.

23. Follow the plan of care to determine if the side rails should be raised or lowered.

24. Recheck that any tubing is secure and in place. If you have any concerns, ask a licensed nursing staff member to check that the IV or other tubing is functioning properly. If the resident has a urinary drainage bag, be sure it is secured below the bladder.

25. Remove, clean, and store equipment in the proper location. Remove soiled linens and discard disposable equipment.

Follow-Up

26. Wash your hands to ensure infection control.

27. Make sure the resident is comfortable and place the call light and personal items within reach.

28. Conduct a safety check before leaving the room. The room should be clean and free from clutter or spills.

29. Wash your hands or use hand sanitizer before leaving the room.

Reporting and Documentation

30. Communicate any specific observations, complications, or unusual responses to the licensed nursing staff. Record this information, along with the care provided, in the chart or EMR.

Turning a Resident in Bed

Turning a resident is an important part of positioning. Some positions, such as the lateral position, require the turning of the resident. You may also need to turn a resident during care (for example, when giving a bed bath or making an occupied bed). A draw sheet can assist you with turning residents, particularly residents who have limited mobility.

Procedure   Turning a Resident in Bed

Rationale

When a resident must remain in bed, turning can help prevent skin breakdown, promote comfort, and prepare residents for care procedures (such as bathing and bed making).

Preparation

1. Ask the licensed nursing staff how this procedure fits into the plan of care, if there are doctor's orders for the procedure, if there are any special instructions or precautions, and if the resident can be moved into the positions required for this procedure.

2. Practice safety by asking for assistance from a coworker.

3. Wash your hands or use hand sanitizer before entering the room.

4. Knock before entering the room.

5. Introduce yourself using your full name and title. Explain that you work with the licensed nursing staff and will be providing care.

6. Greet the resident and ask the resident to state her full name, if able. Then check the resident's identification bracelet.

7. Use Mr., Mrs., or Ms. and the last name when conversing.

8. Explain the procedure in simple terms, even if the resident is not able to communicate or is disoriented. Ask permission to perform the procedure.

9. Bring the necessary equipment into the room. Place the following items in an accessible location:
   - pillows of various sizes, if available and needed
   - folded or rolled towels and blankets
   - trochanter rolls
   - draw sheet
   - padding for skin and bony areas
   - hip abduction wedge

   If you are unsure how to use a positioning device, check with the licensed nursing staff.

(continued)

> **Best Practice**
> An immobile resident, whether in bed or seated in a chair, should be repositioned or turned at least every two hours. Some residents may need to be repositioned or turned more often. Follow the plan of care instructions.

The Procedure

10. Provide privacy by closing the curtains, using a screen, or closing the door to the room.
11. Ask the resident if she has any concerns about turning.
12. Lock the bed wheels and then raise the bed to hip level.

> **Best Practice**
> Disposable gloves are worn only if required for infection prevention and control.

13. Ensure safety during the procedure. If there are side rails, raise and secure the rails on the opposite side of the bed from where you will be working. Lower the rail on the side you are working.
14. Be sure any tubing, such as IV catheters or urinary drainage bags, are not dislodged or kinked during or after positioning.
15. Place the resident's head pillow up against the headboard of the bed to protect the resident's head.
16. Ask the resident to assist as much as possible.

> **Best Practice**
> Consider how close the resident will be to the side rail after being turned.

17. If using a draw sheet to turn the resident toward you, reach over the resident and untuck the side of the draw sheet farthest from you so you can grasp it. The draw sheet may already be on the bed. If the draw sheet is not on the bed, place the draw sheet on the bed below the resident's shoulders and hips.
18. Ask or assist the resident to bend her knees.
19. Cross the resident's arms over her chest.
20. Cross the resident's leg farthest from you over the leg nearest to you.

21. Reach over the resident and support her behind the shoulders with one hand and behind the hip with the other.
22. Using proper body mechanics, roll the resident gently and smoothly toward you. If there is a draw sheet, you can use that to help roll the resident.
23. Bend the resident's upper knee and hip forward slightly into a comfortable position.
24. Place a pillow against the resident's back for support and place a pillow under the resident's top leg, behind the legs, and under the top arm for comfort.
25. Reposition the head pillow under the resident's head and check the neck for proper alignment.

> **Best Practice**
> Be proactive and provide padding to cushion pressure points and to support the natural curves of the body, if needed.

26. Raise the side rail, if used, on the side where you worked. Move to the opposite side of the bed (behind the resident) and lower the side rail. Place your hands under the resident's shoulders and hip.
27. Adjust the shoulder and hips for comfort while the resident lies against a pillow.

> **Best Practice**
> When positioning the resident, push instead of pulling. Pushing is much safer than pulling.

28. To turn a resident away from you, start by repeating steps 10–15.
29. Ask or assist the resident to bend her knees.
30. Cross the resident's arms over her chest.
31. Cross the resident's leg nearest to you over the leg farthest from you.
32. Place one hand under the resident's shoulders and the other hand under the resident's hip.
33. Using proper body mechanics, roll the resident gently and smoothly away from you. If there is a draw sheet, untuck it, or place a draw sheet on the bed to help roll the resident.
34. Bend the resident's upper knee and hip forward slightly into a comfortable position.
35. Reposition the head pillow under the resident's head and check the neck for proper alignment.
36. Place a pillow behind the resident's back to help maintain a side-lying position.

37. Adjust the shoulder and hips for comfort while the resident lies against the pillow.

38. Use pillows to make further body alignments and adjustments and straighten out the resident's clothing, bed linens, and any tubes (Figure 17.15).

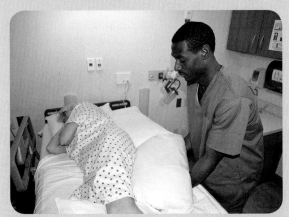

Figure 17.15

39. Check to be sure the bed wheels are locked and lower the bed.

40. Follow the plan of care to determine if the side rails should be raised or lowered.

41. Straighten the resident's clothing and bed linens. Recheck that any tubing is secure and in place. If you have any concerns, ask a licensed nursing staff member to check that the IV or other tubing is functioning properly. If the resident has a urinary drainage bag, be sure it is secured below the bladder.

42. Remove, clean, and store equipment in the proper location. Remove soiled linens and discard disposable equipment.

Follow-Up

43. Wash your hands to ensure infection control.

44. Make sure the resident is comfortable and place the call light and personal items within reach.

45. Conduct a safety check before leaving the room. The room should be clean and free from clutter or spills.

46. Wash your hands or use hand sanitizer before leaving the room.

Reporting and Documentation

47. Communicate any specific observations, complications, or unusual responses to the licensed nursing staff. Record this information, along with the care provided, in the chart or EMR.

Image courtesy of Wards Forest Media, LLC

Procedure   Logrolling

Rationale

Logrolling is a useful technique for safely turning and moving bedridden residents. During logrolling, the resident's body is kept in straight alignment (like a log). Logrolling is typically used for a resident who has had a spinal injury or who must be turned in one movement without twisting. Two healthcare staff members are required to complete the logrolling procedure.

Preparation

1. Ask the licensed nursing staff how this procedure fits into the plan of care, if there are doctor's orders for the procedure, if there are any special instructions or precautions, and if the resident can be moved into the positions required for this procedure.

2. Practice safety by asking for assistance from a coworker.

3. Wash your hands or use hand sanitizer before entering the room.

4. Knock before entering the room.

5. Introduce yourself using your full name and title. Explain that you work with the licensed nursing staff and will be providing care.

6. Greet the resident and ask the resident to state his full name, if able. Then check the resident's identification bracelet.

7. Use Mr., Mrs., or Ms. and the last name when conversing.

(continued)

8. Explain the procedure in simple terms, even if the resident is not able to communicate or is disoriented. Ask permission to perform the procedure.

9. Bring the necessary equipment into the room. Place the following items in an accessible location:
   - pillows of various sizes, if available and needed
   - folded or rolled towels and blankets
   - draw sheet

The Procedure

10. Provide privacy by closing the curtains, using a screen, or closing the door to the room.

11. Lock the bed wheels and then raise the bed to hip level.

12. Ensure safety during the procedure. If there are side rails, raise and secure the rails on the opposite side of the bed from where you will be working. Lower the rail on the side you are working.

13. Be sure any tubing, such as IV catheters or urinary drainage bags, are not dislodged or kinked during or after positioning.

> **Best Practice**
> Disposable gloves are worn only if required for infection prevention and control.

14. Make sure the bed is in the flat position and the resident is in the supine position. If allowed, remove the pillow beneath the resident's head.

15. Stand next to the bed on the side opposite of the way you will turn the resident.

16. Position one of your legs in front of the other and slightly bend your front knee.

17. Move the resident's entire body to the side of the bed nearest to you. Use the draw sheet, if necessary.

18. Place the resident's arms across his chest. Place a pillow lengthwise between the resident's legs to protect the knees.

19. Raise the side rail, if used, on the side where you worked. Move to the other side of the bed and lower the side rail.

20. Stand near the resident's shoulders and chest. A coworker should stand on the same side of the bed near the resident's hips and thighs.

21. Stand with your feet apart and with one foot in front of the other.

22. Ask the resident to hold his body rigid.

23. On the count of three, you and your coworker should roll the resident toward you in a single movement (Figure 17.16A). Use the draw sheet, if necessary or if instructed (Figure 17.16B). Keep the resident's head, spine, and legs aligned.

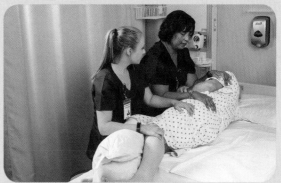

A

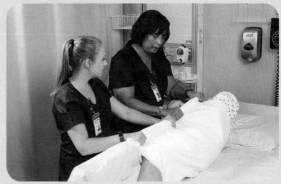

Figure 17.16   B

24. Reposition the pillow under the resident's head and straighten the bed linens.

25. Position the resident to maintain good body alignment in a side-lying position. Use pillows as instructed by the charge nurse or the plan of care.

26. Straighten the resident's clothing, bed linens, and any tubes.

27. Check to be sure the bed wheels are locked and lower the bed.

28. Follow the plan of care to determine if the side rails should be raised or lowered.

29. Straighten the resident's clothing and bed linens. Recheck that any tubing is secure and in place. If you have any concerns, ask a licensed nursing staff member to check that the IV or other tubing is functioning properly. If the resident has a urinary drainage bag, be sure it is secured below the bladder.

30. Place any soiled linens in the appropriate laundry hamper.

Follow-Up

31. Wash your hands to ensure infection control.

32. Make sure the resident is comfortable and place the call light and personal items within reach.

33. Conduct a safety check before leaving the room. The room should be clean and free from clutter or spills.

34. Wash your hands or use hand sanitizer before leaving the room.

Reporting and Documentation

35. Communicate any specific observations, complications, or unusual responses to the licensed nursing staff. Record this information, along with the care provided, in the chart or EMR.

Images courtesy of © Tori Soper Photography

Dangling

In addition to positioning and turning residents, nursing assistants also help residents get out of bed. An important first step prior to a resident moving out of bed to sit or stand is *dangling*, or sitting at the edge of the bed. Dangling helps residents become comfortable in a seated position and is particularly important if residents have been bedridden for a period of time.

Sitting before standing lowers the risk of **orthostatic hypotension**, a condition in which blood pressure falls when a resident stands. Orthostatic hypotension occurs when gravity causes blood to pool in the abdomen and legs, decreasing blood pressure as less blood circulates back to the heart. Orthostatic hypotension is more common in adults ages 65 and older, because special receptors (located near the heart and neck arteries) that sense and regulate blood pressure slow down with age. An older heart may not beat fast enough to make up for a drop in blood pressure. Certain medications may also cause orthostatic hypotension. If orthostatic hypotension does occur, a resident may feel lightheaded or dizzy after standing up, feel weak, experience **syncope** (fainting), and become a fall risk.

Procedure — Dangling at the Edge of the Bed

Rationale

Helping a resident dangle, or sit, at the edge of the bed before getting up promotes safety. It reduces the risk of falling from possible dizziness or fainting due to orthostatic hypotension.

Preparation

1. Ask the licensed nursing staff how this procedure fits into the plan of care, if there are doctor's orders for the procedure, if there are any special instructions or precautions, and if the resident can be moved into the positions required for this procedure.

2. Wash your hands or use hand sanitizer before entering the room.

3. Knock before entering the room.

4. Introduce yourself using your full name and title. Explain that you work with the licensed nursing staff and will be providing care.

5. Greet the resident and ask the resident to state her full name, if able. Then check the resident's identification bracelet.

6. Use Mr., Mrs., or Ms. and the last name when conversing.

7. Explain the procedure in simple terms, even if the resident is not able to communicate or is disoriented. Ask permission to perform the procedure.

8. Place the resident's robe and shoes nearby, if needed.

9. Clear the area of furniture and equipment to provide space to move.

(continued)

The Procedure

10. Provide privacy by closing the curtains, using a screen, or closing the door to the room.

11. Lock the bed wheels and then raise the bed to hip level.

12. Ensure safety during the procedure. If there are side rails, raise and secure the rails on the opposite side of the bed from where you will be working. Lower the rail on the side you are working.

13. Fanfold the linens to the foot of the bed.

14. Ask the resident to move to the edge of the bed or assist the resident, if necessary.

15. Raise the head of the bed slowly so the resident is in a sitting position. Raising the head slowly will help prevent the resident from becoming dizzy or experiencing discomfort.

16. Face the resident and stand at the side of the bed with your feet spread apart and your knees slightly bent to protect your back.

17. Slip one arm behind the resident's shoulders and grasp the far shoulder.

18. Slip your other arm under the resident's knees and rest your hand on the side of the resident's thigh (Figure 17.17).

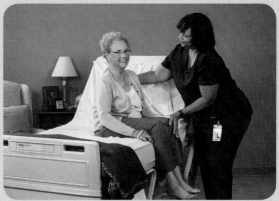

Figure 17.18

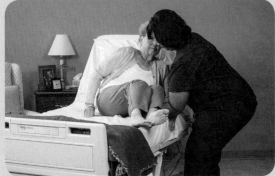

Figure 17.17

19. In a single, smooth, pivoting movement, slide the resident's legs over the side of the bed and move her head and shoulders upward so that the resident sits on the edge of the bed (Figure 17.18).

20. Instruct the resident to hold on to the side of the mattress for support, if needed.

21. Stand in front of the seated resident to block her in case of a fall forward.

22. Do not leave the resident. Provide support, if necessary. Observe the resident and ask how she is feeling.

23. Observe the resident's condition during dangling. Ask how the resident is feeling (for example, dizzy or lightheaded). Check the resident's pulse and respirations. Check for any difficulty breathing and note if the skin is pale or bluish in color (called *cyanosis*).

> **Best Practice**
> A resident may feel dizzy for the first few minutes of dangling, but this feeling should pass. If it doesn't, return the resident to a lying position with the head raised and immediately notify the charge nurse.

24. If the resident is getting out of bed, make sure the resident is stable and feels well enough to continue the procedure.

25. To return the resident to a lying position after dangling, reverse this procedure and position the resident using proper body alignment.

Follow-Up

26. Wash your hands to ensure infection control.

27. Make sure the resident is comfortable and place the call light and personal items within reach.

28. Conduct a safety check before leaving the room. The room should be clean and free from clutter or spills.

29. Wash your hands or use hand sanitizer before leaving the room.

Reporting and Documentation

30. Communicate any specific observations, complications, or unusual responses to the licensed nursing staff. Record this information, along with the care provided, in the chart or EMR.

Images courtesy of © Tori Soper Photography

Transferring a Resident

Transferring residents from their beds to a chair, wheelchair, or stretcher (and back again) is another procedure that requires concentration and safety awareness. Transfers are performed when residents need assistance moving from their beds to sit in a chair or wheelchair (Figure 17.19). Transfers may also be required when a resident must be transported using a wheelchair or stretcher to another part of the facility. Stretchers are used when a resident is not able to sit in a wheelchair for transport.

Transfer sheets, slides, roll boards, and wooden or plastic slide or transfer boards are typically used for transfers between beds and stretchers. As you learned in chapter 16, a *gait belt* (sometimes called a *transfer belt* when used for transfer) is a safety device that nursing assistants can use to move residents who are standing and ambulating. The gait belt is worn by the resident, who may be too weak to support himself or herself, and helps prevent falls. A gait belt should never be used to lift a resident and is contraindicated for residents who have had abdominal surgery. The gait belt also decreases the risk of the nursing assistant sustaining back injuries. Gait belts come in a variety of sizes and materials, such as canvas, nylon, or leather.

Lifts may be used for residents who are extremely overweight, cannot bend their bodies, or are unable to bear weight on their feet. Lifts can be mechanical or electronic (Figure 17.20). Facilities will have policies regarding when and how to use a lift.

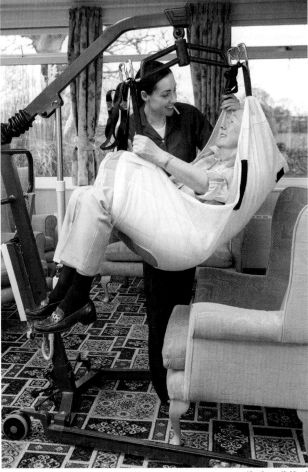

iStock.com/SolStock

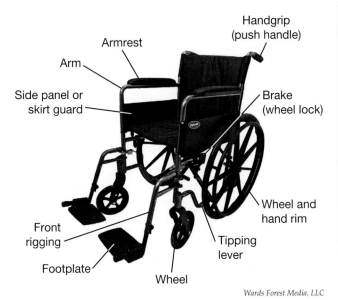

Wards Forest Media, LLC

Figure 17.19 Knowing the parts of a wheelchair can help you provide wheelchair transport.

Figure 17.20 Lifts help transfer residents who are overweight, who cannot bend, or who cannot put any weight on their feet.

Rationale

Transferring a resident in one smooth or pivoting motion minimizes fatigue and promotes safety.

Preparation

1. Ask the licensed nursing staff how this procedure fits into the plan of care, if there are doctor's orders for the procedure, if there are any special instructions or precautions, and if the resident can be moved into the positions required for this procedure.

2. Wash your hands or use hand sanitizer before entering the room.

3. Knock before entering the room.

4. Introduce yourself using your full name and title. Explain that you work with the licensed nursing staff and will be providing care.

5. Greet the resident and ask the resident to state his full name, if able. Then check the resident's identification bracelet.

6. Use Mr., Mrs., or Ms. and the last name when conversing.

7. Explain the procedure in simple terms, even if the resident is not able to communicate or is disoriented. Ask permission to perform the procedure.

8. Bring the necessary equipment into the room. Place the following items in an accessible location:
   - chair or wheelchair
   - a gait belt (in good condition and functional)
   - bath blanket
   - a robe and slippers
   - a pillow, if needed

The Procedure

9. Provide privacy by closing the curtains, using a screen, or closing the door to the room.

10. Lock the bed wheels and then lower the bed to its lowest position.

11. Ensure safety during the procedure. If there are side rails, raise and secure the rails on the opposite side of the bed from where you will be working. Lower the rail on the side you are working.

12. Position the chair or wheelchair next to the bed. If the resident has a weak side, position the chair or wheelchair so the resident can transfer using his stronger side.

13. Stabilize the chair for safety. If transferring the resident into a wheelchair, lock the wheels of the wheelchair and raise the footplates. Be sure the front swivel wheels of the wheelchair are facing forward.

14. Assist the resident to the edge of the bed and to a dangling position.

15. Apply a gait belt around the resident's waist over his clothing, if needed. The buckle of the gait belt should be in the front. Thread the belt through the teeth of the buckle and through the belt's two loops to lock it.

16. Check that the gait belt is snug, but that there is still enough room to place your fingers under the belt.

17. Stand in front of the resident with your feet about 12 inches apart.

18. Place one of your feet between the resident's feet and place your other foot outside one of the resident's feet. This will allow you to lock a sliding resident's knee with your knees.

19. Place your feet so that you have room to pivot them toward the chair.

20. Face the resident and hold on to the gait belt using an underhand grasp for greater safety.

21. Instruct the resident to hold on to your shoulders or arms, but not to put his arms around your neck.

22. Using the gait belt, assist the resident into a standing position. Lift the resident using your arm and leg muscles. Bend your knees and keep your back straight. Do not twist your body.

23. Continue to hold on to the gait belt while the resident gains his balance. Have the resident stand erect with his head up and back straight. Suggest the resident shift his weight from one foot to the other to become comfortable standing before starting the transfer.

24. Face the chair or wheelchair and move your feet toward it as the resident follows, taking baby steps.

25. Once the resident is standing in front of the chair or wheelchair, ask if the resident feels the chair or wheelchair on the back of his legs.

26. Instruct the resident to put his hands on the armrests.

27. Assist the resident into a seated position using proper body mechanics.

28. Position the resident properly. The back and buttocks should be supported by the back of the chair or wheelchair. If there are footrests, place the resident's feet on them. There should be some space between the backs of the knees and calves and the edge of the seat. A small pillow behind the resident's lower back may provide support.

29. Arrange the resident's robe and clothing and cover the resident's legs with a bath blanket. Make sure the bath blanket does not touch the floor or the wheels of the chair.

30. Observe the resident for signs of discomfort or dizziness.

31. If transporting a resident using a wheelchair, push the wheelchair from behind and keep your body close to the chair. When entering an elevator, pull the wheelchair in backward. When leaving an elevator, wait until everyone leaves and then push the open button, turn the wheelchair around, and pull the wheelchair out of the elevator backward.

Follow-Up

32. Make sure that the resident's body is in alignment and that the resident is safe and comfortable.

33. Place the call light and personal items within reach.

34. Conduct a safety check before leaving the room. The room should be clean and free from clutter or spills.

35. Wash your hands or use hand sanitizer before leaving the room.

Reporting and Documentation

36. Communicate any specific observations, complications, or unusual responses to the licensed nursing staff. Record this information, along with the care provided, in the chart or EMR.

Procedure — Transferring to a Chair or Wheelchair Using a Lift

Rationale

Moving a weak or immobile resident with a lift promotes safety and comfort during the transfer process.

Preparation

1. Ask the licensed nursing staff how this procedure fits into the plan of care, if there are doctor's orders for the procedure, if there are any special instructions or precautions, and if the resident can be moved into the positions required for this procedure.

2. Practice safety by asking for assistance from a coworker.

3. Wash your hands or use hand sanitizer before entering the room.

4. Knock before entering the room.

5. Introduce yourself using your full name and title. Explain that you work with the licensed nursing staff and will be providing care.

6. Greet the resident and ask the resident to state his full name, if able. Then check the resident's identification bracelet.

7. Use Mr., Mrs., or Ms. and the last name when conversing.

8. Explain the procedure in simple terms, even if the resident is not able to communicate or is disoriented. Ask permission to perform the procedure.

9. Bring the necessary equipment into the room. Place the following items in an accessible location:
   - lift
   - the appropriate size and type of sling for the resident's weight and size (consult the charge nurse if you are unsure what is appropriate)
   - a chair or wheelchair
   - a robe and slippers
   - a bath blanket

The Procedure

10. Provide privacy by closing the curtains, using a screen, or closing the door to the room.

11. Position the chair or wheelchair next to the bed and stabilize the chair for safety. If transferring the resident into a wheelchair, lock the wheels of the wheelchair and raise the footplates. Be sure the front swivel wheels of the wheelchair face forward.

(continued)

12. Lock the bed wheels and then lower the bed to the lowest position.

13. Ensure safety during the procedure. If there are side rails, raise and secure the rails on the opposite side of the bed from where you will be working. Lower the rail on the side you are working.

14. Roll the resident toward you and position the sling under him. You may need to roll the resident from side to side to maneuver the sling into place beneath him. The lower part of the sling should rest behind the resident's knees, and the upper part should rest beneath the resident's upper shoulders.

15. Position the lift bar and frame over the bed in an open position. Lock the lift's wheels.

16. Attach the sling to the lift following the instructions in the manufacturer's handbook.

17. Make sure the open ends of the lift's hooks that will attach to the sling face away from the resident.

18. Ask the resident to fold his arms across his chest.

> **Best Practice**
> Talk to the resident as you lift him free of the bed. Talking to the resident will help lower anxiety.

19. When the lift holds the resident freely above the bed and is stable, move the resident away from the bed. Your coworker should support the resident's legs.

20. Position the resident above the chair or wheelchair.

21. Gently lower the resident as your coworker guides him into the chair or wheelchair. If the resident is being lowered into a chair, be sure the chair will not move.

22. Make sure the resident's feet and hands are positioned comfortably.

23. Lower the lift's bar so you can easily unhook the sling.

24. Follow your facility's policy to determine if the sling can be left beneath the resident.

25. Cover the resident with a blanket. Make sure the blanket does not touch the floor.

26. Remove, clean, and store equipment in the proper location. Remove soiled linens and discard disposable equipment.

Follow-Up

27. Wash your hands to ensure infection control.

28. Make sure the resident is comfortable and place the call light and personal items within reach.

29. Conduct a safety check before leaving the room. The room should be clean and free from clutter or spills.

30. Wash your hands or use hand sanitizer before leaving the room.

Reporting and Documentation

31. Communicate any specific observations, complications, or unusual responses to the licensed nursing staff. Record this information, along with the care provided, in the chart or EMR.

Procedure | Transferring from a Bed to a Stretcher

Rationale

Transferring a resident in one smooth or pivoting motion promotes safety.

Preparation

1. Ask the licensed nursing staff how this procedure fits into the plan of care, if there are doctor's orders for the procedure, if there are any special instructions or precautions, and if the resident can be moved into the positions required for this procedure.

2. Practice safety by asking for assistance from a coworker.

3. Wash your hands or use hand sanitizer before entering the room.

4. Knock before entering the room.

5. Introduce yourself using your full name and title. Explain that you work with the licensed nursing staff and will be providing care.

6. Greet the resident and ask the resident to state his full name, if able. Then check the resident's identification bracelet.

7. Use Mr., Mrs., or Ms. and the last name when conversing.

8. Explain the procedure in simple terms, even if the resident is not able to communicate or is disoriented. Ask permission to perform the procedure.

9. Bring the necessary equipment into the room. Place the following items in an accessible location:
   - stretcher
   - bath blanket
   - a robe and slippers
   - a pillow, if needed
   - a draw sheet, slide board, or other assistive device, if needed

The Procedure

10. Provide privacy by closing the curtains, using a screen, or closing the door to the room.

11. Lock the bed wheels and then raise the bed to hip level.

12. Ensure safety during the procedure. If there are side rails, raise and secure the rails on the opposite side of the bed from where you will be working. Lower the rail on the side you are working.

13. Position the stretcher alongside the resident's bed. Lock the stretcher wheels.

14. Lower the head of the bed to be as flat as possible. Raise the bed so it is even with the stretcher.

15. Stand on the side of the bed. The stretcher should be between your body and the resident's bed. Your coworker should stand on the other side of the resident's bed.

16. Place a draw sheet, if not already on the bed, under the resident. If the draw sheet is on the bed, untuck it. If the resident is too weak to move his head, adjust the sheet to support the head.

17. Ask the resident to move closer to the edge of the bed and closer to the stretcher, if able.

Best Practice
Ask the resident to do as much of the transfer as possible while assisting with the draw sheet.

18. If the resident is too weak to assist with the transfer, instruct the resident to place his arms across his chest and tuck his chin to his chest to avoid hyperextending his neck.

Best Practice
You can use a plastic or wooden slide board to assist in moving the resident. This device is placed between the bed and stretcher from the resident's back extending from the resident's shoulder to his hips.

19. On the count of three, move or slide the resident gently and smoothly from the bed to the stretcher with the draw sheet or slide board. You will usually transfer the lower body of the resident first and then move the upper body. Some residents will need to be transferred in one motion to prevent injury.

20. Cover the resident with a sheet or bath blanket to ready him for transport. Fasten safety straps, if available.

21. Raise the side rails of the stretcher and release the brake.

22. Position yourself at the head of the stretcher and push the stretcher so that the resident's feet face forward. Keep your body close to the stretcher as you transport the resident to the appropriate location in the healthcare facility.

Follow-Up

23. Make sure that the resident's body is in alignment and that the resident is safe and comfortable.

24. Place the call light and personal items within reach.

25. Conduct a safety check before leaving the room. The room should be clean and free from clutter or spills.

26. Wash your hands or use hand sanitizer before leaving the room.

Reporting and Documentation

27. Communicate any specific observations, complications, or unusual responses to the licensed nursing staff. Record this information, along with the care provided, in the chart or EMR.

How Can Comfort Be Promoted?

Positioning can promote resident relaxation, sleep, and overall comfort. As a holistic nursing assistant, you should use the resident's preferred position for rest, if possible. Follow doctors' orders for turning, if specified. Other suggestions for ensuring resident comfort include the following:

- Obtain comfortable bedding. When working in a long-term care facility, you may be able to use the resident's own bedding, such as a pillow or afghan.

- Straighten or change soiled linens, if necessary (Figure 17.21). Ensure that bedding covering the limbs, particularly the feet and legs, is not too tight and does not irritate or rub the skin (possibly causing decubitus ulcers).

- Adjust positions for maximum support and comfort. Use pillows, blankets, or rolls, as appropriate.

- Remind residents who are more mobile to change their positions often.

- Identify any mechanical sources of discomfort, such as tubes, drains, syringe caps, or other equipment or devices. Remove any items, such as syringe caps, that can be discarded. Alert the licensed nursing staff if residents complain of discomfort related to tubes and drains. Nonfunctioning equipment (for example, alarms that sound without cause) should be repaired.

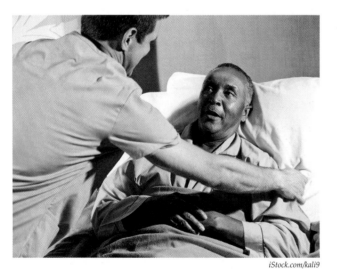

iStock.com/kali9

Figure 17.21 Straightening and changing linens can help promote comfort and preserve a resident's skin integrity.

Using the Key Terms

Complete the following sentences using key terms in this section.

1. A sudden drop in blood pressure can result in fainting, which is also called _____.
2. The stiffening or immobility of a joint is _____.
3. In _____, body parts are placed optimally for efficient use.
4. When residents with _____ stand, their blood pressure falls.
5. A footboard is sometimes used to help prevent _____.
6. _____ prevent external rotation of the hips.

Know and Understand the Facts

7. What are the benefits of good body alignment?
8. Identify two guidelines for helping residents overcome the psychological and social effects of immobility.
9. Describe three body positions that can be used with residents.
10. Identify three resident-handling guidelines to follow when preparing to position a resident.

Analyze and Apply Concepts

11. Why is it important for residents to change positions? How often should positioning be done?
12. Explain how to turn a resident safely.
13. Describe what may happen if a resident stands too quickly. What can be done to prevent this reaction?
14. Describe the steps for using a lift.

Think Critically

Read the following care situation. Then answer the questions that follow.

Today, Lisa will be taking care of Mrs. G, who was admitted to the hospital yesterday for pneumonia. Mrs. G is 85 years old and does not speak English well. Lisa has been asked to transfer Mrs. G from her bed to a wheelchair in preparation for an X-ray. Mrs. G's two daughters are visiting and appear very protective of their mother. They are speaking Spanish to her when Lisa enters the room.

15. What guidelines should Lisa follow when transferring Mrs. G to a wheelchair?
16. What can Lisa do to include Mrs. G's daughters in the transfer process?
17. What two actions should Lisa take to ensure the transfer is performed safely?
18. Identify any issues that may influence the success of this transfer.

Questions to Consider

- Have you ever had an injury that prevented you from walking for a period of time?
- When you were injured, was it difficult to do the things you like to do?
- Did you use crutches or a cane? Did it take time for you to become comfortable using your crutches or cane? How did people react to you? Were they respectful of your problem or were they unwilling to help? How did their treatment make you feel?

Objectives

To promote and support mobility, nursing assistants must understand the importance of ambulation. Some residents may rely on canes, walkers, or crutches to ambulate. As a holistic nursing assistant, you must assist residents in using these devices safely. To achieve the objectives for this section, you must successfully

- **describe** the importance and stages of ambulation;
- **recognize** the limitations residents may have when ambulating;
- **explain** how to assist residents when they ambulate; and
- **identify** the steps needed to assist residents with canes, walkers, and crutches.

Key Terms

Learn these key terms to better understand the information presented in the section.

axilla
ballistic

double pendulum

Why Is Ambulation Important?

Think About This

On average, children first walk independently when they are 11 months old. By adulthood, the average walking speed is about 3.1 miles per hour (mph), though the walking speed for older adults is slower. Walking speed varies depending on a person's height, weight, age, fitness level, effort, and culture. The ground surface and load a person is carrying also influence walking speed.

Ambulation, or the ability to walk around, is essential for achieving optimal well-being. Ambulation improves circulation and muscle tone, preserves lung tissue and airway function, and helps promote muscle and joint mobility. When hospital patients ambulate early during their stays, their lung function improves greatly. In a recent study, patients who increased their walking by at least 600 steps between the first and second 24-hour days in the hospital were discharged approximately two days earlier compared to other patients.

Ambulation requires an action called a **double pendulum**. When a person walks, the leg leaves the ground and swings forward from the hip. This is the first pendulum. When the leg strikes the ground, the heel touches first and rolls through to the toe. This motion is the second pendulum. To walk, the two legs coordinate so that one foot is always in contact with the ground.

Walking differs from running. During walking, one leg is always in contact with the ground, while the other swings. During running, a **ballistic** phase occurs when both feet are off the ground at the same time and the body's momentum moves it forward.

What Are the Stages of Ambulation?

As a nursing assistant, you will usually assist a resident through three stages that lead to ambulation. Nursing assistants play an important role in each of these stages and are responsible for making sure these stages occur safely and appropriately.

The three stages of assisting a resident in ambulating follow:

1. Assist the resident into a dangling position. Dangling after lying in bed avoids orthostatic hypotension, or a drop in blood pressure, and helps prevent potential dizziness and fainting.
2. Assist the resident in standing. The resident may wear a gait belt for support during ambulation.

3. The resident begins ambulating. Sometimes, after the resident stands, it is helpful to assist the resident into a chair to rest prior to ambulating.

If you are helping someone ambulate in his or her home, there are additional safety precautions you should take during ambulation. These include the following:

- Remove any small rugs or electrical cords on the floor, clean up any spills, and move anything that may cause a fall.
- Place nonslip bath mats in the bathroom. Grab bars, a raised toilet seat, and a shower tub seat are also helpful.
- Make sure everyday household items are easily accessible.
- Encourage the use of a backpack, fanny pack, apron, or briefcase to enable the person to carry objects during ambulation.

How Should a Nursing Assistant Assist with Ambulation?

To prepare for any procedure in which you will assist a resident with ambulation, you should be familiar with the abbreviations and acronyms related to resident mobility (Figure 17.22). Further, you should be able to perform the following steps:

1. Ask the resident if he or she is feeling any pain. If the resident is feeling pain, alert the licensed nursing staff about the resident's pain before beginning ambulation.

2. Depending on the resident's level of mobility, use appropriate equipment. Equipment may include a full-body lift; mobile, sit-to-stand lift; or gait belts. These pieces of equipment help reduce the load of a resident's body weight on the healthcare staff. As a nursing assistant, you should know how equipment works and understand the procedure for using it.

3. Gather the appropriate supplies, equipment, and coworkers, if needed.

4. Organize the physical environment and equipment to ensure safe completion of the procedure. Lock the wheels of the bed or chair, put the bed or stretcher at the correct height, and make sure any electronic mobile equipment is charged. Identify and remove any tripping hazards such as electrical cords, throw rugs, and clutter.

5. If other healthcare staff members are needed to conduct a procedure, make sure they know what to do.

6. Tell the resident what actions you expect from him or her.

7. Show the resident what to do and help the resident during the procedure.

8. When assisting residents, use good posture and proper body mechanics.

9. If a resident begins to collapse during ambulation, do not try to carry, hold up, or catch him or her. Rather, assume a broad stance and place your preferred foot slightly ahead of the other and between the resident's legs. Grasp the resident's body firmly at the waist or under the **axilla** (*armpit*), and allow the resident to slide down against your leg (Figure 17.23). Ease the resident slowly to the floor, using your body as an incline. If necessary, lower your body along with the resident's. Remember to always use proper body mechanics.

Abbreviations and Acronyms Related to Resident Mobility	
Abbreviation or Acronym	**Meaning**
amb	ambulation
BR	bed rest
BRP	bathroom privileges
HOB	head of bed
OOB	out of bed
up ad lib	up as desired
W/C	wheelchair

Figure 17.22 Nursing assistants should be familiar with terminology related to mobility.

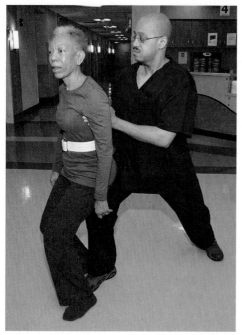

Wards Forest Media, LLC

Figure 17.23 If a resident begins to collapse, grasp the resident around the waist or under the armpits. Let the resident slide down against your leg and ease the resident to the floor.

10. If family members or friends would like to assist with ambulation, they may do so as long as a member of the licensed nursing staff has given permission and as long as each person understands and is comfortable with the procedure. Family members and friends must know how to avoid risks or prevent harm to themselves and the resident. You may need to provide instructions and assistance the first few times family members or friends assist with ambulation. Be sure to show family members and friends what to do if the resident collapses or begins to fall.

When people do not feel well, they often want to stay in bed. Therefore, assisting with mobility is one of the most important responsibilities of holistic nursing assistants. The following procedure provides information about how to help residents move out of their beds and ambulate.

Procedure | Helping a Resident Ambulate

Rationale

Assisting a resident with ambulation can improve the resident's mental and physical health.

Preparation

1. Ask the licensed nursing staff how this procedure fits into the plan of care, if there are doctor's orders for the procedure, if there are any special instructions or precautions, and if the resident can be moved into the positions required for this procedure.

2. Wash your hands or use hand sanitizer before entering the room.

3. Knock before entering the room.

4. Introduce yourself using your full name and title. Explain that you work with the licensed nursing staff and will be providing care.

5. Greet the resident and ask the resident to state her full name, if able. Then check the resident's identification bracelet.

6. Use Mr., Mrs., or Ms. and the last name when conversing.

7. Explain the procedure in simple terms, even if the resident is not able to communicate or is disoriented. Ask permission to perform the procedure.

8. Bring the necessary equipment into the room. Place the following items in an accessible location:
   - a robe, if needed to ensure the resident is not exposed, or properly fitting clothing
   - nonslip, properly fitting, low-heeled footwear
   - a gait belt (in good condition and functional)

The Procedure

9. Provide privacy by closing the curtains, using a screen, or closing the door to the room.

10. If the resident is in bed, lock the bed wheels and then lower the bed to its lowest position.

11. Ensure safety during the procedure. If the resident is in a bed with side rails, raise and secure the rails on the opposite side of the bed from where you will be working. Lower the rail on the side you are working.

12. If the resident is in bed, assist her to a dangling position on the side of the bed. The resident may also be seated in a chair.

13. Help the resident put on nonslip, properly fitting shoes and a robe, if needed.

14. Apply the gait belt around the resident's waist over her clothing, if needed. The buckle of the gait belt should be in the front. Thread the belt through the teeth of the buckle and through the belt's two loops to lock it.

15. Check that the belt is snug, but that there is still enough room for you to place your fingers under the belt.

16. Face the resident and take hold of the gait belt using an underhand grasp for greater safety. The resident may place her hands on your shoulders (Figure 17.24).

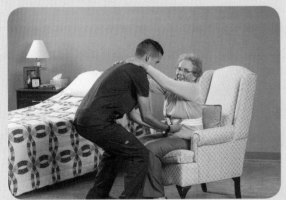
Figure 17.24

17. Using the gait belt, assist the resident to a standing position (Figure 17.25). Lift the resident using your arm and leg muscles. Bend your knees and keep your back straight. Do not twist your body.

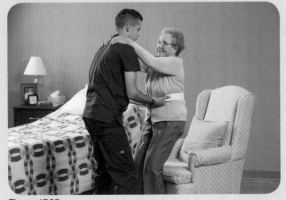
Figure 17.25

18. Continue holding on to the gait belt while the resident gains her balance. Have the resident stand erect with her head up and back straight.

19. Walk behind and to one side of the resident during ambulation.

20. Hold on to the gait belt directly from behind. Watch for signs of possible resident collapse. *Do not attempt to catch a resident who begins to collapse during ambulation. Instead, slowly ease the resident to the floor using your body as an incline.*

21. Determine if the resident has a weak side. If the resident does, position yourself accordingly:

    - If the resident has a weak right side, stand behind and slightly to the right of her (Figure 17.26A).
    - If the resident has a weak left side, stand behind and slightly to the left of her (Figure 17.26B).

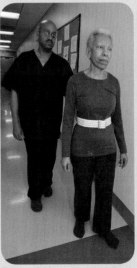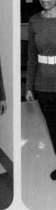
Figure 17.26   **A**   **B**

22. Let the resident set the pace and keep a firm grasp on the gait belt, if used.

23. Encourage the resident to ambulate the ordered distance, but be observant. Watch for signs of resident fatigue. If collapse occurs, follow the steps discussed earlier.

24. When ambulation is complete, help the resident return to her room or bed. Remove the gait belt and the resident's robe and shoes.

(continued)

25. If the resident returns to her bed, check to be sure the bed wheels are locked. Then reposition the resident and ensure the bed is in a low position.

26. Follow the plan of care to determine if the side rails should be raised or lowered.

27. Remove, clean, and store equipment in the proper location. Remove soiled linens and discard disposable equipment.

Follow-Up

28. Wash your hands to ensure infection control.

29. Make sure the resident is comfortable and place the call light and personal items within reach.

30. Conduct a safety check before leaving the room. The room should be clean and free from clutter or spills.

31. Wash your hands or use hand sanitizer before leaving the room.

Reporting and Documentation

32. Communicate any specific observations, complications, or unusual responses to the licensed nursing staff. Record this information, along with the care provided, in the chart or EMR.

Figure 17.24 © Tori Soper Photography, Figure 17.25 © Tori Soper Photography, Figure 17.26 Wards Forest Media, LLC

How Are Assistive Devices Used During Ambulation?

Some residents require assistive devices for ambulation because they can bear a limited amount of weight on their legs and feet. These assistive devices usually include canes, crutches, and walkers. The type of device used depends on how much support is needed.

Canes are particularly useful for residents who have had surgery and are not yet able to maintain balance or who need extra stability. Older adults may use a cane if they have recovered from a stroke and are not yet able to fully ambulate. They may also use a cane if they have arthritis that results in restricted movement.

Crutches are often used by residents who have short-term conditions such as a sprained ankle or broken leg. Crutches can also assist residents with amputations or disabilities because they provide better support over time. Residents need upper body strength to use canes and crutches.

Walkers are helpful for residents who have had surgery on the lower limbs (for example, a hip or knee replacement). During rehabilitation, the walker helps a resident reach the goal of full ambulation. Older adults may also use walkers when they begin to lose their balance or stability and need extra assistance. Walkers are often preferred to canes or crutches because they more evenly distribute the resident's weight and do not require as much upper body strength (although the resident using the walker must still be able to pick it up).

Ambulating with a Cane

Several types of canes help residents ambulate (Figure 17.27). The type of cane chosen depends on the resident's preferred grip, balancing ability, and need.

Canes with a single shaft and a crook neck are known as *C canes*. These canes resemble candy canes and are used for temporary walking impairment. They are available at local pharmacies and usually have a slip-resistant tip.

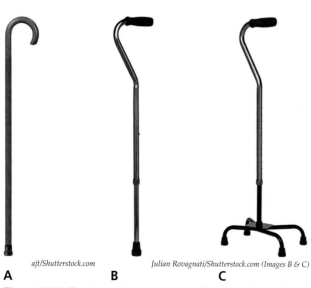

A   **B**   **C**

Figure 17.27 The types of canes include C canes (A), functional grip canes (B), and quad canes (C).

A *functional grip cane* is another type of single-shaft cane. This type of cane has a straight handle for a steadier grip. While the C and functional grip canes provide support, they do not assist with balance. Some canes may also have a slim, contoured handle and may be foldable or collapsible.

The *quad cane* has a base with four prongs, and each prong has a skid-resistant tip. The quad cane offers more stability than a single-shaft cane. It offers support, provides a functional grip, and assists with balance.

To ambulate successfully with a cane, a resident needs a cane that fits well and needs to use the cane properly (Figure 17.28). When a resident stands up straight with the arms at the sides, the top of the cane should be in line with the resident's wrist crease (the wrinkle that separates the arm from the hand). The resident should be able to slightly bend his or her elbow (approximately 15–20°) while using the cane. The resident should always hold the cane with his or her stronger hand (the hand opposite the side that needs more support).

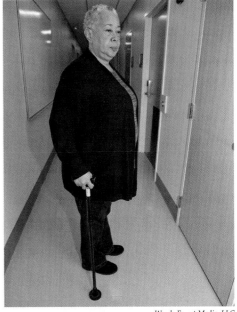

Wards Forest Media, LLC

Figure 17.28 Correct cane fit is important for resident safety. The resident should be able to bend his or her elbow slightly while using the cane.

Procedure Providing Assistance with a Cane

Rationale

Assisting a resident who is ambulating with a cane reduces the chance of injury and promotes safe ambulation by helping the resident achieve balance and giving support.

Preparation

1. Ask the licensed nursing staff how this procedure fits into the plan of care, if there are doctor's orders for the procedure, if there are any special instructions or precautions, and if the resident can be moved into the positions required for this procedure.

2. Wash your hands or use hand sanitizer before entering the room.

3. Knock before entering the room.

4. Introduce yourself using your full name and title. Explain that you work with the licensed nursing staff and will be providing care.

5. Greet the resident and ask the resident to state her full name, if able. Then check the resident's identification bracelet.

6. Use Mr., Mrs., or Ms. and the last name when conversing.

7. Explain the procedure in simple terms, even if the resident is not able to communicate or is disoriented. Ask permission to perform the procedure.

8. Bring the necessary equipment into the room. Place the following items in an accessible location:
   - a robe, if needed to ensure the resident is not exposed, or properly fitting clothing
   - nonslip, properly fitting, low-heeled footwear
   - a cane with one or four tips for added support (free from flaws, cracks, bends, or missing parts)
   - a gait belt (in good condition and functional)

The Procedure

9. Provide privacy by closing the curtains, using a screen, or closing the door to the room.

10. If the resident is in bed, lock the bed wheels and then lower the bed to its lowest position.

11. Ensure safety during the procedure. If the resident is in a bed with side rails, raise and secure the rails on the opposite side of the bed from where you will be working. Lower the rail on the side you are working.

(continued)

Providing Assistance with a Cane (continued)

12. If the resident is in bed, assist her to a dangling position on the side of the bed. The resident may also be seated in a chair.

13. Help the resident put on nonslip, properly fitting shoes and a robe, if needed.

14. Apply the gait belt, if needed. Put the belt around the resident's waist over her clothing with the buckle in the front. Thread the belt through the teeth of the buckle and through the belt's two loops to lock it. Make the belt snug, but leave enough room to place your fingers under the belt.

15. The resident should hold the cane on her stronger side.

16. Face the resident and take hold of the gait belt using an underhand grasp for greater safety.

17. Using the gait belt, assist the resident to a standing position. Lift the resident using your arm and leg muscles. Bend your knees and keep your back straight. Do not twist your body.

18. Continue holding on to the gait belt while the resident gains her balance. Have the resident stand erect with her head up and back straight.

19. Position the cane and stabilize the resident with the cane before ambulation begins.

20. During ambulation, the resident should move the cane forward about 6–10 inches (Figure 17.29).

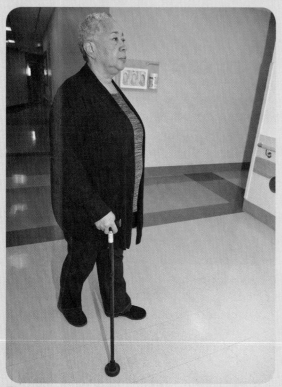

Figure 17.29

21. After moving the cane forward, the resident should follow, first with the weak leg and then with the strong leg.

22. If using a gait belt, stand slightly behind and on the weaker side of the resident to provide additional support as needed.

23. Grasp the gait belt directly from behind using an underhand grip, if needed.

24. Encourage the resident to use handrails, if available.

25. Let the resident set the pace and keep a firm grasp on the gait belt, if used. Encourage the resident to ambulate the ordered distance, but be observant. Watch for signs of resident fatigue or possible collapse. *Do not attempt to catch a resident who begins to collapse during ambulation. Instead, slowly ease the resident to the floor, using your body as an incline.*

26. If it is permissible and if the resident is strong enough, assist the resident with climbing stairs with a cane. Before beginning, check to be sure that the resident can walk safely on flat surfaces.

27. Have the resident grasp the handrail (if possible) with the hand on her weak side. Ask the resident to hold the cane in her opposite, strong hand.

28. The resident should climb each stair using her strong leg first. Once the resident is balanced, she can move the cane up the stair, followed by her weak leg. She can repeat these steps to move up the stairs.

29. To come down stairs, the resident should place the cane on each stair first, followed by her weaker leg and then her stronger leg. Remind the resident to face forward and "go up with the good, down with the bad." When going up stairs, the resident should lead with the stronger leg.

30. When the ambulation is complete, help the resident return to her room or bed. Remove the gait belt, if used, and the resident's robe, cane, and shoes.

31. If the resident returns to her bed, check to be sure the bed wheels are locked. Then reposition the resident and ensure the bed is in the low position.

32. Follow the plan of care to determine if the side rails should be raised or lowered.

33. Remove, clean, and store equipment in the proper location. Remove soiled linens and discard disposable equipment.

Follow-Up

34. Wash your hands to ensure infection control.

35. Make sure the resident is comfortable and place the call light and personal items within reach.

36. Conduct a safety check before leaving the room. The room should be clean and free from clutter or spills.

37. Wash your hands or use hand sanitizer before leaving the room.

Reporting and Documentation

38. Communicate any specific observations, complications, or unusual responses to the licensed nursing staff. Record this information, along with the care provided, in the chart or EMR.

Image courtesy of Wards Forest Media, LLC

Ambulating with a Walker

Some residents need more support with ambulation than a cane can provide. For these residents, a walker is often a better option. A walker lets residents use their arms to take all or some of their weight off their lower body.

A walker must fit the resident properly (Figure 17.30). The handles or top of the walker should be even with the resident's wrist when the resident is standing in an upright position with arms relaxed at the sides. When the resident holds on to the walker, his or her elbows should be bent in a comfortable and natural position. The resident should never stoop over while using the walker.

There are different types of walkers (Figure 17.31). A *standard, pickup walker* is made of lightweight metal and has four solid, rubber-tipped legs, which provide a wider base of support. A resident uses this type of walker when he or she is able to pick up the walker while ambulating.

A *rolling walker,* or *rollator,* has four legs with wheels or casters that roll during ambulation. To provide stability, some rolling walkers have two wheels on the front two legs and no wheels on the back two legs. Some also have four wheels and hand brakes, as well as platforms and pouches to carry personal items. Rolling walkers let residents push walkers rather than lifting them during ambulation. The resident will still need enough strength to lift the walker when needed.

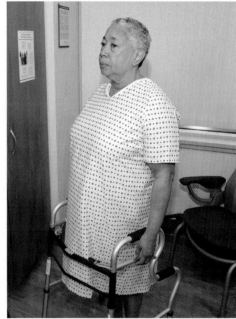

Wards Forest Media, LLC

Figure 17.30 The top of a correctly fitted walker should be even with the wrists.

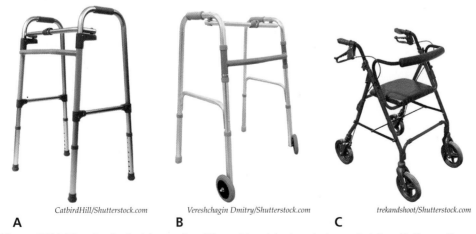

CatbirdHill/Shutterstock.com

A

Vereshchagin Dmitry/Shutterstock.com

B

trekandshoot/Shutterstock.com

C

Figure 17.31 The standard, pickup walker (A) must be picked up during ambulation. Rolling walkers may have two wheels (B) or four wheels (C).

As a resident builds strength using a walker, endurance may improve, and the resident may gradually be able to ambulate for longer periods of time. A resident should never try to climb stairs or use an escalator with a walker. Nursing assistants must closely monitor a resident ambulating with a walker. If the resident appears tired and weak, ambulation must stop to allow the resident time to rest.

Procedure | Providing Assistance with a Walker

Rationale

Assisting a resident with correctly using a walker reduces the chance of injury and promotes safe ambulation.

Preparation

1. Ask the licensed nursing staff how this procedure fits into the plan of care, if there are doctor's orders for the procedure, if there are any special instructions or precautions, and if the resident can be moved into the positions required for this procedure.

2. Wash your hands or use hand sanitizer before entering the room.

3. Knock before entering the room.

4. Introduce yourself using your full name and title. Explain that you work with the licensed nursing staff and will be providing care.

5. Greet the resident and ask the resident to state her full name, if able. Then check the resident's identification bracelet.

6. Use Mr., Mrs., or Ms. and the last name when conversing.

7. Explain the procedure in simple terms, even if the resident is not able to communicate or is disoriented. Ask permission to perform the procedure.

8. Bring the necessary equipment into the room. Place the following items in an accessible location:
   - a robe or properly fitting clothing
   - nonslip, properly fitting, low-heeled footwear
   - a standard or rolling walker
   - gait belt (in good condition and functional)

The Procedure

9. Provide privacy by closing the curtains, using a screen, or closing the door to the room.

10. If the resident is in bed, lock the bed wheels and then lower the bed to its lowest position.

11. Ensure safety during the procedure. If the resident is in a bed with side rails, raise and secure the rails on the opposite side of the bed from where you will be working. Lower the rail on the side you are working.

12. If the resident is in bed, assist her to a dangling position on the side of the bed. The resident may also be seated in a chair.

13. Help the resident put on nonslip, properly fitting shoes and a robe, if needed.

14. Apply the gait belt, if needed. Put the belt around the resident's waist over her clothing with the buckle in the front. Thread the belt through the teeth of the buckle and through the belt's two loops to lock it. Make the belt snug, but leave enough room to place your fingers under the belt.

15. Position the seated resident so she is centered in front of and inside the frame of the walker.

16. Place the walker about one step ahead of the seated resident and make sure the legs of the walker are level on the ground and stable.

17. Have the resident use both hands to grip the top of the walker for support. Then have the resident stand and walk into the walker. The resident should take the first step with her weaker leg. The heel of the foot should touch the ground first, and the foot should flatten.

18. The resident should take her next step with her strong leg. As the resident ambulates, position yourself behind and slightly to the side of her.

19. The resident should step with her weak leg and then with her strong leg again. This sequence should be repeated. Do not hurry the resident.

20. Make sure the resident does not step all the way to the front bar of the walker. Have her take small steps when she turns.

21. Let the resident set the pace and keep a firm grasp on the gait belt, if used.

22. Encourage the resident to ambulate the ordered distance, but be observant. Watch for signs of resident fatigue or possible collapse. *Do not attempt to catch a resident who begins to collapse during ambulation. Instead, slowly ease the resident to the floor, using your body as an incline.*

23. To assist the resident into a sitting position, first make sure the chair is stable. Have the resident stand with her back to the chair (Figure 17.32A). The resident should be close enough to sit down on the chair. Have the resident slide her weaker leg forward and shift her weight to the stronger leg. Have her switch hands from the walker to the arms of the chair and sit down slowly (Figure 17.32B).

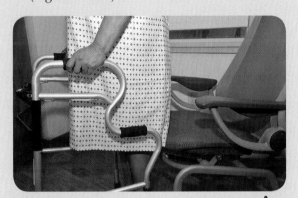

A

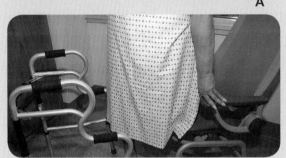

Figure 17.32   B

24. To assist the resident in getting up from a chair, put the walker in front of the chair. Have the resident move forward in the chair, place her hands on the arms of the chair, and push up. She should then move her hands to the grips of the walker. The resident should stand for enough time to gain stability and balance before beginning to ambulate.

25. When ambulation is complete, help the resident return to her room or bed. Remove the gait belt and the resident's robe, walker, and shoes.

26. If the resident returns to her bed, check to be sure the bed wheels are locked. Then reposition the resident and ensure the bed is in the low position.

27. Follow the plan of care to determine if the side rails should be raised or lowered.

28. Remove, clean, and store equipment in the proper location. Remove soiled linens and discard disposable equipment.

Follow-Up

29. Wash your hands to ensure infection control.

30. Make sure the resident is comfortable and place the call light and personal items within reach.

31. Conduct a safety check before leaving the room. The room should be clean and free from clutter or spills.

32. Wash your hands or use hand sanitizer before leaving the room.

Reporting and Documentation

33. Communicate any specific observations, complications, or unusual responses to the licensed nursing staff. Record this information, along with the care provided, in the chart or EMR.

Images courtesy of Wards Forest Media, LLC

Ambulating with Crutches

After an injury or surgical procedure, a patient may need to keep weight off his or her legs or feet. In these cases, the patient may have to use crutches. Crutches are also used for patients with lower limb amputations or disabilities. Crutches are seldom recommended for older adults because they require upper body strength older adults may not have.

Types of Crutches

There are several different types of crutches (Figure 17.33):

- *Standard underarm crutches:* are also called *axillary crutches* and are generally made of wood or aluminum. They can be adjusted for height, have padding on the underarms, and have handholds. These crutches are usually for short-term use.

- *Strutter crutches:* are similar to standard crutches, but have a U-shaped underarm support that distributes weight over a larger area of the skin surface. These crutches also have a larger base. This provides better balance and helps alleviate any possible injury to the nerves and blood vessels in the axilla.
- *Platform crutches:* use the same base as standard crutches, but feature a horizontal, padded armrest. The patient using these crutches straps his or her arms onto each armrest and then maneuvers the crutches.
- *Forearm crutches:* are typically used for patients with disabilities. While these crutches can be used temporarily, they are often selected for long-term use. Forearm crutches can be slipped on and off through a forearm cuff that provides stability and allows for a tighter grip on the handholds. The cuff is usually made of aluminum or plastic and is shaped like a half-circle (open cuff) or complete circle (closed cuff).

Newer, hands-free assistive devices also exist. For example, a knee walker or knee scooter is a wheeled device that supports the injured leg. The knee of the injured leg is placed in a padded seat, and the good leg pushes the scooter. The patient uses the scooter handles to maneuver and make turns.

Guidelines for Using Crutches

Some healthcare facilities do not allow nursing assistants to ambulate a patient with crutches. Facilities that do allow this may have special procedures or training for nursing assistants who help patients with crutches ambulate. Nursing assistants should always check facility policies and procedures before assisting patients ambulating with crutches.

The fit and size of standard crutches are important. Before a patient can ambulate with crutches, the fit and size of the crutches must be deemed appropriate (Figure 17.34). The tops of the crutches (crutch pads) should sit about 1.5 inches below the axilla while the patient stands up straight with shoulders relaxed. The handholds of the crutches should be even with the hips, and the elbows should be able to bend slightly when the handholds are used. The crutch length should equal the distance between the axilla and about 6 inches in front of the patient's shoe. The patient should hold the tops of the crutches tightly to his or her sides, but should never press them into the axilla, which can damage the nerves. The bottoms of the crutches should always have rubber tips.

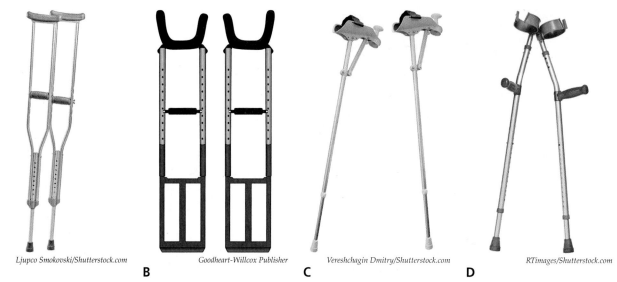

A   *Ljupco Smokovski/Shutterstock.com*
B   *Goodheart-Willcox Publisher*
C   *Vereshchagin Dmitry/Shutterstock.com*
D   *RTimages/Shutterstock.com*

Figure 17.33 The different types of crutches include standard underarm crutches (A), strutter crutches (B), platform crutches (C), and forearm crutches (D).

Before helping a patient ambulate with crutches, check for flaws (cracks in wooden crutches and bends in metal crutches) and tighten all the bolts on the crutches, if appropriate.

Appropriate Gait

It is important to know which crutch walking gait has been ordered by the doctor. The walking gait ordered will affect the instructions you should give. Each gait starts in a tripod position (Figure 17.35). In this position, crutch tips are placed about 4–6 inches to the side and slightly in front of each foot. The strong foot bears the weight of the body. Following are the four types of gaits (Figure 17.36).

- A *four-point gait* is used when both legs have some weight-bearing ability. Start with the tripod position. Then follow the sequence for the four-point gait.

- A *two-point gait* is an alternative to the four-point gait. It is used when both legs can bear some weight. Start with the tripod position and follow the sequence for the two-point gait.

- A *three-point gait* is used when the affected, or injured, leg should bear no weight. Start with the tripod position and follow the sequence for the three-point gait. In the three-point gait, the non-weight-bearing leg should move forward along with the crutches.

- A *swing-through gait* is used when the legs are paralyzed and in braces. Start with the tripod position and follow the sequence for the swing-through gait.

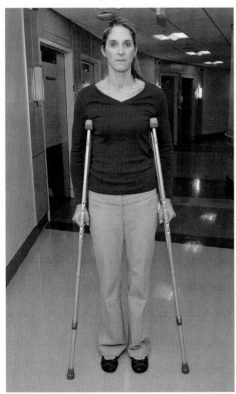

Wards Forest Media, LLC

Figure 17.34 For proper fit, the handholds of crutches should be level with the hips, and the elbows should bend slightly.

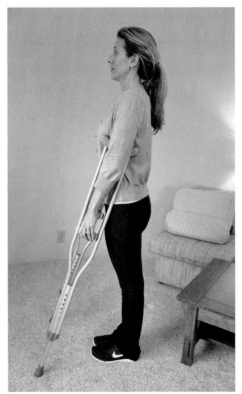

Wards Forest Media, LLC

Figure 17.35 In the tripod position, crutch tips are placed to the side and slightly in front of each foot.

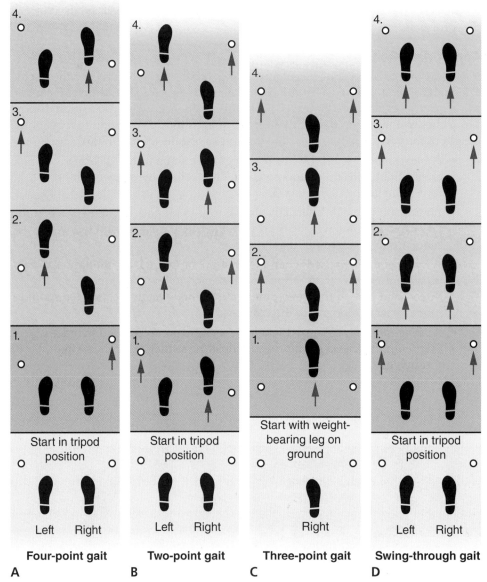

Four-point gait
A

Two-point gait
B

Three-point gait
C

Swing-through gait
D

Figure 17.36 The weight-bearing ability of the legs determines which gait should be used.

Procedure   Providing Assistance with Crutches

Rationale

Assisting patients ambulating with crutches reduces the chance of injury and helps promote safe ambulation.

Preparation

1. Ask the licensed nursing staff how this procedure fits into the plan of care, if there are doctor's orders for the procedure, if there are any special instructions or precautions, and if the patient can be moved into the positions required for this procedure.

2. Wash your hands or use hand sanitizer before entering the room.

3. Knock before entering the room.

4. Introduce yourself using your full name and title. Explain that you work with the licensed nursing staff and will be providing care.

5. Greet the patient and ask the patient to state her full name, if able. Then check the patient's identification bracelet.

6. Use Mr., Mrs., or Ms. and the last name when conversing.

7. Explain the procedure in simple terms, even if the patient is not able to communicate or is disoriented. Ask permission to perform the procedure.

8. Bring the necessary equipment into the room. Place the following items in an accessible location:
   - a robe or properly fitting clothing
   - nonslip, properly fitting, low-heeled footwear
   - gait belt (in good condition and functional)
   - a pair of crutches that have been properly sized and are in working condition

The Procedure

9. Provide privacy by closing the curtains, using a screen, or closing the door to the room.

10. If the patient is in bed, lock the bed wheels and then lower the bed to its lowest position.

11. If the patient is in bed, assist her to a dangling position on the side of the bed. The patient may also be seated in a chair.

12. Help the patient put on nonslip, properly fitting shoes and a robe, if needed.

13. Apply the gait belt, if needed. Put the belt around the patient's waist over her clothing with the buckle in the front. Thread the belt through the teeth of the buckle and through the belt's two loops to lock it. Make the belt snug, but leave enough room to place your fingers under the belt.

14. Ensure the crutches fit properly. Discuss any concerns with the licensed nursing staff.

15. Check that the crutches are in the tripod position. Instruct the patient to use the handholds to absorb her weight. The patient should not place any weight on the axilla.

16. Determine the gait ordered by the patient's doctor and have the patient follow the sequence for that gait.

17. Remind the patient to keep an erect posture and focus on where she is ambulating by looking straight ahead, not at her feet.

18. Walk safely at the side of the patient.

19. Let the patient set the pace and keep a firm grasp on the gait belt, if used.

20. Encourage the patient to ambulate the ordered distance, but be observant. Watch for signs of patient fatigue or possible collapse. *Do not attempt to catch a patient who begins to collapse during ambulation. Instead, slowly ease the patient to the floor, using your body as an incline.*

21. If permissible, a patient may climb stairs using crutches. The patient must have enough strength and flexibility to achieve this. To climb stairs, the patient could hold the handrail with one hand and tuck both crutches under the opposite axilla. When going up stairs, the patient should lead with the strong foot and keep the weak foot raised behind. When going down stairs, the patient should hold the weak foot up in front of the body and hop down each stair on the strong foot, taking one step at a time. To assist, place yourself behind the patient when she is going up stairs and in front of the patient when she is going down stairs.

A patient may also sit on the stairs and inch up or down each step (Figure 17.37). The patient should hold her weak leg out in front of her body and carry both crutches flat against the stairs in the hand opposite the railing. She should scoot her bottom up or down to the next step, using her free hand and strong leg for support.

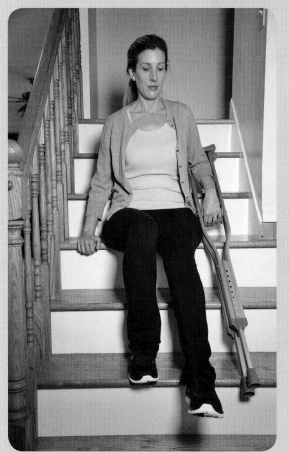
Figure 17.37

(continued)

Providing Assistance with Crutches *(continued)*

22. When ambulation is complete, help the patient return to her room or bed. Remove the gait belt and the patient's robe, crutches, and shoes.

23. If the patient returns to bed, check to be sure the bed wheels are locked. Then reposition the patient and ensure the bed is in the low position.

24. Follow the plan of care to determine if the side rails should be raised or lowered.

25. Remove, clean, and store equipment in the proper location. Remove soiled linens and discard disposable equipment.

Follow-Up

26. Wash your hands to ensure infection control.

27. Make sure the resident is comfortable and place the call light and personal items within reach.

28. Conduct a safety check before leaving the room. The room should be clean and free from clutter or spills.

29. Wash your hands or use hand sanitizer before leaving the room.

Reporting and Documentation

30. Communicate any specific observations, complications, or unusual responses to the licensed nursing staff. Record this information, along with the care provided, in the chart or EMR.

Image courtesy of Wards Forest Media, LLC

Section 17.3 Review and Assessment

Using the Key Terms
Complete the following sentences using key terms in this section.

1. In the _____, the leg swings forward from the hip and then the heel touches and rolls forward to the toe.

2. The _____ phase of running occurs when both feet are off the ground at the same time.

3. If a resident begins to collapse, you should grasp the resident under the _____, or armpit.

Know and Understand the Facts

4. Explain why it is important for residents to ambulate regularly.

5. What are the three stages of ambulation?

6. Identify three safety precautions to follow when helping residents ambulate with assistive devices.

Analyze and Apply Concepts

7. What should a nursing assistant do if a resident collapses during ambulation?

8. Describe the steps to follow when assisting a resident ambulating with a cane.

9. Explain the steps to follow when assisting a resident ambulating with a walker.

10. What steps should be taken to maintain safety when assisting a patient ambulating with crutches?

Think Critically
Read the following care situation. Then answer the questions that follow.

Mrs. B will be going home soon from the hospital. She will have a caregiver look after her once a day when she is home. It is important that Mrs. B walks well with her cane. She dislikes using the cane fitted for her, but is willing to use the cane that belonged to her husband.

11. If Mrs. B's husband's cane is used, what guidelines could help ensure the cane fits Mrs. B properly?

12. How will you know if Mrs. B is capable of ambulating safely with her cane?

13. What instructions about ambulation are important for Mrs. B's caregiver to know?

Objectives

To promote and support mobility, you must understand the importance of rehabilitation and restorative care. The use of assistive devices can positively affect the mobility of residents. To achieve the objectives for this section, you must successfully

- **define** rehabilitation and restorative care;
- **explain** range-of-motion exercises residents may need; and
- **list** the types of assistive devices used for rehabilitation and restorative care.

Key Terms

Learn these key terms to better understand the information presented in the section.

atony	restorative care
embolus	stroke
orthotic	thrombus
prosthetic	

Questions to Consider

- Have you ever had a goal that took a long time to achieve? What challenges or barriers made the goal difficult to achieve? Did any barriers keep you from accomplishing your goal? How did those barriers make you feel?
- What course of action did you take to achieve your long-term goal? If you did you not achieve your goal, did you have to settle for something less? Was that good enough?

What Are Rehabilitation and Restorative Care?

Rehabilitation and restorative care are complementary services that work together to help residents regain lost abilities, maintain abilities, and prevent further loss of abilities. Rehabilitation services help residents maintain, regain, or improve skills that have been lost or impaired because of illness, trauma, or disability. The skills targeted often relate to functions of daily life, such as mobility, speech, or cardiac rehabilitation (in which an exercise program helps strengthen the cardiovascular system). Rehabilitation may be necessary at various ages. Infants and young children may need this type of care if they are born with a physical disability or speech disorder. Adults may receive rehabilitation if they have suffered a serious accident, brain or spine injury, or broken bones; undergone an operation; or been diagnosed with a degenerative disorder.

Restorative care goes beyond rehabilitation. Restorative care has two goals. The first is to preserve and support improvements accomplished by rehabilitation. The second is to offer modifications and adjustments that enable residents to live as independently as possible. Restorative care is intended to increase residents' self-esteem and to help residents achieve and maintain the highest possible physical, mental, and psychosocial function. This type of care provides services designed to improve residents' function significantly in a reasonable and predictable period of time.

Older adults most often require both rehabilitation and restorative care. This care will usually be given after an older adult has suffered a **stroke**, or blockage of a blood vessel in the brain. Older adults who have hip fractures or coronary artery disease or who have been immobile or bedridden will also receive this care.

Rehabilitation and Restorative Care Providers

Rehabilitation and restorative care can be given in hospitals, outpatient clinics, long-term care facilities, residential care facilities, or homes. There are OBRA requirements for the provision of specific rehabilitation and restorative services in nursing facilities.

These services may be provided by the facility, by external providers, or by both. The range of services may include a variety of therapies and activities, which are integrated into a resident's plan of care.

Rehabilitative and restorative care may last only a few weeks or can occur over a long period of time due to the type or chronic nature of the disease or condition. This care typically includes physical therapy, occupational therapy, speech therapy, or activity or recreational therapy. A team that includes doctors, physical therapists, occupational therapists, speech therapists, nurses, and other healthcare providers plan this care.

A doctor must order rehabilitation and restorative care. Once care has been ordered, the healthcare team consults with the resident and often the family to determine a plan of care based on realistic goals. Residents are encouraged to reach these goals on a daily basis. Progressing toward these goals can often be a slow, sometimes frustrating process. Residents and their families are important factors in the success of care. A resident's positive attitude, coping skills, willingness to participate, and family support can make a difference. A resident's age and overall health status can also influence progression.

The healthcare providers involved in rehabilitation and restorative care are critical to the care's success. The physical therapist can provide range-of-motion exercises, muscle strengthening, and general conditioning exercises. Some treatments that physical therapists use include heat and water therapy, electric nerve therapy, traction, and massage therapy. Occupational therapists provide support with ADLs, which include bathing, dressing, cooking, and eating. Occupational therapists also teach residents and their family members how to use assistive devices, such as special eating utensils, for maximum independence. Speech therapists help residents with communication. For example, after a stroke, residents may have difficulty speaking or swallowing. The activity director or recreational therapist provides programs and activities that promote socialization, encourage mobility, and help to improve self-esteem.

The Nursing Assistant's Role

Holistic nursing assistants play an important role in rehabilitation and restorative care. Whenever a resident is not with a physical therapist, occupational therapist, or speech therapist, the resident will usually require follow-up and practice with ADLs (for example, eating, hygiene, communicating, and ambulating) according to the plan of care. Nursing assistants also help by focusing on resident abilities, providing encouragement, celebrating successes, observing resident progress, and providing ongoing documentation. It is important to be familiar with acronyms and abbreviations related to rehabilitation and restorative care (Figure 17.38).

Abbreviations and Acronyms Related to Rehabilitation and Restorative Care	
Abbreviation or Acronym	**Meaning**
AAROM	active-assistive range of motion
ABD	abduction
ADL	activity of daily living
CPM	continuous passive motion
ROM	range of motion

Figure 17.38 It is important to know terminology related to rehabilitation and restorative care.

Why Are Range-of-Motion Activities Important in Rehabilitation and Restorative Care?

The human body is designed for motion and activity. Regular exercise contributes to a healthy body and well-being. Conversely, immobility has a negative effect. A joint that has not been moved sufficiently can begin to stiffen within 24 hours and will eventually become inflexible. Long periods of joint immobility may also negatively affect tendons and muscles. Therefore, regular exercise is very important and has many benefits. Regular exercise helps maintain joint mobility and prevent contractures, **atony** (lack of strength), and atrophy of muscles. It also stimulates circulation to prevent the formation of a **thrombus** (immobile blood clot) or **embolus** (mobile blood clot). Exercise also improves coordination and builds and maintains muscle strength.

Most people move and exercise their joints and muscles by completing ADLs. Some also exercise regularly. When long periods of bed rest or immobility prevent regular exercise or activity, physical and emotional consequences can include the loss of muscle mass or depression. *Range-of-motion (ROM) exercises* can help improve heart and lung function, increase flexibility, improve a resident's mood, and aid a resident in meeting rehabilitation and restorative care goals. Nursing assistants can help residents perform these exercises.

Types of ROM Exercises

There are three types of ROM exercises. Depending on a resident's abilities, one type or a combination of exercises may be used. The resident's doctor determines which ROM exercises are appropriate.

1. **Active range of motion (AROM):** uses the full range of motion of one or more body parts. The resident does not require physical help to perform exercises. Nursing assistants may need to remind or observe the resident to make sure exercises are done correctly.

2. **Active-assistive range of motion (AAROM):** is used when a resident needs help achieving the full range of motion for one or more body parts. This may be because the muscles are too weak or stiff. Nursing assistants help with range of motion by encouraging normal muscle function.

3. **Passive range of motion (PROM):** is used when a resident cannot move one or more body parts. Nursing assistants perform the full range of motion without any help from the resident. Passive exercises will not preserve muscle mass, but they will keep joints flexible.

Active-assistive and passive ROM exercises are performed slowly and gently to avoid hurting the resident or harming joints and bones. If a resident is in pain, the exercises must stop, and the licensed nursing staff should be notified. Sometimes weights are used with active and active-assistive range of motion. Some residents may need to wear a splint or brace to support their limbs during ROM exercises. Parallel bars and gait belts also help provide stability and balance and assist movement.

ROM exercises require people to perform a variety of body movements. Some of these body movements are described in Figure 17.39.

Contraindications for ROM Exercises

It is important to remember that there may be *contraindications* for ROM exercises, or situations in which ROM exercises should not be used. ROM exercises may be contraindicated for residents with heart and respiratory diseases and conditions. This is because heart and respiratory problems may make the heart beat too fast and cause shortness of breath, chest pain, and fatigue. ROM exercises can also put stress on the soft tissues of joints and on bony structures. Therefore, ROM exercises should not be performed if joints are swollen or inflamed or if a muscle or bone near the joint has been injured.

General Guidelines for ROM Exercises

Before you conduct ROM exercises with a resident, you should familiarize yourself with the following general guidelines and with your facility's policies.

Follow a Schedule

To organize ROM exercises, follow the schedule for when they should be done. Discussing the schedule and its importance with residents may make them more willing to participate. Always explain what you are going to do before beginning

Body Movements		
Movement	**Description**	**Example**
Flexion	The act of bending a joint	Bending the arm at the elbow
Extension	The act of straightening a joint	Lowering the arm back down at the elbow
Hyperextension	An exaggerated, or extreme, extension	Moving the arm from the side so that it extends behind the body
Abduction	Lateral (sideways) movement away from the midline (an invisible line running vertically through the body)	Moving the leg away from the body
Adduction	Lateral movement toward the midline of the body	Moving the leg toward the body
Rotation	Turning of a body part around an axis, or fixed point	Rotating the ankle outward so that the foot moves away from the body
Circumduction	Rotating a body part in a complete circle	Moving the pointer finger in a circular motion
Supination	Rotating a body part from the body	Rotating the forearm so that the palm faces upward
Pronation	Rotating a body part toward the body	Rotating the forearm so that the palm faces downward

Figure 17.39 Some body movements involved in ROM activities include flexion, extension, hyperextension, abduction, adduction, rotation, circumduction, supination, and pronation.

any exercise and encourage the resident to help as much as possible. Remember to maintain proper body mechanics to avoid hurting or straining yourself.

ROM exercises should be performed routinely, at least twice daily. Immobile residents must have their joints exercised once every eight hours to prevent contractures. One good time to perform these exercises is during a resident's bath. Doing these exercises as a resident bathes is beneficial because warm water relaxes the muscles and can reduce muscle spasms. Exercising before bedtime is another option. Begin each exercise slowly, using smooth and rhythmic movements appropriate for the resident's condition.

Use the Best Approach

Remove pillows and supportive devices so there are no barriers to movement. Begin with exercises in the neck and work your way down the body. Exercise each joint through its range of motion a minimum of three times (preferably five times). Do not exercise the resident to the point of fatigue. When passively exercising the joints of the arms or legs, make sure you support the extremity involved. Never force a joint to the point of pain and never exercise a reddened or swollen joint. Move each joint until you feel slight resistance. Always return the joint to a neutral position when you have completed the exercise.

Pay Attention

You can cause serious injury if you do not perform ROM exercises properly. Check with the licensed nursing staff for specific instructions or limitations. For example, some facilities do *not* allow nursing assistants to exercise the neck. Remember to only exercise the joints that require exercise. Always stop and notify the licensed nursing staff if the resident complains of pain.

Rationale

Range-of-motion (ROM) exercises are critical for maintaining resident flexibility, preserving movement, and preventing skin inflammation or injury, such as a decubitus ulcer.

Preparation

1. Ask the licensed nursing staff how this procedure fits into the plan of care, if there are doctor's orders for the procedure, if there are any special instructions or precautions, and if the resident can be moved into the positions required for this procedure.
2. Wash your hands or use hand sanitizer before entering the room.
3. Knock before entering the room.
4. Introduce yourself using your full name and title. Explain that you work with the licensed nursing staff and will be providing care.
5. Greet the resident and ask the resident to state her full name, if able. Then check the resident's identification bracelet.
6. Use Mr., Mrs., or Ms. and the last name when conversing.
7. Explain the procedure in simple terms, even if the resident is not able to communicate or is disoriented. Ask permission to perform the procedure.
8. Bring the necessary equipment into the room. Place the following items in an accessible location:
   - towels or bath blankets

The Procedure

9. Provide privacy by closing the curtains, using a screen, or closing the door to the room.
10. Lock the bed wheels and then raise the bed to hip level.
11. Ensure resident safety during the procedure. If there are side rails, raise and secure the rails on the opposite side of the bed from where you will be working. Lower the rail on the side you are working.

> **Best Practice**
> Disposable gloves should be worn only if required for infection prevention and control.

12. Help the resident into the supine position (flat on the back).
13. Fanfold the top linens to the foot of the bed. Expose only the body part being exercised. A bath blanket or towel can be used to cover an exposed body part for modesty or warmth, if desired.
14. Exercising the neck
    - Exercise the neck *only* if your facility allows it and if you have been instructed to do so.
    - Support the resident's head and jaw with both hands (Figure 17.40). The head should be in a neutral position to start.

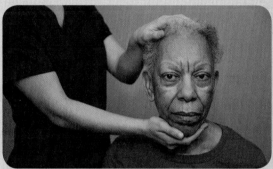

Figure 17.40

- Flexion—bring the head forward (Figure 17.41). Unless contraindicated, the chin should touch the chest.
- Extension—bring the head back (Figure 17.42). Avoid hyperextending the neck, or extending the neck beyond its normal limits.

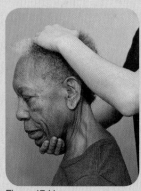 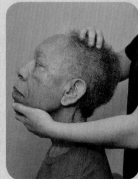

Figure 17.41   Figure 17.42

(continued)

Performing Range-of-Motion Exercises (*continued*)

- Rotation—turn the head from side to side (Figure 17.43).

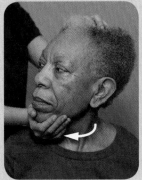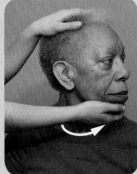

Figure 17.43

- Lateral flexion—move the head to the right and to the left (Figure 17.44).

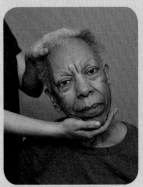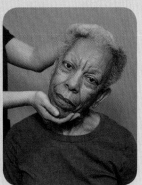

Figure 17.44

Best Practice
When exercising limbs, perform all of the steps listed here on one side of the body. Then move to the other side.

15. Exercising the shoulder
    - Grasp and support the resident's wrist with one hand. Grasp and support the resident's elbow with your other hand.
    - Flexion—raise the arm straight out in front of the resident and over the head (Figure 17.45).
    - Extension—bring the arm down to the side (Figure 17.46).

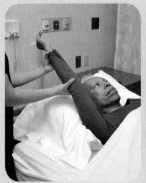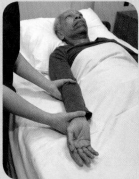

Figure 17.45   Figure 17.46

- Abduction—move the straight arm away from the side of the body (Figure 17.47).
- Adduction—move the straight arm to the side of the body (Figure 17.48).

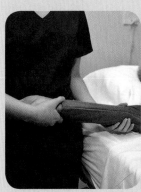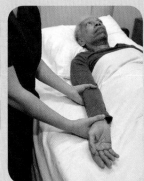

Figure 17.47   Figure 17.48

- Internal rotation—bend the elbow (Figure 17.49). Unless contraindicated, place the elbow at the same level as the shoulder. Move the forearm down toward the body.
- External rotation—move the forearm toward the head (Figure 17.50).

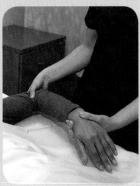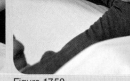

Figure 17.49   Figure 17.50

16. Exercising the elbow
    - Grasp and support the resident's wrist with one hand. Grasp and support the resident's elbow with your other hand.
    - Flexion—bend the arm to touch the same-side shoulder, if possible (Figure 17.51).
    - Extension—straighten the arm (Figure 17.52).

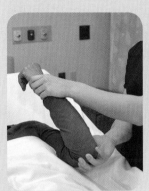

Figure 17.51   Figure 17.52

17. Exercising the forearm
    - Grasp and support the resident's wrist with one hand. Grasp and support the resident's elbow with your other hand.
    - Pronation—turn the hand so the palm is facing down.
    - Supination—turn the hand so the palm is facing up (Figure 17.53).

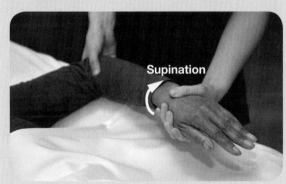

Supination

Figure 17.53

18. Exercising the wrist
    - Hold the resident's wrist with both of your hands.
    - Flexion—bend the hand down (Figure 17.54).
    - Extension—straighten the hand (Figure 17.54).

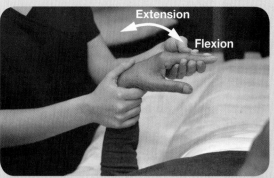

Extension

Flexion

Figure 17.54

- Radial flexion—with the hand straight up, turn the hand toward the thumb approximately 20°, as if the resident is waving.
- Ulnar flexion—with the hand straight up, turn the hand toward the little finger approximately 30°.

19. Exercising the thumb
    - Hold the resident's hand with one hand. Grasp the resident's thumb with your other hand.
    - Abduction—move the thumb out, away from the index finger (Figure 17.55).
    - Adduction—move the thumb in, toward the index finger (Figure 17.56).

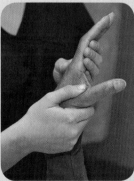

Figure 17.55   Figure 17.56

- Opposition—touch each fingertip with the thumb (Figure 17.57).

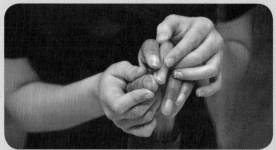

Figure 17.57

(continued)

- Flexion—bend the thumb into the hand (Figure 17.58).
- Extension—move the thumb out to the side of the fingers (Figure 17.59).

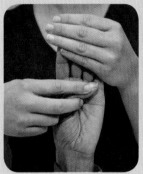
Figure 17.58

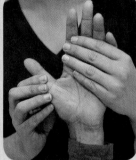
Figure 17.59

20. Exercising the fingers
    - Abduction—spread the fingers and the thumb apart.
    - Adduction—bring the fingers and thumb together (Figure 17.60).

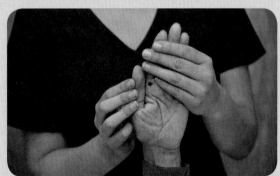
Figure 17.60

- Flexion—curl the fingers up to make a fist (Figure 17.61).
- Extension—open the hand so the fingers, hand, and arm are straight (Figure 17.62).

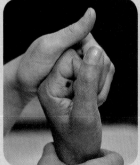
Figure 17.61

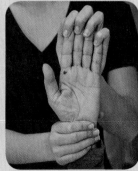
Figure 17.62

21. Exercising the hip
    - Support the leg by placing one hand on top of the resident's thigh and your other hand under the resident's calf.
    - Flexion—raise the leg and bend the knee (Figure 17.63).

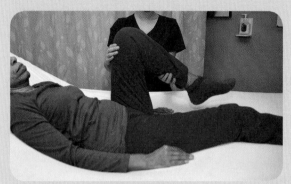
Figure 17.63

- Extension—straighten the leg (Figure 17.64).

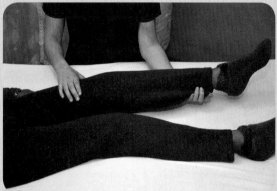
Figure 17.64

- Abduction—move the leg away from the body (Figure 17.65).

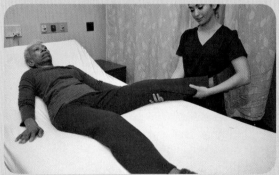
Figure 17.65

- Adduction—move the leg toward the other leg (Figure 17.66).

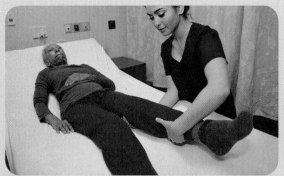
Figure 17.66

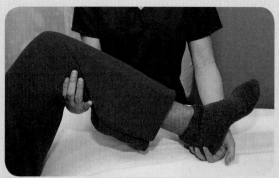
Figure 17.69

- Internal rotation—turn the leg inward (Figure 17.67).

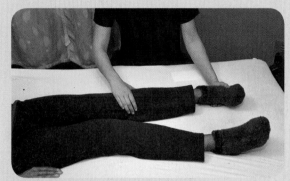
Figure 17.67

- External rotation—turn the leg outward (Figure 17.68).

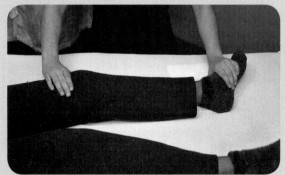
Figure 17.68

22. Exercising the knee
   - Support the knee by placing one hand under the resident's knee and your other hand under the resident's ankle.
   - Flexion—bend the knee (Figure 17.69).

- Extension—straighten the knee (Figure 17.70).

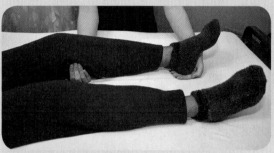
Figure 17.70

23. Exercising the ankle
   - Support the foot and ankle by placing one hand under the resident's foot and your other hand under the resident's ankle.
   - Dorsal flexion—pull the foot forward and push down on the heel at the same time (Figure 17.71).
   - Plantar flexion—turn the foot down or point the toes (Figure 17.72).

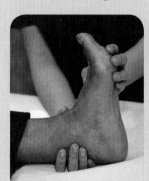
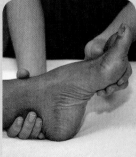
Figure 17.71   Figure 17.72

24. Exercising the foot
   - Support the foot and ankle by placing one hand under the resident's foot and your other hand under the resident's ankle.

(continued)

- Pronation—turn the outside of the foot up and the inside down (Figure 17.73).
- Supination—turn the inside of the foot up and the outside down (Figure 17.74).

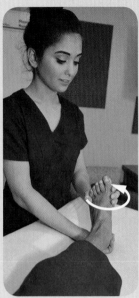 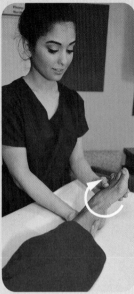

Figure 17.73   Figure 17.74

25. Exercising the toes
- Flexion—curl the toes (Figure 17.75).
- Extension—straighten the toes (Figure 17.76).

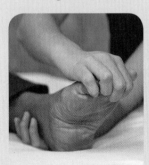 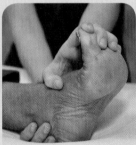

Figure 17.75   Figure 17.76

- Abduction—spread the toes apart (Figure 17.77).

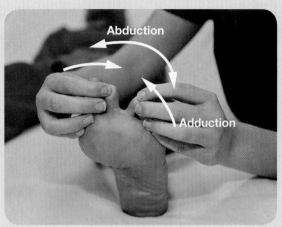

Figure 17.77

- Adduction—pull the toes together.
26. Cover the exposed part of the resident's body and raise the side rail, if used.
27. Go to the other side of the bed and lower the side rail, if it is up.
28. Repeat exercises for the shoulder, elbow, forearm, wrist, fingers, hip, knee, ankle, foot, and toes on the other side of the body. Start with the shoulder and work your way down the body.
29. Check to be sure the bed wheels are locked, then reposition the resident and lower the bed.
30. Follow the plan of care to determine if the side rails should be raised or lowered.
31. Remove, clean, and store equipment in the proper location. Remove soiled linens and discard disposable equipment.

Follow-Up

32. Wash your hands to ensure infection control.
33. Make sure the resident is comfortable and place the call light and personal items within reach.
34. Conduct a safety check before leaving the room. The room should be clean and free from clutter or spills.
35. Wash your hands or use hand sanitizer before leaving the room.

Reporting and Documentation

36. Communicate any specific observations, complications, or unusual responses to the licensed nursing staff. Record this information, along with the care provided, in the chart or EMR.

Images courtesy of Wards Forest Media, LLC

For the past few months, healthcare staff at a local nursing home have encouraged immobile residents to play games and puzzles on tablets. This exercise has improved resident engagement, mobility, and dexterity. Tablets' touch screens, puzzles, and games have helped reeducate residents who have suffered a stroke or have dementia. This way, older adults who are not mobile enough to play active video games can still engage and learn using tablets. The swipe, tap, and slide functionality of the tablet allows these residents to play a game of checkers, even if they cannot pick up a checker piece.

Apply It

1. If you were a nursing assistant at this facility, how might you teach residents to use a tablet, even if they are not familiar with this technology?

2. What strategies could you use to integrate the use of tablets with physical exercises?

What Assistive Devices Help Achieve Independent Living?

Many assistive devices can help people function safely and independently in healthcare facilities and at home. Some devices assist with ambulation, others help with ADLs, and still others make life easier and more enjoyable. Some examples of assistive devices include

- walkers and canes;
- shower chairs;
- grab bars on the side and back of the bathtub or toilet;
- graspers or reachers to lift items up from the floor;
- special eating utensils with built-up handles to help people feed themselves;
- cups with lids and specialized plates with deep centers;
- special combs and brushes;
- shoehorns to help people put on their shoes;
- raised sitting chairs, raised toilet seats, and chair leg extenders (Figure 17.78);
- large-print books and audio books; and
- large clocks, large telephone dials, and flashing lights to signal a telephone ring.

Two other specialized types of assistive devices are prosthetic devices and orthotic devices.

Prosthetic Devices

A **prosthetic** is an artificial device designed to replace a missing body part. Arm and leg prosthetics are attached to the remaining limb and come in a wide variety, enabling different levels of activity. Arm prosthetics include hand and elbow prosthetics. An artificial hand may allow a person to grip objects or may lengthen a missing finger. Elbow prosthetics can provide a movable elbow joint. Lower-limb prosthetics include above-the-knee and below-the-knee devices (Figure 17.79). Prosthetics may use fluid hydraulics or microprocessors to create natural movement or may be made from rubber and wood.

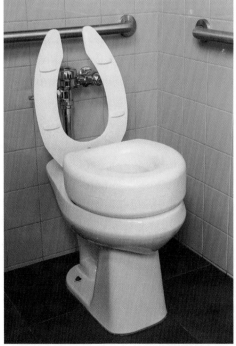

© Tori Soper Photography

Figure 17.78 Raised toilet seats can help prevent falls in the bathroom.

Other prosthetics include *dentures*, which may replace all or some of a person's teeth and gums. Artificial eyes typically consist of glass or plastic prostheses made to look like eyes and placed in the eye sockets. A person with a prosthetic of any kind often undergoes physical therapy to learn how to use the new device.

Orthotic Devices

An **orthotic** is a device that supports, aligns, or corrects a weak, immobile, injured, or deformed body part. Orthotics can improve joint movement or support the spine and other extremities. These devices come into direct contact with the body. Commonly used orthotics include casts, shoe inserts, and splints. Most orthotics can be purchased from a pharmacy and then fitted to the person. Some orthotics are custom made. Custom-made orthotics are fitted by an *orthotist* (orthotics specialist), doctor, or therapist. Uncomfortable orthotics can cause additional problems, so proper fit is very important.

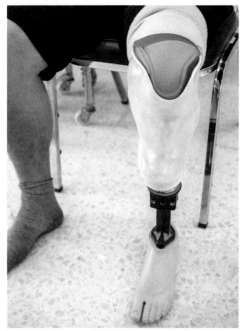

Eakwiphan Smitabhindhu/Shutterstock.com

Figure 17.79 Prosthetic devices can promote function even after a limb or other body part is removed.

Section 17.4 Review and Assessment

Using the Key Terms

Complete the following sentences using key terms in this section.

1. A mobile blood clot is called a(n) _____.
2. _____ assists with any modifications and adjustments residents must make to live as independently as possible.
3. An immobile blood clot is a(n) _____.
4. Rehabilitation often follows a(n) _____, or a blockage of a blood vessel in the brain.

Know and Understand the Facts

5. Describe the difference between rehabilitation and restorative care.
6. Identify two members of the healthcare team who provide rehabilitation or restorative care.
7. What are the three types of range-of-motion exercises?
8. Name six assistive, prosthetic, or orthotic devices.

Analyze and Apply Concepts

9. Why are range-of-motion exercises essential for rehabilitation and restorative care?
10. Explain the steps needed to perform range-of-motion exercises on a resident's shoulder.

Think Critically

Read the following care situation. Then answer the questions that follow.

Han, a nursing assistant, has been asked to do ROM exercises with Mrs. F, a patient recovering from a broken hip. Mrs. F is getting ready to go home in a few weeks, but has not been willing to exercise as much as her doctor thinks she should. She complains of pain and is afraid to do ROM exercises on her own. Her doctor believes she must be adequately healed to be more independent.

11. What should Han do when he meets Mrs. F for the first time?
12. How should Han handle Mrs. F's complaints of pain when doing range-of-motion exercises?

Key Points

Reviewing the key points for this chapter will help you practice more safely and competently as a holistic nursing assistant and will help you prepare for the certification competency examination.

- Proper body mechanics allow you to complete tasks safely and efficiently without straining your muscles or joints.
- Changing residents' positions on a regular basis helps restore body function, prevents deformities, relieves pressure, maintains skin integrity, and helps achieve comfort.
- Ambulation improves circulation and muscle tone, preserves lung tissues and airway function, and safeguards muscle and joint mobility.
- Moving and exercising the joints using range-of-motion (ROM) exercises can increase heart and lung function and improve muscle strength.
- Rehabilitation and restorative care are complementary services that work together to help residents regain lost abilities, maintain abilities, and prevent further loss of abilities.

Action Steps to Holistic Care

Review the information in this chapter. Complete the following activities.

1. Prepare a short paper or digital presentation that describes why body alignment is important and how it is maintained when residents are positioned, turned, dangled, and transferred. Discuss what actions ensure a safe environment for the resident.
2. With a partner, prepare a poster about assisting residents with canes, walkers, and crutches. Include the key steps and the actions that need to be taken to ensure safety.
3. Find two pictures in a magazine, in a newspaper, or online that best represent correct body mechanics. Explain why you selected these images.
4. Research current scientific information about different types of prosthetic and orthotic devices. Write a brief report describing three current facts about prosthetics and orthotics that were not discussed in this chapter.

 Preparing for the Certification Competency Examination

To prepare for the nursing assistant certification competency examination, you will need to know content found in this chapter. This content may be tested in the knowledge (written or oral) and skills (hands-on demonstration) portions of the exam. The following areas will be emphasized:

- body mechanics
- body positions
- procedures for positioning, turning, lifting, and transferring
- supportive equipment and assistive devices
- effects of limited mobility
- safe ambulation
- ambulation with canes, walkers, and crutches
- rehabilitation and restorative care
- passive and active range of motion

These sample test questions are similar to ones you will find on the certification competency exam. See how well you can answer them. Be sure to select the *best* answer.

1. A nursing assistant can help a resident perform active ROM exercises by
   A. instructing the resident about how to perform the exercises
   B. watching the resident perform the exercises
   C. taking the resident outdoors for stimulation
   D. moving the resident to the dining room in a wheelchair

2. Which device is used to maintain proper foot alignment and prevent foot drop?
   A. headboard
   B. backboard
   C. bed board
   D. footboard

(continued)

3. Nursing assistants should lift and move residents on the count of
   A. five
   B. two
   C. three
   D. four

4. A nursing assistant has been asked to lift a resident. Which of the following actions should she take to use proper body mechanics?
   A. She should bend over the resident.
   B. She should push and not pull.
   C. She should stay close to the resident.
   D. She should take small breaks.

5. Which of the following statements is true about range-of-motion (ROM) exercises?
   A. They are performed just once a day.
   B. They are best performed starting from the bottom of the body.
   C. They are often performed during ADLs, such as bathing or dressing.
   D. They require at least 10 repetitions of each exercise.

6. During ambulation, a gait or transfer belt is often
   A. worn around the nursing assistant's waist for back support
   B. used to keep the resident positioned properly
   C. removed before walking
   D. worn around the resident's waist and used to hold on to the resident

7. Mrs. S is a resident who can move on her own with some assistance. What should a nursing assistant do to help her reposition in bed?
   A. assist Mrs. S in bending her knees and pushing up with her feet
   B. keep your knees straight while lifting her up under her arms
   C. use a gait or transfer belt to assist with repositioning
   D. pull the resident up holding one side of the draw sheet at a time

8. Which type of services helps residents maintain, restore, or improve skills and functioning for daily living?
   A. restorative care
   B. rehabilitation
   C. range of motion
   D. prosthetic devices

9. Mrs. A is a new cane user. A nursing assistant is helping her ambulate for the first time. What is an important guideline to ensure safety?
   A. When Mrs. A stands straight, her arms should be rigid at her sides.
   B. Mrs. A's elbow should be fully bent when she is using the cane.
   C. The cane should always be held in Mrs. A's stronger hand.
   D. The cane should always be held in Mrs. A's weaker hand.

10. Which of the following is *not* a principle of proper body mechanics?
    A. narrow base of support
    B. line of gravity
    C. stable center of gravity
    D. proper alignment when standing

11. Mr. O is experiencing shortening and tightening of his wrist due to lack of movement. What is this condition?
    A. atrophy
    B. atony
    C. ankylosis
    D. contracture

12. If a resident is seated in his bed with the head of the bed raised 45°, this position is called
    A. supine position
    B. Fowler's position
    C. Sims' position
    D. lateral position

13. When a limb or joint is moved beyond its normal range of motion, this is called
    A. flexion
    B. distal
    C. proximal
    D. hyperextension

14. A nursing assistant is caring for Ms. T, who is bedridden. How often should Ms. T be repositioned?
    A. every hour
    B. every 15 minutes
    C. every two hours
    D. every three hours

15. Which of the following is an artificial device designed to replace a missing body part?
    A. prosthetic
    B. orthotic
    C. atonic
    D. dystonic

Did you have difficulty with any of the questions? If you did, review the chapter to find the correct answer(s).

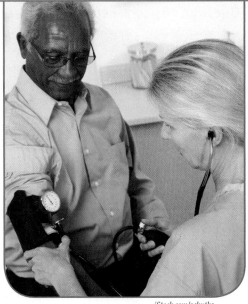
iStock.com/gchutka

Welcome to the Chapter

This chapter provides the knowledge and skills needed to measure the vital signs of temperature, pulse, respirations, and blood pressure. It also contains information about using a pulse oximeter to measure how well oxygen is being carried to body tissues and about measuring height and weight. You will learn to effectively use these skills when providing care and will understand why accuracy in taking, measuring, and recording this information is so important.

The information and procedures presented in this chapter will help you build the knowledge and skills needed to become a holistic nursing assistant. Check with your instructor to ensure these procedures are within your state's regulations for nursing assistant practice. The topics discussed in the chapter are highlighted on the Providing Holistic Care Framework.

You are now ready to start this chapter, *Vital Signs, Height, and Weight*.

Chapter Outline

Section 18.1
Measuring and Recording Vital Signs

Section 18.2
Measuring and Recording Height and Weight

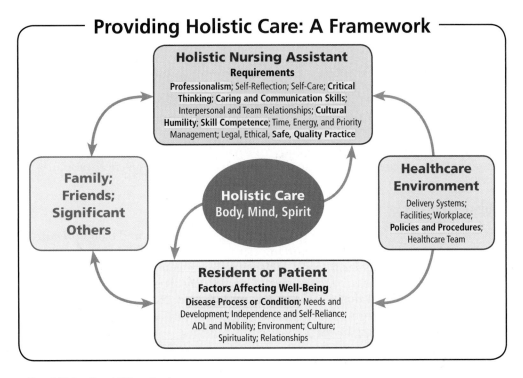

Providing Holistic Care: A Framework

Holistic Nursing Assistant
Requirements
Professionalism; Self-Reflection; Self-Care; **Critical Thinking; Caring and Communication Skills;** Interpersonal and Team Relationships; **Cultural Humility; Skill Competence;** Time, Energy, and Priority Management; Legal, Ethical, **Safe, Quality Practice**

Family; Friends; Significant Others

Holistic Care
Body, Mind, Spirit

Healthcare Environment
Delivery Systems; Facilities; Workplace; **Policies and Procedures;** Healthcare Team

Resident or Patient
Factors Affecting Well-Being
Disease Process or Condition; Needs and Development; Independence and Self-Reliance; ADL and Mobility; Environment; Culture; Spirituality; Relationships

Objectives

To provide the best possible care, you must understand how to take vital signs accurately and effectively. This includes temperature, pulse, respirations, and blood pressure. Vital signs are essential in helping monitor important and necessary information about a resident's condition. To achieve the objectives for this section, you must successfully

- **discuss** the purpose and importance of taking vital signs;
- **identify** the normal and abnormal ranges of vital signs;
- **describe** the locations and methods used to take vital signs;
- **list** the equipment needed to take vital signs;
- **describe** the importance of using a pulse oximeter; and
- **explain** how to measure and record vital signs accurately and effectively.

Key Terms

Learn these key terms to better understand the information presented in the section.

apical pulse	hypotension
apnea	hypoventilation
aural	hypoxia
axillary temperature	probe
bradycardia	radial pulse
bradypnea	stertorous breathing
carotid pulse	stethoscope
Celsius (C)	systolic blood pressure
diastolic blood pressure	tachycardia
dyspnea	tachypnea
Fahrenheit (F)	temporal arteries
hyperventilation	tympanic temperature

As you have learned, *vital signs* are the rates or values of a person's temperature, pulse, respirations, and blood pressure. These signs are considered *vital* because they relate to essential body functions. When vital signs are taken (measured), a resident's height and weight may also be measured and recorded. Vital signs that are not within the normal range give healthcare providers important information about a resident's health and may indicate the presence of a disease, infection, or injury.

Why Are Vital Signs Important?

Taking the vital signs of body temperature, pulse, respirations, and blood pressure are important skills for a holistic nursing assistant to master. Vital signs can help doctors diagnose particular diseases, determine treatments and medications, and evaluate the effectiveness of treatments and medications. For example, a high body temperature can signal that a resident has an infection. If temperature starts to lower once treatment begins, this typically means the body is fighting the infection and the resident is getting better.

The process of taking vital signs is essentially the same for children and adults; however, the preferred method and normal ranges are different. For example, you may use a rectal thermometer to measure a newborn's temperature, but an oral thermometer to measure the temperature of an adult. It can be challenging to keep children still long enough to obtain an accurate measurement.

Vital signs are usually taken in a doctor's office during an exam, during admission to a healthcare facility, or once a day in long-term care facilities (more frequently when necessary). A patient who is very ill in the hospital or who has had surgery may have vital signs taken hourly, often using vital sign machines. Vital signs may also be taken if a patient complains of dizziness, if a patient has nausea or pain, after a patient has an emergency, or before and after a patient takes certain medications. For each vital sign, well-established guidelines help nursing assistants determine whether adults and children are in a normal range.

Facility guidelines impact how vital signs are recorded. Some facilities use paper forms for all residents on a shift and then transfer the measurements to each resident's chart or EMR. Other facilities use a specific form for each resident or enter vital signs into a resident's electronic record immediately.

How Is Temperature Measured and Recorded?

When you take a resident's temperature, you are measuring body heat, including how much body heat is produced and lost. Temperature is recorded in degrees (°) and is measured using either the Fahrenheit or the Celsius scale. The **Fahrenheit (F)** scale is used mostly in the United States. In the Fahrenheit scale, water freezes at 32° and boils at 212°. The **Celsius (C)**, or *centigrade*, scale is used in other parts of the world. In the Celsius scale, water freezes at 0° and boils at 100° (Figure 18.1).

While a resident's body temperature can change over the course of a day due to the dilation and expansion of blood vessels, *pyrexia*, or *fever*, is caused by the body heating up to protect itself. Pyrexia can signal an infection, some other disease process, an injury, or a possible reaction to a medication. Age can also affect temperature. An older person may not adjust as quickly to changes in temperature and may often express feelings of being cold.

Body temperature is regulated by the *hypothalamus*, which is located in the brain. The hypothalamus is the body's internal thermostat. It resets the body to a higher temperature when an infection or illness is present. As you learned in chapter 14, the heat generated defends the body against toxins, causing infection or illness.

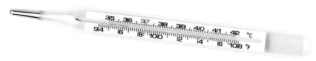

catshila/Shutterstock.com

Figure 18.1 Both the Celsius and Fahrenheit scales are shown on this thermometer.

Locations for Taking Temperature

Temperature can be taken using several different body locations. Temperatures can be

- oral (taken under the tongue, or *sublingually*);
- rectal (taken in the anus);
- axillary (taken under the armpit);
- tympanic (taken in the ear); and
- temporal (taken on the forehead).

Oral Temperatures

Oral temperatures are taken by placing a thermometer under the tongue. This is the most common method of taking a temperature, but is not appropriate for residents who are receiving oxygen, who are coughing or sneezing, who are agitated or comatose, who have had mouth surgery, who may bite the thermometer, or who cannot follow instructions due to cognitive impairment. Taking oral temperature is also inappropriate for children younger than four years of age. When taking an oral temperature, you must know whether a resident has recently eaten, had something to drink, or smoked. You should wait at least 15 minutes (or the time specified by facility policy) after these events before inserting the oral thermometer.

Rectal Temperatures

A *rectal temperature* is taken by placing a thermometer into the anus. The temperatures of infants and small children are often taken rectally. A lubricated thermometer is inserted 1 inch or less into the anus and is held in place for three to five minutes (Figure 18.2). Rectal temperatures should not be taken if a patient has diarrhea, hemorrhoids, rectal bleeding, or rectal surgery. Rectal temperatures are also not advised for residents with certain heart conditions, as taking a rectal temperature can stimulate the vagus nerve and cause a temporary decrease in heart rate and blood pressure. Taking rectal temperature is also inappropriate for patients who cannot follow directions or hold still.

Temporal Artery Temperatures

A *temporal artery temperature* is taken by measuring the temperature of the **temporal arteries**, which are located on each side of the head. Rectal and temporal artery temperatures provide more accurate measurements than temperatures at other sites. As a result, temporal artery temperatures are taken most frequently in medical offices. They are also taken for babies and children, as they can be easier to take than rectal temperatures. If a hat, wig, or bandages have covered the forehead, this can affect the temperature. Use only the area of the forehead that is bare. Also, when using a temporal thermometer (or any medical equipment), be sure to follow the manufacturer's recommendations for use. An improper technique could result in an inaccurate result.

Axillary Temperatures

Axillary temperature is taken by placing a thermometer into the axilla, or armpit. Do not use this location if the resident has had breast or chest surgery. When taking an axillary temperature, note if the resident has recently washed under the arms or put on deodorant. Recent washing and deodorant use can affect the reading. After these events, wait 15 minutes before taking the temperature.

Tympanic Temperatures

A **tympanic temperature** is more difficult to measure because a thermometer must be placed properly in the ear for an accurate reading. Do not use this location if there is drainage from the ear.

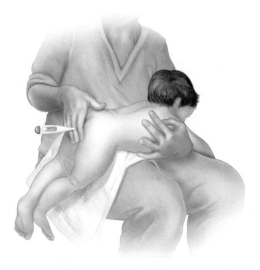

© *Body Scientific International*

Figure 18.2 A rectal thermometer is inserted into the anus and held there for three to five minutes. It should be inserted 1 inch or less into the anus.

If a resident has been sleeping or resting on the ear, this can generate heat. Use the other ear to ensure an accurate reading. Always check that you are using the best and safest location to take a temperature for each resident.

Average Body Temperatures

A resident's temperature may change slightly (by 1°F) during the day due to exertion, how much a resident eats or drinks, and external temperature. The normal, or average, temperature for an adult is 98.6°F (37.0°C), although the average range is 97.0–99.0°F (36.5–37.2°C). The average rectal temperature is approximately 1°F (0.6°C) higher than the average oral temperature, and axillary and temporal artery temperatures can be 1°F (0.6°C) lower. *Hypothermia*, while not seen often, is a body temperature below 95°F (35°C). Average temperature ranges also vary based on a resident's age and the type of thermometer used (Figure 18.3).

Types of Thermometers

Several different types of thermometers help measure temperature. Some thermometers are filled with a liquid that is usually colored alcohol. These are nondigital, or *manual*, thermometers. Some thermometers contain a plastic strip (usually disposable) with liquid crystals that change color to indicate different temperatures. Others are electronic and use digital displays. Healthcare facilities may use any of these temperature devices. No matter what device is used, all types of thermometers have the same purpose. Therefore, it is best to learn about them all.

Nondigital Thermometers

Nondigital thermometers can be used to take oral, rectal, or axillary temperatures. Figure 18.1 earlier in this section shows a nondigital thermometer. These thermometers are tubes filled with a liquid (colored alcohol) that expands and moves up or down in response to heat. The bulb at the end of the thermometer is inserted into the body. The bulb of a rectal thermometer is thicker and broader than the bulb of an oral thermometer. Some thermometers are marked with a colored dot—blue for oral or axillary, and red for rectal.

It is important to correctly place each thermometer and leave it in for the prescribed amount of time. Use the following guidelines based on the type of thermometer:

- **Oral temperatures**: insert the thermometer under the tongue and ask the resident to close his or her mouth completely while breathing through the nose. Leave the thermometer in for three minutes.

Average Ranges of Body Temperature			
Thermometer	Birth to Two Years	Three to Eleven Years	Twelve Years and Older
Oral	Should not be taken	97.0°F–99.5°F (36.1°C–37.5°C)	97.6°F–99.6°F (36.4°C–37.5°C)
Rectal	97.0°F–100.4°F (36.1°C–38.0°C)	97.9°F–100.4°F (36.6°C–38.0°C)	98.6°F–100.6°F (37.0°C–38.1°C)
Tympanic	Should not be taken	98.0°F–99.6°F (36.7°C–37.5°C)	98.6°F–100.4°F (37.0°C–38.0°C)
Axillary	97.5°F–99.3°F (36.4°C–37.4°C)	96.6°F–99.0°F (36.0°C–37.2°C)	96.6°F–98.6°F (35.9°C–37.0°C)
Temporal Artery	98.3°F–100.3°F (36.8°C–37.9°C)	97.8°F–100.1°F (36.5°C–37.8°C)	97.2°F–100.1°F (36.2°C–37.8°C)

Figure 18.3 The average temperature ranges for infants, children, and adults are shown here.

- **Rectal temperatures**: lubricate the thermometer and place it one inch or less into the anus for three to five minutes.
- **Axillary temperatures**: lower the resident's arm completely and leave the thermometer under the armpit for five or more minutes.

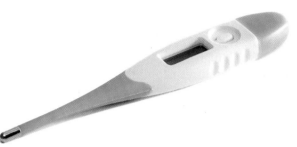

AGorohov/Shutterstock.com

Figure 18.4 A digital thermometer shows temperature on a digital display.

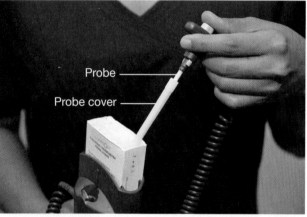

Wards Forest Media, LLC

Figure 18.5 A probe cover protects the probe of the thermometer. A new probe cover should be used for each reading.

Do not shake a thermometer when removing it. To read a nondigital thermometer, look at the thermometer's scale. Be sure the scale is visible so you can determine the level of liquid on the scale. The liquid level denotes the resident's temperature.

Digital Thermometers

Digital thermometers are used to take oral, rectal, axillary, or tympanic temperatures and can take temperature in a few seconds. They are handheld, have a digital display, and are connected to an electronic unit (Figure 18.4). Instead of a bulb, digital thermometers have a **probe**, which measures temperature. The probe of a tympanic thermometer is the tip. Probes are often marked by color—blue for oral or axillary, and red for rectal. The tip of a tympanic thermometer is short and is shaped to fit comfortably inside the external ear canal. Fresh covers should be placed on the probes or tips of digital thermometers and should be discarded after each use (Figure 18.5). Once the probe or tip of the digital thermometer is inserted, the digital display should show the temperature reading in 20–60 seconds.

The type of thermometer, nondigital or digital, you will use will depend on what is available in the healthcare facility where you work. As a nursing assistant, you will follow a specific procedure for taking, measuring, and recording a temperature. When recording a temperature, always identify the type of thermometer used and report any irregularities to the licensed nursing staff.

Procedure   Using an Oral Thermometer—Digital

Rationale

Body temperature that is outside the normal range can be a sign of a disease or condition or the result of an injury. The decision to use an oral thermometer is based on the need for accuracy and the age and condition of the resident. An oral thermometer is accurate for adults, as long as the adult keeps his or her mouth closed during the reading. Always follow the thermometer manufacturer's instructions and facility policy.

Preparation

1. Ask the licensed nursing staff how this procedure fits into the plan of care, if there are doctor's orders for the procedure, if there are any special instructions or precautions, and if the resident can be moved into the positions required for this procedure.

2. Wash your hands or use hand sanitizer before entering the room.

3. Knock before entering the room.

4. Introduce yourself using your full name and title. Explain that you work with the licensed nursing staff and will be providing care.

5. Greet the resident and ask the resident to state his full name, if able. Then check the resident's identification bracelet.

6. Use Mr., Mrs., or Ms. and the last name when conversing.

7. Explain the procedure in simple terms, even if the resident is not able to communicate or is disoriented. Ask permission to perform the procedure.

8. Bring the necessary equipment into the room. Place the following items in an accessible location:
   - a digital thermometer
   - the appropriate probe attachment (the *blue* probe for an oral temperature)
   - disposable probe covers
   - disposable gloves, if appropriate
   - pen and pad, form, or digital device for recording the temperature

9. Be sure the resident has not eaten, had something to drink, smoked, or chewed gum for at least 15 minutes prior to taking the oral temperature.

The Procedure

10. Provide privacy by closing the curtains, using a screen, or closing the door to the room.

11. If the resident is in bed, lock the bed wheels and then raise the bed to hip level.

12. Ensure safety during the procedure. If the resident is in a bed with side rails, raise and secure the rails on the opposite side of the bed from where you will be working. Lower the rail on the side you are working.

13. Position the resident comfortably.

> **Best Practice**
> Let the resident know how long the thermometer will be in place. Instruct the resident not to talk while the reading is being taken.

14. Place a disposable probe cover over the *blue* probe. Start the thermometer and wait until it shows it is ready.

> **Best Practice**
> Disposable gloves are worn only if required for infection prevention and control.

15. Have the resident open his mouth and lift his tongue. Slowly insert the covered probe into the mouth until the tip of the probe touches the base of the mouth under the tongue and to one side (Figure 18.6). Have the resident lower his tongue and close his mouth.

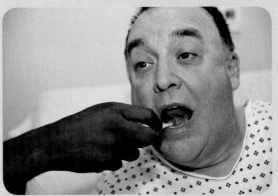
Figure 18.6

16. Hold the probe in place in the mouth until you hear or see the signal that the reading is complete (Figure 18.7).

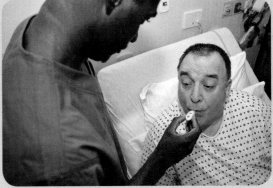
Figure 18.7

17. Remove the thermometer from the resident's mouth and read the temperature on the display screen.

18. Do not touch the used probe cover with your bare hands. Dispose of the probe cover safely in a waste container or per facility policy.

19. If the resident is in bed, check to be sure the bed wheels are locked. Then reposition the resident and lower the bed.

20. Follow the plan of care to determine if the side rails should be raised or lowered.

21. Clean the probe according to facility policy and return the probe to its storage compartment on the thermometer.

(continued)

22. Wash your hands or use hand sanitizer to ensure infection control.

23. Record the temperature on a pad, on a form, or in the electronic record.

24. Return the thermometer to a charging location per facility policy, if appropriate.

Follow-Up

25. Make sure the resident is comfortable and place the call light and personal items within reach.

26. Conduct a safety check before leaving the room. The room should be clean and free from clutter or spills.

27. Wash your hands or use hand sanitizer before leaving the room.

Reporting and Documentation

28. Communicate any specific observations, complications, or unusual responses to the licensed nursing staff.

Images courtesy of Wards Forest Media, LLC

Procedure | Using a Rectal Thermometer—Digital

Rationale

Body temperature that is outside the normal range can be a sign of a disease or condition or the result of an injury. The decision to use a rectal thermometer is based on the need for accuracy and the age and condition of the resident. For example, rectal temperatures can be more accurate than oral temperatures for young children. Always follow the thermometer manufacturer's instructions and facility policy.

Preparation

1. Ask the licensed nursing staff how this procedure fits into the plan of care, if there are doctor's orders for the procedure, if there are any special instructions or precautions, and if the resident can be moved into the positions required for this procedure.

2. Wash your hands or use hand sanitizer before entering the room.

3. Knock before entering the room.

4. Introduce yourself using your full name and title. Explain that you work with the licensed nursing staff and will be providing care.

5. Greet the resident and ask the resident to state her full name, if able. Then check the resident's identification bracelet.

6. Use Mr., Mrs., or Ms. and the last name when conversing.

7. Explain the procedure in simple terms, even if the resident is not able to communicate or is disoriented. Ask permission to perform the procedure.

8. Bring the necessary equipment into the room. Place the following items in an accessible location:
   - a digital thermometer
   - the appropriate probe attachment (the *red* probe for a rectal temperature)
   - disposable probe covers
   - disposable gloves
   - water-soluble lubricating gel
   - tissues or toilet paper
   - pen and pad, form, or digital device for recording temperature
   - sheet or drape

The Procedure

9. Provide privacy by closing the curtains, using a screen, or closing the door to the room.

10. If the resident is in bed, lock the bed wheels and then raise the bed to hip level.

11. Ensure safety during the procedure. If the resident is in a bed with side rails, raise and secure the rails on the opposite side of the bed from where you will be working. Lower the rail on the side you are working.

12. Wash your hands or use hand sanitizer to ensure infection control.

13. Put on disposable gloves.

14. Place a disposable probe cover over the *red* probe. Start the thermometer and wait until it shows it is ready.

15. Assist the resident into a side-lying or lateral position. Have the resident bend her upper leg up to her stomach as far as possible. Help, if needed.

16. If the resident is covered by a drape or top sheet, fold it back to expose the buttocks. Expose only the area necessary for the procedure. Keep the rest of the resident covered to protect her privacy.

17. Apply enough water-soluble lubricating gel (about the size of a quarter) for comfortable entry.

> **Best Practice**
> To lubricate the end of the covered probe, you may put the gel directly on the probe or you may use tissue or toilet paper to apply the lubricant.

18. With one hand, gently raise the upper buttock to expose the anal area.

19. With the other hand, gently insert the rectal probe 1 inch or less into the anus.

20. Hold the probe in place until you hear or see the signal that the reading is complete.

21. Remove the thermometer and read the temperature on the display screen.

22. Dispose of the probe cover safely in a waste container or per facility policy.

23. Wipe the lubricant off the resident and discard the tissue or toilet paper.

24. Clean the probe with alcohol according to facility policy. Return the probe to its storage compartment on the thermometer.

25. Remove and discard your gloves and wash your hands or use hand sanitizer to ensure infection control.

26. Record the temperature on a pad, on a form, or in the electronic record.

27. If the resident is in bed, check to be sure the bed wheels are locked. Then reposition the resident and lower the bed.

28. Follow the plan of care to determine if the side rails should be raised or lowered.

29. Return the thermometer to a charging location per facility policy.

Follow-Up

30. Make sure the resident is comfortable and place the call light and personal items within reach.

31. Conduct a safety check before leaving the room. The room should be clean and free from clutter or spills.

32. Wash your hands or use hand sanitizer before leaving the room.

Reporting and Documentation

33. Communicate any specific observations, complications, or unusual responses to the licensed nursing staff.

Procedure Using an Axillary Thermometer—Digital

Rationale

Body temperature that is outside the normal range can be a sign of a disease or condition or the result of an injury. While axillary temperature is not as accurate as other temperatures, the axilla (*armpit*) can be more easily accessible than other locations. Always follow the thermometer manufacturer's instructions and facility policy.

Preparation

1. Ask the licensed nursing staff how this procedure fits into the plan of care, if there are doctor's orders for the procedure, if there are any special instructions or precautions, and if the resident can be moved into the positions required for this procedure.

2. Wash your hands or use hand sanitizer before entering the room.

3. Knock before entering the room.

4. Introduce yourself using your full name and title. Explain that you work with the licensed nursing staff and will be providing care.

5. Greet the resident and ask the resident to state his full name, if able. Then check the resident's identification bracelet.

6. Use Mr., Mrs., or Ms. and the last name when conversing.

7. Explain the procedure in simple terms, even if the resident is not able to communicate or is disoriented. Ask permission to perform the procedure.

(continued)

8. Bring the necessary equipment into the room. Place the following items in an accessible location:
   - a digital thermometer
   - the appropriate probe attachment (the *blue* probe for an axillary temperature)
   - disposable probe covers
   - disposable gloves, if appropriate
   - a towel
   - pen and pad, form, or digital device for recording temperature

The Procedure

9. Provide privacy by closing the curtains, using a screen, or closing the door to the room.
10. If the resident is in bed, lock the bed wheels and then raise the bed to hip level.
11. Ensure safety during the procedure. If the resident is in a bed with side rails, raise and secure the rails on the opposite side of the bed from where you will be working. Lower the rail on the side you are working.

> **Best Practice**
> Disposable gloves are worn only if required for infection prevention and control.

12. Help the resident remove any clothing to expose his upper arm area.
13. Dry the axilla with the towel.
14. Place a disposable probe cover over the *blue* probe. Start the thermometer and wait until it shows it is ready.
15. Place the covered probe in the center of the axilla.
16. Place the resident's arm across his chest while holding the probe in place (Figure 18.8).

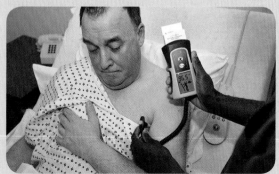

Figure 18.8

Image courtesy of Wards Forest Media, LLC

17. Hold the probe in place in the axilla until you hear or see the signal that the reading is complete.
18. Remove the thermometer from the axilla and read the temperature on the display screen.

> **Best Practice**
> Do not touch the probe cover.

19. Dispose of the probe cover safely in a waste container or per facility policy.
20. Clean the probe with alcohol according to facility policy. Return the probe to its storage compartment on the thermometer.
21. Wash your hands or use hand sanitizer to ensure infection control.
22. Record the temperature on a pad, on a form, or in the electronic record.
23. Assist the resident in replacing and securing his clothing.
24. If the resident is in bed, check to be sure the bed wheels are locked. Then reposition the resident and lower the bed.
25. Follow the plan of care to determine if the side rails should be raised or lowered.
26. Return the thermometer to a charging location per facility policy.

Follow-Up

27. Make sure the resident is comfortable and place the call light and personal items within reach.
28. Conduct a safety check before leaving the room. The room should be clean and free from clutter or spills.
29. Wash your hands or use hand sanitizer before leaving the room.

Reporting and Documentation

30. Communicate any specific observations, complications, or unusual responses to the licensed nursing staff.

Disposable Oral Thermometers

Another type of thermometer is the *disposable oral thermometer* (Figure 18.9). Disposable oral thermometers are used to reduce the risk of cross- or re-infection and to measure the temperature of patients in isolation. They are plastic or paper and are discarded once used. The dots on the thermometer change color to show body temperature.

Tympanic Thermometers

A *tympanic thermometer* measures the temperature of **aural** blood vessels, or blood vessels in the ear. Tympanic temperature is taken on the tympanic membrane, or *eardrum*. Tympanic thermometers are usually battery-operated, are handheld, and have a digital display on the handle (Figure 18.10).

Placement of the tympanic thermometer is very important for getting an accurate reading. In addition, too much wax in the ears can interfere with the reading. Do not use this type of thermometer if the patient has a sore ear, has an ear infection, or has had ear surgery.

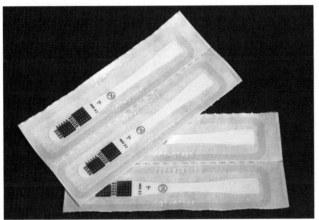

Wards Forest Media, LLC

Figure 18.9 Disposable oral thermometers are used once and then discarded. They help prevent infections from spreading in healthcare facilities.

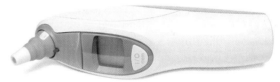

luk/Shutterstock.com

Figure 18.10 Tympanic thermometers are handheld and are inserted into the ear to measure tympanic temperature.

Procedure   Using a Tympanic Thermometer—Digital

Rationale

Body temperature that is outside the normal range can be a sign of a disease or condition or the result of an injury. Tympanic (*ear*) thermometers are another option for taking temperatures. Placement is most important for an accurate reading. Always follow the thermometer manufacturer's instructions and facility policy.

Preparation

1. Ask the licensed nursing staff how this procedure fits into the plan of care, if there are doctor's orders for the procedure, if there are any special instructions or precautions, and if the resident can be moved into the positions required for this procedure.

2. Wash your hands or use hand sanitizer before entering the room.

3. Knock before entering the room.

4. Introduce yourself using your full name and title. Explain that you work with the licensed nursing staff and will be providing care.

5. Greet the resident and ask the resident to state his full name, if able. Then check the resident's identification bracelet.

6. Use Mr., Mrs., or Ms. and the last name when conversing.

7. Explain the procedure in simple terms, even if the resident is not able to communicate or is disoriented. Ask permission to perform the procedure.

(continued)

8. Bring the necessary equipment into the room. Place the following items in an accessible location:
   - a digital tympanic thermometer
   - disposable plastic tympanic covers
   - disposable gloves, if necessary
   - pen and pad, form, or digital device for recording the temperature

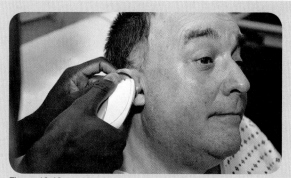
Figure 18.12

The Procedure

9. Provide privacy by closing the curtains, using a screen, or closing the door to the room.

10. If the resident is in bed, lock the bed wheels and then raise the bed to hip level.

11. Ensure safety during the procedure. If the resident is in a bed with side rails, raise and secure the rails on the opposite side of the bed from where you will be working. Lower the rail on the side you are working.

Best Practice
Disposable gloves are worn only if required for infection prevention and control.

12. Check the lens of the tympanic thermometer to make sure it is clean and intact.

13. Position the resident's head so that the ear being used for the procedure is directly in front of you.

14. Place the disposable plastic cover on the tympanic thermometer.

15. For an adult or child, pull the outer ear up and back to open the ear canal (Figure 18.11). For an infant, pull the ear straight back.

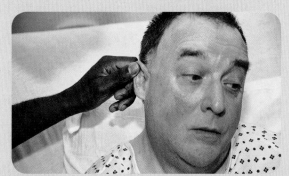
Figure 18.11

16. Gently insert the covered tympanic thermometer into the ear until it seals the ear canal (Figure 18.12).

17. Start the thermometer.

18. Hold the probe in place in the ear until you hear or see the signal that the reading is complete.

19. Remove the thermometer and read the temperature on the display screen.

Best Practice
Do not touch the plastic tympanic cover.

20. Dispose of the plastic tympanic cover safely in a waste container or per facility policy.

21. Clean the tympanic thermometer according to facility policy.

22. Wash your hands or use hand sanitizer to ensure infection control.

23. Record the temperature on a pad, form, or in the electronic record.

24. If the resident is in bed, check to be sure the bed wheels are locked. Then reposition the resident and lower the bed.

25. Follow the plan of care to determine if the side rails should be raised or lowered.

26. Return the thermometer to a charging location per facility policy.

Follow-Up

27. Make sure the resident is comfortable and place the call light and personal items within reach.

28. Conduct a safety check before leaving the room. The room should be clean and free from clutter or spills.

29. Wash your hands or use hand sanitizer before leaving the room.

Reporting and Documentation

30. Communicate any specific observations, complications, or unusual responses to the licensed nursing staff.

Images courtesy of Wards Forest Media, LLC

Temporal Artery Thermometers

Temporal artery thermometers use the surface temperature of the temporal artery to measure body temperature. This type of temperature is often more accurate than an oral temperature because it is not affected by what a patient eats or drinks. Temporal artery thermometers can measure the temperature of arteries on either side of the head using a handheld, infrared scanner with a digital display (Figure 18.13). The device is swept across the forehead to read the patient's temperature.

Sometimes a forehead thermometer strip is also used to measure a patient's temperature at this location (Figure 18.14). These strips contain heat-sensitive liquid crystals that change color to reflect different temperatures.

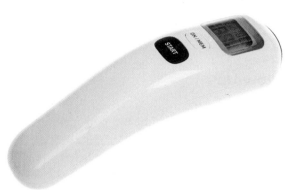

Michael Dechev/Shutterstock.com

Figure 18.13 Temporal artery thermometers measure the temperature of the temporal arteries on either side of the forehead.

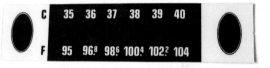

wheatley/Shutterstock.com

Figure 18.14 Forehead thermometer strips change color to indicate body temperature.

Procedure — Using a Temporal Artery Thermometer—Digital

Rationale

Body temperature that is outside the normal range can be a sign of a disease or condition or the result of an injury. The temporal artery thermometer, used on the forehead, can also be used to take a temperature. This thermometer is less invasive than others because it does not need to enter a body cavity. Always follow the thermometer manufacturer's instructions and facility policy.

Preparation

1. Ask the licensed nursing staff how this procedure fits into the plan of care, if there are doctor's orders for the procedure, if there are any special instructions or precautions, and if the resident can be moved into the positions required for this procedure.

2. Wash your hands or use hand sanitizer before entering the room.

3. Knock before entering the room.

4. Introduce yourself using your full name and title. Explain that you work with the licensed nursing staff and will be providing care.

5. Greet the resident and ask the resident to state his full name, if able. Then check the resident's identification bracelet.

6. Use Mr., Mrs., or Ms. and the last name when conversing.

7. Explain the procedure in simple terms, even if the resident is not able to communicate or is disoriented. Ask permission to perform the procedure.

8. Bring the necessary equipment into the room. Place the following items in an accessible location:

   • a temporal artery thermometer

   • a pen and pad, form, or digital device for recording the temperature

The Procedure

9. Provide privacy by closing the curtains, using a screen, or closing the door to the room.

10. If the resident is in bed, lock the bed wheels and then raise the bed to hip level.

(continued)

11. Ensure safety during the procedure. If the resident is in a bed with side rails, raise and secure the rails on the opposite side of the bed from where you will be working. Lower the rail on the side you are working.

> **Best Practice**
> Disposable gloves are worn only if required for infection prevention and control.

12. Position the resident comfortably.
13. Help or have the resident turn so that his forehead faces you.
14. Start the thermometer and wait until it shows it is ready.
15. Place the probe in the middle of the patient's forehead (Figure 18.15A). Then slowly move the thermometer across the forehead toward the ear, stopping in front of the ear (Figure 18.15B).

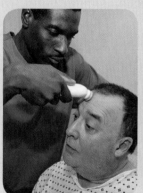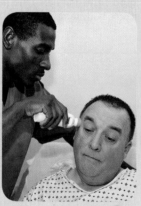

Figure 18.15   **A**   **B**

Images courtesy of Wards Forest Media, LLC

16. Wait until you see or hear the signal that the temperature is complete.
17. Wash your hands or use hand sanitizer to ensure infection control.
18. Record the temperature on a pad, on a form, or in the electronic record.
19. If the resident is in bed, check to be sure the bed wheels are locked. Then reposition the resident and lower the bed.
20. Follow the plan of care to determine if the side rails should be raised or lowered.
21. Clean and store the temporal artery thermometer according to the facility policy.

Follow-Up

22. Make sure the resident is comfortable and place the call light and personal items within reach.
23. Conduct a safety check before leaving the room. The room should be clean and free from clutter or spills.
24. Wash your hands or use hand sanitizer before leaving the room.

Reporting and Documentation

25. Communicate any specific observations, complications, or unusual responses to the licensed nursing staff.

What Is a Pulse?

When you take (measure) a *pulse*, you are feeling or hearing the pressure of blood against the wall of an artery as the heart *beats*, or contracts and relaxes. Pulse is an important vital sign because it shows how well the cardiovascular system is working. It is particularly important if a resident has a heart or respiratory condition.

Pulse Locations

There are several locations in which an artery comes close enough to the surface of the skin that you can feel a pulse (Figure 18.16). Arteries that can be felt through bare skin include the temporal, carotid, apical, brachial, radial, femoral, popliteal, and dorsalis pedis arteries.

The three pulse locations that are most commonly used are the

1. radial artery
2. apical artery; and
3. carotid artery.

Of these three, the radial and apical arteries are used most often. A nursing assistant may also measure pulse at the carotid and brachial arteries.

The **radial pulse** is taken by feeling the radial artery located at the wrist (thumb side of the hand) on bare skin. Two fingers are gently placed on the radial artery to take the pulse. If a resident has an intravenous (IV) catheter in one arm, do not use that arm when taking the pulse.

The **apical pulse** is taken by listening to the apical artery located at the *apex* of the heart (bottom left between the sternum and left nipple). It is usually taken if radial pulse is difficult to count or if a resident is unconscious. This pulse is taken using a **stethoscope**, or a medical device for listening to sounds in the body through bare skin.

The **carotid pulse** is taken by feeling the carotid artery. It is usually taken when a resident is unconscious (for example, during CPR).

The Stethoscope

A stethoscope is used to help measure an apical pulse. It is also used when taking blood pressure, which is discussed later in this section. The stethoscope increases the sound of a pulse and transfers it to the user's ears. A stethoscope is composed of two earpieces; rubber or plastic tubing; a brace, which connects the tubing to the earpieces; a diaphragm, or larger, flat surface that magnifies sound; and a bell on the other side, which can detect fainter sounds (Figure 18.17).

Before using a stethoscope, always disinfect the earpieces, diaphragm, and bell by rubbing them lightly with antiseptic or alcohol wipes. When cleaning the earpieces with alcohol, give the alcohol time to evaporate. Alcohol can be painful in the ear canal. Wipe the tubing if it has come in contact with the resident or bed linen. Place the earpieces firmly in your ear canals. The earpieces should fit snugly and block out any outside sounds. Once the earpieces are in place, rub lightly on

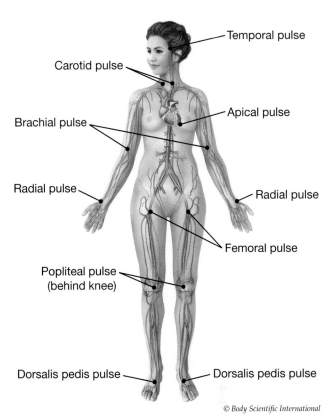

© *Body Scientific International*

Figure 18.16 Pulse can be measured at all of the locations shown here.

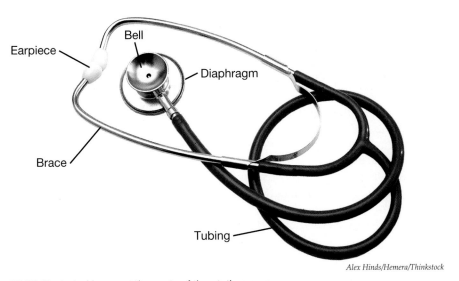

Alex Hinds/Hemera/Thinkstock

Figure 18.17 Illustrated here are the parts of the stethoscope.

the diaphragm and ensure you can hear a sound clearly. If you cannot, rotate the diaphragm and try again. If it still does not work, try this process again with a different stethoscope.

Pulse Rate Measurements

Pulse rate is measured by "feeling" or "hearing" pulse and counting the number of beats in one minute using a watch with a second hand. Pulse rate is reported in *beats per minute*, or *bpm* (for example, *72 beats per minute* or *72 bpm*).

Resting pulse is taken when a resident is breathing normally and resting (sitting in a chair or in bed). The average ranges for normal resting pulse rates are found in Figure 18.18.

Pulse rate can be affected by activity, anxiety, excitement, pain, fever, medications, sleep patterns, and diseases or health conditions. For instance, during exercise, the average person's pulse rate can range from 90 to 120 beats per minute. In contrast, if a person is an athlete, resting pulse can be as low as 40–60 beats per minute. This is because an athlete's body is in such good condition that the heart does not have to work as hard to pump blood.

A pulse that is slow (fewer than 60 beats per minute) is called **bradycardia**. A pulse that is fast (100 beats or more per minute) is called **tachycardia**.

When taking a pulse, remember that you are not only counting the number of beats, but also determining the rhythm (pauses between beats). The rhythm may be described as normal (*regular*) or intermittent (*irregular*). The quality of the pulse can be full (*bounding*) or weak (*thready*). A thready pulse is hard to feel. When you consider all of these factors, you might report a pulse as *82 bpm and regular*.

Pulse is documented in a resident's electronic record or a form provided by the healthcare facility. Any irregularities of the pulse must be reported to the licensed nursing staff.

Average Resting Pulse Rates Per Minute	
Adults	60–100 bpm
Teenagers	60–100 bpm
Children	70–120 bpm
Infants	120–160 bpm

Figure 18.18 Illustrated here are the resting pulse rates for infants, children, teenagers, and adults.

Procedure — Measuring a Radial Pulse

Rationale

Counting a radial pulse is the most common method of measuring heart rate and its quality. A pulse that falls outside the normal range may indicate a health issue, disease, or condition.

Preparation

1. Ask the licensed nursing staff how this procedure fits into the plan of care, if there are doctor's orders for the procedure, if there are any special instructions or precautions, and if the resident can be moved into the positions required for this procedure.

2. Wash your hands or use hand sanitizer before entering the room.

3. Knock before entering the room.

4. Introduce yourself using your full name and title. Explain that you work with the licensed nursing staff and will be providing care.

5. Greet the resident and ask the resident to state her full name, if able. Then check the resident's identification bracelet.

6. Use Mr., Mrs., or Ms. and the last name when conversing.

7. Explain the procedure in simple terms, even if the resident is not able to communicate or is disoriented. Ask permission to perform the procedure.

8. Bring the necessary equipment into the room. Place the following items in an accessible location:

   - a watch or clock with a second hand (not a digital watch)
   - pen and pad, form, or digital device for recording the pulse

The Procedure

9. Provide privacy by closing the curtains, using a screen, or closing the door to the room.

10. If the resident is in bed, lock the bed wheels and then raise the bed to hip level.

11. Ensure safety during the procedure. If the resident is in a bed with side rails, raise and secure the rails on the opposite side of the bed from where you will be working. Lower the rail on the side you are working.

12. Have the resident sit or lie down. Select the hand and arm you use to take the pulse.

Best Practice
If the resident has an intravenous (IV) catheter in one arm, do not use that arm to take the pulse. Also, do not take the pulse on a weak arm. Some residents may have an arm that has been weakened by a stroke.

13. Position the hand and arm so they are well supported and rest comfortably.

14. Locate the radial artery by placing your middle finger and index finger toward the inside of the resident's wrist on the thumb side (Figure 18.19).

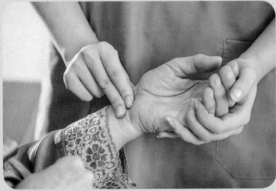
Figure 18.19

Best Practice
Do not use your thumb to feel for pulse. The thumb has its own pulse, which can be confused with the pulse you are taking.

15. Press your fingers gently on bare skin until you feel the pulse. Also, note the rhythm and quality of the pulse.

16. Start taking the pulse when you note the position of the second hand on your watch (Figure 18.20). Count pulse beats for one full minute. Some facilities allow nursing assistants to count the pulse for 30 seconds and multiply the result by two. Follow the facility policy. Counting for one full minute is more accurate, however, and should be done if the pulse rhythm seems weak or irregular.

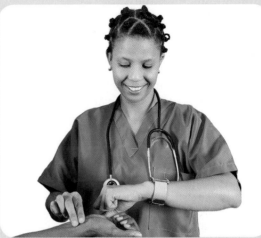
Figure 18.20

17. Record the pulse on a pad, on a form, or in the electronic record.

18. If the resident is in bed, check to be sure the bed wheels are locked. Then reposition the resident and lower the bed.

19. Follow the plan of care to determine if the side rails should be raised or lowered.

Follow-Up

20. Wash your hands to ensure infection control.

21. Make sure the resident is comfortable and place the call light and personal items within reach.

22. Conduct a safety check before leaving the room. The room should be clean and free from clutter or spills.

23. Wash your hands or use hand sanitizer before leaving the room.

Reporting and Documentation

24. Communicate any specific observations, complications, or unusual responses to the licensed nursing staff.

Figure 18.19 Tyler Olson/Shutterstock.com; Figure 18.20 michaeljung/Shutterstock.com

Rationale

Apical pulse is usually taken if you want more information than a radial pulse can provide or if it is not possible to take a radial pulse. A pulse outside the normal range may indicate a health issue, medical disease, or condition.

Preparation

1. Ask the licensed nursing staff how this procedure fits into the plan of care, if there are doctor's orders for the procedure, if there are any special instructions or precautions, and if the resident can be moved into the positions required for this procedure.

2. Wash your hands or use hand sanitizer before entering the room.

3. Knock before entering the room.

4. Introduce yourself using your full name and title. Explain that you work with the licensed nursing staff and will be providing care.

5. Greet the resident and ask the resident to state his full name, if able. Then check the resident's identification bracelet.

6. Use Mr., Mrs., or Ms. and the last name when conversing.

7. Explain the procedure in simple terms, even if the resident is not able to communicate or is disoriented. Ask permission to perform the procedure.

8. Bring the necessary equipment into the room. Place the following items in an accessible location:

   - a stethoscope
   - antiseptic wipes
   - a watch or clock with a second hand (not a digital watch)
   - pen and pad, form, or digital device for recording the pulse rate

The Procedure

9. Provide privacy by closing the curtains, using a screen, or closing the door to the room.

10. If the resident is in bed, lock the bed wheels and then raise the bed to hip level.

11. Ensure safety during the procedure. If the resident is in a bed with side rails, raise and secure the rails on the opposite side of the bed from where you will be working. Lower the rail on the side you are working.

12. Have the resident sit or lie down.

13. Clean the earpieces and diaphragm of the stethoscope with an antiseptic wipe.

14. Warm the diaphragm of the stethoscope by rubbing it in the palms of your hands.

15. Place the earpieces of the stethoscope in your ears.

16. Uncover the left side of the resident's chest. Avoid any overexposure.

17. Place the diaphragm of the stethoscope on the left side of the chest, under the breast, or just below the left nipple (Figure 18.21).

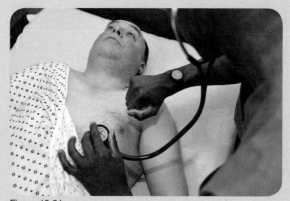

Figure 18.21

> **Best Practice**
> If the heartbeat is difficult to hear, have the resident turn slightly to the left or sit upright.

18. Note the position of the second hand on your watch. Count the heartbeats for one full minute. Note the rhythm and quality.

19. Cover the resident's chest.

20. Record the pulse on a pad, on a form, or in the electronic record.

21. If the resident is in bed, check to be sure the bed wheels are locked. Then reposition the resident and lower the bed.

22. Follow the plan of care to determine if the side rails should be raised or lowered.

What Is the Rate of Respiration?

The *rate of respiration* is the measurement of a resident's breathing cycle (inhalation followed by exhalation). Respiration rate helps determine a resident's level of *blood oxygenation*, or how well oxygen is supplied to body cells. Respiration rate also helps determine if a resident is breathing in a normal range. This provides information about conditions such as asthma, heart disease, and even infections.

Measuring Respirations

To determine the rate of respiration, nursing assistants record the number of full breaths (each rise and fall of the chest) taken in one minute (Figure 18.22). Typically, this involves counting respirations for 15 seconds and multiplying the result by four. Some healthcare facilities require nursing assistants to count respirations for 30 seconds and then multiply the result by two. If respirations are irregular, the nursing assistant should count the number of full breaths for one full minute using a watch with a second hand.

It is best to count respiration rate with no warning immediately after pulse is taken. This way, the resident is breathing as he or she normally would. After taking the pulse, switch to counting respirations without mentioning the change to the resident. A resident who knows his or her respirations are being counted may subconsciously alter his or her breathing, giving the nursing assistant an inaccurate result.

Understanding Respiratory Rates

A normal adult respiration rate is 12–20 breaths per minute. Infants and children breathe much faster. Infants can breathe from 30 to 60 breaths per minute, and children can breathe from 18 to 30 breaths per minute. Respiration can be affected by activity, anxiety, pain, fear, fever, infection, injury, and diseases of the heart and lungs.

Observing how well a resident is breathing (regularity, expansion of the chest, and depth of respiration) is just as important as determining the rate (counting breaths). When counting respirations, also note the following:

- Is the breathing regular or irregular?
- Is the resident experiencing **hyperventilation** (deep, rapid breathing) or **hypoventilation** (slow, shallow breathing)?
- Is the breathing rapid (called **tachypnea**), deep and labored (called **dyspnea**), or unusually slow (called **bradypnea**)?
- Is the breathing noisy like snoring (called **stertorous breathing**)?
- Are there periods of no breathing at all (called **apnea**)?

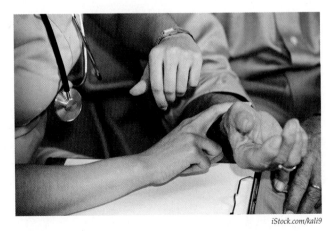

iStock.com/kali9

Figure 18.22 Counting respirations directly after taking pulse can help ensure the resident's breathing is normal.

Rationale

Counting respirations involves measuring the number of inhalations and exhalations in one minute. A respiration rate that falls outside the normal range may indicate a health issue, medical disease, or condition.

Preparation

1. Ask the licensed nursing staff how this procedure fits into the plan of care, if there are doctor's orders for the procedure, if there are any special instructions or precautions, and if the resident can be moved into the positions required for this procedure.

2. Wash your hands or use hand sanitizer before entering the room.

3. Knock before entering the room.

4. Introduce yourself using your full name and title. Explain that you work with the licensed nursing staff and will be providing care.

5. Greet the resident and ask the resident to state his or her full name, if able. Then check the resident's identification bracelet.

6. Use Mr., Mrs., or Ms. and the last name when conversing.

7. Explain the procedure in simple terms, even if the resident is not able to communicate or is disoriented. Ask permission to perform the procedure.

8. Bring the necessary equipment into the room. Place the following items in an accessible location:
   - a watch or clock with a second hand (not a digital watch)
   - a pen and pad, form, or digital device for recording the respiration rate

The Procedure

9. Provide privacy by closing the curtains, using a screen, or closing the door to the room.

10. If the resident is in bed, lock the bed wheels and then raise the bed to hip level.

11. Ensure safety during the procedure. If the resident is in a bed with side rails, raise and secure the rails on the opposite side of the bed from where you will be working. Lower the rail on the side you are working.

12. Have the resident sit or lie down.

13. The best time to count respirations is immediately after counting pulse rate. It is best not to tell residents you are counting respirations. When residents know their breathing is being observed, they may alter their breathing patterns.

> **Best Practice**
> Depending on which pulse was taken, keep your fingers on the wrist or keep the stethoscope on the chest while counting respirations.

14. Begin counting respirations when the chest rises. Each rise and fall of the chest counts as one respiration. Note the regularity and depth of respirations, the expansion of the chest, and any pain or difficulty breathing.

15. Note the position of the second hand on your watch and count respirations for one full minute. Some facilities allow nursing assistants to count respirations for 15 seconds and multiply the result by four or count respirations for 30 seconds and multiply the result by two. Follow the facility policy. Counting respirations for one full minute should be done if the respiration is irregular.

16. Notify the licensed nursing staff immediately if the resident complains of pain or difficulty breathing.

17. Record the respiration rate on a pad, on a form, or in the electronic record.

18. If the resident is in bed, check to be sure the bed wheels are locked. Then reposition the resident and lower the bed.

19. Follow the plan of care to determine if the side rails should be raised or lowered.

Follow-Up

20. Wash your hands to ensure infection control.

21. Make sure the resident is comfortable and place the call light and personal items within reach.

22. Conduct a safety check before leaving the room. The room should be clean and free from clutter or spills.

23. Wash your hands or use hand sanitizer before leaving the room.

Reporting and Documentation

24. Communicate any specific observations, complications, or unusual responses to the licensed nursing staff.

Using a Pulse Oximeter

Another way to measure how well oxygen is being used in the body is to determine oxygen saturation in the blood. A *pulse oximeter* is used to measure blood oxygenation. It is commonly used when vital signs are being measured and is also used to measure oxygen effectiveness for a resident receiving oxygen.

A pulse oximeter is applied to the finger (or sometimes the earlobe or toe). It uses infrared light that passes through the body tissue of the finger. A pulse oximeter's digital display will show the amount of oxygen in the blood as a percentage (Figure 18.23). A normal reading is 95 percent to 100 percent oxygen in the blood. A reading below 85 percent is too low and is called **hypoxia** (lack of adequate oxygen in the body). The notation used for recording oxygen saturation in the blood is SpO_2.

Using a pulse oximeter has minimal risks. If improperly placed, the pulse oximeter may give an inaccurate reading. If a pulse oximeter is used continuously, pay attention to the skin around and under the device and check for possible irritation.

Respirations (rate, regularity, and depth) and pulse oximeter percentages are recorded on a form provided by the healthcare facility or in the electronic record. Any irregularities must be reported to the licensed nursing staff.

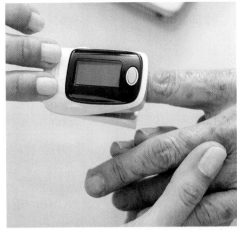

Click and Photo/Shutterstock.com

Figure 18.23 The pulse oximeter is placed on the finger and measures oxygen saturation in the blood.

How Is Blood Pressure Measured?

Blood pressure is the force of blood pushing against the body's arterial walls. Measuring blood pressure is important. If a resident has **hypotension** (blood pressure that is too low), the body may not be getting enough oxygen and nutrients. Conversely, *hypertension* (blood pressure that is too high) may place too much pressure on the walls of the arteries (Figure 18.24). This pressure can cause a stroke or other cardiovascular problems. High or low blood pressure can also signal or cause certain diseases and conditions, such as heart disease, kidney damage or failure, various injuries, or dizziness.

Measuring Blood Pressure

A blood pressure reading is made up of two pressure levels, which are measured as the heart beats. The first is **systolic blood pressure**, which is pressure when the heart muscle contracts and pushes blood through the artery. The second is **diastolic blood pressure**, which is pressure when the heart muscle relaxes. These pressure levels are measured using a stethoscope and a sphygmomanometer.

Both pressure levels are measured in *millimeters of mercury (mmHg)*. Systolic blood pressure is the higher number and the first beat heard (as a tapping sound) and measured (as 120 mmHg, for example). Diastolic blood pressure is the lower number and is the last beat heard and measured (as 80 mmHg, for example). For someone with these measurements, blood pressure would be recorded as the fraction 120/80 mmHg. The average ranges of normal blood pressure for adults, children, and infants can be found in Figure 18.25.

> **Think About This**
>
> The Centers for Disease Control and Prevention recently reported that 75 million American adults (29 percent) have high blood pressure. This means that about one in every three adults has hypertension. Approximately one-half (54 percent) of those with high blood pressure have their condition under control.

Blood Pressure Classification			
Hypotension	**Normal**	**Elevated**	**Hypertension**
<90/60 mmHg	90–120/60–80 mmHg	120–129/<80 mmHG	**Stage 1:** 130–139/80–90 mmHG **Stage 2:** >140/90 mmHg

Figure 18.24 Blood pressure measurements are important indicators of health and may indicate or cause certain diseases or conditions.

Average Blood Pressure Measurements		
Age	***Systolic* Pressure**	***Diastolic* Pressure**
Adult	100–130	60–90
Teenager	94–134	64–84
Children	100–120	60–74
Infant	70–90	50–64

Figure 18.25 These ranges represent the average blood pressures for adults, teenagers, children, and infants.

Knowing Factors That Affect Blood Pressure

> **Remember**
>
> *Ability is what you're capable of doing. Motivation determines what you do. Attitude determines how well you do it.*
>
> Lou Holtz, coach

Many factors can affect blood pressure. These factors include the following:

- **Diet**: diets high in salt and fat may lead to higher blood pressure.
- **Weight**: being overweight can lead to higher blood pressure.
- **Exercise**: systolic blood pressure may be higher if a resident does not exercise or exercised right before blood pressure was taken.
- **Race**: African-American individuals tend to have a higher occurrence of high blood pressure and at an earlier age compared to Caucasians or people of Hispanic descent.
- **Time of day**: blood pressure may be lower in the morning than later in the day and may be higher after a meal.
- **Position**: blood pressure may be higher if a resident is lying down and lower if a resident is standing up.
- **Cigarettes and alcohol**: using cigarettes and alcohol can increase blood pressure.
- **Drugs or medications**: some medications and drugs can make blood pressure higher or lower.
- **Stress, fear, or pain**: blood pressure may be higher if a resident is experiencing stress, fear, or pain.

Becoming a Holistic Nursing Assistant

Taking Vital Signs

To provide holistic care when measuring and recording vital signs, you can use the following guidelines:

- Be knowledgeable about the function of and the normal ranges for different vital signs.
- Demonstrate skill and proficiency.
- Ensure accurate measurements. Repeat the measurement if you are unsure of a reading. Explain to the resident that you want to take an accurate reading.
- Ask a member of the licensed nursing staff for help if you have trouble measuring a vital sign. *Never* make up a reading.
- Quickly report any abnormal results to the licensed nursing staff.
- When appropriate, give residents choices about the procedure. For example, you might let the resident choose the arm used to measure blood pressure or choose whether to sit up or lie down.
- Know that vital signs can be variable and are unique to each resident, the resident's environment, and factors of daily living such as diet and exercise.
- Maintain a professional and patient attitude when taking vital signs. Never show frustration or concern if you are having difficulty measuring a vital sign or if a vital sign is not in a normal range.

Apply It

1. Would any of these guidelines be challenging for you to follow? Explain your answer.
2. From your personal perspective, which guidelines would require more attention or practice on your part?

Taking a Resident's Blood Pressure

Blood pressure can be measured manually or electronically, depending on the equipment available. Both ways are accurate; however, electronic devices reduce potential human error as long as they are checked regularly for accuracy. Equipment may be movable, on a wall mount, or part of an electronic vital sign monitoring machine.

When taking a resident's blood pressure, be sure to check the equipment, make sure the resident is relaxed, and ensure you feel prepared to perform the procedure. Avoid using an arm with an IV catheter, cast, wound, or injury to take blood pressure. Residents who have undergone a mastectomy should not have blood pressure taken on the same side as the breast removal.

It is important to recheck a blood pressure reading if you are not sure the measurement is accurate or if you cannot hear the sounds clearly. You should recheck blood pressure if you suspect an error or faulty equipment, if you notice a change in the resident's normal blood pressure, or if the reading is the first occurrence of high or low blood pressure for that resident. If retaking a blood pressure, be sure the blood pressure cuff is completely deflated with all of its air released. Wait one minute before retrying. Also check the stethoscope to be sure it is working correctly and is placed in the correct location. Be sure the earpieces are properly located in your ears.

When taking a manual blood pressure measurement, you will need a stethoscope and a *sphygmomanometer* (*sphygm/o* = pulse; *man/o* = pressure; *-meter* = measure). Before beginning, check that the stethoscope is in working order. There are two main types of sphygmomanometers used to measure blood pressure (Figure 18.26):

1. **Manual aneroid sphygmomanometer**: is movable and has a round dial and a needle that points to the numbers. You will need to use a stethoscope when using this device.

2. **Electronic sphygmomanometer**: has a digital display and is found in many healthcare facilities. You will not need a stethoscope when using this device.

A sphygmomanometer has two parts: the measuring device and the cuff. When applying a blood pressure cuff, check that it is the right size. Cuffs come in various sizes—pediatric, small adult, adult, and large adult (Figure 18.27). If the cuff is too small or too large, the blood pressure reading will not be accurate. The inflatable part of the cuff should cover two-thirds of the distance from the elbow to the shoulder. You should be able to fit your fingers between the closed cuff and the skin. No matter what type of device you use, be sure it is in working order before taking blood pressure.

Before taking blood pressure, have residents relax or rest for a few minutes (five minutes). This will help you get a reading that is most normal for the resident. The blood pressure reading may not be accurate if the resident has just been exercising, is in pain, is feeling anxious, or has recently had physical therapy. If possible, wait at least 30 minutes after these events before taking a routine blood pressure measurement. Also make sure the area in which blood pressure is taken is quiet. This will help you hear through the stethoscope and better ensure accuracy of the measurement.

Taking blood pressures can seem challenging at first, but practice helps build confidence and will improve your ability to hear through the stethoscope and take accurate readings.

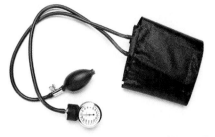

A

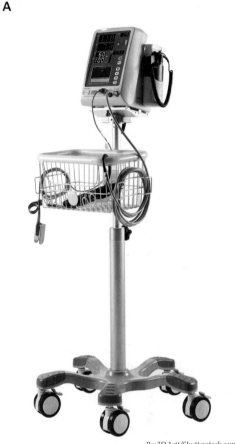

B

Figure 18.26 Both manual (A) and electronic (B) sphygmomanometers can be used to measure blood pressure.

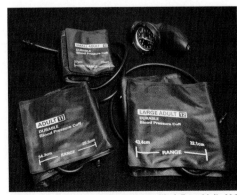

Figure 18.27 Using the appropriate cuff is important for getting an accurate measurement.

Rationale

Blood pressure measures the force of blood pushing against the body's arterial walls. A blood pressure reading outside the normal range may indicate a disease or health issue.

Preparation

1. Ask the licensed nursing staff how this procedure fits into the plan of care, if there are doctor's orders for the procedure, if there are any special instructions or precautions, and if the resident can be moved into the positions required for this procedure.

2. Wash your hands or use hand sanitizer before entering the room.

3. Knock before entering the room.

4. Introduce yourself using your full name and title. Explain that you work with the licensed nursing staff and will be providing care.

5. Greet the resident and ask the resident to state his full name, if able. Then check the resident's identification bracelet.

6. Use Mr., Mrs., or Ms. and the last name when conversing.

7. Explain the procedure in simple terms, even if the resident is not able to communicate or is disoriented. Ask permission to perform the procedure.

8. Bring the necessary equipment into the room. Place the following items in an accessible location:

   - a sphygmomanometer
   - an appropriately sized cuff (pediatric, small adult, adult, or large adult)
   - a stethoscope, if using a manual sphygmomanometer
   - antiseptic wipe(s)
   - a pen and pad, form, or digital device for recording the blood pressure

The Procedure: Manual Device

9. Provide privacy by closing the curtains, using a screen, or closing the door to the room.

10. Clean the cuff with an antiseptic wipe or cover with a disposable paper cover.

11. Have the resident rest quietly and lie comfortably on the bed or sit in a chair. Make sure the room is quiet.

12. When appropriate, let the resident choose which arm he wants you to use for taking blood pressure and whether he wants to sit up or lie down.

13. If the resident is in bed, lock the bed wheels and then raise the bed to hip level. If he is on an examining table, stand next to him or sit in a chair in front of him so you can get a clear view of the dial.

14. Clean the earpieces of the stethoscope with an antiseptic wipe and warm the diaphragm with your hands before cleaning it with antiseptic wipes.

15. Position the resident's arm so it rests level with the heart with the palm turned upward. Provide support, if needed (Figure 18.28).

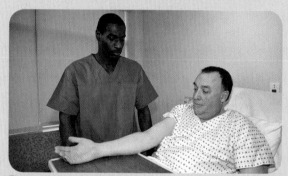

Figure 18.28

> **Best Practice**
> Expose the upper arm so that you can place the cuff on bare skin.

16. Unroll the blood pressure cuff and loosen the valve on the bulb of the sphygmomanometer by turning it counterclockwise (Figure 18.29).

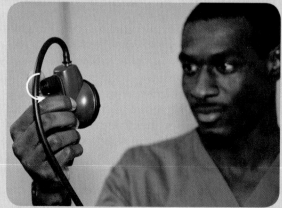

Figure 18.29

17. Squeeze the cuff to expel any remaining air.
18. With your fingertips, locate the brachial artery at the inner aspect of the elbow (Figure 18.30).

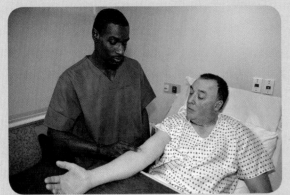
Figure 18.30

19. Wrap the cuff smoothly and snugly around the exposed arm about 1 inch above the elbow. Do not wrap the cuff around clothing. Make sure the cuff is not too snug (Figure 18.31).

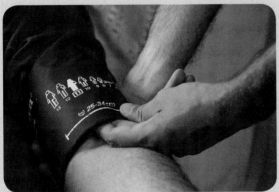
Figure 18.31

20. Place the center of the cuff, usually marked with an arrow, above the brachial artery. (Figure 18.32).

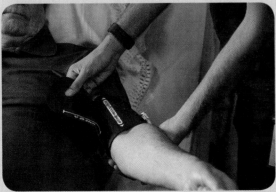
Figure 18.32

21. Close the valve on the bulb of the sphygmomanometer by turning it clockwise. Be careful not to turn it too tightly.
22. Place the earpieces of the stethoscope in your ears.
23. Find the brachial pulse.
24. Place the warmed diaphragm of the stethoscope over the brachial artery.
25. If using a manual aneroid sphygmomanometer, keep the measuring scale level with your eyes.
26. Inflate the cuff to 180 mmHg. You should not be able to hear the resident's pulse. If you do, inflate the cuff to 200 mmHg.

> **Best Practice**
> The stethoscope diaphragm should be held firmly against the skin close to the cuff, but should not be placed under the cuff (Figure 18.33).

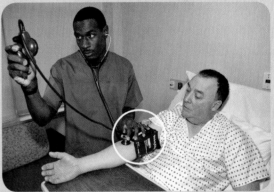
Figure 18.33

27. Deflate the cuff by slowly turning the valve on the bulb of the sphygmomanometer counterclockwise at an even rate of 2–4 millimeters per second.
28. Listen carefully while the cuff is deflating. Note the dial reading when you hear the first sound (beat). This is the systolic blood pressure.
29. Continue deflating the cuff slowly and evenly. Note the dial reading when the sound (beat) disappears. This is the diastolic blood pressure.
30. Remove the stethoscope earpieces from your ears. Completely deflate the cuff and remove it from the arm.

(continued)

31. Record the blood pressure on a pad, on a form, or in the electronic record.

32. Report abnormal results to the appropriate licensed nursing staff member immediately.

33. Return the cuff to its case or wall mount.

34. Clean the earpieces and diaphragm of the stethoscope with antiseptic wipes.

35. Return the stethoscope and cuff case (if appropriate) to their storage locations.

36. If the resident is in bed, check to be sure the bed wheels are locked. Then reposition the resident and lower the bed.

37. Follow the plan of care to determine if the side rails should be raised or lowered.

The Procedure: Electronic Device

38. Provide privacy by closing the curtains, using a screen, or closing the door to the room.

39. Bring the electronic blood pressure unit near the resident and plug it into a source of electricity.

40. Clean the cuff with an antiseptic wipe or cover with a disposable paper cover.

41. Have the resident rest quietly and lie comfortably on the bed or sit in a chair.

42. If the resident is in bed, lock the bed wheels and then raise the bed to hip level. If he is on an examining table, stand next to him or sit in a chair in front of him so you can get a clear view of the digital display.

43. Remove any restrictive clothing from the resident's arm. Ask the resident which arm he would prefer, if appropriate.

44. Locate the *Power* switch and turn on the machine.

45. Squeeze any excess air out of the blood pressure cuff.

46. Connect the cuff to the connector hose.

47. Wrap the cuff smoothly and snugly around the resident's exposed arm. Do not wrap the cuff around clothing. Make sure the cuff is not too snug.

48. Make sure the arrow marked on the outside of the cuff is correctly placed over the brachial artery.

49. Make sure the connector hose between the cuff and the machine is not kinked.

50. Press the *Start* button. The cuff should begin to inflate and then deflate as the reading is being taken.

51. You will see or hear a signal when the reading is complete.

52. If you are taking periodic, automatic measurements, set the machine for the designated frequency of blood pressure measurements. The upper and lower alarm limits for systolic, diastolic, and mean blood pressure readings are set according to facility policy.

53. Record the blood pressure on a pad, on a form, or in the electronic record.

54. Report abnormal results to the licensed nursing staff immediately.

55. Clean the tubing and cuff with an antiseptic wipe. Discard the disposable sleeve, if used.

56. Remove the machine and place it in its appropriate storage location.

57. If the cuff is to remain on the arm between blood pressure readings, loosen it. Remove the cuff at least every two hours and rotate to the other arm, if possible. Evaluate the skin for redness or irritation. Report any abnormal observations to the licensed nursing staff.

58. If the resident is in bed, check to be sure the bed wheels are locked. Then reposition the resident and lower the bed.

59. Follow the plan of care to determine if the side rails should be raised or lowered.

Follow-Up

60. Wash your hands to ensure infection control.

61. Make sure the resident is comfortable and place the call light and personal items within reach.

62. Conduct a safety check before leaving the room. The room should be clean and free from clutter or spills.

63. Wash your hands or use hand sanitizer before leaving the room.

Reporting and Documentation

64. Communicate any specific observations, complications, or unusual responses to the licensed nursing staff.

Figure 18.28 Wards Forest Media, LLC; Figure 18.29 Wards Forest Media, LLC; Figure 18.30 Wards Forest Media, LLC; Figure 18.31 © Tori Soper Photography; Figure 18.32 © Tori Soper Photography; Figure 18.33 Wards Forest Media, LLC

Using the Key Terms

Complete the following sentences using key terms in this section.

1. Low blood pressure is called _____.
2. In the _____ scale, water freezes at 0° and boils at 100°.
3. _____ is a pulse slower than 60 beats per minute.
4. To measure the _____, you would listen to the heartbeat at the apex of the heart using a stethoscope.
5. In the _____ scale, water freezes at 32° and boils at 212°.
6. _____ is the pressure of blood against the arteries when the heart contracts.
7. To measure the _____, you would feel the radial artery located on the inside of the wrist.
8. _____ is a pulse faster than 100 beats per minute.
9. _____ is the pressure of blood against the arteries when the heart relaxes.
10. _____ is described as rapid, shallow breathing.
11. A(n) _____ is measured by placing a thermometer into the ear.
12. _____ is abnormally slow breathing.

Know and Understand the Facts

13. Describe two reasons why vital signs are measured.
14. Identify the locations where a pulse can be measured.
15. List the equipment needed to measure a blood pressure.
16. An adult has a blood pressure of 140/95 mmHg. Is this within the normal range?

Analyze and Apply Concepts

17. What should a nursing assistant do if a vital sign does not seem to be accurate?
18. What should a nursing assistant do if a vital sign is significantly higher or lower than it was when taken at an earlier time?
19. What equipment is needed to take a rectal temperature?
20. Which steps must always be performed to ensure blood pressure is measured accurately?
21. List two important descriptions that should be recorded when measuring a pulse.

Think Critically

Read the following care situation. Then answer the questions that follow.

Seiji, a nursing assistant at the city rehabilitation facility, was taking Mr. L's vital signs. When Seiji finished, he realized that Mr. L's vital signs were very different from those taken the day before. Yesterday, Mr. L's blood pressure and pulse were much lower. Seiji used a different sphygmomanometer and stethoscope, so he thought that may be the problem.

22. What is the first action Seiji should take?
23. Should Seiji let the charge nurse know about the change? If so, what should he say?
24. What should Seiji record in Mr. L's chart or electronic record?

Questions to Consider

- How often do you weigh yourself? Are you happy with your weight? If you are not, what changes would you like to make? How would you go about making these changes?
- Do you keep track of your height? For what reasons do you measure your weight and height?

Objectives

To provide the best possible care, you must understand how to measure height and weight accurately and effectively for ambulatory, wheelchair-bound, and bedridden residents. These skills provide essential information for monitoring a resident's condition. To achieve the objectives for this section, you must successfully

- **describe** why height and weight measurements are important to know when providing care; and
- **demonstrate** the skills needed to measure height and weight accurately and effectively for ambulatory, wheelchair-bound, and bedridden residents.

Key Terms

Learn these key terms to better understand the information presented in the section.

body mass index (BMI)   malnutrition
ideal body weight (IBW)

Why Is It Important to Measure Height and Weight?

Height and weight are usually measured on admission to a healthcare facility, during a resident's stay, and during a patient visit to a doctor's office. The frequency of these measurements (daily, weekly, or monthly) depends on doctors' orders for a health condition or disease. For example, a resident with kidney disease or congestive heart failure (CHF) may need to be weighed daily to help determine if he or she has *edema* (retention of fluid in the body tissues). If a patient is admitted to a healthcare facility, the facility's policy will also dictate how often measurements are taken. A baseline height and weight measurement is also usually taken.

Height and weight measurements enable healthcare staff to monitor a resident's health and determine nutritional status and medication dosages. The relationship between height and weight is also important because it can indicate a resident's overall health status. Height and weight are used to calculate ideal body weight (IBW) and body mass index (BMI). **Ideal body weight (IBW)** is the healthiest weight for an individual. **Body mass index (BMI)** is a number that determines whether a resident is a healthy weight, overweight, or underweight. This number is calculated by dividing weight in kilograms (kg) by height in meters (m) squared. These calculations help a doctor plan calorie intake, protein, and fluid needs for a resident.

Measuring Height

Height can be measured in two ways. If a resident is able to walk, you can use an upright, *balance scale* to measure height. If a resident is bedridden, you will need to use a tape measure. Height should be recorded in feet (') and inches (") or in centimeters (cm), depending on facility policy.

If a resident is able to walk, have the resident stand very straight on the center of the scale with arms and hands down at his or her sides. Lower the height bar until it rests on the top of the head. Read the height at the movable part of the ruler.

If a resident is bedridden, use a tape measure. If allowed, have the resident lie on his or her back, as straight as possible with arms straight at the sides and legs extended. Straighten and tighten the bedsheet. With the help of another healthcare staff member, extend the tape measure along the resident's side from the top of the head to the bottom of the heel (Figure 18.34). Measure the distance between the two points.

Measuring Weight

A resident's weight is often used to calculate medication dosage. As a result, accurate measurement is essential. Weight can also indicate certain conditions, such as **malnutrition** (poor nourishment) or edema. There are different ways of measuring weight. Weight can be measured using an upright balance or a digital scale for ambulatory residents (Figure 18.35). Chair and wheelchair scales may also be used. A hydraulic digital body lift or sling scale, a scale built into a bed, or a digital pad placed under the wheels of a bed can be used if a resident is bedridden (Figure 18.36).

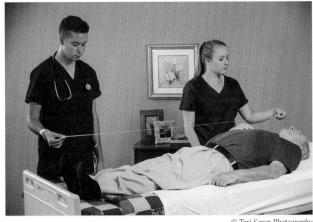

© Tori Soper Photography

Figure 18.34 To measure the height of a bedridden resident, use a tape measure.

Weight should be measured at the same time each day. The resident should wear the same or similar clothing each time, and the same scale should be used, if possible. Be sure the resident has urinated before measurement. Always factor in additional items that may add weight, such as shoes, casts, catheters, colostomy bags, or other bodily devices. Weight can be measured when a resident is standing, sitting, or lying in bed. Weight should be measured in pounds (lbs) or in kilograms (kg), depending on facility policy.

If using a balance or digital scale for a standing resident, have the resident stand straight on the center of the scale with arms and hands down at his or her sides. If using a balance scale, move the weights on the balanced scale bar to zero. Move the lower and upper weights until the balance pointer is in the middle. Add the amounts shown on the two bars together to determine weight.

If using a lift or bed scale, be sure to follow the facility policy and instructions for the equipment. You will need another healthcare staff member to assist in this procedure.

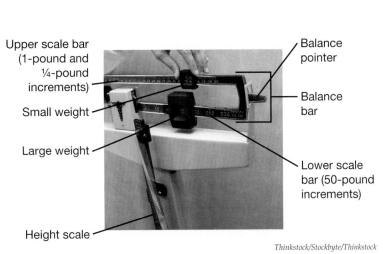

Thinkstock/Stockbyte/Thinkstock

Figure 18.35 A balance scale is used to measure weight. It can also measure height.

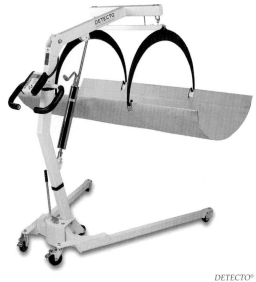

DETECTO®
www.Detecto.com

Figure 18.36 This is an example of a bed scale that can be used to weigh bedridden residents.

Rationale

Height and weight measurements are used to calculate medication dosages and determine nutritional needs. Therefore, nursing assistants must measure and record height and weight accurately and according to facility policy.

Preparation

1. Ask the licensed nursing staff how this procedure fits into the plan of care, if there are doctor's orders for the procedure, if there are any special instructions or precautions, and if the resident can be moved into the positions required for this procedure.

2. Wash your hands or use hand sanitizer before entering the room.

3. Knock before entering the room.

4. Introduce yourself using your full name and title. Explain that you work with the licensed nursing staff and will be providing care.

5. Greet the resident and ask the resident to state his or her full name, if able. Then check the resident's identification bracelet.

6. Use Mr., Mrs., or Ms. and the last name when conversing.

7. Explain the procedure in simple terms, even if the resident is not able to communicate or is disoriented. Ask permission to perform the procedure.

8. Ambulatory residents can walk to a scale placed in a central location within the facility. Bring the following items to the scale:
   - paper towel
   - a pen and pad, form, or digital device for recording the height and weight

The Procedure

9. Provide privacy by closing the curtains, using a screen, or closing the door to the room.

10. Place a paper towel on the scale platform.

11. Raise the height bar above the level of the resident's head.

12. Help the resident remove her shoes or slippers and stand on the scale platform.

13. Ask the resident to stand up straight on the center of the scale with arms and hands down at her sides.

14. Lift the height bar, extend the arm, and then lower the arm until it rests on top of the resident's head (Figure 18.37).

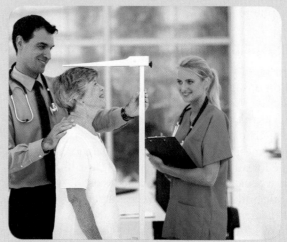

Figure 18.37

15. Read the height at the movable part of the ruler (Figure 18.38).

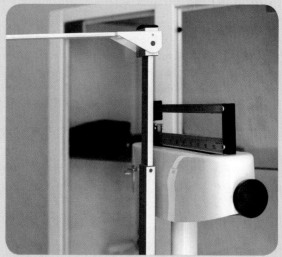

Figure 18.38

16. Record the height on a pad, on a form, or in the electronic record.

17. Raise the height bar above the level of the resident's head. When it reaches a safe height, lower the arm and then return the height bar to its starting point.

18. Ask the resident to stand straight again with arms and hands at her sides.

19. Move the weights on the balanced scale bar to zero.

20. Move the lower and upper weights until the balance pointer is in the middle.

> **Best Practice**
> Move the large weight 50 pounds at a time until the weight bar falls. Then back the large weight up 50 pounds. Finally, move the small weight until the scale is balanced.

21. Add the amounts shown on the two bars together to determine the resident's weight (Figure 18.39).

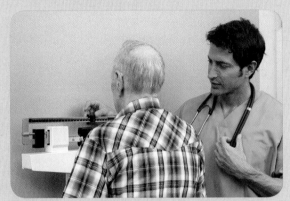

Figure 18.39

22. Record the weight on a pad, on a form, or in the electronic record.

23. Help the resident step off the scale platform.
24. Assist the resident in putting on her shoes or slippers.
25. Remove and discard the paper towel from the scale platform.
26. Assist the resident safely back to her room or bed.
27. If the resident is in bed, check to be sure the bed wheels are locked. Then reposition the resident and lower the bed.
28. Follow the plan of care to determine if the side rails should be raised or lowered.

Follow-Up

29. Wash your hands to ensure infection control.
30. Make sure the resident is comfortable and place the call light and personal items within reach.
31. Conduct a safety check before leaving the room. The room should be clean and free from clutter or spills.
32. Wash your hands or use hand sanitizer before leaving the room.

Reporting and Documentation

33. Communicate any specific observations, complications, or unusual responses to the licensed nursing staff.

Figure 18.37 michaeljung/Shutterstock.com; Figure 18.38 iStock.com/Paolo_Toffanin; Figure 18.39 iStock.com/inhauscreative

---

Procedure   Measuring the Height of Bedridden Residents

Rationale

Height measurements must be accurate for bedridden residents. The height measurement may be used when calculating medication dosages and assessing a resident's nutritional needs.

Preparation

1. Ask the licensed nursing staff how this procedure fits into the plan of care, if there are doctor's orders for the procedure, if there are any special instructions or precautions, and if the resident can be moved into the positions required for this procedure.
2. Wash your hands or use hand sanitizer before entering the room.
3. Knock before entering the room.
4. Introduce yourself using your full name and title. Explain that you work with the licensed nursing staff and will be providing care.
5. Greet the resident and ask the resident to state his full name, if able. Then check the resident's identification bracelet.
6. Use Mr., Mrs., or Ms. and the last name when conversing.
7. Explain the procedure in simple terms, even if the resident is not able to communicate or is disoriented. Ask permission to perform the procedure.

(continued)

8. Bring the necessary equipment into the room. Place the following items in an accessible location:

   - a tape measure
   - a pen and pad, form, or digital device for recording the height

9. You will need another person to assist in this measurement. Ask a coworker to help.

The Procedure

10. Provide privacy by closing the curtains, using a screen, or closing the door to the room.

11. Lock the bed wheels and then raise the bed to hip level.

12. Ensure safety during the procedure. If there are side rails, raise and secure the rails on the opposite side of the bed from where you will be working. Lower the rail on the side you are working.

13. If allowed, have the resident lie on his back, as straight as possible, with his arms straight against his sides.

> **Best Practice**
> Straighten and tighten the bedsheet.

14. Extend the tape measure along the side of the resident from the top of his head to the bottom of his heel.

15. Measure the distance between the two points.

16. Record the height on a pad, on a form, or in the electronic record.

17. Check to be sure the bed wheels are locked, then reposition the resident and lower the bed.

18. Follow the plan of care to determine if the side rails should be raised or lowered.

Follow-Up

19. Wash your hands to ensure infection control.

20. Make sure the resident is comfortable and place the call light and personal items within reach.

21. Conduct a safety check before leaving the room. The room should be clean and free from clutter or spills.

22. Wash your hands or use hand sanitizer before leaving the room.

Reporting and Documentation

23. Communicate any specific observations, complications, or unusual responses to the licensed nursing staff.

Procedure — **Weighing Bedridden Residents Using a Hydraulic Digital Lift or Sling Bed Scale**

Rationale

Weight measurements must be accurate for bedridden residents. The weight measurement may be used to calculate medication dosages and assess a resident's nutritional needs.

Preparation

1. Ask the licensed nursing staff how this procedure fits into the plan of care, if there are doctor's orders for the procedure, if there are any special instructions or precautions, and if the resident can be moved into the positions required for this procedure.

2. Wash your hands or use hand sanitizer before entering the room.

3. Knock before entering the room.

4. Introduce yourself using your full name and title. Explain that you work with the licensed nursing staff and will be providing care.

5. Greet the resident and ask the resident to state her full name, if able. Then check the resident's identification bracelet.

6. Use Mr., Mrs., or Ms. and the last name when conversing.

7. Explain the procedure in simple terms, even if the resident is not able to communicate or is disoriented. Ask permission to perform the procedure.

8. Bring the necessary equipment into the room. Place the following items in an accessible location:
   - a bed scale with the appropriate sling and attachments
   - a pen and pad, form, or digital device for recording the weight
9. You will need another person to assist in this measurement. Ask a coworker to help.

The Procedure

10. Provide privacy by closing the curtains, using a screen, or closing the door to the room.
11. Lock the bed wheels and then raise the bed to hip level.
12. Ensure safety during the procedure. If there are side rails, raise and secure the rails on the opposite side of the bed from where you will be working. Lower the rail on the side you are working.
13. To ensure the measurement is accurate, balance the bed scale with the sling attached following the manufacturer's instructions.
14. Help the resident roll to one side. Position the sling beneath the resident's body lengthwise behind the shoulders, thighs, and buttocks. Be sure the sling is smooth.
15. Roll the resident back onto the sling and ensure the sling is correctly positioned under the shoulders, thighs, and buttocks.
16. Center the bed scale over the bed. Carefully lower the weighting arms of the scale and attach them securely to the sling bars.
17. Instruct the resident to keep her arms to her sides while she is being weighed.
18. Raise the sling so the resident's body and the sling hang freely over the bed (Figure 18.40).

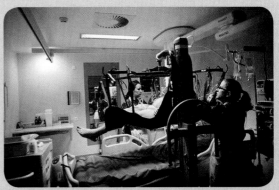

Figure 18.40

19. Adjust the weights until the balance bar hangs freely on the end or read the digital display screen.
20. Record the weight on a pad, on a form, or in the electronic record.
21. Lower the resident back onto the bed and remove the sling.
22. Check to be sure the bed wheels are locked, then reposition the resident and lower the bed.
23. Follow the plan of care to determine if the side rails should be raised or lowered.

Follow-Up

24. Wash your hands to ensure infection control.
25. Make sure the resident is comfortable and place the call light and personal items within reach.
26. Conduct a safety check before leaving the room. The room should be clean and free from clutter or spills.
27. Wash your hands or use hand sanitizer before leaving the room.

Reporting and Documentation

28. Communicate any specific observations, complications, or unusual responses to the licensed nursing staff.

Practicing Safety

Always be aware of safety issues when measuring a resident's height and weight, particularly if a resident is frail or has problems with fainting or dizziness. Pay attention to infection control by washing your hands before and after these procedures. Document each procedure accurately and in a timely fashion. Notify the licensed nursing staff if there are any irregularities with your measurements.

Healthcare Scenario
Bed Scales

A community hospital and health center recently purchased a new bed scale. Everyone is excited because the bed scale allows healthcare staff members to weigh bedridden residents easily. The bed scale has a digital display, has a mat attached to the mattress, and is powered by a simple electrical cord. The bed scale can be left on the bed beneath the resident, if desired.

Apply It

1. What is the most important step a nursing assistant should take when using a new piece of equipment?
2. List the safety concerns that should be addressed when using this equipment.
3. What actions should be taken to promote resident comfort while using this device?

Section 18.2 Review and Assessment

Using the Key Terms

Complete the following sentences using key terms in this section.

1. The healthiest weight for an individual is known as _____.
2. _____ is calculated by dividing weight in kilograms by height in meters squared.
3. An abnormal weight measurement can indicate _____, or lack of proper nourishment.

Know and Understand the Facts

4. Describe one purpose of measuring height.
5. Describe one purpose of measuring weight.
6. What steps can be taken to ensure safety when weighing a resident with a bed scale?
7. What steps should be taken to be sure a resident's weight is accurate?

Analyze and Apply Concepts

8. What equipment should you assemble to measure the height of an ambulatory resident?
9. How do you measure weight using an upright, balance scale?
10. Explain how to measure the height of a bedridden resident.

Think Critically

Read the following care situation. Then answer the questions that follow.

Jessica and Juana, two nursing assistants, have been asked to weigh Mr. G using a bed scale. Mr. G was just admitted, is in pain, and has never been weighed with a bed scale. He is very overweight and tells Jessica he is embarrassed about his recent weight gain. As Jessica and Juana start to position Mr. G, Mr. G starts to cry and moan and says he does not want to be weighed.

11. How could Jessica and Juana respond to Mr. G using holistic communication skills?
12. Which is the best action for Jessica and Juana to take? Should they weigh Mr. G no matter what he does or says? Should they come back later and weigh Mr. G when he calms down? Should they tell the charge nurse? Explain your choice.

Key Points

Reviewing the key points for this chapter will help you practice more safely and competently as a holistic nursing assistant and will help you prepare for the certification competency examination.

- Vital signs include temperature, pulse, respirations, and blood pressure. Vital signs provide information about health and the possible presence of a disease, infection, or injury.

- Body temperature is a person's body heat in degrees.

- Pulse measures the pressure of blood against the wall of an artery as the heart beats; it is an indicator of how well the cardiovascular system is working.

- Rate of respirations is a measurement of breathing. It indicates the quality of gas exchange and the cycle of inhalation followed by exhalation in the lungs.

- Blood pressure measures the force of blood against the body's arterial walls.

- Height and weight are used to determine medication dosage and nutritional status and can indicate overall health status.

Action Steps to Holistic Care

Review the information in this chapter. Complete the following activities.

1. With a partner, practice the procedure for measuring a radial pulse. Take turns practicing the procedure and evaluating each other's performance. Note any steps in the procedure that your partner performed incorrectly or forgot. Afterwards, review the procedure to reacquaint yourself with any steps you may have performed inaccurately or forgotten.

2. Prepare a short paper or digital presentation describing how nursing assistants can ensure safe, accurate measurements when taking blood pressures.

3. With a partner, write a song or a poem about counting respirations. Include the normal adult range, when it is done, and actions to take if the rate is high or low.

4. Research the importance of a pulse oximeter for taking vital signs. Write a brief report describing three current facts not discussed in the chapter.

Preparing for the Certification Competency Examination

To prepare for the nursing assistant certification competency examination, you will need to know content found in this chapter. This content may be tested in the knowledge (written or oral) and skills (hands-on demonstration) portions of the exam. The following areas will be emphasized:

- normal ranges of vital signs across the life span
- purpose of taking vital signs and the factors affecting these measurements
- ways of measuring and recording body temperature pulse (radial and apical), and respirations
- use of a pulse oximeter
- ways of measuring and recording blood pressure and any related precautions and contraindications
- ways of measuring and recording height and weight
- the importance of identifying and reporting abnormal findings

These sample test questions are similar to ones you will find on the certification competency exam. See how well you can answer them. Be sure to select the *best* answer.

1. A nursing assistant took Mrs. G's blood pressure this morning and found that it was 165/110 mmHg, much higher than yesterday's measurement. What should the nursing assistant do next?
   A. take the blood pressure again and record only the second measurement
   B. take the blood pressure again and share both measurements with the charge nurse
   C. record only the blood pressure taken
   D. take blood pressure later in the day

2. Where should the stethoscope be placed for taking an apical pulse?
   A. above the diaphragm and sternum
   B. at the apex (bottom right) of the heart
   C. below the diaphragm and sternum
   D. at the apex (bottom left) of the heart

3. What is the medical term for high blood pressure?
   A. hypertension   C. hypotension
   B. hypotachia   D. hypertachia

(continued)

4. When is the best time to count respirations?

   A. right before measuring temperature
   B. right after measuring blood pressure
   C. right after measuring pulse
   D. right before measuring pulse

5. Which of the following pulse rates is in the normal range for an adult?

   A. 52 bpm
   B. 70 bpm
   C. 125 bpm
   D. 105 bpm

6. According to Mr. L's chart, he has a temperature of 100.6°F. What does this mean?

   A. His body temperature is low, indicating hypothermia. He should have his temperature taken again in the next few hours.
   B. His body temperature is in the normal range. No further action is required.
   C. His body temperature is high, indicating fever. He should have his temperature taken again in the new few hours.
   D. His body temperature is high, indicating fever. He should have his temperature taken again tomorrow.

7. Ms. V just ate breakfast. How long should a nursing assistant wait before measuring her oral temperature?

   A. 1–3 minutes
   B. 5–10 minutes
   C. 10–15 minutes
   D. 15–20 minutes

8. What is the level of blood pressure called when the heart muscle relaxes?

   A. embolic blood pressure
   B. diastolic blood pressure
   C. systolic blood pressure
   D. sclerotic blood pressure

9. Oxygen saturation in the blood is measured using a

   A. pulse oximeter
   B. sphygmomanometer
   C. stethoscope
   D. probe

10. How should a resident stand on a balance scale while his height is being measured?

    A. on the center of the scale with his arms at his sides
    B. facing the nursing assistant
    C. on the center of the scale with his arms raised
    D. at the back of the scale looking forward

11. Mr. A's blood pressure is usually 128/88 mmHg. A nursing assistant just measured his blood pressure. Which of the following results might mean Mr. A. has stage 2 hypertension?

    A. 152/98 mmHg
    B. 136/82 mmHg
    C. 128/78 mmHg
    D. 130/80 mmHg

12. Where is tympanic temperature taken?

    A. the axilla
    B. the anus
    C. the ear
    D. the forehead

13. Mrs. D's weight must be measured today. She is ambulatory, so the nursing assistant can use a balance scale. He should do all of the following except

    A. ask the resident to stand straight with her arms above her head
    B. move the weights on the balance scale bar to zero
    C. move the lower and upper weights until the balance pointer is in the middle
    D. add the amounts shown on the two bars to determine weight

14. A nursing assistant is taking rectal temperature for a baby. What must the nursing assistant remember about thermometer placement?

    A. The thermometer should be inserted 1½ inches into the anus and held in place for three to five minutes.
    B. The thermometer should be inserted 1 inch or less into the anus and held in place for three to five minutes.
    C. The thermometer should be inserted 1 inch or less into the anus and held in place for two minutes.
    D. The thermometer should be inserted 2 inches into the anus and held in place for five minutes or longer.

15. Ms. S has not been feeling well this morning. She states that she feels short of breath. The nursing assistant takes her pulse and it is 98. What is the medical term for a fast heart rate?

    A. bradycardia
    B. apnea
    C. dyspnea
    D. tachycardia

Did you have difficulty with any of the questions? If you did, review the chapter to find the correct answer(s).

Welcome to the Chapter

Physical examinations (PEs) are an important part of care, and holistic nursing assistants are often responsible for preparing the patient, equipment, and supplies required for a physical examination. Physical examinations are conducted on an annual basis to check body system function and assess overall well-being. Examinations are also conducted on an as-needed basis to evaluate specific complaints or injuries. The comprehensive annual physical examination, the well-woman exam, the well-man exam, and the well-baby exam will be discussed.

Collecting specimens is another important responsibility of holistic nursing assistants. Specimens may be collected for diagnostic purposes or as part of a physical exam. The testing and analysis of specimens such as sputum, urine, and stool provide information for determining body system function, the presence of diseases and conditions, and monitoring well-being and the healing process.

The information and procedures presented in this chapter will help you build the knowledge and skills needed to become a holistic nursing assistant. Check with your instructor to ensure these procedures are within your state's regulations for nursing assistant practice. The topics discussed in the chapter are highlighted on the Providing Holistic Care Framework.

You are now ready to start this chapter, *Physical Examination and Specimen Collection*.

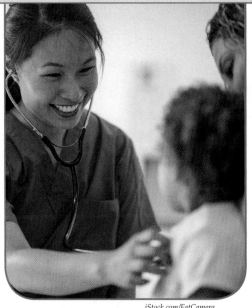
iStock.com/FatCamera

Chapter Outline

Section 19.1
Physical Examination

Section 19.2
Specimen Collection

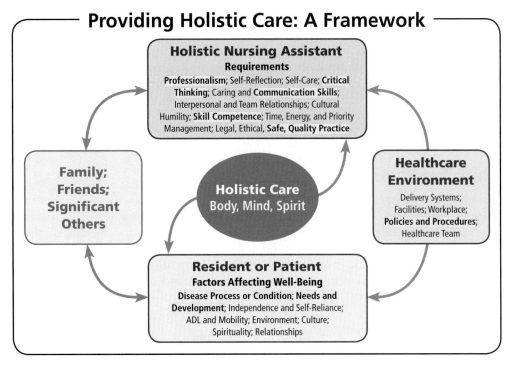

Providing Holistic Care: A Framework

Holistic Nursing Assistant
Requirements
Professionalism; Self-Reflection; Self-Care; **Critical Thinking**; Caring and **Communication Skills**; Interpersonal and Team Relationships; Cultural Humility; **Skill Competence**; Time, Energy, and Priority Management; Legal, Ethical, **Safe, Quality Practice**

Family; Friends; Significant Others

Holistic Care
Body, Mind, Spirit

Healthcare Environment
Delivery Systems; Facilities; Workplace; **Policies and Procedures**; Healthcare Team

Resident or Patient
Factors Affecting Well-Being
Disease Process or Condition; Needs and Development; Independence and Self-Reliance; ADL and Mobility; Environment; Culture; Spirituality; Relationships

Questions to Consider

- Think about the last time you had a physical examination. What was the reason for the examination?
- Do you wish you had known anything before, during, or after the examination?
- Were you nervous, worried, or uncomfortable about the examination? What would have made you feel more comfortable?

Objectives

Preparing the patient, equipment, and supplies for a physical examination is an important responsibility of holistic nursing assistants. Physical examinations are usually performed annually to check body systems, function, and the status of a person's well-being. Physical examinations may also be performed on a more frequent, specific schedule (such as for a well-baby exam) or on an as-needed basis to evaluate a specific complaint or injury. To achieve the objectives for this section, you must successfully

- **discuss** the purpose of conducting physical examinations;
- **describe** the different types and importance of physical examinations;
- **identify** needed equipment and the draping procedures used to prepare patients for physical examinations; and
- **explain** the procedure to prepare for physical examinations.

Key Terms

Learn these key terms to better understand the information presented in the section.

auscultation	otoscope
inspection	palpation
laryngeal mirror	percussion
ophthalmoscope	speculum

When and Where Are Physical Examinations Performed?

A *physical examination (PE)* is performed to determine the status or condition of a patient's body systems and functions. Depending on the patient, some examinations (such as well-woman and well-man exams) may be performed annually. Well-baby examinations may be scheduled more frequently to monitor an infant's growth and development. Additional examinations may be performed to evaluate a specific complaint or monitor a chronic disease.

Physical examinations usually take place in doctors' offices or clinics. When performed in a hospital or long-term care facility, a physical examination may occur in a patient's room or in an examining room. In such cases, nursing assistants may prepare the room and patient for a physical examination. Other healthcare staff members may be responsible for these tasks in a doctor's office.

Remember

If you love living, you try to take care of the equipment.

Sally Rand, American actress

How Are Physical Examinations Performed?

Prior to a physical examination, patients provide information related to their health history, current medications and supplements, past surgeries and hospitalizations, and relevant family medical history. This information may be documented by the patient or by the nursing assistant, who enters the information into the patient's electronic record. In some cases, patients must also provide information regarding their nutrition, exercise, sleep patterns, mental status or mood (for example, feelings of depression), and pain.

A physical examination is performed by a doctor, nurse practitioner, or physician assistant. These licensed healthcare providers review the patient's health history and information before beginning the examination.

Before the examination, vital signs are usually measured by a nursing assistant or medical assistant. Sometimes the healthcare provider will take vital signs. Other evaluations of body functions, called *health screening tests*, are also performed. These tests may include checking cholesterol levels, testing for osteoporosis, conducting Pap smears for female patients, and conducting prostate cancer screening for male patients. In a comprehensive exam, the healthcare provider examines each body system, starting at the patient's head and moving toward the feet. This is called a *head-to-toe examination*. If a head-to-toe examination is unnecessary, the healthcare provider may examine only a specific body system.

During a head-to-toe examination, the licensed healthcare provider may use the following methods to discover clues and information about the status of body structures and functions (Figure 19.1):

1. **Inspection**: the visual examination of a body part (for example, looking at the color of the skin or observing any bruising or discoloration)

2. **Palpation**: the use of the hands to feel an object (for example, feeling a lump or mass in the body to determine its location, size, shape, or hardness)

3. **Percussion**: the method of placing one hand on the surface of the patient's body and then striking or tapping a finger on that hand with the index finger or middle finger of the opposite hand to examine underlying body structures (for example, checking for fluid in the lungs or abdominal cavity)

4. **Auscultation**: the method of listening to the internal sounds of the body (for example, using a stethoscope to listen to lung sounds and the heartbeat)

What Types of Physical Examinations Are Performed?

There are several types of physical examinations:

- comprehensive annual physical examinations, which usually include routine health screenings
- preemployment physical examinations
- travel physical examinations, which may include specific immunizations
- well-woman, well-man, and well-baby exams
- physical examinations needed to perform special diagnostic procedures or to examine specific body parts or functions

A physical examination may also be performed to screen for a disease, to evaluate a medical problem such as a respiratory issue or an injury, to update vaccinations, or to provide coaching for a healthier lifestyle.

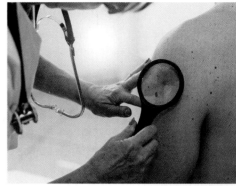

thodonal88/Shutterstock.com

A

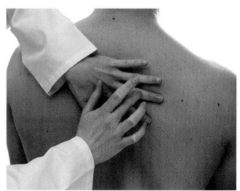

JPC-PROD/Shutterstock.com

B

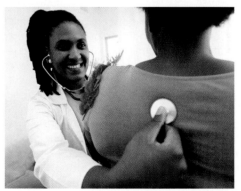

Ocskay Bence/Shutterstock.com

C

iStock.com/Henk Badenhorst

D

Figure 19.1 Doctors use inspection (A), palpation (B), percussion (C), and auscultation (D) to examine body structures and functions.

Annual Adult Physical Exams

Think About This

According to a recent analysis, annual physical examinations last an average of 23 minutes. How time is spent during the examination depends on the doctor or other licensed healthcare provider. Physical examinations can vary in price from free to several hundred dollars, depending on the patient's insurance coverage.

An *annual physical examination* is an opportunity to evaluate body system function and any diseases or conditions. This exam may reveal a previously undiagnosed disease or condition, even if the patient has not experienced any noticeable signs or symptoms. Early diagnosis of a disease or condition, such as type 2 diabetes or cancer, may lead to a better prognosis, particularly if treatment begins without delay. The following tests or procedures may be performed during an annual physical examination:

- assessment of vital signs
- routine laboratory tests, such as a complete blood count (CBC), urinalysis, and chest X-ray
- electrocardiogram (ECG or EKG)
- blood cholesterol tests
- screening tests to identify diseases such as diabetes and colon or lung cancer
- tests to monitor cardiovascular health, the bone mineral density of female patients (DEXA scan), vision, hearing, and skin health

Vaccines are also offered during the annual physical exam. As you learned in chapter 14, vaccines are administered according to specific immunization guidelines and schedules. A patient may receive an annual flu shot and pneumococcal vaccine. A shingles, or herpes zoster, vaccine may be administered if the patient is at high risk or is over 60 years of age.

Well-Woman Exams

In addition to an annual physical exam, women should also have a yearly *well-woman examination.* A gynecologist, primary care provider, or other appropriate licensed healthcare provider may perform the well-woman exam as a separate exam or during an annual comprehensive physical examination. The well-woman examination includes a pelvic examination, Pap smear, and clinical breast exam. After a woman reaches 50 years of age, a mammography is also included as part of this exam. Additional tests for sexually transmitted infections (STIs) may be performed, and healthcare providers and their patients will often discuss lifestyle behaviors.

Culture Cues
Reasons People Avoid Physical Examinations

Annual physical examinations are part of US healthcare culture. Still, many people choose not to have annual examinations. People may make this choice due to financial reasons, values, culture, history, or even body image. Some people believe the body will heal itself, making physical examinations unnecessary. Others see visiting the doctor as a sign of weakness and avoid physical examinations unless they are very ill. Some patients experience a condition known as *white coat syndrome*, in which blood pressure rises above the normal range in a doctor's office, but not in other settings. Fear of receiving negative test results, discussing or showing certain body parts, or sharing intimate details may keep these and other people from scheduling an examination. Some people who may not have good health habits do not want a "lecture" about their health practices. Still other people simply do not want to see a doctor. Adult men, in particular, see the doctor less often than women do. Men often see themselves as strong and may not be as concerned about their health. They may believe they are not vulnerable to health risks.

Apply It

1. Have you ever encountered someone who did not want to go to the doctor? If so, what was the person's reason?

2. What are some possible consequences of avoiding physical examinations?

3. What approaches or strategies can encourage people to schedule a physical examination?

Pelvic Examination

An annual *pelvic examination* is recommended for women 21 years of age and older. It includes an inspection of the external genitalia, the use of a medical instrument called a **speculum** to examine the vagina and cervix, and the manual palpation of the uterus and ovaries (using two gloved and lubricated fingers) to be sure they feel normal. Women over 40 years of age usually have a *rectovaginal examination*, which identifies signs of possible tumors behind the uterus, on the walls of the vagina, or in the rectum. This examination can also provide information about the tone and alignment of the pelvic organs.

A *Pap smear* is performed as part of the pelvic exam and determines if there are any abnormal cells that may lead to cancer in the cervix. During a Pap smear, cells are scraped from the outer and inner lining of the cervix for testing. Between the ages of 30 and 64, women need a Pap smear every three years or a combination of a Pap smear and HPV screening every five years. (You learned about HPV in chapter 9.) Women who have had total hysterectomies not due to cervical cancer or who are past the age of 65 do not require Pap smears.

Clinical Breast Exam

Clinical breast exams are recommended for all women over age 40. They are recommended even earlier for women who have a family history of or risk factors for breast cancer or breast diseases such as fibrocystic breast disease. Some licensed healthcare providers prefer to perform a clinical breast exam as part of the annual well-woman exam, regardless of a patient's age. Women younger than 40 years of age should observe their breasts for any changes and perform monthly *breast self-examinations (BSEs)* several days after menstruation.

A clinical breast exam begins with external inspection of the breasts. The patient raises her arms above her head, and the breasts are observed for any dimpling, inversion of the nipples (the nipples turning in, not out), soreness, redness, rash, or swelling. The healthcare provider then palpates the breasts with the pads of three middle fingers for evidence of lumps or thickening. The healthcare provider palpates from the bottom of the breast to the collarbone and under each armpit (Figure 19.2). The patient then lies down, and the same exam is performed again. The nipples are also squeezed for any discharge.

Mammography

Mammography is the process of X-raying the breasts for cancer (Figure 19.3). Annual mammography exams, called *mammograms*, are recommended for women beginning at age 40 until age 75. A woman with risk factors for breast cancer may require more frequent mammograms.

There are two types of mammograms: screening mammograms and diagnostic mammograms. *Screening mammograms* are appropriate for women who have no signs or symptoms of breast disease or cancer. A screening mammogram usually consists of two or more X-rays of each breast. The X-rays may reveal tiny nodules that sometimes indicate the presence of breast cancer. *Diagnostic mammograms* check for cancer after a lump or other sign of cancer has been found during the screening mammogram. This procedure takes longer because more X-rays are needed.

In the United States, *digital mammography* allows electronic images of the breasts to be stored in the patient's EHR. Digital mammography is advantageous because the electronic images can be enhanced,

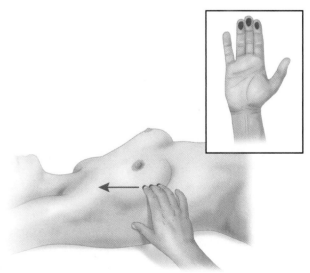

© *Body Scientific International*

Figure 19.2 In a clinical breast exam, the healthcare provider palpates the breast using three fingers. The healthcare provider starts at the bottom of the breast and moves toward the collarbone.

magnified, or manipulated. *Three-dimensional (3-D) mammography*, also called *digital breast tomosynthesis (DBT)*, is a new type of digital mammography that creates images of thin slices of the breast from different angles. When these images are compiled, they create a detailed image of the breast as a whole.

Laboratory Tests

During a well-woman exam, laboratory tests are usually conducted to detect infections or viruses and STIs. Women younger than 25 years of age are usually screened for chlamydia and gonorrhea. After age 25, women receive this screening if they are at high risk or may have been exposed to an STI.

Well-Man Exams

In addition to an annual comprehensive physical examination, men also receive a *well-man examination*. A primary care provider, urologist, or other appropriate licensed healthcare provider may perform the well-man exam during the annual comprehensive physical examination or as a separate exam. The well-man exam includes a prostate cancer screening; testicular, penis, and hernia exams; discussions about lifestyle behaviors; and testing for STIs.

Prostate Cancer Screening

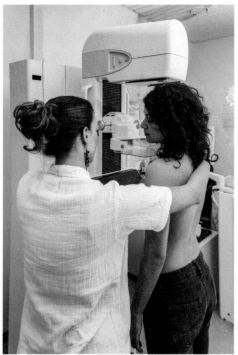

iStock.com/choja

Figure 19.3 A mammography machine takes X-rays of the breasts to screen for breast cancer.

The *prostate-specific antigen (PSA) serologic assay* is the most common test used to diagnose prostate cancer. The test is usually combined with a *digital rectal examination*, in which the healthcare provider gently inserts a lubricated, gloved finger into the rectum to feel the size of the prostate and identify any questionable areas. These tests are not routinely performed for men under 50 years of age unless there are symptoms of prostate disease or cancer. Men who are 50 years of age or older (African-Americans in particular) are at higher risk for prostate disease or cancer and should have this screening performed annually.

Testicular, Penis, and Inguinal Hernia Exams

During this exam, the penis is inspected for any sores, rashes, swelling, or ulcers. The testicles are palpated for lumps, changes in size, tenderness, pain, and the presence of an *inguinal hernia* (when part of the intestine sticks out through a weak spot in the abdominal wall). The presence of an inguinal hernia is determined by palpation.

Laboratory Tests

Laboratory tests are usually performed to check for viruses and STIs. Men who are sexually active may be tested for chlamydia, gonorrhea, HPV, genital herpes, or HIV/AIDS.

Well-Baby Exams

Well-baby exams begin one month after birth when the mother and infant visit the pediatrician, primary care provider, or other appropriate licensed healthcare provider for the exam. Regular exams are scheduled at various milestones throughout the first year of the baby's life (Figure 19.4).

A baby's weight is an integral part of the exam and one of the most important measurements. Weight is an indicator of adequate nutrition and growth and is used to calculate medication dosages, if needed. As a holistic nursing assistant, you may be asked to weigh a baby. The following are important guidelines for weighing a baby:

1. Practice hand hygiene and provide privacy for the baby and mother.
2. Check the baby's identity.
3. Use a baby scale and place a paper cover on the scale (Figure 19.5).

Well-Baby Exam Milestones	
Milestone	**Examination**
One month	• The baby is weighed and measured. • A physical exam checks the head, heart, lungs, eyes, ears, mouth, body, abdomen (umbilical stump), genitals, and movement of limbs. • Immunizations are given.
Two months	• The baby is weighed and measured. • A physical exam is performed. • The shape of the head, reflexes, and muscle tone are checked. • Immunizations are given.
Four months	• The baby is weighed and measured. • A physical exam is performed. • Head control and emerging teeth are checked. • Immunizations are given.
Six months	• The baby is weighed and measured. • A physical exam is performed. • Response to sound and muscle control when sitting up are checked. • Immunizations are given.
Nine months	• The baby is weighed and measured. • A physical exam is performed. • Response to sound, new teeth, and shape of head are checked. • Any needed immunizations are given.
One year	• The baby is weighed and measured. • A physical exam is performed. • Language ability is checked. The baby should be able to speak several words, such as *mama* and *dada*. • The ability to walk and feed self with hands is checked. • Any needed immunizations are given.

Figure 19.4 Well-baby exams begin at one month and continue until the end of the first year.

4. Adjust the scale to zero.
5. Undress the baby, remove the diaper, and clean the baby, if needed.
6. Place the baby on the center of the scale.
7. Keep one hand on the baby to prevent the baby from falling.
8. Move the weight bar to the correct weight until the scale balances.
9. When done, place the baby on a safe surface, diaper, and dress.
10. Ensure the baby is given to the mother or placed in a safe location.
11. Remove and discard the paper cover and clean and store the scale.
12. Report weight and any other observations about the baby.

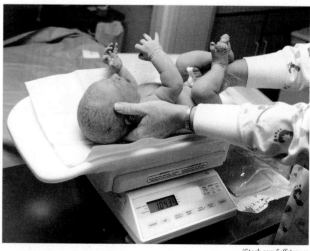

iStock.com/jeffstrauss

Figure 19.5 Before placing a baby on the scale, always place a paper cover beneath the baby.

How Do Nursing Assistants Prepare a Patient for an Examination?

In advance of a physical examination, nursing assistants are responsible for preparing the exam room and gathering the needed equipment. Exam rooms can be found in a doctor's office, hospital, or long-term care facility. A physical exam can also be performed in the patient's or resident's room. Depending on the type of examination, various equipment and screening tools may be needed:

- thermometer
- sphygmomanometer to measure blood pressure
- stethoscope to measure blood pressure, heart and lung sounds, and pulse
- tongue depressor to examine the throat
- **otoscope** to examine the ears (Figure 19.6A)
- **ophthalmoscope** to examine the eyes (Figure 19.6B)
- flashlight to examine pupils for dilation
- eye chart for vision screening
- **laryngeal mirror** to examine the mouth, tongue, and teeth (Figure 19.6C)
- tuning fork to test hearing (Figure 19.6D)
- percussion or reflex hammer to tap body parts to test reflexes (Figure 19.6E)
- vaginal speculum to examine the vagina and other parts of the female reproductive system (Figure 19.6F)
- nasal speculum
- sheets or drapes to cover the patient
- disposable covering for the examination table
- containers for soiled instruments, gloves, tissues, and disposable covering and drapes
- disposable gloves
- lubricant
- alcohol wipes
- cotton-tipped applicators
- specimen containers and labels
- tissues
- paper towels

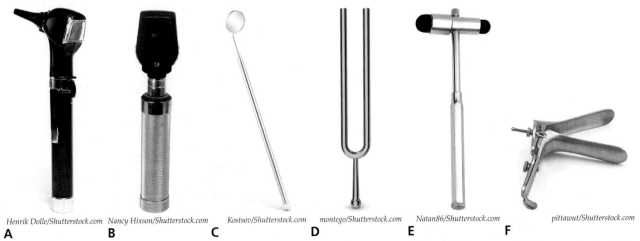

Henrik Dolle/Shutterstock.com *Nancy Hixson/Shutterstock.com* *Kostsov/Shutterstock.com* *montego/Shutterstock.com* *Natan86/Shutterstock.com* *pittawut/Shutterstock.com*

A   **B**   **C**   **D**   **E**   **F**

Figure 19.6 For a physical examination, a healthcare provider may need an otoscope (A), ophthalmoscope (B), laryngeal mirror (C), tuning fork (D), reflex hammer (E), and vaginal speculum (F).

Many different positions and draping are used to prepare for physical examinations. You learned about some of these positions in chapter 17. The type of examination determines the positions and draping used. In some examinations, the patient stands on the floor or sits on the examining table. Draping is important to prevent unnecessary exposure of the patient's body, to keep the patient comfortable, and to prevent chilling. The positions discussed in the sections that follow may be used.

Dorsal Recumbent Position

Dorsal recumbent position is used to examine the vagina or rectum. The patient lies flat on his or her back with the knees bent and feet flat on the table (Figure 19.7). A drape is placed in a diamond shape that covers the chest and perineal area (between the anus and scrotum on males and between the anus and vaginal opening on females).

Lithotomy Position

Lithotomy position is used to examine the vagina. The patient lies on her back, and her hips and buttocks are brought to the corners of the table (Figure 19.8). Her legs are bent, and her feet are placed in padded stirrups. A drape is placed in a diamond shape that covers the body, but not the head.

Fowler's Position

Fowler's position is often used to examine the legs and feet. The patient is seated on the table with the backrest at a 45° angle (Figure 19.9). The legs are extended flat on the table. A drape should cover the legs.

Knee-Chest Position

Knee-chest position is used to examine the rectum. The patient kneels on the table with buttocks raised (Figure 19.10). The head remains on the table, the arms are extended above the head, and the elbows are bent. The head is turned to one side. A pillow under the head may provide comfort. A drape covers the back and legs.

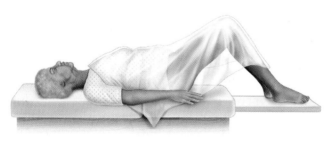

© Body Scientific International

Figure 19.7 In dorsal recumbent position, the drape should cover the chest and perineal area.

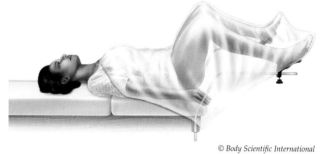

© Body Scientific International

Figure 19.8 In lithotomy position, the drape should cover the body, but not the head.

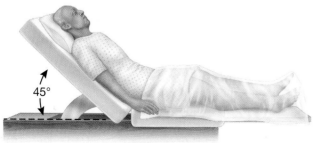

© Body Scientific International

Figure 19.9 In Fowler's position, the drape should cover the legs.

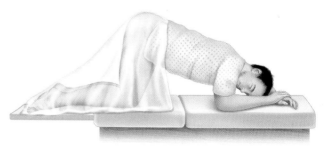

© Body Scientific International

Figure 19.10 In knee-chest position, the drape should cover the back and legs.

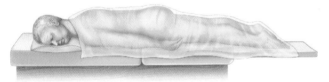

© Body Scientific International

Figure 19.11 In prone position, the drape should cover the shoulders and legs.

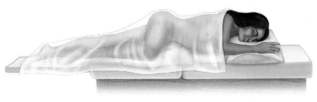

© Body Scientific International

Figure 19.12 In Sims' position, the drape should extend from the shoulders to the toes.

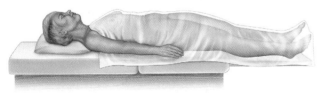

© Body Scientific International

Figure 19.13 In supine position, the drape should extend under the armpits to the toes.

Prone Position

Prone position is used to examine the spine and legs. The patient lies on his or her abdomen with arms and hands to each side (Figure 19.11). The head is turned to one side. A drape extends from the shoulders to the legs and may cover the feet.

Sims' Position

Sims' position is usually used to examine the rectum and sometimes the vagina. It is a left side-lying position (Figure 19.12). The patient's left arm is bent and behind the back, while the right arm can be positioned comfortably resting on the table or pillow. The upper knee is bent, raised toward the chest, and supported by a pillow. A pillow under the bottom of the foot should make sure the toes do not touch the table. A drape extends from the shoulders to the toes.

Supine Position

Supine position is used to examine the front of the body and breasts. The patient lies flat on his or her back with the arms at each side (Figure 19.13). A drape extends from under the armpits to the toes.

When a physical examination is complete, a doctor, nurse practitioner, or physician assistant reviews the results. Recommendations are given for treatments and follow-up visits.

Rationale

Appropriate positioning and draping provides comfort and promotes a safe and accurate physical examination. Proper draping also provides privacy by limiting exposure to only the body part, or parts, being examined.

Preparation

1. Ask the licensed nursing staff how this procedure fits into the plan of care, if there are doctor's orders for the procedure, if there are any special instructions or precautions, and if the patient can be moved into the positions required for this procedure.

2. Wash your hands or use hand sanitizer before entering the room.

3. Bring the necessary paperwork or chart. If electronic health records are used, prepare the appropriate screen using a digital device.

4. Cover the examining table with a disposable sheet.

5. Prepare the equipment and instruments needed for the specific exam. Lay out the equipment and instruments for easy access during the examination. Make sure you understand any specific approaches the healthcare provider likes to use during the examination (for example, the location of certain equipment). Ensure there are adequate supplies in the room.

6. Prepare the drapes necessary for the exam.

7. Approach the patient and introduce yourself using your full name and title. Explain that you work with the licensed nursing staff and will be providing care.

8. Bring the patient into the examining room. If in an office or clinical facility, bring the patient in from a waiting room. The examination may also take place in the patient's room (especially if in a long-term care facility).

9. Encourage the patient to use the bathroom before the examination.

10. Measure the patient's height and weight if the scale is outside the examining room.

The Procedure

11. Provide privacy by closing the curtains, using a screen, or closing the door to the room.

12. Have the patient remove only the clothes required by the examination.

13. Ask the patient to put on a gown. Explain whether the gown should be tied in the front or the back of the body and where clothes may be stored, if necessary. Assist, if needed. If the patient does not need assistance, step out of the room until the patient has indicated he is ready.

14. Be sure there is adequate lighting. Some exams require additional lighting, particularly if performed in a patient's room.

15. Measure the patient's vital signs, as instructed. Measure the patient's height and weight if the scales are in the examining room.

16. Record the vital signs, height, and weight on a pad, on a form, or in the electronic record.

17. Help the patient onto the examining table, if appropriate.

18. If a special position is needed for the examination, prepare the patient for the necessary position and explain why it is required.

19. Make sure the patient is safe and comfortable. Do not leave the patient alone in the room once he is positioned.

20. Drape the patient for the examination. Ensure warmth and show respect for privacy.

> **Best Practice**
> The equipment used to examine an infant or child may be the same as the equipment used for an adult patient, only smaller. Always be sure the infant or child is positioned safely. You may need to have the parent help if the child will not cooperate.

Follow-Up

21. Provide assistance during the examination, as requested. Wear disposable gloves as required for infection prevention and control.

22. After an examination of the vagina or rectum, provide the patient with tissues to clean off the lubricant used during the examination.

23. Assist with dressing, if appropriate. Ensure the patient's safety and comfort.

> **Best Practice**
> Respond to any questions the patient may have to the best of your ability. If you cannot answer a question, refer the question to the appropriate healthcare provider.

(continued)

Preparing for an Examination (*continued*)

24. Remove, clean, and store equipment in the proper location. Remove soiled linens and discard disposable equipment. Send a speculum or other equipment to the supply area for sterilization.

25. Wash your hands or use hand sanitizer before leaving the room.

Reporting and Documentation

26. Communicate any specific observations, complications, or unusual responses to the licensed nursing staff.

Section 19.1 Review and Assessment

Using the Key Terms

Complete the following sentences using key terms in this section.

1. The visual examination of a body part is _____.
2. A(n) _____ is a medical instrument used to examine the ears.
3. Using the hands to feel for a lump or mass in the body is an example of _____.
4. During a well-woman exam, a medical instrument called a(n) _____ is used to examine the vagina.
5. _____ is the act of listening to the internal sounds of the body with a stethoscope.
6. When examining the eyes, doctors use a medical instrument called a(n) _____.
7. The _____ is a medical instrument used to examine the mouth, teeth, and tongue.
8. _____ is the act of placing one hand on the surface of the body and striking or tapping a finger on that hand with the index finger of the other hand.

Know and Understand the Facts

9. Describe one purpose of conducting an annual physical examination.
10. Identify two types of examinations.
11. List three screenings or tests that are part of a well-woman exam.
12. Identify two pieces of equipment typically used for physical examinations.

Analyze and Apply Concepts

13. Explain how to drape a patient for the knee-chest and lithotomy positions.
14. What are three measurements a healthcare provider may take in a well-baby exam?
15. Discuss four responsibilities a nursing assistant may have when preparing a patient for a physical examination.

Think Critically

Read the following care situation. Then answer the questions that follow.

Ms. I is a frail, 75-year-old resident at the long-term care facility where you work. This morning, she was crying and complaining about trouble breathing and itching on her abdomen and under her breasts. When you give Ms. I care, you notice a rash in those areas. When Ms. I urinates, her urine is cloudy and slightly brown. Ms. I's doctor is coming to see her this morning. When he arrives, he decides to conduct a physical examination in the exam room down the hall.

16. What is the first thing you should do to prepare for the physical examination?
17. What exam equipment do you think the doctor will need?
18. How should you position and drape Ms. I?
19. What safety measures will be most important for the physical examination?

Objectives

Collecting specimens is an important responsibility for holistic nursing assistants. The testing and analysis of specimens such as sputum, urine, and stool offer information about whether body systems are functioning properly. Test results can also be used by a doctor or other healthcare provider to determine if a resident's condition is improving. Testing and analysis are usually performed in a clinical laboratory, either in a facility or at another location by specially trained staff. To achieve the objectives for this section, you must successfully

- **explain** the purpose and importance of collecting specimens;
- **identify** the types of specimens and the tests used for analysis;
- **discuss** why accurate specimen collection is essential; and
- **demonstrate** the procedures for collecting sputum, urine, and stool specimens.

Key Terms

Learn these key terms to better understand the information presented in the section.

glucometer

guaiac test

occult blood

point-of-care testing (POCT)

specimens

sputum

Questions to Consider

- Have you ever had to provide a specimen as part of a physical examination, procedure, or to prepare for surgery? For example, have you been asked to give a doctor or nurse a small quantity of urine for analysis?
- When providing a specimen, did you understand how to ensure the specimen was taken properly and did not become contaminated? Were the instructions clear? If they were not, what might the doctor or nurse have said or done differently?

What Is the Purpose and Importance of Collecting Specimens?

Specimens are samples of a bodily substance. They are collected so that specific tests can be done to provide information about a resident's health. Commonly collected specimens include **sputum** (a blend of saliva and mucus that is also called *phlegm*), urine, and stool. Specimens are tested and analyzed for several important reasons:

- Specimen analysis is an essential health screening tool utilized during a comprehensive physical examination.
- Specimens can be tested to determine the presence of a specific pathogen. For example, if a urinary tract infection (UTI) is suspected, a urine specimen can help with diagnosis.
- Testing specimens can help identify the type of treatment needed (for example, the antibiotic to destroy a pathogen found).
- The results of specimen testing provide critical information prior to a procedure or surgery, particularly if results are outside the normal range.

Specimen collection can occur in the place where a resident is receiving care. This is called **point-of-care testing (POCT)**. For example, a nursing assistant may use a medical instrument called a **glucometer** to measure blood sugar in a resident's room. Other specimens may need to go to a clinical laboratory.

Specimens are sent to a laboratory in special, labeled containers with laboratory *requisition forms* (or *laboratory slips*) that contain specific information about the resident and the test requested. A licensed nursing staff member or the laboratory completes the requisition form. The form contains the resident's full name, sex, and date of birth; the type of test requested; an identifier (such as a resident ID or Social Security number); and other information needed by the facility and laboratory.

When results are returned from the laboratory, they will be reported within certain ranges. Results are usually communicated as *positive* (indicating the presence of an infection or disease) or *negative* (indicating that results are within normal range). The use of these terms can be confusing for residents. Some residents may think that *negative* results are "bad," when negative results actually indicate a good outcome. If a resident is confused, inform a licensed nursing staff member so he or she can follow up with the resident. It is *not* within a nursing assistant's scope of practice to explain test results to a resident.

Valid test results depend on accurate specimen collection. Because important decisions are made based on test results, the results must be accurate. Valid results also depend on the proper and accurate labeling and handling of specimens. Information must be printed on specimen container labels. Hand hygiene must be used effectively to avoid introducing pathogens, procedures for specimen collection must be performed accurately and according to facility policy, and specimens must be properly labeled and handled effectively.

How Are Common Specimens Best Collected?

Three main specimens are used for testing and analysis: sputum, urine, and stool (*feces*). There is a standard method and purpose for collecting each specimen (Figure 19.14).

Sputum Specimens

As a nursing assistant, you will likely care for residents with respiratory infections or diseases such as bronchitis, COPD, pneumonia, and tuberculosis. A *sputum specimen* is collected to detect an infection or determine if a known infection is improving or gone. A nursing assistant or respiratory therapist may collect a sputum specimen. Sputum is collected when a resident coughs. The sputum specimen is sent to a laboratory and placed in a dish or plate containing special material (called a *culture media*). The specimen is allowed to grow on the culture media. If the specimen does not grow, the results are negative, and there is no infection. If the specimen does grow, the results are positive, and further analysis identifies the pathogen.

Specimen Collection			
Specimen Type	**Collection Method**	**Tests**	**Purpose**
Sputum	Coughing	Routine sputum culture	To detect an infection and identify any pathogens (bacteria, viruses, or fungi)
Urine	Urination; removal from urinary catheter	Dipstick; urine straining; routine urinalysis; midstream clean catch for urine culture; 24-hour urine specimen collection	To diagnose diseases, monitor disease status or body system function, and detect the presence of medications and drugs
Stool	Feces; colostomy or ileostomy bag	Fecal occult blood test; stool culture; stool DNA test with immunochemical test	To detect blood in the stool, detect the presence of an infection, and screen for and diagnose diseases (such as colorectal cancer)

Figure 19.14 The three common specimens that are collected and tested are sputum, urine, and stool.

Rationale

Sputum specimens are typically collected when a resident has a respiratory disease or condition. Sputum is expelled from the lungs or bronchial tubes by coughing.

Preparation

1. Ask the licensed nursing staff how this procedure fits into the plan of care, if there are doctor's orders for the procedure, if there are any special instructions or precautions, and if the resident can be moved into the positions required for this procedure.

2. Wash your hands or use hand sanitizer before entering the room.

3. Knock before entering the room.

4. Introduce yourself using your full name and title. Explain that you work with the licensed nursing staff and will be providing care.

5. Greet the resident and ask the resident to state her full name, if able. Then check the resident's identification bracelet.

6. Use Mr., Mrs., or Ms. and the last name when conversing.

7. Explain the procedure in simple terms, even if the resident is not able to communicate or is disoriented. Ask permission to perform the procedure.

8. Bring the necessary equipment into the room. Place the following items in an accessible location:

   - sputum specimen container and lid (Figure 19.15)

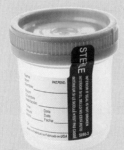

Figure 19.15

   - label
   - disposable gloves
   - cup of water
   - emesis basin
   - paper towel

- tissues
- completed laboratory requisition form
- specimen transport bag with a biohazard label, if needed (Figure 19.16)

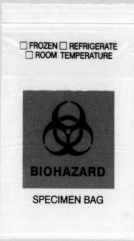

Figure 19.16

9. Ask the licensed nursing staff if PPE should be worn during the procedure. If you need a face mask or other PPE, don these items according to the procedures in chapter 15. If the resident is in isolation, put on PPE before entering the room. Otherwise, put on PPE in the resident's room.

10. Complete the label by printing the resident's name and room number, the time and date of the specimen collection, and the doctor's name. Place the label on the specimen container (Figure 19.17). Some labels may request additional information, such as birth date or other identifiers. Be sure the name on the label matches the resident's identification.

> Helen Johns
> Room 117
> 0630, 8/15/2017
> Dr. Lynton

Figure 19.17

Best Practice

It is best to collect sputum specimens in the early morning, before the resident has had anything to eat or drink.

(continued)

The Procedure

11. Provide privacy by closing the curtains, using a screen, or closing the door to the room.

12. Lock the bed wheels and then raise the bed to hip level.

13. Ensure safety during the procedure. If there are side rails, raise and secure the rails on the opposite side of the bed from where you will be working. Lower the rail on the side you are working.

14. Wash your hands or use hand sanitizer to ensure infection control.

15. Put on disposable gloves and any other PPE, as required by the licensed nursing staff.

16. Position the resident in Fowler's position or have the resident sit on the side of the bed. These positions make it easier for the resident to cough.

17. Ask the resident to rinse her mouth with water and spit into the emesis basin.

Best Practice

A steam-like mist may be used to loosen sputum prior to collection. A resident who is well hydrated prior to the collection may find it easier to cough because the fluids will help thin out the sputum.

---

18. Give the resident the sputum specimen container. Instruct her not to touch the inside of the container or lid. Place the lid on top of a paper towel on the overbed table.

19. Have the resident take three deep breaths with her mouth open and then cough deeply to bring up sputum. Ask the resident to shield her mouth with a tissue, using her other hand, while coughing. Collect 1–2 tablespoons of sputum, unless otherwise instructed.

20. Put the lid on the sputum specimen container immediately.

21. Remove and discard your gloves.

22. Wash your hands or use hand sanitizer to ensure infection control.

23. Put on a new pair of disposable gloves.

24. Double-check that the specimen identified on the label matches the specimen collected.

25. Attach the requisition form to ensure the specimen container is complete and ready for transport to the laboratory. Make sure the lid is tightly placed on the container.

26. Place the sputum specimen container in a specimen transport bag. Use a biohazard bag or label, if needed. Do not let the specimen container touch the outside of the bag

27. Check to be sure the bed wheels are locked, then reposition the resident and lower the bed.

28. Follow the plan of care to determine if the side rails should be raised or lowered.

29. Offer the resident a glass of water and an emesis basin to cleanse the mouth. An ambulatory resident can do this in the bathroom.

30. Remove, clean, and store equipment in the proper location. Remove soiled linens and discard disposable equipment.

Follow-Up

31. Remove and discard your gloves.

32. Wash your hands to ensure infection control.

33. Make sure the resident is comfortable and place the call light and personal items within reach.

34. Conduct a safety check before leaving the room. The room should be clean and free from clutter or spills.

35. Wash your hands or use hand sanitizer before leaving the room.

36. Send or take the labeled sputum specimen container to the laboratory or another assigned location with the requisition form. Sputum must be tested before it begins to dry.

Reporting and Documentation

37. Communicate any specific observations, complications, or unusual responses to the licensed nursing staff. Record this information, along with the procedure, in the chart or EMR.

Figure 19.15 © Tori Soper Photography; Figure 19.16 iStock.com/lpkoe

Urine Specimens

After blood, urine is the second-most collected specimen. Urine specimens are tested in three ways:

1. observation of clarity, color, and odor
2. dipstick examination
3. microscopic examination in a laboratory

Urine Clarity, Color, and Odor

As a nursing assistant, you may be asked to observe a resident's urine for clarity, color, and odor. Healthy urine is usually transparent, amber in color, and odorless. The more hydrated a resident is, the clearer urine will be. Conversely, if a resident is dehydrated, urine will be concentrated and orange in color.

Most changes in urine color are temporary and caused by food colors or medications. An abnormal urine color may, however, indicate the presence of a disease or condition. For example, red urine usually indicates the presence of blood in the urine (called *hematuria*). Cloudy urine with pus or mucus might signal a UTI. A foul odor, such as a fishy smell, may be a sign of a bladder infection. Observing urine can also detect the presence of sugar (*glycosuria*), ketones, or protein.

Dipsticks

Nursing assistants may also be asked to test a urine specimen using a *dipstick reagent*, or *test strip* (Figure 19.18). This is considered a point-of-care test (POCT). The dipstick is a thin, plastic strip saturated in chemicals that detect indicators of a disease or condition. The chemical strip reacts to the presence of particular substances by changing color. This test typically reveals if urine is concentrated or acidic or has abnormal amounts of protein, ketones, bilirubin, sugar, and white or red blood cells (evidence of blood). When using a dipstick, follow the instructions on the dipstick package and report the results to the licensed nursing staff.

Microscopic Examination of Urine

Urine specimens may be tested microscopically. In this examination, specimens or cultures are viewed through a microscope to identify substances in the urine. For these tests, a sufficient amount of urine must be collected. The urine specimen container should be 1/3 to 1/2 full. After the specimen is collected, the container should be placed in a location determined by facility policy. These specimens are usually picked up by the clinical laboratory staff.

Types of Urine Specimens

There are three types of urine specimens that nursing assistants may need to collect:

- **Routine specimens**: are used to identify any abnormalities in different components of the urine. Once a specimen is collected, routine urinalysis detects chemicals and medications in the urine, identifies the presence of infection, and can help diagnose diseases (such as diabetes). Routine urinalysis is usually performed as part of a physical examination, on admission to a hospital, or prior to surgery.

- **Midstream specimens**: are also called *clean-catch specimens* and are free from pathogens. Before collection, the perineal area is cleansed with disposable wipes or washcloths with soap and water (Figure 19.19). Then, the specimen is collected midway through urination after a short stream of urine has exited the urethra. This keeps microorganisms from the skin of the vagina or penis from contaminating the specimen. The last stream of urine is not collected. The collection container is considered sterile. Midstream specimens are used to identify an infection as well as such conditions as kidney stones.

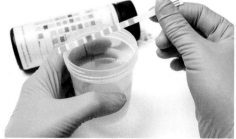

iStock.com/AlexRaths

Figure 19.18 A dipstick reagent contains chemicals that change color depending on the presence of particular substances in the urine.

- **Twenty-four-hour specimens**: are usually used to check kidney function. All urine expelled over a full 24-hour period is collected. The urine is stored in a container kept in ice (Figure 19.20).

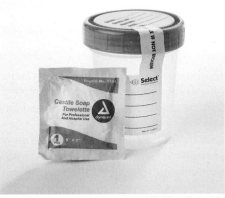

© Tori Soper Photography

Figure 19.19 A urine collection kit consists of a specimen container and wipe.

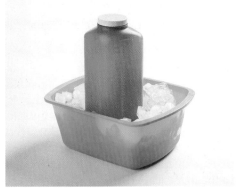

© Tori Soper Photography

Figure 19.20 A 24-hour collection container should be placed in ice.

Procedure | Collecting Urine Specimens

Rationale

Urine specimens help detect functional abnormalities in the urinary system, diseases, or infections. They can also identify the presence of chemicals and medications in the body. Proper collection of urine specimens is necessary to get accurate results. Various methods, including routine collection, midstream collection, and 24-hour collection, are used.

Preparation

1. Ask the licensed nursing staff how this procedure fits into the plan of care, if there are doctor's orders for the procedure, if there are any special instructions or precautions, and if the resident can be moved into the positions required for this procedure.

2. Wash your hands or use hand sanitizer before entering the room.

3. Knock before entering the room.

4. Introduce yourself using your full name and title. Explain that you work with the licensed nursing staff and will be providing care.

5. Greet the resident and ask the resident to state his full name, if able. Then check the resident's identification bracelet.

6. Use Mr., Mrs., or Ms. and the last name when conversing.

7. Explain the procedure in simple terms, even if the resident is not able to communicate or is disoriented. Ask permission to perform the procedure.

The Procedure: Routine Urine Specimen

8. Bring the necessary equipment into the room. Place the following items in an accessible location:
   - urinary hat (Figure 19.21)

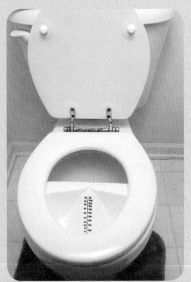

Figure 19.21

- bedpan or urinal and cover
- disposable gloves
- urine specimen container and lid
- label
- urine graduate
- completed laboratory requisition form
- specimen transport bag with a biohazard label, if needed
- pen and form or digital device for recording the intake and output (I&O)
- paper towel

9. Complete the label by printing the resident's name and room number, the time and date of the specimen collection, and the doctor's name. Place the label on the specimen container. Some labels may request additional information, such as birth date or other identifiers. Be sure the name on the label matches the resident's identification.

10. Provide privacy by closing the curtains, using a screen, or closing the door to the room.

11. Wash your hands or use hand sanitizer to ensure infection control.

12. Put on disposable gloves.

13. Have the resident urinate into a urinary hat placed in the front half of the toilet, into a bedpan, or into a urinal. The first urination of the morning is best for this test because the urine is usually concentrated.

14. Ask the resident not to have a bowel movement or to put toilet paper into the urine specimen. Provide a bag or waste container for the toilet paper.

15. If the resident used a bedpan or urinal, cover it and take it into the bathroom. If measuring the resident's I&O, pour the urine from the bedpan or urinal into a clean graduate (Figure 19.22).

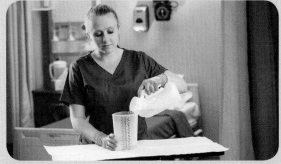

Figure 19.22

16. Remove and discard your gloves.

17. Wash your hands or use hand sanitizer to ensure infection control.

18. Put on a new pair of gloves.

19. Note the total urine output amount and record it on the paper or electronic intake and output form.

20. Place a paper towel on a flat surface.

21. Remove the lid from the urine specimen container and place it, inside facing up, on the paper towel. Carefully pour about 120 mL of the urine directly from the graduate into the specimen container. If I&O is not measured, you may pour the urine directly from the urinal into the specimen container (Figure 19.23). To avoid contamination, do not touch the inside of the specimen container or lid.

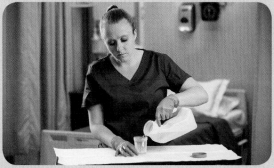

Figure 19.23

22. Put the lid on the specimen container. Double-check that the specimen identified on the label matches the specimen collected. Make sure the lid is tightly placed on the container.

23. Attach the requisition form to ensure the specimen container is complete and ready for transport to the laboratory.

24. Place the specimen container in a specimen transport bag. Use a biohazard bag or label, if needed. Do not let the specimen container touch the outside of the bag.

25. Empty the rest of the urine into the toilet.

26. Remove, clean, and store equipment in the proper location. Remove soiled linens and discard disposable equipment.

27. Remove and discard your gloves.

28. Wash your hands or use hand sanitizer to ensure infection control.

29. Put on a new pair of gloves.

30. Assist the resident with hand washing, and hygiene, as needed.

31. If the resident is in bed, check to be sure the bed wheels are locked, then reposition the resident and lower the bed.

32. Follow the plan of care to determine if the side rails should be raised or lowered.

(continued)

The Procedure: Midstream Urine Specimen

33. Bring the necessary equipment into the room. Place the following items in an accessible location:

    - midstream specimen kit, packaged in a sterile wrapper (including specimen container, label, disposable wipes, and disposable gloves)
    - several washcloths
    - soap
    - disposable gloves
    - completed laboratory requisition form
    - specimen transport bag with a biohazard label, if needed

34. Complete the label by printing the resident's name and room number, the time and date of the specimen collection, and the doctor's name. Place the label on the specimen container. Some labels may request additional information, such as birth date or other identifiers. Be sure the name on the label matches the resident's identification.

35. Provide privacy by closing the curtains, using a screen, or closing the door to the room.

36. Wash your hands or use hand sanitizer to ensure infection control.

37. Put on disposable gloves.

38. Assist the resident to the bathroom or provide a bedside commode, bedpan, or urinal.

> **Best Practice**
> Explain the procedure, and if appropriate, allow the resident to collect the specimen. Otherwise, assist the resident with the procedure.

39. Have the resident cleanse the perineal area with disposable wipes or a washcloth, soap, and warm water. Provide assistance, if needed.

    A. **Female**: Use one hand to separate the labia with a wipe. This hand is now contaminated and should not touch anything sterile. Hold a wipe in the other hand and clean down the urethral area from front to back. Use a clean wipe for each wipe. Keep the labia separated to collect the urine specimen.

    B. **Male**: Hold the penis with one hand. If the penis is not circumcised, pull back the foreskin. The hand holding the penis is now contaminated and should not touch anything sterile. Clean the penis in a circular motion starting at the urethral opening. Start at the center and work outward. Use a clean wipe for each wipe. Keep holding the penis until the urine specimen is collected.

40. Remove and discard your gloves.

41. Wash your hands or use hand sanitizer to ensure infection control.

42. Open the midstream specimen kit on the bathroom counter or on the overbed table. Open the packaging and keep the contents on top of the sterile wrapper.

43. Put on a new pair of gloves.

44. Open the specimen container and place the lid on the sterile wrapper, with the inside of the lid facing up. Open the wipes in the kit.

45. Make sure the toilet paper and specimen container are within reach.

46. Instruct the resident to start a stream of urine and then stop urinating.

47. Have the resident hold the specimen container, if able, to catch the next stream of urine. Hold the specimen container yourself if the resident is unable.

48. After obtaining the specimen, remove the container before the flow of urine stops. The specimen should contain only urine that passes during the middle of urination.

49. Put the lid on the specimen container immediately. Do not allow anything to touch the inside of the container. Make sure the lid is tightly placed on the container.

50. Double-check that the specimen identified on the label matches the specimen collected.

51. Attach the requisition form to ensure the specimen container is complete and ready for transport to the laboratory.

52. Place the specimen container in a specimen transport bag. Use a biohazard bag or label, if needed. Do not let the specimen container touch the outside of the bag.

53. Remove, clean, and store equipment in the proper location. Remove soiled linens and discard disposable equipment.

54. Remove and discard your gloves.

55. Wash your hands or use hand sanitizer to ensure infection control.

56. Put on a new pair of gloves.

57. Assist the resident with hand washing and hygiene, as needed.

58. If the resident is in bed, check to be sure the bed wheels are locked, then reposition the resident and lower the bed.

59. Follow the plan of care to determine if the side rails should be raised or lowered.

The Procedure: 24-Hour Urine Specimen

60. Bring the necessary equipment into the room. Place the following items in an accessible location:
    - a 24-hour urine collection container
    - pan and ice
    - label
    - disposable gloves
    - urinary hat
    - sign for the room to indicate a 24-hour urine collection
    - completed laboratory requisition form
    - pen and form or digital device for recording the collection and I&O

61. Complete the label by printing the resident's name and room number, the time and date of the specimen collection, and the doctor's name. Place the label on the specimen container. Some labels may request additional information, such as birth date or other identifiers. Be sure the name on the label matches the resident's identification.

62. Place the 24-hour urine collection container in the bathroom in a pan of ice.

63. Post a sign over the bed or in the bathroom about the specimen collection, as instructed by the licensed nursing staff.

64. Provide privacy by closing the curtains, using a screen, or closing the door to the room.

65. Wash your hands or use hand sanitizer to ensure infection control.

66. Put on disposable gloves.

67. Be sure the resident understands that, for the next 24 hours, all urine needs to be saved and poured into the designated container in the bathroom.

68. Before collection begins, the resident should urinate and discard the urine. This will ensure the bladder is completely empty and marks the start of the 24-hour collection. Note the date and time on the appropriate form or in the electronic record.

69. Have the resident urinate into the urinary hat in the toilet. Ask the resident not to put toilet paper into the pan and to notify you when done. If the resident is not ambulatory, collect the urine from the bedside commode, bedpan, or urinal.

70. If the resident is on I&O, measure all the urine and record it before pouring it into the 24-hour collection container.

71. Maintain fresh ice in the pan under the specimen container.

72. At the end of the 24 hours, have the resident urinate one more time and pour the urine into the container.

73. Double-check that the specimen identified on the label matches the specimen collected. Make sure the lid is tightly placed on the container.

74. Attach the requisition form to ensure the specimen container is complete and ready for transport to the laboratory.

75. Remove the sign about the 24-hour urine collection from the room.

76. Remove and discard your gloves. Perform hand hygiene and put on a new pair of gloves.

77. Assist the resident with hand washing and hygiene, as needed.

78. Check to be sure the bed wheels are locked, then reposition the resident and lower the bed.

79. Follow the plan of care to determine if the side rails should be raised or lowered.

80. Remove, clean, and store equipment in the proper location. Remove soiled linens and discard disposable equipment.

Follow-Up

81. Remove and discard your gloves.

82. Wash your hands to ensure infection control.

83. Make sure the resident is comfortable and place the call light and personal items within reach.

84. Conduct a safety check before leaving the room. The room should be clean and free from clutter or spills.

(continued)

85. Wash your hands or use hand sanitizer before leaving the room.
86. Send or take the labeled urine specimen containers to the laboratory with the requisition form or store the specimen according to instructions from the licensed nursing staff.

Reporting and Documentation

87. Communicate any specific observations, complications, or unusual responses to the licensed nursing staff. Record this information, along with the procedure, in the chart or EMR.

Figure 19.21 iStock.com/robeo; Figure 19.22 © Tori Soper Photography; Figure 19.23 © Tori Soper Photography

Think About This

Colorectal cancer is the third most common cancer and the second leading cause of cancer-related death in the United States. It affects both men and women ages 50 and older. Sixty percent of colorectal cancer cases could be avoided with regular screening.

Urine Specimen Straining

Occasionally, urine specimens need to be strained. Urine straining is usually done when a resident has kidney or bladder stones that need to be retrieved for testing. Urine is collected and strained through a strainer. It continues to be strained until all stones have been collected or until a licensed nursing staff member ends the collection. The stones are put into a container and sent to the laboratory per facility policy.

Stool Specimens

Stool (*feces*) specimens help detect blood in the stool, identify possible infections, and screen for colon cancer. Three different tests may be performed to examine stool specimens. One is the fecal **occult blood** test, which detects blood in the stool. Stool specimens may also be used to screen for and diagnose possible infection. A third test examines stool specimens for signs of colon cancer or the presence of noncancerous *polyps*, or growths.

Procedure | Collecting a Stool Specimen

Rationale

Proper collection of a stool specimen is necessary to ensure accurate screening and diagnosis.

Preparation

1. Ask the licensed nursing staff how this procedure fits into the plan of care, if there are doctor's orders for the procedure, if there are any special instructions or precautions, and if the resident can be moved into the positions required for this procedure.
2. Wash your hands or use hand sanitizer before entering the room.
3. Knock before entering the room.
4. Introduce yourself using your full name and title. Explain that you work with the licensed nursing staff and will be providing care.
5. Greet the resident and ask the resident to state her full name, if able. Then check the resident's identification bracelet.
6. Use Mr., Mrs., or Ms. and the last name when conversing.
7. Explain the procedure in simple terms, even if the resident is not able to communicate or is disoriented. Ask permission to perform the procedure.
8. Bring the necessary equipment into the room. Place the following items in an accessible location:
   - disposable specimen pan
   - bedpan and cover or commode
   - disposable gloves
   - stool specimen container and lid
   - label
   - toilet paper
   - wooden tongue blade
   - plastic bag or waste container for disposal
   - completed laboratory requisition form
   - specimen transport bag with a biohazard label, if needed

9. Complete the label by printing the resident's name and room number, the time and date of the specimen collection, and the doctor's name. Place the label on the specimen container. Some labels may request additional information, such as birth date or other identifiers. Be sure the name on the label matches the resident's identification.

The Procedure

10. Provide privacy by closing the curtains, using a screen, or closing the door to the room.

11. Wash your hands or use hand sanitizer to ensure infection control.

12. Put on disposable gloves.

13. If the resident is ambulatory, have her use the toilet in the bathroom. Ask the resident to urinate first and flush the toilet. Then ask the resident to stand. Place a disposable specimen pan in the back half of the toilet. Ask the resident to have a bowel movement into the specimen pan.

14. If the resident is not ambulatory, have her use a bedside commode or bedpan and urinate first. Discard the urine. If the resident uses a bedside commode, place a disposable specimen pan in the back half of the bucket. Then instruct the resident to have a bowel movement into the disposable specimen pan or into the bedpan.

15. Provide a plastic bag or waste container to dispose of toilet paper.

16. If a bedside commode or bedpan was used, cover the disposable specimen pan or bedpan and take it into the bathroom.

17. Use a wooden tongue blade to remove about 2 teaspoons of stool from the bedpan or disposable specimen pan (Figure 19.24). Observe the stool for color, amount, and quality. The sample should be about the size of a walnut. Try to remove stool from two different places. Include any pus, mucus, or blood present in the stool.

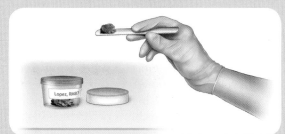

Figure 19.24

18. Put the lid on the specimen container. Make sure the lid is tightly placed on the container.

19. Double-check that the specimen identified on the label matches the specimen collected.

20. Attach the requisition form to ensure the specimen container is complete and ready for transport to the laboratory.

21. Place the specimen container in a specimen transport bag. Use a biohazard bag or label, if needed. Do not let the specimen container touch the outside of the bag.

22. Wrap the wooden tongue blade in toilet paper. Discard it in a plastic bag or waste container. Empty the remaining stool into the toilet.

23. Remove and discard your gloves. Perform hand hygiene and put on a new pair of gloves.

24. Assist the resident with hand washing and hygiene, as needed.

25. Check to be sure the bed wheels are locked, then reposition the resident and lower the bed.

26. Follow the plan of care to determine if the side rails should be raised or lowered.

27. Remove, clean, and store equipment in the proper location. Remove soiled linens and discard disposable equipment.

Follow-Up

28. Remove and discard your gloves.

29. Wash your hands to ensure infection control.

30. Make sure the resident is comfortable and place the call light and personal items within reach.

31. Conduct a safety check before leaving the room. The room should be clean and free from clutter or spills.

32. Wash your hands or use hand sanitizer before leaving the room.

33. Send or take the labeled stool specimen container to the laboratory with the requisition form or store the specimen according to instructions from the licensed nursing staff.

Reporting and Documentation

34. Communicate any specific observations, complications, or unusual responses to the licensed nursing staff. Record this information, along with the procedure, in the chart or EMR.

Image courtesy of © Body Scientific International

Fecal Occult Blood Test (FOBT)

The *fecal occult blood test (FOBT)*, or **guaiac test**, is a POCT that can be performed at the bedside. The resident should avoid certain foods (such as red meat, horseradish, and broccoli) and medications (such as aspirin, ibuprofen, and vitamin C supplements) three days prior to the test. This will help prevent inaccurate results.

To perform a FOBT, you will need a *Hemoccult kit*. The Hemoccult kit contains a *Hemoccult slide*, which has front and back portions covered with a paper flap and a developer solution. During a FOBT, a stool sample is applied to special guaiac paper on the front of the Hemoccult slide. Then the back flap of the Hemoccult slide is opened, and the developer solution is applied to the back side of the paper. This solution creates a chemical reaction that indicates the presence of occult blood.

Nursing assistants may not be allowed to perform this test in some states or facilities. If nursing assistants are allowed to perform this test, they should follow facility policy and package directions, along with these general steps:

1. Practice hand hygiene and standard precautions.
2. Ensure privacy and check the resident's identification.
3. Provide an explanation of the procedure you will be performing.
4. Secure a Hemoccult kit, paper towel, and wooden tongue blade. Open the Hemoccult kit.
5. Label the outside of the Hemoccult slide with the resident's name, the date, and the time the specimen was collected.
6. Place a paper towel on a flat surface. Open the front flap of the Hemoccult slide, exposing the guaiac paper.
7. Using the wooden tongue blade, collect a small amount of stool from a fresh stool specimen.
8. Smear a small amount of stool in Box A on the Hemoccult slide (Figure 19.25).
9. Repeat the procedure using stool from a different part of the stool specimen. Smear the stool in Box B on the Hemoccult slide.
10. Close the front flap of the Hemoccult slide and turn the slide over to the reverse side.
11. Open the back flap of the Hemoccult slide. Apply two drops of the developer solution to each box on the guaiac paper and wait 30–60 seconds before reading the results (Figure 19.26). If the slide turns blue, occult blood is present in the stool (considered *guaiac positive*). If the slide does not change color, there is no occult blood in the stool (considered *guaiac negative*).

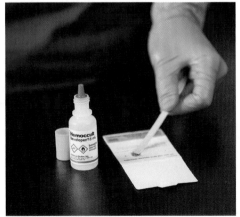

© *Tori Soper Photography*

Figure 19.25 A small amount of stool should be smeared on the Hemoccult slide using a wooden tongue blade.

12. Dispose of the Hemoccult slide in the appropriate container, according to the facility's policy.

13. Report the results to the licensed nursing staff and document the results and care given in the chart or EMR.

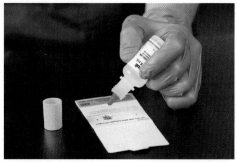

© Tori Soper Photography

Figure 19.26 The developer solution is applied to the Hemoccult slide to help detect occult blood.

Section 19.2 Review and Assessment

Using the Key Terms

Complete the following sentences using key terms in this section.

1. A(n) _____ is a medical instrument used to measure blood sugar levels.
2. An FOBT is used to detect _____, or very small amounts of blood in stool.
3. Collecting a specimen at a resident's bedside while the resident is receiving care is an example of _____.
4. _____ is a blend of saliva and mucus.
5. The _____ is a diagnostic procedure used to detect fecal occult blood.
6. Sputum, urine, and stool are examples of _____.

Know and Understand the Facts

7. Explain why specimen collection is important.
8. Identify and describe three types of specimens that are collected.
9. Why is a sputum specimen collected?
10. Why is a midstream urine specimen collected?
11. Identify two reasons why accurate specimen collection is essential.

Analyze and Apply Concepts

12. Explain how to position and assist a resident when collecting a sputum specimen.
13. Describe how to clean a female resident for a midstream urine specimen collection.
14. Explain the steps to collect a stool specimen.
15. Describe the guidelines for performing an FOBT.

Think Critically

Read the following care situation. Then answer the questions that follow.

Mrs. Z was admitted to a long-term care facility last week. She is not happy about being in the facility and hopes to leave soon. She has mild dementia and a slight limp from a stroke last year. She is an anxious woman who does not often smile and frequently complains about her health. Today, Mrs. Z says she is experiencing itching and burning when she urinates. Mrs. Z's stomach has been upset for days, and she is sure she is bleeding when she has a bowel movement. Mrs. Z and her daughter want to know what you are going to do about her pain and concerns. The daughter has already called Mrs. Z's doctor.

16. What should you tell Mrs. Z you are going to do about her pain and concerns?
17. What should you be observing, given Mrs. Z's complaints?
18. If the doctor orders an FOBT and midstream urine specimen for Mrs. Z, how should you prepare Mrs. Z for specimen collection?

Key Points

Reviewing the key points for this chapter will help you practice more safely and competently as a holistic nursing assistant and will help you prepare for the certification competency examination.

- Physical examinations help determine the status of body systems and screen for and diagnose diseases. Annual physical examinations, well-woman exams, well-man exams, and well-baby exams are all examples.

- Specimens may be collected as part of a health screening, or to determine the presence of pathogens or necessary treatments. Valid test results depend on accurate specimen collection.

- The three most commonly collected specimens are sputum, urine, and stool. Sputum is collected when a resident coughs. Urine can be collected as a routine specimen, midstream specimen, or 24-hour specimen. Some urine specimens need to be strained. Stool is collected and tested in a fecal occult blood test (FOBT) or using a stool DNA test.

Action Steps to Holistic Care

Review the information in this chapter. Complete the following activities.

1. With a partner, select one type of physical examination. Prepare a poster that illustrates four facts patients and the public should know.

2. With a partner, write a song or a poem about the process used to drape a patient for a physical examination. Include the reasons why this information is important.

3. Find two pictures in a magazine, in a newspaper, or online depicting a physical examination. Describe the type of exam, any nonverbal communication shown, and discuss what message is being conveyed about the exam.

4. Research and write a brief report describing three current facts about urine specimen collection not covered in the chapter.

5. Create a poster or digital presentation that describes each of the specimen collections discussed in the chapter. Include when, why, and how each specimen is collected, and any best practice guidelines the nursing assistant should follow to ensure accuracy.

Preparing for the Certification Competency Examination

To prepare for the nursing assistant certification competency examination, you will need to know content found in this chapter. This content may be tested in the knowledge (written or oral) and skills (hands-on demonstration) portions of the exam. The following areas will be emphasized:

- preparation for physical examinations
- specimen collection
- standard precautions during specimen collection
- specimen sources
- tests used to examine specimens
- specimen collection procedures for sputum, urine, and stool
- accurate documentation

These sample test questions are similar to ones you will find on the certification competency exam. See how well you can answer them. Be sure to select the *best* answer.

1. Which medical instrument is used to examine the ears?

   A. ophthalmoscope
   B. glucometer
   C. otoscope
   D. speculum

2. If a doctor uses her hands to feel a body part, she is performing

   A. palpation
   B. percussion
   C. inspection
   D. observation

3. A nursing assistant helping Dr. James with a physical examination wants to be sure the patient, Mrs. E, is comfortable. What is the best approach the nursing assistant can take?

   A. make sure Mrs. E dresses and undresses herself
   B. double-drape Mrs. E to maintain her privacy
   C. stand behind Dr. James so Mrs. E can hear the instructions
   D. make sure the drape covers Mrs. E properly and keeps her warm

4. What makes a dipstick urine test different from other urine tests?

   A. The dipstick is checked every hour for 24 hours.
   B. The dipstick test uses a chemical strip that changes color.
   C. The dipstick test is done in a sterile environment.
   D. Urine is only collected from a urinary catheter.

5. Which position is necessary for a well-woman exam?

   A. Fowler's position
   B. supine position
   C. knee-chest position
   D. lithotomy position

6. Sputum is collected when a resident

   A. urinates
   B. coughs
   C. sneezes
   D. blinks

7. A resident was just told his test results were negative. What does this mean?

   A. The test results were within normal range.
   B. The test results were not within normal range.
   C. The test results were unclear.
   D. The test results need to be repeated.

8. How do nursing assistants use a biohazard bag when collecting specimens?

   A. Nursing assistants use it to store equipment.
   B. Nursing assistants put the specimen container in it for storage.
   C. Nursing assistants put the specimen container in it for transport.
   D. Nursing assistants use it to dispose of unused items.

9. Mr. J has been experiencing rectal bleeding, and the doctor wants to examine him. Which position will be necessary?

   A. prone position
   B. supine position
   C. Sims' position
   D. Fowler's position

10. How does the procedure for midstream urine collection differ from that of routine collection?

    A. The container is sterile.
    B. Only the last part of the stream is saved.
    C. The perineal area must be cleansed.
    D. Midstream collection is done only in the morning.

11. Which of the following is the one way to detect if there is blood in the stool?

    A. midstream collection
    B. stool DNA test
    C. fecal occult blood test
    D. stool culture

12. Which of the following is an important part of a well-man examination?

    A. prostate cancer screening
    B. blood pressure
    C. cholesterol test
    D. DEXA scan

13. What might a nursing assistant do to retrieve a kidney or bladder stone from urine?

    A. culture the urine
    B. strain the urine
    C. store the urine
    D. heat the urine

14. Ms. J is going to her first mammogram. Which type of mammogram is she likely to receive?

    A. diagnostic
    B. DEXA scan
    C. screening
    D. manual

15. Mr. L is having a 24-hour urine collection. What is the most important action to ensure an accurate test result?

    A. The container should be shaken.
    B. The container should have a lid.
    C. The container should be kept warm.
    D. The container should be kept iced.

Did you have difficulty with any of the questions? If you did, review the chapter to find the correct answer(s).

CHAPTER 20
Creating a Safe, Restful Environment

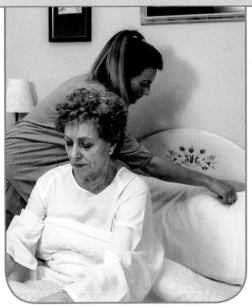

David Pereiras/Shutterstock.com

Chapter Outline

Section 20.1
The Call System and Respecting Personal Items

Section 20.2
Making Beds

Section 20.3
Promoting Comfort, Relaxation, Rest, and Sleep

Welcome to the Chapter

This chapter provides information about the environment of a room in a healthcare facility. You will learn about typical room arrangements in hospitals and long-term care facilities, call light use, and ways to respond to requests. Holistic nursing assistants can promote residents' feelings of security by respecting and safeguarding personal items.

Various types of beds are used in healthcare facilities, and nursing assistants must know how to make an occupied, unoccupied (closed and open), and surgical bed. In this chapter, you will learn about the importance of promoting comfort by establishing an environment that is relaxing, is restful, and encourages sleep. One way to create a relaxing and restful environment is to give residents back rubs.

The information and procedures presented in this chapter will help you build the knowledge and skills needed to become a holistic nursing assistant. Check with your instructor to ensure these procedures are within your state's regulations for nursing assistant practice. The topics discussed in the chapter are highlighted on the Providing Holistic Care Framework.

You are now ready to start this chapter, *Creating a Safe, Restful Environment*.

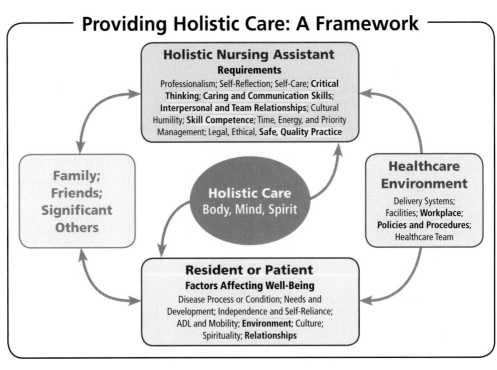

Providing Holistic Care: A Framework

Holistic Nursing Assistant
Requirements
Professionalism; Self-Reflection; Self-Care; **Critical Thinking; Caring and Communication Skills; Interpersonal and Team Relationships**; Cultural Humility; **Skill Competence**; Time, Energy, and Priority Management; Legal, Ethical, **Safe, Quality Practice**

Holistic Care
Body, Mind, Spirit

Family; Friends; Significant Others

Healthcare Environment
Delivery Systems; Facilities; **Workplace; Policies and Procedures;** Healthcare Team

Resident or Patient
Factors Affecting Well-Being
Disease Process or Condition; Needs and Development; Independence and Self-Reliance; ADL and Mobility; **Environment**; Culture; Spirituality; **Relationships**

Objectives

To provide the best possible care, you must know how rooms in healthcare facilities are arranged. It is also critical to know how call systems function and how to respond to calls. You will need to respect and safeguard residents' personal items. To achieve the objectives for this section, you must successfully

- **describe** the equipment typically found in a patient's or resident's room;
- **explain** how communication call systems function;
- **demonstrate** how to respond to communication call systems; and
- **identify** the best way to respect and safeguard personal items.

Key Terms

Learn these key terms to better understand the information presented in the section.

traction   ward

Questions to Consider

- Think about the last time you visited some place new. Did you feel out of place or lost? Did you experience any feelings of fear, confusion, or insecurity?
- What helped you feel better? Did anyone help you? If so, what did he or she say or do?

When people are hospitalized or admitted to a long-term care facility, they enter a different and unfamiliar environment. Not only will residents have to communicate with strangers, but the facility will look very different from home. The facility may be very noisy and have unfamiliar sounds and smells. Holistic nursing assistants who are familiar with the organization of residents' rooms will be best able to help residents feel comfortable. When residents are comfortable, a safe, healing environment can be best achieved.

Long-term care facilities must comply with OBRA requirements that care and services enhance each resident's quality of life and that each resident is treated with dignity and respect.

What Do Rooms Look Like in a Healthcare Facility?

Rooms in healthcare facilities are often arranged in a similar manner. Most healthcare facilities do not have a lot of space, so rooms are designed as efficiently as possible. Room arrangements must be conducive to both the healthcare providers and the patient or resident.

Historically, healthcare facilities did not offer private rooms. Instead, several patients received care in the same **ward**, or large room (Figure 20.1). The use of wards maximized limited space.

Today, rooms in a healthcare facility are designed to be attractive. They have pictures on the walls and are painted in therapeutic colors. Rooms are private or semiprivate. A private room holds only one resident or patient, and a semiprivate room holds two residents or patients. Rooms often include separate bathrooms with safety modifications (such as handrails) and a small closet or wardrobe to store personal items. Residents and patients must be able to easily hang, store, and remove their personal items.

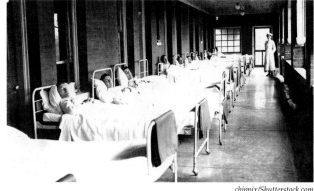

chippix/Shutterstock.com

Figure 20.1 Historically, healthcare facilities housed patients in wards. A ward was a large room that contained several patients.

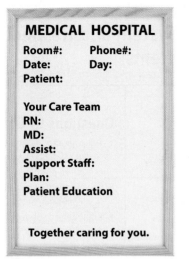

MEDICAL HOSPITAL

Room#:   Phone#:
Date: Day:
Patient:

Your Care Team
RN:
MD:
Assist:
Support Staff:
Plan:
Patient Education

Together caring for you.

Figure 20.2 A communication board contains important information about a patient and his or her care.

Room Equipment

For the most part, rooms in a healthcare facility all include similar equipment. Each room has a bed, which is sometimes called a *hospital bed* due to its style and function (not to the type of facility). A movable *overbed table* is used for personal care and can hold a meal tray. The overbed table should not be used for placing dirty or contaminated items or supplies, such as used dressings or containers holding any type of drainage without a barrier such as a paper towel. A *bedside stand*, which may be movable or built into the wall, usually holds personal items and has room on top for a telephone. Personal items and supplies may also be stored inside the stand. One or two chairs are normally located next to the bed. On the wall opposite the bed, there may be a communication board, which contains important information that is updated each shift (Figure 20.2). Most rooms also have a television.

Many rooms have equipment or lighting attached to the wall behind the bed. For example, in some facilities, oxygen and blood pressure equipment are installed in the wall above or beside the bed. Additional equipment may also be kept in the room. Communication systems or call lights are placed near or on the bed to enable communication between the resident or patient and healthcare providers. Other equipment or supplies may be needed on a continuous basis due to a resident's or patient's disease or condition. These supplies may include extra towels or blankets, **traction** equipment (weights, pulleys, and tape that help treat muscular and skeletal disorders), a blood pressure machine, or a bedside commode for residents or patients who cannot easily walk to the bathroom.

Privacy

Rooms in a healthcare facility have features that ensure privacy. Privacy curtains enclose the area around the bed. A half curtain may provide privacy between two residents or patients in a room, or a full curtain may surround each personal area. In some private rooms, a curtain near the doorway may maintain privacy from people in the hallway (Figure 20.3). When there are no curtains, screens are used.

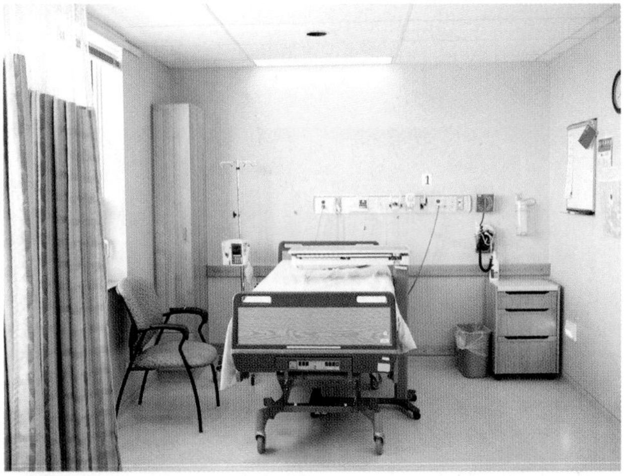

Figure 20.3 Like most rooms in a healthcare facility, this room contains a chair, overbed table, bedside stand, and privacy curtain.

Long-Term Care Facility Rooms

Because residents in long-term care facilities often stay in facilities for an extended period of time, they usually have more personal items than hospital patients. A room in a long-term care facility may be designed to look like a typical bedroom in a home (Figure 20.4). Residents have the right to retain and use personal items, including furnishings, as space permits and as long as items do not infringe on the rights, health, and safety of other residents.

Why Are Call Lights Important?

Call lights make up a communication system that residents use to let nursing staff know when they have a particular need or desire. As you learned in chapter 16, answering a call light promptly helps ensure resident safety. Answering a call light quickly can prevent residents from wandering, becoming confused, or unsafely getting out of bed. A call light should always be within a resident's reach.

The Call Light Communication System

Call lights are part of a communication system that electronically connects each resident to the nursing staff. There are many types of communication systems, and they can be wired or wireless (Figure 20.5). Call lights are found in resident rooms, and emergency call lights are also found in resident bathrooms, usually near the toilet (Figure 20.6).

The call light communication system has an *alert and response cycle*. The *alert* occurs when a resident presses the call light. When this happens, a signal goes to a device that displays the room number at the nurses' station. An alert light or sound, such as a ring or buzz, may also be activated. Sometimes the alert may cause a light to turn on above or on the side of the door to the resident's room and may be accompanied by a ringing sound outside the room. In some facilities, staff members carry mobile electronic devices, such as pagers or cell phones, which receive the alert (Figure 20.7).

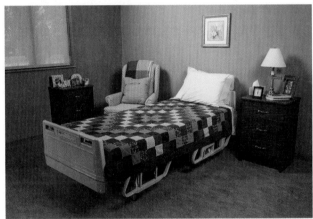

© Tori Soper Photography

Figure 20.4 In a long-term care facility, a resident's room may be arranged to look like a typical bedroom with storage and furnishings.

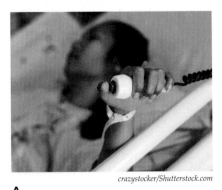

crazystocker/Shutterstock.com

A

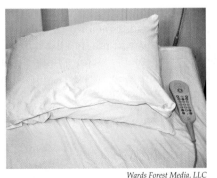

Wards Forest Media, LLC

B

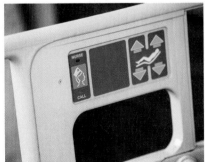

© Tori Soper Photography

C

Figure 20.5 There are many types of call lights, including traditional call light buttons (A), remote call lights (B), and call lights on beds (C).

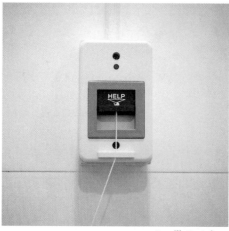

pattang/Shutterstock.com

Figure 20.6 Emergency call light buttons are found in the bathrooms.

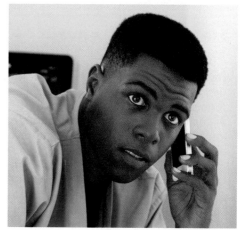

Rocketclips, Inc./Shutterstock.com

Figure 20.7 Some healthcare facilities provide staff members with mobile electronic devices for receiving call light alerts.

The *response* part of the cycle occurs when a staff member answers the call light by intercom or phone call, responds to a page, or goes to the room to see what is needed. Once the staff member who answers is in the room, the call light should be turned off. This communication system is similar to the system of calling a flight attendant on an airplane.

It is important to orient residents and patients to the call light system, especially after first admission. To orient residents and patients, show them where the call light is located and how to use it. The call light should always be available and easily accessible. If a resident or patient cannot use a call light, check with the licensed nursing staff, the plan of care, and facility policy on how to best respond to the resident's needs.

Timely Response

When a call light goes on, the closest member of the nursing staff should respond immediately. The resident using the call light is communicating a need he or she believes is important. The resident may need pain relief or assistance going to the bathroom. The longer it takes the nursing staff to respond to the call light, the more unsafe the situation may become, increasing the risk of possible falls or injury. Responding to call lights quickly promotes safety and decreases the chance of a fall. A quick response also increases satisfaction with care.

Frequent Call Light Use

Sometimes it may seem like a resident uses a call light too often or unnecessarily. Frequent call light use may be the result of fear or anxiety, past experiences with long wait times, or boredom. Answering frequent call lights might frustrate nursing staff members and cause them to label the resident a "pest." It is important not to label a resident this way or fall into the trap of not responding. This approach can put the patient or resident at risk for a fall or injury. No matter how many times there is a call, remember that the resident is in need. It is your responsibility to respond and deliver safe, quality care.

The Impact of Rounding

As you learned in chapter 12, nursing staff members in some facilities conduct *rounds*, which involve going into residents' rooms to monitor their diseases or conditions. Rounds give staff members more time at a resident's bedside. They increase awareness of present or potential needs. Rounding can reduce unnecessary call light use, as residents know they will interact with the staff periodically throughout each shift.

Becoming a Holistic Nursing Assistant
Answering Call Lights

Following specific guidelines for answering resident calls can help you provide holistic care. These guidelines will also improve the quality of care, ensure resident safety and comfort, and reduce the number of unnecessary calls.

When you answer a call light, do so quickly and according to facility policy and procedure. If the call comes from a resident's bathroom, consider it an emergency and respond immediately. Be courteous when responding to the call. Many call lights now have an intercom that allows nursing staff members to talk to the resident. If you use the intercom, make sure you can be heard. Do not rely exclusively on the intercom to respond to a resident's needs. If the call comes from a bathroom, never use the intercom. Go directly to the room.

When you enter a resident's room, be polite and attentive to the resident's requests. If you feel the resident is a nuisance or has inconvenienced you, your body language may tell the resident how you feel. Be sure your nonverbal communication is as considerate as your words.

The following guidelines can help you respond well to and reduce a resident's need to use the call light:

- Observe the resident's position and ask if the resident is comfortable. Reposition the resident, if needed.
- Make sure the call light is accessible to the resident. For example, if a resident has a weak left arm and hand, place the call light on his or her right, or stronger, side.

- Put the telephone, TV remote control, and bed light switch within the resident's reach.
- Place the overbed table next to the bed, if needed.
- Position the tissue box and drinking water so they can be easily reached.
- Put the waste container next to the bed.
- Ask about the resident's pain level. If the resident is experiencing pain, notify the licensed nursing staff immediately.

Prior to leaving the room, ask the resident if there is anything else you can do before you go. Be sincere and show interest in the resident's response. If appropriate, remind the resident that you (or another member of the nursing staff) will be back again to check on him or her during your shift.

Apply It

1. A resident has used the call light five times in the last hour. When you answered the last call light, the resident requested ice for his water and help picking up a piece of paper he could not reach. When the call light goes on for the sixth time, what should you do?

2. What actions can you take to help lessen a resident's frequent use of the call light?

How Can a Nursing Assistant Safeguard Personal Items?

Patients and residents often bring personal items into hospitals and long-term care facilities. Patients are usually discouraged from bringing personal items for short-term hospital stays, but still may bring some items with them. In long-term care facilities, where stays are much longer, residents typically have many personal items.

Personal items may include clothing, jewelry, handbags and wallets, photos, books, and plants or gifts received during a resident's stay. These items are very important and become a critical part of a resident's or patient's personal space. Residents and patients may be concerned about the security of their personal items in different and unfamiliar environments. This is particularly true for older adults. For example, a female resident may hold her handbag close while walking or keep it with her in bed.

As a holistic nursing assistant, be sure to respect personal items. These items are special and irreplaceable to residents. It is your duty and responsibility to keep them safe. Do not move a resident's personal items without reason. If you have to move a personal item, do so carefully so it will not fall or break. Ask for permission if you need to go through a resident's personal items in the bedside stand or closet. Do not go through a resident's handbag or wallet. If you need something from the wallet or handbag, ask the resident or a family member to retrieve it or follow the appropriate facility policy.

As you learned in chapter 5, safeguarding a resident's personal items begins at admission and continues until transfer or discharge. During admission, an inventory of all clothing and personal items is completed according to facility policy (Figure 20.8). Residents in long-term care facilities often have more items than hospital patients do. These items must be labeled with dignity (on the insides of clothing or shoes) with the resident's name and room number. Labeling items on the inside prevents the resident from feeling like a child. It also preserves the resident's privacy if the resident chooses not to share his or her name and room number with others. Any valuable or expensive items may be placed in the facility safe.

During transfer or discharge, you should assist in collecting and packing personal items. Return any valuable items that have been kept in the facility's safe. Carry personal items to the personal or transportation vehicle or move them to the new unit, if appropriate.

How Can Nursing Assistants Promote a Healing Environment?

One of your most important responsibilities as a holistic nursing assistant is to promote and maintain a healing environment. A *healing environment* is one that fosters the individual rights of residents and humanizes their experience. Part of promoting a healing environment is understanding how rooms are arranged, responding to call lights, and respecting personal items. As you learned in chapters 3 and 16, federal and state laws, regulations, and standards also protect patient and resident rights and outline care requirements. The following guidelines reflect these laws, regulations, and standards and will help you promote a safe, healing environment for residents:

- Always try to accommodate resident preferences.

- Organize the room in a manner that ensures resident safety.

- Maintain cleanliness in the resident's room and during procedures. If you see something on the floor, pick it up using gloves or a paper towel. Always wash your hands after throwing something away. This is also a safety precaution.

- Ensure proper temperature and ventilation in resident rooms. OBRA regulations require that room temperature be kept between 71°F and 81°F. Older adults may want the room to be on the warm side of that range. Keeping the door open or opening a window can provide sufficient ventilation, if appropriate.

- Reduce odors in resident rooms. Proper ventilation can help prevent odors from becoming an issue. Odor control may be needed after elimination, during dressing changes, and if there are soiled linens.

Remember

I've learned that people will forget what you said, people will forget what you did, but people will never forget how you made them feel.

Maya Angelou,
American author and poet

Inventory of Personal Effects

RESIDENT'S NAME	ROOM NO.	DATE OF ADMISSION

CONTACT LENSES	DENTURES Full: Upper ☐ Lower ☐ Partial: Upper ☐ Lower ☐

EYE GLASSES	HEARING AID

JEWELRY	WATCH

ITEM LIST

NUMBER	ITEM	DESCRIPTION
	Bathrobe	
	Belt	
	Blouse	
	Brush	
	Cane or crutches	
	Coat	
	Dress	
	Furniture	
	Gloves	
	Handkerchief	
	Hat	
	Housecoat	
	Necktie	
	Nightgown	
	Pajamas	
	Pants	
	Prosthesis	
	Purse	
	Radio	
	Razors	
	Shirts	
	Shoes	
	Skirts	
	Slippers	
	Socks	
	Stockings	
	Sweater	
	Television (model and serial number)	
	Underpants	
	Undershirt	
	Walker	
	Wallet	
	Wheelchair (model and serial number)	
	Other:	

I have read and agree that this is an accurate list of my personal belongings.

NURSE'S SIGNATURE	DATE	RESIDENT'S OR GUARDIAN'S SIGNATURE	DATE

Figure 20.8 An inventory lists a resident's personal items. This list helps nursing assistants keep track of and safeguard resident belongings.

- Keep noise to a minimum. A quiet environment promotes healing. Residents can use headphones to watch television or listen to music.
- Ensure that enough safe electrical outlets are available to prevent the use of extension cords.
- Provide sufficient lighting so that residents can read easily and function even with impaired vision. Lighting should not be so glaring that it is uncomfortable.
- Make sure residents are able to use the telephones in their rooms comfortably. If a room is shared, place the telephone so that a conversation can occur without being overheard.
- Ensure that any seating in the room is at the right height to support residents and allows for easy wheelchair transfer.
- Keep the room free from clutter and allow enough space for the resident to get up and ambulate or freely maneuver with ambulation equipment.
- Take into consideration any physical disabilities. For example, you may need to provide adaptive devices for reaching for or picking up items.
- Above all, be respectful and treat residents with dignity.

Section 20.1 Review and Assessment

Using the Key Terms

Complete the following sentences using key terms in this section.

1. _____ equipment is used to help treat muscular and skeletal disorders.
2. A(n) _____ is a room in which several patients are given care.

Know and Understand the Facts

3. List three types of equipment in a typical room in a healthcare facility.
4. How is equipment in a resident's room usually arranged?
5. Explain the primary functions of a call light.
6. Why should the communication board be updated at the beginning of each shift?

Analyze and Apply Concepts

7. Explain when and how to respond to a call light.
8. What can be done if a resident seems to be overusing the call light system?
9. Identify two ways to safeguard and respect personal items.
10. List four guidelines for promoting a healing environment.

Think Critically

Read the following care situation. Then answer the questions that follow.

Mr. L has been in the rehabilitation facility for two weeks after bilateral knee-replacement surgery. He is 55 years old and very impatient about his recovery. Mr. L has a wife who is not well, and his children live in other states. He is usually very active and works in a high-level management position. Mr. L uses a walker now, but is in a lot of pain and does not move about his room very much. He seems anxious about his slow recovery, and his attitude has become very negative. He uses his call light a lot, making requests that seem unnecessary to the staff. You are his nursing assistant today and have answered his call light at least four times this morning.

11. Why do you think Mr. L is using the call light system so frequently?
12. What could you say to Mr. L to lessen his need to use the call light?

Objectives

Making beds is an important part of the nursing assistant's responsibility to provide personal care. In this section, you will learn about the different types of beds in healthcare facilities and appropriate bed-making procedures related to each. To achieve the objectives for this section, you must successfully

- **describe** the different types of beds commonly found in healthcare facilities; and
- **demonstrate** how to make an occupied, unoccupied, and surgical bed.

Key Terms

bath blanket   disposable protective pad

draw sheet

Questions to Consider

- Think about the last time you were sick and had to stay in bed. What was it like to be in bed all day or even several days?
- Did you find your bed linens uncomfortable after a while? How did you feel after eating in bed? Did crumbs you could not get rid of press against your skin?
- Did you have a fever, and did it cause you to sweat and leave your sheets and pillowcase damp? Did you feel different after your linens were changed?

What Types of Beds Are Used in Healthcare Facilities?

Many brands of beds are used in healthcare facilities. Some types of specialty beds are made for patients over 500 pounds or eliminate pressure points. Two different bed types allow a resident's position to be changed in bed. These types are electric and manual (Figure 20.9). An *electric bed* can be raised or lowered and can reposition the head and foot. Controls for an electric bed may be at the side of the bed, in a hand controller, or sometimes at the foot of the bed. This type of bed allows residents to control their positions. *Manual beds* are not used as frequently as electric beds. A crank mechanism is used to change the position of a manual bed and is located at the end of the bed. For safety reasons, the crank mechanism must be in the down position when not in use.

Beds are usually movable and have wheels at each corner. These wheels can be locked or unlocked using a foot lever by each wheel or a lever under the bed near the wheels (Figure 20.10). Beds are equipped with a mattress that may be covered with plastic. As you learned in chapter 16, a mattress must fit on the bed frame well to prevent possible entrapment. Regular monitoring of the resident, according to facility policy, can also help prevent entrapment.

Beds in hospitals are equipped with side rails only at the top of the bed or at the top and bottom of the bed. Some beds may have side rails that span the full length of each side of the bed (Figure 20.11). Beds in some long-term care facilities may not have side rails or may have an ambulatory assist rail. Side rails can be raised or lowered with a release lever. These levers are located at different places on the bed, depending on the bed's brand.

Because different brands of beds may be used in the same facility, take time to locate all lock and release levers each time you deliver care. This will help you feel comfortable working with the bed and maintaining safety.

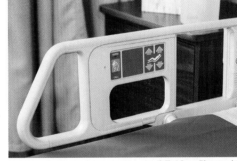

© Tori Soper Photography

A

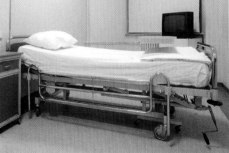

iStock.com/Lebazele

B

Figure 20.9 An electric bed can be adjusted using controls on the side or foot of the bed (A). A manual bed can be adjusted using a crank at the end of the bed (B).

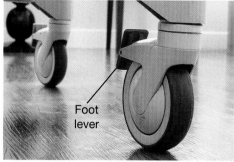

Foot lever

Figure 20.10 Each bed wheel has a foot lever that locks or unlocks it.

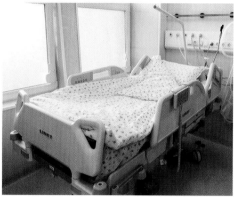

A

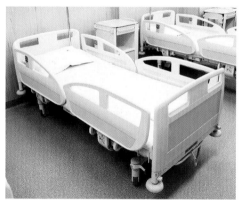

B

Figure 20.11 Many beds have side rails that may span only the top of the bed (A) or the full length of the bed (B).

What Is the Proper Way to Make a Bed?

As a nursing assistant, you will be making beds daily. In some cases, you will be making *occupied beds*, or beds with residents in them, because residents are *bedridden*, meaning they cannot get in or out of bed. If a resident is bedridden, you will need to change the linens while the resident is still in bed. You also need to know how to make *unoccupied* and *surgical beds*. Unoccupied beds can be made closed or open. If a bed will not be occupied for an extended period of time, it should be made *closed* with the top linens pulled up. A closed bed may also be made in preparation for a new admission. *Open* beds have the top linens pulled down because they will soon be occupied. If a resident has left her bed for the day, the bed should be remade open. An open bed promotes comfort and allows the resident to get in and out of bed with ease.

When a patient comes into a room after surgery, a surgical bed should be prepared. A surgical bed has linens opened lengthwise (Figure 20.12). This allows the patient to be transferred safely and comfortably from the stretcher to the bed after a surgery or procedure.

Linens

Before you begin making a bed, familiarize yourself with the linens you will be using. Some healthcare facilities use only bottom and top flat sheets to make beds; however, many facilities now use a fitted bottom sheet and flat top sheets. In addition to flat and fitted sheets, blankets, and pillowcases, you may use the following special types of linens and bed coverings:

- **Draw sheet**: also called a *pull sheet*, *turning sheet*, or *lift sheet*, this sheet is either smaller in size than a regular-size flat sheet or is a flat sheet folded in half. It is placed lengthwise over the middle of the bottom sheet. A draw sheet has several uses. It can keep the mattress and bottom sheets dry and can be used to turn or move a resident in bed.

- **Bath blanket**: this regular-size blanket is usually made from cotton or another absorbent material and is used to keep residents warm during a bed bath. It may also be used as a protective covering to maintain resident modesty and warmth during various procedures.

- **Disposable protective pad**: sometimes called an *incontinence pad*, this small, often multilayered, leakproof, highly absorbent pad is made from washable cotton or a disposable, paperlike material. It is placed under a resident's buttocks and on top of the draw sheet. Disposable protective pads are used to promote the comfort of incontinent residents, absorb drainage, and prevent the bed from becoming soiled during procedures.

Mitered Corners

When making a bed, a flat or fitted bottom sheet may be used, depending on facility preference. If a flat sheet is used, maintain resident skin integrity by making the bed with mitered corners. This ensures the flat sheet is tucked securely and neatly under the mattress. Figure 20.13 details the process of making a mitered corner.

Pillowcases

Changing a pillowcase is an important part of making a bed. Residents place their heads on pillowcases while resting and while sleeping during the night. They may lie facedown on their pillowcases and will sometimes cough or sneeze on their pillowcases. As a result, the pillowcase is a breeding ground for pathogens. Changing the pillowcase routinely and when it appears to be soiled is essential for infection prevention and control.

To change a pillowcase when the resident is in bed, ask the resident to raise his or her head and assist, if needed. The resident may have more than one pillow on his or her bed. If possible, leave a pillow under the resident's head while you change another pillowcase. If there is only one pillow, keep the resident flat in bed after removing it to avoid neck injury. Discard the used pillowcase in the laundry hamper. To maintain infection prevention and control, do not shake the pillowcase or pillow and do not let them touch your scrubs.

There are two ways a pillowcase can be changed (Figures 20.14). There is no best method. Oftentimes nursing assistants select the method that is easiest or most comfortable, or simply continue using the method they were first taught.

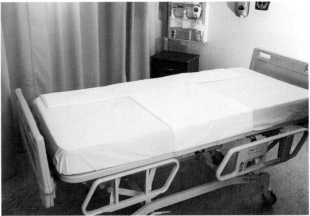

© Tori Soper Photography

Figure 20.12 A surgical bed is made to allow for safe transfer after a surgery or procedure.

Mitered Corners

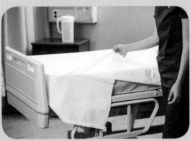
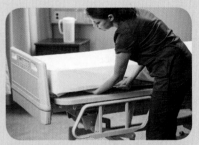

A. Tuck the top of the flat sheet underneath the head of the mattress and the bottom of the sheet underneath the foot of the mattress. The sides of the sheet should remain untucked.

B. Start at one corner of the bed. Grasp the hem of the sheet with one hand, approximately a foot in from the end of the bed, and pull it up vertically, creating a triangle. Place the triangle on top of the mattress.

C. Tuck the hanging, or bottom, part of the sheet underneath the mattress with both hands.

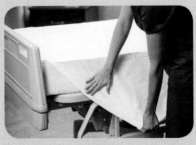
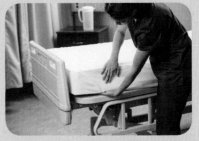

D. Lift the triangle corner of the sheet off the mattress with one hand and tightly pull it down toward the floor. Smooth out any wrinkles with your other hand.

E. Tuck the sheet under the mattress tightly with one hand, while smoothing out the mitered corner with the other hand. Miter each corner of the bed.

© Tori Soper Photography

Figure 20.13 Mitered corners should be used with a flat bottom sheet, top sheet, and bedspread.

Method 1		Method 2

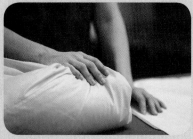 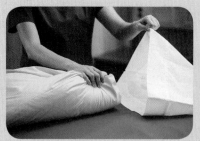 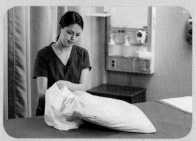

A. Lay the pillow and pillowcase on a flat surface. With one hand, fold the pillow at one end.

B. Open the pillowcase with the other hand.

A. Lay the pillow on a flat surface. With one hand, grasp the outside of the pillowcase's closed end and the middle of the pillow's short side.

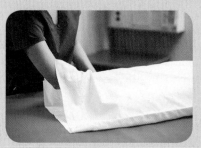 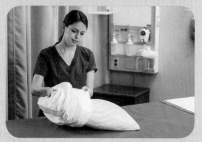

C. Insert the pillow.

D. Fit the corners of the pillow into the corners of the pillowcase.

B. While holding the pillowcase and pillow, use your other hand to bring the pillowcase over the pillow.

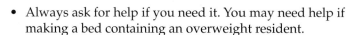

© Tori Soper Photography

Figure 20.14 The two methods for changing a pillowcase are illustrated here.

Guidelines for Bed Making

Whether you are making an open, closed, or surgical bed, the following guidelines can help you provide holistic care and promote safety:

- Pay attention to the condition of the bed. Are the linens very wrinkled or in disarray? Are the linens soiled? If so, remake the bed with fresh, clean linens.

- Always ask for help if you need it. You may need help if making a bed containing an overweight resident.

- If residents have dressings, tubes, or an IV catheter, be sure not to dislodge these devices when changing the linens.

- Be mindful of fragile skin as you move a resident in bed and make sure the skin is not scraped or bruised.

- Make sure the bed linen is not too tight around and on top of the feet, particularly if the resident is an older adult. To prevent this from happening, create a *toe pleat*. Fold the linen at the top of the resident's feet. Then grasp the fold and lift it gently so the resident can move his or her feet freely (Figure 20.15).

- Always follow facility policy and consider safety and comfort during and after bed-making procedures.

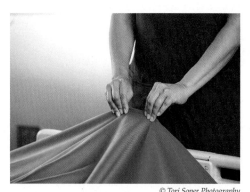

© Tori Soper Photography

Figure 20.15 A toe pleat can prevent bed linens from being too tight around and on top of the feet.

Rationale

An occupied bed is made when a resident is not able or permitted to be out of bed. Making an occupied bed provides an opportunity to observe the resident's skin integrity. Alert the licensed nursing staff if you observe any redness, sores, or decubitus ulcers.

Preparation

1. Ask the licensed nursing staff how this procedure fits into the plan of care, if there are doctor's orders for the procedure, if there are any special instructions or precautions, and if the resident can be moved into the positions required for this procedure.

2. Wash your hands or use hand sanitizer before entering the room.

3. Knock before entering the room.

4. Introduce yourself using your full name and title. Explain that you work with the licensed nursing staff and will be providing care.

5. Greet the resident and ask the resident to state his full name, if able. Then check the resident's identification bracelet.

6. Use Mr., Mrs., or Ms. and the last name when conversing.

7. Explain the procedure in simple terms, even if the resident is not able to communicate or is disoriented. Ask permission to perform the procedure.

8. Bring the necessary equipment into the room. Place the following items in an accessible location:
   - laundry hamper
   - 1 bath blanket
   - 1 bottom sheet (flat or fitted)
   - 1 top, flat sheet
   - 1 cotton draw sheet, if needed
   - 1 disposable protective pad, if needed
   - 1 bedspread, if used
   - 2 blankets
   - pillowcases, depending on how many pillows are being used

> **Best Practice**
> Once you bring linens into a room, the linens cannot be used for another resident, not even a roommate. Never bring in more linens than you need. Remove any unused linens, as they are considered contaminated (dirty).

The Procedure

9. Provide privacy by closing the curtains, using a screen, or closing the door to the room.

10. Lock the bed wheels and then raise the bed to hip level.

11. Ensure safety during the procedure. If there are side rails, raise and secure the rails on the opposite side of the bed from where you will be working. Lower the rail on the side you are working.

> **Best Practice**
> Disposable gloves are worn only if required for infection prevention and control.

12. Arrange the clean linens in the order they will be used.

13. Remove the call light from the bed.

14. Make sure the bed is flat, unless otherwise indicated by the plan of care.

15. Loosen the top linens from the foot of the bed.

> **Best Practice**
> Never shake any linens, whether they are clean or dirty. Shaking them can spread pathogens.

16. Place the bath blanket over the top linens (blanket and top sheet).

17. Ask the resident to hold the top edge of the bath blanket or tuck it under the resident's shoulders.

18. Remove the top linens from under the bath blanket. Be careful not to expose the resident.

19. Place the top linens in the laundry hamper.

20. Make the bed one side at a time. If the mattress has slipped out of place, ask a coworker to help you move it to the head of the bed before continuing.

(continued)

Making an Occupied Bed (continued)

21. Ask the resident to turn toward the side of the bed farthest from you and grasp the side rail, if used.

22. Help the resident turn, if necessary. Keep the resident covered with the bath blanket.

23. Move the pillow with the resident and adjust it under the head for comfort.

24. Starting at the head of the bed, loosen the soiled bottom linens. Remove and dispose of the disposable protective pad, if used.

25. Roll the soiled bottom linens toward the resident and tuck them against his back (Figure 20.16).

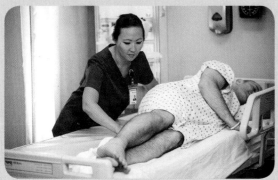

Figure 20.16

26. Place a clean bottom sheet on top of the mattress. If using a fitted bottom sheet, pull the corners of the sheet tightly and smoothly over the corners of the mattress. Smooth the sheet and tuck it tightly under the top and side of the mattress. If using a flat sheet, place the center fold next to the resident. The narrow hem should come to the foot edge of the mattress. Tuck the top of the sheet under the head of the mattress. Make a mitered, or square, corner and tuck the sheet under the side of the mattress working toward the foot of the bed.

27. If used, position the draw sheet with the center fold next to the resident. Tuck it under the mattress.

28. Ask the resident to roll toward you and over all of the soiled linens. Assist the resident, if needed. Move the pillow and bath blanket with the resident.

29. Raise and secure the side rail, if used. Then go to the opposite side rail and lower it.

30. Remove the soiled bottom linens by rolling the edges inward and toward you. Put the soiled linens in the laundry hamper.

Best Practice
Never allow soiled linens to touch your scrubs.

31. Pull the clean bottom sheet into place as quickly as possible (Figure 20.17). If using a fitted bottom sheet, pull the corners of the sheet tightly and smoothly over the corners of the mattress. Smooth the sheet and tuck it tightly under the top and side of the mattress. If using a flat sheet, tuck the sides under the mattress at the head and foot of the bed. Make a mitered corner at each end. Pull the sheet tight and tuck it under the mattress from top to bottom.

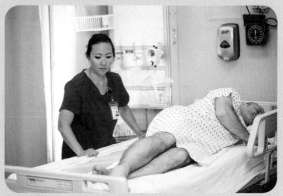

Figure 20.17

32. If used, pull the draw sheet tight and tuck it in. Place an a disposable protective pad on top of the draw sheet and under the resident's buttocks, if needed.

33. Ask the resident to lie on his back in the center of the bed. Assist him into this position if he cannot move himself.

34. Change the pillowcases and place the pillows under the resident's head. Discard the used pillowcases in the laundry hamper.

Best Practice
When changing pillowcases, help the resident move his head, if needed. Have the resident raise his head when you remove the pillow and help, if needed. When the pillow is removed, keep the resident flat in bed to avoid neck injury.

35. Place the clean top sheet over the resident.

36. Remove the bath blanket. Discard the bath blanket in the laundry hamper.

37. Place the blanket and bedspread (if used) on the resident. Tuck these in at the bottom of the bed and make mitered corners.

38. If needed, create room for the toes by making toe pleats in the top linens.

39. Once the resident is positioned comfortably, lower the bed.

40. Follow the plan of care to determine if the side rails should be raised or lowered.

Follow-Up

41. Wash your hands to ensure infection control.

42. Make sure the resident is comfortable and place the call light and personal items within reach.

43. Conduct a safety check before leaving the room. The room should be clean and free from clutter or spills.

44. Wash your hands or use hand sanitizer before leaving the room.

Reporting and Documentation

45. Communicate any specific observations, complications, or unusual responses to the licensed nursing staff. Record this information, along with the care provided, in the chart or EMR.

Images courtesy of © Tori Soper Photography

Procedure | Making an Unoccupied Bed

Rationale

An unoccupied bed may be made open or closed. A closed bed is made with the top linens pulled to the head of the bed. An open bed is made with the top linens fanfolded at the foot of the bed.

Preparation

1. Wash your hands or use hand sanitizer before entering the room.

2. If the room is occupied, knock before entering. If you know the room is vacant, skip ahead to step 7.

3. Introduce yourself using your full name and title. Explain that you work with the licensed nursing staff and will be providing care.

4. Greet the resident and ask the resident to state his or her full name, if able. Then check the resident's identification bracelet.

5. Use Mr., Mrs., or Ms. and the last name when conversing.

6. Explain the procedure in simple terms, even if the resident is not able to communicate or is disoriented. Ask permission to perform the procedure.

7. Bring the necessary equipment into the room. Place the following items in an accessible location:
   - laundry hamper
   - 1 bottom sheet (flat or fitted)
   - 1 top sheet

- 1 cotton draw sheet, if needed
- 1 disposable protective pad, if needed
- 1 bedspread, if used
- 2 blankets
- pillowcases, depending on how many pillows are being used
- mattress pad, if used (Figure 20.18)

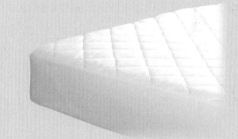

Figure 20.18

The Procedure

8. Lock the bed wheels and then raise the bed to hip level or a comfortable working level. Lower the side rails, if used.

> **Best Practice**
> Disposable gloves are worn only if required for infection prevention and control.

(continued)

9. Arrange the clean linens in the order they will be used.

10. Remove the soiled linens by rolling the edges inward. Deposit them in the laundry hamper.

> **Best Practice**
> Never allow soiled linens to touch your scrubs.

11. If the mattress has slid down, move it back to the head of the bed.

12. To conserve time and energy, work on one side of the bed until that side is complete. Then go to the other side of the bed.

13. If used, place the mattress pad even with the top of the mattress and unfold it. Pull the corners of the mattress pad tightly and smoothly over the corners of the mattress.

14. Place the bottom sheet on top of the mattress pad. Unfold the sheet lengthwise. The center fold should be in the middle of the bed, and the hem stitching should face the mattress pad. The small hem should be at the foot of the bed.

15. If using a fitted bottom sheet, pull the corners of the sheet tightly and smoothly over the corners of the mattress. Smooth the sheet and tuck it tightly under the top and side of the mattress. If using a flat sheet, make a mitered corner. Tuck the sheet in at the head of the bed and along the side of the bed to the foot. Repeat this step on the other side of the bed.

16. If used, place a draw sheet on the bed (Figure 20.19). Tuck it under the mattress. Place a disposable protective pad on top of and in the center of the draw sheet.

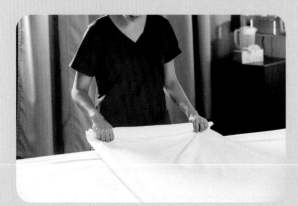

Figure 20.19

17. Unfold and apply the top sheet with the wrong side up. Place the hem even with the upper edge of the mattress and the center fold in the center of the bed.

18. Keeping the blanket centered, spread it over the top sheet and foot of the mattress. Do the same with the bedspread, if used.

19. Tuck the top sheet, blanket, and bedspread (if used) under the mattress at the foot of the bed.

20. If making a closed bed, make a mitered corner at the foot of the bed and tuck in the sides of the top sheet, blanket, and bedspread, if used (Figure 20.20). Fold the top sheet back over the blanket to make an 8-inch cuff at the head of the bed.

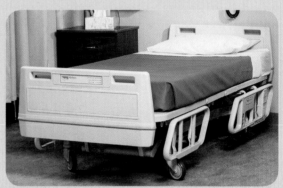

Figure 20.20

21. If making an open bed, do not tuck in the sides of the bedspread (if used), blanket, and top sheet. Instead, face the head of the bed and grasp these linens with both hands. Fanfold the bed linens to the foot of the bed (Figure 20.21). Smooth the hanging sheet on both sides of the bed.

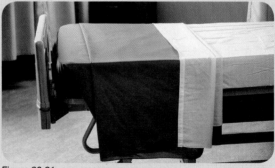

Figure 20.21

22. Insert the pillows into the pillowcases.

23. Place the pillows at the head of the bed. The open ends of the pillowcases should face away from the door.

24. Check to be sure the bed wheels are locked, then lower the bed to its lowest position.

Follow-Up

25. Wash your hands to ensure infection control.

26. Place the call light on the bed.

27. Replace the bedside stand next to the bed if it was moved to make the bed.

28. Place the chair in its assigned location.

29. Place the overbed table over the foot of the bed, opposite the chair.

30. Take the laundry hamper to the proper location.

31. Conduct a safety check before leaving the room. The room should be clean and free from clutter or spills.

32. Wash your hands or use hand sanitizer before leaving the room.

Reporting and Documentation

This is an accepted, standard procedure. It does not need to be reported or documented.

Figure 20.19 Luisa Leal Photography/Shutterstock.com; Figure 20.20 © Tori Soper Photography; Figure 21.21 © Tori Soper Photography

Procedure | Making a Surgical Bed

Rationale

Properly arranging bed linens can promote ease in quickly and smoothly moving a patient from a stretcher into bed after a surgery or procedure.

Preparation

1. Wash your hands or use hand sanitizer before entering the room. You do not need to knock, as the room will be unoccupied.

2. Bring the necessary equipment into the room. Place the following items in an accessible location:
   - laundry hamper
   - 1 bottom sheet (flat or fitted)
   - 1 top sheet
   - 1 draw sheet, if needed
   - disposable protective pad, if needed
   - 1 bedspread, if used
   - 2 blankets
   - pillowcases, depending on how many pillows are being used
   - mattress pad, if used

The Procedure

3. Lock the bed wheels and then raise the bed to hip level or a comfortable working level.

> **Best Practice**
> Disposable gloves are worn only if required for infection prevention and control.

4. Arrange the clean linens in the order they will be used.

5. Strip the bed and deposit any used linens in the laundry hamper.

6. Wash your hands or use hand sanitizer to ensure infection control.

7. Make the bottom layer of the bed like an unoccupied, closed bed. Start by placing the mattress pad, if used, even with the top of the mattress and unfolding it. Pull the corners of the mattress pad tightly and smoothly over the corners of the mattress.

8. Place the bottom sheet on top of the mattress pad. Unfold the sheet lengthwise. The center fold should be in the middle of the bed, and the hem stitching should face the mattress pad. The small hem should be at the foot of the bed.

9. If using a fitted bottom sheet, pull the corners of the sheet tightly and smoothly over the corners of the mattress. Smooth the sheet and tuck it tightly under the top and side of the mattress. If using a flat sheet, make a mitered corner. Tuck the sheet in at the head of the bed and along the side of the bed to the foot.

10. If used, place a draw sheet on the bed. Tuck it under the mattress. Place a disposable protective pad on top and in the center of the draw sheet, if needed.

11. Make the top layer of the bed like an unoccupied, closed bed, but do not tuck in the bottom sheet, blanket(s), and bedspread. Start by unfolding and applying the top sheet with the wrong side up. Place the hem even with the upper edge of the mattress so the center fold is in the center of the bed.

(continued)

12. Keeping the blanket centered, spread it over the top sheet and foot of the mattress. Do the same with the bedspread, if used.

13. Fold the top linens back from the foot of the bed and onto the bed, even with the edge of the mattress.

14. Fanfold the top linens lengthwise away from the side of the bed where the stretcher will be placed. (The stretcher is usually positioned on the side of the bed nearest the door.) This leaves that side of the bed open to receive the patient.

15. Put the pillowcases on the pillows according to procedure and place the pillows upright against the headboard. This will help prevent the patient's head from hitting the headboard during transfer from the stretcher to the bed.

16. Leave the wheels of the bed locked and raise the bed to its highest position.

17. Leave both side rails down.

18. Move furniture away from the bed to make room for the stretcher.

Follow-Up

19. Place the call light on the bedside stand or under the pillow until the patient comes to the room.

20. Return the laundry hamper to the proper location.

21. Conduct a safety check before leaving the room. The room should be clean and free from clutter or spills.

22. Wash your hands or use hand sanitizer before leaving the room.

Reporting and Documentation

This is an accepted, standard procedure. It does not need to be reported or documented.

Section 20.2 Review and Assessment

Using the Key Terms

Complete the following sentences using key terms in this section.

1. A(n) _____ can be used to help turn a resident in bed.

2. A highly absorbent _____ is often used to absorb drainage and prevent the bed from becoming soiled.

3. _____ keep residents warm during a bed bath.

Know and Understand the Facts

4. Explain two reasons why properly making a bed is important for providing care.

5. Describe three different types of linens used when making beds.

6. Identify three important guidelines for making beds.

7. What is a toe pleat and why is it important?

Analyze and Apply Concepts

8. Describe the differences between making an occupied and unoccupied bed.

9. When should an unoccupied bed be made?

10. Explain the steps for making a surigcal bed.

Think Critically

Read the following care situation. Then answer the questions that follow.

Farah has been asked to make Mrs. G's bed. Mrs. G has diabetes and is quite overweight. She is bedridden today after a procedure to clean a wound on her leg. The wound now has a dressing, and Mrs. G also has an IV catheter. Farah knows she will need to make an occupied bed.

11. Which steps of the bed-making procedure should Farah be especially aware of when making Mrs. G's bed?

12. How should Farah handle Mrs. G's IV catheter and dressing as she makes the bed?

13. Given that Mrs. G has diabetes and is overweight, are there any special steps Farah should take during and after the bed-making procedure?

Objectives

Promoting comfort, relaxation, rest, and sleep is an essential part of a holistic nursing assistant's responsibility. In this section, you will learn how comfort, relaxation, rest, and sleep significantly improve the quality of a resident's experience and contributes to the healing process and wellness. To achieve the objectives for this section, you must successfully

- **discuss** how comfort, relaxation, rest, and sleep contribute to healing and better health;
- **describe** ways holistic nursing assistants can promote and provide comfort, relaxation, rest, and sleep; and
- **demonstrate** how and when to give appropriate and effective back rubs.

Key Terms

Learn these key terms to better understand the information presented in the section.

dysrhythmia   hallucinations

fatigue   sleep deprivation

Questions to Consider

- Sleep is an important part of maintaining a healthy life balance. How many hours do you sleep each night? Do you get too little, too much, or just the right amount of sleep?
- If you do not get enough sleep, what keeps you from sleeping? Is lack of sleep a recent development or something you have experienced your whole life? Have your sleeping patterns affected your life while awake?
- If you want to change your sleeping patterns, what could you do differently?

When patients and residents are comfortable, feel relaxed, and have enough rest and sleep, they heal and achieve a sense of well-being more quickly and effectively. Therefore, it is essential that holistic nursing assistants demonstrate sensitivity to and promote the kind of environment that achieves these outcomes.

How Do Nursing Assistants Provide Comfort?

There are two aspects of comfort in healthcare. The first is the resident's feeling of comfort. The second is the actions the holistic nursing assistant takes to promote and give comfort. Comfort is usually a personal experience learned over time. Residents may find comfort in an object, the presence of family and friends, a particular food, or the memory of good health. For those who have chronic pain, a period of being pain free can bring comfort. To promote and give comfort, holistic nursing assistants must learn what is comfortable for others.

In the early 1990s, a nursing theorist named Katharine Kolcaba developed the *Theory of Comfort*. She found that comfort exists in three forms: relief, ease, and transcendence. *Relief* occurs when comfort needs are met, and the resident experiences a sense of relief. *Ease* is a feeling of contentment or peace (for example, after resolving a stressful issue). *Transcendence* takes place when residents rise above challenges to achieve comfort (for example, by learning how to walk again after a paralyzing stroke).

Comfort is experienced in different dimensions. It can be physical, spiritual, sociocultural, and environmental. To promote and give comfort, holistic nursing assistants must observe levels of comfort. They can do this by asking residents what is comfortable for them, being sensitive to any culturally relevant issues related to comfort, identifying and performing actions that promote comfort, and asking if actions achieve the desired levels of comfort.

In chapter 9, you learned about the importance of relieving pain to achieve comfort. Helping residents with pain relief is an important part of holistic care and will promote comfort. Some pain-relief approaches for residents include

- being sensitive to and aware of residents experiencing pain during care;
- keeping the licensed nursing staff informed of resident pain levels;
- making use of relaxation activities, deep breathing, and comfortable positioning; and
- providing massages and range-of-motion exercises, as appropriate.

How Can Nursing Assistants Promote Relaxation?

Relaxation is another important aspect of healing. Relaxing reduces stress hormones and provides a healthy internal and external environment.

Relaxation is a personal experience. What some people find relaxing may not be relaxing for others. For example, some people find exercise relaxing, while others think it is tiring and stressful. However relaxation is achieved, it is an essential part of wellness. Residents coping with a disease or condition may find it challenging to relax. When a resident is seriously ill or in pain, relaxation can seem impossible. Still, it is important for holistic nursing assistants to promote relaxation.

Some pain-relief approaches, such as deep breathing and soothing music, can help a resident relax. One technique is *mindful presence*, the practice of checking your body for thoughts and feelings of stress and then consciously letting go of these stressful feelings and thoughts. Many people also find yoga or meditation relaxing. As a holistic nursing assistant, you can relax by showing residents you feel grateful for each day, laughing out loud, giving a reassuring smile, and simply providing a human touch. These actions may result in residents feeling relaxed as well. In response, residents may sigh, let out a deep breath, sit back, loosen their shoulders, and laugh and smile back at you (Figure 20.22).

Why Are Rest and Sleep Important?

There is a difference between rest and sleep, and both rest and sleep are essential to health, well-being, and relaxation. *Rest* can occur at any time and is usually the result of **fatigue** (extreme tiredness). In contrast, *sleep* is necessary for survival and must occur daily. Sleep restores the body's energy, helps repair muscle tissue, and releases hormones that promote growth in children and young adults.

Circadian Rhythm

The body has a natural sleep-wake cycle called *circadian rhythm*. Circadian rhythm is controlled by structures in the brain that help regulate sleepiness and wakefulness over 24 hours. Circadian rhythm responds to light, causing people to sleep when it is dark and be awake when it is light. Depending on circadian rhythm, some people are "morning people," while others are more productive in the evening. As people age, their circadian rhythm can change, and people may develop sleep problems or disorders. Travel across times zones can disrupt circadian rhythm and cause jet lag. It may take the body a few days to adjust to a new time zone or overcome the temporary fatigue caused by jet lag. People who have vision problems and cannot detect light may also have trouble sleeping due to disrupted circadian rhythm.

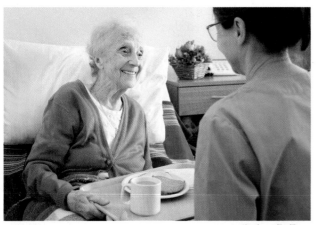

iStock.com/FredFroese

Figure 20.22 If you are relaxed, residents may follow your lead and seem more comfortable in their environment.

Sleep Deprivation

When people get too little sleep, they may experience **sleep deprivation**. Recent research has found that one in three adults does not get the recommended seven hours of sleep each night (Figure 20.23). When people get too little sleep, they usually need even more sleep to make up for loss of sleep. Insufficient sleep causes a person to be drowsy and makes it difficult to concentrate. Ongoing sleep deprivation can lead to impaired memory and unsafe physical performance. It can generate mood swings and **hallucinations** (visual, verbal, or physical perceptions that are not real, but are mistaken for reality). Sleeping problems are common among people with heart disease, diabetes, Alzheimer's disease, stroke, cancer, and mental disorders such as depression and schizophrenia. Sleep deprivation can increase a person's risk for obesity, headaches, and epileptic seizures.

Recommended Hours of Sleep by Age Group	
Age Group	**Recommended Hours of Sleep**
Infants	16–18
Toddlers	11–12
School-age children	10
Adolescents	9–10
Adults	7–8

Figure 20.23 Recommended hours of sleep are highest during childhood. Adults should get 7–8 hours of sleep each night.

Sleep Stages

The quality of sleep is important to health. Sleep quality is associated with how much time a person spends in the *REM (rapid eye movement)* stage of sleep. There are five stages of sleep: four stages of nonREM (NREM) sleep and one stage of REM sleep, which is the most restorative. During sleep, a person goes through each of the five stages of sleep and then keeps cycling through them. The number of sleep cycles a person has and the lengths of the sleep stages can be affected by a person's age; the time of day or night; recent amounts of sleep, exercise, and stress; and environmental conditions (such as room temperature and lighting).

A full sleep cycle lasts about 90–110 minutes. The first cycle of sleep contains a short REM stage with longer periods of deeper sleep (stages 3 and 4). As people sleep longer, they experience longer REM stages and shorter periods of deep sleep. Specific events occur during each stage of the sleep cycle (Figure 20.24).

NREM Stage 1

Stage 1 is the lightest stage of sleep, in which people feel they are drifting in and out of sleep. In this stage, people can be awakened easily. If awakened, some people experience sudden muscle contractions or jump as if startled. In this stage, the body begins to slow down and relax. Little time is spent in stage 1.

NREM Stage 2

The second stage of sleep is still considered light sleep; however, brain activity, heart rate, and breathing start to slow down. The body continues to relax in preparation for deeper sleep in later stages.

NREM Stage 3

Deep sleep begins in stage 3. The brain's electrical activity is very slow, although there are some bursts of activity. A person awakened during this stage will likely feel groggy, be confused, and have difficulty focusing.

NREM Stage 4

The deepest stage of the sleep cycle is stage 4. Stages 3 and 4 typically last 5–15 minutes each, but are about one hour long in the first sleep cycle. The body begins its repairs during stage 4 of sleep. It is usually difficult to wake someone from deep sleep. There is no eye movement or muscle activity during this stage. Children may experience night terrors, bedwetting, or sleep walking during deep sleep.

Think About This

According to the National Highway Traffic Safety Administration, driver fatigue is responsible for approximately 100,000 police-reported auto accidents, 1,550 deaths, and 71,000 injuries each year in the United States. If a person feels drowsy while driving and can't stop yawning, he or she is experiencing driver fatigue, is likely not driving safely, and needs to pull over.

Remember

Take rest; a field that has rested gives a bountiful crop.
Ovid, Roman poet

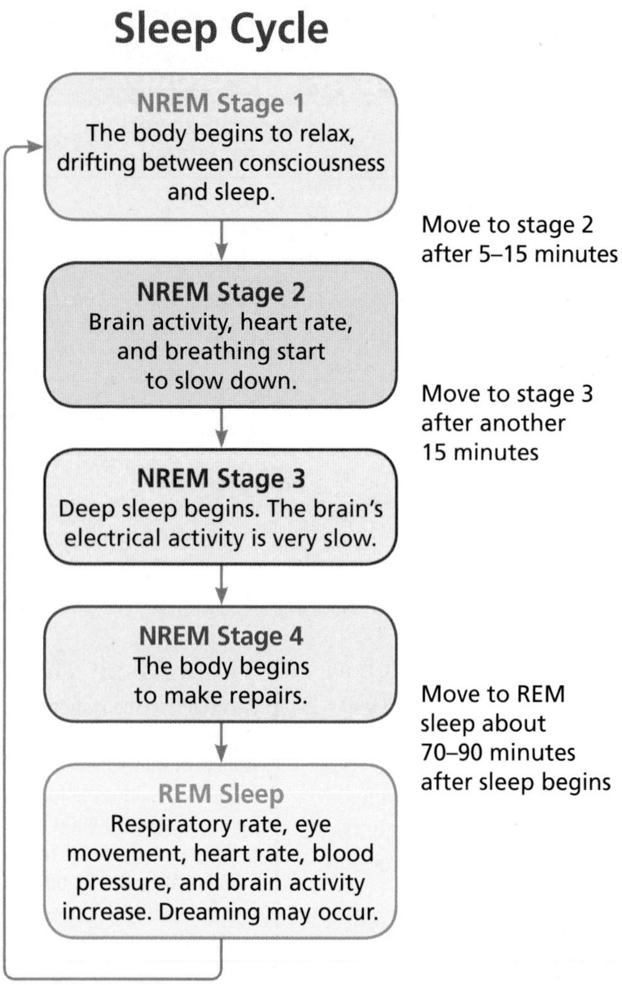

Sleep Cycle

NREM Stage 1
The body begins to relax, drifting between consciousness and sleep.

Move to stage 2 after 5–15 minutes

NREM Stage 2
Brain activity, heart rate, and breathing start to slow down.

Move to stage 3 after another 15 minutes

NREM Stage 3
Deep sleep begins. The brain's electrical activity is very slow.

NREM Stage 4
The body begins to make repairs.

Move to REM sleep about 70–90 minutes after sleep begins

REM Sleep
Respiratory rate, eye movement, heart rate, blood pressure, and brain activity increase. Dreaming may occur.

Figure 20.24 There are five stages of sleep. These five stages cycle repeatedly as long as a person is asleep.

REM Sleep

The fifth stage of sleep is *REM sleep* or *active sleep*. During this stage, people can dream. Breathing is rapid and irregular, the eyes jerk, heart rate and blood pressure rise, and brain activity increases until it is similar to wakefulness. The muscles in the arms and legs become periodically paralyzed, possibly to prevent people from acting out their dreams. If awakened from REM sleep, people will often be able to describe their dreams.

REM sleep happens often throughout the night. It first occurs about 70–90 minutes after sleep begins and lasts for about 10 minutes. REM sleep happens again as sleep continues, and the final period of REM lasts about one hour.

Healthy Sleep Habits

Good sleep habits can help people get the sleep they need. Some good sleep habits include the following:

- Set a regular schedule for going to sleep and waking up.
- Limit the number and length of naps during the day. A short nap may be restful and help meet sleep requirements, but too many naps can interfere with the ability to sleep at night.
- Avoid large meals, caffeinated drinks (coffee or tea), chocolate, and soft drinks. Some medications may also cause sleeplessness.
- Relax before bed and sleep in a comfortable, quiet, and dark environment with a temperature conducive to sleep.
- Use restful activities such as warm baths, deep breathing, and activities associated with relaxation to help induce sleep.
- Pursue activities such as reading or listening to music if you cannot fall asleep.
- Exercise during the day, but not five to six hours before going to sleep.

Sleep Disorders

Nearly 70 million people in the United States have sleep disorders. The most common sleep disorders are insomnia, sleep apnea, narcolepsy, and restless legs syndrome (RLS). All of these sleep disorders can have significant effects on residents and their mobility, ability to manage ADLs, and general health and well-being.

Insomnia

Insomnia is a sleep disorder characterized by the inability to fall or stay asleep. One in 10 US adults has *chronic insomnia*, which is defined as one episode of sleeplessness each week. Between 20 and 30 percent of adults experience temporary insomnia at any given time. Sleep medications may be prescribed to treat insomnia, but insomnia is best managed by healthy sleep habits.

Sleep Apnea

Interrupted breathing during sleep is called *sleep apnea* or *obstructive sleep apnea*. Sleep apnea may cause periodic gasping, snorting, or snoring. For about 10–20 seconds, a person may struggle to breathe. Blood oxygen will decrease, and the person will

Think About This

There is some evidence that lavender essential oil has chemical properties that can lower heart rate, decrease blood pressure, and help a person fall asleep faster. Lavender essential oil can be applied to the skin, put in bathwater, or used in aromatherapy. Care should always be taken, as the substance may interact with prescribed medications, diseases, or conditions. If in a healthcare facility, always check with the licensed nursing staff before considering the use of lavender essential oil.

wake up enough to resume breathing. This may occur many times during the sleep cycle, leaving people with feelings of irritability and depression and a morning headache.

People with sleep apnea have increased risks for stroke or heart attack. Sleep apnea may be the result of obesity and can be treated through losing weight or sleeping on the side. A *continuous positive airway pressure (CPAP) machine* can increase pressure on the throat and prevent it from collapsing (Figure 20.25). Surgery may be prescribed to treat sleep apnea in some cases. People with sleep apnea should not take sleep medications that prevent them from waking during the night. In the United States, approximately 12–18 million people have sleep apnea, and one-quarter of these people are middle-age men.

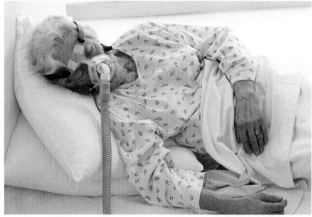

JPC-PROD/Shutterstock.com

Figure 20.25 The CPAP machine helps treat sleep apnea by preventing the throat from collapsing.

Narcolepsy

Severe daytime sleepiness with uncontrollable, sometimes sudden periods of sleep is called *narcolepsy*. Signs of narcolepsy include sudden loss of voluntary muscle control and feelings of weakness ranging from slurred speech to collapse, hallucinations, or sleep paralysis. Episodes of narcolepsy are sometimes called *sleep attacks*. These attacks may last several seconds or minutes during the day. After episodes end, recovery is usually rapid. Narcolepsy often develops during childhood and is considered a genetic disease because it occurs more frequently in families. A brain injury or neurological disease may also cause narcolepsy.

Narcolepsy affects an estimated 1 in 2,000 people in the United States. It is usually treated with prescription medications, such as stimulants or antidepressants. These medications help people avoid falling asleep at inappropriate times. Scheduled naps are also helpful.

Restless Legs Syndrome (RLS)

Restless legs syndrome (RLS) causes an unpleasant creeping, crawling, and prickling sensation in the legs and feet. This feeling makes people want to move their legs to find relief. One in 10 people in the United States have RLS, which is usually inherited. Constant leg movements, aches, and pains can make it challenging to fall and stay asleep, leading to insomnia. Symptoms can occur at any age, but RLS is more common among older adults. RLS can often be relieved with prescription medications.

How Can Nursing Assistants Promote a Comfortable Environment?

A comfortable, relaxing, and restful environment helps promote healing. Providing this environment is an important part of giving holistic care. Holistic nursing assistants can create a healing environment by providing books or magazines to read, suggesting social activities of interest, encouraging residents to spend time with family members, turning on a favorite television program, playing music, repositioning residents, or suggesting a nap. Keeping noise levels down is also an important part of promoting a comfortable environment. Regular exposure to a noisy environment can lead to hearing impairment and loss and hypertension.

Helping residents feel relaxed is particularly important in the evening, before residents go to bed. Holistic nursing assistants can help create a relaxing, restful environment by providing evening, or *p.m. care*, or giving a back rub.

The duties of evening or p.m. care are performed in the evening hours when a resident is getting ready to sleep. Evening care typically includes taking routine vital signs, if ordered; assisting with elimination and measuring output; helping residents

Remember

Sleep is that golden chain that ties health and our bodies together.

Thomas Dekker,
English playwright

Think About This

The relative intensity of sound is measured using units called *decibels*. Prolonged exposure to sounds over 85 decibels may cause hearing loss. According to the National Institute of Occupational Safety and Health, the following decibel measurements are associated with these common sounds:

- 140 decibels = jet taking off
- 120 decibels = ambulance siren
- 90 decibels = hair dryer
- 60 decibels = normal conversation
- 30 decibels = whisper

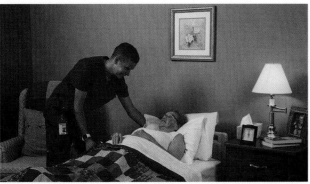

© Tori Soper Photography

Figure 20.26 Evening care helps get a resident ready to go to bed. Evening care should promote relaxation and comfort at the end of the day.

wash their faces, comb their hair, and perform oral care; and assisting in changing soiled gowns or pajamas. Other duties include straightening bed linens; changing soiled sheets or blankets; arranging pillows and assistive devices for a comfortable position; and providing fresh drinking water, unless the patient or resident is NPO (*nothing by mouth*) for an ordered procedure or surgery the next day (Figure 20.26).

Giving a *back rub*, if appropriate, is another common nursing assistant responsibility. A back rub should *not* be performed without permission from the doctor or licensed nursing staff; if the resident refuses; or if there are burns on the back, rib or spinal fractures, pulmonary embolism, or open wounds. If the resident has hypertension or **dysrhythmia** (abnormal heart rhythm), measure the resident's pulse and blood pressure to be sure it is safe to give a back rub. Back rubs can be given during morning or a.m. care, during evening or p.m. care, after a bath, or after changing a position.

Maintaining privacy during care is essential. For example, close the curtains around the resident. While giving care, talk with residents about the day's activities and experiences. Ask residents about any health or treatment gains they have made, any problems they have encountered, their feelings, and any pain. Report residents' answers (particularly related to pain levels and difficulty sleeping) to the licensed nursing staff and document pertinent items. Some residents may want to listen to music, read, or watch television prior to sleeping. Remember that leaving the lights or any electronics on can disturb the sleep cycle. Make sure radio or television volumes are at a reasonable level and that controls are in reach. Also ask if the resident would like any other personal items nearby.

Evening care helps promote physical and emotional well-being at the end of the day. Be gentle and talk in soft tones when giving care. Wash your hands or use hand sanitizer before and after any activities, as well as when you enter and leave the room. You may need to wear gloves, if appropriate, to ensure infection control.

Procedure   Giving a Back Rub

Rationale

Back rubs stimulate circulation to the skin and muscles, relieve muscle tension and stiffness, promote comfort and relaxation, help relieve pain, and offer nursing assistants an opportunity to observe the resident's skin for any redness or decubitus ulcers.

Preparation

1. Ask the licensed nursing staff how this procedure fits into the plan of care, if there are doctor's orders for the procedure, if there are any special instructions or precautions, and if the resident can be moved into the positions required for this procedure.

2. Wash your hands or use hand sanitizer before entering the room.

3. Knock before entering the room.

4. Introduce yourself using your full name and title. Explain that you work with the licensed nursing staff and will be providing care.

5. Greet the resident and ask the resident to state his full name, if able. Then check the resident's identification bracelet.

6. Use Mr., Mrs., or Ms. and the last name when conversing.

7. Explain the procedure in simple terms, even if the resident is not able to communicate or is disoriented. Ask permission to perform the procedure.

8. Bring the necessary equipment into the room. Place the following items in an accessible location:

   • a basin of warm water (100–105°F)

   • 1 hand towel

- 2 bath towels
- 1 bath blanket
- body lotion (one the resident has used before or one that will not irritate the skin)
- disposable gloves
- laundry hamper

Cover the bedside stand with the hand towel and then place the needed equipment and linens on top of the bedside stand.

The Procedure

9. Provide privacy by closing the curtains, using a screen, or closing the door to the room.

> **Best Practice**
> You should explain the procedure to the resident before starting. During the back rub, however, you may not want to talk with the resident. Silence can help create a relaxing environment. Pay special attention to the resident's behavior, attitude, responses to the procedure, and interactions with you.

10. Lock the bed wheels and then raise the bed to hip level.

11. Ensure safety during the procedure. If there are side rails, raise and secure the rails on the opposite side of the bed from where you will be working. Lower the rail on the side you are working.

> **Best Practice**
> Disposable gloves are worn only if required for infection prevention and control.

12. Place the lotion bottle in the basin of warm water.

13. Make sure the room is a comfortable temperature. Dim the lights, if appropriate.

14. Cover the resident with the bath blanket. If possible, ask the resident to hold the bath blanket while you fanfold the bed linens to the foot of the bed. Be sure the resident is not exposed.

15. If permitted, help the resident turn to the prone position. Otherwise, move him to a side-lying position facing away from you. Use whichever position is most comfortable and appropriate for the resident.

16. Expose the resident's back. Keep the rest of the body covered with the bath blanket.

17. Check the skin for signs of redness. Pay special attention to the coccyx (*tailbone*) and bony areas.

18. Pour a small amount of lotion into the palm of your hand. Rub your hands together and use friction to continue warming the lotion.

19. Keep your knees slightly bent and your back straight to maintain good body mechanics. Apply the warm lotion to the resident's back.

20. Starting from the sacral area, make small, circular motions with the palms of your hands (Figure 20.27). Stroke upward on both sides of the spine and be sure to always apply pressure *away* from the spine. Move your hands up to the back of the neck.

21. Next, use firm, smooth strokes across and around the shoulders. Move down the upper arms, applying less pressure than on the shoulders.

22. Finally, using a circular motion, move your hands from the shoulders down the sides of the back to the buttocks.

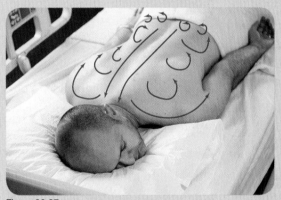

Figure 20.27

> **Best Practice**
> Massage gently and move slowly to help the resident relax. Ask if you are applying too much or too little pressure during the back rub. Do not massage painful or red areas and stop if the resident complains of numbness or tingling in the arms and legs or if the lotion causes a rash or feeling of itchiness.

23. Repeat the procedure for three to five minutes, adding more warm lotion as needed. Complete the back rub by providing long, gentle strokes up from the lower back to the base of the neck and down again several times.

(continued)

Giving a Back Rub (continued)

24. After completing the back rub, gently remove any excess lotion and pat the resident's skin dry with the bath towel.

25. Close or change the resident's gown or pajama top. Remove the bath blanket, straighten the linens, and tighten the bottom sheet.

26. Check to be sure the bed wheels are locked, then reposition the resident and lower the bed.

27. Follow the plan of care to determine if the side rails should be raised or lowered.

28. Remove, clean, and store equipment in the proper location. Remove soiled linens and discard disposable equipment.

Follow-Up

29. Wash your hands to ensure infection control.

30. Make sure the resident is comfortable and place the call light and personal items within reach.

31. Conduct a safety check before leaving the room. The room should be clean and free from clutter or spills.

32. Wash your hands or use hand sanitizer before leaving the room.

Reporting and Documentation

33. Communicate any specific observations, complications, or unusual responses to the licensed nursing staff. Record this information, along with the care provided, in the chart or EMR.

Image courtesy of © Tori Soper Photography

Section 20.3 Review and Assessment

Using the Key Terms

Complete the following sentences using key terms in this section.

1. An irregular heart rhythm is called _____.
2. _____ is a deficiency of the recommended hours of sleep.
3. Perceptions that are not real, but are mistaken for reality, are _____.
4. _____ is a feeling of extreme tiredness.

Know and Understand the Facts

5. Describe two ways sleep contributes to health.
6. Discuss three actions holistic nursing assistants can take to promote and provide comfort and relaxation.
7. What are the five stages of the sleep cycle?
8. Describe one sleep disorder.

Analyze and Apply Concepts

9. Discuss why rest and sleep are particularly important for older residents.
10. What are the responsibilities of providing evening or p.m. care?
11. Describe two best practices for performing a back rub.

Think Critically

Read the following care situation. Then answer the questions that follow.

Joe, a 22-year-old college student, was in a traumatic motorcycle accident. He has a concussion, second-degree burns on his arms, and numerous lacerations. He also fractured his right arm, right hip, right femur, and left ankle. After spending several weeks in the hospital, he was recently transferred to a rehabilitation facility. He has made great progress; however, his arm and leg are in casts and are not very mobile. He is depressed about his immobility and complains frequently that he cannot sleep at night, and is too uncomfortable to rest or relax during the day.

12. What do you know about rest and sleep that might help Joe?
13. What are three actions you could take to help Joe rest and sleep?

Key Points

Reviewing the key points for this chapter will help you practice more safely and competently as a holistic nursing assistant and will help you prepare for the certification competency examination.

- As a nursing assistant, you must promote and maintain a healing environment in the resident's room and create an atmosphere that fosters residents' rights and humanizes their experiences.
- Call lights should always be available and easily accessible for the resident. Answer the call light immediately, no matter how frequently it is used.
- Respect and keep residents' personal items safe.
- Healthcare facilities have beds that can be repositioned electronically or manually. Bed wheels can be locked and unlocked with a foot lever.
- Occupied, unoccupied, and surgical beds must be made according to procedure. When making a bed, consider safety, ask for help, and take special care with residents who have dressings, tubes, IV catheters, or fragile skin.
- Promoting comfort, rest, relaxation, and sleep is necessary for healing and well-being.

Action Steps to Holistic Care

Review the information in this chapter. Complete the following activities.

1. Prepare a short paper or digital presentation that describes how call systems should be used to ensure a safe environment for residents.
2. Research recently developed call light technology and create a poster or digital presentation outlining two new types of technology. Explain how this technology is used and how it might improve response time and patient or resident satisfaction.
3. With a partner, prepare a poster about making occupied, unoccupied, and surgical beds. Include the key steps and actions that ensure safety.
4. Practice the procedures for making a mitered corner and properly replacing a pillowcase. When you have finished, review your textbook to ensure the procedure was executed properly. If you made a mistake, repeat the procedure until you can execute it accurately.
5. Find one picture in a magazine, in a newspaper, or online that you believe best represents a safe, comfortable resident's room. Explain why you selected the image.

 Preparing for the Certification Competency Examination

To prepare for the nursing assistant certification competency examination, you will need to know content found in this chapter. This content may be tested in the knowledge (written or oral) and skills (hands-on demonstration) portions of the exam. The following areas will be emphasized:

- preparation of a room
- communication to meet resident needs
- fall prevention
- safety and security of personal items
- occupied, unoccupied, and surgical bed making
- comfort, relaxation, rest, and adequate sleep
- evening, or p.m., care
- ways to perform a back rub

These sample test questions are similar to ones you will find on the certification competency exam. See how well you can answer them. Be sure to select the *best* answer.

1. Excessive tiredness and sudden muscle weakness during the day are symptoms of
   - A. insomnia
   - B. narcolepsy
   - C. RLS
   - D. sleep apnea

2. The type of bed that residents can control themselves is a(n)
   - A. manual bed
   - B. electronic bed
   - C. occupied bed
   - D. motorized bed

(continued)

3. What kind of cycle does the call light system operate?

   A. receive and relate
   B. alert and respond
   C. notify and respond
   D. listen and act

4. What can a nursing assistant do to avoid spreading pathogens when handling linens?

   A. keep linens close to his or her uniform
   B. avoid shaking linens out when placing them on the bed
   C. give dirty linens to another nursing assistant after removing them
   D. put clean linens on top of the dirty laundry hamper

5. A nursing assistant fanfolds the top linens to the foot of the bed when making a(n)

   A. surgical bed
   B. occupied bed
   C. open, unoccupied bed
   D. closed, occupied bed

6. In his room, Mr. H has many personal items that sometimes get in the way of providing care. What should a nursing assistant do to safeguard these items and provide a comfortable environment for Mr. H?

   A. ask the family members to take many of these items home
   B. store the items in the resident's closet so they don't get in the way
   C. ask Mr. H if you can move his items and have him decide where
   D. while Mr. H is sleeping, move his items to other spots in the room

7. When a call light goes off from the bathroom, what should a nursing assistant do first?

   A. immediately go to that bathroom
   B. call the resident on the intercom
   C. ask another staff member to check the room
   D. check that resident's chart

8. Which of the following actions will help make residents' rooms more comfortable?

   A. offering residents drinking water often
   B. talking with residents about their families and friends
   C. keeping the room at a comfortable temperature
   D. conversing with residents during morning care

9. When a nursing assistant was making beds in room 2, he brought in too many linens. What should he do with the unused, clean linens?

   A. use them for another bed in the room
   B. use them for the next room
   C. put them back in the linen closet
   D. discard them in the laundry hamper

10. What is the most important consideration when working with beds?

    A. bed cleanliness   C. bed safety
    B. bed comfort   D. bed location

11. Mrs. W was admitted to the hospital two days ago. She is frightened about her stay and very concerned about her small children. She uses the call light often for seemingly unnecessary requests. What can a nursing assistant do to lessen her need to use the call light?

    A. ask if she needs anything else before leaving the room
    B. gently assure her that her children will be fine
    C. ask her roommate to talk with her
    D. keep the television on to distract and entertain her

12. One primary purpose of an overbed table is to

    A. stack linens
    B. place meal trays
    C. place dressings
    D. place the resident's chart

13. A nursing assistant wants to be sure he properly safeguards a resident's personal items. What should he do?

    A. inventory the items and label them, if needed
    B. put the items neatly and safely in the closet
    C. help the resident put the items in a favorite place
    D. ask the family to take most of the items home

14. What is the rationale for making a surgical bed?

    A. cleanliness   C. quality
    B. comfort   D. ease of transfer

15. To efficiently make a closed or open, unoccupied bed, a nursing assistant should

    A. start from the top
    B. do one side at a time
    C. start from the bottom
    D. ask someone to help him or her

Did you have difficulty with any of the questions? If you did, review the chapter to find the correct answer(s).

Welcome to the Chapter

In this chapter, you will learn two important daily responsibilities of holistic nursing assistants: assisting with personal hygiene and grooming. Typically, these responsibilities often start with a.m. care, or *morning care*. They may include shampooing, brushing, and combing hair; shaving; providing oral and denture care; giving fingernail and foot care; and performing perineal care. Assistance with dressing, undressing, and changing a hospital gown (especially if the patient has an IV catheter) may also be needed. In addition to a.m. care, some residents will also require a complete or partial bed bath or assistance with a tub bath or shower. At times, a therapeutic whirlpool or sitz bath may be ordered by a doctor.

A holistic nursing assistant must also care for residents' skin. This chapter includes procedures related to maintaining the skin's integrity, such as the use of warm moist compresses, warm soaks, an aquathermia pad, cold moist compresses, and ice packs.

The information and procedures presented in this chapter will help you build the knowledge and skills needed to become a holistic nursing assistant. Check with your instructor to ensure these procedures are within your state's regulations for nursing assistant practice. The topics discussed in the chapter are highlighted on the Providing Holistic Care Framework.

You are now ready to start this chapter, *Assisting with Personal Hygiene.*

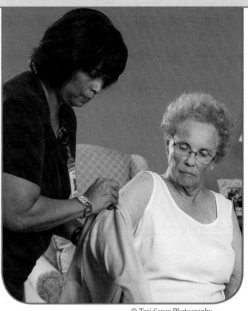
© Tori Soper Photography

Chapter Outline

Section 21.1
Bathing, Grooming, and Dressing

Section 21.2
Caring for the Skin

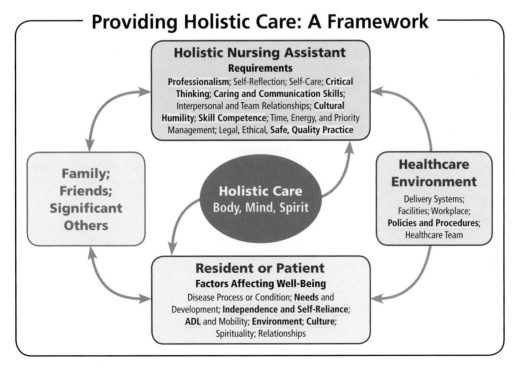

Providing Holistic Care: A Framework

Holistic Nursing Assistant
Requirements
Professionalism; Self-Reflection; Self-Care; **Critical Thinking; Caring and Communication Skills**; Interpersonal and Team Relationships; **Cultural Humility; Skill Competence**; Time, Energy, and Priority Management; Legal, Ethical, **Safe, Quality Practice**

Holistic Care
Body, Mind, Spirit

Family; Friends; Significant Others

Healthcare Environment
Delivery Systems; Facilities; Workplace; **Policies and Procedures**; Healthcare Team

Resident or Patient
Factors Affecting Well-Being
Disease Process or Condition; **Needs** and Development; **Independence and Self-Reliance; ADL** and Mobility; **Environment; Culture**; Spirituality; Relationships

Bathing, Grooming, and Dressing

Questions to Consider

- Has someone ever had to help you with your daily hygiene or grooming, such as bathing, brushing your teeth, or dressing and undressing? If so, how did it feel to rely on someone else for an activity you usually do yourself?
- If you have not ever had help with daily hygiene or grooming, imagine what the experience might be like. How do you think it would make you feel?
- What actions could someone take to help another person accept and feel good about receiving assistance with daily hygiene?

Objectives

Helping residents maintain their personal hygiene and grooming is an important caring and health-promoting responsibility of holistic nursing assistants. While performing these responsibilities, nursing assistants should help residents be as independent as possible. To achieve the objectives for this section, you must successfully

- **describe** the principles of personal hygiene and grooming and their importance in daily care;
- **identify** ways to promote independence during personal hygiene and grooming;
- **demonstrate** personal hygiene and grooming responsibilities; and
- **perform** the steps for providing oral and dental care, fingernail and foot care, and perineal care.

Key Terms

Learn these key terms to better understand the information presented in the section.

emesis basin	podiatrist
hemorrhoids	sitz bath
hygiene	skin integrity
perineal care	therapeutic
perineum	whirlpool

Remember

Hygiene is two-thirds of health.

Lebanese Proverb

Hygiene is routine actions such as bathing that promote and maintain cleanliness and health. Personal hygiene and grooming are essential to promoting healing and providing an environment of cleanliness, relaxation, and comfort. They also help maintain a resident's physical and emotional well-being and enhance quality of life by helping residents look and feel their best.

What Are Personal Hygiene and Grooming Responsibilities?

When providing care to residents, nursing assistants have several personal hygiene and grooming responsibilities. These responsibilities include morning care, bathing, hair care and shaving, oral care, fingernail and foot care, dressing or undressing, and perineal care. **Perineal care** is care of the **perineum**, or the area between the thighs (including the coccyx, pubis, anus, urethra, and external genitals). In this section, you will learn about these responsibilities and the procedures for performing them properly.

Morning Care

Morning care, or *a.m. care*, is one of the first daily activities of a holistic nursing assistant. Morning care is usually performed in the early morning hours, when residents first awake. The purpose of morning care is to promote physical and emotional health at the start of the day.

Morning care duties typically include taking vital signs; assisting with elimination and measuring output; collecting specimens ordered by the doctor; helping residents wash their faces, comb their hair, and perform oral care; and if necessary, changing soiled bed clothes. Other duties include straightening bed linens, changing soiled sheets or blankets, providing fresh drinking water, and arranging the bedside for breakfast (Figure 21.1). Some female residents may also ask for assistance with the application of makeup, such as face powder or lipstick. Morning care may not include arranging the bedside for breakfast if the resident is going to the dining room or is NPO (*nothing by mouth*) due to an ordered procedure or surgery. If residents are going to the dining room, a holistic nursing assistant may need to assist them.

While hygiene and grooming activities are essential during morning care, the morning is not the only time this type of care is needed. Some residents may also require assistance with toileting or washing their hands and face before lunch and dinner. They may need oral care after a meal or require perineal care at other times during the day.

Use these general guidelines when performing morning care. Wash your hands or use hand sanitizer prior to and after providing care, as well as when you enter and leave the room. This will help ensure infection control. Maintain a clean, safe environment while providing personal hygiene and grooming care. Once linens and gowns are taken out of the linen closet for a resident, they cannot be used for another resident unless they are washed first. Never use equipment that is intended for one resident on another resident without cleaning or disinfecting the equipment first. Never reuse soiled towels or linens. Always throw away disposable items after use.

Bathing

Bathing is one of the most important parts of personal hygiene and grooming. It helps maintain cleanliness and keeps residents free from perspiration, irritation, and possible bacterial growth. Baths can also be pleasant, relaxing, and **therapeutic** (healing). They provide an opportunity for the nursing assistant to observe a resident's **skin integrity** (condition of the skin) and look for signs of breakdown. During bathing, you can also observe a resident's level of hydration and muscle and joint movement. While bathing the whole body may not be possible on a daily basis, it is important that the resident's hands, face, and genital areas are washed every day and as needed throughout the day.

Some residents are mobile enough to use a shower or take a tub bath. Showers and tub baths promote skin cleanliness and healing and control odors. During a shower or tub bath, the condition of a resident's skin can be observed to promote healing. Some residents need a shower chair so they can sit in the shower. A chair may also be used as a fall-prevention strategy in case a resident gets tired during the shower. To ensure safety, place a nonslip bath mat or towel on the floor where the resident will step out of the shower. If the resident is taking a tub bath, place a towel in the tub so the resident can sit on it. All necessary towels, soap, and hygiene items should be within easy reach. Turn on the shower and adjust the water temperature or fill the tub half-full of water at a temperature of 100–105°F (the average water temperature for a tub bath or shower), or as directed by the licensed nursing staff. Make sure the grab bars in the shower and tub are easily accessible and that the resident knows where they are. Do not leave the resident unattended.

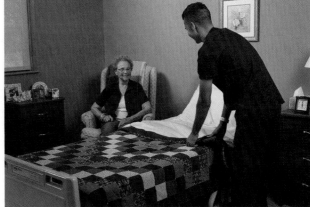

© Tori Soper Photography

Figure 21.1 One example of morning care is straightening a resident's bed linens.

Bathing Residents with Limited Mobility

For residents who are not able to get out of bed or wash themselves, a doctor may order a *total bed bath*. During a total bed bath, the entire body is washed by a nursing assistant using washcloths and warm, soapy water in a washbasin. Some facilities use liquid, no-rinse soap for a total bed bath. At times, a total bed bath may be too exhausting for a resident. Instead, a *partial bed bath* may be given. A partial bed bath involves washing the face, hands, axilla, genitalia, back, and buttocks. The nursing assistant may provide only part of the bath for residents who can perform some bathing tasks themselves. A resident's ability to bathe independently can change daily.

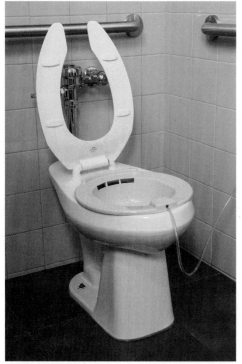

© Tori Soper Photography

Figure 21.2 In a sitz bath, a resident soaks up to the hips. This helps cleanse and relieve pain in the perineal area.

As a nursing assistant, ask and also observe the extent to which residents can perform their own bed baths. If a resident is able to do a partial bed bath, prepare the resident, water, washcloths, and towels and provide privacy during bathing. During a partial bed bath, it may be appropriate to leave the room while the resident bathes. Be sure to keep residents safe, wash your hands or use hand sanitizer, and replace your gloves when you return.

One alternative to a traditional bed bath is a *towel bath*. In a towel bath, a resident is bathed using a prepared, warm, moist bath towel. The resident is massaged through the towel, which has been immersed in no-rinse soap solution. Upon completion, the resident is dried with a bath blanket.

Another alternative to the bed bath is a *bag bath*. A bag bath is performed using a series of 10 washcloths. The washcloths are moistened with a no-rinse cleanser, placed in a bag, and warmed in a microwave, according to specific instructions. Bag baths are available for purchase or can be assembled using the facility's washcloths and no-rinse cleanser. During a bag bath, each washcloth should be used for a different body area (for example, one for the face, eyes, ears, and neck). Used washcloths should be discarded into a bath basin. The next body part should be washed with a fresh cloth, and so on. Once the bath is complete, the resident should be dried with a bath blanket.

Using Sitz Baths and Whirlpools

Some baths, such as sitz baths and whirlpools, are considered to be therapeutic. A **sitz bath** is a treatment in which a resident soaks in warm water up to his or her hips (Figure 21.2). This helps

---

Becoming a Holistic Nursing Assistant
The Personal Experience of Hygiene Care

Caring for another person's body is a very personal activity. To the resident, you may be a stranger. As a stranger, you have a duty to be conscious of your approach, style, and communication (both verbal and nonverbal). Be sure you have a resident's permission to give care. You must also be aware of how and where you touch others. When caring for a resident's body, maintain professional boundaries and do not expose the resident or invade personal space. Respect that this is a private experience for the resident.

People can become frustrated and impatient when they are no longer able to care for themselves. Holistic caregiving requires that you safely promote independence and support personal and cultural

desires and needs. It is important to talk with residents while giving care. Share information about the care being given and pay attention to your verbal and nonverbal communication and the responses you get during care.

Apply It

1. As a holistic nursing assistant, what can you do to maintain professional and personal boundaries during personal hygiene or grooming care?

2. Explain what actions a holistic nursing assistant can take to provide comfort and relaxation during care.

promote healing for soreness and irritation. It also reduces burning from diseases and conditions such as diarrhea, **hemorrhoids** (inflamed veins around the anus or inside the rectum), and vaginal infections. If giving a sitz bath, refer to the plan of care to determine the appropriate water temperature. A sitz bath generally lasts 10–20 minutes. Always note the time the sitz bath begins. Make sure the resident is comfortable and provide warmth by placing a blanket around the resident's shoulders and over the legs, if needed. Check on the resident every five minutes during the bath to ensure safety. Stay with the resident if he or she is feeling weak or not steady.

A **whirlpool** is a bathtub that uses small jets to move warm water (Figure 21.3). The resident places his or her entire body or a body part into the tub for treatment. The motion from the warm, moving water helps decrease swelling and inflammation, eases muscle spasms and pain, and promotes healing. The resident may bathe or sit in the whirlpool as long as instructed or directed by the plan of care. Always ensure comfort and safety.

No matter what type of bath is ordered, encourage residents to do as much of it themselves as they can. It is important to always keep residents warm and safe and maintain privacy. When helping with a bath, use excellent body mechanics as you turn and position the resident. If the resident is extremely overweight or unconscious, be sure to ask for assistance, if needed.

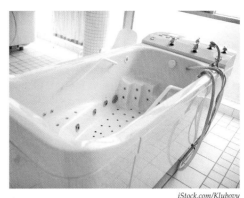

iStock.com/Klubovy

Figure 21.3 A whirlpool contains jets that move warm water to treat areas of the body.

Procedure   Giving a Total or Partial Bed Bath

Rationale

Bed baths cleanse the skin, control odor, and promote healing. They also give nursing assistants an opportunity to observe skin integrity. A total bed bath is given when an entire bath must be performed for the immobile resident. Partial bed baths are given to residents who cannot perform parts of the bath independently or who cannot tolerate a total bed bath.

Preparation

1. Ask the licensed nursing staff how this procedure fits into the plan of care, if there are doctor's orders for the procedure, if there are any special instructions or precautions, and if the resident can be moved into the positions required for this procedure.

2. Wash your hands or use hand sanitizer before entering the room.

3. Knock before entering the room.

4. Introduce yourself using your full name and title. Explain that you work with the licensed nursing staff and will be providing care.

5. Greet the resident and ask the resident to state her full name, if able. Then check the resident's identification bracelet.

6. Use Mr., Mrs., or Ms. and the last name when conversing.

7. Explain the procedure in simple terms, even if the resident is not able to communicate or is disoriented. Ask permission to perform the procedure.

Best Practice
To promote relaxation, be sure the room is at a comfortable temperature for the resident and that there are no drafts. Turn on the resident's favorite music at a low volume, if desired.

8. Bring the necessary equipment into the room. Place the following items in an accessible location:
   - bath blankets
   - disposable protective pad
   - disposable gloves
   - laundry hamper
   - clean bed linens

   Place the following items on a chair next to the bed:
   - several washcloths and hand towels
   - 2–3 bath towels
   - 2 clean gowns

   (continued)

Arrange the towels, linens, and gowns in the order they will be used. Then place a hand towel on the overbed table. Place the following equipment and linens on the hand towel:

- washbasin
- liquid soap (no-rinse, if appropriate)
- personal hygiene products, such as deodorant and lotion
- cotton-tipped applicators

The Procedure

9. Provide privacy by closing the curtains, using a screen, or closing the door to the room.

10. Lock the bed wheels and then raise the bed to hip level.

11. Ensure safety during the procedure. If there are side rails, raise and secure the rails on the opposite side of the bed from where you will be working. Lower the rail on the side you are working.

12. Wash your hands or use hand sanitizer to ensure infection control.

> **Best Practice**
> Before beginning the bath, ask if the resident needs to use a bedpan or urinal. Also remove any jewelry except a wedding ring. Place jewelry in a safe and secure place.

13. Put on disposable gloves.

14. Loosen and pull the bed linens out from under the mattress. Let them hang on all four sides of the bed.

15. Fanfold the bedspread and blanket to the foot of the bed, but leave the top sheet covering the resident.

16. Place the bath blanket over the top sheet. If possible, have the resident hold the bath blanket while you pull the top sheet out from under the bath blanket. If you will not be changing the bed linens, fanfold the top sheet to the foot of the bed. If you will be changing the bed linens, place the soiled top sheet in the laundry hamper.

17. Keep the resident covered with the bath blanket as you remove her gown and put it in the laundry hamper.

18. Fill the washbasin about two-thirds full of warm water. Check the water temperature. It should be 100–105°F. The water should feel comfortably warm to your elbow. You

may also ask the resident to feel the water temperature, but always check yourself first.

19. Place the washbasin on the overbed table, which should be covered with a hand towel. Be sure the washcloths and towels are easy to reach.

> **Best Practice**
> Bathing starts at the top of the body. Begin with the face and proceed to the bottom of the body, section by section.

20. Check the position of the bed and resident. Position the resident so she is on the side of the bed closest to you. If necessary and permitted, adjust the bed so the resident is in a Fowler's position. Place a dry towel across her chest under the chin and another under her head.

21. Make a bath mitt with a washcloth (Figure 21.4).

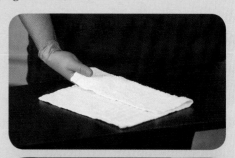

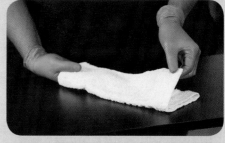

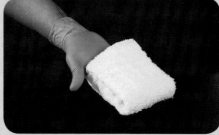

Figure 21.4

22. Wet the bath mitt using only water, not soap. If the resident requests soap, keep the soap away from her eyes. Gently wash each eye from the inner corner to the outer corner (Figure 21.5). To prevent infection, use a different, clean part of the mitt for each swipe.

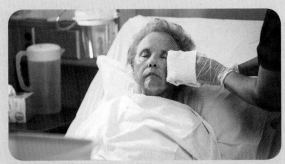
Figure 21.5

23. Wash the entire face, ears, and neck with a new bath mitt. Rinse sufficiently to remove any soap used. Gently pat-dry the face, ears, and neck with a dry towel.

> **Best Practice**
> Before washing each arm, place a dry towel under it.

24. Support the arm farthest from you. Wash the shoulder, axilla, arm, hand, and fingers with soap and water using a clean bath mitt. Wash the axilla thoroughly. Rinse and dry well.
25. Apply deodorant, unless directed otherwise.
26. Apply lotion to the resident's arm and hand, unless directed otherwise. Gently massage the lotion in a circular motion with the palm of your hand.

> **Best Practice**
> Always warm lotion in your gloved hands before placing it on the resident.

27. Rinse and dry the resident's hand well with a clean towel. Keep the resident warm by placing the dry arm under the bath blanket.
28. Support the arm nearest to you. Wash, rinse, dry, and apply lotion to the shoulder, axilla, arm, hand, and fingers using the same procedure.
29. Place a dry bath towel across the resident's chest and fold the bath blanket down to the pubic area.

> **Best Practice**
> Never expose the resident. During the bath, observe the resident for redness, sores, or irritation on the skin, especially under breast tissue and skin folds or on bony prominences. Take extra care around any dressings or catheters. Always check with the resident to be sure you are not rubbing too hard.

30. Lift the dry bath towel slightly and wash, rinse, and dry the chest and abdominal areas. Wash the navel and any creases in the skin with cotton-tipped applicators.
31. Apply lotion to the skin, unless directed otherwise. Gently massage the lotion in a circular motion with the palm of your hand.
32. Pull the bath blanket up and over the bath towel. Then remove the bath towel from beneath the bath blanket.
33. Lower the bed and raise the side rails for safety. Give the resident the call light.
34. Empty, rinse, and refill the washbasin about two-thirds full of warm water. Check the water temperature. It should be 100–105°F. The water should feel comfortably warm to your elbow. You may also ask the resident to feel the water temperature, but always check yourself first.
35. Place the washbasin on the overbed table.

> **Best Practice**
> If needed, remove your gloves and wash your hands before emptying the washbasin. Practice hand hygiene and put on a new pair of gloves after replacing the washbasin on the overbed table.

36. Place a dry towel under the resident's leg farthest from you. Be sure the genitalia are not exposed. Support the thigh and leg. Wash, rinse, and dry the thigh and leg well.
37. Apply lotion according to the plan of care. If lotion is used, gently massage it in a circular motion with the palm of your hand.
38. Wash, rinse, dry, and apply lotion to the thigh and leg nearest you using the same procedure. Then cover both legs with the bath blanket.
39. Expose the foot and thigh nearest you and bend the knee. Place the washbasin on top of a towel near the foot to be washed. Support the knee and place the resident's foot in the water (Figure 21.6). Using a bath mitt, wash and clean between the toes and under the toenails. Remove the foot from the water, then rinse and dry it well.

(continued)

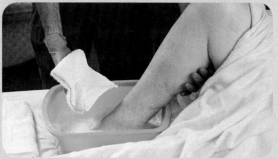

Figure 21.6

40. Apply lotion according to the plan of care. If lotion is used, gently massage it in a circular motion with the palm of your hand. To prevent fungal infection, do not put lotion between the toes.

41. Wash, rinse, dry, and apply lotion to the other foot using the same procedure.

Best Practice
Observe the toenails and the skin between the toes for redness and cracks.

42. Remove the washbasin and the towel.

43. Cover the resident's legs and feet with the bath blanket.

44. Lower the bed and raise the side rails for safety. Give the resident the call light.

45. Place any soiled linens in the laundry hamper.

46. Empty, rinse, and refill the washbasin about two-thirds full of warm water. Check the water temperature. It should be 100–105°F. The water should feel comfortably warm to your elbow. You may also ask the resident to feel the water temperature, but always check yourself first.

47. Help the resident turn onto her side. Her entire back and buttocks should be exposed. Place a towel lengthwise next to her back. Wash, rinse, and dry the back of the neck, back, and buttocks (Figure 21.7).

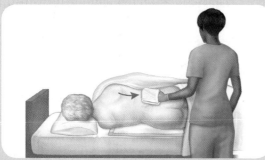

Figure 21.7

48. Give the resident a back rub with warmed lotion (following the back rub procedure in chapter 20).

49. Help the resident turn onto her back with a towel under her buttocks and upper legs.

50. Lower the bed and raise the side rails for safety. Give the resident the call light.

51. Empty, rinse, and refill the washbasin about two-thirds full of warm water. Check the water temperature. It should be 100–105°F. The water should feel comfortably warm to your elbow. You may also ask the resident to feel the water temperature, but always check yourself first.

52. If there is no urinary catheter, offer the resident a clean, soapy washcloth to wash the genital area. If the resident cannot do this, perform perineal care, as outlined in the perineal care procedure later in this section.

53. Help the resident put on a clean gown or other clothing, as appropriate.

54. Check to be sure the bed wheels are locked, then reposition the resident and lower the bed.

55. Follow the plan of care to determine if the side rails should be raised or lowered.

56. Remove, clean, and store equipment in the proper location. Remove soiled linens and discard disposable equipment.

Follow-Up

57. Remove and discard your gloves.

58. Wash your hands to ensure infection control.

59. Make sure the resident is comfortable and place the call light and personal items within reach.

60. Conduct a safety check before leaving the room. The room should be clean and free from clutter or spills.

61. Wash your hands or use hand sanitizer before leaving the room.

Reporting and Documentation

62. Communicate any specific observations, complications, or unusual responses to the licensed nursing staff. Record this information, along with the care provided, in the chart or EMR.

Figure 21.4 © Tori Soper Photography; Figure 21.5 © Tori Soper Photography; Figure 21.6 © Tori Soper Photography; Figure 21.7 © Body Scientific International

Hair Care

Another personal hygiene and bathing responsibility that nursing assistants have is shampooing, brushing, and combing residents' hair. People have different types of hair, and hair may be affected by age, genetics, medications, and skin conditions.

Knowing Hair Types

Hair can be fine, medium, coarse, wiry, or frizzy, depending on hair's thickness and a person's genetics. Hair may also be straight, curly, kinky (tightly coiled), or wavy.

Over time, a person's hair thins. Genetics, hormones, environmental factors, and lifestyle habits all influence hair thinning. Hair loss can also occur due to iron deficiency, poor diet, thyroid imbalance, or chemotherapy. Baldness (*alopecia*) is progressive hair thinning. About 40 percent of women will experience female-pattern hair loss by the time they reach menopause, and about 50 percent of men experience male-pattern hair loss by the age of 50. Baldness varies and usually becomes apparent after a person has lost 50 percent of his or her hair.

With age, hair turns gray or white due to changes in melanin (pigment) production in the hair follicles. *Canities* is the term used for gray hair. Gray hair usually develops due to age and stress, though the cause is different for each individual. Nevertheless, most people 75 years of age or older have varying amounts of gray hair. Men tend to become grayer at a younger age than women.

Think About This

On average, hair grows 1/2 inch per month. A person can lose between 40 and 150 strands of hair per day. Combing hair daily results in better blood circulation. In addition, hair health is influenced by good nutrition. Eating eggs, fish (such as salmon), carrots, green vegetables, and vitamins D and C will make a difference.

Understanding Hair Conditions

Various hair conditions may affect hair care. The scalp may have lesions such as cuts, ulcerations or sores, scabs, or blisters. Itching may be associated with a lesion. If a resident has lesions on the scalp, be careful and gentle when providing hair care.

While some shedding of dead skin cells is normal, *dandruff* can occur due to excessive flaking of dead skin cells from the scalp and is usually accompanied by redness and irritation. Dandruff is often a result of frequent exposure to extreme temperature variations (heat or cold) or certain triggers such as stress.

Lice are parasites that crawl and can be spread by close human contact. The type of lice found on the head is called *Pediculus humanus capitis*. Head lice attach their eggs to the base of the hair shaft on the scalp, usually around and behind the ears and near the neckline. Symptoms of head lice include a sense of something moving in

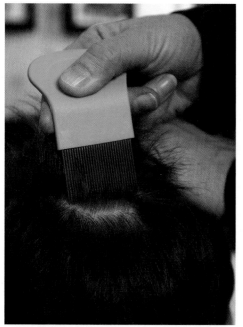

Figure 21.8 Combing the hair to check for lice is an important step in treating head lice.

vichni/Shutterstock.com

the hair, itching, and sores on the head due to excessive scratching (which can lead to infection). Treatment includes over-the-counter or prescription medications. When using these products, carefully follow the instructions provided. Supplemental treatment for head lice usually includes combing the hair to check for lice every two to three days for two to three weeks (Figure 21.8).

Shampooing Hair

Hair care is different for each type of hair. For dry hair, extra moisture is needed daily, and monthly conditioning is recommended. Hair that is oily due to overactive oil-producing glands requires a shampoo designed to remove oil and hydrate the hair and scalp.

Some residents in your care will be able to shampoo their own hair while showering. Others may require assistance during their shower or bath, but be able to wash their hair independently. For others who are bedridden, alternative shampoos may be used. Alternative shampoos include dry shampoo (in the form of a spray or powder) and liquid, no-rinse shampoo that does not require water.

Some residents in your care will be immobile and will need to have their hair shampooed in bed. The following procedure describes the steps for providing assistance with hair care when a resident is nonambulatory. This includes shampooing, combing, or brushing the hair.

Procedure | Providing Assistance with Hair Care

Rationale

Shampooing hair promotes cleanliness and comfort. The scalp is stimulated during shampooing, and this improves circulation.

Preparation

1. Ask the licensed nursing staff how this procedure fits into the plan of care, if there are doctor's orders for the procedure, if there are any special instructions or precautions, and if the resident can be moved into the positions required for this procedure.

2. Wash your hands or use hand sanitizer before entering the room.

3. Knock before entering the room.

4. Introduce yourself using your full name and title. Explain that you work with the licensed nursing staff and will be providing care.

5. Greet the resident and ask the resident to state his full name, if able. Then check the resident's identification bracelet.

6. Use Mr., Mrs., or Ms. and the last name when conversing.

7. Explain the procedure in simple terms, even if the resident is not able to communicate or is disoriented. Ask permission to perform the procedure.

8. Bring the necessary equipment into the room. Place the following items in an accessible location:
   - shampoo basin or tray; if inflatable, have the basin or tray ready (Figure 21.9)

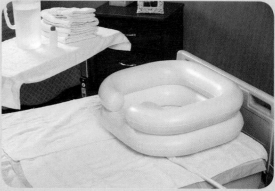

Figure 21.9

   - catch basin to collect used water
   - 2 bath blankets
   - waterproof pillow cover

- disposable protective pads or clean plastic trash bag
- a small washbasin, liquid soap, and antiseptic
- disposable gloves

Place the following items on the overbed table:

- 2 bath towels
- several washcloths
- shampoo and conditioner
- pitcher of warm water (100–105°F)
- washbasin with warm water (100–105°F) to refill the pitcher
- brush (without metal prongs that can damage the hair and scalp)
- comb (large-tooth comb for wet hair; avoid metal combs or combs with broken teeth that can tear individual hair strands and damage the scalp)
- several cotton balls or 2 × 2 gauze bandages
- hair dryer, if available
- personal hair products, if needed or desired
- handheld mirror

The Procedure

9. Provide privacy by closing the curtains, using a screen, or closing the door to the room.

10. Lock the bed wheels and then raise the bed to hip level.

11. Ensure safety during the procedure. If there are side rails, raise and secure the rails on the opposite side of the bed from where you will be working. Lower the rail on the side you are working.

12. Wash your hands or use hand sanitizer to ensure infection control.

13. Put on disposable gloves.

14. Carefully comb, brush, or gently use your fingers to remove any tangles from the resident's hair prior to shampooing.

> **Best Practice**
> Observe and report signs of skin breakdown, such as lesions or any other skin conditions, as you prepare to shampoo the hair.

15. Gently place a cotton ball or a 2 × 2 gauze bandage in each ear canal to prevent the entry of water.

16. Loosen the resident's gown at the neck.

17. Help the resident into a supine position and then lower the head of the bed.

18. Cover the resident with the bath blanket. Fanfold the top bed linens to the foot of the bed. Make sure the resident is not exposed.

19. Remove the pillow from under the resident's head and gently place the resident's head on the bed.

20. Place the disposable protective pad or plastic trash bag and then a towel on the bed beneath the resident's head and upper body.

21. Remove the pillowcase and replace it with the waterproof cover.

22. Place the pillow with the waterproof cover beneath the resident's shoulders so the resident's head is tilted slightly backward.

23. Place a bath towel around the resident's head and shoulders. There should be enough padding to provide comfort and prevent water leakage.

24. Raise the resident's head and slide the shampoo tray or basin under it. Be sure the basin tubing is connected to the catch basin.

25. Place a protective pad on the floor near the head of the bed. Put the catch basin on top of the pad.

26. Place a washcloth over the resident's eyes.

27. Check the water to be sure it is at a warm, but safe, temperature.

28. Using the pitcher, pour enough water to wet the hair (Figure 21.10). When needed, refill the pitcher using the washbasin filled with warm water.

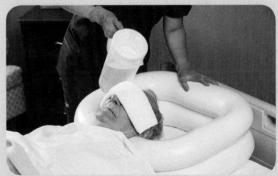

Figure 21.10

29. Apply a small amount of shampoo to your hands and begin forming a lather. With both hands, apply the shampoo to the scalp using a massaging motion. Apply the shampoo from the scalp outward to the ends of the hair strands, and from the front to the back of the head. Lift the resident's head gently to shampoo the back of the head.

(continued)

Providing Assistance with Hair Care
(continued)

> **Best Practice**
> Use your fingertips, *not* your fingernails. Be extremely careful if there are lesions on the scalp.

30. Rinse the resident's hair thoroughly, pouring warm water from the pitcher. Rinse from the hairline and work down to the ends of the hair strands. When needed, refill the pitcher using the washbasin filled with warm water. Check the water temperature.

31. If appropriate, apply conditioner and rinse thoroughly.

32. Remove and discard your gloves. Put on another pair of disposable gloves.

33. Dry the resident's forehead, ears, and neck with a clean bath towel. Remove the cotton balls or 2 × 2 gauze bandages from each ear canal.

34. Carefully remove the shampoo basin or tray and set it on the chair next to the bed. Be sure there is a dry bath towel under the resident's head.

35. Raise the head of the bed 60–90°, if appropriate.

36. Dry the resident's hair with a clean bath towel by blotting, not by rubbing.

37. If the hair is wet, comb it to remove tangles and then style the hair. Part the hair in sections. Comb each section separately using a downward motion and comb from underneath to remove any tangles (Figure 21.11). If the resident is able, have him move his head so you can get all angles. If the resident is unable, support his head while moving it.

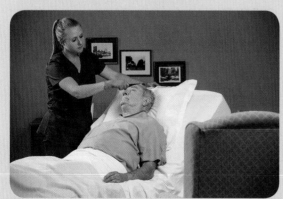
Figure 21.11

> **Best Practice**
> Hair is fragile when it is wet. Do not brush wet hair because brushing can damage the hair. Instead, use a comb.

38. Brush the hair if it is dry and not tangled. Be slow and gentle. Have the resident move his head so you can get all angles. If the resident is unable, support his head while moving it.

> **Best Practice**
> To prevent hair loss, do not brush or pull the hair too much during drying or styling. If caring for a resident undergoing chemotherapy, use a child or baby hair brush with softer bristles.

39. Style the resident's hair neatly. If a resident has long hair, suggest a loose braid to prevent snarls, knots, or tangles. Use a hair dryer only if available and permitted.

40. Remove the towel and let the resident use the handheld mirror, if desired, to view the hair. If a hair salon or barber shop is available in the facility, ask the resident if he might want to visit in the future.

41. Remove all equipment and used towels from the bed.

42. Assist with changing the resident's gown if it got wet during the procedure.

43. Remove the bath blanket and replace the linens.

44. Remove the waterproof cover, replace it with a clean pillowcase, and put the pillow under the resident's head.

45. Check to be sure the bed wheels are locked, then reposition the resident and lower the bed.

46. Follow the plan of care to determine if the side rails should be raised or lowered.

47. Remove, clean, and store equipment in the proper location. Clean the brush and comb in the bathroom. Use the washbasin of warm water and a small amount of liquid soap. You may also use a small amount of antiseptic. Quickly tap the brush or comb in the filled washbasin and then rinse with cool, running water. Let the brush and comb air-dry and then put them away. Remove soiled linens and discard disposable equipment.

Shaving

Many men choose to shave daily, while others shave less regularly. Factors such as the condition of the skin, the texture of the hair, and hair growth patterns can make shaving challenging for men. The skin products and razors used are typically based on personal preference. Heavier beard growth, irritations, acne, and skin or razor bumps (*ingrown hairs*) are often problems. Preshaving oil or shaving cream with aloe can soften skin and hair and help prevent irritation, nicks, cuts, and razor bumps and burns. Leaving a little hair growth during shaving helps avoid razor bumps. *Electric razors* are less irritating than blades and should be used if the resident is taking anticoagulant medications (*blood thinners*). If a blade is used, a *safety razor* with a single or double blade is better than multiblade brands (Figure 21.12).

Some men like to use aftershave lotion and toner. These products tighten the skin and narrow the pores. Lotions and toners containing alcohol should be avoided, as they can dry the skin. When helping a resident shave, you may recommend a barber or stylist if these services are available in the healthcare facility. You may also suggest that family members assist with shaving or trimming the mustache or beard. If you are asked to help a male resident with grooming, be sure to practice infection control and follow these guidelines:

- Make sure any dentures are in place before you begin.

- Before using a safety razor, soften the beard by wetting washcloths in a basin of warm water. Use the washcloths as compresses by gently laying them on the resident's face. Then generously apply shaving cream or gel to the areas that will be shaved. Rinse the razor often in the warm water while shaving and be sure all of the shaving cream is gone when shaving is completed and the skin is rinsed thoroughly.

- Before using an electric razor, ask the resident if he prefers a dry shave or one with preshave lotion. If lotion is desired, apply it liberally to the areas that will be shaved.

- Hold the skin tight with the fingers of one hand and shave in the direction of hair growth (Figure 21.13). Start under the sideburns and work downward over the cheeks. Shave the chin carefully. Work downward on the neck under the chin. When shaving the chin or under the nose, ask the resident to hold that part of the skin tight. If there is facial hair, maintain the mustache or beard line.

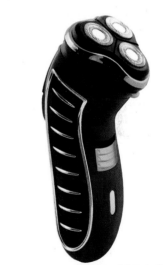

GzP_Design/Shutterstock.com

A

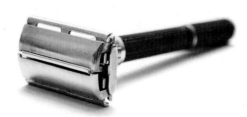

Paolo Querci/Shutterstock.com

B

Figure 21.12 An electric razor (A) should be used if a resident is taking blood thinners. If a blade is used, safety razors (B) are the safest option.

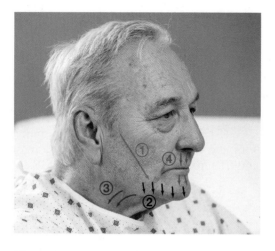

1. Start at the sideburns and shave in downward strokes to the jawline.
2. Use short, downward strokes along the jawline.
3. Carefully shave the neck using gentle, downward strokes.
4. Use short strokes to shave above and below the lips.

Figure 21.13 Always shave in the direction of hair growth.

- Shave lightly to prevent nicks or cuts. If a nick or cut occurs, apply pressure with a small piece of facial tissue. This will help the blood clot at the site. Remove and dispose of the tissue at the end of shaving once the bleeding has stopped. Report any nicks or cuts to the licensed nursing staff after you finish shaving.

- Take care not to shave over any skin sores, moles, growths, acne, or bruises on the face.

- Use a fine-tooth comb to straighten mustache hairs. Use a wide-tooth comb for a wet beard. Once dry, beards can be brushed. Wax or balm can be applied to the mustache or beard. Apply aftershave lotion or powder, if desired.

- Make sure any used razor blades are discarded in the sharps container.

Oral and Denture Care

To give oral care, a nursing assistant should be familiar with the structures of the mouth and teeth. These structures were discussed in chapter 8.

At birth, humans have 20 deciduous teeth (commonly called *baby teeth*), which are eventually replaced by 32 permanent (*adult*) teeth. Some residents do not have all of their natural teeth. They may have bridges, partial dentures, or full dentures, which contain false teeth to replace missing teeth (Figure 21.14). A *bridge* fills a gap between teeth. Bridges are anchored to the permanent teeth. *Partial dentures* have a plastic base or metal structure that attaches to missing teeth. Partial dentures may be removable and are held in place by clasps that hook onto natural teeth. *Full*, or *complete, dentures*, replace all natural teeth on the upper, lower, or both parts of the gums. Full dentures are plastic and are shaped and colored to look like natural teeth and gums. They are made to fit to the resident's mouth and stay in place by forming a suction seal on top of the natural gums.

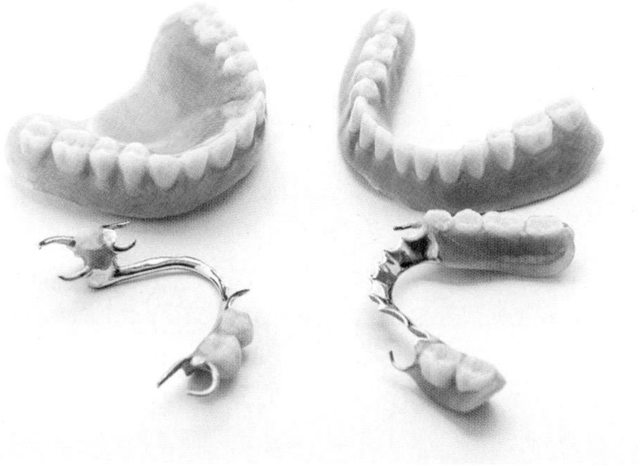

Dentures that have been properly cared for typically last about five years. As people age, their bones and gums age too, which may cause dentures to become loose. This can worsen over time, resulting in an inability to chew well and in food being caught

Bunwit Useree/Shutterstock.com

Figure 21.14 Partial dentures replace some missing teeth and often have a metal or plastic base. Full dentures replace all natural teeth on the upper, lower, or both gums.

between the gums and dentures. Because of these difficulties, residents may not receive adequate nutrients, which may cause lack of healing and weight loss. Poorly fitting dentures can also cause mouth and gum irritation, sores, and infections. Sometimes dentures can get tiny cracks, which need to be repaired to maintain the integrity of the dentures.

Oral care and teeth cleaning are a critical part of daily hygiene. They ensure that the mouth is fresh, that the teeth and gums remain healthy, and that the resident experiences no bad tastes from illnesses or medications. Good oral care can help prevent dental cavities or *caries* (tooth decay that damages the hard surface of the teeth), *halitosis* (bad breath), *gingivitis* (gum disease), and *periodontitis* (infection of the gums and bones that support the teeth).

Oral care may be needed as often as every two hours if the resident is unable to take fluids by mouth. Routine teeth cleaning consists of daily brushing and flossing in the morning and evening and after eating. Flossing is important, as it removes up to 80 percent of the film that hardens into plaque, which can stick to the teeth and become difficult to remove. Rinsing the mouth is also essential. If a resident wears dentures, dentures must be cleaned properly and correctly stored if they are not being worn.

Procedure — Providing Oral Care

Rationale

Oral care is an essential part of daily hygiene. Performing oral care helps reduce bacteria, provides moisture, freshens the mouth, makes food taste better, and cleans the teeth.

Preparation

1. Ask the licensed nursing staff how this procedure fits into the plan of care, if there are doctor's orders for the procedure, if there are any special instructions or precautions, and if the resident can be moved into the positions required for this procedure.
2. Wash your hands or use hand sanitizer before entering the room.
3. Knock before entering the room.
4. Introduce yourself using your full name and title. Explain that you work with the licensed nursing staff and will be providing care.
5. Greet the resident and ask the resident to state her full name, if able. Then check the resident's identification bracelet.
6. Use Mr., Mrs., or Ms. and the last name when conversing.
7. Explain the procedure in simple terms, even if the resident is not able to communicate or is disoriented. Ask permission to perform the procedure.

8. Bring the necessary equipment into the room. Some of these items may already be in the bedside stand or bathroom. Place a paper towel, towel, or disposable protective pad on the overbed table as an infection-control barrier before placing the following items:
   - soft-bristled toothbrush (always use soft-bristled for older adults)
   - toothpaste (with an American Dental Association seal)
   - mouthwash
   - pitcher of fresh, cool water
   - several disposable cups
   - spoon or tongue blade
   - disposable gloves
   - **emesis basin**, which should be small and kidney shaped (Figure 21.15)
   - 2 washcloths
   - 2–3 towels
   - 2 face masks, if needed
   - dental floss

> **Best Practice**
> Replace a toothbrush every three to four months. Replace it sooner if the bristles become frayed.

(continued)

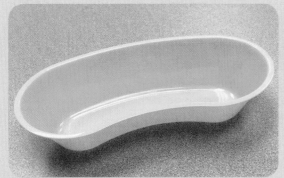

Figure 21.15

The Procedure

9. Provide privacy by closing the curtains, using a screen, or closing the door to the room.

10. If the resident is able to sit in a chair, assist her to a chair and then place the overbed table with the equipment and linens in a comfortable position so she may brush her teeth.

11. If the resident is in bed and needs assistance, lock the bed wheels and then raise the bed to hip level.

12. Ensure safety during the procedure. If there are side rails, raise and secure the rails on the opposite side of the bed from where you will be working. Lower the rail on the side you are working.

13. Raise the head of the bed to at least 60–90° and ensure there is sufficient lighting to perform the procedure.

14. Wash your hands or use hand sanitizer to ensure infection control.

15. Put on disposable gloves.

16. Spread a towel across the resident's chest to protect her clothing and the top linen.

17. Fill a disposable cup half-full with water and half-full with mouthwash and mix with a spoon or tongue blade.

18. Have the resident take a mouthful from the cup and swish the mixture in her mouth.

19. Hold the emesis basin underneath the resident's chin so she can spit the mixture into the basin. Wipe the resident's mouth and chin dry.

20. Fill a disposable cup half-full with water. Wet the toothbrush in the water.

21. Put toothpaste on the wet toothbrush. If the resident is able, let her brush her own teeth. If she cannot, brush her teeth for her.

   A. Hold the brush at a 45° angle to the gum (Figure 21.16).

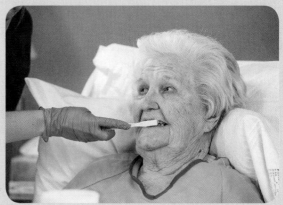

Figure 21.16

   B. Starting at the back of the mouth, use gentle, circular motions to brush the outer surfaces, inner surfaces, and chewing surfaces of the teeth (Figure 21.17).

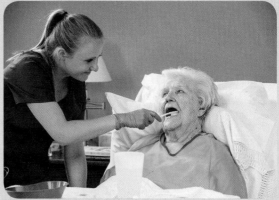

Figure 21.17

   C. To clean the inside surfaces of the front teeth, tilt the brush vertically and make several up-and-down strokes.

   D. Brush the tongue to remove bacteria and keep the breath fresh, but do not brush so far back that gagging occurs.

22. During brushing, have the resident spit toothpaste and excess saliva into the emesis basin, as needed (Figure 21.18).

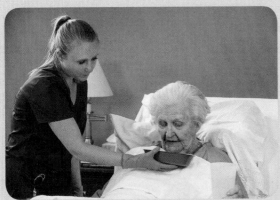
Figure 21.18

23. When finished, help the resident rinse the toothpaste out of her mouth using the mouthwash solution or fresh water and the emesis basin. Then wipe her mouth.

24. If the resident is able, let her floss her teeth. If she is not able, floss her teeth for her. Put on a face mask before beginning, if needed.

Best Practice
If the resident will floss independently, you may need to show her the proper way to floss.

A. Cut a piece of floss 18 inches long.

B. Wrap the ends of the floss around the middle finger of each hand. Place the other fingers out of the way and hold the dental floss stretched tight between the middle fingers (Figure 21.19).

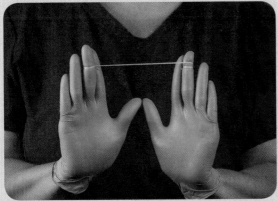
Figure 21.19

C. Ask the resident to open her mouth.

D. Gently insert the floss between each pair of teeth. Do not press the floss into the gum. Slide the floss around both sides of each tooth. Discard the floss when completed.

E. When finished, offer the resident the mouthwash solution or fresh water to rinse the mouth.

Best Practice
Alert the licensed nursing staff if you observe complaints of pain or sensitivity, sores on the lips or mouth, cracked or bleeding lips or gums, bad breath that does not improve after oral care, or chipped or cracked teeth.

25. If the resident is in bed, check to be sure the bed wheels are locked. Then reposition the resident and lower the bed. If the resident is in a chair, help her back to bed, if desired.

26. Follow the plan of care to determine if the side rails should be raised or lowered.

27. Remove, clean, and store equipment in the proper location. Remove soiled linens and discard disposable equipment.

Follow-Up

28. Remove and discard your gloves.

29. Wash your hands to ensure infection control.

30. Make sure the resident is comfortable and place the call light and personal items within reach.

31. Conduct a safety check before leaving the room. The room should be clean and free from clutter or spills.

32. Wash your hands or use hand sanitizer before leaving the room.

Reporting and Documentation

33. Communicate any specific observations, complications, or unusual responses to the licensed nursing staff. Record this information, along with the care provided, in the chart or EMR.

Figure 21.15 Rachael Woznick; Figure 21.16 © Tori Soper Photography; Figure 21.17 © Tori Soper Photography; Figure 21.18 © Tori Soper Photography; Figure 21.19 © Tori Soper Photography

Procedure | Cleaning and Storing Dentures

Rationale

Cleaning and properly storing dentures is an essential part of daily hygiene. Cleaning dentures keeps them intact, freshens the mouth, removes remaining food particles that can cause irritation, and reduces lingering bacteria on the dentures.

Preparation

1. Ask the licensed nursing staff how this procedure fits into the plan of care, if there are doctor's orders for the procedure, if there are any special instructions or precautions, and if the resident can be moved into the positions required for this procedure.
2. Wash your hands or use hand sanitizer before entering the room.
3. Knock before entering the room.
4. Introduce yourself using your full name and title. Explain that you work with the licensed nursing staff and will be providing care.
5. Greet the resident and ask the resident to state his full name, if able. Then check the resident's identification bracelet.
6. Use Mr., Mrs., or Ms. and the last name when conversing.
7. Explain the procedure in simple terms, even if the resident is not able to communicate or is disoriented. Ask permission to perform the procedure.
8. Bring the necessary equipment into the room. Put a paper towel, towel, or disposable protective pad on the overbed table as an infection-control barrier before placing the following items:
   - toothbrush or denture brush
   - denture cup and lid, labeled with the resident's name and room number (Figure 21.20)

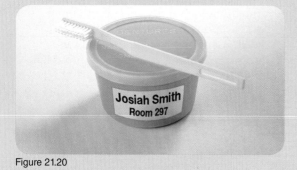

Figure 21.20

- toothpaste or denture cleaner
- disposable cups
- emesis basin
- washcloths
- mouthwash
- denture solution
- several towels
- several packets of 2 × 2 gauze bandages
- oral swabs
- disposable gloves

The Procedure

9. Provide privacy by closing the curtains, using a screen, or closing the door to the room.
10. If the resident is able to sit in a chair, assist him to a chair and then place the overbed table with the equipment and linens in a comfortable position so he may clean his dentures.
11. If the resident is in bed and needs assistance, lock the bed wheels and then raise the bed to hip level.
12. Ensure safety during the procedure. If there are side rails, raise and secure the rails on the opposite side of the bed from where you will be working. Lower the rail on the side you are working.
13. Raise the head of the bed, if permitted.
14. Wash your hands or use hand sanitizer to ensure infection control.
15. Put on disposable gloves.
16. Spread a towel across the resident's chest to protect his clothing and the top linen.
17. Place a washcloth in the bottom of the emesis basin.
18. Ask the resident to remove his dentures and place them in the emesis basin.
19. If the resident cannot remove his dentures, ask him to open his mouth. Remove his dentures for him.
    A. **Upper dentures**: grasp the upper denture firmly using a 2 × 2 gauze bandage. Ease the denture downward and forward and then remove it from the mouth.
    B. **Lower dentures**: grasp the lower denture firmly using a new 2 × 2 gauze bandage. Ease the denture upward and forward and then remove it from the mouth.

20. Place the dentures in the emesis basin on top of the washcloth. Never carry the dentures in your hands. Take the emesis basin, toothbrush or denture brush, and toothpaste or denture cleaner to the sink. Place the basin next to the sink.

21. If the resident wears full dentures, clean the resident's oral cavity after the dentures are removed. Clean the resident's oral cavity with oral swabs and half-strength mouthwash.

22. Place a washcloth in the bottom of the clean sink to protect the dentures from breaking or scratching in case they fall. *Do not place the dentures in the sink.*

23. Take one denture out of the emesis basin. Apply toothpaste or denture cleaner to the denture. Wet the toothbrush by immersing it in clean, running water. Make sure to brush away from you (Figure 21.21). Hold the denture low in the sink. With the denture in the palm of your hand, brush all surfaces until they are clean. Then rinse the denture thoroughly using cool, running water. Repeat the same procedure for a second denture.

> **Best Practice**
> Hot water can damage dentures and cause them to lose their shape.

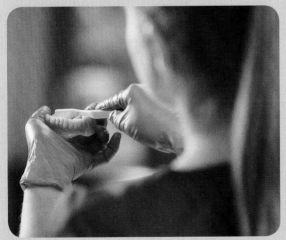

Figure 21.21

> **Best Practice**
> Be sure to check the dentures for any cracks. Report cracks to the licensed nursing staff.

24. If the dentures will be stored, fill the labeled denture cup with cool water, mouthwash, or denture solution. Place the dentures in the cup and close the lid.

> **Best Practice**
> Always store dentures in liquid when they are out of the resident's mouth.

25. Leave the labeled denture cup with clean solution on the bedside stand, where it can be easily reached.

26. Check that the dentures are moist if reinserting them. If the resident is able, ask him to put the dentures back into his mouth. Assist, if needed. Check that the dentures fit correctly.

27. Remove and discard your gloves after either storing the dentures or inserting them into the resident's mouth.

28. Wash your hands or use hand sanitizer to ensure infection control.

29. Put on a new pair of gloves.

30. If the resident is in bed, check to be sure the bed wheels are locked. Then reposition the resident and lower the bed. If the resident is in a chair, help him back to bed, if desired.

31. Follow the plan of care to determine if the side rails should be raised or lowered.

32. Remove, clean, and store equipment in the proper location. Use disinfectant to clean the emesis basin. Remove soiled linens and discard disposable equipment.

Follow-Up

33. Remove and discard your gloves.

34. Wash your hands to ensure infection control.

35. Make sure the resident is comfortable and place the call light and personal items within reach.

36. Conduct a safety check before leaving the room. The room should be clean and free from clutter or spills.

37. Wash your hands or use hand sanitizer before leaving the room.

Reporting and Documentation

38. Communicate any specific observations, complications, or unusual responses to the licensed nursing staff. Record this information, along with the care provided, in the chart or EMR.

Images courtesy of © Tori Soper Photography

Fingernail Care

As you learned in chapter 8, fingernails and toenails are composed of protein, keratin, and epithelial cells. The hard surface of the nail is the *nail plate* (Figure 21.22). The *cuticle* is the band of tissue at the sides and base of the nail plate. The *nail root* anchors the nail plate. The pink color of the nail comes from blood vessels directly underneath the nail plate. Nails need oxygen because they are composed of living cells and tissue.

Cuticle
A thin lip of dead skin cells surrounds the edge of the nail plate.

Nail Plate
The nail plate is the hard "shell" at the end of the finger or toe.

Root
The nail extends from a matrix, or root, at the top of the nail plate. The edge is visible as the lunule, or whitish half-moon on the nail plate.

Nail Groove
The nail is embedded in a fold of skin at the sides and base near the root.

Nail Bed
Capillaries in the sensitive nail bed below the nail plate provide nutrients for the nail growth at the root.

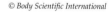

© Body Scientific International

Figure 21.22 Each nail includes a nail plate, cuticle, and nail root.

Procedure   Providing Fingernail Care

Rationale

Routine fingernail care promotes cleanliness and helps prevent irritation or infection from torn or bleeding cuticles, cracked fingernails, or dirt under the fingernails. Smooth fingernails also prevent the skin from breaking if residents scratch themselves.

Preparation

1. Ask the licensed nursing staff how this procedure fits into the plan of care, if there are doctor's orders for the procedure, if there are any special instructions or precautions, and if the resident can be moved into the positions required for this procedure.

2. Wash your hands or use hand sanitizer before entering the room.

3. Knock before entering the room.

4. Introduce yourself using your full name and title. Explain that you work with he licensed nursing staff and will be providing care.

5. Greet the resident and ask the resident to state his full name, if able. Then check the resident's identification bracelet.

6. Use Mr., Mrs., or Ms. and the last name when conversing.

7. Explain the procedure in simple terms, even if the resident is not able to communicate or is disoriented. Ask permission to perform the procedure.

8. Bring the necessary equipment into the room. Place a paper towel, towel, or disposable protective pad on the overbed table as an infection-control barrier before placing the following items:

- washbasin with warm water (100–105°F)
- 1–2 emery boards
- nail clipper
- orangewood stick, if permitted
- 2–3 hand towels
- disposable protective pad
- several washcloths
- lotion
- disposable gloves
- soap

The Procedure

9. Provide privacy by closing the curtains, using a screen, or closing the door to the room.

10. If the resident is able to sit in a chair, assist him to a chair. Place the overbed table with the equipment and linens in a comfortable position so he may care for his fingernails. You may need to assist with clipping fingernails and using the emery board. Ask if the resident would like his fingers and hands massaged after care, if permitted.

11. If the resident is in bed, lock the bed wheels and then raise the bed to hip level.

12. Ensure safety during the procedure. If there are side rails, raise and secure the rails on the opposite side of the bed from where you will be working. Lower the rail on the side you are working.

13. Raise the head of the bed.

14. Wash your hands or use hand sanitizer to ensure infection control.

15. Put on disposable gloves.

16. Place the overbed table in front of the resident with the washbasin of warm water. Check the water temperature. It should be 100–105°F. The water should feel comfortably warm to your elbow. You may also ask the resident to feel the water temperature, but always check yourself first. Add a small amount of soap to the washbasin.

17. Help the resident comfortably position his fingers in the washbasin to soak. If appropriate, use a rolled-up towel to support his wrists. Cover the resident's hands and the washbasin with a dry hand towel to retain the heat.

18. Soak the resident's fingernails for approximately 5–10 minutes. If needed, remove the resident's hands and add more warm water.

19. Wash the resident's hands, cleaning under the fingernails.

20. If permitted, push the cuticles back gently with a washcloth or the dull end of an orangewood stick. Clean under each nail with an orangewood stick. Wipe the orangewood stick after cleaning each nail.

21. Remove the washbasin and dry the resident's hands thoroughly.

22. Use a nail clipper to cut the fingernails straight across, if permitted. Do not clip below the tips of the fingers (Figure 21.23).

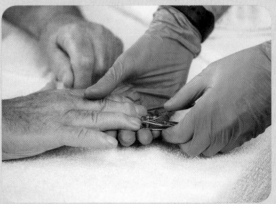

Figure 21.23

> **Best Practice**
> Be very careful not to accidentally clip or damage the skin surrounding the fingernail.

23. Shape and smooth the fingernails with an emery board.

24. Apply lotion and gently massage the resident's fingers and hands. Remove extra lotion with a towel.

> **Best Practice**
> Alert the licensed nursing staff if you observe loose nails or dry, reddened, or irritated areas.

25. If the resident is in bed, check to be sure the bed wheels are locked. Then reposition the resident and lower the bed. If the resident is in a chair, help him back to bed, if desired.

26. Follow the plan of care to determine if the side rails should be raised or lowered.

(continued)

27. Remove, clean, and store equipment in the proper location. Disinfect the nail clippers. Remove soiled linens and discard disposable equipment.

Follow-Up

28. Remove and discard your gloves.

29. Wash your hands to ensure infection control.

30. Make sure the resident is comfortable and place the call light and personal items within reach.

31. Conduct a safety check before leaving the room. The room should be clean and free from clutter or spills.

32. Wash your hands or use hand sanitizer before leaving the room.

Reporting and Documentation

33. Communicate any specific observations, complications, or unusual responses to the licensed nursing staff. Record this information, along with the care provided, in the chart or EMR.

Image courtesy of © Tori Soper Photography

Foot Care

Think About This

Every day, your fingernails grow 0.1 millimeter. Your toenails grow 1 millimeter per month. Nails grow faster in the summer than in the winter. The middle fingernail grows the fastest, and the slowest-growing nail is the thumbnail.

As they age, residents may have more difficulty with their feet and toenails. For example, toenails may become thick and yellow, unattractive, and harder to keep clean and trimmed. Problems with the feet include calluses and corns. *Calluses* are hard, rough areas on the skin caused by repeated friction or rubbing, potentially from wearing poor-fitting shoes or walking barefoot over a long period (Figure 21.24A). Calluses normally appear on the heel or ball of the foot. The skin becomes thick and less sensitive. *Corns* are small patches of thickened, dead skin with a central core. Corns often form on the tops and sides of the feet (Figure 21.24B). They may be caused by lack of cushioning on the foot or by a *bunion* (swelling on the joint of the big toe). Corns can become infected if they break when the feet are enclosed in shoes, creating a moist environment perfect for bacterial growth. Some over-the-counter treatments are available for these foot problems. A **podiatrist** is a doctor who specializes in foot health.

Special foot care should be given to residents who have diabetes or peripheral vascular disease (PVD). Usually, a podiatrist will regularly check these residents' feet. Diabetes and PVD can lead to serious nerve damage, or *peripheral neuropathy*, which causes a loss of pain, heat, and cold sensitivity in the feet. The feet may also

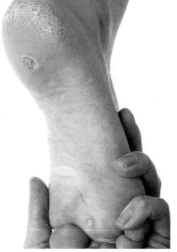

Arve Bettum/Shutterstock.com

A

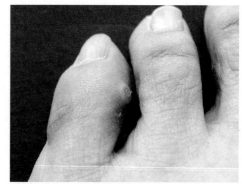

Songrit Kamolmarttayakul/Shutterstock.com

B

Figure 21.24 Calluses (A) are rough areas of skin caused by friction. Corns (B) are patches of thickened, dead skin with a central core.

become numb, which can result in unnoticed sores and swelling of the feet. For these residents especially, daily foot care is essential. The following are helpful guidelines for providing foot care:

- To promote good blood circulation, have the resident elevate his or her feet when sitting. The resident should wiggle his or her toes and move the ankles up and down for five minutes two to three times daily. The legs should never be crossed for long periods.

- Carefully check the feet for signs of irritation, cuts, swelling, or blisters.

- Wash the feet daily and fully dry them, especially between the toes.

- Use skin lotion on the tops and bottoms of the feet. Never put lotion between the toes, as this can cause fungal growth.

- Trim the toenails straight across and file the edges with an emery board or nail file, if permitted.

- Encourage residents to wear comfortable shoes. Check the insides of shoes before residents put them on. Ensure the lining is smooth and there are no objects inside. Socks should also be worn, and residents should never walk barefoot.

- Protect the feet from hot and cold. Do not put feet into very hot water. Always test the temperature of water first. Never use hot water bottles, heating pads, or electric blankets on the feet.

Procedure   Providing Foot Care

Rationale
Routine foot care promotes cleanliness and helps prevent infections and foot odor.

Preparation

1. Ask the licensed nursing staff how this procedure fits into the plan of care, if there are doctor's orders for the procedure, if there are any special instructions or precautions, and if the resident can be moved into the positions required for this procedure.

2. Wash your hands or use hand sanitizer before entering the room.

3. Knock before entering the room.

4. Introduce yourself using your full name and title. Explain that you work with the licensed nursing staff and will be providing care.

5. Greet the resident and ask the resident to state his full name, if able. Then check the resident's identification bracelet.

6. Use Mr., Mrs., or Ms. and the last name when conversing.

7. Explain the procedure in simple terms, even if the resident is not able to communicate or is disoriented. Ask permission to perform the procedure.

8. Bring the necessary equipment into the room. Place a paper towel, towel, or disposable protective pad on the overbed table as an infection-control barrier before placing the following items:

- washbasin or foot bath with warm water (100–105°F)
- 1–2 emery boards, nail clipper, and orangewood stick, if permitted
- 2–3 hand towels
- several washcloths
- disposable protective pad
- lotion
- disposable gloves
- soap

The Procedure

9. Provide privacy by closing the curtains, using a screen, or closing the door to the room.

10. If the resident is able to sit in a chair, assist her to a chair. Place a disposable protective pad on the floor in front of the chair.

11. If the resident is in bed, lock the bed wheels and then raise the bed to hip level.

(continued)

12. Ensure safety during the procedure. If there are side rails, raise and secure the rails on the opposite side of the bed from where you will be working. Lower the rail on the side you are working.

13. Raise the head of the bed.

14. Wash your hands or use hand sanitizer to ensure infection control.

15. Put on disposable gloves.

16. Place the washbasin or foot bath with warm water on top of the protective pad. Check the water temperature. It should be 100–105°F. The water should feel comfortably warm to your elbow. You may also ask the resident to feel the water temperature, but always check yourself first. Add a small amount of soap to the washbasin or foot bath.

17. Help the resident comfortably position each foot in the washbasin or foot bath to soak. Each foot may need to be soaked separately if the resident is lying in bed. If the resident is sitting in a chair, both feet can be soaked at the same time.

18. Make sure the feet are completely covered by the water. Cover the feet and washbasin with a dry hand towel to retain heat.

19. Soak the feet for approximately 10–15 minutes. If needed, remove the feet and add more warm water.

20. Lift one foot out of the washbasin at a time and wash the entire foot. Clean between the toes and under the toenails with a soapy washcloth.

21. Rinse off all soap, especially between the toes.

> **Best Practice**
> The feet should be inspected for redness, cracks, or breaks in the skin, especially around the toenails. If observed, immediately report these to the licensed nursing staff.

22. Push the cuticles back gently with a washcloth or the dull end of an orangewood stick, if permitted.

23. Remove the washbasin or foot bath and dry the feet thoroughly, especially between the toes.

24. Use a nail clipper to cut the toenails, if permitted. Do not cut below the tips of the toes. Trimming the toenails is always easier after they have been soaked or bathed.

25. Shape and smooth any rough toenail edges with an emery board.

26. Apply lotion to the tops and soles of the feet and gently massage it into the skin (Figure 21.25). Do not apply between the toes. Gently remove any excess lotion with a dry, clean towel.

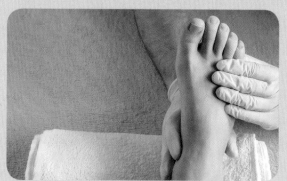

Figure 21.25

27. Remove and discard your gloves.

28. Wash your hands or use hand sanitizer to ensure infection control.

29. Put on a new pair of gloves.

30. If the resident is in bed, check to be sure the bed wheels are locked. Then reposition the resident and lower the bed. If the resident is in a chair, help her back to bed, if desired.

31. Follow the plan of care to determine if the side rails should be raised or lowered.

32. Remove, clean, and store equipment in the proper location. Disinfect the nail clippers. Remove soiled linens and discard disposable equipment.

Follow-Up

33. Remove and discard your gloves.

34. Wash your hands to ensure infection control.

35. Make sure the resident is comfortable and place the call light and personal items within reach.

36. Conduct a safety check before leaving the room. The room should be clean and free from clutter or spills.

37. Wash your hands or use hand sanitizer before leaving the room.

Reporting and Documentation

38. Communicate any specific observations, complications, or unusual responses to the licensed nursing staff. Record this information, along with the care provided, in the chart or EMR.

Perineal Care

Perineal care (sometimes called *peri care*) is the process of cleaning the genitals, or *external organs*, of the female and male reproductive systems, the urethral opening, and the anus. Perineal care is important, as it can prevent infections, skin breakdown, and possible odor. Perineal care is part of daily hygiene. It is also performed after elimination for residents who are immobile or who cannot provide this care for themselves. Perineal care is also necessary each time a resident is incontinent. Residents who have a catheter will require catheter care in addition to perineal care (see chapter 23).

Procedure   Providing Female and Male Perineal Care

Rationale
Proper perineal care promotes cleanliness, provides comfort, and reduces the potential for infections.

Preparation

1. Ask the licensed nursing staff how this procedure fits into the plan of care, if there are doctor's orders for the procedure, if there are any special instructions or precautions, and if the resident can be moved into the positions required for this procedure.
2. Wash your hands or use hand sanitizer before entering the room.
3. Knock before entering the room.
4. Introduce yourself using your full name and title. Explain that you work with the licensed nursing staff and will be providing care.
5. Greet the resident and ask the resident to state his or her full name, if able. Then check the resident's identification bracelet.
6. Use Mr., Mrs., or Ms. and the last name when conversing.
7. Explain the procedure in simple terms, even if the resident is not able to communicate or is disoriented. Ask permission to perform the procedure.
8. Bring the necessary equipment into the room. Place a paper towel, towel, or disposable protective pad on the overbed table as an infection-control barrier before placing the following items:
   - washbasin
   - bath blanket
   - disposable gloves
   - soap
   - disposable protective pad
   - several washcloths
   - several hand towels
   - bedpan or urinal
   - laundry hamper

The Procedure: Female Perineal Care

9. Provide privacy by closing the curtains, using a screen, or closing the door to the room.
10. Lock the bed wheels and then raise the bed to hip level.
11. Ensure safety during the procedure. If there are side rails, raise and secure the rails on the opposite side of the bed from where you will be working. Lower the rail on the side you are working.
12. Wash your hands or use hand sanitizer to ensure infection control.
13. Put on disposable gloves.
14. Position the resident on her back, if possible. Place the disposable protective pad under the resident's buttocks.
15. Cover the resident with a bath blanket. If possible, have the resident hold the bath blanket while you fanfold the bed linens to the foot of the bed. Be sure the resident is not exposed.
16. Offer the resident a bedpan or urinal. If the resident uses the bedpan or urinal, empty the contents and wash the bedpan or urinal. Remove and discard your gloves after assisting with toileting.
17. Wash your hands or use hand sanitizer to ensure infection control.
18. Put on a new pair of gloves.
19. Fill the washbasin with warm water. Check the water temperature. It should be 100–105°F. The water should feel comfortably warm to your elbow. You may also ask the resident to feel the water temperature, but always check yourself first.
20. Ask the resident to bend her knees and separate her legs.

(continued)

> **Best Practice**
> If the resident cannot bend her knees and separate her legs, access the perineal area from a lateral, or side-lying, position with the knees bent.

21. Move the linens down to the foot of the bed to expose only the perineal area. Keep the legs covered.
22. Wet a washcloth in the washbasin and apply a small amount of soap.

> **Best Practice**
> Soap can be difficult to rinse from a female's perineal area. Use a small amount to avoid leaving residue, which can be irritating.

23. Gently separate the labia with one hand. Keep the labia separated as much as possible during the procedure.
24. Wash the outer folds of the labia (*labia majora*) and the inner folds (*labia minora*) using single, downward strokes from top to bottom or front to back (Figure 21.26).

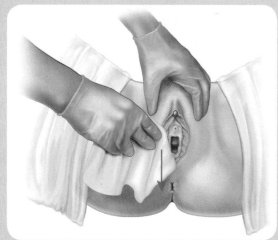

Figure 21.26

25. With each downward stroke, turn the washcloth to a clean side or get a new washcloth. You will use several washcloths during this procedure. Avoid placing your fingers on an area after washing it.
26. Use a new washcloth with a small amount of soap to clean from the clitoris to the anus (down the center).

27. Fill the washbasin with fresh, warm water. Change your gloves, if needed.
28. Using fresh water and a clean washcloth, rinse the area thoroughly.
29. Gently pat the area dry with a towel.
30. Turn the resident onto her side away from you.
31. Apply soap to a wet washcloth.
32. With one hand, lift the upper buttock to expose the anus. Wash the anal area using gentle, front-to-back strokes from the vagina to the anus (Figure 21.27).

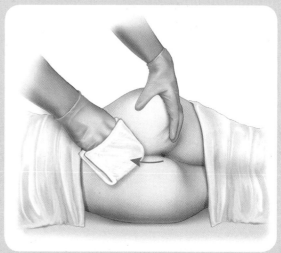

Figure 21.27

33. Rinse and gently pat the area dry.
34. Reposition the resident so she is lying on her back.
35. Remove and dispose of the protective pad.
36. Remove and discard your gloves.
37. Wash your hands or use hand sanitizer to ensure infection control.
38. Put on a new pair of gloves.
39. Replace the top covers and remove the bath blanket.
40. Check to be sure the bed wheels are locked and then lower the bed.
41. Follow the plan of care to determine if the side rails should be raised or lowered.
42. Remove, clean, and store equipment in the proper location. Remove soiled linens and discard disposable equipment.

The Procedure: Male Perineal Care

43. Provide privacy by closing the curtains, using a screen, or closing the door to the room.

Images courtesy of © Body Scientific International

44. Lock the bed wheels and then raise the bed to hip level.

45. Ensure safety during the procedure. If there are side rails, raise and secure the rails on the opposite side of the bed from where you will be working. Lower the rail on the side you are working.

46. Wash your hands or use hand sanitizer to ensure infection control.

47. Put on disposable gloves.

48. Position the resident on his back, if possible. Place the disposable protective pad under the resident's buttocks.

49. Cover the resident with a bath blanket. If possible, have the resident hold the bath blanket while you fanfold the bed linens to the foot of the bed. Be sure the resident is not exposed.

50. Offer the resident a bedpan or urinal. If the resident uses the bedpan or urinal, empty the contents and wash the bedpan or urinal. Remove and discard your gloves after assisting with toileting.

51. Wash your hands or use hand sanitizer to ensure infection control.

52. Put on a new pair of gloves.

53. Fill the washbasin with warm water. Check the water temperature. It should be 100–105°F. The water should feel comfortably warm to your elbow. You may also ask the resident to feel the water temperature, but always check yourself first.

54. Ask the resident to bend his knees and separate his legs.

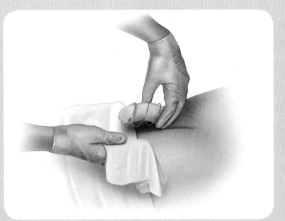

Figure 21.28

> **Best Practice**
> If the resident cannot bend his knees and separate his legs, access the perineal area from a lateral, or side-lying, position with the knees bent.

55. Move the linens down to the foot of the bed to expose only the perineal area. Keep the legs covered.

56. Wet a washcloth in the washbasin and apply a small amount of soap.

57. Gently lift and hold the penis in one hand. Start at the tip of the penis (meatus) and wash on each side in a circular motion down the shaft of the penis to the base (Figure 21.28).

58. If the penis is not circumcised, carefully pull back the foreskin while washing, rinsing, and drying the penis. If the foreskin will not retract, report this to the licensed nursing staff.

59. Lift and wash the scrotum. Also wash the inner thighs.

60. Fill the washbasin with fresh, warm water. Change your gloves, if needed.

61. Using fresh water and a clean washcloth, rinse the area thoroughly.

62. Gently pat the area dry with a towel.

63. Turn the resident onto his side away from you.

64. Apply soap to a wet washcloth.

65. Wash the anal area using gentle, front-to-back strokes.

66. Rinse and gently pat the area dry.

67. Reposition the resident so he is lying on his back.

68. Remove and dispose of the protective pad.

69. Remove and discard your gloves.

70. Wash your hands or use hand sanitizer to ensure infection control.

71. Put on a new pair of gloves.

72. Replace the top covers and remove the bath blanket.

73. Check to be sure the bed wheels are locked and then lower the bed.

74. Follow the plan of care to determine if the side rails should be raised or lowered.

75. Remove, clean, and store equipment in the proper location. Remove soiled linens and discard disposable equipment.

(continued)

Follow-Up

76. Remove and discard your gloves.

77. Wash your hands to ensure infection control.

78. Make sure the resident is comfortable and place the call light and personal items within reach.

79. Conduct a safety check before leaving the room. The room should be clean and free from clutter or spills.

80. Wash your hands or use hand sanitizer before leaving the room.

Reporting and Documentation

81. Communicate any specific observations, complications, or unusual responses to the licensed nursing staff. Record this information, along with the care provided, in the chart or EMR.

Dressing and Undressing

As a nursing assistant, you will often assist in dressing and undressing residents. A person's clothing is often reflective of his or her personal preferences and image. Thus, it is very helpful for residents to choose what to wear and to select clothing for maximum comfort. Encourage residents to be as independent as possible during dressing and undressing by helping only with buttons, snaps, or shoes, if needed. Clothing with zippers, Velcro™ fasteners, elastic waistbands, and slip-on shoes can make it easier for residents to maintain some independence when dressing. Shoes or slippers should fit well and have nonskid soles (not gum or rubber soles) or strips. This helps maintain safety so that residents do not slip or trip.

Procedure | Dressing and Undressing

Rationale

Residents in your care may require assistance during dressing and undressing. Your role in assisting is to ensure these activities are performed safely.

Preparation

1. Ask the licensed nursing staff how this procedure fits into the plan of care, if there are doctor's orders for the procedure, if there are any special instructions or precautions, and if the resident can be moved into the positions required for this procedure.

2. Wash your hands or use hand sanitizer before entering the room.

3. Knock before entering the room.

4. Introduce yourself using your full name and title. Explain that you work with the licensed nursing staff and will be providing care.

5. Greet the resident and ask the resident to state her full name, if able. Then check the resident's identification bracelet.

6. Use Mr., Mrs., or Ms. and the last name when conversing.

7. Explain the procedure in simple terms, even if the resident is not able to communicate or is disoriented. Ask permission to perform the procedure.

8. Bring the necessary equipment into the room. Place the following items in an accessible location:
   - bath blanket, as needed
   - disposable gloves, if needed
   - laundry hamper
   - clothes, arranged in the order they will be put on

The Procedure: Dressing

9. Provide privacy by closing the curtains, using a screen, or closing the door to the room.

10. Lock the bed wheels and then raise the bed to hip level.

11. Ensure safety during the procedure. If there are side rails, raise and secure the rails on the opposite side of the bed from where you will be working. Lower the rail on the side you are working.

12. Assist the resident to a Fowler's position. Determine how high to raise the head of the bed based on resident comfort. If the resident is mobile, she may be dressed in a chair or while sitting on the edge of the bed.

13. If the resident is in bed, fanfold the top linens to the foot of the bed. Cover the resident with a bath blanket, as needed, for warmth, dignity, and privacy.

14. If the resident wears a bra, ask her to put her arms through the straps and then place her breasts in the breast cups. Ask the resident to lean forward, assisting as needed. Bring the sides of the bra together in the back and close the fasteners. Adjust, if needed.

15. To put on upper garments that open in the back, slip the clothing over the resident's hands (weak side first). Move the clothing up the arms and position it on the shoulders. Close the garment and any fasteners in the back.

16. To put on upper garments that open in the front, slide the clothing onto the weak or painful arm and shoulder first (Figure 21.29A). Bring the garment around the resident's back. Ask the resident to lower her head and shoulders so she can slide her stronger arm through the garment more easily (Figure 21.29B). Close the garment and any fasteners in the front.

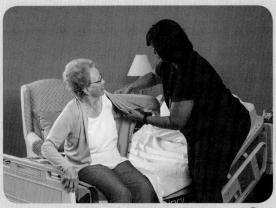

B

17. To put on upper garments that slip over the head, put the neck of the garment over the resident's head. Slide the resident's weaker arm and shoulder into the garment. Raise the resident's head and shoulders and pull the garment toward the waist. Slide the arm and shoulder of the stronger arm through the garment. Close any fasteners.

18. Slide the resident's underwear and then pants over the feet and up the legs (Figure 21.30). Start with the weak or painful side first. Ask the resident to bend at the knees and lift her buttocks off the bed. Assist, if needed. Grasp the top of the garment with both hands and slide the garment over the resident's hips and buttocks toward the waist. Close any fasteners. If the resident is unable to assist, roll her from side to side to dress the lower body.

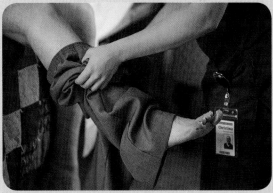

Figure 21.30

19. Pull the resident's socks or stockings up over each foot. Adjust until the length of the sock or stocking is smooth.

20. If the resident will be leaving her bed, put nonskid footwear on her feet and secure any fasteners. If she will be staying in bed, do not put on shoes.

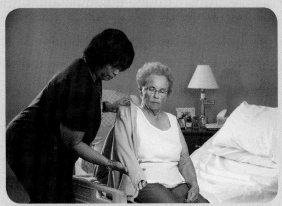

Figure 21.29

A

(continued)

21. If the resident is staying in bed, replace the top bed linens. Discard the bath blanket, if used, in the laundry hamper.

22. Check to be sure the bed wheels are locked, then reposition the resident and lower the bed.

23. Follow the plan of care to determine if the side rails should be raised or lowered.

The Procedure: Undressing

24. Provide privacy by closing the curtains, using a screen, or closing the door to the room.

25. Lock the bed wheels and then raise the bed to hip level.

26. Ensure safety during the procedure. If there are side rails, raise and secure the rails on the opposite side of the bed from where you will be working. Lower the rail on the side you are working.

> **Best Practice**
> Disposable gloves are worn only if required for infection prevention and control.

27. Assist the resident to a Fowler's position. Determine how high to raise the head of the bed based on resident comfort. If the resident is mobile, she may be undressed in a chair or while sitting on the edge of the bed.

28. If the resident is in bed, fanfold the top linens to the foot of the bed. Cover the resident with a bath blanket, as needed, for warmth, dignity, and privacy.

29. Raise the resident's head and shoulders or turn her slightly to the side away from you. This will make it easier to undo fasteners.

30. Pull the clothing to the resident's sides.

31. Remove the clothing from the resident's arms.

32. If the clothing does not open in the back, bring the clothing up to the resident's neck and remove over her head.

> **Best Practice**
> Remember to remove clothing from the stronger arm first and then from the weaker arm. Do not force or overextend the arms.

33. Remove the resident's shoes and socks or stockings.

34. Undo clothing fasteners and remove the resident's belt. Ask the resident to lift her buttocks, assisting, if needed.

35. Grasp the top of the garment with both hands and slide the pants over the resident's buttocks and down toward the knees. If the resident is unable to assist, have her roll from side to side as you lower the pants. Slide the pants down the legs. Remove the clothing from the stronger leg first and then from the weaker leg. Never force or overextend the legs.

> **Best Practice**
> Never pull, push, or otherwise roughly handle the resident when putting on or removing clothes.

36. Replace the top linens. Discard the bath blanket, if used, in the laundry hamper.

37. Check to be sure the bed wheels are locked, then reposition the resident and lower the bed.

38. Follow the plan of care to determine if the side rails should be raised or lowered.

Follow-Up

39. Wash your hands to ensure infection control.

40. Make sure the resident is comfortable and place the call light and personal items within reach.

41. Conduct a safety check before leaving the room. The room should be clean and free from clutter or spills.

42. Wash your hands or use hand sanitizer before leaving the room.

Reporting and Documentation

43. Communicate any specific observations, complications, or unusual responses to the licensed nursing staff. Record this information, along with the care provided, in the chart or EMR.

Images courtesy of © Tori Soper Photography

When delivering care, you may be asked to change a hospital gown for a patient who has an IV catheter. This needs to be done carefully so the IV catheter insertion and tubing are not dislodged and so the IV pole remains in place. The procedure that follows should be used when the IV is hanging on an IV pole and gowns with snaps or Velcro™ at the sleeves and shoulders are not available. When an IV is running through an electric pump, a gown with snaps or Velcro™ at the sleeves and shoulders will be required.

Procedure — Changing a Hospital Gown with an IV Catheter

Rationale

A patient's hospital gown should be changed daily and whenever it becomes wet or soiled. Special care should be taken when the patient has an IV catheter.

Preparation

1. Ask the licensed nursing staff how this procedure fits into the plan of care, if there are doctor's orders for the procedure, if there are any special instructions or precautions, and if the patient can be moved into the positions required for this procedure.

2. Wash your hands or use hand sanitizer before entering the room.

3. Knock before entering the room.

4. Introduce yourself using your full name and title. Explain that you work with the licensed nursing staff and will be providing care.

5. Greet the patient and ask the patient to state his full name, if able. Then check the patient's identification bracelet.

6. Use Mr., Mrs., or Ms. and the last name when conversing.

7. Explain the procedure in simple terms, even if the patient is not able to communicate or is disoriented. Ask permission to perform the procedure.

8. Bring the necessary equipment into the room. Place the following items in an accessible location:
   - bath blanket
   - 2 clean gowns
   - disposable gloves
   - laundry hamper

The Procedure

9. Provide privacy by closing the curtains, using a screen, or closing the door to the room.

10. Lock the bed wheels and then raise the bed to hip level.

11. Ensure safety during the procedure. If there are side rails, raise and secure the rails on the opposite side of the bed from where you will be working. Lower the rail on the side you are working.

12. Wash your hands or use hand sanitizer to ensure infection control.

13. Put on disposable gloves.

14. Assist the patient to a Fowler's position. Determine how high to raise the head of the bed based on patient comfort.

15. Cover the patient with a bath blanket and fanfold the top bed linens to the foot of the bed.

16. If the patient is wearing a gown without snaps or fasteners at the neck, undo the gown ties at the neck and free the gown from underneath the body.

17. Slip the gown down the patient's arms. Make sure the bath blanket stays in place.

18. Remove the gown from the patient's arm without the IV catheter and tubing. Move the gown across the patient's chest and lay it next to the other arm.

19. Gather the sleeve of the arm with the IV catheter so there is no pull or pressure on the IV tubing. Slide the gown over the IV site and tubing (Figure 21.31A).

20. Carefully remove the patient's arm and hand from the sleeve.

21. Keep the sleeve gathered and slide your hand along the tubing to the IV bag. Remove the IV bag from the IV pole (Figure 21.31B). Never disconnect the IV tubing from its insertion site or the IV bag.

> **Best Practice**
> Never lower the bag of IV fluid below the arm while changing the gown.

(continued)

Changing a Hospital Gown with an IV Catheter *(continued)*

22. Slide the IV bag and tubing through the sleeve (Figure 21.31C). Hang the IV bag back on the pole.

23. To put a clean gown on the patient, gather the sleeve of the gown that will go on the arm with the IV catheter.

24. Remove the IV bag from the pole (Figure 21.31D). Slide the sleeve over the IV bag and tubing at the shoulder part of the gown. Hang the IV bag back on the pole.

25. Slide the gathered sleeve over the IV tubing, the patient's hand and arm, and the IV site. Slide the sleeve onto the patient's shoulder.

26. Put the patient's other arm through the opposite sleeve and fasten the gown.

27. Replace the top linens and remove the bath blanket.

28. Check to be sure the bed wheels are locked, then reposition the patient and lower the bed.

29. Follow the plan of care to determine if the side rails should be raised or lowered.

30. Remove, clean, and store equipment in the proper location. Remove soiled linens and discard disposable equipment.

Follow-Up

31. Remove and discard your gloves.

32. Wash your hands to ensure infection control.

33. Make sure the patient is comfortable and place the call light and personal items within reach.

34. Conduct a safety check before leaving the room. The room should be clean and free from clutter or spills.

35. Wash your hands or use hand sanitizer before leaving the room.

Reporting and Documentation

36. Communicate any specific observations, complications, or unusual responses to the licensed nursing staff. Record this information, along with the care provided, in the chart or EMR.

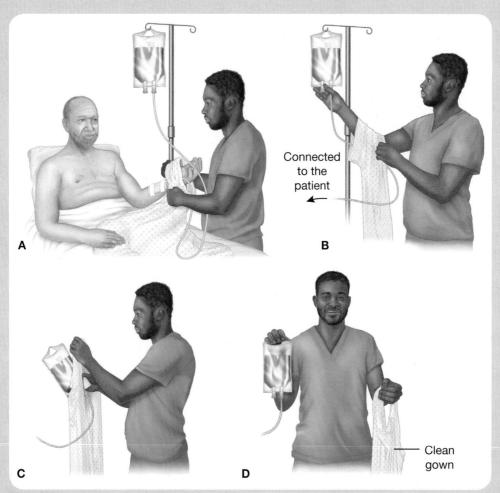

Connected to the patient ←

A

B

Clean gown

C

D

Figure 21.31

Image courtesy of © Body Scientific International

Using the Key Terms

Complete the following sentences using key terms in this section.

1. A(n) _____ is a type of bathtub used for therapeutic purposes.
2. Swollen, inflamed veins found around the anus are called _____.
3. _____ is routine actions that promote and maintain cleanliness and health.
4. A(n) _____ is a small, kidney-shaped bowl often used during oral care.
5. The _____ is the area between the thighs, spanning the coccyx, pubis, anus, urethra, and external genitals.
6. A doctor who specializes in diagnosing and treating foot diseases is a(n) _____.
7. A(n) _____ is a therapeutic bath in which the resident's perineum and buttocks are soaked in warm water.
8. Therapies that have a healing effect on the body and mind are known as _____.
9. When skin is intact and without irritation, it has good _____.
10. The procedure performed to cleanse the perineum is called _____.

Know and Understand the Facts

11. List three reasons why personal hygiene and grooming are important.
12. What are two guidelines a holistic nursing assistant should follow to perform safe fingernail care?
13. Identify two important actions a holistic nursing assistant should take when giving oral care.
14. What special care considerations are important for performing foot care?

Analyze and Apply Concepts

15. Identify two ways a holistic nursing assistant can encourage independence during personal hygiene and grooming.
16. Describe how to bathe the arm of a resident with limited mobility.
17. A resident is not able to wash her own hair. Describe the steps needed to best assist her with hair care.
18. Explain how to perform female perineal care.
19. What is one best practice for changing the hospital gown of a patient with an IV catheter?

Think Critically

Read the following care situation. Then answer the questions that follow.

Mrs. D is 80 years old and was admitted to the hospital last night with pneumonia. She has diabetes, PVD, and arthritis. You have been assigned to help her with personal hygiene and grooming this morning. Mrs. D is having difficulty breathing and has an IV catheter. She is also stiff from her arthritic joints. When you enter Mrs. D's room, you find that she is sleeping. She has a strong body odor, her hair is tangled, and she has very long, dirty fingernails.

20. If you could perform only one personal hygiene procedure, which would be the most important?
21. What steps would you need to take to perform the procedure?
22. What actions can you take to help Mrs. D be more comfortable when providing care?
23. Given Mrs. D's current condition, describe five safety and quality care issues you would need to be aware of when performing her personal hygiene and grooming.

Questions to Consider

- The next time you are with friends or family members, observe their skin. Look at their faces, arms, or legs. How would you describe their skin texture (smooth or rough), tone, and integrity? Is their skin dry or oily? Does their skin have marks such as freckles, moles, bumps, pimples, or a rash?
- Compare your skin with the skin of a person you are observing. What are the similarities and differences?
- How healthy do you think the person's skin is? How healthy is your skin? What makes the skin look healthy or unhealthy?

Objectives

Preserving skin integrity is one of the most important aspects of personal hygiene and grooming. Keeping skin clean, dry, and free from irritation, inflammation, damage, or injury ensures that pathogens cannot easily break through the skin's surface. In particular, it is important to observe the skin of older adults in your care on a continuous basis. Caring for residents' skin conscientiously can influence quality of life. Using hot or cold therapies may also relax residents and reduce pain or swelling. To achieve the objectives for this section, you must successfully

- **explain** the importance of maintaining skin integrity;
- **describe** how heat and cold applications can help and harm the skin;
- **demonstrate** safe skin care when using hot and cold therapies.

Key Terms

Learn these key terms to better understand the information presented in the section.

anticoagulants

compresses

cryotherapy

cyanotic

gangrene

hydration

pallor

tepid

thermotherapy

How Do Skin Types Differ?

The skin is the largest organ in your body and is the body part that best reflects your health. For example, dry skin can be a sign of dehydration.

Skin types can be categorized as normal, dry, oily, or combination. A person's skin type depends on

- the water content of the skin, which affects elasticity;
- oiliness, which affects texture; and
- sensitivity.

Skin type can change over time due to personal care, cosmetics used, environment, medications taken, hormones, and aging. Each skin type usually requires specialized care. See Figure 21.32 for a comparison of skin types.

What Factors Promote Skin Integrity?

Several actions can help maintain the integrity of the skin so that skin remains healthy and undamaged and retains its normal functions. These actions are especially important for older skin, which is at greater risk for tears, cuts, and bruises:

- **Eat a healthy diet.** Eating a well-rounded diet that includes fruits, vegetables, whole grains, and lean protein is important for skin health. Vitamins A, D, C, and E, in particular, promote healthy skin.
- **Stay hydrated.** Men should drink about 15 cups (3.7 liters) of fluids each day. Women should drink about 11 cups (2.7 liters) each day.

Think About This

The thickest skin on your body is 1.4 inches deep and can be found on the soles of your feet. The thinnest skin is on your eyelids and is 0.02 millimeters deep.

Characteristics of Skin Types	
Type	**Characteristics**
Normal	• Radiant complexion • Balance between dryness and oiliness • Few blemishes • Little sensitivity • Barely visible pores
Dry	• Dry, rough complexion with more visible lines • Less elastic • Red, inflamed, peeling, and cracking skin • Scaly, itchy patches • Invisible pores
Oily	• Shiny and dull colored • Increased tendency to develop blackheads, pimples, and other blemishes • Enlarged pores
Combination	• Dry and oily in different areas; may have an oily T-zone (nose, forehead, and chin) • Increased tendency to develop blackheads • Larger-than-normal pores

Figure 21.32 These four skin types have different characteristics and require different care.

- **Maintain good skin care habits**. Cleanse the skin every morning and night (Figure 21.33). Always wash your hands before touching your face. Do not overuse skin products, as they can cancel out each other's benefits. Keep makeup brushes fresh and clean.

- **Sufficiently hydrate the skin**. Using moisturizer helps keep skin hydrated. Moisturizer is best applied when the skin is damp so that surface moisture is drawn into the skin.

- **Use sunscreen**. Wear broad spectrum sunscreen that protects against UVA and UVB rays and has an SPF of 30 or higher. Apply sunscreen every two to three hours when in the sun.

- **Live a balanced life**. Make exercise part of your daily activities, sleep seven to eight hours each night, and manage stress using healthy strategies such as mindful meditation and yoga.

- **Do not smoke**. Smoking significantly advances the aging of skin and causes drooping, wrinkles, lines, and broken surface blood vessels (Figure 21.34). Smoking also causes changes in the fiber and moisture of the skin, increases the risk of burns, and reduces blood flow to the epidermis by causing blood vessels to narrow. Reduced blood flow decreases the amount of oxygen carried to the skin.

Think About This
Studies have shown that, by the age of 70, a person who has smoked 30 cigarettes a day has added the equivalent of 14 years to his or her skin. Skin aging can take the form of lines around the eyes called *crow's feet* and multiple vertical lines around the mouth called *smoker's lines*.

How Can Nursing Assistants Help Maintain Skin Integrity?

There are many ways nursing assistants can help maintain the skin integrity of residents. These ways include giving excellent skin care and being vigilant about observing the skin, particularly when caring for older adults and residents with diabetes. You should also be especially careful with residents taking **anticoagulants**

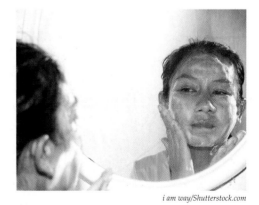

i am way/Shutterstock.com

Figure 21.33 Skin should be cleansed twice a day: in the morning and at night.

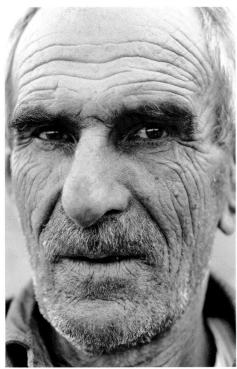
Zurijeta/Shutterstock.com

Figure 21.34 Smoking causes skin to age faster and develop more wrinkles and lines.

(medications that prevent blood clot formation) and steroid medications, which cause bruising to occur more easily. Any changes in the skin must be reported immediately to the licensed nursing staff. Following are several actions you should take as part of your care:

- Avoid giving residents long baths, as these can remove oils from the skin. Use warm, rather than very hot, water.
- Use mild cleansers rather than strong soaps. Strong soaps have ingredients that can remove oil from the skin.
- Gently pat the skin dry after a bath or shower. This leaves some moisture on the skin.
- Regularly moisturize the skin, especially if it is dry. Do not put lotion between the toes, where fungus can grow. Give a very light massage, if appropriate, while applying lotion.
- If the resident is incontinent, use disposable protective pads. These can be removed and replaced more easily than linens.
- Keep linens neat and wrinkle free. Make sure linens are free from food crumbs and any other items that can place pressure on the skin.
- Keep the skin clean and dry. If the skin is covered with urine or feces due to incontinence, clean the skin immediately with mild soap and water and gently pat the area dry. Wear disposable gloves for infection control.
- Avoid dragging or pulling the resident during positioning. Friction can cause the skin to become red or irritated and experience shearing or tearing.

Pressure Points and Decubitus Ulcers

Residents who are immobile due to illness, who are in wheelchairs, or who need to use assistive devices are more vulnerable to changes in skin integrity. As you learned in chapter 9, certain areas of the body are more likely to be at risk for reduced skin integrity than others. These areas are called *pressure points* and can be found where skin covers the bony areas of the body. Pressure points are in constant danger of being exposed to continuous pressure, and when the skin is compromised, *decubitus ulcers* (also called *bedsores* or *pressure sores*) can develop. The severity of decubitus ulcers ranges from stage 1 to stage 4 (as illustrated in Figure 9.6). As the image shows, in stage 1, the skin is somewhat red. Stage 4 is characterized by deep skin damage, exposed muscle and bone, necrotic tissue formation, and bleeding ulcers. The best way to detect decubitus ulcers and ensure skin integrity is to observe the skin carefully while performing personal hygiene activities, grooming, and any other procedures.

Observation of the Skin

When observing the skin, always be sure there is sufficient bright light. Notice whether the skin is cool, warm, hot, moist, or dry. Look at the color of the skin, lips, and nail beds. Report to the licensed nursing staff if you observe any of the following:

- The skin has a **pallor** (unusually pale color), is flushed (red), or is **cyanotic** (blue due to insufficient oxygen).
- There are new abrasions, tears, bruises, rashes, and blisters.
- A blister has opened.
- There are new lumps and swollen or tender areas.
- There is new or increased drainage or bleeding.
- You smell unusual odors.

- The resident complains of itching or burning or is scratching or rubbing an area excessively.
- The scalp is flaky, itchy, or sore.
- Head lice are present.

Regularly check the skin for red areas, irritation, or skin breakdown at pressure points. Observe the following areas, which are illustrated in Figure 9.7, closely:

- toes, heels, ankles, and knees
- elbows and shoulder blades
- spine, especially the area around the tailbone
- back of the head over the ears
- nose and ears, if a resident is using an oxygen cannula

Also check areas where body parts rub together, especially if the resident is obese:

- under the breasts
- between the folds of the abdomen
- between the buttocks
- between the thighs

If you notice red skin, immediately remove whatever is causing the pressure. Do not massage the area. Recheck the skin in 15 minutes. If the redness is gone, you do not need to take any other action. If the redness does not disappear after 15 minutes, talk with the licensed nursing staff about ways to provide relief.

Change a resident's position every two hours. When possible, and with a doctor's order, help residents ambulate and perform range-of-motion exercises. In all cases, pressure points should be kept dry and clean. Any ulcers should be cleaned and dressed with bandages, and wet or creased dressings and bandages should be changed according to the plan of care.

How Are Heat Applications Beneficial?

The use of heat to increase circulation and ease pain is called **thermotherapy**. Thermotherapy can be very beneficial to residents and can promote healing. Heat has many healing qualities. It opens or dilates blood vessels, which increases the circulation of oxygen and nutrients and reduces pain. Heat is very effective at relaxing muscles and also improves flexibility and lessens spasms. Heat applications on the surface of the skin are used to treat chronic injuries or later-stage acute injuries, such as dislocation of a joint or contusion. Heat can also be used to treat arthritis and tendonitis, ease headaches and muscle tension, and warm up the muscles before exercise. Heat should be avoided after exercise and during the acute phase of an injury.

In healthcare facilities, a doctor will determine the appropriateness of using heat applications. Care should be taken if the resident cannot feel the heat of the application; is sensitive to heat; or has infections, tumors, open wounds, or stitches. Physical therapists often apply heat applications, but some heat applications are applied by nursing assistants, based on a doctor's order and the plan of care. Heat applications may include warm, moist **compresses** (pads); warm soaks; and an aquathermia pad.

Types of Heat Applications

Heat applications can be moist or dry. Moist heat is usually preferred because it penetrates the skin more effectively and is less drying. Heat applications can include heating pads, heat wraps, and compresses or soaks. Sitz baths and the whirlpool tub are also considered heat applications. Heat applications that can raise body temperature include hot baths, saunas, steam baths, and hot showers. Some commercial, premoistened heat compresses are available and are packaged in foil. The *aquathermia pad*, or *K-pad*, provides dry heat to promote skin circulation by

Think About This
Because the body does not have a natural mechanism to remove scar tissue, scars form on the skin after a wound is completely healed. After an injury to the skin, tissue is often discolored and lacks sweat glands and hair.

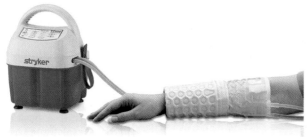

Copyright © 2017 Stryker

Figure 21.35 The aquathermia pad increases skin circulation in the body part to which it is applied.

applying a constant temperature to a body part for a specified period of time (Figure 21.35). Distilled water is used. When aquathermia pads are used, they should have a flannel cover or a barrier to prevent pads from directly touching the skin. Do not use pins and be sure the tubing and the pad are level with the heating unit. The tubing should never hang below the bed. The pad should be checked for leaks and should be in good operating condition.

Care Considerations for Heat Applications

Several important care considerations need to be followed to ensure heat applications are helpful and not harmful:

- Practice safety when working with water. Prevent or clean up spills on or near the resident and your work area.
- Make sure the heat application is warm, not hot. Maintain a consistent temperature, if possible.
- Apply heat for 15–20 minutes, unless the doctor orders a shorter or longer time, and check every five minutes to see how well the resident's skin tolerates the heat application. Heat applications may be applied more than once a day, depending on the doctor's order.
- Never apply a heat application directly to the resident's skin. Always provide a wrapping, such as a cover, or place a barrier between the heat application and the skin.
- If using an aquathermia pad, set the temperature as directed by the licensed nursing staff. Check the skin underneath the pad for redness, swelling, or blisters. Stop the treatment and remove the pad if redness, swelling, or blisters appear or if the resident complains of pain, discomfort, or decreased sensation. Immediately notify the licensed nursing staff. Refill the heating unit if distilled water drops below the full line.
- Maintain resident **hydration** (a sufficient amount of fluid in body tissues), proper resident body position, and comfort during treatment with heat applications.

Further treatment may be required after a heat application. For example, dressings may need to be reapplied to the affected area. Review the procedures for changing dressings in chapter 15.

Procedure | Using Warm, Moist Compresses

Rationale
The safe and proper application of warm, moist compresses promotes healing and eases pain.

Preparation
1. Ask the licensed nursing staff how this procedure fits into the plan of care, if there are doctor's orders for the procedure, if there are any special instructions or precautions, and if the resident can be moved into the positions required for this procedure.

2. Wash your hands or use hand sanitizer before entering the room.
3. Knock before entering the room.
4. Introduce yourself using your full name and title. Explain that you work with the licensed nursing staff and will be providing care.
5. Greet the resident and ask the resident to state his full name, if able. Then check the resident's identification bracelet.
6. Use Mr., Mrs., or Ms. and the last name when conversing.

7. Explain the procedure in simple terms, even if the resident is not able to communicate or is disoriented. Ask permission to perform the procedure.

8. Bring the necessary equipment into the room. Place a paper towel, towel, or disposable protective pad on the overbed table as an infection-control barrier before placing the following items:
   - washbasin
   - several gauze pads
   - 2–3 washcloths and hand towels
   - bath towel
   - plastic wrap, ties, tape, and rolled gauze, if needed
   - bath blanket
   - disposable protective pad
   - disposable gloves
   - laundry hamper

The Procedure

9. Provide privacy by closing the curtains, using a screen, or closing the door to the room.

10. Lock the bed wheels and then raise the bed to hip level.

11. Ensure safety during the procedure. If there are side rails, raise and secure the rails on the opposite side of the bed from where you will be working. Lower the rail on the side you are working.

12. Position the resident properly for the procedure. The proper position will depend on the body part receiving the warm, moist compress.

13. Place a disposable protective pad under the body part that will receive the warm, moist compress and use the bath blanket to cover any other exposed areas.

14. Fill the washbasin one-half to two-thirds full of warm water. Check the water temperature. It should be 100–105°F. The water should feel comfortably warm to your elbow. You may also ask the resident to feel the water temperature, but always check yourself first.

15. Wash your hands or use hand sanitizer to ensure infection control.

16. Put on disposable gloves.

17. Use a washcloth or gauze pad as a compress for the skin. Place the compress in the warm water and squeeze out any excess moisture.

18. Observe the application site for inflammation and skin color. Alert the licensed nursing staff if the skin is red or inflamed. Proceed only by direction.

19. Apply the compress to the body part. Note the time of application.

20. Cover the compress with plastic wrap and then a bath towel. You may also secure the bath towel in place with ties, tape, or rolled gauze. Follow instructions from the licensed nursing staff. Never put tape on the resident's skin.

21. Place the call light and personal items within reach. Place a glass of fresh water on the overbed table, if permitted.

22. Check to be sure the bed wheels are locked, then lower the bed.

23. Follow the plan of care to determine if the side rails should be raised or lowered. Unscreen the resident or open the door to the room, if appropriate.

24. Remove and discard your gloves.

25. Wash your hands or use hand sanitizer to ensure infection control.

26. Check on the resident every five minutes (Figure 21.36). Treatments usually last no longer than 20 minutes, unless otherwise ordered by the doctor.

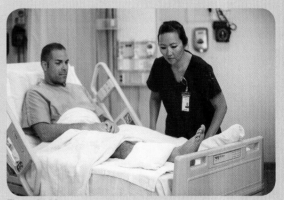

Figure 21.36

Best Practice
Observe and check the following: Is the compress warm enough or too hot? Is there pain or burning at the site? Does the resident feel weak, faint, or drowsy? If there are any problems or complications, remove the application and report to the licensed nursing staff.

(continued)

27. When it is time to remove the warm, moist compress, lock the bed wheels and then raise the bed to hip level.

28. Ensure safety during the procedure. If there are side rails, raise and secure the rails on the opposite side of the bed from where you will be working. Lower the rail on the side you are working.

29. Wash your hands or use hand sanitizer to ensure infection control.

30. Put on disposable gloves.

31. Carefully remove the compress. Note the time the compress is removed. Observe the resident's response to the application.

32. Appropriately discard the compress. Remove the protective pad and change any wet linens. Assist with any further treatment as instructed by the licensed nursing staff.

33. Check to be sure the bed wheels are locked, then reposition the resident and lower the bed.

34. Follow the plan of care to determine if the side rails should be raised or lowered.

35. Remove, clean, and store equipment in the proper location. Remove soiled linens and discard disposable equipment.

Follow-Up

36. Remove and discard your gloves.

37. Wash your hands to ensure infection control.

38. Make sure the resident is comfortable and place the call light and personal items within reach.

39. Conduct a safety check before leaving the room. The room should be clean and free from clutter or spills.

40. Wash your hands or use hand sanitizer before leaving the room.

Reporting and Documentation

41. Communicate any specific observations, complications, or unusual responses to the licensed nursing staff. Record this information, along with the care provided, in the chart or EMR.

Image courtesy of © Tori Soper Photography

Procedure | Using Warm Soaks

Rationale

The safe and proper application of warm soaks promotes healing and eases pain. Warm soaks increase blood flow to the affected area.

Preparation

1. Ask the licensed nursing staff how this procedure fits into the plan of care, if there are doctor's orders for the procedure, if there are any special instructions or precautions, and if the resident can be moved into the positions required for this procedure.

2. Wash your hands or use hand sanitizer before entering the room.

3. Knock before entering the room.

4. Introduce yourself using your full name and title. Explain that you work with the licensed nursing staff and will be providing care.

5. Greet the resident and ask the resident to state his full name, if able. Then check the resident's identification bracelet.

6. Use Mr., Mrs., or Ms. and the last name when conversing.

7. Explain the procedure in simple terms, even if the resident is not able to communicate or is disoriented. Ask permission to perform the procedure.

8. Bring the necessary equipment into the room. Place a paper towel, towel, or disposable protective pad on the overbed table as an infection-control barrier before placing the following items:
   - washbasin or an arm or foot bath
   - disposable protective pad
   - bath blanket
   - several hand towels
   - disposable gloves

The Procedure

9. Provide privacy by closing the curtains, using a screen, or closing the door to the room.

10. If the resident is in bed, lock the bed wheels and then raise the bed to hip level.

11. Ensure safety during the procedure. If there are side rails, raise and secure the rails on the opposite side of the bed from where you will be working. Lower the rail on the side you are working.

12. Wash your hands or use hand sanitizer to ensure infection control.

13. Put on disposable gloves.

14. Position the resident and body part for the procedure. If the resident cannot get out of bed, the soak may take place in bed. The soak may also take place out of bed, with the resident seated at the edge of the bed or in a chair.

15. Use a bath blanket to cover any exposed areas and provide warmth.

16. Fill the washbasin half-full with warm water. Check the water temperature. The water should feel comfortably warm to your elbow. You may also ask the resident to feel the water temperature, but always check yourself first.

17. Put a disposable protective pad under the washbasin to catch any spills.

18. Place the affected body part into the warm water. Pad the edge of the washbasin with a towel. Note the time of the application.

19. Place the call light and personal items within reach. Place a glass of fresh water on the overbed table, if permitted.

20. If the resident is in bed, check to be sure the bed wheels are locked, then lower the bed. Follow the plan of care to determine if the side rails should be raised or lowered. If the resident is sitting in a chair or on the edge of the bed, be certain all safety precautions are in place. Unscreen the resident or open the door to the room, if appropriate.

21. Remove and discard your gloves.

22. Wash your hands or use hand sanitizer to ensure infection control.

23. Check on the resident every five minutes. Treatments usually last no longer than 15–20 minutes, unless otherwise ordered by the doctor. The water may have to be changed to maintain the desired warmth.

Best Practice
Observe and check the following: Is the water warm enough or too hot? Is there pain or burning? Does the resident feel weak, faint, or drowsy? If there are any problems or complications, remove the application and report to the licensed nursing staff.

24. When the warm soak is complete, lock the bed wheels and then raise the bed to hip level if the resident is in bed.

25. Ensure safety during the procedure. If there are side rails, raise and secure the rails on the opposite side of the bed from where you will be working. Lower the rail on the side you are working.

26. Wash your hands or use hand sanitizer to ensure infection control.

27. Put on disposable gloves.

28. Remove the body part from the warm water and pat it dry with a clean hand towel (Figure 21.37). Note the time the soak was stopped. Assist with any further treatment as instructed by the licensed nursing staff.

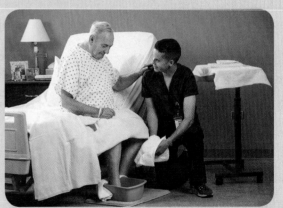
Figure 21.37

29. Discard the water. Remove the protective pad and change any wet linens.

30. If the resident is in bed, check to be sure the bed wheels are locked. Then reposition the resident and lower the bed.

31. Follow the plan of care to determine if the side rails should be raised or lowered.

32. Remove, clean, and store equipment in the proper location. Remove soiled linens and discard disposable equipment.

(continued)

Follow-Up

33. Remove and discard your gloves.

34. Wash your hands to ensure infection control.

35. Make sure the resident is comfortable and place the call light and personal items within reach.

36. Conduct a safety check before leaving the room. The room should be clean and free from clutter or spills.

37. Wash your hands or use hand sanitizer before leaving the room.

Reporting and Documentation

38. Communicate any specific observations, complications, or unusual responses to the licensed nursing staff. Record this information, along with the care provided, in the chart or EMR.

Image courtesy of © Tori Soper Photography

When Are Cold Applications Useful?

Cryotherapy is the use of cold applications to reduce swelling and ease pain and is typically recommended for acute injuries. Cold applications are most effective when applied early and often during the first 24–48 hours after an injury. They decrease blood flow to the injury, lessening inflammation and swelling (*edema*).

Cryotherapy is most effective for sprains, bumps, bruises, and soft-tissue injuries. Cold applications cause *vasoconstriction* (the shrinking of blood vessels), which decreases blood flow to an area. This slows the demand for oxygen and reduces inflammation, muscle contractions and spasms, and swelling. Cold applications can slow or stop bleeding and ease pain. They cannot, however, decrease swelling that is already present.

In healthcare facilities, a doctor will determine when to use cold applications. Physical therapists often apply cold applications, but nursing assistants may apply some cold applications based on a doctor's order and the plan of care. Cold applications can include cold, moist compresses and different types of ice packs (Figure 21.38). An *ice cap*, an ice pack used specifically for the head, has a wide opening so it can be filled easily with ice chips. Another specialized ice pack is the *ice collar*, a narrow bag filled with ice that curves to fit the neck.

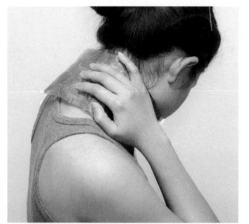
Praisaeng/Shutterstock.com

Figure 21.38 Ice packs come in many shapes and sizes and can be applied to various parts of the body.

Healthcare Scenario
Warm Soak Safety

A recent online news article told the story of Mr. W, who is 79 years old and a resident at a local healthcare facility. The nursing assistant caring for Mr. W was in a rush when she provided a warm soak for his feet, as ordered per his plan of care. Mr. W is diabetic, and warm soaks are an important part of his foot care. The nursing assistant prepared the warm soak, but did not feel the temperature of the water. She only asked Mr. W if the water was okay. Mr. W has PVD from diabetes and has little sensitivity to hot and cold. He put his feet in the water and said it was fine. Mr. W did not remove his feet until the nursing assistant returned 10 minutes later. When the nursing assistant came into the room, she found that Mr. W's skin was red and blistered.

Apply It

1. What did the nursing assistant do wrong?

2. What proper procedure should the nursing assistant have followed?

3. What should the nursing assistant do when she sees Mr. W's skin after the warm soak?

Other cold applications include a **tepid** (slightly warm) sponge bath and a hypothermia blanket, which is a mattress pad through which a continuous stream of very cold water flows. The hypothermia blanket can only be applied by the licensed nursing staff. The goal of these applications is to lower body temperature.

Several important care considerations need to be observed to ensure cold applications are helpful and not harmful:

- Practice safety when working with water. Prevent or clean up spills on or near the resident and your work area.
- Apply cold compresses to injured areas for no more than 20 minutes at a time or as long as ordered by the doctor. The cold application can be removed for 10 minutes and then reapplied for 10 minutes. Check every five minutes to see how well the resident's skin tolerates the cold application.
- Always cover the rest of the resident if he or she feels cold during the application.
- Always wrap ice packs in a thin covering such as a towel before applying them to the resident's body.
- Immediately stop a cold application if the resident complains of numbness or if the skin appears white or spotty.
- Stop the cold application if the resident complains of burning pain. Burning pain can indicate a lack of blood supply to the skin, called *ischemia*, which can lead to necrosis.
- Check for signs of *frostbite*, a condition in which the skin becomes too cold or frozen, red, and numb (Figure 21.39). *Frostnip* is the first stage of frostbite and can be treated by warming the skin. Severe frostbite can cause infection and **gangrene** (decay of body tissue) and can possibly require amputation.
- Maintain proper resident body position and comfort during treatment with cold applications.

Further treatment may be required after a cold application. For example, dressings may need to be reapplied to the affected area. Review the procedures for changing dressings in chapter 15.

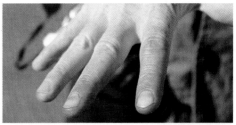

tome213/Shutterstock.com

A

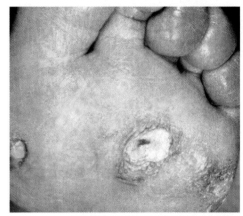

Clinical Photography, Central Manchester University Hospitals NHS Foundation Trust, UK/Science Source

B

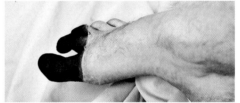

iStock.com/powerofforever

C

Figure 21.39 Frostbite develops in three stages. In frostnip (A), the skin appears red. In the second stage of frostbite (B), skin turns pale. In the most severe stages of frostbite (C), all layers of skin are affected.

Procedure | Using Cold, Moist Compresses

Rationale

Cold, moist compresses help reduce swelling and bruising and ease pain when an acute injury occurs.

Preparation

1. Ask the licensed nursing staff how this procedure fits into the plan of care, if there are doctor's orders for the procedure, if there are any special instructions or precautions, and if the resident can be moved into the positions required for this procedure.

2. Wash your hands or use hand sanitizer before entering the room.

3. Knock before entering the room.

4. Introduce yourself using your full name and title. Explain that you work with the licensed nursing staff and will be providing care.

5. Greet the resident and ask the resident to state her full name, if able. Then check the resident's identification bracelet.

6. Use Mr., Mrs., or Ms. and the last name when conversing.

(continued)

7. Explain the procedure in simple terms, even if the resident is not able to communicate or is disoriented. Ask permission to perform the procedure.

8. Bring the necessary equipment into the room. Place a paper towel, towel, or disposable protective pad on the overbed table as an infection-control barrier before placing the following items:
   - large basin with ice
   - small basin with cold water
   - several small towels and washcloths
   - gauze pads (appropriate size for the area receiving application)
   - bath towel
   - bath blanket
   - disposable protective pad
   - disposable gloves, if needed

The Procedure

9. Provide privacy by closing the curtains, using a screen, or closing the door to the room.

10. If the resident is in bed, lock the bed wheels and then raise the bed to hip level.

11. Ensure safety during the procedure. If there are side rails, raise and secure the rails on the opposite side of the bed from where you will be working. Lower the rail on the side you are working.

12. Position the resident and body part for the procedure. The proper position will depend on the body part receiving the cold, moist compress. If the resident cannot get out of bed, the cold, moist compress may be used in the bed. The cold, moist compress may also be used out of bed, with the resident seated on the edge of the bed or in a chair.

13. Place a disposable protective pad under the body part that will receive the cold, moist compress and use the bath blanket to cover any other exposed area and provide warmth.

14. Pour the cold water from the small basin into the large basin with ice.

15. Use a washcloth or gauze pad as a compress for the skin. Place the compress in the cold water and thoroughly wring out the compress to remove excess moisture.

16. Gently apply the compress to the body part and wrap it with a towel (Figure 21.40). Work as quickly as possible to prevent temperature change. Note the time of the application.

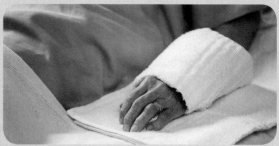

Figure 21.40

17. Change the compress frequently. Continue the treatment as ordered, usually for 20 minutes.

> **Best Practice**
> Ask the resident about the temperature of the compress. Is it too cold? Does the resident feel numb or have any burning pain? Check often for red or pale skin. If there are any problems or complications, remove the application and report to the licensed nursing staff.

18. Appropriately discard each compress. Remove the protective pad and change any wet linens. Assist with any further treatment as instructed by the licensed nursing staff.

19. If the resident is in bed, check to be sure the bed wheels are locked. Then reposition the resident and lower the bed.

20. Follow the plan of care to determine if the side rails should be raised or lowered.

21. Remove, clean, and store equipment in the proper location. Remove soiled linens and discard disposable equipment.

Follow-Up

22. Wash your hands to ensure infection control.

23. Make sure the resident is comfortable and place the call light and personal items within reach.

24. Conduct a safety check before leaving the room. The room should be clean and free from clutter or spills.

25. Wash your hands or use hand sanitizer before leaving the room.

Reporting and Documentation

26. Communicate any specific observations, complications, or unusual responses to the licensed nursing staff. Record this information, along with the care provided, in the chart or EMR.

Image courtesy of © Tori Soper Photography

Procedure Using Ice Packs

Rationale
Ice packs can help reduce swelling and ease pain.

Preparation

1. Ask the licensed nursing staff how this procedure fits into the plan of care, if there are doctor's orders for the procedure, if there are any special instructions or precautions, and if the resident can be moved into the positions required for this procedure.

2. Wash your hands or use hand sanitizer before entering the room.

3. Knock before entering the room.

4. Introduce yourself using your full name and title. Explain that you work with the licensed nursing staff and will be providing care.

5. Greet the resident and ask the resident to state his or her full name, if able. Then check the resident's identification bracelet.

6. Use Mr., Mrs., or Ms. and the last name when conversing.

7. Explain the procedure in simple terms, even if the resident is not able to communicate or is disoriented. Ask permission to perform the procedure.

8. Bring the necessary equipment into the room. Place a paper towel, towel, or disposable protective pad on the overbed table as an infection-control barrier before placing the following items:

    - 1 ice pack (ice bag, ice collar, ice glove, or ready-to-use disposable cold pack depending on the affected body part)
    - flannel cover
    - ties, tape, or rolled gauze
    - ice chips or crushed ice, if needed
    - large spoon, cup, or ice scooper, if needed
    - paper towels
    - bath blanket
    - disposable protective pad
    - disposable gloves, if needed

The Procedure

9. Provide privacy by closing the curtains, using a screen, or closing the door to the room.

10. If the resident is in bed, lock the bed wheels and then raise the bed to hip level.

11. Ensure safety during the procedure. If there are side rails, raise and secure the rails on the opposite side of the bed from where you will be working. Lower the rail on the side you are working.

12. Position the resident and body part for the procedure. The ice pack may be used in bed or while the resident is seated at the edge of the bed or in a chair.

13. Place a disposable protective pad under the body part that will receive the ice pack and use the bath blanket to cover any exposed areas to provide warmth.

14. If you are not using a disposable cold pack, fill an ice pack one-half full of crushed ice or ice chips using a spoon, cup, or ice scooper.

15. Remove excess air from the ice pack by twisting or squeezing it.

16. Place the cap or stopper on the ice pack tightly. Check for any leaks.

17. Dry the ice pack with towels. Place the ice pack in its cover.

18. Apply the ice pack to the body part. Note the time of application.

19. Secure the ice pack with ties, tape, or rolled gauze, if needed. Never apply tape to the resident's skin.

20. Place the call light and personal items within reach. Place a glass of fresh water on the overbed table, if permitted.

21. If the resident is in bed, check to be sure the bed wheels are locked, then lower the bed. Follow the plan of care to determine if the side rails should be raised or lowered. If the resident is sitting in a chair or on the edge of the bed, be certain all safety precautions are in place. Unscreen the resident or open the door to the room, if appropriate.

22. Check on the resident every five minutes. Treatments usually last no longer than 20 minutes, unless ordered by the doctor. Change the ice pack if the ice starts melting.

> **Best Practice**
> Ask the resident about the temperature of the compress. Is it too cold? Does the resident feel numb or have any burning pain? Check often for red or pale skin. If there are any problems or complications, remove the application and report to the licensed nursing staff.

(continued)

23. When the ice pack application is complete, lock the bed wheels and then raise the bed to hip level if the resident is in bed. Ensure safety during the procedure. If there are side rails, raise and secure the rails on the opposite side of the bed from where you will be working. Lower the rail on the side you are working.

24. Remove the ice pack and pat the body part dry with a clean hand towel. Note the time the ice pack was removed. Assist with any further treatment as instructed by the licensed nursing staff.

25. Discard the water from the ice pack. Remove the protective pad and change any wet linens.

26. If the resident is in bed, check to be sure the bed wheels are locked. Then reposition the resident and lower the bed.

27. Follow the plan of care to determine if the side rails should be raised or lowered.

28. Remove, clean, and store equipment in the proper location. Remove soiled linens and discard disposable equipment.

Follow-Up

29. Wash your hands to ensure infection control.

30. Make sure the resident is comfortable and place the call light and personal items within reach.

31. Conduct a safety check before leaving the room. The room should be clean and free from clutter or spills.

32. Wash your hands or use hand sanitizer before leaving the room.

Reporting and Documentation

33. Communicate any specific observations, complications, or unusual responses to the licensed nursing staff. Record this information, along with the care provided, in the chart or EMR.

Section 21.2 Review and Assessment

Using Key Terms

Complete the following sentences using key terms in this section.

1. _____ is the use of cold applications to reduce swelling and ease pain.
2. _____ skin is blue in color due to insufficient oxygen.
3. A sufficient amount of fluid in body tissues is called _____.
4. _____ is unusually pale-colored skin.

Know and Understand the Facts

5. Identify four strategies for maintaining skin integrity.
6. When is it appropriate to use a heat application?
7. Describe three different heat applications.
8. Describe two different cold applications.

Analyze and Apply Concepts

9. Explain how heat and cold applications can be helpful and harmful.
10. Discuss the steps for applying a warm, moist compress to a resident's ankle.
11. Discuss the steps for applying an ice pack to a resident's arm.

Think Critically

Read the following care situation. Then answer the questions that follow.

During Mrs. J's bath yesterday, her nursing assistant Iman noticed that Mrs. J's skin bruised more easily even though she was very gentle. Mrs. J's lips have a bluish color, and her skin is pale. Yesterday, Mrs. J hit her arm getting out of bed. The arm is swollen, and Mrs. J states it is painful. The doctor ordered cold, moist compresses for 15 minutes, three times a day. Mrs. J is assigned to Iman today.

12. When Iman noticed the changes in Mrs. J's skin, what should she have done?
13. What is the rationale for using cold applications to help Mrs. J?

Key Points

Reviewing the key points for this chapter will help you practice more safely and competently as a holistic nursing assistant and will help you prepare for the certification competency examination.

- Personal hygiene and grooming promote healing and physical and emotional well-being; create an environment of cleanliness, relaxation, and comfort; and help improve quality of life.

- Personal hygiene responsibilities include morning care; bathing; shampooing, brushing, and combing hair; shaving; oral and denture care; fingernail and foot care; and perineal care. Nursing assistants may also assist with dressing and undressing residents and changing the hospital gown of a patient with an IV catheter.

- Maintaining skin integrity keeps the skin healthy. Nursing assistants must be vigilant about observing the skin and immediately reporting any changes to the licensed nursing staff.

- Heat applications increase circulation, raise skin temperature, relax muscles, and ease pain. Cold applications are typically recommended for acute injuries because they decrease blood flow to the injury and reduce inflammation and swelling.

Action Steps to Holistic Care

Review the information in this chapter. Complete the following activities.

1. Select one personal hygiene procedure from this chapter. Prepare a short paper or digital presentation that identifies and describes the four most important practices in the procedure. Include one that promotes comfort and one that ensures safety.

2. Select one of the following age groups: pregnant mothers, babies, teenagers, adults under age 35, or older adults over age 65. Prepare a poster that illustrates three facts people in this age group should know to keep their skin healthy.

3. Find four pictures in a magazine, in a newspaper, or online: two that demonstrate good skin integrity and two that depict poor skin integrity. Describe each image and explain why it was selected.

4. Select one cultural, ethnic, or religious group and describe its beliefs about personal hygiene and grooming. List two ways holistic nursing assistants can respect those beliefs when providing care.

 ## Preparing for the Certification Competency Examination

To prepare for the nursing assistant certification competency examination, you will need to know content found in this chapter. This content may be tested in the knowledge (written or oral) and skills (hands-on demonstration) portions of the exam. The following areas will be emphasized:

- principles of daily hygiene and grooming, including independence and self-reliance during these activities
- personal hygiene and grooming within a plan of care
- bathing, including a sitz bath and whirlpool
- hair care and shampooing, brushing, and combing hair
- shaving of male residents
- oral and denture care
- nail and foot care and important actions for residents with particular diseases and conditions
- dressing and undressing and changing gowns for patients with IV catheters
- skin integrity and the complications and effects of inadequate skin care
- applications of heat and cold

These sample test questions are similar to ones you will find on the certification competency exam. See how well you can answer them. Be sure to select the *best* answer.

1. To what angle should the head of the bed be raised for oral care?
   - A. at least 20°
   - B. at least 45°
   - C. at least 15°
   - D. at least 60°

2. Unless otherwise ordered by the doctor, a warm, moist compress is usually applied for
   - A. 25 minutes
   - B. 15 minutes
   - C. 10 minutes
   - D. 5 minutes

(continued)

3. Mrs. D recently had a stroke, and her left side is paralyzed. When helping Mrs. D dress, which arm should the nursing assistant put into the sleeve of her pajama top first?

   A. right arm
   B. stronger arm
   C. stable arm
   D. weaker arm

4. A nursing assistant is providing a foot bath for Mr. G, a diabetic. Which of the following should the nursing assistant do?

   A. soak Mr. G's feet for at least 40 minutes
   B. use enough water to cover Mr. G's ankles
   C. make sure the water is not too hot
   D. strongly rub Mr. G's feet with a towel after the bath

5. One of the most important responsibilities holistic nursing assistants have when providing personal hygiene and grooming is

   A. discarding all dirty linens immediately
   B. encouraging resident independence and self-reliance
   C. giving clear instructions
   D. have residents' families help as much as possible

6. A new nursing assistant has been asked to wash Mrs. F's hair. She reviews the procedure for rinsing out shampoo and finds that she should

   A. start at the hairline and move down the strands of hair
   B. start from the bottom of the hair and work up to the top strands
   C. rinse from side to side and then rinse the hairline
   D. start in the middle of the scalp and move toward the hairline

7. When giving a total bed bath, the nursing assistant should

   A. start with the arms and then wash the legs and the rest of the body
   B. start with the abdomen, wash the arms and legs, and then wash the rest of the body
   C. start with the feet and work up the body to the face
   D. start at the top of the body, beginning with the face

8. Which of the following is an important guideline for giving foot care?

   A. apply lotion to the toes and feet and massage briskly
   B. apply lotion to the feet, toes, and between the toes
   C. apply lotion to the tops and soles of the feet, but not between the toes
   D. apply lotion to the tops and soles of the feet and between the toes

9. When performing female perineal care, a nursing assistant should

   A. place her fingers on the areas being washed
   B. wash the labia using downward strokes from top to bottom
   C. wash from the thighs in toward the labia
   D. wash the labia using upward strokes from bottom to top

10. When observing the skin of an older, frail, female resident, where should the nursing assistant look first?

    A. under the breasts
    B. between the legs
    C. around the neck and ears
    D. at the elbows and tailbone

11. One possible harmful effect of cold applications is

    A. frostbite
    B. cyanosis
    C. edema
    D. pallor

12. Which of the following is an important guideline for shaving?

    A. put a cool compress on the face and then shave in the direction of hair growth
    B. put a warm compress on the face and then shave opposite the direction of hair growth
    C. put a warm compress on the face and then shave in the direction of hair growth
    D. put a cool compress on the face and then shave opposite the direction of hair growth

13. What is the difference between a whirlpool and a sitz bath?

    A. A sitz bath is usually part of a total bed bath.
    B. A whirlpool has jets that swirl the water.
    C. A whirlpool is usually part of a total bed bath.
    D. A sitz bath has jets that swirl the water.

14. Yesterday, the doctor diagnosed Mrs. I with a sprained ankle. His order is to apply

    A. warm, moist compresses
    B. warm soaks
    C. a heating pad
    D. cold, moist compresses

15. Which of the following is included in a.m. care?

    A. oral care
    B. warm, moist compresses
    C. whirlpool
    D. cold, moist compresses

Did you have difficulty with any of the questions? If you did, review the chapter to find the correct answer(s).

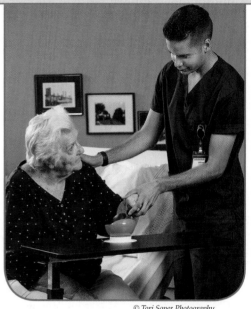

CHAPTER 22

Healthy Eating and Nutritional Challenges

Welcome to the Chapter

In chapters 8 and 9, you learned about the structure and function of the *gastrointestinal system*, which provides the foundation for understanding nutrition and the importance of healthy eating. In this chapter, you will focus on the nutrients and foods that make up a well-balanced, healthy diet at different stages of life (called *life cycle nutrition*). You will also learn about the factors that can determine food preferences and about the influence of tradition and culture on food selection. You will become familiar with different eating and weight disorders, and therapeutic diets doctors may order for residents.

As a holistic nursing assistant, you will be responsible for helping residents during mealtime. You may need to feed residents or help them with their meals, sometimes with adaptive and assistive eating devices. You will also need to understand and be comfortable with alternative feeding therapies and eating problems, which may include dysphagia, choking, and aspiration.

The information and procedures presented in this chapter will help you build the knowledge and skills needed to become a holistic nursing assistant. Check with your instructor to ensure these procedures are within your state's regulations for nursing assistant practice. The topics discussed in the chapter are highlighted on the Providing Holistic Care Framework.

You are now ready to start this chapter, *Healthy Eating and Nutritional Challenges*.

© Tori Soper Photography

Chapter Outline

Section 22.1
Life Cycle Nutrition

Section 22.2
Therapeutic Diets and Nutritional Support

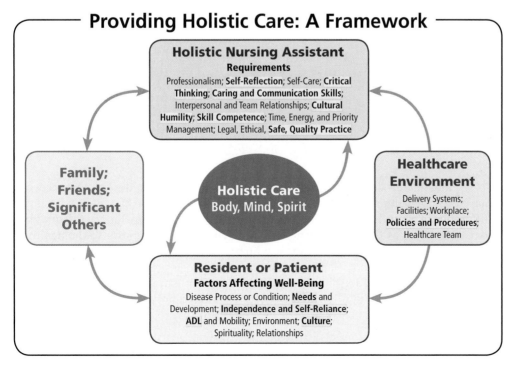

Providing Holistic Care: A Framework

Holistic Nursing Assistant
Requirements
Professionalism; **Self-Reflection**; Self-Care; **Critical Thinking; Caring and Communication Skills;** Interpersonal and Team Relationships; **Cultural Humility; Skill Competence;** Time, Energy, and Priority Management; Legal, Ethical, **Safe, Quality Practice**

Family; Friends; Significant Others

Holistic Care
Body, Mind, Spirit

Healthcare Environment
Delivery Systems; Facilities; Workplace; **Policies and Procedures;** Healthcare Team

Resident or Patient
Factors Affecting Well-Being
Disease Process or Condition; **Needs** and Development; **Independence and Self-Reliance; ADL** and Mobility; Environment; **Culture;** Spirituality; Relationships

Questions to Consider

- Consider the foods that you eat regularly. Do you eat healthfully? If you do not, what foods do you eat that are not good for you? Why do you eat these foods? Is it because they are easy to obtain? Do they taste so good you can't give them up? Are these foods eaten as part of a family tradition?
- In addition to the foods you eat regularly, do you snack? What snacks do you eat, and when do you eat them? Would you consider your snacks healthy? Why?
- If you were asked to change your diet and eat foods that are better for you, how would you respond? Would you be able to make the change? What obstacles would keep you from making this change?

Objectives

Nutrition is an essential need that all human beings share. No one can live very long without the proper nutrients needed to nourish the body. People's eating patterns and food selections are usually based on their likes and dislikes. These preferences typically come from people's experiences with food, family traditions, and cultural preferences. A healthy diet is key to living well, properly growing, and having a long life. A healthy diet includes several nutrients, and different amounts are required during different stages in the life cycle. People who have eating or weight disorders or conditions related to eating may not get proper nutrition or eat healthfully. Eating conditions and disorders can lead to serious illnesses and sometimes death. To achieve the objectives for this section, you must successfully

- **discuss** the factors that influence and the reasons behind individual food preferences and food selection;
- **identify** the components of a healthy diet;
- **explain** what nutrients are;
- **identify** how recommended dietary allowances (RDAs) and recommended amounts in each food group change at different stages of the life cycle;
- **describe** different eating disorders and conditions, including obesity and weight loss in seniors; and
- **describe** how eating disorders and conditions impact the body.

Key Terms

Learn these key terms to better understand the information presented in the section.

botanicals
calories
carbohydrates
dietary fats
eating disorder
electrolytes
herbals
hydrated
international units (IUs)
legumes

malabsorption
metabolism
minerals
nutrition
obesity
proteins
Recommended Dietary Allowances (RDAs)
sedentary
triglycerides
vitamins

As a holistic nursing assistant, you need to understand the importance of nutrition and its impact on health and well-being. Good nutrition can make a positive difference in growth and development and can significantly influence the quality of people's lives as they age. Eating healthfully is a key contributor to the healing process and a vital ingredient for those who have chronic illnesses such as diabetes. Without appropriate food selection, residents with diabetes can experience metabolic imbalances. Good nutrition should also be an important part of *your* daily life. When you eat healthfully, you will have the energy needed to provide safe, quality care.

Why Do People Have Different Food Preferences?

People's patterns of food selection and food preferences are usually based on their life habits, which are learned as a result of experience and life condition. Often, people do not consider whether a certain food is "good for them." What matters is how hungry people are, what people like or even "love" to eat, or what people feel like eating at a certain time. Often, liking or "loving" a food that feels "comforting" is the deciding factor in how people think and feel about their food preferences.

People's food preferences begin to develop during childhood (Figure 22.1). These preferences are shaped by a family's access to food, dietary traditions, finances, and ethnic or religious origins. Preferences are also shaped by age, diseases or conditions, medications taken, and even the aroma of food. Knowledge of **nutrition**, which encompasses ingesting foods that maintain the health of the body, also influences food preferences (Figure 22.2).

People may also select foods based on their food allergies or sensitivities, physical disabilities that might prevent them from chewing or swallowing normally, the amount of time people have, financial resources, or special diets. Foods may be selected based on how they are advertised or arranged in the food market. Some people cannot afford the foods they like. Other people may not have sufficient time to cook and may purchase more accessible "fast" foods. "Comfort" foods may be chosen to make people feel better. These "comfort" foods may or may not be good for people, but feel and taste "good" when eaten.

Eating patterns, which describe how often and how fast people eat, are similarly affected by experience. These patterns begin to develop during childhood and usually become more established as people become adults. To understand your eating patterns, ask yourself when you eat during the day. Are you distracted while you are eating? Do you eat slowly or quickly? Do you eat more in the morning or in the evening? Do you snack during the day, or do you "raid" the refrigerator during the night? Do you eat while working or driving? These eating patterns become habits, guide your choice of foods, influence how you eat foods, can affect your digestion, and can cause weight disorders.

Think About This

Once you start eating, it takes about 20 minutes for your body to feel physically full. This is the amount of time needed for signals between your gastrointestinal system and the brain to let you know you are full. If a person eats too fast, this feeling of fullness may occur after he or she has overeaten.

Remember

To eat is a necessity, but to eat intelligently is an art.

François de La Rochefoucauld, French author

How Do Foods Fuel the Body?

Eating a healthy diet means including the proper amounts of essential *nutrients* (substances needed for normal body function) in your diet.

The essential nutrients are carbohydrates, dietary fats (lipids), proteins, vitamins, minerals, and water. These nutrients are required for **metabolism**, which is the chemical process by which nutrients are converted into energy. During the process

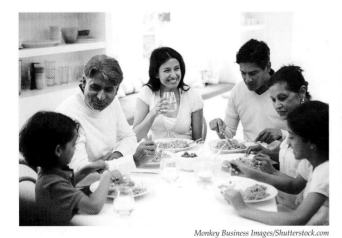

Monkey Business Images/Shutterstock.com

Figure 22.1 Family and culture have a significant impact on a person's eating patterns and food selections.

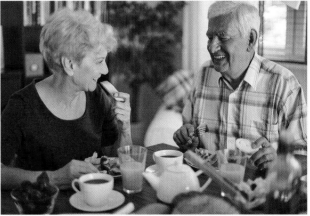

gpointstudio/Shutterstock.com

Figure 22.2 Knowledge of nutrition enables people to make healthful food choices.

Culture Cues

Food Traditions

Cultural and religious groups typically have unique food traditions. Some traditional foods are served on holidays, celebrations, special occasions, or feast days. Many cultures also have customs that outline how and when food should be eaten and that identify accepted or prohibited foods. Some foods are eaten to convey a person's social status, and some foods are symbolic and represent maintaining health and attaining a long life. Food practices are not followed by all families and individuals in a culture; however, many people do maintain all or some parts of their cultural or religious eating traditions.

As a holistic nursing assistant, you must be aware of and sensitive to residents' food traditions. Some food traditions promote residents' treatments, and other food traditions are barriers to residents' treatments. If you are not sure about a resident's food traditions, you can check the plan of care. You can also ask the resident what eating traditions or customs he or she practices.

Apply It

1. What traditional foods and food aromas do you remember from your childhood?
2. List the foods that are special to your family traditions, culture, or religion.
3. Describe any cultural or religious food traditions your family has. Do you maintain your family's cultural or religious food traditions? If you do, describe any challenges you have encountered in keeping these traditions.
4. Describe any cultural or religious food traditions that your friends follow. In what ways do these traditions differ from yours? How do you feel about the differences?
5. If a resident's family brings in foods that are part of the resident's culture, but that are not part of the resident's prescribed diet, what do you think would be the best action to take?

of metabolism, **calories** (units of energy) in food and fluids combine with oxygen to release energy that the body needs to function properly. Metabolism is also important for building, maintaining, and repairing body tissues.

Metabolic Rate and Physical Activity

The body relies on metabolism to get the energy it needs to carry out basic functions and perform tasks. A person's *metabolic rate* is the number of calories the body uses to carry out its basic functions. Factors such as biological sex, body size and composition, and age all affect how calories are used (or *burned*). It is estimated that metabolic rate accounts for 70 percent of the calories burned daily. The remaining 30 percent of calories are burned through the normal processes of digesting, absorbing, transporting, and storing food consumed and through physical activity. General guidelines for the number of calories needed daily are based on age and activity levels. As illustrated in Figure 22.3, a person's activity level can be described as **sedentary** (inactive), *moderately active*, or *active* according to the National Institutes of Health (NIH).

Calorie Guidelines by Sex, Age, and Activity Levels

		Activity Level		
Sex	**Age**	**Sedentary**	**Moderately Active**	**Active**
Female	19–30	2000 calories	2000–2200 calories	2400 calories
	31–50	1800 calories	2000 calories	2200 calories
	51+	1600 calories	1800 calories	2000–2200 calories
Male	19–30	2400 calories	2600–2800 calories	3000 calories
	31–50	2200 calories	2400–2600 calories	2800–3000 calories
	51+	2000 calories	2200–2400 calories	2400–2800 calories

Figure 22.3 Calorie needs depend on sex, age, and activity levels.

Energy Balance

Determining how best to consume and burn calories requires understanding *energy balance*. The energy *in* (calories from food and fluids) should balance the energy *out* (metabolic rate and the calories burned as a result of body functions and physical activity). While energy does not have to be balanced every day, it must be balanced over time for the body to maintain a healthy weight:

- If energy (calories) *in* equals energy (calories) *out*, weight stays the same.
- If energy (calories) *in* is greater than energy (calories) *out*, weight is gained.
- If energy (calories) *in* is less than energy (calories) *out*, weight is lost.

Calories that are consumed, but not used, are stored in a person's fat cells as **triglycerides**. Energy from triglycerides may later be released as needed between meals. If people consume more calories than they are able to burn, they will likely have high levels of triglycerides, leading to a condition known as *hypertriglyceridemia*. This condition can be detected by a blood test.

As you review the different nutrients, remember that *life cycle nutrition* means people have different nutritional needs based on their ages, life events (such as pregnancy and breast-feeding), body types, and levels of physical activity. Children, for example, have established nutritional requirements for healthy growth and development.

What Are the Essential Nutrients?

Essential nutrients are needed for the body to function normally and must be consumed through foods and fluids. Essential nutrients are carbohydrates, dietary fats (lipids), proteins, vitamins, minerals, and water. While it is important for the body to receive adequate daily nutrition, sometimes this does not happen. **Malabsorption** can occur if the intestine fails to take in essential nutrients and fluids and transfer them to the bloodstream. Malabsorption can result from intestinal diseases, infections, inflammation, trauma, surgery, or nutritional deficiencies and can lead to weight loss and dehydration. This condition must be corrected, as it can lead to serious outcomes if essential nutrients are not consumed daily.

Carbohydrates

Carbohydrates are the body's main source of energy and contain carbon, hydrogen, and oxygen. They are considered a *macronutrient* because large amounts of carbohydrates need to be obtained from food for the body to function properly. There are three types of carbohydrates found in food: starches, which are also known as *complex carbohydrates*; sugars, which are also known as *simple carbohydrates*; and fiber (Figure 22.4):

- **Starch**: is found in vegetables, such as potatoes; in dried beans, such as kidney or pinto beans; and in grains, such as oats, rice, pasta, or bread. There are two types of grains: *whole grains*, which contain the entire grain kernel, and *refined grains*, which have had part of the kernel removed. Often, refined grains are enriched with vitamins and iron.
- **Sugar**: naturally occurs in milk and fruit and can also be added to foods during canning or baking. Sugar has different names. For example, *lactose* is sugar found in milk, *fructose* is fruit sugar, and *sucrose* is table sugar. Molasses, honey, and corn syrup are also sugars.
- **Fiber**: is found only in fruits, vegetables, whole grains, nuts, and **legumes** (plants with pods that contain edible seeds). Dietary fiber cannot be digested, so the majority of it passes through and out of the body. Fiber is important for digestive health, however. Fiber helps a person feel full after eating and assists with elimination. While there are many fiber supplements available, fiber should be ingested as part of a person's daily diet.

Think About This

Artificial sweeteners are often used as replacements for sugar because they are typically lower in calories. Because artificial sweeteners are 100 times more intense than sugars, they are only needed in small amounts. Most artificial sweeteners cannot be metabolized by the body and pass through the body without being digested. There are six artificial sweeteners approved by the US Food and Drug Administration (FDA). These include aspartame, saccharin, and stevia. Stevia is a popular sweetener that comes from the stevia plant. It is generally recognized by the FDA as a safe food additive and tabletop sweetener.

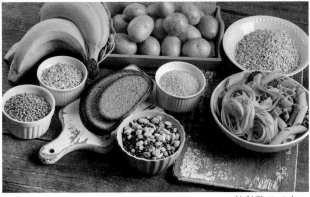

Figure 22.4 Illustrated here are some examples of carbohydrates. Carbohydrates can be found in grains, vegetables (such as potatoes), dried beans, fruits (such as bananas), and nuts, among other foods.

Carbohydrates, while important for a healthy diet, need to be selected wisely to achieve the best nutrition and to maintain a caloric balance. Foods with added sugars and refined grains, such as white flour, white bread, and white rice, should be avoided. Rather, it is recommended that fruits, vegetables, and whole grains be chosen.

Dietary Fats

Dietary fats are also macronutrients that provide energy for the body. They are composed of carbon, hydrogen, and oxygen. Dietary fats, which are also called *lipids*, perform several essential body functions; assist in the absorption of vitamins A, D, E, and K; and help food taste better. Dietary fats are found in nearly all foods, and fats are often added during cooking. It is important to recognize that dietary fat does not necessarily turn into body fat.

There are three different types of fats: saturated fats, *trans* fats, and unsaturated fats. The saturation of a fat is based on the chemical bonds that make up its fatty acid molecular structure (Figure 22.5):

- **Saturated fats**: are packed with hydrogen molecules and are therefore considered "solid" fats. Saturated fats are found in animal and dairy products, such as meats, butter, cream, and cheese. In liquid form, saturated fats can be found in coconut and palm oils. Eating too many saturated fats has been found to raise total blood cholesterol levels and *low-density lipoprotein (LDL)*, or bad cholesterol, levels. High cholesterol levels can increase the risk of cardiovascular disease. Too much saturated fat may also increase the risk of type 2 diabetes.

- *Trans* **fats**: also called *trans-fatty acid*, *trans* fats are usually found in foods that are chemically processed using partially hydrogenated vegetable oil (oil with added hydrogen to extend shelf life). *Trans* fat can be found in cakes or cookies containing shortening, margarine, and foods fried with partially hydrogenated oil. *Trans* fats increase the risk of cardiovascular disease because they can lower levels of *high-density lipoproteins (HDLs)*, or good cholesterol, and increase levels of LDLs, or bad cholesterol.

- **Unsaturated fats**: include monounsaturated fats (omega-9 fatty acids) and polyunsaturated fats (omega-3 and -6 fatty acids). Unsaturated fats are found in olive, canola, safflower, peanut, and corn oils; most nuts; mayonnaise; and avocados. Omega-3 fatty acids are found in salmon, tuna, trout, mackerel, sardines, herring, and flaxseed. Unsaturated fats improve cholesterol levels and decrease the risk of cardiovascular disease and type 2 diabetes.

Proteins

Proteins are the third macronutrient. They are major contributors to energy production. Proteins can be found in every cell of the body and are the main builders of body tissue. Proteins also promote growth and repair. Proteins are vital to cell structure and

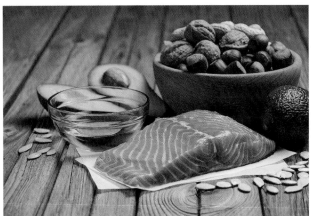

Figure 22.5 Some examples of foods containing unsaturated dietary fats are oil, fish, avocados, and nuts.

function, carry oxygen and enzymes, and supply nitrogen needed for genetic substances. Proteins also help with the balance of needed fluids and **electrolytes**, which are substances that carry electrical charges when dissolved in water.

Proteins are chemically structured as *amino acids*. The body needs 20 amino acids, eight of which are considered *essential* because the body cannot synthesize them on its own. The eight essential amino acids are histidine, isoleucine, leucine, lysine, methionine, phenylalanine, threonine, tryptophan, and valine. These amino acids must be ingested through a person's diet. Proteins are found in eggs, milk, soybeans, meat, poultry, seafood, vegetables, grains, processed soy products, nuts, and seeds (Figure 22.6).

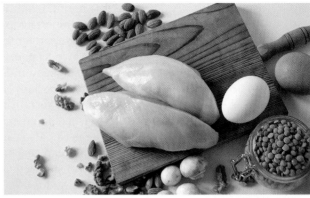

valoshka/Shutterstock.com

Figure 22.6 Meats and poultry are rich in protein, as are eggs, nuts, and seeds.

Vitamins

Vitamins are organic compounds that are important for the development and growth of cells and are needed for the body to function properly. For the most part, essential vitamins cannot be produced by the body. As a result, they must be ingested from foods in a person's diet or from vitamin supplements.

Types of Vitamins

There are 13 vitamins. Four vitamins are *fat soluble*, and the remaining vitamins are *water soluble*. Fat-soluble vitamins (vitamins A, D, E, and K) can be dissolved in fat and stored in the body. Water-soluble vitamins (B complex vitamins and vitamin C) dissolve in water, cannot be stored in the body, and are easily eliminated. The B complex vitamins are comprised of eight B vitamins (B_1, B_2, B_3, B_5, B_6, B_7, B_9, and B_{12}). A lack of sufficient intake or the excessive intake of some vitamins can pose certain risks. Some vitamins can also have harmful interactions with medications.

Recommended Dietary Allowances (RDAs)

Vitamins have specific functions and benefits and can be found in a variety of food sources. There are **Recommended Dietary Allowances (RDAs)**, or recommended levels of intake, as well as *upper intake levels (ULs)* for each vitamin. Ingesting more than the UL for a vitamin leads to an excess of the needed vitamin. Consistent with life cycle nutrition, RDAs are different for each life stage.

RDAs designate the amount that should be ingested using metric units and **international units (IUs)**. IUs are based on international standards. One IU for a substance results in a specific biological effect. Metric units are based on the metric system. The *metric system*, which was developed in the late 1700s, standardized measurement in Europe and today is the primary system of measurement throughout the world. The metric system has three main units of measurement: the *meter* for length, the *gram* for weight or mass, and the *liter* for liquid volume. Prefixes are added to the names of these units to indicate their amounts based on measures of 10. For example, 1,000 meters is 1 kilometer.

While the United States does use the metric system for some measurements, it has not adopted the metric system as its official system of measurement. Instead, *US customary units* include inches and feet, which measure length; pounds and ounces, which measure weight; and pints, quarts, and gallons, which measure liquid volume. There was an attempt in the late 1980s to achieve "metrification" in the United States by passing the Omnibus Trade and Competitiveness Act. The Act designated the metric system as the preferred system of measurement for trade and commerce; however, compliance was voluntary. As a result, both metric units and US customary units are used in healthcare. For example, metric units are typically used for measuring medication doses or for liquid measurement. The US customary

Think About This

US customary units are not unlike the British Imperial System of measurement. Both systems use English units with Roman and Anglo-Saxon roots. For example, the Romans used the number 12 as their base number for conversions. US customary units and the British Imperial System both use the *foot*, which can be divided into 12 inches. Some US customary and British Imperial measurements developed out of convenience. For example, early Saxon kings used the sashes or girdles they wore around their waists for measurement. Other measurements came as a result of a royal decree. For example, the *yard* is believed to result from a decree by King Henry I, who said a yard should be the distance between the tip of his nose and the end of his outstretched thumb. The length of a *furlong* (a unit of distance) was established by early Tudor rulers and amounted to 220 yards. In the sixteenth century, Queen Elizabeth I declared the mile to be 5,280 feet, not the traditional Roman mile of 5,000 feet. This made the mile exactly 8 furlongs long, or 1 mile as we know it.

unit of the pound is used for measuring a resident's weight. Because both systems are used, it is important to know both systems and the conversions between them. For example, it is important to know that 1 meter is equal to 3.28 feet. More information about these two systems (the metric system and US customary units) and their conversions can be found in Appendix A.

RDAs are important benchmarks for vitamin intake, and lack of sufficient vitamin intake can pose certain risks. For example, older adults can develop vitamin D deficiency when aging skin does not synthesize vitamin D as efficiently. More time spent indoors can also cause inadequate intake of this vitamin. Excessive intake of some vitamins can also have negative effects. For example, too much vitamin C can cause an upset stomach and kidney stones. Too much vitamin B_3 (called *niacin*) can cause flushing and redness of the skin. Some vitamins can also interfere with clinical tests and have harmful interactions with medications (for example, vitamins E and K for residents taking blood thinners).

Minerals

Minerals are inorganic substances found in the body. Minerals in food do not directly add to the body's source of energy, but they do function as regulators and assist in metabolism. There are more than 50 minerals, and 25 are considered essential for the body to function properly. Some of the essential minerals are calcium, sodium, iron, potassium, magnesium, fluorine, and zinc.

Vitamin and Mineral Supplements

It is important to understand vitamin and mineral supplementation and ways supplementation is used. The majority of people in the United States take one or more dietary supplements daily. Most supplements include vitamins and minerals, but can also include **herbals** (substances containing herbs), **botanicals** (plant-based substances), and enzymes. Supplements are usually available as tablets, capsules, powders, drinks, or energy bars and can be purchased over-the-counter at retail stores. Some examples of supplements are echinacea, St. John's wort, turmeric, or *probiotics* (microbes that stimulate the growth of beneficial microorganisms, such as intestinal flora). All of these supplements are meant to add to a person's daily diet, not to take the place of healthy food selections. Supplements are *not* medicine.

The FDA provides specific regulations for dietary supplements and dietary ingredients. These regulations are not the same as regulations for prescription or over-the-counter medications. According to these regulations, suppliers of dietary supplements must ensure that supplements are safe and that the labels are not misbranded (are "truthful and not misleading"). It is important to know what supplements residents have taken or are taking during a hospital stay or in a long-term care facility. Some supplements may adversely affect the medications and diets ordered for the resident. Supplements may put residents at increased risk for consuming more than the RDA for a vitamin or mineral.

Water

Water makes up 55 to 60 percent of the body's total weight. On a daily basis, people lose a great deal of water just by breathing, sweating, and eliminating. Staying **hydrated**, or having sufficient fluids, is critical for all age groups (Figure 22.7). It is particularly important for people who live in a hot climate, routinely exercise, decrease the amounts they drink, or have difficulty swallowing liquids. Sufficient hydration improves a person's energy, mood, and clarity in thinking. Even the smallest amount of *dehydration*, or lack of sufficient fluids, can significantly slow down the body's metabolism and result in serious changes to the thermoregulatory and metabolic functions and cardiovascular and central nervous systems. One simple way to assess hydration is to check the color of your urine. If your urine is pale yellow, you are adequately hydrated. If the color of your urine is closer to dark yellow or orange, you may need to drink more fluids.

Think About This

The CDC recently reported that 9 out of 10 people in the United States receive a good amount of essential nutrients and vitamins, including vitamin D for bone health and iron to avoid anemia. While the status of overall nutrition in the United States is adequate, some population groups, such as non-Hispanic African-Americans and Mexican-Americans, have low levels of vitamin D, which place them at risk for soft, brittle bones.

Think About This

You have probably heard that a person must drink eight 8-ounce glasses of water daily. What does this mean? The Institute of Medicine (IOM) recommends that adequate intake (AI) of fluids for men is approximately 15 cups (3.7 liters) of total fluids daily. The AI for women is about 11 cups (2.7 liters) daily. Eight 8-ounce glasses of water daily is 1.9 liters. Clearly, this is not enough to meet the AI for men or women.

Fluid intake includes all of the beverages a person consumes. Even fruits and vegetables contain water. The temperature of the fluid ingested is important. Lukewarm fluids are easier for the body to digest than hot or cold beverages.

How Do People Choose Safe and Healthy Foods?

Both MyPlate and the *Dietary Guidelines for Americans* help people choose healthy foods in appropriate amounts. Choosing nutritious foods is critical to consuming all essential nutrients. When selecting foods, people can use food labels to determine the nutrients in a food. Food safety is also important to ensure foods do not cause disease or injury.

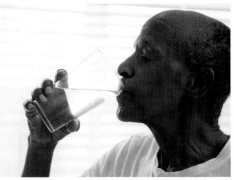
wavebreakmedia/Shutterstock.com

Figure 22.7 Hydration improves energy, mood, and thinking. It is essential to the body's functions.

MyPlate

To ensure adequate nutrition and ingestion of all essential nutrients, people should eat the recommended daily intake for each of the five main food groups. These food groups are fruits, vegetables, grains, protein, and dairy, as illustrated by the MyPlate logo in Figure 22.8. *MyPlate* is a government resource that helps people learn about food groups, the proper proportions of the different food groups in a healthy diet, and food selections.

MyPlate offers the following guidelines for selecting foods from the five food groups:

- **Fruits**: Vary food selections and pick potassium-rich fruits, such as bananas, orange juice, prunes and prune juice, dried peaches, and apricots. If choosing canned fruits, select fruits that are canned with 100 percent fruit juice or water instead of syrup.

- **Vegetables**: Vegetables are categorized into five groups: dark green vegetables, starchy vegetables, red and orange vegetables, beans and peas, and other vegetables. For the best nutrition, pick any vegetable or 100 percent vegetable juice. Vegetables selected can be raw, cooked, fresh, frozen, canned, dried, or dehydrated.

- **Grains**: Grains are divided into two groups: whole grains and refined grains. Whole grains contain the entire grain kernel. In refined grains, the bran and germ of the grain kernel have been removed. This improves the grain's shelf life, but removes dietary fiber. Refined grains include white rice and bread. Instead of selecting refined grains, select whole grains, such as whole-wheat flour, bulgur (cracked wheat), oatmeal, whole cornmeal, and brown rice. Some grains are enriched with vitamins and the mineral iron. Some people are *gluten sensitive* or *gluten intolerant*. These people have an abnormal immune response to gluten during digestion and cannot eat food products containing wheat, barley, or rye. These people can, however, eat grains such as rice, corn, or millet.

- **Protein**: Eat meat, poultry, seafood, beans and peas, eggs, processed soy products, nuts, and seeds. Select lean or low-fat meat and poultry. While people who are vegetarians do not eat meat, they can still select beans and peas, processed soy products, and nuts and seeds.

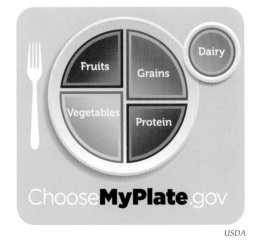
USDA

Figure 22.8 MyPlate is a food guidance system designed to help people make healthy nutritional choices.

- **Dairy**: This food group includes all liquid milk products and foods made from milk. Select fat-free or low-fat milk, yogurt, and cheese, as well as calcium-fortified soy milk. Some people are *lactose intolerant*, which means they have trouble digesting milk products. These people will need to drink or eat low-lactose or lactose-free milk products or soy beverages.

The *serving* or *portion size* of a food is important to achieving a healthy diet. Small servings or portions help reduce the number of calories consumed. When people are on special diets, the servings or portion sizes identified must be strictly followed. Figure 22.9 shows guidelines for servings and portion sizes in the five food groups.

Dietary Guidelines for Americans

In addition to MyPlate, the US government (Department of Health and Human Services) also provides the *Dietary Guidelines for Americans*. The *Dietary Guidelines for Americans* offers the following guidance:

- Carbohydrates should account for 45 to 65 percent of a person's total daily intake. When selecting carbohydrates, people should limit calories from added sugar in foods such as soft drinks and desserts.
- Eat 25 to 30 grams of fiber each day. Most people consume about one-half of what is recommended. Sources of fiber that contain 5 grams or more per serving are recommended.
- Fats should be restricted to less than 30 percent of a person's daily caloric intake, and saturated fats should account for less than 10 percent. Replace saturated fats with monounsaturated or polyunsaturated fats and avoid *trans* fats.
- Select a variety of protein, including at least 8 ounces of cooked seafood per week. Young children need less than this amount, depending on their ages and calorie needs.
- At least one-half of all grains consumed should be whole grains.
- During pregnancy, select foods that have the vitamins and minerals needed for a healthy pregnancy. Most doctors ask pregnant women to take daily prenatal vitamins and mineral supplements in addition to a healthy diet.

Food Labels

When purchasing foods, some people use *food labels* to assess a food's nutrient content. The 1990 Nutrition Labeling and Education Act (NLEA) requires most foods to include labels showing nutritional information. This Act led to the development

> **Remember**
>
> *If you can't pronounce it, don't eat it.*
>
> Michael Pollan, American author, journalist, activist, and professor

Serving and Portion Size Guidelines	
Food Group	**Guidelines**
Fruits	In general, 1 cup is equal to 1 cup of fruit, 1 cup of 100-percent fruit juice, or 1/2 cup of dried fruit.
Vegetables	In general, 1 cup is equal to 1 cup of raw or cooked vegetables, 1 cup of 100-percent vegetable juice, or 2 cups of raw leafy greens.
Grains	In general, 1 ounce-equivalent is equal to 1 slice of bread, 1 cup of ready-to-eat cereal, or 1/2 cup of cooked rice, cooked pasta, or cooked cereal.
Protein	In general, 1 ounce-equivalent is equal to 1 ounce of meat, poultry, or fish; 1/4 cup cooked beans; 1 egg; 1 tablespoon of peanut butter; or 1/2 ounce of nuts or seeds.
Dairy	In general, 1 cup is equal to 1 cup of milk, yogurt, or soy milk (soy beverage); 1 1/2 ounces of natural cheese; or 2 ounces of processed cheese.

Figure 22.9 Understanding portion sizes is vital to getting adequate nutrition.

of the Nutrition Facts label. According to the NLEA, food labels must be adhered to every canned, boxed, or packaged food sold. These labels provide information about how food products meet RDAs and dietary guidelines.

In 2016, Nutrition Facts labels were updated to reflect new, scientific information (Figure 22.10). In June 2017, the FDA moved the compliance date for the new Nutrition Facts label to a future date. Some manufacturers, however, have proceeded toward implementing the new label.

Food labels are important to review, as they offer information that people need to determine if they want to consume a food product. Food labels also enable comparison between two foods. Food labels are helpful to review when you are caring for residents who are on special diets or have dietary restrictions.

The following is the best way to read a food label:

1. Always start at the top of the food label. This information defines a single serving size and lists the total number of servings in the food item.

2. Check the total number of calories *per serving*. Remember that the number of servings eaten affects the number of calories consumed. Foods that are low in calories might have 60 calories per serving, while foods that are high in calories might have 400 calories or more per serving.

3. Look at the nutrients in the food. These nutrients include fat, sugar, dietary fiber, protein, calcium, iron, and other vitamins and minerals. On a food label, the term *total carbohydrate* encompasses all three types of carbohydrates. This is the number you should pay attention to if you are counting carbohydrates.

4. Examine the % Daily Value (DV) for each nutrient. These values are determined by public health experts and tell you what percentage of the recommended daily amount for each nutrient a single serving contains. For example, if you want to eat less saturated fat or sodium, choose foods with lower % DVs (5 percent or less) for saturated fat and sodium. If you want to consume more fiber or protein, look for higher % DVs (20 percent or more) for these nutrients.

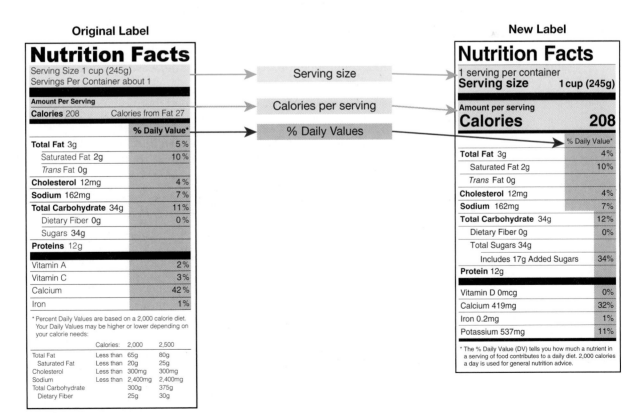

Figure 22.10 The Nutrition Facts label provides information about the nutrients in a food and how the food meets RDAs.

Food Safety

Food safety is another important aspect of healthy eating and dietary awareness. During the preparation and consumption of food, there is a risk for *foodborne illnesses*, which are diseases caused by pathogens or chemicals (such as pesticides) that contaminate food. There are more than 250 different foodborne illnesses, which can be caused by bacteria (for example, botulism and *E. coli*), by viruses (norovirus and hepatitis), or by parasites (trichinosis and toxoplasmosis).

In a foodborne illness, a pathogen enters the body with food that is ingested. As a result, symptoms are gastrointestinal in nature and include cramping, nausea, vomiting, and diarrhea. Sometimes the symptoms are mild, and other times they can be severe. Infants, seniors, people with weak immune systems, and pregnant women are at greater risk for acquiring foodborne illnesses and having severe symptoms.

Think About This

Annually, there are approximately 48 million cases of foodborne illness. This means that one in six people get sick each year. These illnesses result in an estimated 128,000 hospitalizations and 3,000 deaths.

In the United States, government laws regulate food ingredients and food additives, dietary supplements, agricultural chemicals, and water. Some government agencies are also responsible for setting food safety standards, conducting needed inspections, guaranteeing standards are met, maintaining a strong enforcement program to handle those who do not comply with standards, and providing food education. Biotechnology is emerging in agriculture and food processing, and many crops and food are being genetically modified using growth hormones and genetic-marker-assisted breeding. As a result, new safeguards are always needed. The government agencies involved in food safety include

- the US Department of Agriculture (USDA);
- the Food and Drug Administration (FDA);
- the Centers for Disease Control and Prevention (CDC);
- the Environmental Protection Agency (EPA); and
- the US Department of Health and Human Services (HHS).

Recently, the Food Safety Modernization Act (FSMA) was enacted to strengthen the food safety system. The FSMA authorizes the FDA to focus more time on preventing foodborne illnesses than on reacting to food safety issues after they occur.

At the individual level, there are general guidelines you can follow daily to avoid foodborne illness. These include the following:

- Wash your hands and the surfaces used for food often.
- Prevent cross-contamination. After using a knife, wash it before using it to cut other food.
- Cook food to its proper temperature. Use a food thermometer to check.
- Promptly refrigerate foods.
- Do not eat unpasteurized (raw) milk, cheese, and juices or raw or undercooked animal foods, such as seafood, meat, poultry, and eggs.

What Can Happen When People Are Not Eating Healthfully?

Remember

Eat like you love your body.

Lailah Gifty Akita, author and founder of the Smart Youth Volunteers Foundation

Unfortunately, it is not always easy to eat healthfully. Not only do people deal with their own food preferences, selections, and patterns, but people are also bombarded with food products through advertisements and the arrangement of food products at food markets. Some foods are good for people, and some are not. Only the dietary aware consumer can understand this difference.

Overweight, Obesity, and Underweight

Nutrition is a human need and is based on personal choices. Due to the many factors already discussed, however, many people in the United States make choices that result in being overweight or even obese. The United States is now facing an

Healthcare Scenario

Obesity

The CDC recently released statistical information that more than one-third (36.5 percent) of US adults are obese. Obesity is more common among middle-age adults ages 40–59 (40.2 percent) and older adults ages 60 or older (37.0 percent) than among younger adults ages 20–39 (32.3 percent). Approximately 17 percent (or 12.7 million) children and teens ages 2–19 are obese.

Apply It

1. Why do you think so many adults are obese? What might be one reason obesity is more common among middle-age and older adults?
2. If you were asked to help people who are obese, what would you suggest they do to decrease their weight?
3. Why do you think so many children and teens are obese?
4. Name two factors that you think contribute to childhood obesity.

obesity epidemic, which is considered a significant health problem. **Obesity** is a health condition characterized by a body weight much greater than what is considered healthy for a certain height. Not only are adults affected, but childhood obesity is also a problem. Being obese results in serious diseases, such as diabetes and cardiovascular conditions.

A common way to measure if a person is underweight, at a healthy weight, overweight, or obese is to use *body mass index* or *BMI*. BMI is a calculation of a person's body fat based on an adult man's or woman's height (in meters) and current weight (in kilograms). To calculate BMI, divide a person's weight in kilograms by his or her height in meters squared [weight/(height)^2]. You can also calculate BMI using pounds and inches (Figure 22.11).

- A BMI less than 18.5 falls within the *underweight* range.
- A BMI between 18.5 and 24.9 indicates a healthy weight.
- A BMI between 25.0 and 29.9 falls within the *overweight* range.
- A BMI of 30.0 or higher falls within the *obese* range.

How to Calculate Body Mass Index	
Measurement Units	**Formula and Calculation**
Kilograms and meters (or centimeters)	**Formula:** weight (kg)/[height (m)]^2 In the metric system, the formula for BMI is weight in kilograms divided by height in meters squared. Since height is commonly measured in centimeters, divide height in centimeters by 100 to obtain height in meters. **Example:** Weight = 68 kg, Height = 165 cm (1.65 m) **Calculation:** 68 ÷ (1.65)^2 = 24.98
Pounds and inches	**Formula:** weight (lb)/[height (in)]^2 × 703 Calculate BMI by dividing weight in pounds (lb) by height in inches (in) squared and multiplying by a conversion factor of 703. **Example:** Weight = 150 lbs, Height = 5′5″ (65″) **Calculation:** [150 ÷ (65)^2] × 703 = 24.96

Courtesy of the Centers for Disease Control and Prevention

Figure 22.11 BMI determines the health of a person's weight based on weight compared to height.

Obesity is frequently divided into three categories:

- class 1 obesity, which includes a BMI between 30.0 and 34.9
- class 2 obesity, which includes a BMI between 35.0 and 39.9
- class 3 obesity, which includes a BMI of 40.0 or higher and is sometimes categorized as *extreme* or *severe obesity*

Consider, as an example, a woman whose height is 5′5″ and who weighs 165 pounds. The woman's BMI is 27.5, which places her in the overweight category (25.0–29.9). To achieve a healthy weight, this woman would need to aim for a weight between 111 and 150 pounds or for a BMI between 18.5 and 24.9. Note that BMI is interpreted differently for children and teens due to their continuing developmental height and weight changes.

While the obesity epidemic affects many people in the United States, being underweight is also a serious condition. Some people, particularly seniors, may become underweight and frail because they do not eat enough or have a diet lacking in essential nutrients. They may lack appetite and have a reduced sense of taste. Limited mobility, physical changes, tooth and mouth problems, poorly fitting dentures, and changes in the social environment can also decrease appetite and result in weight loss. Normal weight loss can happen over time; however, sudden, rapid, unintentional, and unexplained weight loss usually indicates an underlying disease and needs to be treated by a doctor. Ways to respond to residents who are overweight or underweight are discussed in the next section of this chapter.

Eating Disorders

In chapter 9, diseases and conditions of the gastrointestinal (GI) system were discussed. You learned about gastroesophageal reflux disease (GERD), peptic ulcers, gallbladder disease, and diverticulitis. In this chapter, you will learn about eating disorders, including anorexia nervosa, binge-eating disorder, and bulimia nervosa.

Some people can become preoccupied with their weights. These people may be at a normal weight, but see themselves as overweight or even obese and have feelings of shame or anxiety about their body sizes and shapes. As a result, these people may develop dysfunctional eating behaviors as a way to deal with their perceptions of their bodies. A pattern of these behaviors can result in an **eating disorder**. An eating disorder is not an eating preference, but is considered a serious illness.

How Eating Disorders Develop

Eating disorders affect both males and females; however, rates among females are twice that of males. These disorders typically occur during the teen years or young adulthood, although they can also appear during childhood or later in life. The prevalence of eating disorders is alarming. In a national survey, four out of 10 people indicated they had suffered or knew someone who suffered from an eating disorder.

Often, changes in eating patterns are hidden and are not discovered until the eating disorder is out of control. Some people may start to eat smaller portions, eat more slowly to reduce intake, or even say, "I am not hungry." Others may engage in secretive behaviors, such as hiding food to be eaten later or going to the bathroom to *purge* (evacuate food from the body) after eating.

Several factors may trigger an eating disorder. Factors may be genetic, such as early puberty or obesity that runs in the family. Other factors may be physical or sexual abuse. Sometimes a person may start dieting, get out of control, and not be able to stop. Eating disorders are also associated with some personality characteristics, including perfectionism, high achievement, and low self-esteem. Certain sports or activities that emphasize body weight (for example, ballet or gymnastics) can also promote an intense focus on eating and weight gain and cause dysfunctional eating patterns.

Three common eating disorders are anorexia nervosa (self-starvation), binge-eating disorder (BED), and bulimia nervosa (bingeing and purging).

Think About This

If you are interested in knowing your BMI, use the adult BMI calculator on the CDC website. Fill in your height and weight and calculate your results. You can also determine your BMI by finding your height and weight in the BMI index table on the National Heart, Lung, and Blood Institute website.

Think About This

Recent evidence shows that there is a physical relationship between the brain and the intestines. This is called the *brain-gut interaction*. The lower intestine, which houses normal flora (bacteria), produces chemicals that pass through the intestinal walls and enter the blood circulating to the brain. These chemicals can cause brain disturbances associated with inflammatory bowel disease, obesity, and eating disorders.

Anorexia Nervosa

Anorexia nervosa is an intense fear of gaining weight or becoming fat. This is not the same as being underweight or being unable to maintain a normal weight. Anorexia nervosa is characterized by the following behaviors:

- being persistent about constantly losing weight
- eating only small quantities of food (Figure 22.12)
- portioning out food and eating very slowly
- frequently weighing to check for weight gain
- denying that extreme weight loss is a serious problem

Medical symptoms associated with anorexia nervosa include lack of menstruation, brittle hair and nails, constipation, muscle weakness, coldness, and tiredness. When anorexia nervosa is more severe, osteoporosis and low blood pressure can occur. Anorexia nervosa can also lead to heart malfunction, resulting in a heart attack or multiorgan failure.

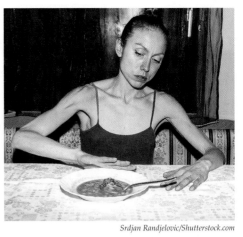

Srdjan Randjelovic/Shutterstock.com

Figure 22.12 People with anorexia nervosa eat only small quantities of food, leading to underweight. Underweight has many negative health consequences.

Binge-Eating Disorder (BED)

Binge-eating disorder (BED) is a condition in which a person loses control and excessively overeats. The behaviors associated with BED include feeling compelled to eat, not being able to stop eating even after the feeling of hunger subsides, not feeling satisfied, and going back and forth for more food. People who have BED do not engage in any compensatory behaviors to ease their guilt after bingeing. Rather, feelings of guilt and shame about the bingeing episode lead to more binge eating. As a result of these behaviors, people who have BED are usually overweight or obese, which places them at higher risk for cardiovascular disease.

Bulimia Nervosa

Bulimia nervosa is a condition characterized by recurring episodes of binge eating and purging. After binge eating, people who have bulimia nervosa seek to prevent weight gain by purging. Purging can involve forced vomiting, the use of laxatives and enemas, the use of diuretics, fasting, excessive exercise, or a combination of these behaviors. People with bulimia nervosa have distorted perceptions of their bodies and want to lose weight, regardless of whether they are at a normal weight or are overweight due to bingeing. Bingeing and purging are usually done secretly and are often done due to feelings of shame and disgust. This cycle can occur several times a week or as often as many times a day.

There are symptoms associated with bulimia nervosa. Bulimia nervosa can lead to a chronic sore throat, acid reflux or GERD, and GI distress resulting from the use of too many laxatives. When the cycle of bingeing and purging becomes chronic, symptoms such as worn tooth enamel and decaying teeth, severe dehydration, and electrolyte imbalance may occur.

Treatment Used for Eating Disorders

Treatments for eating disorders are designed to respond to individual issues and concerns. Treatment approaches include counseling to ensure adequate nutrition, therapy (individual or family), medical supervision, and sometimes medications (for example, antidepressants). When an eating disorder is severe, hospitalization can provide the care needed to correct electrolyte imbalance and malnutrition. In some cases requiring treatment, eating is monitored and possibly supplemented to ensure a person is getting adequate nutrition.

Using the Key Terms

Complete the following sentences using the key terms in this section.

1. The units of energy in food and fluids are called _____.
2. A(n) _____ is a plant-based substance found in some supplements.
3. The chemical process by which nutrients are converted into energy in the body is called _____.
4. _____ is a condition characterized by a BMI of 30.0 or higher.
5. A person who leads an inactive lifestyle may be described as _____.
6. _____ are substances that carry electrical charges when dissolved in water.
7. The reduced ability of the intestine to take in essential nutrients and fluids is called _____.
8. _____ are calories stored in a person's fat cells.

Know and Understand the Facts

9. What are two factors that influence individual food preferences and selection?
10. Identify the food groups that should be part of a healthy diet.
11. List the six essential nutrients and explain why each nutrient is important.
12. Explain the purpose of RDAs.
13. What is the serving and portion size for grains?
14. Identify three eating disorders and describe the differences between them.

Analyze and Apply Concepts

15. Explain how MyPlate and the *Dietary Guidelines for Americans* impact your diet.
16. List three changes you might need to make to improve your diet.
17. Why is it important to read food labels?
18. Explain why someone might be overweight or underweight.
19. Discuss how a sedentary lifestyle can influence a person's caloric intake.
20. Describe how you might be able to tell if a person has bulimia nervosa.

Think Critically

Read the following care situation. Then answer the questions that follow.

Joanie, a typically active 13-year-old, has seemed more tired lately and has not been interested in the after-school events she usually enjoys. The only activity she still seems motivated to attend is gymnastics. Joanie has been involved with gymnastics for two years and hopes to be in the Olympics one day. There is a new gymnastics coach this year, and Joanie seems to like and want to please her. In the past, Joanie has been slightly overweight for her age and height and has been somewhat self-conscious about it. Over the past three months, she has gotten much thinner—thinner than she should be. Joanie has stopped taking lunch to school, seems pickier than usual at dinnertime, and does not ask for her favorite snacks. She has asked for smaller portions because she says the coach wants all of the girls on the gymnastics team to be lean.

21. What do you think happened that changed Joanie's eating behaviors?
22. Do you think Joanie might be developing an eating disorder? If so, which one? Why?
23. If you were Joanie's parent, what might you say to her? What might you say to Joanie's coach?
24. What food groups and servings should Joanie be consuming to eat healthfully?

Objectives

In addition to healthful eating, the location and way people eat meals are also important. This is particularly true for those who are not feeling well or who have acute or chronic conditions or diseases. Optimal environments and conditions for eating help promote healing for these people. Residents will often eat therapeutic diets (special foods needed due to a disease or condition) ordered by their doctors. Residents may also need alternative feeding therapies, such as feeding tubes, due to surgery or dysphagia (difficulty swallowing). It is essential that holistic nursing assistants understand the reasons for and the importance of these diets and alternative feeding therapies. Some residents may also need assistance with eating. Providing assistance may involve totally feeding residents, providing assistive eating devices, or simply serving the meal tray at the bedside or in the facility dining room. Residents may have eating challenges, such as the risk of aspiration (inhalation of food or liquid), due to age or disease. Each meal should be treated as a special time essential to the body's function, the capacity to heal, and the realization of optimal wellness. To achieve the objectives for this section, you must successfully

- **identify** environments and approaches that promote optimal eating;
- **explain** the reasons behind and care considerations for selected diets, including therapeutic diets;
- **discuss** the responsibilities of nursing assistants in assisting residents who require alternative feeding therapies;
- **describe** challenges of eating and ways to help residents avoid or overcome them;
- **recognize** different types of adaptive eating equipment (assistive eating devices) and their functions; and
- **demonstrate** how to assist with eating effectively and record food intake.

Key Terms

Learn these key terms to better understand the information presented in the section.

alternative feeding therapy
aspirate
dysphagia
enteral

parenteral
patent
therapeutic diets

Questions to Consider

- Have you ever been on a special diet? Have you had to stay away from certain foods because they gave you a stomachache or because you were allergic to them? What did that feel like?
- How have the diets you've tried affected your daily eating patterns? Have you been able to stay on a diet for the length of time needed? If you were, what helped you stay on the diet? If you were not, what obstacles did you face?
- Were you able to overcome any obstacles to staying on your diet? What strategies or approaches did you use?

What Promotes Optimal Eating?

Mealtimes should be special—not just with family and friends or when celebrating a holiday, but at *all* times. Eating is not just physically essential; it is also a significant part of each person's day. People should enjoy the sheer act of eating and should experience joy as they interact and socialize with others during mealtime. This enjoyment should always be present, regardless of whether someone is at home, is in a restaurant, is in a dining room at a long-term care facility, is confined to bed, or is using alternative feeding therapies. The dining experience, resident preparation, and the atmosphere set all help make the eating process optimal (Figure 22.13).

Remember

One cannot think well, love well, sleep well, if one has not dined well.

Virginia Woolf,
English writer and modernist
in the twentieth century

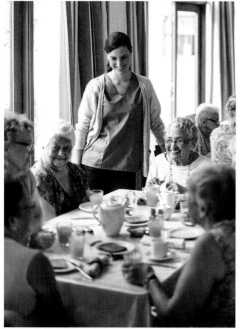

Figure 22.13 As a nursing assistant, you can help make the eating experience enjoyable and healing for residents in your care.

iStock.com/shapecharge

The Dining Experience

In healthcare facilities, the dining experience is more routine than what people experience at home. Meals occur at specific times each day, and foods are chosen by dietitians based on the ordered diet. As discussed in chapter 4, *dietitians* are responsible for creating special diets that residents require due to an illness or disease. They also help residents adjust to new diets, learn about diets, and make dietary changes (with a doctor's order), when needed. The dietary department in a healthcare facility also has other staff members who help order; cook; and deliver food, drinks, and healthy supplements. It is always important that the food prepared is appropriate for each resident. Some residents will require **therapeutic diets** that promote healing. Other residents will be able to select their meals from a buffet line or prepared menu. Long-term care facilities are required to ensure that meals meet individual needs, follow special diets, contain all of the appropriate nutrients, are prepared in a way that is appetizing with suitable seasoning, and are accompanied by a variety of beverages.

Preparation

Residents are prepared for their meals prior to eating and particularly during morning or a.m. care. Preparation includes personal hygiene or before-meal hygiene and oral and denture care (as discussed in

---

Becoming a Holistic Nursing Assistant
Mindful Eating

Eating more carefully and thoughtfully, without interruption and distractions, has been shown to help people make better food choices and more effectively digest the food eaten. This is called *mindful eating*. Mindful eating involves being fully aware of what is happening within and around you when you are eating. Mindful eating allows you to choose your food well and fully smell, see, and taste the food.

The following questions can help you assess how mindfully you eat. Read the questions and consider your answers:

- Before you eat, do you ask yourself if you are really hungry?
- Do you consider whether your hunger is emotional or physical? You may *feel* hungry (emotional), but not physiologically *need* food (physical).
- When your hunger is emotional, do you do some other activity to replace the feeling of hunger?
- Do you sit in a chair at a dining table when you eat? Do you avoid eating casually on a sofa or lounge chair?
- Do you make sure there are no interruptions or distractions while you are eating?
- Do you pay attention to proper portion sizes?

- If your portion size is too big, are you able to eat less?
- When you are eating, do you eat slowly? Remember that it takes 20 minutes after eating for your body to feel full.
- Do you pay attention to what you eat by looking at the food?
- Do you take small bites?
- Do you chew the food well?
- When you are eating, do you stop and taste the food?
- When you are finished eating, do you take the time to think about the experience and how you felt about the food you ate?

Apply It

1. Consider your answers to the questions about mindful eating. How many questions did you answer with "yes"?
2. Which questions did you answer with "no"? What obstacles prevent you from "being present" at mealtime in these ways? How can you overcome these obstacles?
3. What did you learn from answering these questions? What lessons can you include in your care to help residents eat more mindfully?

---

chapter 21). This preparation not only offers residents an opportunity to feel refreshed, but also gives nursing assistants the opportunity to determine if residents have any problems with dentures or sores in the mouth that may prevent chewing or swallowing. If a resident is going to the dining room, he or she will need to dress appropriately. Residents may be able to dress independently or may need assistance. If a resident has eyeglasses or a hearing aid, be sure they are in place and functional. Some residents may need time to pray prior to eating.

Atmosphere

In long-term care facilities, residents usually eat in dining rooms, assuming they are physically mobile, can ambulate using assistive devices, or can be transported by wheelchair. Residents may like to sit with particular people during mealtimes or may choose to sit alone (often to decrease noise and stimulation or to learn how to eat independently). This is important information for nursing assistants to learn, since holistic nursing assistants can use this information to make mealtime a pleasant experience. If a patient is in a hospital or if a resident is bedridden in a long-term care facility, the meal is brought to the patient's or resident's room and served on a tray. In any atmosphere, the patient or resident should be encouraged to eat mindfully, or to pay attention during the meal (Figure 22.14).

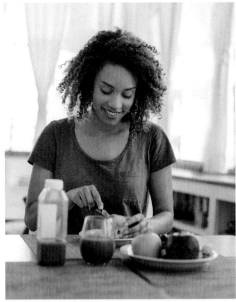

iStock.com/andresr

Figure 22.14 Eating mindfully involves paying attention to your meal and surroundings while eating. Mindful eating makes meals more enjoyable and helps people make better food choices.

What Nutritional Assistance Is Available for Residents?

As you have learned, not everyone is overweight or obese. Some people, particularly seniors, are underweight or malnourished. Seniors are vulnerable to malnutrition due to the aging process, as metabolic rate and lean body mass decline. Nutritional needs change, and degenerative diseases and conditions influence nutritional intake and metabolism. Seniors' appetites may change as a result of a diminished sense of smell, alterations in taste, and sometimes challenges with chewing and swallowing. The significance or severity of weight loss is an important factor to consider for seniors. *Significant weight loss* constitutes losing 1–2 pounds in one week and 5 pounds in one month. Weight loss becomes *severe* when a resident loses even more weight in this time frame. For example, losing 3 pounds in one week is considered severe weight loss.

Licensed nursing staff members and dietitians usually conduct a *nutritional status assessment* to determine a resident's plan of care and assess how well a resident eats and drinks. This assessment also identifies any eating and swallowing problems a resident has, any recent weight changes, and any complaints about meals and eating.

As a holistic nursing assistant, you can follow the plan of care to assist residents with nutritional support. You can also provide nutritional support and help residents get adequate nutrition by being aware of any special diets, as ordered; recording weight on a daily basis; and ensuring skin integrity. You can provide small, frequent meals that are dense in calories; increase intake of appropriate beverages and snacks if the resident is not eating sufficiently or needs more frequent meals (for example, a resident with diabetes); and add supplemental nutrition drinks as recommended by a doctor or dietitian.

Supplemental Nutrition Drinks

Supplemental nutrition drinks provide a balance of protein, carbohydrates, and fat. Supplemental nutrition drinks must not interfere with medications being given. Supplemental nutrition drinks fall into two categories: shakes or formulas. *Shakes* are usually fortified with vitamins and use sugar to improve taste. *Formulas* are typically given to those who have specific diseases, such as cancer or chronic obstructive pulmonary disease (COPD). Formulas can be consumed orally, but are often delivered via feeding tubes, and must be ordered by a doctor. Another option for providing supplemental nutrition through a drink is a fruit smoothie, which is food based. Fruit smoothies tend to have fewer added sugars and are less processed.

No matter what supplemental nutrition drink is ordered by the doctor and included in a resident's plan of care, be aware of its content. Read the food label. Supplemental nutrition drinks usually have 10–20 grams of protein and no more than 40 grams of carbohydrates in an 8-ounce drink. Pay attention to the number of calories in the drink. If the drink is a meal replacement, it should contain no more than 400 calories. Be wary of supplemental nutrition drinks after a full meal. A drink may be too filling for the resident and contain too many calories, making it unhelpful to reaching specific nutritional goals. No matter which drink is used, know that supplements by themselves do not replace the nutrients provided by actual food sources (Figure 22.15).

Therapeutic Diets

Therapeutic diets are commonly seen in healthcare facilities. A resident may be admitted with a therapeutic diet, or a therapeutic diet may be ordered by a doctor during a resident's stay. The goal of therapeutic diets is to maintain residents' intake of essential nutrients while adjusting foods appropriate to a specific disease, condition, or procedure. When possible, a resident's cultural food preferences are considered. Recently, *liberalized diets* have become more common. Liberalized diets are used by doctors and dietitians to find more creative ways of managing diseases through diet. The goal of liberalized diets is to improve resident compliance and increase enjoyment. In a liberalized diet, the basics of a therapeutic diet remain; however, individualized decisions about foods within the diet are explained, and assistance is provided to help residents make wise nutritional choices.

A variety of therapeutic diets are prescribed for different reasons (rationales). Each therapeutic diet has specific requirements. Following are some diets you will often encounter.

Regular Diet

A *regular diet* is ordered when there are no food restrictions for a resident. This diet includes a variety of foods from all of the food groups. Regular diets may be adjusted by changing foods due to allergies or changing the consistency of food to make it pureed or soft.

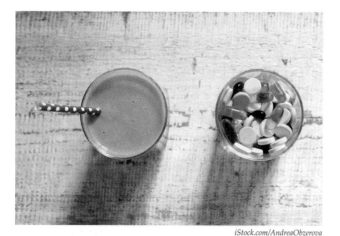

Figure 22.15 Supplementary nutrition drinks and vitamin and mineral supplements are two examples of supplementation used in healthcare facilities.

Soft Diet

A *soft* or *mechanical soft diet* is ordered when a resident has difficulty chewing or swallowing due to weakness or dental difficulties. Some conditions that might contribute to weakness or dental difficulties include poorly fitting dentures; chemotherapy; radiation to the head or neck; radiation to the abdomen, which can cause digestive problems; and a sore mouth. Soft and mechanical soft diets are sometimes used to relieve stomach or intestinal discomfort. They can also help residents transition from liquids to a regular diet and determine tolerance.

Soft and mechanical soft diets include foods that are easy to chew and swallow. Some examples of foods are tender, juicy meats; soup; eggs; pudding; custard; and smooth yogurt or ice cream. A soft or mechanical soft diet limits or eliminates foods such as raw fruits and vegetables, chewy breads, and tough meats, which are hard to chew and swallow. For this diet, foods can be softened using machines or devices that cook or mash them. Canned or soft-cooked fruits and vegetables can be used. Foods should be varied according to taste preferences and ease of chewing and swallowing.

Full Liquid Diet

A *full liquid diet* is ordered when residents transition from clear liquids to a soft diet and when residents have undergone special procedures or GI surgery. This diet may also be ordered for residents who have certain chewing or swallowing problems.

A full liquid diet includes a variety of liquid foods, including cream soups (strained), pureed meats, bland vegetables and white potatoes, custard-style yogurt, pudding, plain ice cream, sherbet, sorbet, coffee, tea, cream, carbonated beverages, fruit and vegetable juices, milk, milkshakes, cream of wheat or rice cereal, mild seasonings, margarine, sugar, syrup, jelly, and honey. No other foods are allowed on this diet. High-protein, high-calorie supplements fortified with vitamins and minerals may also be ordered. If a resident is lactose intolerant, then milk products may be substituted with lactose-free liquid products.

Clear Liquid Diet

A *clear liquid diet* is ordered prior to certain tests, medical procedures, or surgeries that require the gastrointestinal system to be free from food. This diet is also ordered for residents with certain digestive problems, such as nausea, vomiting, or diarrhea.

A clear liquid diet includes water (plain, carbonated, or flavored); fruit juices; lemonade; broth; plain gelatin; tea or coffee without milk or cream; strained tomato or vegetable juice; sports drinks; honey or sugar; hard candy, such as lemon drops or peppermint rounds; and ice pops without milk. Clear liquid diets do *not* provide sufficient calories and nutrients; therefore, they should not be continued for more than a few days.

Bland Diet

A *bland diet* is ordered to help treat ulcers, heartburn, nausea, vomiting, diarrhea, and gas. It may also be ordered after stomach or intestinal surgery.

A bland diet includes foods that are soft, not spicy, and low in fiber. Some foods included in a bland diet are milk and other dairy products (low-fat or fat-free only); cooked, canned, or frozen vegetables; fruit juices and vegetable juices; weak tea; breads, crackers, and pasta made with refined white flour; hot cereals, such as cream of wheat; lean, tender meats (such as poultry, whitefish, and shellfish) that are steamed, baked, or grilled with no added fat; creamy peanut butter; pudding and custard; eggs; tofu; and soup (broth).

A resident who is on a bland diet should not consume spicy, fried, or raw foods; strong cheeses; seeds; nuts; whole grains; cured or smoked meats; alcohol; or beverages with caffeine. A resident on a bland diet should also

- eat small meals often during the day;
- chew food slowly and well;
- stop smoking cigarettes; and
- not eat within two hours of bedtime.

Low-Sodium Diet

A *low-sodium diet* is ordered for residents who have kidney problems. This diet is ordered to lower the amount of salt consumed (to less than 1 teaspoon daily) because the kidneys cannot effectively filter sodium. Excess sodium causes fluid retention and swelling (edema). A low-sodium diet is also helpful for residents with heart diseases, as it reduces excess sodium and fluid buildup in the bloodstream and helps the heart pump more effectively.

A low-sodium diet includes reduced amounts of heavily processed foods such as hot dogs, sausage, ham, prepackaged meats, canned vegetables and soups, and

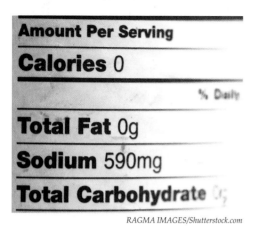

Amount Per Serving	
Calories 0	
	% Daily
Total Fat 0g	
Sodium 590mg	
Total Carbohydrate	

RAGMA IMAGES/Shutterstock.com

Figure 22.16 Sodium content is listed on food labels for foods and fluids. The American Heart Association recommends that people eat no more than 1500 mg of sodium per day.

frozen prepared meals. Fresh or frozen beef, lamb, poultry, or fish; eggs or egg substitutes; milk, yogurt, or ice cream; fresh and frozen vegetables without sauces; and fresh potatoes are some of the foods that can be included in this diet. Carefully reading food labels provides information about sodium content (Figure 22.16).

Cardiac or Heart-Healthy Diet

A *cardiac* or *heart-healthy diet* is ordered for residents who have cardiovascular diseases or who are at risk for cardiac problems. Some people use this diet to promote overall health and weight loss.

A cardiac or heart-healthy diet includes heart-healthy foods such as whole grains, fiber, fruits, and vegetables. This diet prohibits some types of fat, sodium, cholesterol, and sometimes caffeine. Typically, this diet cuts out the consumption of egg yolks, bacon, luncheon meats, cheese, high-fat milk, high-fat red meat, and bakery products. The diet usually restricts sodium intake to 2000–4000 mg daily. In this diet, snacks may consist of fruits, such as apples or grapes.

Diabetic or Carbohydrate-Controlled Diet

A *diabetic* or *carbohydrate-controlled diet* is ordered for residents who have diabetes. Residents on this diet eat three meals daily at regular times to ensure steady blood sugar levels. This diet matches food intake with insulin needs by balancing healthy carbohydrates, such as fruits, vegetables, and grains; fiber-rich foods; proteins; and monounsaturated and polyunsaturated fats. Saturated fats, *trans* fats, and cholesterol are avoided, and sodium is limited to less than 2300 mg daily.

Diabetic diets are developed according to resident needs. Meal plans may be based on specific methods, such as preparing a plate with one-half nonstarchy vegetables (such as carrots); one-quarter protein (such as tuna); and one-quarter of a whole-grain item or starchy food. Another method involves counting carbohydrates and eating the same amount each day to control blood sugar. An exchange list system with categories based on carbohydrate, protein, and fat content may also be used. Each serving in a category has about the same amount of carbohydrates, proteins, fats, and calories. One other method is the *glycemic index*. This method ranks carbohydrate-containing foods by their effect on blood sugar levels.

Renal Diet

A *renal diet* is ordered for residents who have kidney damage or disease. Declining kidney function is progressive and permanent. Damage to the kidneys makes the kidneys less able to filter waste products, fluids, and nutrients (such as phosphorus and potassium) from the blood. Excessive amounts of these substances can build up in the blood. The renal diet has to be carefully managed.

The renal diet includes restrictions to the following four components:

- **Proteins**: animal proteins, such as eggs, milk, meat, poultry, and fish, are eaten. These proteins are rich in essential amino acids and are proteins of "high biological value."
- **Phosphorus**: care is taken with milk, cheese, yogurt, ice cream, pudding, custard, cocoa, dried beans, nuts, seeds, whole-grain breads and cereals, bran, chocolate, caramel, dried fruits, and beer.
- **Potassium**: care is taken with fruits and vegetables, milk products, meats, whole grains, dry beans, and salt substitutes.
- **Sodium and fluid**: care is taken with table salt, bouillon cubes, potato chips, salted nuts, bacon, hot dogs, cold cuts, cheese, canned soup and vegetables, pretzels, and fast food.

High-Fiber Diet

A *high-fiber diet* is ordered for residents who have chronic constipation, irritable bowel syndrome, or an elevated risk for colon cancer. Foods that are high in fiber should also be part of a regular diet, as fiber is good for the colon and is also heart healthy.

A high-fiber diet includes approximately 20–25 grams of fiber daily. This amount can be obtained by eating five or more servings of fruits and vegetables and between four and six servings of whole-grain breads or cereals. The AI for fluid intake is important and should also be consumed daily. Residents on this diet should minimize restaurant meals and processed foods, which are low in fiber.

Low-Fiber Diet

A *low-fiber diet* is ordered when a resident is experiencing GI problems, such as abdominal pain, diarrhea, and diverticulitis. This diet is also ordered when a resident has an intestinal stricture or obstruction.

A low-fiber diet includes a fiber intake below 10 grams each day. This diet should only be used for the short term until GI problems are resolved.

Alternative Feeding Therapies

Some residents are not able to eat food through their mouths. As a result, these residents require nutrition to be delivered using an **alternative feeding therapy**. Alternative feeding therapies can be given by **parenteral** (by way of the veins) or **enteral** (by way of the gastrointestinal system) means. Residents may be unable to eat food through their mouths due to a specific disease or condition, such as cancer, surgery, oral trauma, eating disorders, frailness, or unconsciousness. Parenteral nutrition provides nutrients such as sugar, carbohydrates, proteins, and electrolytes, to the body via an intravenous (IV) line (see chapter 23). Enteral nutrition delivers a formula (usually commercially prepared) through feeding tubes. The formula contains proteins, carbohydrates, fats, vitamins, and minerals. Feeding tubes are located at different places in the GI system. Some tubes are inserted, and others are surgically placed, depending on the doctor's order, the function of the GI system, and the length of time the tube will be used. The insertion of the tube may be performed by a doctor or by the licensed nursing staff, depending on the type of tube.

The different types of feeding tubes include the following (Figure 22.17):

- **Nasogastric (NG) tubes**: are inserted through the nose and run down the esophagus into the stomach.

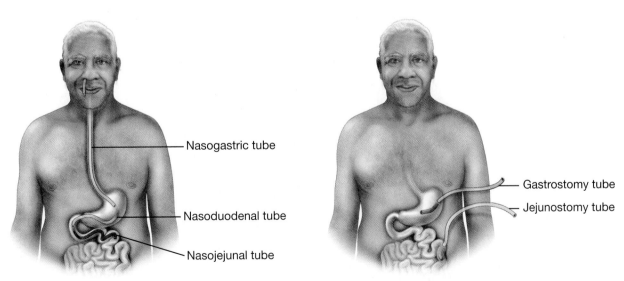

Nasogastric tube

Nasoduodenal tube

Nasojejunal tube

Gastrostomy tube

Jejunostomy tube

© *Body Scientific International*

Figure 22.17 The nasogastric, nasoduodenal, and nasojejunal feeding tubes are inserted through the nose. The gastrostomy and jejunostomy feeding tubes are surgically placed.

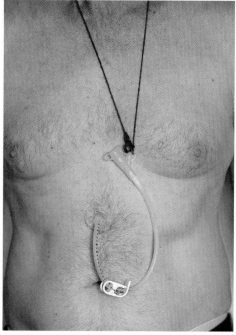

Figure 22.18 A lanyard or some other device is used to ensure the tube is not dislodged.

iStock.com/Lighthousebay

- **Nasoduodenal (ND) tubes**: are inserted through the nose and end in the first portion of the small intestine (duodenum). These tubes bypass the stomach, which can help residents who have stomachs that don't empty well, who are chronically vomiting, or who **aspirate** (inhale) stomach contents into their lungs.

- **Nasojejunal (NJ) tubes**: are inserted through the nose and end in the second portion of the small intestine (jejunum).

- **Gastrostomy (G) tubes**: are surgically inserted through the abdominal wall into the stomach. These tubes are most commonly used for residents who receive enteral nutrition for a long period of time. A G tube may consist of a long tube, sometimes called a *percutaneous endoscopic gastronomy (PEG)* tube, and a skin-level button device (Figure 22.18). When a button device is used, an extension tube is attached for feeding and then removed on completion of the feeding.

- **Jejunostomy (J) tubes**: are surgically placed directly into the intestine.

In some states, nursing assistants can be delegated the responsibility of giving tube feedings and removing NG tubes. Always check to be sure this responsibility is within your scope of practice and is documented in your job description. Be sure that you know how to use the appropriate equipment, that you have had training in the procedure, and that you have reviewed the procedure with the licensed nursing staff.

Following are general information and guidelines that holistic nursing assistants should be aware of when caring for residents receiving enteral nutrition:

- Tube feeding may be continuous or scheduled. If scheduled, tube feedings are usually given four times a day (8–12 ounces over 30 minutes). If a continuous pump is used, the feeding may be given slowly over a 24-hour period (with a certain amount being given each hour). If feedings are given on a continuous schedule, regularly check the level of the formula. The formula level should continually decrease as the feeding occurs. If this is not occurring, alert the licensed nursing staff.

- Formula should be given at room temperature. Cold fluids can cause cramping. Open formula can last only eight hours at room temperature.

- Tube feedings may be given with a syringe or from a feeding bag (Figure 22.19).

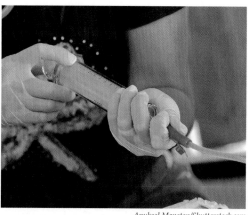

Anukool Manoton/Shutterstock.com

A

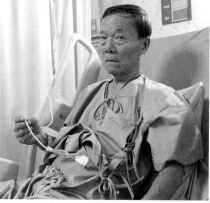

stockphoto mania/Shutterstock.com

B

Figure 22.19 Tube feedings can be delivered via a syringe (A) or a feeding bag (B).

- During tube feeding, the head of the resident's bed should be elevated at least 30–45°, or as specified in the care plan. If tube feedings are scheduled for certain times, make sure the head of the bed remains elevated for at least one hour after each feeding is completed.
- Licensed nursing staff members will regularly check a feeding tube's placement to be sure the feeding tube is **patent** (open) and to determine if the feeding tube has moved out of place or been tugged loose due to regular movement or care delivery. Licensed nursing staff members will also check to see if the resident is restless, confused, or disoriented. As a nursing assistant, you will need to be observant and notice if the tube does not look like it is correctly placed. If the tube looks displaced, immediately notify the licensed nursing staff.
- Regularly check the outer part of the feeding tube to be sure it is not bent or obstructed in any way.
- Always check the area around the feeding tube and its insertion. Notify the licensed nursing staff if it seems to be pulled out or if there is any skin irritation.
- Check for redness, swelling, drainage, or odor around or from the tube insertion site.
- During tube feeding, notify the licensed nursing staff immediately if there is nausea or bloating; abdominal distention (a swollen abdomen); complaints of pain or discomfort during the feeding; coughing, gagging, or vomiting during the feeding; respiratory distress; increased pulse rate; flatulence; diarrhea; or constipation.
- To improve a resident's comfort and hygiene, provide frequent oral and nasal care. Lubricate the lips often, as dryness is common. It is helpful to offer a mouth rinse every two hours. If appropriate, suggest that the resident suck on a lemon drop or chew sugarless gum.

Adaptive and Assistive Eating Equipment

Adaptive and *assistive eating equipment* includes devices and products that aid residents who want to remain as independent as possible during meals. These types of equipment include special plates and bowls, *utensils* (tools for eating), utensil holders, cups and mugs, and thickening fluids for residents who have **dysphagia** (difficulty swallowing). Signs of dysphagia include food spilling out of the mouth and coming up through the nose, coughing or choking during or after swallowing, complaining that food will not go down or feels stuck in the throat, and avoiding foods that require chewing or have a certain texture or temperature. Some examples of adaptive and assistive eating equipment include the following:

- adaptive and nonskid plates and bowls that prevent foods from slipping off or moving due to the force of eating utensils (Figure 22.20A)
- weighted knives, forks, and spoons that help hands remain steady (Figure 22.20B)
- utensil holders (clips, straps, and foam handles) that help residents achieve better grip
- cup holders, weighted mugs, nonslip bases, and no-spill lids that help prevent spills

Additionally, commercial thickening fluids, if needed, can aid safe swallowing and prevent aspiration. Commercial thickening products can be added to most hot and cold liquids without affecting taste. These products are important, as the consistencies of liquids can ease swallowing. The thicker a liquid is, the less risk there is of choking. Figure 22.21 lists four liquid consistencies and examples for each.

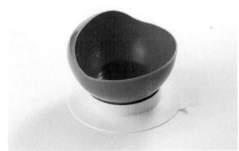

© Tori Soper Photography

A

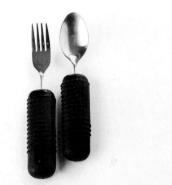

© Tori Soper Photography

B

Figure 22.20 This nonskid bowl (A) will not move while a resident is eating. Weighted utensils (B) are easier to grip than other utensils.

Liquid Consistencies	
Level of Consistency	**Description**
Extremely thick	Puddinglike; holds shape and can be served with a spoon
Moderately thick	Honeylike; will not flow freely, but will run off a spoon
Medium thick	Nectarlike; does not hold shape and will run off a spoon
Thin	Free-flowing liquids, such as water, soda, coffee, or juice

Figure 22.21 The consistency of a liquid can influence the ease of swallowing.

What Are the Nursing Assistant's Responsibilities in Assisting Residents with Meals?

As a holistic nursing assistant, you will be asked to assist residents with their meals. In some cases, you will assist by preparing residents for meals and helping residents to the dining room. In other cases, you will serve the meal tray, set it up at the bedside, and help feed the resident. Other important responsibilities will be ensuring that residents on therapeutic diets get the correct meal, that required foods are sufficiently consumed, and that some residents eat on time.

When caring for residents, you should always practice good hygiene by washing your hands or using hand sanitizer, as appropriate. You must also ensure resident safety. One of the most important aspects of caring for residents during mealtime is preventing aspiration. You can use the following guidelines to help prevent aspiration:

- Provide a brief rest before eating.
- Sit the resident upright in a chair. If the resident is confined to bed, elevate the backrest to a sitting position.
- Slightly flex the resident's head to achieve a chin-down position. This is helpful for reducing aspiration and some types of dysphagia. Swallowing studies may be ordered by the doctor to determine which residents are most likely to benefit from this position.
- Adjust the rate of feeding and the sizes of bites to a resident's tolerance. Do not force or rush the feeding.
- Provide small, bite-sized portions of food.
- Alternate between liquid and solid foods.
- Vary the placement of food in the mouth. Be aware if there is weakness on either side of the face. Always place food in the strongest side of the mouth.
- Check the thickness of food and liquid to be sure it can be tolerated without choking or gagging. For example, some residents best swallow thickened liquids.
- Check to see if residents are on medications that may make them sleepy. Drowsiness may put residents at a higher risk for aspiration. Provide a 30-minute rest period prior to feeding time; a rested person will likely have less difficulty swallowing.

Nursing assistants are also responsible for recording the resident's meal intake. This information is recorded using a form provided by the healthcare facility or in the electronic record (Figure 22.22).

For the most part, keeping residents independent and self-reliant is always encouraged. Going to the dining room to eat meals is not only important for social interaction, but also helps promote and encourage better nutrition. The procedure that follows focuses on assisting residents eating in their rooms—in bed, by the bedside in a chair, or in a wheelchair. Many of the steps in the procedure also apply to assisting a resident in the dining room.

DIETARY INTAKE RECORD

Month	Year

Directions:

1. For each meal, record the **total percentage** of food the resident consumed in the **TOP** portion of the box.
2. For each meal, record the **total fluids (in ml's)** the resident consumed in the **BOTTOM** portion of the box.
3. If resident was offered snacks, indicate **refusal** or **percentage consumed**.

DAY	1	2	3	4	5	6	7	8	9	10	11	12	13	14	15
BREAKFAST															
Snack AM															
LUNCH															
Snack PM															
DINNER															
Snack HS															

DAY	16	17	18	19	20	21	22	23	24	25	26	27	28	29	30	31
BREAKFAST																
Snack AM																
LUNCH																
Snack PM																
DINNER																
Snack HS																

FOOD INTAKE	FLUID INTAKE	SNACK INTAKE
0% = Consumed none or only bites (but less than 25%)	1 oz. Cup = 30 ml	R = Refused
25% = Consumed 1/4 of all item(s)	4 oz. Cup = 120 ml	0% = Consumed none or only bites (but less than 25%)
50% = Consumed 1/2 of all item(s)	5 oz. Cup = 150 ml	25% = Consumed 1/4 of all item(s)
75% = Consumed 3/4 of all item(s)	6 oz. Cup/Bowl = 180 ml	50% = Consumed 1/2 of all item(s)
100% = Consumed all item(s)	8 oz. Cup/Bowl = 240 ml	75% = Consumed 3/4 of all item(s)
		100% = Consumed all item(s)

Resident Name	ID#	Room #	Doctor

Figure 22.22 An intake form like this one records the foods and fluids a resident consumes.

Procedure | Assisting with Meals in the Room

Rationale

Residents receive adequate nutrition when they consume the proper amounts of essential nutrients from a variety of food groups. Due to diseases or conditions, some residents require assistance to eat comfortably and consume sufficient amounts of their meals.

Preparation

1. Ask the licensed nursing staff how this procedure fits into the plan of care, if there are doctor's orders for the procedure, if there are any special instructions or precautions, and if the resident can be moved into the positions required for this procedure.
2. Wash your hands or use hand sanitizer before entering the room.
3. Knock before entering the room.
4. Introduce yourself using your full name and title. Explain that you work with the licensed nursing staff and will be providing care.
5. Greet the resident and ask the resident to state his full name, if able. Then check the resident's identification bracelet.
6. Use Mr., Mrs., or Ms. and the last name when conversing.
7. Explain the procedure in simple terms, even if the resident is not able to communicate or is disoriented. Ask permission to perform the procedure.

> **Best Practice**
> To promote comfort during the meal, be sure the room is free from unpleasant odors.

8. Bring the necessary equipment into the room. Place the following items in an accessible location:
   - disposable gloves, if needed
   - a cloth or paper clothing protector to prevent soiling during the meal
   - adaptive and assistive eating devices (as needed)
   - pen and pad, form, or digital device for recording meal intake
   - supplies for before-meal hygiene, if needed

> **Best Practice**
> Always check to be sure adaptive and assistive eating devices are usable. If they are not, notify the licensed nursing staff immediately.

The Procedure

9. Provide privacy by closing the curtains, using a screen, or closing the door to the room.

> **Best Practice**
> Before starting, ask the resident if he needs to use the toilet, bedpan, or urinal.

10. If the resident will be eating in bed and if you will be assisting, lock the bed wheels and then raise the bed to hip level. Raise the head of the bed and adjust for comfort in eating. If appropriate, help the resident to a sitting position at the side of the bed or to a chair. If the resident is not dressed, help the resident put on a robe and slippers.
11. Ensure safety during the procedure. If there are side rails, raise and secure the rails on the opposite side of the bed from where you will be working. Lower the rail on the side you are working.

> **Best Practice**
> Disposable gloves are worn only if required for infection prevention and control.

12. Provide before-meal hygiene. If the resident is ambulatory, hygiene can be performed in the bathroom. If the resident is not ambulatory, provide supplies for washing the hands and face, brushing teeth, or using mouth rinse. Assist the resident as needed.

13. Confirm that the name on the meal tray matches the name of the resident.

14. Clear the overbed table before placing the meal tray. Check the meal tray to make sure that all appropriate foods are there and represent the correct diet. If any foods that should be on the tray are missing, get them or ask to have them brought in, if appropriate.

15. If the resident is in bed, place a cloth or paper clothing protector over the resident's chest to prevent the resident's clothing from becoming soiled with food during the meal.

16. Sit at eye level next to the resident.

17. Prepare the meal tray. Depending on the situation, you may need to help with
    - opening milk cartons;
    - removing utensils from their wrappers;
    - buttering bread;
    - cutting up meat; or
    - seasoning food to the resident's taste (not to yours).

18. If the resident can handle finger foods, arrange the plate so these are in reach.

19. If the resident has poor eyesight or limited vision, describe the foods being served. If the resident is feeding himself, help the resident locate the food on the plate by describing where foods are in terms of a clockface (Figure 22.23).

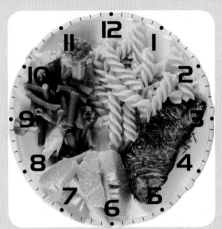

Figure 22.23

20. If a resident cannot see the tray at all and needs assistance, name each mouthful of food as you offer it.

21. If a resident is weak or paralyzed on one side, feed the resident on the strong side, not on the side that is weak or paralyzed.

22. Alternate between solid foods and liquids. Offer liquids frequently between bites. Do not rush the feeding. Serve the food in order of resident preference.

23. Allow the resident enough time for chewing and swallowing. Encourage residents to swallow twice between each bite. Check the mouth to see if it is empty before offering more foods or fluids.

(continued)

Assisting with Meals in the Room (*continued*)

24. Provide a straw for liquids if the resident cannot drink from a cup or glass. Provide a different straw for each liquid. If the resident is weak, provide a short straw.

> **Best Practice**
> Residents with dysphagia usually do not use straws. They may take thickened liquids with a spoon.

25. Encourage the resident to eat as much as possible. Approaches or techniques you can use to help include
    - using verbal cues, such as short and simple phrases, to prompt the resident;
    - demonstrating or acting out what you want the resident to do;
    - placing your hand over the resident's hand for guidance (Figure 22.24); and
    - praising successes along the way.

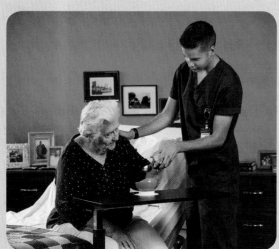

Figure 22.24

26. Using a napkin, wipe the resident's hands, face, and mouth as needed during and at the end of the meal. Discard the napkin when done.

27. Once the resident has finished eating, remove the meal tray. Be sure to note how much was eaten and which foods the resident consumed. Identify which foods were not eaten. If a particular food was not eaten, ask the resident why.

28. Provide for privacy. Assist with post-meal hygiene by having the resident wash his hands and perform oral care. Assist as needed.

29. The amount of food eaten should be recorded according to facility policy using a form provided by the healthcare facility or in the electronic record. Some policies require that you note the portion of the total meal consumed. Other policies require the percentage of the food eaten. Whatever method is used, the amount of food eaten will be converted into calories by the licensed nursing staff or a dietitian. Always inform the licensed nursing staff if less than 75 percent (two-thirds) of a meal is eaten.

30. If the resident is in bed, check to be sure the bed wheels are locked. Then reposition the resident and lower the bed.

31. Follow the plan of care to determine if the side rails should be raised or lowered.

32. Take the used meal tray to the meal cart.

33. Remove, clean, and store equipment in the proper location. Remove soiled linens and discard disposable equipment.

Follow-Up

34. Wash your hands to ensure infection control.

35. Make sure the resident is safe and comfortable and place the call light and personal items within reach.

36. Conduct a safety check before leaving the room. The room should be clean and free from clutter or spills.

37. Wash your hands or use hand sanitizer before leaving the room.

Reporting and Documentation

38. Communicate any specific observations, complications, or unusual responses to the licensed nursing staff. Record this information, along with the care provided, in the chart or EMR.

Figure 22.23 Oleksandra Naumenko/Shutterstock.com; GzP_Design/Shutterstock.com;
Figure 22.24 © Tori Soper Photography

Using the Key Terms

Complete the following sentences using the key terms in this section.

1. A feeding tube that is open may also be described as _____.
2. Parenteral and enteral feeding techniques are types of _____.
3. _____ are eating plans that cause healing.
4. _____ feeding delivers nutrients by way of the gastrointestinal system.
5. To _____ means to inhale a foreign object while eating.
6. A person who has difficulty or discomfort when swallowing is experiencing _____.
7. _____ feeding delivers nutrients by way of the veins.

Know and Understand the Facts

8. Identify two factors that help promote optimal eating.
9. What is mindful eating and how can it be accomplished?
10. Describe two therapeutic diets and explain why they are ordered.
11. Describe three responsibilities nursing assistants have when they assist with alternative feeding therapies.
12. What are supplemental nutrition drinks and when are they used?
13. Identify two challenges residents may encounter when eating.
14. Describe two different adaptive or assistive eating devices and explain their functions.

Analyze and Apply Concepts

15. What three steps should be taken to prepare a resident for a meal?
16. Identify one eating challenge a resident may face and describe two ways to avoid or overcome it.
17. Describe three important principles nursing assistants should keep in mind when assisting residents with meals.
18. Explain how to record food intake.

Think Critically

Read the following care situation. Then answer the questions that follow.

You are taking care of Mr. M today. Mr. M is a frail, 78-year-old man who was admitted last week to the long-term care facility where you work. Mr. M had been living at home with his sister for the last five years. Mr. M has been falling recently when ambulating, so he has several bruises on his arms. He is unstable when walking and has moderate-to-severe arthritis in his hands and hips. This is the first time you will be taking care of Mr. M. Mr. M's chart states that he is alert and communicative. When you entered Mr. M's room this morning, you found him sleepy, very groggy, and unwilling to participate in his morning care. It is now time for Mr. M's noontime meal.

19. What is the first thing you should do before serving Mr. M's meal?
20. Mr. M will be eating lunch. How will you know whether Mr. M should go to the dining room, stay in his room to eat at his bedside, or stay in bed to eat?
21. What will you need to consider when preparing Mr. M for his meal?
22. What should you do to prevent any eating challenges Mr. M may have (for example, Mr. M choking on his food, since he seemed so groggy)?

Key Points

Reviewing the key points for this chapter will help you practice more safely and competently as a holistic nursing assistant and will help you prepare for the competency certification examination.

- Calories provide the energy the body needs to function properly and build, maintain, and repair body tissues. There are six essential nutrients needed for a healthy diet: carbohydrates, dietary fats, proteins, vitamins, minerals, and water.
- MyPlate and the *Dietary Guidelines for Americans* provide guidance concerning what types of foods people should eat. Reading food labels and maintaining food safety are important for healthy eating and optimal nutrition.
- Nursing assistants must understand the reasons for and importance of therapeutic diets.
- Residents may need assistance with eating, including feeding residents, providing adaptive and assistive eating devices, or simply preparing meal trays at the bedside or in the facility dining room. Some residents will require alternative feeding therapies, such as tube feeding.

Action Steps to Holistic Care

Review the information in this chapter. Complete the following activities.

1. Select one set of guidelines or a procedure about assisting with meals in this chapter. Prepare a short paper or digital presentation that describes the top three most important practices for assisting with eating, including one that promotes comfort and one that assures safety.
2. With a partner, write a song or a poem about one nutrient. Include why the nutrient is important to body function and what foods contain it.
3. With a partner, prepare a poster that illustrates one eating disorder or condition. Include at least four facts that residents and the public should know about the disorder.
4. Research one therapeutic diet. Write a brief report that describes one new, science-based fact.

 Preparing for the Certification Competency Examination

To prepare for the nursing assistant certification competency examination, you will need to know content found in this chapter. This content may be tested in the knowledge (written or oral) and skills (hands-on demonstration) portions of the exam. The following areas will be emphasized:

- principles of nutrition
- essential nutrients, basic food groups, and RDAs
- serving and portion sizes
- personal, cultural, religious, and medical conditions requiring diet variations
- situational factors that influence or interfere with adequate intake
- contributory factors that influence age-related dietary problems
- therapeutic diets and their rationales
- alternate feeding methods
- care needed to assist in meeting dietary needs
- care for residents unable to obtain adequate nutrition independently
- the importance of observing and recording food intake

These sample test questions are similar to ones you will find on the certification competency exam. See how well you can answer them. Be sure to select the *best* answer.

1. Which of the following is a fat-soluble vitamin?
   A. vitamin C
   B. vitamin A
   C. vitamin B_6
   D. vitamin B_{12}

2. Mr. J recently had a mild heart attack and is on dialysis. Which therapeutic diet would doctors most likely order for Mr. J?
   A. bland diet
   B. clear liquid diet
   C. soft diet
   D. renal diet

3. Which of the following is the major function of protein?

   A. storage in body tissue
   B. building of body tissue
   C. absorption of fats
   D. synthesis of minerals

4. Susie is overweight and spends a lot of time raiding the refrigerator in the kitchen during the night. Which of the following eating disorders does she most likely have?

   A. cachexia nervosa
   B. dysphagia nervosa
   C. binge-eating disorder
   D. anorexia nervosa

5. Which of the following is an important responsibility holistic nursing assistants have when they provide care during enteral feeding?

   A. keeping the resident occupied during the feeding
   B. providing frequent oral and nasal care
   C. making sure the bed linens are not wrinkled
   D. letting the family know when the feeding occurs

6. A nursing assistant is taking care of Mrs. D, who has become dehydrated after vomiting all morning from a mild stomach virus. Mrs. D can now tolerate a clear liquid diet. To begin the process of hydration, how much liquid should the nursing assistant encourage Mrs. D to drink today?

   A. 11 cups   C. 14 cups
   B. 8 cups   D. 10 cups

7. A common calculation to determine if a person is underweight, at a healthy weight, overweight, or obese is to use which of the following?

   A. a balance scale   C. a digital scale
   B. the FDA   D. BMI

8. Which of the following are units of measurement in the metric system?

   A. feet, meter, and mile
   B. meter, gram, and liter
   C. liter, ounce, and dram
   D. pound, ounce, and meter

9. Units of energy that combine with oxygen to release energy the body needs are called

   A. carbohydrates   C. calories
   B. vitamins   D. minerals

10. A nursing assistant has been asked to assist Mrs. L with her eating. Mrs. L is independent, but her hands tremble when she holds her fork. What might the nursing assistant do to help?

    A. leave Mrs. L alone to eat
    B. go ahead and feed Mrs. L her main meal
    C. have Mrs. L wait until her family returns
    D. have Mrs. L try an assistive utensil

11. Which of the following are the three types of carbohydrates found in food?

    A. starch, sugars, and fiber
    B. minerals, fiber, and fats
    C. starch, fats, and sugars
    D. fiber, minerals, and water

12. Mrs. H is able to eat independently, but is not mobile enough to leave her bed. She sometimes has trouble swallowing. What position should the head of Mrs. H's bed be in during eating?

    A. lateral
    B. Trendelenburg
    C. Fowler's or semi-Fowler's
    D. Sims'

13. If a resident has dysphagia, which consistency of liquid is best consumed to avoid choking?

    A. moderately thick
    B. extremely thick
    C. thin
    D. medium thick

14. A nursing assistant at a local long-term care facility knows she should practice food safety. Which of the following is a guideline she should follow?

    A. She should be sure the resident's diet is correct.
    B. She should record all the foods the resident eats.
    C. She should look at all food labels carefully.
    D. She should wash her hands and food-preparation and eating surfaces often.

15. Mr. D likes to eat a large breakfast early in the morning and is always upset when his meal tray comes late. This is an example of

    A. a therapeutic diet
    B. religious tradition
    C. food preferences
    D. alternative nutrition

Did you have difficulty with any of the questions? If you did, review the chapter to find the correct answer(s).

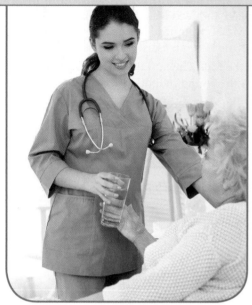

Africa Studio/Shutterstock.com

Chapter Outline

Section 23.1
Maintaining Hydration

Section 23.2
Assisting with Elimination

Welcome to the Chapter

As you learned in chapters 8 and 9, regulating hydration and eliminating waste are functions of the urinary and gastrointestinal systems. As a nursing assistant, you will ensure residents maintain hydration and assist them with elimination needs. You may be asked to keep track of the fluids residents drink and lose through elimination. For ill patients and frail residents, maintaining hydration is critical to promoting healing and achieving optimal wellness. At times, residents do not drink enough fluids or have an illness or condition that prevents them from maintaining hydration. In these cases, parenteral IV infusion may be ordered.

Nursing assistants also assist residents with their elimination needs, including using a bedpan, urinal, bedside commode, or toilet. Nursing assistants provide catheter and ostomy care, empty urinary drainage bags, and change colostomy bags. Inserting suppositories and rectal tubes and administering soapsuds and commercial enemas may be additional responsibilities.

The information and procedures presented in this chapter will help you build the knowledge and skills needed to become a holistic nursing assistant. Check with your instructor to ensure these procedures are within your state's regulations for nursing assistant practice. The topics discussed in the chapter are highlighted on the Providing Holistic Care Framework.

You are now ready to start this chapter, *Hydration and Elimination*.

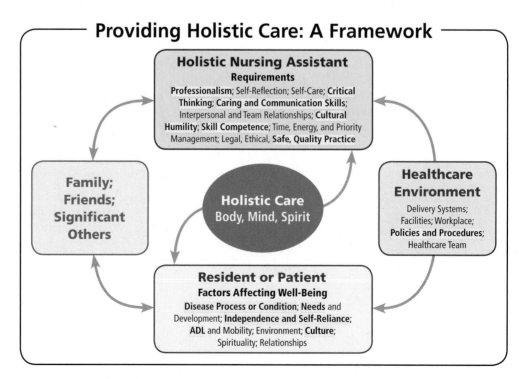

Providing Holistic Care: A Framework

Holistic Nursing Assistant
Requirements
Professionalism; Self-Reflection; Self-Care; **Critical Thinking; Caring and Communication Skills**; Interpersonal and Team Relationships; **Cultural Humility; Skill Competence**; Time, Energy, and Priority Management; Legal, Ethical, **Safe, Quality Practice**

Family; Friends; Significant Others

Holistic Care
Body, Mind, Spirit

Healthcare Environment
Delivery Systems; Facilities; Workplace; **Policies and Procedures**; Healthcare Team

Resident or Patient
Factors Affecting Well-Being
Disease Process or Condition; Needs and Development; Independence and Self-Reliance; ADL and Mobility; Environment; **Culture**; Spirituality; Relationships

Objectives

To help residents maintain hydration and fluid balance, you must pay attention to the fluids residents drink and the fluids lost through perspiration or sweat. Other factors that affect fluid balance include the consumption of salty food (which causes water retention) and vegetables and fruit that contain water. Maintaining fluid balance also requires awareness of elimination. Constipation may be a sign that a resident is not drinking enough fluids, while diarrhea causes the loss of fluids and important electrolytes. Keeping track of residents' ingestion and elimination is an important responsibility of a nursing assistant. To achieve the objectives for this section, you must successfully

- **discuss** the importance of hydration and the consequences of dehydration;
- **describe** how nursing assistants care for residents receiving parenteral IV infusion;
- **demonstrate** how to empty urinary drainage bags; and
- **measure** and **record** intake and output (I&O).

Questions to Consider

- Think about the last time you were extremely thirsty. Do you remember why you were thirsty? Maybe you were outside in very hot weather, had been exercising a lot, or were sick and had a high fever.
- What were the physical signs of your thirst? How did you feel?
- What did you do to satisfy your thirst? How much did you have to drink to feel better? How long did it take for you to feel hydrated?

Key Terms

Learn these key terms to better understand the information presented in the section.

constipation

dehydration

diarrhea

graduate

void

Why Is It Important to Stay Hydrated?

In chapter 22, you learned about the importance of water consumption and hydration. Adequate fluid intake is essential for the body systems to function properly. Fluids in the body moisten tissues in the eyes, nose, and mouth; protect organs; regulate body temperature; lubricate joints; and flush toxins from the body.

Some people may have too much fluid in the body, perhaps due to a particular disease or condition (for example, kidney disease). Excess fluid can lead to *edema*, or swelling in the body tissue. Other people do not take in enough fluids, which can lead to **dehydration**, or lack of adequate fluids in the body tissue.

Dehydration

Dehydration can happen very quickly. Even minor dehydration, such as a loss of 2 percent of body fluids, can decrease body function. Infants, children, and older adults have the highest risks for dehydration.

Dehydration occurs when the body lacks adequate body fluids due to decreased consumption, excessive perspiration, or a disease or injury. This creates an imbalance in the body's systems and can become so severe it leads to death. Adults may experience dehydration if they consume insufficient fluids due to lack of access, inability to consume fluids, dysphagia (difficulty swallowing), or unconsciousness. Exposure to excessive or long-lasting heat, exercise, or a high fever may cause dehydration. Constant vomiting, excessive **diarrhea** (frequent, watery stools), and extreme skin injuries such as burns can also cause significant loss of fluids.

Urine Color Chart

TRANSPARENT
You're drinking a lot of water

PALE STRAW COLOR
You're well hydrated

TRANSPARENT YELLOW
Normal

DARK YELLOW
Drink water soon

AMBER OR HONEY
Your body isn't getting
enough water

SYRUP OR BROWN ALE
Drink a lot of
water immediately

Figure 23.1 Urine color is a good indicator of a person's level of hydration.

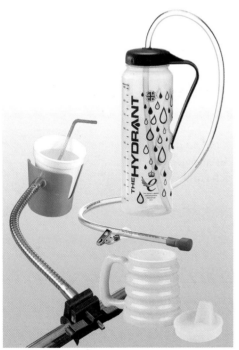

Figure 23.2 Assistive devices such as a clip-on drink holder, hand-to-hand mug, and hydrant water bottle make it easier for residents to maintain hydration.

The first signs of dehydration are increased thirst and a dry mouth. Some people also experience dizziness and may feel weak or fatigued. As dehydration becomes more severe, the tongue may become swollen, and heart palpitations may begin. Some people may have headaches, become confused, and faint. Advanced dehydration can cause chest pain, difficulty breathing, inability to sweat, **constipation** (infrequent, hard, dry stools), and a noticeable decrease in urinary output. Urine becomes more concentrated due to the lack of fluid and becomes dark yellow or orange in color (Figure 23.1).

In many cases, increasing the amount and variety of fluids and water-concentrated fruits and vegetables, such as oranges, tomatoes, and pineapple, can increase fluid intake to prevent dehydration. As a holistic nursing assistant, you can verbally remind residents to drink plenty of fluids during and between meals. Provide fresh drinking water at the bedside and suggest and provide a variety of beverages within a resident's diet restrictions. Also remind residents to avoid caffeinated beverages, as caffeine has a *diuretic* effect that increases urine output.

When dehydration becomes severe or when a resident experiences challenges drinking fluids, use assistive drinking devices such as cups with long spouts to help boost intake (Figure 23.2). Some residents may be totally unable to consume sufficient fluids or may be so dehydrated they need fluid replacement quickly. A doctor may order *parenteral IV infusion* (infusion by way of the veins) for these residents. IVs may also infuse, or *administer*, specific medications.

Parenteral IV Infusion

Parenteral IV infusion restores fluids and electrolytes and ensures adequate intake of fluids. In parenteral IV infusion, fluid is administered through a closed system consisting of a bag of fluid, tubing, and a needle or catheter (Figure 23.3). The bag of fluid hangs on a pole above the patient's head, and the pole may be attached to the head of the bed or stand next to the bed. When the bag of fluid is hanging, gravity aids the flow of the fluid.

Tubing attaches the bag to a *catheter* with a needle that is inserted into the body. The catheter is usually inserted into a peripheral vein in the patient's arm (Figure 23.4). It can sometimes be inserted into the leg, foot, or scalp. Catheters are inserted by the licensed nursing staff. In some facilities, an *IV pump* is used. An IV pump is a medical device that delivers fluids into a patient's body in a controlled manner. IV pumps improve the accuracy and continuity of IV infusions by allowing licensed nursing staff members to program infusion rates and volume.

The type and amount of IV fluid is ordered by the doctor and is infused at an appropriate rate based on the condition. For example, an IV fluid may consist of saline with a percentage of dextrose (*sugar*) and vitamins or electrolytes, such as potassium chloride. The IV fluid drips at a prescribed rate from the bag through the tubing and catheter into the vein. Some patients may be able to drink fluids while undergoing parenteral IV infusion, and others may be NPO (*nothing by mouth*).

While the IV infusion is being administered, licensed nursing staff members ensure that the IV remains a closed system; however, the tubes and catheters need to be patent (remain open), and the flow rate must be accurate. Licensed nursing staff members also maintain a record of IV fluid intake and monitor the insertion site. Members of the licensed nursing staff will also increase or reduce the flow rate based on the doctor's orders, change the bag of fluid, and change the dressings that keep the IV catheter secure. Many times, a protective device (with a clear covering) is placed over the needle or catheter to secure it and provide a better view of the insertion. Patients are instructed to avoid disturbing, twisting, or bending the tubing or dressing, which can prevent fluid from flowing into the vein. Patients are also asked to report any pain, burning, or swelling at the IV site or blood in the tubing. A patient receiving an IV infusion should be monitored continuously for signs of dehydration. Patients should also be monitored for signs of fluid overload, such as elevated blood pressure, weight gain, edema, or difficulty breathing.

A nursing assistant can assist the licensed nursing staff with these responsibilities by performing the following:

- Frequently observe the IV site for possible signs of *infiltration* (swelling at or around the IV site due to IV fluid leaking into the body). Infiltration can occur at any time, but is more common one to two hours after the IV catheter is first inserted. Observe for puffiness or swelling, hot or cold skin, and pale or reddened skin at the site of the needle or catheter (Figure 23.5). If these signs are observed, alert the licensed nursing staff immediately.

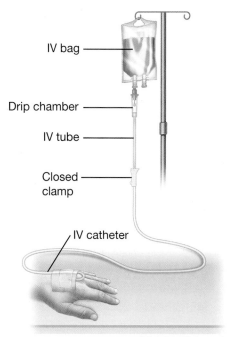

Figure 23.3 The closed IV system consists of an IV bag, tubing, and catheter. Fluid flows through a clear, plastic drip chamber. This chamber prevents air from entering the IV tubing and regulates IV flow rate. The clamp is used to start and stop the IV solution and control the amount of fluids entering the vein.

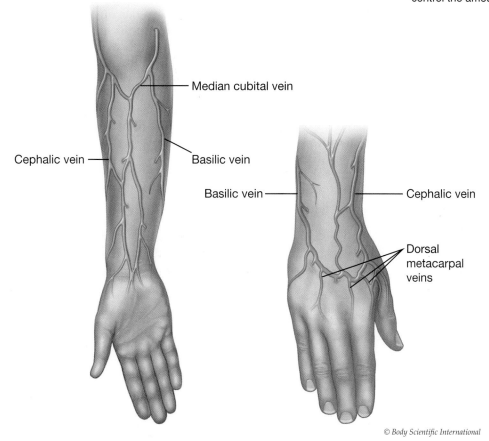

Figure 23.4 Some common IV insertion sites in the arm include the cephalic vein, median cubital vein, basilic vein, and dorsal metacarpal veins.

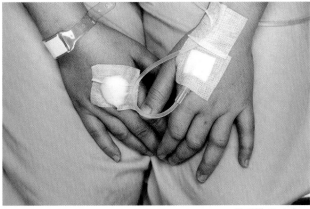

Toa55/Shutterstock.com

Figure 23.5 Always observe around or at the IV site for possible signs of infiltration (swelling).

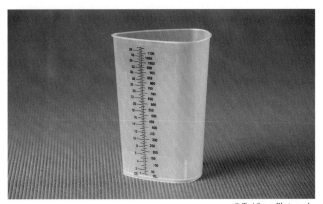

© Tori Soper Photography

Figure 23.6 A graduate measures urine and drainage output.

- Regularly monitor the IV system to make sure the IV fluid bag remains above the patient's heart and there is no fluid leaking from or kinks in the tubing or at the IV site. Check for blood in the tubing and ensure there is enough fluid in the bag. Remind the resident to keep the extremity with the IV lowered so blood does not flow back. If you observe any problems, alert the licensed nursing staff immediately.

- Respond if the patient complains of discomfort, such as pain or burning at or near the site. Other symptoms may be systemic (for example, fever, itching, shortness of breath, chest pain, irregular pulse, or a drop in blood pressure). Alert the licensed nursing staff immediately.

- Ensure the security of the dressing and maintain the position of the tubing and the extremity in which the IV needle or catheter is inserted. This is especially important during personal hygiene and ADLs.

How Are Intake and Output Recorded?

Given the importance of hydration, extreme care needs to be taken if recording fluid intake and urinary output is ordered. This is especially true for residents in long-term care facilities. In chapter 22, you learned how to record meal intake. In this chapter, you will learn how to measure the *intake and output (I&O)* of fluids.

Fluid intake includes all oral fluids, IV fluids, and tube feedings. *Output* includes any urine that is **voided** (expelled from the body) and urine from a urinary drainage bag. Emesis (vomit), diarrhea, colostomy bag drainage, and any other drainage (such as from wounds) are also considered output. I&O is measured on a 24-hour schedule using a **graduate**, or a container with a measurement scale for fluids and for some drainage (Figure 23.6). A urinary hat is also used to measure output and

Standard Volumes for Intake and Output		
Item	**Volume in Ounces (oz)**	**Volume in Milliliters (mL)**
Drinking glass	8 oz	240 mL
Cup	8 oz	240 mL
Teacup	6 oz	180 mL
Styrofoam cup	6 oz	180 mL
Popsicle	3 oz	90 mL
Ice cube	Melts to 1/2 the original volume	

Figure 23.7 Standard measurements will help you accurately record fluid intake.

has a measurement scale. IV fluid bags and drainage bags often have their own measurement scales. Before measuring I&O, you should ask the licensed nursing staff for the standard measurements of glasses and dishes used by the facility (Figure 23.7). In some facilities, these measurements are listed on the I&O form or can be obtained from the nursing or dietary departments.

An *I&O form* can be paper or electronic and is used in facilities to record the intake and output amounts (Figure 23.8). I&O is recorded throughout each shift. At the end of each shift, I&O is subtotaled. Recording continues during the next shift. All subtotals are added together for a total I&O at the end of the shift that completes the 24-hour recording period.

Remember

Fast is fine, but accuracy is everything.

Wyatt Earp, Arizona deputy sheriff and marshal

Intake & Output Form

Resident Name: _____   Room #: _____

Date: _____   Floor #: _____

	Intake			Output			
				Urine		Gastric	
	By mouth	Tube	Parenteral	Voided	Catheter	Emesis	Suction
Time 7–3							
Total							
Time 3–11							
Total							
Time 11–7							
Total							
24-Hour Total							
24-Hour Grand Total • Intake				24-Hour Grand Total • Output			

Figure 23.8 This sample I&O form records total intake and output during a 24-hour recording period.

Rationale

Careful and accurate measurement of intake and output (I&O) is essential to maintaining the body's fluid balance. This is particularly true for residents who may be dehydrated or who have a specific disease or condition.

Preparation

1. Ask the licensed nursing staff how this procedure fits into the plan of care, if there are doctor's orders for the procedure, if there are any special instructions or precautions, and if the resident can be moved into the positions required for this procedure.

2. Wash your hands or use hand sanitizer before entering the room.

3. Knock before entering the room.

4. Introduce yourself using your full name and title. Explain that you work with the licensed nursing staff and will be providing care.

5. Greet the resident and ask the resident to state his or her full name, if able. Then check the resident's identification bracelet.

6. Use Mr., Mrs., or Ms. and the last name when conversing.

7. Explain the procedure in simple terms, even if the resident is not able to communicate or is disoriented. Ask permission to perform the procedure.

8. Bring the necessary equipment into the room. Place the following items in an accessible location:

   - disposable gloves
   - pen and form or digital device for recording the I&O
   - appropriate measuring containers and graduate
   - urinary hat, bedpan, or urinal
   - disposable protective pad
   - antiseptic swab(s)
   - paper towel

The Procedure: Measuring Oral Fluid Intake

9. Provide privacy by closing the curtains, using a screen, or closing the door to the room.

10. Wash your hands or use hand sanitizer to ensure infection control.

> **Best Practice**
> Disposable gloves are worn only if required for infection prevention and control.

11. For each container, note the amount of liquid that the resident was served. Pour the remaining liquid (that was not consumed) into a measuring cup or graduate. Keep the graduate level. Measure the amount left in each container at eye level.

> **Best Practice**
> Fluids are measured and recorded in fluid ounces (oz), milliliters (mL), or cubic centimeters (cc). One mL equals 1 cc. One fluid ounce is equal to 30 mL or 30 cc.

12. Subtract each amount measured from the full amount the resident was served. Note each amount. These are the amounts the resident actually drank.

13. Add all of the amounts together to get the total amount of liquid the resident drank. Immediately record this amount on the intake side of the I&O form.

14. All other intake, such as from IV fluids or liquids given by tube, will also need to be measured. Ask the licensed nursing staff who is responsible for this measurement.

The Procedure: Measuring Urinary Output

15. Provide privacy by closing the curtains, using a screen, or closing the door to the room.

16. Wash your hands or use hand sanitizer to ensure infection control.

17. Put on disposable gloves.

18. If the resident is ambulatory, place a urinary hat in the commode or toilet. Instruct the resident to urinate into the hat, not into the commode or toilet (Figure 23.9). Each resident will have his or her own personal urinary hat.

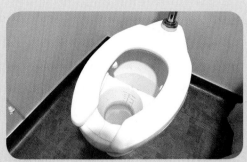
Figure 23.9

19. Ask the resident not to put toilet paper into the commode or toilet. Provide a bag or waste container for the toilet paper. Also instruct the resident *not* to remove the urinary hat. Ask the resident to use a call light to indicate if the urinary hat needs to be emptied.

20. If the resident is in bed, a bedpan, urinal, or urinary catheter with a drainage bag may be used to collect urine.

Best Practice
Sometimes urine can remain in the handle of a urinal. Be sure this amount is poured out for measurement.

21. To empty a urinary drainage bag, place a disposable protective pad on the floor underneath the drainage bag and place a graduate on top of the protective pad. Clean the tubing with an antiseptic swab, open the drain at the bottom of the bag, and empty the urine into a graduate. When emptying the drainage bag, make sure that the urine does not splash and that the drainage tube does not touch the sides of the graduate (Figure 23.10).

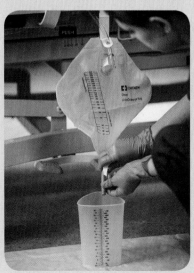
Figure 23.10

22. Close the drain on the urinary drainage bag.

23. Wipe the drain on the urinary drainage bag with an antiseptic swab or according to facility policy. Replace the drain in the holder on the urinary drainage bag. Note the color, odor, clarity, or presence of any particles in the urine.

24. Place a paper towel on a level surface and put the graduate used to measure output on top of the paper towel. If a bedpan or urinal were used, carefully pour the urine into the graduate (Figure 23.11). Always measure the amount of urine at eye level (Figure 23.12). Make note of this amount.

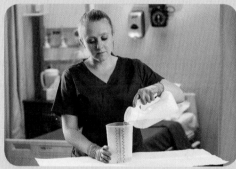
Figure 23.11

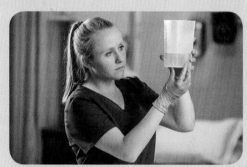
Figure 23.12

25. Always dispose of urine in the toilet. Avoid splashes. Carefully rinse the graduate and pour the rinse water into the toilet as well.

26. All other output, such as the contents of a colostomy drainage bag, will also need to be measured. Ask the licensed nursing staff who is responsible for this measurement.

27. Remove, clean, and store equipment in the proper location. Remove soiled linens and discard disposable equipment.

28. Remove and discard your gloves.

29. Wash your hands to ensure infection control.

30. Record the urine output amount on the paper or electronic I&O form. At the end of your shift, or as ordered, record the total urine output amount on the output side of the I&O form.

(continued)

Measuring and Recording Fluid Intake and Urinary Output (continued)

31. Whether the resident ambulated to the bathroom or remained in bed, check to be sure the bed wheels are locked, then reposition the resident and lower the bed.

32. Follow the plan of care to determine if the side rails should be raised or lowered.

Follow-Up

33. Make sure the resident is comfortable and place the call light and personal items within reach.

34. Conduct a safety check before leaving the room. The room should be clean and free from clutter or spills.

35. Wash your hands or use hand sanitizer before leaving the room.

Reporting and Documentation

36. Communicate any specific observations, complications, or unusual responses to the licensed nursing staff. Record this information, along with the care provided, in the chart or EMR.

Figure 23.9 Karin Hildebrand Lau/Shutterstock.com; Figure 23.10 © Tori Soper Photography; Figure 23.11 © Tori Soper Photography; Figure 23.12 © Tori Soper Photography

Section 23.1 Review and Assessment

Using the Key Terms

Complete the following sentences using key terms in this section.

1. The lack of adequate body fluids is called _____.
2. A(n) _____ is a container used to measure intake and output.
3. Output includes urine that is _____, or expelled from the body.
4. Bowel movements characterized by frequent, watery stools are called _____.
5. _____ is a condition characterized by infrequent, hard, dry stools.

Know and Understand the Facts

6. Identify three reasons why hydration is important.
7. Describe two consequences of dehydration.
8. List three ways nursing assistants can assist the licensed nursing staff with parenteral IV infusions.

Analyze and Apply Concepts

9. What two actions must a nursing assistant take to measure input accurately?
10. Explain the steps needed to empty a urinary drainage bag.
11. A nursing assistant needs to record fluid intake for a resident who drank one full, 8-ounce glass of water. How many cubic centimeters should she record on the I&O form?

Think Critically

Read the following care situation. Then answer the questions that follow.

Ms. A, who is 78 years old, just had hip-replacement surgery and has been transferred to the hospital where you work. She is very restless and is moving around in bed quite a bit. The doctor ordered parenteral IV infusion for the rest of the day and a full liquid diet when Ms. A asks to eat. Ms. A can drink beverages if she wants. She has a urinary catheter with a half-full urinary drainage bag. When you enter the room, it looks like she has had one-half of a glass of water.

12. Describe what you should check to make sure Ms. A's IV catheter and urinary drainage bag are correctly placed.
13. You will need to measure Ms. A's I&O during your shift. List the steps you will take to measure her input.
14. You will be checking Ms. A's output at the end of your shift. Explain what you will need to do to take an accurate measurement.

Objectives

Urinary and bowel elimination are essential body processes and key functions of the urinary and gastrointestinal systems. Some diseases and conditions may cause these systems to malfunction, resulting in elimination difficulties or conditions. These conditions not only affect fluid balance and body functions, but they can also be quite embarrassing for residents. Holistic nursing assistants provide care and support residents by assisting with elimination problems such as incontinence, diarrhea, and constipation. Nursing assistants also provide care for residents with urinary catheters and ostomy bags. To achieve the objectives for this section, you must successfully

- **discuss** the process of urinary and bowel elimination, including potential problems and care considerations;
- **explain** how to record bowel movements;
- **demonstrate** the ability to safely and effectively assist residents with elimination using a toilet, bedside commode, bedpan, or urinal;
- **perform** catheter and colostomy care;
- **show** how to insert a suppository or rectal tube and change a drainage bag; and
- **describe** the process of bladder and bowel retraining.

Key Terms

Learn these key terms to better understand the information presented in the section.

defecate	motility
enema	ostomy
flatus	stoma
hernia	suppositories
impaction	

Questions to Consider
- Have you ever been constipated due to the food you ate or medications you took?
- If you have been constipated, was it uncomfortable? Were you hesitant to talk about your elimination problems because you felt self-conscious or embarrassed?
- Were you able to ease your level of discomfort? What did you do?

How Can Nursing Assistants Help with Urinary Elimination?

On average, a person urinates 800–2000 cc every 24 hours, which requires six to eight trips to the bathroom. When a resident has limited mobility, holistic nursing assistants may need to frequently assist him or her with elimination needs.

Urine is a waste product produced by the kidneys that passes through the bladder to the urethra, where it is expelled from the body. Urine is composed primarily of water (91–96 percent), organic compounds, and some solid materials (about 59 grams, or a little over 2 ounces per person). Changes in the normal composition of urine are usually due to medications, urinary disorders, infection, or diet. For example, protein and glucose are not found in healthy urine. The presence of these substances indicates a potential health issue such as diabetes.

Some residents have mobility challenges that make it difficult to use the bathroom and may need to get up during the night to void (called *nocturia*). These residents may need assistance getting to the toilet or may use a bedside commode. Residents who are unable to ambulate may use bedpans for urinary and bowel elimination needs. There are two types of bedpans: a standard bedpan and a fracture bedpan.

Think About This

Sometimes urine can have an unusual color or odor. Often, color change indicates dehydration, but sometimes dehydration is not the cause. Certain foods can also affect the color of urine. For example, beets can give urine a reddish tint; rhubarb can make it dark brown or even black; blackberries can turn it pink; and carrots, carrot juice, and vitamin C can color it orange. The smell of urine can also change as a result of diet. Asparagus, for example, contains *asparagine*, an amino acid that changes the chemical composition of urine and creates a distinct odor.

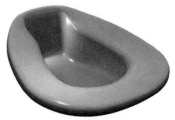

Dani Simmonds/Shutterstock.com

Figure 23.13 A standard bedpan is placed under the resident for the collection of urine and stool.

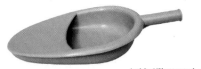

ArtMari/Shutterstock.com

Figure 23.14 A fracture bedpan is better for residents who have limited mobility.

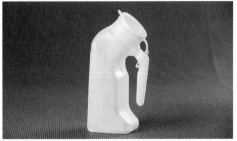

© Tori Soper Photography

Figure 23.15 A urinal includes an opening, neck portion, and bottle portion.

Both types are usually plastic. Metal bedpans must be warmed (with warm water) and dried before use. A *standard bedpan* fits the contour of the buttocks and has a shallow bowl that collects urine and stool (Figure 23.13). A *fracture bedpan* is used when a resident has limited mobility, casts, traction, missing limbs, or spinal cord injuries or surgeries. It is flatter and has a lower collection pan to make placement under the buttocks easier and more comfortable (Figure 23.14). For women, bedpans should always be placed under the anus and urethra to prevent spillage onto the bed. Men will typically use a bedpan for bowel elimination and a urinal for urinary elimination. If a bedpan is used, it should be placed under the anus, and the penis should be placed so that urine streams directly into the bedpan. Bedpans can be uncomfortable, so correctly positioning residents to reduce discomfort is important.

Men who have limited mobility may use a handheld urinal for urinary elimination while in bed. Urinals are usually plastic and have a narrow opening and long neck that leads to a bottle-shaped container for collecting the urine (Figure 23.15). The penis is placed in the neck of the urinal and positioned so the urine stream goes directly into the bottle portion. A urinal may be used when a resident is lying down, sitting up, or standing.

As a nursing assistant, your primary responsibility is to provide support and ensure a safe process and environment for the resident. You should always be aware of any potential problems during urinary elimination and any abnormal conditions, such as a change in urine color, urgency, burning, painful or difficult urination (*dysuria*), and abnormal amount of urine (as in *oliguria*, a small amount of urine, and *polyuria*, an excessive amount of urine). Good infection control and prevention procedures should always be followed, as urine and stool may contain pathogens.

Procedure   Assisting to a Toilet or Bedside Commode

Rationale

Residents who are ambulatory may need assistance to the toilet. A bedside commode is used for residents who have limited mobility.

Preparation

1. Ask the licensed nursing staff how this procedure fits into the plan of care, if there are doctor's orders for the procedure, if there are any special instructions or precautions, and if the resident can be moved into the positions required for this procedure.

2. Wash your hands or use hand sanitizer before entering the room.

3. Knock before entering the room.

4. Introduce yourself using your full name and title. Explain that you work with the licensed nursing staff and will be providing care.

5. Greet the resident and ask the resident to state his full name, if able. Then check the resident's identification bracelet.

6. Use Mr., Mrs., or Ms. and the last name when conversing.

7. Explain the procedure in simple terms, even if the resident is not able to communicate or is disoriented. Ask permission to perform the procedure.

8. Bring the necessary equipment into the room. Place the following items in an accessible location:

   - bedside commode with the container in place, if needed
   - toilet seat extension, if needed
   - disposable gloves
   - bath blanket
   - resident's robe and slippers

- gait belt, if appropriate
- washbasin
- soap
- towels
- disinfectant spray or wipes
- toilet paper, if needed
- pen and form or digital device for recording the I&O

The Procedure: Assisting to the Toilet

9. Provide privacy by closing the curtains, using a screen, or closing the door to the room.

> **Best Practice**
> Make sure the bathroom contains toilet paper and a clean hand towel or paper towels.

10. Lock the bed wheels. Raise the head of the bed and lower the bed, if needed.

11. Ensure safety during the procedure. If there are side rails, raise and secure the rails on the opposite side of the bed from where you will be working. Lower the rail on the side you are working.

12. Wash your hands or use hand sanitizer to ensure infection control.

13. Put on disposable gloves.

14. Help the resident dangle at the edge of the bed and put on his robe and slippers, if needed or desired.

15. Help the resident stand and walk to the bathroom. Be safe. If appropriate, put on a gait belt for ambulation.

16. Remove and adjust the resident's clothing so he can sit comfortably on the toilet. Use a toilet seat extension, if needed (Figure 23.16).

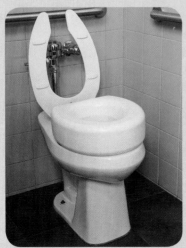

Figure 13.16

17. If the resident is on I&O, place a urinary hat in the toilet and ask the resident not to put toilet paper in the toilet. Provide a bag or waste container for the toilet paper. Ask the resident not to flush the toilet.

18. If the resident can be safely left alone, place the toilet paper and call light within his reach. Instruct him to use the call light when he is finished. Remove and discard your gloves. Wash your hands or use hand sanitizer before leaving the room.

19. If the resident cannot be left alone, stay in the bathroom to ensure safety.

20. If you left the room, return to the room when the resident uses the call light or within five minutes to check on the resident. Wash your hands or use hand sanitizer to ensure infection control. Put on disposable gloves.

21. Assist with wiping and with perineal care, as needed.

> **Best Practice**
> Remember to wipe from front to back and use a new piece of toilet paper for each wipe.

22. Remove and discard your gloves.

23. Wash your hands or use hand sanitizer to ensure infection control.

24. Put on a new pair of disposable gloves.

25. Help the resident put on new briefs or undergarments, if worn. Change the resident's gown, if needed. Change gloves, if needed.

26. Help the resident wash his hands.

27. Help the resident back to bed and remove his robe and slippers, if worn.

28. Check to be sure the bed wheels are locked, then reposition the resident and lower the bed.

29. Follow the plan of care to determine if the side rails should be raised or lowered.

30. Return to the bathroom. Observe the urine for color, odor, and clarity. Check the stool for unusual appearance or odor.

31. If I&O is being monitored, measure the urinary output or the amount of liquid stool. Record the amount of output on the paper or electronic I&O form.

32. If there was a bowel movement, record it in the form provided by the healthcare facility or in the electronic record.

(continued)

33. If a urinary hat was used, empty its contents into the toilet. Avoid splashes. Carefully rinse the urinary hat and pour the rinse water into the toilet as well. Then flush the toilet.

34. Using disinfectant spray or wipes, clean and then dry the urinary hat according to facility policy. Store the clean urinary hat in the proper location.

The Procedure: Assisting with a Bedside Commode

35. Provide privacy by closing the curtains, using a screen, or closing the door to the room.

36. Place the commode next to the bed (Figure 23.17). If the commode has wheels, lock them.

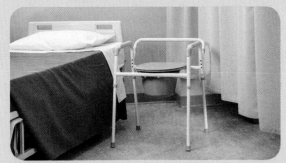

Figure 23.17

37. Lock the bed wheels. Raise the head of the bed and lower the bed, if needed.

38. Ensure safety during the procedure. If there are side rails, raise and secure the rails on the opposite side of the bed from where you will be working. Lower the rail on the side you are working.

39. Wash your hands or use hand sanitizer to ensure infection control.

40. Put on disposable gloves.

41. Remove the resident's undergarments or briefs. Help the resident dangle at the edge of the bed and put on his slippers.

42. Using proper body mechanics, assist the resident onto the bedside commode. Use a gait belt, if needed. Be sure the resident's gown or any clothing is out of the way.

> **Best Practice**
> To ensure warmth and privacy, cover the resident's lap and shoulders with bath blankets.

43. If the resident is on I&O, ask him *not* to put toilet paper in the commode. Provide a bag or waste container for the toilet paper.

44. If the resident can be safely left alone, place the toilet paper and call light within his reach. Instruct him to use the call light when he is finished. Follow the plan of care to determine if the side rails should be raised or lowered. Remove and discard your gloves. Wash your hands or use hand sanitizer before leaving the room.

45. If the resident cannot be left alone, stay in the room to ensure safety.

46. If you left the room, return to the room when the resident uses the call light or within five minutes to check on the resident. Wash your hands or use hand sanitizer to ensure infection control. Put on disposable gloves.

47. Assist with wiping and with perineal care, as needed. Cover the commode.

> **Best Practice**
> Remember to wipe from front to back and use a new piece of toilet paper for each wipe.

48. Remove and discard your gloves.

49. Wash your hands or use hand sanitizer to ensure infection control.

50. Put on a new pair of disposable gloves.

> **Best Practice**
> Use an odor neutralizer according to facility policy.

51. Help the resident back to bed. Remove the resident's slippers and help him put on new briefs or undergarments, if worn. Change the resident's gown, if needed. Ensure the resident is safely positioned in bed.

52. Fill the washbasin with enough warm water to cover the wrists. Check the water temperature. It should be 100–105°F. The water should feel comfortably warm to your elbow. You may also ask the resident to feel the water temperature, but always check yourself first.

53. Place the washbasin and some towels on the bedside stand.

54. Help the resident wash his hands.

55. Remove the washbasin and used towels. Straighten or change the bed linens, as needed.

56. Check to be sure the bed wheels are locked, then reposition the resident and lower the bed.

57. Follow the plan of care to determine if the side rails should be raised or lowered.

58. Remove the container from the bedside commode. Take the container to the bathroom. Observe the resident's urine for color, odor, and clarity. Check the stool for unusual appearance or odor.

59. If I&O is being monitored, measure the urinary output or the amount of liquid stool. Record the amount of output on the paper or electronic I&O form.

60. If there was a bowel movement, record it in the form provided by the healthcare facility or in the electronic record.

61. Empty the contents of the container into the toilet. Avoid splashes. Carefully rinse the container and pour the rinse water into the toilet as well.

62. Using disinfectant spray or wipes, clean and then dry the container and the bedside commode according to facility policy.

63. Put the clean bedside commode back in the appropriate storage location.

Follow-Up

64. Remove and discard your gloves.

65. Wash your hands to ensure infection control.

66. Make sure the resident is comfortable and place the call light and personal items within reach.

67. Conduct a safety check before leaving the room. The room should be clean and free from clutter or spills.

68. Wash your hands or use hand sanitizer before leaving the room.

Reporting and Documentation

69. Communicate any specific observations, complications, or unusual responses to the licensed nursing staff. Record this information, along with the care provided, in the chart or EMR.

Images courtesy of © Tori Soper Photography

Procedure | Assisting with a Standard or Fracture Bedpan

Rationale

Proper bedpan use provides a safe means of urinary and bowel elimination for residents who are not able to ambulate to the bathroom.

Preparation

1. Ask the licensed nursing staff how this procedure fits into the plan of care, if there are doctor's orders for the procedure, if there are any special instructions or precautions, and if the resident can be moved into the positions required for this procedure.

2. Wash your hands or use hand sanitizer before entering the room.

3. Knock before entering the room.

4. Introduce yourself using your full name and title. Explain that you work with the licensed nursing staff and will be providing care.

5. Greet the resident and ask the resident to state her full name, if able. Then check the resident's identification bracelet.

6. Use Mr., Mrs., or Ms. and the last name when conversing.

7. Explain the procedure in simple terms, even if the resident is not able to communicate or is disoriented. Ask permission to perform the procedure.

8. Bring the necessary equipment into the room. Place the following items in an accessible location:
   - standard or fracture bedpan
   - toilet paper
   - bedpan cover, disposable pad, or towel
   - disposable protective pad
   - disposable gloves
   - washbasin
   - soap
   - washcloth(s)
   - towel(s)
   - bath blanket
   - waste container or plastic bag
   - laundry hamper
   - disinfectant spray or wipes
   - pen and form or digital device for recording the I&O

(continued)

Assisting with a Standard or Fracture Bedpan (continued)

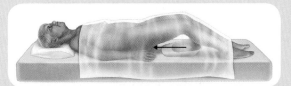

Figure 23.19

The Procedure

9. Provide privacy by closing the curtains, using a screen, or closing the door to the room.

10. Lock the bed wheels and then raise the bed to hip level.

11. Ensure safety during the procedure. If there are side rails, raise and secure the rails on the opposite side of the bed from where you will be working. Lower the rail on the side you are working.

12. Wash your hands or use hand sanitizer to ensure infection control.

13. Put on disposable gloves.

14. Fold the top linens back and raise the resident's gown. Keep it out of the way of the bedpan.

15. Ask the resident to bend her knees and put her feet flat on the mattress.

16. Ask the resident to raise her hips. If necessary, slip your hand under the lower part of the resident's back to help.

17. Put a disposable protective pad on the bed under the resident's hips. Then position the bedpan under the buttocks.

   A. **Standard bedpan**: position a standard bedpan like a regular toilet seat. The buttocks should be placed on the wide, rounded shelf, and the open end should point toward the foot of the bed (Figure 23.18).

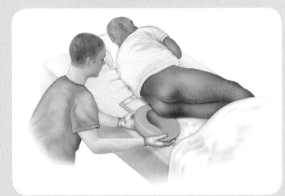

Figure 23.18

   B. **Fracture bedpan**: position a fracture bedpan by having the resident lift her hips. The thin edge of the bedpan should face the head of the bed. Place the bedpan under the resident's buttocks (Figure 23.19).

18. If the resident is unable to lift her hips, roll her onto her side so she faces away from you. Place the bedpan against the resident's buttocks. Then have the resident roll to her back with the bedpan underneath her.

> **Best Practice**
> For comfort and safety, properly position the bedpan under the resident.

19. Put a bath blanket over the resident. Raise the head of the bed or prop pillows behind the resident's back for comfort.

20. If I&O is being measured, ask the resident not to put toilet paper in the bedpan. Provide a bag or waste container for the toilet paper.

21. If the resident can be safely left alone, place the toilet paper and call light within her reach. Instruct her to use the call light when she is finished. Follow the plan of care to determine if the side rails should be raised or lowered. Remove and discard your gloves. Wash your hands or use hand sanitizer before leaving the room.

22. If the resident cannot be left alone, stay in the room to ensure safety.

23. If you left the room, return to the room when the resident uses the call light or within five minutes to check on the resident. Wash your hands or use hand sanitizer to ensure infection control. Put on disposable gloves.

> **Best Practice**
> To maintain skin integrity, do not allow a resident to sit on the bedpan for more than five minutes without checking on him or her.

24. Assist with wiping and with perineal care, as needed.

Images courtesy of © Body Scientific International

25. Remove and discard your gloves.
26. Wash your hands or use hand sanitizer to ensure infection control.
27. Put on a new pair of disposable gloves.
28. Help the resident raise her hips or roll to the side so you can remove the bedpan. Also remove and discard the protective pad at this time. Practice safety and ask for assistance, if necessary.
29. Cover the bedpan immediately with a bedpan cover, disposable pad, or towel. Place the bedpan on top of a paper towel in a secure place.
30. Remove and discard your gloves.
31. Wash your hands or use hand sanitizer to ensure infection control.
32. Put on a new pair of disposable gloves.

33. Fill the washbasin with enough warm water to cover the wrists. Check the water temperature. It should be 100–105°F. The water should feel comfortably warm to your elbow. You may also ask the resident to feel the water temperature, but always check yourself first.
34. Help the resident wash her hands.
35. Remove the washbasin and used towels. Place the used towels in the laundry hamper.
36. Help the resident put on clean briefs or other undergarments, if worn. Change the resident's gown, if needed.
37. Cover the resident with the top linens and remove the bath blanket, placing it in the laundry hamper. Straighten or change the bed linens, as needed.

38. Check to be sure the bed wheels are locked, then reposition the resident and lower the bed.
39. Follow the plan of care to determine if the side rails should be raised or lowered.
40. Take the bedpan to the bathroom. Check the stool and urine for unusual appearance or odor.
41. Empty the contents of the bedpan into the toilet. Avoid splashes. Carefully rinse the bedpan and pour the rinse water into the toilet as well.
42. Using disinfectant spray or wipes, clean and then dry the bedpan and cover according to facility policy. Store the clean bedpan and cover in the appropriate storage location.
43. Remove and discard your gloves.
44. Wash your hands to ensure infection control.
45. If I&O is being monitored, measure the urinary output or the amount of liquid stool. Record the amount of output on the paper or electronic I&O form.
46. If there was a bowel movement, record it in the form provided by the healthcare facility or in the electronic record.

Follow-Up

47. Make sure the resident is comfortable and place the call light and personal items within reach.
48. Conduct a safety check before leaving the room. The room should be clean and free from clutter or spills.
49. Wash your hands or use hand sanitizer before leaving the room.

Reporting and Documentation

50. Communicate any specific observations, complications, or unusual responses to the licensed nursing staff. Record this information, along with the care provided, in the chart or EMR.

Procedure Assisting with a Urinal

Rationale

Proper urinal use provides a safe means of urinary elimination for residents who are not able to ambulate to the bathroom.

Preparation

1. Ask the licensed nursing staff how this procedure fits into the plan of care, if there are doctor's orders for the procedure, if there are any special instructions or precautions, and if the resident can be moved into the positions required for this procedure.

2. Wash your hands or use hand sanitizer before entering the room.

3. Knock before entering the room.

4. Introduce yourself using your full name and title. Explain that you work with the licensed nursing staff and will be providing care.

5. Greet the resident and ask the resident to state his full name, if able. Then check the resident's identification bracelet.

6. Use Mr., Mrs., or Ms. and the last name when conversing.

7. Explain the procedure in simple terms, even if the resident is not able to communicate or is disoriented. Ask permission to perform the procedure.

8. Bring the necessary equipment into the room. Place the following items in an accessible location:

   - handheld urinal and cover
   - disposable gloves
   - disposable protective pad, if needed
   - washbasin
   - soap
   - towel
   - disinfectant spray or wipes
   - pen and form or digital device for recording the I&O

The Procedure

9. Provide privacy by closing the curtains, using a screen, or closing the door to the room.

10. Ensure safety during the procedure. If there are side rails, raise and secure the rails on the opposite side of the bed from where you will be working. Lower the rail on the side you are working.

11. Wash your hands or use hand sanitizer to ensure infection control.

12. Put on disposable gloves.

13. Give the urinal to the resident. If assistance is needed, position the urinal so that the resident's penis is well inside the opening. Make sure the urinal does not spill. You may need to put a disposable protective pad under the resident.

14. If the resident can be safely left alone, place the call light within his reach. Instruct him to use the call light when he is finished. Ask the resident not to place the urinal on the overbed table or bedside stand when he is finished. This would contaminate those surfaces. Follow the plan of care to determine if the side rails should be raised or lowered. Remove and discard your gloves. Wash your hands or use hand sanitizer before leaving the room.

15. If the resident cannot be left alone, stay in the room to ensure safety.

> **Best Practice**
> If the resident is in bed, do not leave the urinal in place longer than is needed. The hard plastic of the urinal could damage the soft flesh of the penis.

16. If you left the room, return to the room when the resident uses the call light. Wash your hands or use hand sanitizer to ensure infection control. Put on disposable gloves.

17. Assist with any needed cleansing and with perineal care, as needed.

18. Remove the urinal and cover it. Place the urinal on top of a paper towel in a secure place.

19. Remove and discard your gloves.

20. Wash your hands or use hand sanitizer to ensure infection control.

21. Put on a new pair of disposable gloves.

22. Fill the washbasin with enough warm water to cover the wrists. Check the water temperature. It should be 100–105°F. The water should feel comfortably warm to your elbow. You may also ask the resident to feel the water temperature, but always check yourself first.

23. Help the resident wash his hands.

24. Remove the washbasin and used towels.

25. Help the resident put on clean briefs or other undergarments, if worn. Change the resident's gown, if needed.

26. Straighten or change the bed linens, as needed.

27. Check to be sure the bed wheels are locked, then reposition the resident and lower the bed.

28. Follow the plan of care to determine if the side rails should be raised or lowered.

29. Take the urinal to the bathroom. Observe the urine for color, odor, and clarity.

30. If the resident is on I&O, measure the urinary output or the amount of liquid stool, if applicable. Record the amount of output on the paper or electronic I&O form.

31. Empty the contents of the urinal into the toilet. Avoid splashes. Carefully rinse the urinal and pour the rinse water into the toilet as well.

32. Using disinfectant spray or wipes, clean and then dry the urinal according to facility policy. Store the clean urinal and cover in the appropriate storage location.

Follow-Up

33. Remove and discard your gloves.

34. Wash your hands to ensure infection control.

35. Make sure the resident is comfortable and place the call light and personal items within reach.

36. Conduct a safety check before leaving the room. The room should be clean and free from clutter or spills.

37. Wash your hands or use hand sanitizer before leaving the room.

Reporting and Documentation

38. Communicate any specific observations, complications, or unusual responses to the licensed nursing staff. Record this information, along with the care provided, in the chart or EMR.

How Do Nursing Assistants Assist with Urinary Catheters?

Some patients and residents experience problems with urinary elimination (for example, an inability to eliminate urine, which can cause bladder distention). Urinary elimination problems may be caused by surgery, childbirth, blockage, or certain diseases and conditions. When problems occur, a *urinary catheter* is usually used to eliminate urine from the body. An *indwelling urinary catheter* (catheter left inside the bladder) is inserted into the urethra and passes into the urinary bladder. It is held in place by a balloon inflated after insertion. Some residents may require a *suprapubic catheter*, which is surgically inserted into the bladder through the abdominal wall just above the pubic area. This type of catheter is used when a resident has a urethral obstruction or injury or prostate cancer.

Gravity allows urine in the urinary bladder to flow into the catheter tubing and empty into a drainage bag outside the body. The urinary drainage bag should always be positioned below the bladder. This is important even when the resident is ambulating. When a resident is in bed, the urinary drainage bag can be attached to the lower bedframe of a resident's bed or to the side of a wheelchair or chair. The urinary drainage bag should not be attached to a movable part of the bed, should be clear of any wheels, and should never touch or rest on the floor.

Catheter Care

Nursing assistants are responsible for providing proper catheter care every eight hours, or as often as required by facility policy. Proper catheter care can help prevent *catheter-associated urinary tract infections (CAUTIs)*. Catheter care involves regularly cleansing the perineum and the area around the catheter, checking the catheter and drainage bag for leaks or kinks that can obstruct the flow of urine, making sure the resident is not lying on the catheter, and observing any other problems related to the catheter.

Holistic nursing assistants should be aware of how catheter use affects residents physically and emotionally. Residents may worry about their body image, since an artificial device has been inserted to help them eliminate. They may also be embarrassed

Think About This

Between 15 and 25 percent of hospitalized patients need urinary catheters during their hospital stays. According to the CDC, approximately 75 percent of UTIs reported in hospitals are associated with urinary catheter use. In long-term care facilities, 1 to 3 million serious infections occur annually. A UTI is one of the most common infections a resident will acquire.

by having their urine visible and captured in a bag. Many residents may also be experiencing pain. Consider these factors when providing care and offer residents your support and understanding. If residents are in pain, alert the licensed nursing staff.

Nursing assistants in many facilities use commercially prepared catheter care kits. A catheter care kit includes disposable gloves, a disposable protective pad, and applicators with antiseptic solution. In facilities that do not provide catheter care kits, nursing assistants use clean washcloths and mild soap in place of applicators and antiseptic. The same procedure is used whether or not a kit is available.

Procedure   Providing Catheter Care

Rationale

Proper catheter care ensures consistent hygiene, maintains skin integrity, and helps prevent CAUTIs.

Preparation

1. Ask the licensed nursing staff how this procedure fits into the plan of care, if there are doctor's orders for the procedure, if there are any special instructions or precautions, and if the resident can be moved into the positions required for this procedure.
2. Wash your hands or use hand sanitizer before entering the room.
3. Knock before entering the room.
4. Introduce yourself using your full name and title. Explain that you work with the licensed nursing staff and will be providing care.
5. Greet the resident and ask the resident to state his or her full name, if able. Then check the resident's identification bracelet.
6. Use Mr., Mrs., or Ms. and the last name when conversing.
7. Explain the procedure in simple terms, even if the resident is not able to communicate or is disoriented. Ask permission to perform the procedure.
8. Bring the necessary equipment into the room. Place the following items in an accessible location:
   - catheter care kit, if available
   - disposable gloves
   - bath blanket
   - washcloths
   - soap
   - towels
   - washbasin, if used
   - disposable protective pad
   - plastic bag
   - laundry hamper

> **Best Practice**
> Always be sensitive to the resident's privacy, culture, and sensitivities when performing catheter care.

The Procedure: Male Catheter Care

9. Provide privacy by closing the curtains, using a screen, or closing the door to the room.
10. Lock the bed wheels and then raise the bed to hip level.
11. Ensure safety during the procedure. If there are side rails, raise and secure the rails on the opposite side of the bed from where you will be working. Lower the rail on the side you are working.
12. Wash your hands or use hand sanitizer to ensure infection control.
13. Put on disposable gloves.
14. Position the resident on his back, if possible.
15. Cover the resident with the bath blanket. Without exposing the resident, fanfold the top linens to the foot of the bed.

> **Best Practice**
> Catheter care is performed after providing perineal care. Remove and discard your gloves once perineal care is complete. Wash your hands to ensure infection control and put on a new pair of gloves before beginning catheter care.

16. Check the catheter insertion area for crusting, lesions, discharge, or anything abnormal. Notify the licensed nursing staff if you observe any of these conditions.

17. Open the catheter kit. Remove the disposable protective pad from the kit. If there is no kit, use the protective pad you brought into the room. Place the protective pad under the resident's buttocks.

18. Remove the applicators from the kit. The applicators are covered with an antiseptic solution. If there is no kit, fill the washbasin with warm water (between 100–105°F). The water should feel comfortably warm to your elbow. You may also ask the resident to feel the water temperature, but always check yourself first. Instead of an applicator, you will use a washcloth and soap.

19. Using a circular motion, apply the antiseptic solution to the entire catheter insertion area. If there is no kit, use a clean part of the washcloth for each cleansing stroke.

20. If the male resident has not been circumcised, gently pull the foreskin of the penis back. Apply antiseptic solution to the area where the catheter is inserted into the penis or clean it using the washcloth and soap.

Best Practice
Work from the cleanest area of the penis to the dirtiest.

21. Hold the catheter tubing near the opening of the penis. This will help prevent pulling or tugging as you clean the catheter.

22. Using a circular motion, clean the catheter. Start near the penis and move down the catheter about 4 inches (Figure 23.20). If using a washcloth, use a clean part of the washcloth.

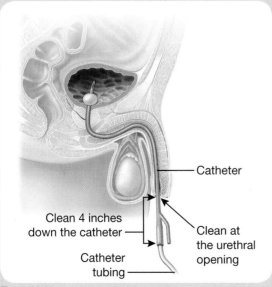

Clean 4 inches down the catheter — Catheter

Clean at the urethral opening

Catheter — Catheter tubing

Figure 23.20

23. Moving from front to back, pat the perineal area dry.

24. Secure the catheter and tubing to the resident's upper thigh using a product approved by the facility or as directed by the licensed nursing staff. Leave some slack in the catheter tubing. Coil the remaining tubing and be sure it is not under the resident, twisted, or bent.

25. Secure the drainage bag to the bottom of the bedframe using the bag ties (Figure 23.21). The drainage bag should always be secured below the resident and should never be secured to a movable part of the bed or near the wheels.

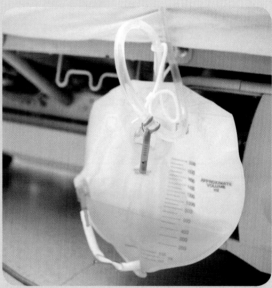

Figure 23.21

26. Remove the disposable protective pad. Cover the resident with the top linens. Remove the bath blanket.

27. Change the resident's gown or other clothing, as appropriate.

28. Check to be sure the bed wheels are locked, then reposition the resident and lower the bed.

Best Practice
If any part of the catheter comes apart, clean the catheter and tubing ends with an antiseptic pad and reconnect them. Alert the licensed nursing staff.

29. Follow the plan of care to determine if the side rails should be raised or lowered.

(continued)

Figure 23.20 © Body Scientific International; Figure 23.21 iStock.com/P_Wei

Providing Catheter Care *(continued)*

30. Remove, clean, and store equipment in the proper location. Remove soiled linens and discard disposable equipment.

The Procedure: Female Catheter Care

31. Provide privacy by closing the curtains, using a screen, or closing the door to the room.

32. Lock the bed wheels and then raise the bed to hip level.

33. Ensure safety during the procedure. If there are side rails, raise and secure the rails on the opposite side of the bed from where you will be working. Lower the rail on the side you are working.

34. Wash your hands or use hand sanitizer to ensure infection control.

35. Put on disposable gloves.

36. Position the resident on her back, if possible.

37. Cover the resident with the bath blanket. Without exposing the resident, fanfold the top linens to the foot of the bed.

Best Practice
Catheter care is often performed after providing perineal care. Remove and discard your gloves once perineal care is complete. Wash your hands to ensure infection control and put on a new pair of gloves before beginning catheter care.

38. Check the catheter insertion area for crusting, lesions, discharge, or anything abnormal. Notify the licensed nursing staff if you observe any of these conditions.

39. Open the catheter kit. Remove the disposable protective pad from the kit. If there is no kit, use the protective pad you brought into the room. Place the protective pad under the resident's buttocks.

40. Remove the applicators from the kit. The applicators are covered with an antiseptic solution. If there is no kit, fill the washbasin with warm water (between 100–105°F). The water should feel comfortably warm to your elbow. You may also ask the resident to feel the water temperature, but always check yourself first. Instead of an applicator, you will use a washcloth and soap.

41. Separate the labia with one gloved hand.

42. Use your other hand to pick up an applicator or washcloth. Cleanse the perineal area from front to back to prevent fecal matter or bacteria from moving upward into the vaginal canal or urethra. Use a new applicator or a clean part of the washcloth for each cleansing stroke.

43. Begin at the center of the perineal area and then cleanse each side. After each stroke, discard the used applicator in a plastic bag. If using a washcloth, use a clean part of the washcloth for each stroke.

44. Hold the catheter tubing near the opening of the urethra. This will help prevent pulling or tugging as you clean the catheter.

45. Clean the catheter in a circular motion from the meatus down the catheter about 4 inches (Figure 23.22). Do this two or three times. If using a washcloth, use different parts of the washcloth each time.

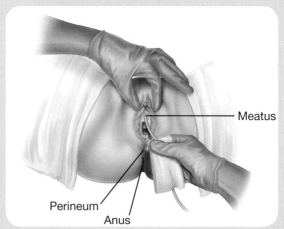

Figure 23.22

46. Moving from front to back, pat the perineal area dry.

47. Secure the catheter and tubing to the resident's upper thigh using a product approved by the facility or as directed by the licensed nursing staff. Leave some slack in the catheter tubing. Coil the remaining tubing and be sure it is not under the resident, twisted, or bent.

48. Secure the drainage bag to the bottom of the bedframe using the bag ties. The drainage bag should always be secured below the resident and should never be secured to a movable part of the bed.

49. Remove the disposable protective pad. Cover the resident with the top linens. Remove the bath blanket.

Image courtesy of © Body Scientific International

50. Change the resident's gown or other clothing, as appropriate.

51. Check to be sure the bed wheels are locked, then reposition the resident and lower the bed.

> **Best Practice**
> If any part of the catheter comes open or apart, clean the catheter and tubing ends with an antiseptic pad and reconnect them. Alert the licensed nursing staff.

52. Follow the plan of care to determine if the side rails should be raised or lowered.

53. Remove, clean, and store equipment in the proper location. Remove soiled linens and discard disposable equipment.

Follow-Up

54. Remove and discard your gloves.

55. Wash your hands to ensure infection control.

56. Make sure the resident is comfortable and place the call light and personal items within reach.

57. Conduct a safety check before leaving the room. The room should be clean and free from clutter or spills.

58. Wash your hands or use hand sanitizer before leaving the room.

Reporting and Documentation

59. Communicate any specific observations, complications, or unusual responses to the licensed nursing staff. Record this information, along with the care provided, in the chart or EMR.

Procedure — Changing a Urinary Drainage Bag

Rationale

Periodically changing a resident's urinary drainage bag promotes cleanliness, prevents possible blockage, and helps ensure infection control.

Preparation

1. Ask the licensed nursing staff how this procedure fits into the plan of care, if there are doctor's orders for the procedure, if there are any special instructions or precautions, and if the resident can be moved into the positions required for this procedure.

2. Wash your hands or use hand sanitizer before entering the room.

3. Knock before entering the room.

4. Introduce yourself using your full name and title. Explain that you work with the licensed nursing staff and will be providing care.

5. Greet the resident and ask the resident to state his full name, if able. Then check the resident's identification bracelet.

6. Use Mr., Mrs., or Ms. and the last name when conversing.

7. Explain the procedure in simple terms, even if the resident is not able to communicate or is disoriented. Ask permission to perform the procedure.

8. Bring the necessary equipment into the room. Place a paper towel, towel, or disposable protective pad on the overbed table as an infection-control barrier before placing the following items:
   - new drainage bag and tubing
   - sterile package containing cap and plug
   - catheter clamp
   - disposable gloves
   - antiseptic wipes
   - 2 disposable protective pads
   - paper towels
   - graduate
   - bedpan
   - bath blanket
   - pen and form or digital device for recording the I&O

The Procedure

9. Provide privacy by closing the curtains, using a screen, or closing the door to the room.

10. Lock the bed wheels and then raise the bed to hip level.

(continued)

11. Ensure safety during the procedure. If there are side rails, raise and secure the rails on the opposite side of the bed from where you will be working. Lower the rail on the side you are working.

12. Wash your hands or use hand sanitizer to ensure infection control.

13. Put on disposable gloves.

14. Position the resident on his back, if possible. Place the disposable protective pad under the resident's buttocks.

15. Cover the resident with the bath blanket. Without exposing the resident, fanfold the top linens to the foot of the bed.

16. Fold the bath blanket to form a triangle on the side of the drainage bag. Turn the triangle up over the resident, exposing the catheter and drainage bag tubing.

17. Clamp the catheter to prevent urine from draining into the drainage tubing.

18. Let the urine below the clamp drain into the drainage bag.

19. Place a protective pad under the resident's leg at the site where the catheter and drainage bag tubing connect.

20. Open the antiseptic wipes and place them on the paper towels on the overbed table.

21. Open the package with the sterile cap and catheter plug. Do not let anything touch the sterile cap or catheter plug.

22. Attach the new drainage bag to the bedframe. Lay the end of the new drainage bag tubing on top of the protective pad on the bed.

23. Disconnect the catheter from the old drainage bag tubing. Do not allow anything to touch the end of the catheter.

24. Hold the sterile catheter plug, but do *not* touch the end that goes inside the catheter.

25. Insert the sterile catheter plug into the end of the catheter. If the end of the catheter touches anything, wipe it with an antiseptic wipe before inserting the plug.

26. Place the sterile cap on the end of the old drainage bag tubing. Do *not* touch the end of the tubing.

27. Remove the cap from the end of the new drainage bag tubing (Figure 23.23A).

28. Remove the sterile plug from the catheter.

29. Insert the end of the new drainage bag tubing into the catheter.

30. Remove the clamp from the catheter (Figure 23.23B).

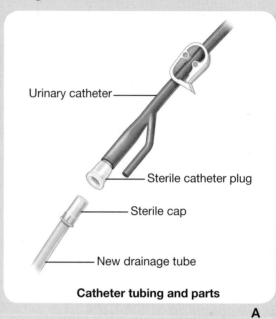

Urinary catheter

Sterile catheter plug

Sterile cap

New drainage tube

Catheter tubing and parts

A

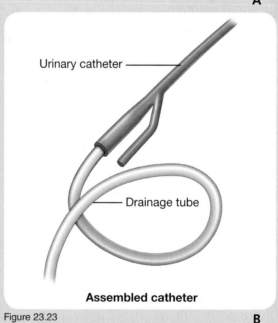

Urinary catheter

Drainage tube

Assembled catheter

Figure 23.23

B

31. Coil and secure the remaining tubing. Be sure it is not twisted or bent.

32. Remove the old drainage bag from the bedframe and place it in the bedpan.

33. Remove and discard the protective pad.

34. Cover the resident with the top linens and remove the bath blanket.

35. Check to be sure the bed wheels are locked, then reposition the resident and lower the bed.

Images courtesy of © Body Scientific International

36. Follow the plan of care to determine if the side rails should be raised or lowered.
37. Take the old drainage bag and tubing to the bathroom.
38. Open the clamp at the bottom of the old drainage bag and allow the urine to drain into the graduate. After the bag is empty, close the clamp.
39. Measure the amount of urine in the graduate. Make note of this amount or record it on the I&O form.
40. Discard the old drainage bag and tubing according to facility policy.
41. Remove, clean, and store equipment in the proper location. Remove soiled linens and discard disposable equipment.

Follow-Up

42. Remove and discard your gloves.
43. Wash your hands to ensure infection control.
44. Make sure the resident is comfortable and place the call light and personal items within reach.
45. Conduct a safety check before leaving the room. The room should be clean and free from clutter or spills.
46. Wash your hands or use hand sanitizer before leaving the room.

Reporting and Documentation

47. Communicate any specific observations, complications, or unusual responses to the licensed nursing staff. Record this information, along with the care provided, in the chart or EMR.

Leg Bags

A *leg bag* may be used as an alternative to the urinary drainage bag when the resident is ambulatory (Figure 23.24). A leg bag is smaller than a drainage bag. It is attached with Velcro™ or elastic straps to the upper thigh, but is low enough on the thigh that gravity will help urine flow into the leg bag. Routinely alternating the thigh that holds the leg bag will help maintain skin integrity. Leg bags come in different sizes and can be hidden by clothing.

Attaching a Leg Bag

The procedure for attaching a leg bag is the same as the procedure for changing a urinary drainage bag. Once you have connected the new leg bag to the catheter, fasten the straps of the leg bag comfortably around the resident's thigh. Make sure the straps are not too tight. Secure the catheter to the thigh using a facility-approved product or as directed by the licensed nursing staff, and be careful not to pull or tug the catheter. Leave some slack in the tubing. Check the catheter and leg bag regularly to be sure the tubing is not twisted or bent.

Emptying a Leg Bag

Leg bags should be emptied when they are half-full or at least twice a day. Before emptying a leg bag, wash your hands and put on disposable gloves. The bag may be emptied into the toilet or another specified container, such as a graduate if I&O is being measured. Undo the straps or Velcro™ attaching the leg bag and be sure the catheter is not being pulled. Open the clamp on the leg bag to allow urine to drain. Never touch the tip of the bag while the urine is being emptied. When the bag is empty, close the clamp. Remove and discard your gloves and wash your hands.

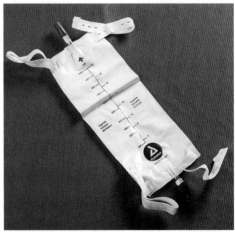

© Tori Soper Photography

Figure 23.24 Leg bags allow ambulatory residents more freedom and independence.

Replacing a Leg Bag with a Urinary Drainage Bag

When a resident will be staying in bed for a long period of time (for example, at night), the leg bag should be removed and replaced with a larger urinary drainage bag. To remove a leg bag and attach a new, urinary drainage bag, follow these guidelines:

1. Practice proper hand hygiene. Wash your hands and wear disposable gloves during the procedure, as appropriate.

2. Place a disposable protective pad on the bed. Attach a urinary drainage bag to the bedframe.

3. Safely help the resident lie on the bed. Keep the resident comfortable and covered, as appropriate.

4. Expose the catheter and leg bag. Clamp the catheter to prevent urine from draining into the tubing and let the urine drain from below the clamp into the leg bag.

5. Disconnect the catheter from the leg bag. If you touch the end of the catheter, use antiseptic wipes to clean it.

6. Hold the sterile catheter plug and do *not* touch the end that goes inside the catheter. Insert the sterile catheter plug into the end of the catheter. Place the sterile cap on the end of the old leg bag tubing and place the leg bag in a bedpan.

7. Remove the cap from the end of the new drainage bag tubing. Then remove the sterile plug from the catheter and insert the end of the drainage tubing into the catheter.

8. Remove the clamp from the catheter and coil the drainage tubing on the bed. Secure the tubing to the bottom bed linens.

9. Take the bedpan with the leg bag to the bathroom. Open the bottom of the leg bag and let the urine drain into the toilet or into a graduate if urine needs to be measured.

10. Clean and dry or discard equipment, according to facility policy.

How Should Nursing Assistants Help Residents with Incontinence?

Urinary incontinence is the loss of bladder control. Women are more likely than men to experience incontinence due to the stressors of pregnancy and childbirth and the structure of the female urinary tract. People over age 50 are also more likely to be incontinent due to age-related weakening of the bladder muscles. Some lifestyle factors also increase the risk of incontinence. These factors include too much alcohol or caffeine; side effects from certain medications; chronic constipation and UTIs; kidney or bladder stones; damage to the bladder muscles due to pregnancy, childbirth, or surgery; an enlarged prostate; diabetes; stroke; Parkinson's disease; and cancer. Some people also experience incontinence in the later stages of Alzheimer's disease and other types of dementia. Physical disabilities that prevent a person from reaching the bathroom can also lead to incontinence. For example, a person with a physical disability may encounter obstacles along the way to the bathroom or not be able to remove clothing quickly enough.

Symptoms of incontinence can range from mild to severe and may be temporary or permanent. There are three types of urinary incontinence:

1. **Stress incontinence**: occurs when certain types of physical activity, such as coughing, sneezing, or laughing, stress the weak sphincter muscle that holds urine, causing urine to leak.

2. **Urge incontinence**: also called an *overactive bladder (OAB)*, occurs when the bladder muscle contracts with enough force to override urethral sphincter muscles, causing involuntary loss of urine.

3. **Overflow incontinence**: occurs when the bladder is not completely emptied, causing the remaining urine to leak at a later time. This may be due to urinary obstructions, weak sphincter muscles, or certain conditions or disorders. This is sometimes called *dribbling*.

People can reduce their risk of urinary incontinence by maintaining a healthy weight, eliminating spicy or acidic foods, taking part in regular physical activity, limiting caffeine and alcohol consumption, and avoiding smoking.

The goal of treating urinary incontinence is to help residents increase bladder control. For example, the plan of care may have residents engage in pelvic-floor muscle training, such as daily Kegel exercises; bladder retraining; or *biofeedback* (the use of relaxation, visualization, or other cognitive control techniques to control muscle tension and other body functions). Other ways to increase bladder control include adjusting diet and fluid intake, scheduling regular bathroom breaks, and using incontinence products as needed (Figure 23.25).

Caring for residents who are incontinent requires empathy, support, and patience. Guidelines for caring for these residents include the following:

- Reassure residents to help reduce feelings of embarrassment and guilt (Figure 23.26).

- Show respect and compassion for the resident's loss of dignity.

- Plan your care so you are not rushed for time and ask for help when needed.

- To prevent embarrassment, do not use the term *diaper* when referring to incontinence briefs. Some residents may resist and feel angry about using incontinence briefs or other incontinence products.

- Learn to apply and remove incontinence briefs correctly. Follow the manufacturer's instructions and facility policy. Applying briefs improperly can cause skin breakdown due to rubbing. For example, do not "double brief," or insert a bladder pad inside the incontinence brief. Ask the licensed nursing staff if you need clarification or further instruction.

- Perform careful perineal care after every episode of incontinence. Clean the skin with mild soap and water. Rinse the skin well and gently pat it dry. If residents have very dry skin, use soap-free skin cleansers that do not cause dryness or irritation.

- Maintain skin integrity by keeping the skin clean and dry. Frequently check for wetness or soiling and remove briefs whenever they are soiled. Check the skin daily for decubitus ulcers. Also look for blisters, sores, or lesions. Report any skin changes or issues to the licensed nursing staff.

- Change bed linens and clothing immediately after an incontinence episode and use pillows or foam padding to prevent skin irritation.

- Use a skin sealant or moisture barrier, if ordered. These products can provide a protective barrier to the skin. Reapply the cream or ointment after you clean and dry the skin according to the plan of care. Do *not* use baby powder.

- Reduce the resident's intake of fluids in the late afternoon and evening to help prevent incontinence overnight, if instructed by the licensed nursing staff. Residents should never be without fluids completely, unless they are NPO.

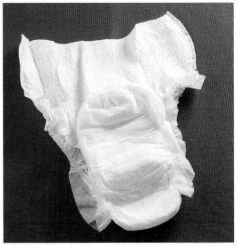

Figure 23.25 Incontinence briefs can be used for residents with urinary incontinence to prevent them from soiling their clothes or bed linens.

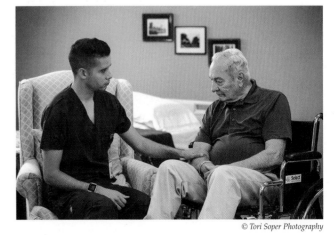

Figure 23.26 When caring for residents who are incontinent, be sure to show empathy. Listen to residents and be supportive.

How Can Nursing Assistants Address Bowel Elimination Needs?

Stool, or *feces*, is a waste product produced from digestion and metabolism. It is expelled from the large intestine via the anus and is composed primarily of undigested food. Stool also contains bacteria, dead cells, and mucus.

Most people have their own definition of a regular bowel movement. Typical stool is brown in color because of the presence of *bilirubin* (found in bile). Bilirubin is produced through the breakdown of hemoglobin and is an important digestive product. The Bristol Stool Chart indicates some standard sizes, shapes, and consistencies for stool (Figure 23.27). While stool size is an important factor to observe, stool consistency can be more helpful in identifying gastrointestinal diseases or disorders. For example, watery stool over a long period may indicate a GI disease or disorder or can be stress related. Helpful bacteria found in the intestines give stool its normal odor. If stool has a fouler odor, this may be due to a change in diet, some vitamins, medications, food allergies, an infection, or a disease that causes malabsorption (such as inflammatory bowel disease or blood in the stool).

The number of bowel movements a person has each day may vary. Usually, it takes three days for food ingested to be digested and expelled via defecation. Therefore, a healthy individual may **defecate** (have a bowel movement) from three times a day to once every three days. On average, most people defecate once or twice a day.

Any change in stool or bowel habits (color, size, shape, smell, or frequency of bowel movements) is important and should be reported to the licensed nursing staff. A change in stool color can signal dietary change, the use of medications, or possible diseases or conditions:

- **Red stool**: can be caused by naturally or artificially colored foods or blood.
- **Orange stool**: can be caused by red or orange foods and some medications.
- **Green stool**: can be caused by green foods or iron supplements.
- **Black stool**: can be caused by vitamins that contain iron or other medications. Stool that is black, sticky (*tarry*), and foul smelling may indicate the presence of blood in the stool, which is a serious condition.

Bristol Stool Chart		
Type 1	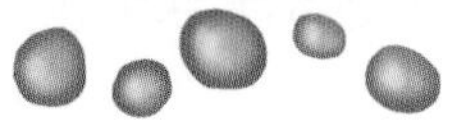	Separate, hard lumps like pellets; hard to pass
Type 2	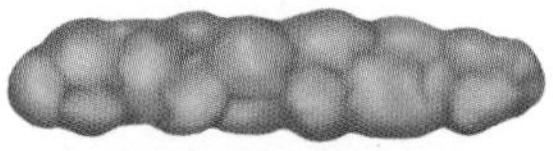	Sausage-shaped, but lumpy
Type 3	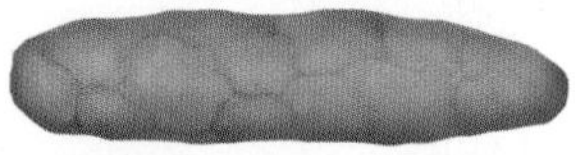	Like a sausage, but with cracks on the surface
Type 4	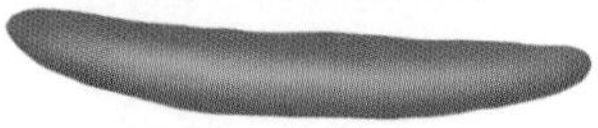	Like a sausage or snake, smooth and soft
Type 5	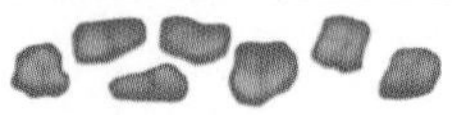	Soft blobs with clear-cut edges; easy to pass
Type 6	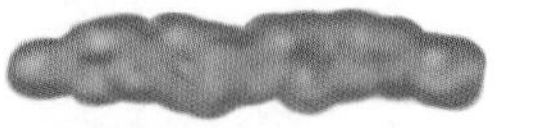	Fluffy pieces with ragged edges; a mushy stool
Type 7	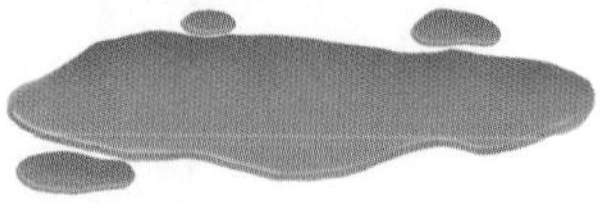	Watery with no solid pieces; entirely liquid

© *Body Scientific International*

Figure 23.27 The Bristol Stool Chart categorizes the consistency of stool.

- **Gray stool**: may also be clay colored or pale. It can be the result of some diagnostic tests, but may also indicate a blockage in the flow of bile or liver disease.

Recording Bowel Movements

Careful observation and accuracy are essential when recording bowel movements. Nursing assistants measuring I&O must always wash their hands to ensure infection control and wear disposable gloves. A good source of light will be needed to observe the stool. Examine bowel movements closely before disposing of stool, so that details can be reported and documented accurately. If necessary, use a disposable stick or tongue blade to examine the stool more closely. The following observations, signs, and symptoms should be reported to the licensed nursing staff immediately:

- excessive **flatus** or *gas*
- diarrhea or constipation
- undigested food
- blood or mucus in the stool
- unusual color, particularly black or dark green
- foul-smelling stool

Your ability to provide comfort and understanding as you give care will be critical to the way patients and residents respond. As you give care, be sure to maintain skin integrity, provide proper hygiene, and achieve an odor-free environment. This approach will influence your ability to promote healing and prevent infection.

The procedures in this chapter are helpful for patients and residents who experience significant discomfort due to elimination problems. These procedures may also be used to prepare residents for surgery, deal with the effects of surgery, or prepare residents for diagnostic procedures. Performing these procedures with skill will help alleviate pain due to excessive flatus or evacuate the bowels for a resident who has an **impaction** (blockage of hard stool in the rectum). If these procedures are preparing a resident for surgery or a diagnostic procedure, the resident may be very anxious and fearful about the outcome of the surgery or diagnostic procedure. Be patient and do not rush. Be positive and establish a calm, helpful environment.

Procedure | Inserting a Rectal Tube

Rationale

A rectal tube and its connected bag are used to help relieve flatus, which can build up in the lower intestine. This procedure is usually performed once every 24 hours until the flatus is relieved.

Preparation

1. Ask the licensed nursing staff how this procedure fits into the plan of care, if there are doctor's orders for the procedure, if there are any special instructions or precautions, and if the resident can be moved into the positions required for this procedure.

2. Wash your hands or use hand sanitizer before entering the room.

3. Knock before entering the room.

4. Introduce yourself using your full name and title. Explain that you work with the licensed nursing staff and will be providing care.

5. Greet the resident and ask the resident to state her full name, if able. Then check the resident's identification bracelet.

6. Use Mr., Mrs., or Ms. and the last name when conversing.

7. Explain the procedure in simple terms, even if the resident is not able to communicate or is disoriented. Ask permission to perform the procedure.

8. Bring the necessary equipment into the room. Place a paper towel, towel, or disposable protective pad on the overbed table as an infection-control barrier before placing the following items:
   - disposable rectal tube with connected flatus bag (Figure 23.28)
   - disposable gloves
   - tissue or toilet paper
   - lubricating gel
   - disposable protective pad
   - bath blanket
   - small piece of tape
   - washcloth or cleansing wipe

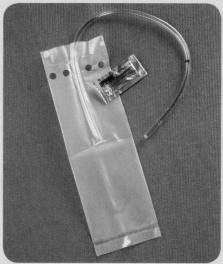

Figure 23.28

The Procedure

9. Provide privacy by closing the curtains, using a screen, or closing the door to the room.

10. Lock the bed wheels and then raise the bed to hip level.

11. Ensure safety during the procedure. If there are side rails, raise and secure the rails on the opposite side of the bed from where you will be working. Lower the rail on the side you are working.

12. Wash your hands or use hand sanitizer to ensure infection control.

13. Put on disposable gloves.

14. Cover the resident with the bath blanket. Without exposing the resident, fanfold the top linens to the foot of the bed.

15. Help the resident turn onto her left side. Bend her right knee toward her chest to place her in Sims' position.

16. Expose the resident's buttocks by raising the lower corner of the blanket covering the anal area.

17. Squeeze lubricating gel onto a tissue or toilet paper. Then rub the gel on the tip of the rectal tube. Be sure the lubricant does not clog the opening at the end of the tube. (This step is not necessary if the rectal tube is prelubricated.)

18. With one hand, lift the upper buttock to expose the anus. Gently insert the rectal tube 2–4 inches into the rectum.

19. Use a small piece of tape or another product according to facility policy or the plan of care to attach the rectal tube to the resident's buttocks. This will help hold the tube in place. Remind the resident to lay still and not dislodge the rectal tube.

20. If the resident can be safely left alone, place the call light within her reach. Instruct her to use the call light, if needed. Follow the plan of care to determine if the side rails should be raised or lowered. Remove and discard your gloves. Wash your hands or use hand sanitizer before leaving the room.

21. If the resident cannot be left alone, stay in the room to ensure safety.

22. If you left the room, return to the room when the resident uses the call light or after 20 minutes to check on the resident. You may check more often, as appropriate, to monitor the resident's condition. Wash your hands or use hand sanitizer to ensure infection control. Put on disposable gloves.

23. Ask the resident if she was able to pass flatus and if she is feeling relieved. Check for drainage.

24. Slowly remove the rectal tube from the rectum.

25. After removing the rectal tube, cleanse the anal area from front to back using a washcloth moistened with warm water or a cleansing wipe. Assist with any additional hygiene care, as needed.

26. Check to be sure the bed wheels are locked, then reposition the resident and lower the bed.

27. Follow the plan of care to determine if the side rails should be raised or lowered.

28. Remove, clean, and store equipment in the proper location. Remove soiled linens and discard disposable equipment.

Follow-Up

29. Remove and discard your gloves.

30. Wash your hands to ensure infection control.

31. Make sure the resident is comfortable and place the call light and personal items within reach.

32. Conduct a safety check before leaving the room. The room should be clean and free from clutter or spills.

33. Wash your hands or use hand sanitizer before leaving the room.

Reporting and Documentation

34. Communicate any specific observations, complications, or unusual responses to the licensed nursing staff. Record this information, along with the care provided, in the chart or EMR.

Image courtesy of © Tori Soper Photography

Special attention and care may be required if residents experience acute or chronic diarrhea, constipation, or fecal incontinence. *Fecal* or *bowel incontinence* may be the result of diarrhea, constipation, or sometimes muscle or nerve damage. It is the accidental leaking or passing of solid or liquid stool or mucus, usually due to the inability to hold in a bowel movement. Some residents may not be aware if they have passed stool in their underwear. Age is a risk factor for fecal incontinence, as are diseases or conditions such as dementia. Fecal incontinence can be very embarrassing for residents, so special care and attention are needed. Excellent hygiene and the maintenance of skin integrity are particularly essential.

Diarrhea

Diarrhea is a condition in which liquid stool is expelled frequently from the body. Diarrhea occurs when food and waste move so rapidly through the gastrointestinal system that the large intestine does not absorb fluids from either substance before expulsion. Diarrhea causes frequent bowel movements, sometimes up to 20 or more per day.

More than 250,000 people are admitted into US hospitals due to diarrhea each year. While diarrhea is often short term, it can become chronic or cause serious complications that may lead to death. Some causes of acute diarrhea are infection, parasites, tainted food, some diseases and medications, and bowel and gastrointestinal **motility** (movement) disorders. Certain diseases, such as celiac disease and inflammatory bowel disease (IBS), may cause chronic diarrhea.

Symptoms associated with diarrhea may include fever of 102°F or higher, nausea, vomiting, and abdominal pain. Blood or pus may be present in the stool, depending on the cause of diarrhea. Complications of diarrhea may include mild to severe dehydration, lack of adequate nutrition, and extreme weight loss. The treatment goal is to manage dehydration and nutrition through sufficient oral intake (to provide more bulk to the stool), supplements, or replacement parenteral IV infusion. Medications may be ordered by the doctor to slow down or stop the diarrhea.

Constipation

Constipation is a condition characterized by difficult and infrequent bowel movements. Infrequent bowel movements can result in major or minor blockages in the intestines, and when a resident is constipated, food and waste move more slowly through the gastrointestinal system. Constipation can be short term or chronic. Risk factors for constipation include advancing age; pregnancy; a low-fiber diet; dehydration; limited physical activity; certain medications, and particularly pain medications; or diseases such as multiple sclerosis, Parkinson's disease, or an eating disorder.

Symptoms of constipation may include a bloated feeling, swollen abdomen, feeling that there is a blockage in the rectum, or inability to empty the bowel. Straining during elimination, having lumpy or hard stool, bleeding during a bowel movement, and needing to press on the abdomen or use a finger to remove stool are also signs of constipation. Constipation is defined as fewer than three bowel movements in a week. Complications of constipation include internal or external hemorrhoids (Figure 23.29), **hernia** (protrusion of an organ through the wall of the body cavity or structure that contains it), *anal fissure* (a break or tear in the lining of the anal canal), *colitis* (inflammation of the large intestine), and laxative dependency. Bowel impaction, obstruction, and rectal prolapse (in which a small amount of the rectum protrudes from the anus) are other serious complications.

Procedures used to determine the cause of constipation include physical and rectal examinations, a *barium enema* (an X-ray procedure in which liquid containing a metallic substance is injected into the lower colon to coat its lining), and a *sigmoidoscopy* (examination of the sigmoid area of the colon). The

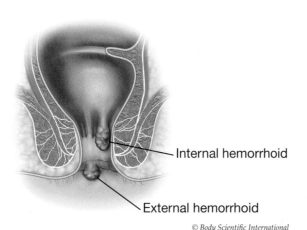

Internal hemorrhoid

External hemorrhoid

© Body Scientific International

Figure 23.29 Hemorrhoids are swollen veins in the tissue of the anus. Internal hemorrhoids form inside the anal canal. External hemorrhoids form around the opening of the anus.

Healthcare Scenario
Constipation Remedies

A recent journal article discussed the benefits of treating constipation using integrative or alternative remedies in addition to typical methods of treatment. One alternative suggestion included taking a *probiotic* (capsule containing bacteria that help the intestines stay healthy). Acupressure was also recommended to relax the abdomen, ease discomfort, and stimulate regular bowel movements. The article also suggested using homeopathy, massage, yoga, aromatherapy, and herbal therapy (such as eating chamomile and dandelion) to stimulate bowel movement, if permitted by the plan of care and facility policy.

Apply It

1. Have you or someone you know used an integrative or alternative treatment for constipation? What was the experience like?

2. Research one of the alternative treatments suggested. How effective is it for treating constipation?

treatment goal for chronic constipation usually begins with encouraging residents to increase fiber intake, exercise, not ignore the urge to have a bowel movement, and take time on the toilet without being distracted or feeling rushed. Laxatives, fiber supplements, stimulants, lubricants, stool softeners, **suppositories** (small, meltable cones that are inserted into a body passage), and enemas may also be helpful. Some treatments are available over the counter, but some must be prescribed by a doctor. If a resident is in a healthcare facility, any treatment must be ordered by the doctor. Surgery may be recommended if there is a blockage, fissure, or *stricture* (narrowing of the lining of the anal canal).

Procedure Inserting a Rectal Suppository

Rationale

A rectal suppository is used primarily to stimulate bowel elimination. A suppository may also be used to administer medications that relieve pain and promote healing.

Preparation

1. Ask the licensed nursing staff how this procedure fits into the plan of care, if there are doctor's orders for the procedure, if there are any special instructions or precautions, and if the resident can be moved into the positions required for this procedure.
2. Wash your hands or use hand sanitizer before entering the room.
3. Knock before entering the room.
4. Introduce yourself using your full name and title. Explain that you work with the licensed nursing staff and will be providing care.
5. Greet the resident and ask the resident to state his full name, if able. Then check the resident's identification bracelet.
6. Use Mr., Mrs., or Ms. and the last name when conversing.
7. Explain the procedure in simple terms, even if the resident is not able to communicate or is disoriented. Ask permission to perform the procedure.
8. Bring the necessary equipment into the room. Place a paper towel, towel, or disposable protective pad on the overbed table as an infection-control barrier before placing the following items:
   - suppository, as ordered (Figure 23.30)
   - disposable gloves
   - toilet paper
   - lubricating gel
   - bedpan and cover or bedside commode, if needed
   - disposable protective pad
   - bath blanket

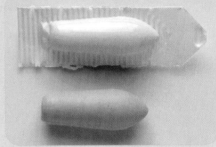
Figure 23.30

The Procedure

9. Provide privacy by closing the curtains, using a screen, or closing the door to the room.
10. Lock the bed wheels and then raise the bed to hip level.
11. Ensure safety during the procedure. If there are side rails, raise and secure the rails on the opposite side of the bed from where you will be working. Lower the rail on the side you are working.
12. Wash your hands or use hand sanitizer to ensure infection control.
13. Put on disposable gloves.
14. Cover the resident with a bath blanket. Fanfold the linens to the foot of the bed and place a disposable protective pad under the resident's buttocks.
15. Help the resident turn onto his left side. Bend the resident's right knee toward his chest to place him in Sims' position.
16. Unwrap the suppository.

(continued)

17. Expose the resident's buttocks by raising the lower corner of the blanket covering the anal area.

18. With one hand, lift the upper buttock to expose the anus.

19. Apply a small amount of lubricating gel to the anus and suppository.

20. Gently insert the suppository into the rectum about 2 inches beyond the anal sphincter (Figure 23.31). Wipe any excess lubricant from the anal area.

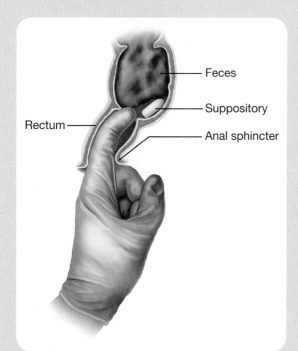

Feces

Suppository

Rectum

Anal sphincter

Figure 23.31

21. Encourage the resident to relax by taking slow, deep breaths until he feels the need to have a bowel movement (may take 5 to 20 minutes).

Best Practice
Explain to the resident that the suppository will melt into liquid due to body heat and that he may feel this occurring. Assure the resident that it may feel unusual, but is expected.

22. If the resident can be safely left alone, place the call light within his reach. Instruct him to use the call light when he feels the need to have a bowel movement. Follow the plan of care to determine if the side rails should be raised or lowered. Remove and discard your gloves. Wash your hands or use hand sanitizer before leaving the room.

23. If the resident cannot be left alone, stay in the room to ensure safety.

24. If you left the room, return to the room when the resident uses the call light or every five minutes to check on the resident. Wash your hands or use hand sanitizer to ensure infection control. Put on disposable gloves.

25. Assist the resident to the bathroom or bedside commode or position the resident on a bedpan.

26. Provide privacy. When the resident is finished, assist him back to bed and with hygiene, as needed.

27. Check to be sure the bed wheels are locked, then reposition the resident and lower the bed.

28. Follow the plan of care to determine if the side rails should be raised or lowered.

29. Check the stool for any unusual appearance. If you see anything abnormal, alert the licensed nursing staff immediately.

30. Discard the stool in the toilet or follow any special instructions, such as saving stool for a sample.

31. Remove, clean, and store equipment in the proper location. Remove soiled linens and discard disposable equipment.

Follow-Up

32. Remove and discard your gloves.

33. Wash your hands to ensure infection control.

34. Make sure the resident is comfortable and place the call light and personal items within reach.

35. Conduct a safety check before leaving the room. The room should be clean and free from clutter or spills.

36. Wash your hands or use hand sanitizer before leaving the room.

Reporting and Documentation

37. Communicate any specific observations, complications, or unusual responses to the licensed nursing staff. Record this information, along with the care provided, in the chart or EMR.

Figure 23.30 Lukasz Siekierski/Shutterstock.com;
Figure 23.31 © Body Scientific International

Enemas

Sometimes a suppository is not enough to initiate a bowel movement. In this case, an **enema** may be needed. Different types of enemas include

- *cleansing enemas*, which introduce tap water, water with soapsuds, or saline into the rectum and colon via the anus;
- *retention enemas*, which use oil to soften and lubricate the stool for easy elimination; and
- commercial or small-volume disposable enemas.

When giving an enema, nursing assistants usually use a disposable enema kit. The disposable enema kit contains an enema bag with tubing, clamp, and disposable protective pad (Figure 23.32).

Enemas can be uncomfortable for anyone, but especially for older adults. Residents may already be uncomfortable from constipation, and the positioning needed to effectively administer the enema can increase discomfort. Residents may also experience cramping when the enema solution flows into the rectum and colon. Working slowly and patiently and providing support by checking with the resident during the procedure can make the experience more comfortable and tolerable.

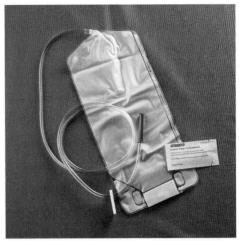

© Tori Soper Photography

Figure 23.32 The enema bag, tubing, and clamp shown here are part of a disposable enema kit.

Procedure | Administering an Enema

Rationale

An enema is used to aid bowel elimination or to prepare the resident for certain surgeries or diagnostic procedures.

Preparation

1. Ask the licensed nursing staff how this procedure fits into the plan of care, if there are doctor's orders for the procedure, if there are any special instructions or precautions, and if the resident can be moved into the positions required for this procedure.
2. Wash your hands or use hand sanitizer before entering the room.
3. Knock before entering the room.
4. Introduce yourself using your full name and title. Explain that you work with the licensed nursing staff and will be providing care.
5. Greet the resident and ask the resident to state her full name, if able. Then check the resident's identification bracelet.
6. Use Mr., Mrs., or Ms. and the last name when conversing.
7. Explain the procedure in simple terms, even if the resident is not able to communicate or is disoriented. Ask permission to perform the procedure.

8. Bring the necessary equipment into the room. Place the following items in an accessible location:
   - disposable enema kit or prepacked enema, as ordered
   - enema solution (1000 ml for adults)
   - IV pole
   - disposable gloves
   - water-soluble lubricant
   - bath blanket
   - disposable protective pad

   Collect the following items, as needed:
   - bedpan and cover or bedside commode
   - urinal
   - nonskid slippers
   - toilet paper
   - paper towels
   - towels, soap, and washbasin

The Procedure: Cleansing Enema

9. Prepare the enema solution, as ordered, in the bathroom or utility room.

(continued)

10. Close the clamp on the enema bag tubing. Fill the enema bag with the amount of enema solution ordered. Seal the enema bag.

11. Unclamp the enema tubing. Run a small amount of enema solution through the tubing to eliminate air and warm the tube. Check the temperature of the enema solution to be sure it is not too warm. Clamp the tubing. Bring the prepared enema bag into the room.

12. Hang the enema bag on the IV pole next to or on the bed. The enema bag should hang 18 inches above the mattress. Hanging the enema bag any higher could cause the resident pain.

13. Provide privacy by closing the curtains, using a screen, or closing the door to the room.

14. Lock the bed wheels and then raise the bed to hip level.

15. Ensure safety during the procedure. If there are side rails, raise and secure the rails on the opposite side of the bed from where you will be working. Lower the rail on the side you are working.

16. Wash your hands or use hand sanitizer to ensure infection control.

17. Put on disposable gloves.

18. Cover the resident with a bath blanket. Fanfold the linens to the foot of the bed and place a disposable protective pad under the resident's buttocks.

19. Help the resident turn onto his left side. Bend the resident's right knee toward his chest to place him in Sims' position.

20. Expose the resident's buttocks by raising the lower corner of the blanket covering the anal area.

21. Lubricate the enema tubing 2–4 inches from the tip.

22. Expose the resident's anus by lifting the resident's upper buttock. Gently insert the enema tubing 2–4 inches into the rectum (Figure 23.33). If the resident complains of pain, if you meet resistance, or if there is bleeding, stop and immediately report this to the licensed nursing staff.

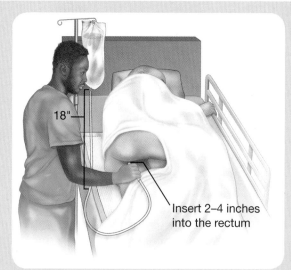

18"

Insert 2–4 inches into the rectum

Figure 23.33

23. Unclamp the enema tubing and let the solution flow slowly. Ask the resident to take slow, deep breaths to relax. Explain that this will help relieve any cramps caused by the enema.

24. When most of the solution has flowed into the rectum, close the clamp before the enema bag is empty. This will prevent air from entering the bowel.

25. Hold toilet paper around the enema tubing and against the anus. Slowly withdraw the tubing. Wrap the tubing in paper towels and place it in the empty enema kit container.

26. Ask the resident to squeeze his buttocks so he holds the solution in the rectum for as long as possible.

27. When the resident is no longer able to hold the solution or when the urge to have a bowel movement is insistent, assist the resident to the bedpan, bedside commode, or bathroom. If the resident will be using a bedpan, raise the head of the bed. Put toilet paper where it can easily be reached. If the resident uses the bathroom, stay nearby to help, if needed, and ask the resident not to flush the toilet. Make sure the call light is within the resident's reach.

28. Remove and discard your gloves.

29. Wash your hands or use hand sanitizer to ensure infection control.

30. Check on the resident every few minutes.

31. While the resident is using the bedpan, bedside commode, or toilet, dispose of the enema equipment according to facility policy.

32. Wash your hands or use hand sanitizer to ensure infection control.

Image courtesy of © Body Scientific International

33. Put on a new pair of gloves.

34. When the resident has finished using the bedpan, bedside commode, or toilet, assist the resident back to bed, if needed. Assist with hygiene care.

35. If the resident is in bed, remove the disposable protective pad and bath blanket. Change any soiled linens and cover the resident with the top linens.

36. Check to be sure the bed wheels are locked, then reposition the resident and lower the bed.

37. Follow the plan of care to determine if the side rails should be raised or lowered.

38. Remove and discard your gloves.

39. Wash your hands or use hand sanitizer to ensure infection control.

40. Put on a new pair of gloves.

41. Remove, clean, and store equipment in the proper location. Remove soiled linens and discard disposable equipment.

The Procedure: Commercial Enema

42. Provide privacy by closing the curtains, using a screen, or closing the door to the room.

43. Lock the bed wheels and then raise the bed to hip level.

44. Ensure safety during the procedure. If there are side rails, raise and secure the rails on the opposite side of the bed from where you will be working. Lower the rail on the side you are working.

45. Wash your hands or use hand sanitizer to ensure infection control.

46. Put on disposable gloves.

47. Cover the resident with a bath blanket. Fanfold the linens to the foot of the bed and place a disposable protective pad under the resident's buttocks.

48. Help the resident turn onto her left side. Bend the resident's right knee toward her chest to place her in Sims' position.

49. Open the box and remove the enema. Place the solution container in warm water, if instructed.

50. Expose the resident's buttocks by moving linens away from the anal area.

51. Remove the cover from the prelubricated enema tip. Gently squeeze the container to make sure the container tip is open.

52. With one hand, raise the resident's upper buttock to expose the anus.

53. Ask the resident to take a deep breath through her mouth and let it out. As the resident lets out her breath, gently insert the enema tip 2 inches into the rectum (Figure 23.34).

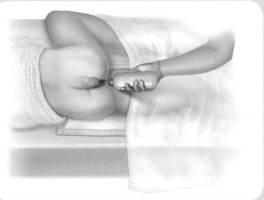

Figure 23.34

54. Gently squeeze the bottom of the enema container and roll the container until almost all of the solution goes into the rectum. A small amount should remain in the container.

55. Remove the enema tip from the anus and place the container in the box.

56. Ask the resident to hold the solution in her rectum for 20 minutes, or as long as possible. Ask her to signal you when she has an insistent urge to defecate.

57. If the resident can be safely left alone, be sure she is positioned safely and place the call light within her reach.

58. If the resident cannot be left alone, stay in the room to ensure safety.

59. Discard the enema container. Remove and discard your gloves. Wash your hands or use hand sanitizer to ensure infection control.

60. If you left the room, return to the room when the resident uses the call light.

(continued)

61. Help the resident to the bedpan, bedside commode, or bathroom. If the resident will be using the bedpan, raise the head of the bed. Put toilet paper where it can easily be reached. If the resident uses the bathroom, stay nearby to help, if needed, and ask the resident not to flush the toilet. Make sure the call light is within the resident's reach.

62. Check on the resident every few minutes.

63. Wash your hands or use hand sanitizer to ensure infection control.

64. Put on a new pair of gloves.

65. When the resident has finished using the bedpan, bedside commode, or toilet, assist with hygiene care.

66. If the resident is in bed, remove the disposable protective pad and bath blanket. Change any soiled linens and cover the resident.

67. Check to be sure the bed wheels are locked, then reposition the resident and lower the bed.

68. Follow the plan of care to determine if the side rails should be raised or lowered.

69. Remove, clean, and store equipment in the proper location. Remove soiled linens and discard disposable equipment.

Follow-Up

70. Remove and discard your gloves.

71. Wash your hands to ensure infection control.

72. Make sure the resident is comfortable and place the call light and personal items within reach.

73. Conduct a safety check before leaving the room. The room should be clean and free from clutter or spills.

74. Wash your hands or use hand sanitizer before leaving the room.

Reporting and Documentation

75. Communicate any specific observations, complications, or unusual responses to the licensed nursing staff. Record this information, along with the care provided, in the chart or EMR.

Ostomies and Stoma Care

Bowel elimination problems can have a significant effect on residents' lives. Some examples of bowel elimination problems include diverticulitis, Crohn's disease, colon cancer, severe obstruction, and trauma or injury to the large intestine. Should any of these problems occur, a surgical procedure called an **ostomy** may be required. An ostomy procedure creates a **stoma**, or an artificial opening, between the surface of the abdomen and the intestine. This stoma allows waste to be eliminated (Figure 23.35). An *ostomy bag* is applied to the stoma to collect waste. If the stoma extends between

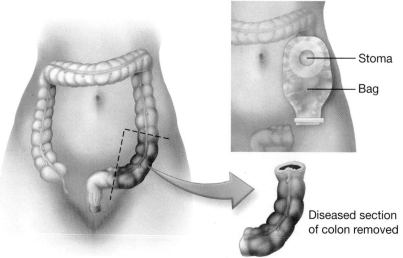

Stoma

Bag

Diseased section of colon removed

© *Body Scientific International*

Figure 23.35 An ostomy procedure creates a stoma, through which waste is eliminated. An ostomy bag is applied to the stoma to collect the waste.

the surface of the abdomen and the large intestine, the procedure is called a *colostomy*. If the stoma extends between the surface of the abdomen and the ileum, the procedure is called an *ileostomy*. When extensive removal of the intestine is required, the stoma is usually permanent. In other cases, the intestine simply needs to rest due to infections, diseases, or surgical procedures within the GI system. When this occurs, the stoma is often temporary. Whether permanent or temporary, a colostomy or ileostomy can be very traumatic and embarrassing for residents. Residents may worry about soiling themselves or about odor. Being patient and supportive is an important responsibility for a holistic nursing assistant.

Nursing assistants are responsible for caring for the stoma and emptying and changing the ostomy bag. As part of hygiene, the stoma must be cleaned and the ostomy bag changed daily, if not more often. The ostomy bag itself will need to be emptied during the day and should never be more than one-third full. Some residents may empty their bags themselves. Others may need assistance.

When providing ostomy care, you will need several pieces of equipment (Figure 23.36):

- correctly sized, clean ostomy bag (sometimes called an *appliance* or *pouch*)
- skin barrier that adheres to the stoma and protects the skin from stoma output
- clamp or clip to open and close the bag (may be attached to the bag)
- clean ostomy belt, if used (to secure the bag against the body)

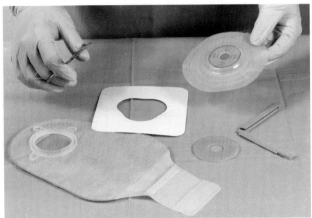

Sherry Yates Young/Shutterstock.com

Figure 23.36 When caring for a stoma, you will need an ostomy bag, skin barrier, and clamp, among other equipment.

Procedure | Providing Ostomy Care

Rationale
Regular care keeps the skin around a stoma clean and prevents irritation and breakdown from contact with stool.

Preparation

1. Ask the licensed nursing staff how this procedure fits into the plan of care, if there are doctor's orders for the procedure, if there are any special instructions or precautions, and if the resident can be moved into the positions required for this procedure.
2. Wash your hands or use hand sanitizer before entering the room.
3. Knock before entering the room.
4. Introduce yourself using your full name and title. Explain that you work with the licensed nursing staff and will be providing care.
5. Greet the resident and ask the resident to state his full name, if able. Then check the resident's identification bracelet.
6. Use Mr., Mrs., or Ms. and the last name when conversing.
7. Explain the procedure in simple terms, even if the resident is not able to communicate or is disoriented. Ask permission to perform the procedure.
8. Bring the necessary equipment into the room. Place a paper towel, towel, or disposable protective pad on the overbed table as an infection-control barrier before placing the following items:
   - correctly sized, clean ostomy bag with skin barrier
   - clamp or clip, if needed
   - clean ostomy belt, if used
   - adhesive remover, if needed
   - antiseptic wipes
   - disposable protective pads
   - disposable gloves
   - small trash bag

(continued)

- bath blanket
- 4 × 4 gauze pads or toilet paper
- washcloths
- towels
- washbasin with warm water
- soap or cleaning agent, as ordered
- bedpan and cover
- graduate
- deodorant, if used

The Procedure

9. Provide privacy by closing the curtains, using a screen, or closing the door to the room.

10. Lock the bed wheels and then raise the bed to hip level.

11. Ensure safety during the procedure. If there are side rails, raise and secure the rails on the opposite side of the bed from where you will be working. Lower the rail on the side you are working.

12. Wash your hands or use hand sanitizer to ensure infection control.

13. Put on disposable gloves.

14. Position the resident on his back, if possible. Place a disposable protective pad under the resident's buttocks.

15. Cover the resident with a bath blanket. Without exposing the resident, fanfold the top linens and move clothing to expose the stoma.

16. Place another protective pad alongside the resident's body and cover the resident with the bath blanket from the waist down.

17. Remove the clamp at the bottom of the ostomy bag and let the stool drain into a graduate. Make sure the drain and the end of the bag do not touch the graduate. Avoid any splashing of the stool or drainage.

18. Wipe the open end of the ostomy bag with an antiseptic wipe, following facility policy. Fold the end of the ostomy bag and close it with the clamp.

19. Note the color, amount, consistency, and odor of the stool and measure the stool and drainage, if recording I&O.

20. Empty the stool and drainage into the toilet or bedpan.

21. Remove and discard your gloves.

22. Wash your hands or use hand sanitizer to ensure infection control.

23. Put on a new pair of gloves.

24. Disconnect the ostomy bag from the ostomy belt, if used. Remove and inspect the belt. If the belt is soiled, dispose of it according to facility policy.

25. Remove the ostomy bag and skin barrier by gently stretching the skin and pulling the ostomy bag away from the skin. Use warm water or adhesive remover, if necessary.

26. Place the ostomy bag in the bedpan and cover the bedpan. Neutralize any odor, following facility policy.

27. Remove any stool or drainage by gently wiping the stoma with a 4 × 4 gauze pad or toilet paper (Figure 23.37). Discard the dirty gauze pads and your gloves in a disposable trash bag.

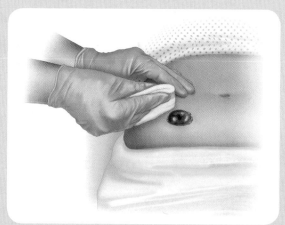

Figure 23.37

28. Wash your hands or use hand sanitizer to ensure infection control.

29. Put on a new pair of gloves.

30. Wash the stoma and the skin around it using a 4 × 4 gauze pad or washcloth mitt, soap, and water or a cleansing agent (as ordered).

31. Rinse and thoroughly dry the skin around the stoma.

32. Observe the stoma and the skin around the stoma. Immediately report any skin irritation, breakdown, or bleeding to the licensed nursing staff.

33. Apply the correctly sized skin barrier, according to the manufacturer's instructions (Figure 23.38).

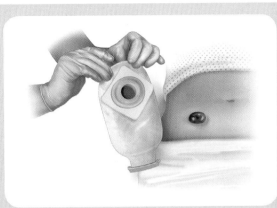

Figure 23.38

34. Position the clean ostomy belt, if used.

35. Remove the adhesive backing from the ostomy bag. The opening of the ostomy bag should be the correct size for the stoma.

36. Make sure the drain or end of the bag is pointing downward and then center the bag over the stoma.

37. Gently press around the edges of the ostomy bag to seal it to the skin. If used, add deodorant to the bag.

> **Best Practice**
> Make sure the skin around and under the ostomy bag is smooth and wrinkle free.

38. Close the ostomy bag at the bottom using the clamp or clip.

39. Attach the ostomy belt, if used, to the ostomy bag. Make sure the belt is not too tight. You should be able to slide two fingers underneath it.

40. Remove the protective pads and change any soiled linen. Remove the bath blanket and replace the top linens.

41. Check to be sure the bed wheels are locked, then reposition the resident and lower the bed.

42. Follow the plan of care to determine if the side rails should be raised or lowered.

43. Remove, clean, and store equipment in the proper location. Remove soiled linens and discard disposable equipment.

Follow-Up

44. Remove and discard your gloves.

45. Wash your hands to ensure infection control.

46. Make sure the resident is comfortable and place the call light and personal items within reach.

47. Conduct a safety check before leaving the room. The room should be clean and free from clutter or spills.

48. Wash your hands or use hand sanitizer before leaving the room.

Reporting and Documentation

49. Communicate any specific observations, complications, or unusual responses to the licensed nursing staff. Record this information, along with the care provided, in the chart or EMR.

Image courtesy of © Body Scientific International

What Are Bladder and Bowel Retraining?

Bladder or *bowel retraining* may be ordered by the doctor to help residents gain greater independence and self-reliance with elimination problems such as incontinence or constipation. Generally, retraining includes changing the diet, tracking elimination to determine individual patterns, scheduling toileting to increase the time between visits, determining any obstacles to toileting, modifying any medications contributing to the issue, learning pelvic-floor exercises, and rehabilitating muscles when possible.

Bladder and bowel retraining require persistence and concentration by residents. Retraining may continue up to three months or more before any progress is made. Retraining orders are written by the doctor, and guidance is given by the licensed nursing staff. Assistance and support, as needed by residents, are usually provided by nursing assistants if retraining occurs in a long-term care facility. The following are instructions often given to residents for bladder and bowel retraining.

> **Remember**
> *The greatest power is often simple patience.*
> E. Joseph Cossman, businessman and entrepreneur

Becoming a Holistic Nursing Assistant

Assisting with Elimination Needs

Residents who need assistance with elimination needs may feel uncomfortable and self-conscious about nursing assistants seeing and touching their genitals. They may also be embarrassed about what is happening and feel shame. Holistic nursing assistants can follow these guidelines to make this difficult time more pleasant, helpful, and comfortable:

- Be aware of your own feelings of comfort when assisting with elimination.
- Be sensitive to and compassionate about a resident's situation and feelings. Remind the resident that you are there to help.
- Some residents are more comfortable than others in expressing their feelings. Be sensitive to how open a resident is when you ask questions about the resident's feelings.
- Encourage the resident to ask questions and ask the resident to share any changes he or she might be experiencing.

- Assure the resident experiencing diarrhea and constipation that everyone has had these conditions at one time or another, so there is no reason to feel ashamed.
- Answer call lights immediately, particularly if a resident is having elimination problems (such as diarrhea or incontinence).
- If a resident is having trouble urinating, put his or her hands in warm water or turn on the faucet so the resident can hear running water.
- Create a relaxing environment.
- Touch the resident gently and carefully when giving care.
- Never rush when giving care.

Apply It

1. Think about each of these guidelines. What are your feelings about elimination and elimination problems?
2. Are there any guidelines you might have trouble following as a holistic nursing assistant? Explain your answer.

Bladder Retraining Instructions for Residents

- Keep a toileting diary. Log how often you urinate, when you have the urge to urinate, and if and when you leak each day. Maintain this diary throughout retraining and routinely review it with your doctor.

- Visit the toilet before you go to bed at night and empty your bladder as soon as you get up in the morning. This starts your retraining schedule daily. Using your diary, schedule regular toileting visits, but add 15 minutes to the end of each interval. If you usually go to the bathroom every hour, plan to urinate every one hour and 15 minutes. Sit on the toilet or stand and try to urinate, whether you have to urinate or not. Increase the time between each toileting visit by 15 minutes until you reach three to four hours between each visit. Follow the schedule while you are awake. At night, go to the toilet only if you awaken and find it necessary.

- Every time you feel an urge to urinate, wait five minutes before going. Increase that time gradually by 10 minutes, until you can delay it for at least three to four hours. Distract yourself if you have a strong urge to urinate. If you are standing, try to sit down and relax. Use deep breathing, count backward, or talk with someone to distract yourself. Visit the toilet when you can't wait any longer. Thereafter, return to your next scheduled toilet visit. Repeat this process every time you feel the urge to urinate.

- Learn Kegel exercises to strengthen muscles for starting and stopping the flow of urine. To do a Kegel exercise, squeeze, or *contract*, the muscles you normally use to stop the flow of urine. Hold the contraction for five seconds and then relax for five seconds. Gradually increase to contract the muscles every 10 seconds, with 10 seconds of rest in between. Work up to three sets of 10 contractions daily. If you do these daily, you will be more successful. Use your diary to keep track of your daily Kegel exercises.

- Limit beverages that increase urination. This includes caffeinated drinks such as sodas, coffee, and tea. Drink less before bedtime.

Bowel Retraining Instructions for Residents

- Set a regular time for daily bowel movements. The time should be convenient and fit with your daily schedule. The best time is 20 to 40 minutes after a meal because eating stimulates bowel activity.

- Change your diet to help create soft, bulky stool. Eat high-fiber foods such as whole grains, fresh vegetables, and beans. Try to drink 2–3 liters of fluid daily, unless your doctor advises against this. Some people find drinking warm prune juice or fruit nectar helpful.

- Use products that have *psyllium* (fiber made from husks of plant seeds), which adds bulk to the stool. These products can be found in retail stores, usually under a commercial name.

- Use daily digital stimulation to trigger a bowel movement. If able, insert a lubricated finger into the anus. Move the finger in a circle until the sphincter muscle relaxes. This may take a few minutes. After stimulation, sit in your normal position on the toilet, commode, or bedpan. Maintain privacy and try to relax. Contracting your stomach muscles and bending forward while bearing down can help increase pressure to evacuate the bowel. If you do not have a bowel movement within 20 minutes, repeat the process.

- You doctor may order a suppository or an enema to help stimulate the bowels. Results usually take about 30 minutes.

- Use Kegel exercises to help strengthen your pelvic rectal muscles. See the bladder retraining guidelines for instructions for performing these exercises.

- If you need to strengthen your rectal sphincter, your doctor may recommend *biofeedback*. A monitoring electrode will be placed on the abdomen, and a plug will be inserted into the rectum. This plug is attached to a computer that displays a graph of your rectal and abdominal muscle contractions as you squeeze them around the plug. The display provides feedback regarding the strength of these muscle contractions and will help you increase the intensity of your contractions.

To be most effective, many of these action items may be done together to make a total program. Know that residents will have both good and bad days. The key to success is to keep trying.

Using the Key Terms

Complete the following sentences using key terms in this section.

1. A blockage of hard stool in the rectum is called _____.
2. _____ is gas or air in the gastrointestinal tract that can be expelled via the anus.
3. In a(n) _____, liquid is inserted into the rectum to clean the intestines.
4. A(n) _____ is a protrusion of an organ through the wall of a body cavity.
5. When residents _____, they have a bowel movement.
6. A(n) _____ is a surgically created opening on the abdomen through which stool is eliminated.
7. A(n) _____ is a small, meltable cone that is inserted into a body passage.
8. The surgical procedure that creates an opening in the abdominal wall is a(n) _____.
9. _____, or the contraction of muscles, moves substances through the GI system.

Know and Understand the Facts

10. Describe how the color of urine and stool can indicate the condition of the body.
11. Identify two problems residents can have with elimination and how nursing assistants can assist.
12. What are three actions that can be taken for bladder retraining?
13. Discuss two reasons why performing catheter care is important.
14. What are the three differences in helping a resident use the toilet versus using a bedside commode?

Analyze and Apply Concepts

15. Explain how to record bowel movements.
16. Describe the steps needed to help a resident use a bedpan.
17. What steps would a nursing assistant follow to empty an ostomy bag?
18. Describe the steps for performing catheter care on a female.
19. What are two important steps when inserting a suppository?
20. If you were giving instructions to a new nursing assistant about helping a resident use a bedside commode, what three actions would be important to include?

Think Critically

Read the following care situation. Then answer the questions that follow.

Mr. L is 26 years old and has just been transferred from the ICU. He was in a motorcycle accident and has a broken leg and arm and a severe injury to his abdomen that required a temporary colostomy. He also has a urinary catheter. Mr. L is able to dangle on the side of the bed with assistance and is on a soft diet. He is on I&O. His girlfriend is with him most of the time and likes to help as much as she can. You are working the day shift, and Mr. L is one of five patients assigned to you today.

21. Describe the procedure for caring for Mr. L's catheter. Identify two areas of special concern, given Mr. L's condition.
22. Describe the procedure for caring for Mr. L's stoma. Identify two areas of special concern, given Mr. L's condition.
23. Are there any specific safety or care problems you might encounter when taking care of Mr. L?
24. What actions can you take to include Mr. L's girlfriend in his care?

Key Points

Reviewing the key points for this chapter will help you practice more safely and competently as a holistic nursing assistant and will help you prepare for the certification competency exam.

- Measuring and recording a resident's intake and output (I&O) provides important indicators about the amount of fluids consumed.
- Nursing assistants work closely with the licensed nursing staff to help monitor IV catheters during parenteral IV infusions.
- A urinary catheter may need to be inserted or a surgical procedure called an *ostomy* may be required to aid in elimination.
- Maintaining proper hygiene and skin integrity are essential while providing aid during toileting, measuring and recording bowel movements, providing catheter and colostomy care, changing drainage bags, and supporting bladder and bowel retraining.
- Elimination problems can be difficult, painful, and embarrassing. Holistic nursing assistants should try to make residents' experiences more pleasant and comfortable.

Action Steps to Holistic Care

Review the information in this chapter. Complete the following activities.

1. Select one procedure you learned in this chapter. Prepare a short paper or digital presentation that identifies and describes the three most important practices. Include one that promotes comfort and one that ensures safety.
2. With a partner, select one elimination problem. Prepare a poster that illustrates at least four facts about the problem.
3. Find two pictures in a magazine, in a newspaper, or online that advertise treatments or medications for people with elimination problems. Describe each image and explain why it was selected.
4. Research current scientific information about incontinence. Write a brief report describing two current facts about incontinence and incontinence solutions.
5. Create an instructional handout for residents discussing the guidelines for bladder and bowel retraining. Along with instructions for retraining, also include a section for fellow nursing assistants discussing strategies for assisting and supporting residents during these processes.

✓ Preparing for the Certification Competency Examination

To prepare for the nursing assistant certification competency examination, you will need to know content found in this chapter. This content may be tested in the knowledge (written or oral) and skills (hands-on demonstration) portions of the exam. The following areas will be emphasized:

- hydration, the consequences of dehydration, and situational factors that influence adequate intake
- sources of fluid intake and output
- fluid restrictions
- calculations for accurate intake and output
- factors that contribute to elimination practices and problems
- care for residents who are incontinent
- catheter and ostomy care
- rectal tubes, suppositories, and enemas
- bladder and bowel retraining programs

These sample test questions are similar to ones you will find on the certification competency exam. See how well you can answer them. Be sure to select the *best* answer.

1. A nursing assistant is observing a resident who has an IV catheter. To detect infiltration, she should observe the skin around the catheter for
   A. swelling
   B. dehydration
   C. warmth
   D. sweating

2. Which of the following describes the frequent expulsion of liquid stool from the body?
   A. CAUTI
   B. constipation
   C. GERD
   D. diarrhea

(continued)

3. Ms. J has had diarrhea all night, and a nursing assistant had to change her linens three times. When Ms. J has diarrhea again, what should the nursing assistant do first?

   A. sigh and quickly help her go to the toilet
   B. tell her he will be right back
   C. quietly change her linens and gown and help her wash
   D. assure her he understands and is happy to help

4. Mrs. O has a catheter. Why should the nursing assistant keep the urinary drainage bag secured to the bed below her?

   A. so that the weight of the bag can cause urine to drain
   B. so that the force of gravity can allow urine to drain
   C. to keep the drainage bag out of the way
   D. so the family does not see Mrs. O's urine

5. A nursing assistant is measuring intake for Mr. G. What should the nursing assistant do?

   A. monitor for dehydration
   B. measure for specific gravity
   C. keep the container at eye level
   D. check the pH of the urine

6. Kegel exercises are used to

   A. control excessive diarrhea
   B. retrain the bladder and bowels
   C. help close a stoma
   D. alleviate cramping and pain

7. When a nursing assistant is administering a cleansing enema, the bag should be

   A. below the resident for best drainage
   B. at the same height as the resident
   C. above the resident for best flow
   D. anywhere that is convenient

8. A new nursing assistant is providing catheter care for Mr. J. What should he do to help prevent a CAUTI?

   A. keep the tubes unkinked
   B. not pull on the tubes
   C. check for a foreskin
   D. keep the tubes coiled

9. A severe complication of constipation is

   A. impaction
   B. hernia
   C. hemorrhoid
   D. incontinence

10. A nursing assistant is taking care of Mr. D, who has had a colostomy. She will be providing ostomy care. When she removes his pouch, what is the first action she should take?

    A. gently cleanse the area around the stoma
    B. provide perineal care, if it is needed
    C. place a protective shield on the stoma
    D. measure the size of his stoma

11. Ms. A has not been feeling well. She refused her breakfast and lunch, and does not want to drink any fluids. Which of the following are the first signs of dehydration?

    A. dry mouth and increased thirst
    B. fainting and chest pains
    C. swollen tongue and headache
    D. confusion and heart palpitations

12. A nursing assistant was emptying the bedpan for Mrs. L. When she saw the color of Mrs. L's stool, she notified the licensed nursing staff immediately. Which of the following colors requires this response?

    A. orange
    B. yellow
    C. black
    D. green

13. I&O is measured in

    A. liters
    B. milliliters
    C. grams
    D. milligrams

14. A new nursing assistant is aware that, when caring for residents with elimination problems, he should

    A. ignore the residents so they are not embarrassed
    B. put on residents' favorite music so they can relax
    C. be patient, reassuring, and supportive
    D. make sure residents wear double-padded briefs to prevent accidents

15. A nursing assistant observes that Mr. J's urine is amber. What might this mean?

    A. He is bleeding.
    B. He has a urinary tract infection.
    C. He is dehydrated.
    D. He has a kidney stone.

Did you have difficulty with any of the questions? If you did, review the chapter to find the correct answer(s).

CHAPTER 24 Disabilities, Cognitive Disorders, and Mental and Emotional Health

Welcome to the Chapter

In this chapter, you will learn about disabilities, including vision, hearing, or speech impairments; congenital and genetic disorders; and disability caused by trauma or injury. You will also explore cognitive disorders, such as delirium and dementia. You will examine how cognitive disorders impact daily living. Learning about these disabilities and disorders will help you understand how you can assist those affected.

As you read this chapter, you will learn what mental and emotional health are and how they are influenced by developmental, social, and environmental factors. You will become familiar with emotional health concerns and mental health conditions, including anxiety disorders, trauma- and stress-related disorders, depressive disorders, substance-use disorders, personality disorders, and schizophrenia spectrum disorder. You will also learn about risk factors and responses to self-harm and suicide. This knowledge will help you understand the responsibilities holistic nursing assistants have when providing care.

The information presented in this chapter will help you build the knowledge and skills needed to become a holistic nursing assistant. The topics discussed in the chapter are highlighted on the Providing Holistic Care Framework.

You are now ready to start this chapter, *Disabilities, Cognitive Disorders, and Mental and Emotional Health.*

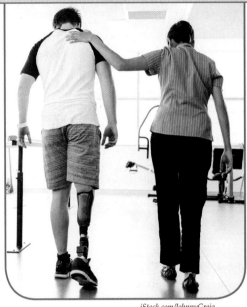

iStock.com/JohnnyGreig

Chapter Outline

Section 24.1
Disabilities and Cognitive Disorders

Section 24.2
Emotional Health Concerns and Mental Health Conditions

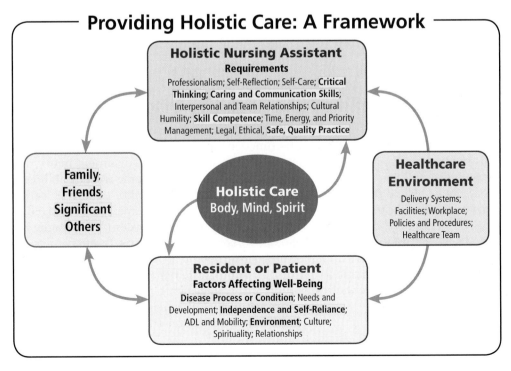

Providing Holistic Care: A Framework

Holistic Nursing Assistant
Requirements
Professionalism; Self-Reflection; Self-Care; **Critical Thinking; Caring and Communication Skills;** Interpersonal and Team Relationships; Cultural Humility; **Skill Competence;** Time, Energy, and Priority Management; Legal, Ethical, **Safe, Quality Practice**

Family; Friends; Significant Others

Holistic Care
Body, Mind, Spirit

Healthcare Environment
Delivery Systems; Facilities; Workplace; Policies and Procedures; Healthcare Team

Resident or Patient
Factors Affecting Well-Being
Disease Process or Condition; Needs and Development; **Independence and Self-Reliance;** ADL and Mobility; **Environment;** Culture; Spirituality; Relationships

Questions to Consider

- Think about a person you know who has experienced significant changes in his or her ability to walk, speak, hear, or see. Maybe this person had an accident and now needs to use crutches or a wheelchair. Maybe the person has a hard time hearing. How do you think these changes impacted the person's daily life?
- What emotions and feelings did this person have after realizing the extent of the change to his or her life? What did the person do to adjust?
- Were the adjustment strategies effective, or did the person have to make modifications? What could you have done to help?

Objectives

Experiencing disability is a life-changing event. Losing the ability to speak or having a traumatic injury can make living life very challenging. For example, just holding a conversation with someone or walking to the refrigerator can be demanding. This is also true for cognitive disorders such as dementia. When a person has Alzheimer's disease (a form of dementia), memory loss interferes with the rhythm of daily life and makes it difficult to complete simple tasks. This is not only frustrating; it can be discouraging. Learning how to best help people with disabilities and cognitive disorders is essential to providing safe, quality care. To achieve the objectives for this section, you must successfully

- **discuss** the difficulties associated with vision, hearing, and speech impairments;
- **explain** the impact of congenital disorders, heredity, and developmental disorders;
- **identify** issues related to trauma, injury, and paralysis;
- **describe** the dimensions, behaviors, and challenges of delirium and dementia; and
- **examine** the care that residents who have disabilities and cognitive disorders require.

Key Terms

Learn these key terms to better understand the information presented in the section.

acuity	neural tube
cerebral palsy (CP)	paralysis
cues	paranoia
cystic fibrosis (CF)	retinal detachment
delusions	scoliosis
hydrocephalus	spina bifida (SB)
intoxication	ventilator
legal blindness	

What Are Disabilities and Cognitive Disorders?

In this section of the chapter, you will examine disabilities and cognitive disorders. A *disability* is a limitation of a person's function. Disability can occur due to aging, a disease process, congenital or genetic disorders, developmental disorders, injury, or trauma. Disabilities affect one or more body systems, and people with disabilities may not be able to fully function in all activities. Some disabilities you will learn about are vision, hearing, and speech impairments; Down syndrome; spina bifida (SB), cystic fibrosis (CF); cerebral palsy (CP); autism spectrum disorder (ASD); fragile X syndrome (FXS); traumatic brain injury (TBI); spinal cord injury (SCI); and paralysis.

A *cognitive disorder* is a limitation on a person's ability to remember, learn, process and understand information, and display appropriate behavior in social settings. Cognitive disorders are the result of organic changes in the brain. Some cognitive disorders are reversible, and others are permanent. Reversible cognitive disorders are treatable and are usually called *delirium*. Delirium may be caused by a medical condition (such as electrolyte imbalance) or by **intoxication** (a condition resulting from the overuse of a prescription medication or drug). Progressive, permanent cognitive disorders are called *dementia*. Types of dementia include Alzheimer's disease (AD), Lewy body dementia, and dementia caused by HIV/AIDS.

In chapters 8 and 9, you learned about the anatomy, physiology, diseases, and conditions of the body systems. You also learned about signs and symptoms, congenital and genetic disorders, and limitations due to injury. In the following sections, you will further explore the impact of various diseases, disorders, and conditions that cause disability. You will become familiar with the care considerations you need to know to assist residents with disabilities.

How Can Nursing Assistants Best Assist Those with Vision Impairment or Loss?

People who have *vision impairments* have difficulty seeing due to changes or conditions of the eye. Vision impairment is especially common among older adults. As a nursing assistant, you will encounter many residents with vision impairments. You may care for some residents who have vision loss. Learning to meet the needs of these residents is important to providing safe, quality care.

Refractive Errors

Refractive errors are eye conditions that cause changes in visual **acuity** (*clearness*) and can result in disability if left uncorrected. Refractive errors occur when the length of the eye, the shape of the cornea, or the lens of the eye changes. These changes often occur due to aging, though some refractive errors are present at a young age. There are four common types of refractive errors:

- **Myopia (nearsightedness)**: a person has clear near vision and blurry far vision.

- **Hyperopia (farsightedness)**: a person has blurry near vision and clear far vision.

- **Presbyopia**: an older person cannot focus on a single, close object or page of text.

- **Astigmatism**: causes problems with focus.

The first symptom of a refractive error is blurred vision. Other symptoms include haziness, sensitivity to glare, squinting, double vision, or headaches. Optometrists and ophthalmologists diagnose refractive errors after comprehensive eye examinations. During the examination, a person's vision is compared to the standard of 20/20 vision. With 20/20 vision, a person can look at an eye chart and clearly see predetermined letters and numbers at the 20/20 size (Figure 24.1). A person who has 20/40 vision can only see predetermined letters and numbers at the 20/40 size, which is larger.

People who have refractive errors often use vision-correction devices, including the following:

- **Eyeglasses**: Eyeglass lenses are prescribed to correct refractive errors and make a person's vision as close to 20/20 as possible. People who have both near- and farsightedness may have *bifocal* or *progressive lenses* that accommodate both errors. People who have more than one refractive error may also choose to use two pairs of eyeglasses.

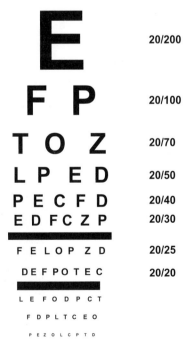

Figure 24.1 A person with 20/20 vision can see the letters at the 20/20 level without correction.

- **Contact lenses**: Contact lenses are also prescribed to correct refractive errors and help people achieve 20/20 vision. Contact lenses are shaped to fit and sit on the surface of the eye to provide clearer vision. Some people wear contact lenses all day, but not while sleeping (as tears do not bring enough oxygen to the eye when the eyelids are closed). Extended-wear contact lenses can be worn all of the time until they need to be changed. Some eye conditions prevent people from wearing contact lenses, and not all people find contact lenses convenient or comfortable to wear.

Another option for treating refractive errors is *refractive surgery*. Refractive surgery permanently reshapes the cornea and restores the eye's ability to focus, thus bringing vision closer to 20/20.

Low Vision and Vision Loss

Low vision is different from a refractive error. People with low vision may have partial blindness, have blurry vision, have poor night vision or tunnel vision, see only shadows, or not be able to distinguish shapes or objects. Low vision interferes with a person's ability to perform ADLs. Unlike refractive errors, low vision cannot be corrected by eyeglasses, contact lenses, medications, or surgeries. Vision loss can result in **legal blindness**, which is described as a refractive error of 20/200 even after vision correction. People who have *total blindness* cannot see even light. In the absence of vision, touch is the most important sense.

Low vision or vision loss can occur at birth, be caused by injury to the brain or eyes, or result from emergencies such as **retinal detachment** (separation of the retina from the back of the eye). Low vision and vision loss can also be caused by a disease (for example, diabetic retinopathy), a stroke, tumors or inflammation in the optic nerve, surgery (such as removal of the eyeball), and aging.

Three vision-related diseases and conditions that can lead to low vision or vision loss are cataracts, glaucoma, and macular degeneration (Figure 24.2). You learned about these diseases and conditions in chapter 9.

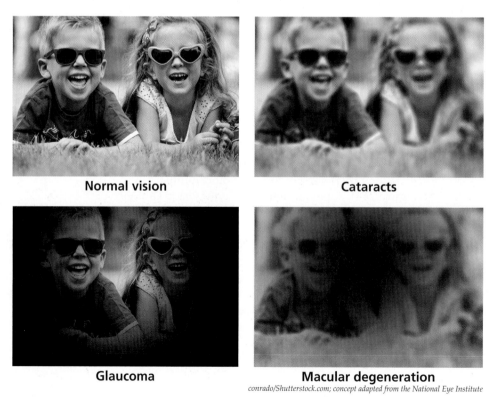

Normal vision

Cataracts

Glaucoma

Macular degeneration

conrado/Shutterstock.com; concept adapted from the National Eye Institute

Figure 24.2 Cataracts, glaucoma, and macular degeneration affect eyesight and can lead to severe vision impairment or loss.

Care Considerations for Vision Impairment or Loss

As a nursing assistant, you will care for residents with vision impairments ranging from refractive errors to legal blindness. The most important parts of caring for a resident with vision impairment or loss are maintaining a safe environment and helping the resident retain self-esteem and have a life that still includes enjoyable activities.

Caring for Eyeglasses

Eyeglasses should be washed at least once a day or whenever they are dirty. To wash eyeglasses, hold the frames by gripping the piece that crosses the bridge of the nose (Figure 24.3). Gently rub the lenses using warm, soapy water. Let the lenses air-dry and then wipe them with a soft, clean, lint-free cloth. Never wipe dry lenses with an abrasive cloth, such as paper towels, tissues, or napkins, as these can scratch the surface. If using a spray or cleanser, select one made for eyeglasses.

Once the eyeglasses are clean, give them back to or place them on the resident. Be sure eyeglasses are placed appropriately and ask if they are comfortable. Eyeglasses should be stored in a strong, sturdy case to protect against scratching, bending, or breaking. Always remind residents where eyeglasses are stored. Make sure that eyeglasses are easily accessible and that residents wear them when they get out of bed. When laying eyeglasses down, put them in a safe, secure place and fold them flat with the frame (not lens) side down.

Caring for Contact Lenses

Practice hand hygiene before handling contact lenses to remove dirt, oils, and lotions and then dry hands with a lint-free towel. When cleaning contact lenses, put the lenses in the palm of your hand and gently rub each lens with the index finger of the other hand (Figure 24.4). Use the special care solutions, cleaners, and drops designated for the contact lenses and never let the tips of the solution bottles touch other surfaces. Do not use tap water directly on the lenses. Every time the lens case is used, clean it with a sterile solution or hot tap water and let it air-dry. Replace the lens case every three months. Check with the licensed nursing staff regarding the placement of lenses in a resident's eyes. Always act according to facility policy and scope of practice.

Caring for Ocular Prostheses

An *ocular prosthesis*, or *prosthetic eye*, is fitted to the inner eye socket and is held in place by the upper and lower eyelids (Figure 24.5). An ocular prosthesis should be cleaned daily. Before inserting or removing an ocular prosthesis, check with the licensed nursing staff and be sure you are acting according to facility policy and scope of practice. When removing an ocular prosthesis, take care and place it in a plastic container filled with lukewarm water and padded with sterile gauze to prevent scratching. Rinse the eye socket with saline and warm water. To clean the ocular prosthesis, practice hand hygiene and use a soft brush with mild soap or the ordered cleaner and lukewarm water. Then rinse the prosthesis with clear water. If a resident does not wear the prosthesis overnight, the prosthesis should be cleaned; stored in a dry, closed container; and cleaned again before insertion.

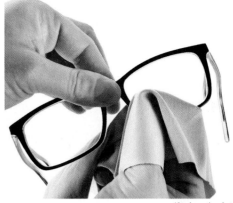
iStock.com/s-cphoto
Figure 24.3 When cleaning eyeglasses, be sure to hold them by the piece that crosses the bridge of the nose. Do not hold them by the arms or lenses.

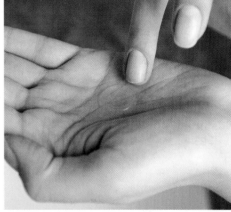
iStock.com/agrobacter
Figure 24.4 Contact lenses should be cleaned in the palm of your hand using the index finger of your other hand.

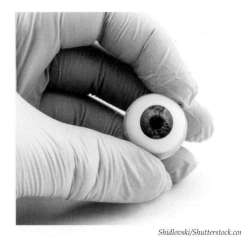
Shidlovski/Shutterstock.com
Figure 24.5 An ocular prosthesis is a false eye that is inserted into the eye socket.

Supporting and Promoting Self-Reliance and Independence

Self-reliance and independence are important and must be supported for residents who have vision impairments. Some residents who have vision impairments may not ask for help and may believe vision impairment or loss is an inevitable result of aging. As a result, these residents may stay in their rooms, be less active or social, and fall (often causing bruising or injury). Residents may also be embarrassed, angry, or lonely. As a holistic nursing assistant, recognize these feelings and be compassionate and patient. Respond by helping residents be as self-reliant and independent as safely possible. Encourage residents to participate in social activities and interact with others. It is important to remember that, if a resident has a vision impairment, procedures may take longer and require ongoing verbal instructions. Use a normal tone of voice, but be sure the resident can hear what you are saying.

Ensuring Safety

Residents who have vision impairments or loss may experience difficulty becoming oriented to new settings and maintaining mobility. Providing orientation to every new setting and having residents touch the areas surrounding them (especially handrails) will provide a sense of comfort and help residents not hit or fall over objects. When helping a resident ambulate, offer your arm or hand, walk one step ahead of the resident, provide verbal directions, and alert the resident to any obstacles along the way. If a resident needs to go up or down stairs, walk one step ahead of the resident, provide instructions for going up or down, and be sure the resident is holding onto the railing. Other safety measures for residents with vision impairments include good lighting, a room that is neat and free from clutter, and an accessible call light. Make sure that residents who have glasses wear them.

Assisting with Eating and Drinking

Assisting with eating and drinking is important for making mealtimes pleasant and easy. Helping residents perform hand hygiene is essential, as residents may want to feel or touch their food. When helping a resident eat, identify each eating utensil and explain where it is placed. Also explain the position of the food on the plate. Use the hands of the clock to identify food locations. For example, you could say that the carrots are at 6:00. Cut up larger pieces of food so they are easier to manage and do not overfill cups or glasses. When helping residents drink, tell them how full the glass is. Have residents use their index fingers to feel the glass and liquid level.

Helping with Daily Activities

Many assistive devices can be used to help residents who have vision impairments with daily activities, such as reading and recreational and leisure activities. Some of these devices include large-print books and magazines, magnifying glasses, audio clocks and books, spoken computer programs, writing aids (such as templates and bold-lined paper), and devices discussed in previous chapters. A resident with legal blindness may use *Braille*, a system of raised dots that can be read with the fingers. Residents with legal blindness may also rely on a guide dog (Figure 24.6), if allowed by facility policy.

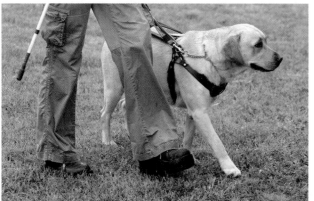

Belish/Shutterstock.com

Figure 24.6 Guide dogs can help people with vision loss navigate new spaces and avoid danger.

How Should Nursing Assistants Assist Those with Hearing Impairment or Loss?

Hearing impairments are characterized by reduced hearing. Many factors can lead to hearing impairment or loss. In chapter 8, you learned about the anatomy of the ear. The structures of the ear receive and convert vibrations into sound waves, which are interpreted by the brain.

The intensity of sound is measured in *decibels (dB)*. The least audible sound is 0 dB, a whisper is 30 dB, and a normal conversation is 60 dB. Sounds between 80 and 90 dB (the sound of a power lawn mower) increase risk for hearing impairment or loss, and injury to the ear occurs at 120 dB (to compare, the sound of a jet engine taking off is 140 dB). The duration of sound at a certain decibel is also important. At the most, a person should be exposed to sounds between 80 and 90 dB eight hours a day; a person should be exposed to a sound of 115 dB for 15 minutes or less. A rapid loss of 30 dB or more of hearing ability is considered sudden hearing loss and requires immediate attention from a doctor.

Lengthy exposure to loud noises is a key factor that causes hearing impairment. Other factors that can lead to hearing impairment include certain medications, illnesses (such as hypertension or an ear infection), head trauma, heredity, and aging.

Hearing impairment can be permanent or reversible. Permanent hearing impairment occurs when there is damage to the inner ear or nerves. Reversible hearing impairment occurs when sound waves cannot reach the inner ear. An example of reversible hearing impairment is a punctured eardrum, which can be helped by treatment or surgery.

Signs and Symptoms of Hearing Impairment

People who have hearing impairments live daily with signs and symptoms that usually get worse over time. Hearing impairments can have a significant impact on quality of life and contribute to anxiety and depression. Coping with symptoms can be a daily challenge. Symptoms of hearing impairment include the following:

- not understanding words in a conversation or over the phone, especially when there is background noise
- asking others to speak more loudly and slowly
- turning up the volume of the television or radio
- hearing muffled words and sounds (for example, *s* and *f* may be hard to distinguish)
- experiencing ringing, roaring, or hissing sounds (called *tinnitus*)

Tests used to diagnose hearing impairments include a physical examination, screening, the use of a tuning fork, and audiometer testing conducted by an audiologist (Figure 24.7). In audiometer testing, a person indicates whether he or she can hear a range of tones and sounds transmitted through headphones.

The levels of hearing impairment are mild, moderate, severe, and profound. In *mild hearing impairment*, a person has difficulty hearing every word in the presence of background noise. A person who has *moderate hearing impairment* needs words to be repeated during conversations and has a hard time keeping up without a hearing aid. *Severe hearing loss* makes it hard to hear a conversation without a powerful hearing aid and the use of lip reading. In *profound hearing impairment*, a person is very hard of hearing and relies on lip reading and *American Sign Language (ASL)*. ASL is the primary language of people who are deaf and uses hand signs combined with facial expressions and body postures.

Aids for Hearing Impairments

Treatment options depend on the cause and severity of hearing impairment. Treatment may be as simple as the removal of earwax blockage or may involve surgery or cochlear implants. *Cochlear implants* amplify sounds directly into the ear canal and bypass any damaged or dysfunctional parts of the inner ear.

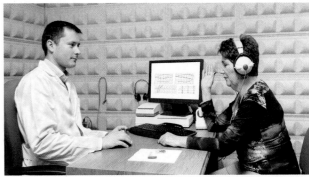

iStock.com/Maica

Figure 24.7 In audiometer testing, a person indicates whether he or she can hear certain sounds.

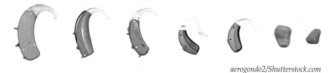

Figure 24.8 Hearing aids come in different shapes and sizes. They can be placed behind the ear, in the ear, or in the ear canal.

aerogondo2/Shutterstock.com

A *hearing aid* (a small, electronic device worn in or behind the ear) can help those whose inner ears are damaged due to disease, aging, injury, noise, or certain medications (Figure 24.8). A hearing aid cannot restore hearing, but it can make sounds stronger and result in better hearing. The greater the hearing impairment is, the more amplification is needed.

A hearing aid is composed of a microphone, amplifier, and speaker. The aid receives sound through the microphone, which converts sound waves into signals that are transmitted to the amplifier. The amplifier increases the power of the signals and sends them to the ear.

There are two types of hearing aids. *Analog hearing aids* convert sound waves into electrical signals, which are then amplified. *Digital hearing aids* convert sound waves into numerical codes (like the binary code of a computer) and then amplifies them. Hearing aids are placed in various parts of the ear (Figure 24.9).

Care Considerations for Hearing Impairment or Loss

As a nursing assistant, you will care for many residents who have hearing impairments. You should use the following considerations and guidelines when taking care of these residents:

- Turn off background noise when conversing.
- Position yourself so you are facing the resident.
- Never stand over the resident. If a resident is in a wheelchair, position yourself at the same level.
- Gain the resident's attention before talking.
- Speak clearly and do not shout.

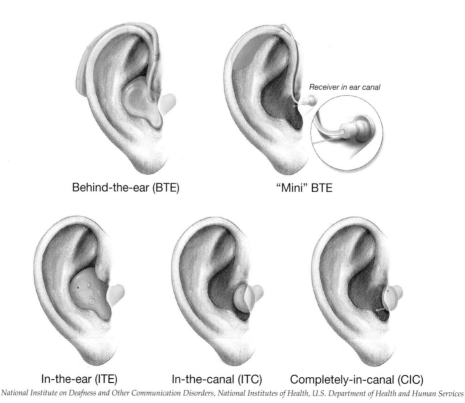

Behind-the-ear (BTE)   "Mini" BTE

Receiver in ear canal

In-the-ear (ITE)   In-the-canal (ITC)   Completely-in-canal (CIC)

National Institute on Deafness and Other Communication Disorders, National Institutes of Health, U.S. Department of Health and Human Services

Figure 24.9 Hearing aids can fit behind the ear, in the ear, or in the ear canal.

- Provide proper maintenance and care of hearing aids. Keep hearing aids away from heat and moisture and clean hearing aids per the manufacturer's instruction. Advise residents to avoid hair-care products when wearing hearing aids. Turn hearing aids off when they are not in use and immediately replace dead batteries.

- Use assistive listening devices, such as TV-listening systems or telephone-amplifying devices. Internet telephone services can also help residents hear phone calls.

How Can Nursing Assistants Help Those with Speech Impairment or Loss?

Speech impairments affect residents' abilities to communicate. Speech impairment or loss usually results from damage or injury to the part of the brain that controls language. One speech impairment you have already learned about is *aphasia*, which is an inability to understand and use words. Aphasia may be caused by a stroke, brain tumor, brain injury, infection, or dementia. The severity and scope of aphasia, from mild to severe, depends on the extent of damage and the area of the brain affected. There are four common types of aphasia:

- **Expressive aphasia (*nonfluent*)**: residents know what they want to say, but have difficulty communicating with others.
- **Receptive aphasia (*fluent*)**: residents can hear a voice or read, but may not understand the meanings of words. Residents take language literally and do not understand meanings, which disrupts speech.
- **Anomic aphasia**: residents struggle to find the right words to speak or write.
- **Global aphasia**: residents have difficulty speaking and understanding words and are unable to read or write. This type of aphasia is the most severe and often occurs after a stroke.

Speech and language therapy can help residents improve their abilities to communicate, restore as much language as possible, and find other methods of communication. The recovery of language skills is often a slow process and starts early after impairment or loss.

As a nursing assistant, you will provide care for residents with varying levels of speech impairment. The following considerations and guidelines will help you take care of these residents:

- Speak slowly and calmly.
- Use simple sentences.
- Use gestures and point to objects.
- Give the resident time to communicate.

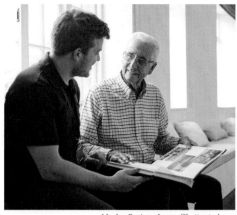

Monkey Business Images/Shutterstock.com

Figure 24.10 Books of words, illustrations, and photos can help residents communicate.

- Do not finish the resident's sentences or correct errors.
- Check the resident's comprehension and summarize what you have said.
- Eliminate any distracting noises.
- Ensure that paper and pencils or pens are available, if needed and appropriate.
- Write one word, write a short sentence, or use a gesture to help explain a procedure or direction.
- Help the resident create a book of words, illustrations, and photos to assist with communication (Figure 24.10).

Which Disabilities Are Due to Congenital and Genetic Disorders?

Some disabilities develop due to congenital or genetic disorders. *Congenital disorders* are caused by problems during fetal development prior to birth. Some of these disorders can be observed at birth. Others may be detected later in a person's life (for example, in the case of a congenital heart defect). *Genetic disorders* develop due to changes or mutations in the normal sequence of a person's DNA. A genetic disorder can be a mutation of one or multiple genes.

Congenital and genetic disorders that can cause disability include Down syndrome, spina bifida (SB), and cystic fibrosis (CF). Knowing about these disorders will help you understand how they affect the abilities and functions of those who have them.

Down Syndrome

Down syndrome is a genetic disorder in which a baby is born with an extra full or partial copy of chromosome 21. The presence of this extra genetic material results in developmental changes related to brain and body development. Two risk factors for Down syndrome are a mother over 35 years of age and a history of Down syndrome in the family. Many couples choose to have genetic screenings during pregnancy to determine if Down syndrome is a possible outcome for the baby. Life expectancy for people with Down syndrome has improved over the years, and today, a person with Down syndrome will often live to 60 years of age and have a full life. Many people with Down syndrome establish relationships, marry, and develop skills to work with some assistance (Figure 24.11).

Children who have Down syndrome have distinctive facial and body features, including a flat face; small ears; slanted eyes; a small mouth; and a short neck, arms, and legs. Children with Down syndrome experience physical disabilities related to poor muscle tone and loose joints. These disabilities can be improved with physical therapy. Down syndrome also causes intellectual disabilities and respiratory, cardiac, GI, and hearing problems. As a result, children with Down syndrome need speech, physical, and occupational therapy. Counseling can help the child and family deal with socioemotional issues.

Adults who have Down syndrome experience premature aging and may show symptoms of early-onset Alzheimer's disease (occurring before age 65). Symptoms can include a decline in the ability to pay attention, less interest in social activities and interaction, changes in coordination, fearfulness, irritability, and memory loss.

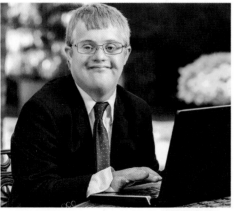

iStock.com/karelnoppe

Figure 24.11 Many people with Down syndrome live full lives as they manage their disabilities.

Spina Bifida (SB)

Spina bifida (SB) is a congenital disorder that results in incomplete development of the spinal cord. SB has genetic and environmental risk factors, including a history of developmental changes in the **neural tube** (structure from which the nervous system develops) and folic acid (vitamin B$_9$) deficiency, which can result in an incomplete spinal cord at birth. The severity of SB is affected by the size and location of the incomplete spinal cord development, the presence of skin covering the affected area, and any protrusion of the spinal nerves.

At birth, visible signs of SB include an abnormal clump of hair or fat, a small dimple, or a birthmark on the baby's back. The most severe form of SB results in a *myelomeningocele*, which occurs when vertebrae in the lower or middle back do not cover and protect the spinal cord. The spinal cord may protrude through the vertebrae, forming a sac that may or may not be covered by skin (Figure 24.12). This area, especially if not covered by skin, is at increased risk for infection.

Common impairments associated with SB are leg muscle weakness and paralysis, bowel and bladder problems, **hydrocephalus** (a condition of fluid in the brain), seizures, developmental changes in the feet, and **scoliosis** (a condition of a spine curved sideways). Most people with SB can walk for short distances, but need assistive devices such as braces, canes, crutches, and wheelchairs for longer distances. Some people with SB may experience challenges related to learning and emotional health due to physical disabilities. Most adults who have SB can live until 35 or 40 years of age. With more recent treatment methods, some adults with SB live 60 or more years.

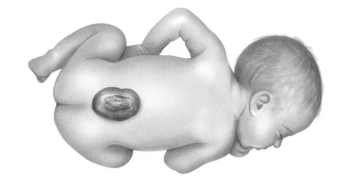

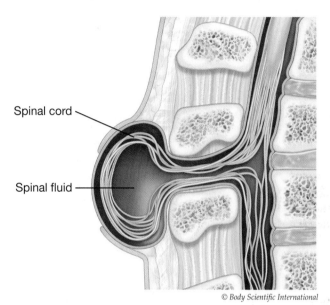

© *Body Scientific International*

Figure 24.12 Babies born with SB may have a myelomeningocele, or a place where the spinal cord protrudes through the spine.

Several treatments can help ease symptoms and improve quality of life for people with SB. These treatments include surgery to close the sac of a myelomeningocele, a surgically placed ventricular shunt to drain fluid from the brain into the abdomen, the management of paralysis and bladder and bowel problems, physical therapy and exercises that aid in walking, and the use of braces or crutches. Some people also benefit from behavioral therapy and assistance with any learning challenges.

Cystic Fibrosis (CF)

Cystic fibrosis (CF) is a genetic disorder that changes how the body makes mucus and sweat. In the United States, all states screen newborns for CF; however, symptoms of CF may not immediately appear. Symptoms of CF vary, but typically include very thick mucus that affects the respiratory system, causes congestion in the lungs, and makes breathing difficult. CF also affects the GI system. It causes difficult digestion and salty sweat that interferes with electrolytes and results in a lack of sufficient perspiration. Other symptoms of CF are constipation and stomach pain; low bone density; and wide, rounded (*clubbed*) fingertips. The average life expectancy for people with CF is 37 years, but some people with CF live into their 40s and 50s. Several treatments help ease symptoms and improve the quality of life for people with CF:

- Daily postural drainage and percussion help mucus drain from the airways in the lungs. People with CF sit and lie in different positions (postural drainage) to make it easier for mucus to drain, and tapping on the chest (percussing) triggers a productive cough.

- Inhaled medications can reduce inflammation.
- Physical therapy increases the strength of the lungs.
- Aerobic exercise also increases strength, though people with CF should ingest extra salt if there is excessive sweating.

What Are Developmental Disabilities?

Developmental disabilities are a group of conditions that occur during a child's development and result in physical, learning, language, or behavioral impairment. These disabilities affect people throughout their lifetimes. In this section, you will learn about and examine the effects of several developmental disabilities, including cerebral palsy (CP), autism spectrum disorder (ASD), and fragile X syndrome (FXS). Knowing about these disabilities will help you understand how they affect the individuals who have them.

Cerebral Palsy (CP)

Cerebral palsy (CP) is a nonprogressive disability that affects movement, muscle tone, and posture. It is typically caused by damage to the developing fetal brain and is one of the most common causes of chronic childhood disability. Risk factors for CP include infections during pregnancy (such as rubella, or German measles); birth injuries; limited or poor oxygen supply to the baby's brain before, during, and immediately after birth; and prematurity. Rh blood incompatibility (in which the mother has a negative Rh factor and the baby has a positive Rh factor) is also a risk factor. In a second or later pregnancy, this incompatibility can cause a buildup of antibodies in the mother to attack the baby's red blood cells. CP can also develop during early childhood as a result of brain injury due to severe illness (such as meningitis), extensive physical trauma, or serious dehydration. If CP develops during early childhood, it will usually appear by age two or three. Life expectancy with CP depends on the severity of the disorder. People with mild CP can have the same life expectancy as the general population.

The physical disabilities associated with CP vary. A person with CP may have some combination of abnormal posture, impaired mobility, muscle rigidity and stiffness, abnormal reflexes and involuntary movements, and imbalance of the eye muscles (Figure 24.13). People with CP may also have swallowing problems, epilepsy, vision or hearing impairments, intellectual disabilities, or learning disorders.

The goal of CP treatment is to maximize abilities and physical strength, prevent complications, and improve quality of life. Specific treatments vary, but usually include physical and speech therapy; the use of assistive equipment, such as special shoes, crutches, *orthotics* (artificial devices such as splints and braces), casts, special seats, walkers, and wheelchairs; massage therapy; yoga and breathing exercises; biofeedback; medications; surgery; and pain relief. Some people with CP also benefit from behavioral therapy and occupational therapy, which promotes independent living.

Autism Spectrum Disorder (ASD)

Autism spectrum disorder (ASD) is a developmental disability that can cause considerable social, communication, and behavioral challenges. ASD includes a wide range, or *spectrum*, of symptoms and levels of disability.

A person with ASD does not exhibit any distinguishing physical characteristics, but ASD does affect how a person communicates, behaves, and learns. The signs of ASD begin in early childhood

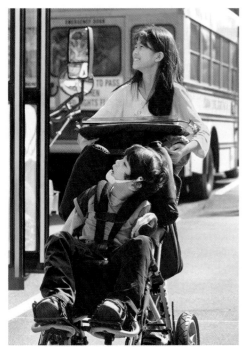

Figure 24.13 CP can result in impaired mobility, depending on the severity of the disorder.

and last throughout life. Signs and symptoms that may be observed in children or adults include the following:

- having trouble relating to or not having interest in others
- avoiding eye contact and wanting to be alone
- repeating or echoing communicated words or phrases
- repeating words or phrases in place of normal language
- repeating actions over and over again
- having trouble understanding other people's feelings or sharing feelings
- generally preferring not to be held or cuddled
- struggling to express needs using typical words or emotions

There is a wide range of skill levels among people with ASD. Some people with ASD need a great deal of assistance, while others do not. Treatments for ASD include behavioral and communication approaches (such as auditory training); music, occupational, and physical therapy; dietary changes (such as removing certain foods from a child's diet or using vitamin or mineral supplements); and medications to manage symptoms such as lack of focus or possible depression.

Fragile X Syndrome (FXS)

Fragile X syndrome (FXS) is a genetic disorder caused by a change in the fragile X mental retardation 1 (FMR1) gene. This gene makes fragile X mental retardation protein (FMRP), which is needed for normal brain development. There is no cure for FXS, and males with FXS often have mild to severe intellectual disability. Females with FXS can have average intelligence, but may experience some degree of intellectual disability. ASD also occurs more frequently with people who have FXS.

Signs and symptoms of FXS may include developmental delays (such as missing a milestone for sitting or walking), trouble learning new skills, lack of eye contact, and difficulty paying attention. People with FXS may also be very active, flap their hands, and speak without thinking.

Treatment for FXS includes a variety of therapies that help with walking, talking, and other forms of communication. Medications may be used to help control behavioral issues, such as lack of focus or activity.

How Can Nursing Assistants Deliver Care After Trauma and Injury?

Trauma and injury can have a significant impact on a person's physical and cognitive abilities. Many parts of the body can be damaged due to injury. Soft tissues and organs can be injured, and neurological and skeletal damage can lead to *amputation* (the loss of a portion or all of an arm or a leg). These injuries are considered emergencies, and the goal of treatment is restoration and rehabilitation of function.

Two types of serious injury you will encounter as a nursing assistant are traumatic brain injury (TBI) and spinal cord injury (SCI). These injuries can result in loss of consciousness or a coma, partial or total paralysis, and the need to use a mechanical **ventilator** to breathe.

Traumatic Brain Injury (TBI)

Traumatic brain injury (TBI) is an acute and acquired injury to the brain. TBI can be caused by a vehicular accident, a bullet from a firearm, a fall, carbon monoxide or lead poisoning, tumors, infections, a stroke, and *deceleration injuries* (in which the brain hits the inside of the skull, causing contusion and swelling). Hypoxia can also cause TBI due to lack of oxygen in the brain. Anyone can experience a TBI, but young adults and older adults are especially at risk. According to recent information from the CDC, TBI is responsible for 30 percent of all injury-related deaths and for the majority of disabilities.

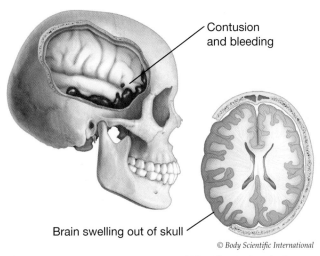

Contusion and bleeding

Brain swelling out of skull

© Body Scientific International

Figure 24.14 Increased pressure and bleeding in the skull can increase the severity of a brain injury.

Levels of TBI

After a TBI, the extent of brain injury may not become apparent until several days, weeks, or months later. Brain injury usually leads not only to physical disabilities, but also to mental and cognitive impairments, headaches, difficulty thinking, memory loss, changes in attention, mood swings, and personality changes. TBI can affect high-level cognitive functions and can also result in a coma. It can lead to limited function or paralysis of the arms and legs, loss of cognition, and abnormal speech or language patterns. TBI can also cause secondary brain injuries due to bleeding in the skull, increased pressure and fluid in the skull, and infection in the case of an open-head injury (Figure 24.14).

TBIs range from mild to severe, depending on loss of consciousness and level of confusion. Different scales determine and categorize the outcomes of TBI and impact on the body. Areas that may be assessed include motor responses (from fully obeying commands to not responding), verbal responses (from being alert to making no sounds), and eye opening (from spontaneous eye opening to no eye opening at all). Some scales also assess levels of consciousness, ranging from mild TBI to brain death (Figure 24.15). Scales provide a consistent way to determine levels of consciousness and outcomes.

Treatment for TBI

Treatment depends on the level and severity of TBI. After a TBI, immediate care such as surgery and other interventions may occur to reduce bleeding and swelling. As brain function improves, a person may experience confusion and disorientation, lack of attention, agitation and nervousness, and difficulty sleeping. Recovery is often not consistent—some days are better than others. Recovery is usually long and challenging. The effects of TBI can be overwhelming for a patient and his or her family. The goal of treatment is always to provide support and maximize function and independence.

Levels of Consciousness	
Level	**Status**
Mild TBI	A person experiences loss of consciousness and confusion lasting fewer than 30 minutes.
Moderate disability	A person experiences loss of consciousness lasting longer than 30 minutes and experiences physical and cognitive disabilities, but is still able to live independently.
Severe disability	A person is conscious, but is dependent on others for care.
Vigil coma	A person has minimal consciousness, but follows a sleep/wake cycle and opens and closes the eyes.
Vegetative state	A person is in a true coma or altered state of consciousness, has no voluntary responses to pain stimuli, and does not move the limbs except for reflex movements. The person's pupils do not respond to light. The coma can be reversed, but not if there is severe brain damage.
Persistent vegetative state	A person's eyes may be open, but the person displays no interaction with the environment.
Brain death	A person exhibits no brain function.

Figure 24.15 TBI can lead to different levels of consciousness, ranging from mild TBI to brain death.

Spinal Cord Injury (SCI)

Spinal cord injury (SCI) is damage to any part of the spinal cord, vertebrae, discs, nerves, or ligaments located at the end of the spine. SCI is equally as traumatic as TBI and usually causes permanent changes such as **paralysis** (loss of function and feeling) at the site of the injury. SCI is often accompanied by dysfunction in other body systems affected by that site (for example, loss of bladder or bowel control).

SCI can be caused by a fall, a blow to the back from a vehicular accident or sports injury, a bullet from a firearm, or a knife wound that severs the spinal cord. Other, nontraumatic causes of SCI include changes in bone density or structure, cancer, or degeneration of the vertebral discs due to aging. Damage can also occur if there is inflammation, bleeding, or swelling from fluid around the spinal cord.

Signs and Symptoms of SCI

The signs and symptoms of SCI include extreme pain or pressure in the neck, head, or back; weakness; numbness; loss of movement and sensation; spasms; difficulty breathing or coughing; loss of bladder or bowel control; and changes in sexual function.

The location and severity of the SCI will determine how much arm or leg control is lost. An injury to the neck (the cervical area of the spinal column) can affect arm movement and respiratory ability and all the functions below the site of the injury. An injury to the thoracic or lumbar part of the spinal column can affect the trunk, legs, bowel and bladder control, and sexual function (Figure 24.16).

Becoming a Holistic Nursing Assistant
Caring for a Patient in a Coma

After a TBI, some patients may experience a *coma*, or a state of prolonged unconsciousness. Some patients will be in a coma for a short period of time. Others may remain unconscious for a longer period of time or may not regain consciousness. Whatever level of consciousness a patient has, it is important to provide safe, quality care and be aware of the following guidelines:

- **Learn how to effectively communicate with those in a coma:** Establish a calm, supportive, and respectful environment when caring for someone in a coma. Remember that all patient rights apply to someone in a coma. Never talk about, around, or above someone in a coma. Rather, talk with the patient, even if you receive no response. Observe for small changes over time. Changes can be very subtle, such as a small movement of a finger or toe, a quick noise, or the opening or closing of eyes. When the eyes are open, the patient may be able to see and track movements.

- **Assume hearing is the last sense to go:** Always knock when entering the room and tell the patient who you are. Never leave a room without telling the patient you are leaving. Speak in a normal voice and tone, keep sentences short, and do not shout. You may read, sing, or play the patient's favorite music, as appropriate. If there is too much

noise in the room (for example, a television), turn off the source of the noise. Touch can be helpful, but be sure to tell patients you are going to touch them. Hold patients' hands as you talk with them. If appropriate, massage their arms, legs, hands, and feet.

- **Know that patients in comas may be feeling pain:** As you care for patients in comas, you can ask whether they are in pain. Patients may be able to answer using minimal communication. You can also observe for signs of pain, such as tears in the eyes. Always ask for permission to do a procedure, even if the patient cannot respond. Introduce yourself and let the patient know what you are doing step by step. Other helpful approaches include displaying personal photos in the room and keeping a comments book in the room so caregivers and family members can record any observed changes. Remember that, during recovery, there is much to do and learn. Know that patience is truly a virtue.

Apply It

1. What challenges would you face in providing holistic care to someone who is not conscious? How could you overcome these challenges?

2. What personal skills do you have that might help you care for a patient in a coma effectively?

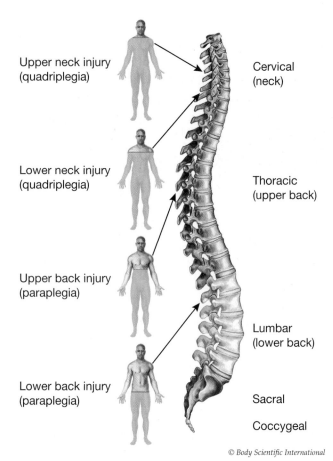

Upper neck injury (quadriplegia)

Lower neck injury (quadriplegia)

Upper back injury (paraplegia)

Lower back injury (paraplegia)

Cervical (neck)

Thoracic (upper back)

Lumbar (lower back)

Sacral

Coccygeal

© Body Scientific International

Figure 24.16 The location of an SCI determines what parts of the body are affected.

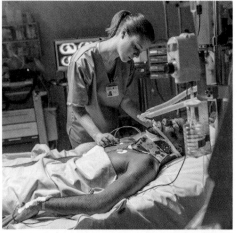

iStock.com/simonkr

Figure 24.17 Mechanical ventilators aid a patient's breathing. This aid can be extremely important for a patient who has experienced an SCI.

SCI severity is classified in terms of its "completeness." A SCI is complete when all movement and feeling are lost below the injury. If only some function or sensation below the injury is lost, the SCI is incomplete. Paralysis is classified according to what areas are affected. *Quadriplegia* (also called *tetraplegia*) is paralysis of the arms, trunk, legs, and pelvic organs. *Paraplegia* is paralysis of the trunk, legs, and pelvic organs. *Hemiplegia* is paralysis on one side of the body.

Treatment for SCI

Treatment for SCI starts with immediate and emergency attention to the injury. Initial care immobilizes the patient to prevent further injury, manages shock, and reduces complications. Surgery may also be performed, if needed.

Immediately after SCI, treatment focuses on correcting respiratory dysfunction, if needed. SCI can affect movement and sensation in the diaphragm and in the muscles of the chest wall and abdomen. As a result, a patient who has experienced SCI may be placed on a *mechanical ventilator* to support breathing (Figure 24.17). Before mechanical ventilation, the patient is *intubated*, which means an endotracheal (ET) tube is inserted into the trachea through the mouth or a *tracheostomy* (surgical opening in the trachea). The mechanical ventilator is attached to the ET tube. In some cases, the ventilator does all or most of the breathing for the patient. In other cases, the patient does some breathing. The ventilator is eventually removed through a slow process called *weaning*. A ventilator is set to the needs of the patient. If breathing patterns change, alarms will sound to notify caregivers.

Licensed nursing staff members have total responsibility for caring for patients with SCI. Nursing assistants can assist by providing proper care, accurate observation, and immediate reports of any changes to the licensed nursing staff. The care given by nursing assistants may include

- being alert to the ventilator alarm and reporting it immediately;
- monitoring vital signs, as ordered, to ensure they remain stable (Figure 24.18);
- assisting the licensed nursing staff with suctioning (removing secretions and mucus from) the ET tube and managing enteral feedings or IV catheters;
- performing routine oral and skin care;
- alerting the licensed nursing staff if the patient is or appears to be in pain;
- abiding by facility restraint procedures, if needed, to prevent the patient from pulling out or dislodging the tubes;
- ensuring a safe environment;
- providing positioning and range-of-motion (ROM) activities, as directed;
- keeping all equipment clean.

Patients on a mechanical ventilator are not able to speak. As such, you should establish a method of communication, if the patient is conscious. A method of communication might be lip reading, blinking the eyes when asked questions that require a yes or no (for example, one blink for yes and two blinks for no), pointing, using a picture board, or writing messages.

SCI cannot be reversed. After immediate intervention, longer-term treatment centers on preventing further injury and helping people have full and active lives. Lifestyle changes after SCI might include changes in diet and fluids to prevent dehydration, weight loss, bladder and bowel retraining (discussed in chapter 23), heightened attention to skin care to prevent decubitus ulcers, and pain relief. Patients who have experienced SCI may need assistance with mobility to prevent deep vein thrombosis (DVT) and issues with muscle spasticity (uncontrolled tightening or movement) or flaccidity (lack of muscle tone). Changes in sexual function and depression due to impairment may also be a concern and will require intervention.

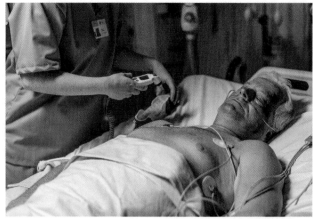
iStock.com/simonkr

Figure 24.18 One major responsibility of nursing assistants is taking regular vital signs. This is very important to caring for a patient who has experienced an SCI.

Often, medications are used to treat the effects of SCI. Sometimes devices can provide electrical stimulation to help control arm and leg muscles, aid patients in reaching and gripping objects, and assist with walking. A new technology called *robotic gait training* is being used for ambulation retraining.

Care Considerations for TBI and SCI

As a nursing assistant, you will care for patients who have experienced TBI and SCI. Patients who have experienced TBI or SCI may need assistive equipment to help with mobility and ADLs. For example, ramps, wide doors, special sinks, grab bars, driving equipment, and vehicle modifications promote greater independence and a safe environment. Computer adaptations and aids such as voice recognition and voice-controlled devices make communication easier after a TBI or SCI.

There are many ways to provide safe, quality care to those with TBI and SCI. For example, you may take vital signs; perform good skin and oral care; observe monitors, IV catheters, and tubes for possible changes or dysfunction; provide wound care; and help with mobility to prevent DVT. In addition to performing these tasks, you will also need to be aware of and sensitive to the feelings of those in your care. In just one day, one hour, or one minute, the life of a person with a TBI or SCI drastically changes. A person becomes someone he or she does not know and is faced with possibly indefinite disability. This is a difficult experience for everyone involved. The help you provide can aid the injured patient and his or her family with recovery. Understand that a period of grief and mourning will follow injury. A patient will initially be in denial and disbelief, and these feelings are often followed by sadness and anger. The hopeful outcome is acceptance. Trained caregivers and support groups can help the patient and his or her family.

Paralysis is a common result of TBI and SCI. As a holistic nursing assistant, you will care for patients who have varying levels of paralysis and who may be in a wheelchair. Patients may use electronic wheelchairs, some of which have the ability to climb stairs and travel over rough ground. As you deliver care to these patients, follow these guidelines:

- Consider your own perceptions and assumptions about patients who are paralyzed and who need to use a wheelchair.
- Always focus on the patient in your care and not on the disability.
- Consider each patient's special needs, as patients will have different capabilities.

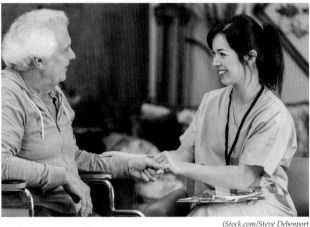

Figure 24.19 When talking with a patient in a wheelchair, sit down so you can maintain level eye contact.

iStock.com/Steve Debenport

- Be respectful. Never talk down to a patient or pat a patient on the head. Speak to the patient directly, and if the conversation lasts longer than a few minutes, find a seat so you can have level eye contact with the patient (Figure 24.19).
- Always ask a patient if assistance is needed before attempting to help. Do not rob a patient of his or her independence.
- If a patient is not sitting in his or her wheelchair, be sure the wheelchair is nearby.
- Never hang or lean on a wheelchair. Remember that a wheelchair is an important part of a patient's personal life space.

As you care for patients who have experienced TBI or SCI, you will work with professionals involved in TBI or SCI treatment. These professionals include neurosurgeons; orthopedic surgeons; physiatrists (doctors who specialize in physical medicine); licensed nursing staff; psychologists; dietitians; physical, occupational, and recreational therapists; and social workers. Many of these caregivers will have specialized training to help those with TBI and SCI.

What Is Delirium, and What Are Its Challenges?

As you learned earlier in this chapter, a *cognitive disorder* is characterized by difficulty thinking, remembering, learning, processing and understanding information, and displaying appropriate behavior in public settings. Cognitive disorders are the result of organic changes in the brain. Some cognitive disorders are reversible, and others are permanent. Reversible or treatable cognitive disorders are called *delirium*.

Delirium is usually caused by acute medical conditions, such as meningitis, urinary tract infections (UTIs), electrolyte imbalances, metabolic and endocrine disorders, and heatstroke. Delirium can also be caused by medications and intoxication or withdrawal from a substance. All of these conditions either disrupt the brain's ability to create and use energy or alter chemical messengers in the brain and nervous system. One type of delirium, known as *delirium not otherwise specified (NOS)*, can result from sensory deprivation (lack of sensory stimulation) or follow the use of general anesthesia. Older adults are most at risk for delirium.

Delirium is dramatic because of its sudden appearance. A person with delirium is confused; has a distorted sense of time; and experiences severe attention, memory, language, and perception problems.

The symptoms of delirium and dementia overlap, which sometimes causes difficulty determining the difference. The difference is that delirium, when treated effectively, will last no longer than one month after the onset of symptoms. If left untreated, delirium can cause more serious and permanent brain damage. Care considerations are similar to those discussed for residents with dementia.

How Can Nursing Assistants Care for Residents with Dementia?

Progressive, permanent cognitive disorders are known as *dementia*. Dementia is not a particular disease, but is rather a range of symptoms that begin slowly and gradually get worse. The most common form of dementia is *Alzheimer's disease (AD)*, followed by vascular dementia. *Vascular dementia* is caused by an acute event, such as a stroke, in which blood flow to the brain is interrupted. It can also develop more gradually over time due to very small blockages or the slowing of blood flow.

Symptoms of vascular dementia will appear more suddenly than symptoms of AD. There is no direct cause for AD. Factors that contribute to the development of AD include genetics, lifestyle, and other environmental factors. *Lewy body dementia* and *frontotemporal dementia* are two other forms of dementia. Some dementias are linked to diseases and disorders such as TBI or Parkinson's disease.

Dementia is caused by damage to brain cells. Once damaged, brain cells do not effectively communicate with each other, causing changes in thinking, behavior, and feelings. This damage can occur in different parts of the brain. For example, in AD, cells in the brain's center for learning and memory (hippocampus) are the first to be damaged. As a result, memory loss is one of AD's earliest symptoms.

Nonmodifiable risk factors for dementia are age and family history. Risk factors that can be modified are hypertension and atherosclerosis, obesity (managed by good nutrition and exercise), alcohol and nicotine use, diabetes, depression, and sleep apnea.

Signs and Symptoms of Dementia

The signs and symptoms of dementia vary greatly and include cognitive, psychological, and physical changes. As time passes, symptoms become more pronounced. For example, AD is characterized by three stages of progressing symptoms (Figure 24.20). Residents with AD usually live four to eight years after diagnosis, though some residents can live up to 20 years. Many times, people who have dementia do not recognize its symptoms. Symptoms of dementia are instead noticed and pointed out by family members or significant others.

Cognitive Changes

Cognitive changes progress over the course of dementia. Some of these cognitive changes include the following:

- memory loss (demonstrated by asking repeatedly for the same information, misplacing objects, and not remembering where one is)
- decreased ability to reason or problem-solve (demonstrated by working with numbers incorrectly or taking much longer to complete tasks)
- difficulty handling tasks such as reading and driving

Think About This

According to the World Health Organization (WHO), 47 million people worldwide have dementia, and there are 9.9 million new cases annually. Alzheimer's disease (AD) is the most common form of dementia and may contribute to 60–70 percent of cases. In the United States, more than 5 million people are living with AD, and this number will likely triple by 2050.

Stages of Alzheimer's Disease (AD)	
Stage	**Symptoms**
Early-stage or mild	The resident is able to function independently, but may have memory lapses (for example, may not remember new names or forget material just read). The resident may also have problems planning or organizing information.
Middle-stage or moderate	This stage is the longest. Continuing damage to brain cells causes difficulty doing daily activities, frustration, and anger. Memory loss, confusion, and restlessness continue, and the resident may wander and become lost. Personality and mood changes may lead to repetitive and compulsive behaviors such as hand wringing. During this stage, more aggressive behavior may occur such as biting, hitting, or swearing. This is also the stage where there may be sexual aggression. Physical changes include trouble controlling bladder and bowel functions and alterations in sleep patterns.
Late-stage or severe	The resident is no longer able to effectively interact with the environment, carry on a normal conversation, or control movements (sitting, walking, and eventually swallowing). The resident may still communicate at a very basic level, but experiences great memory and cognitive losses. The resident needs full-time care for all ADLs, including bathing, dressing, oral hygiene, and toileting. This stage can lead to coma and death, usually from a respiratory infection.

Figure 24.20 The symptoms of AD progress through three stages.

- lack of ability to plan and organize and poor judgment (demonstrated by overspending money or making unneeded purchases)
- confusion about time and dates and disorientation related to time and location
- trouble communicating, finding appropriate words, and following or joining a conversation
- distinct changes in coordination and motor function

Psychological Changes

Psychological changes include alterations in personality and mood that can lead to resistance, anxiety, agitation, **delusions** (irrational beliefs), hallucinations (false or distorted sensory experiences), and **paranoia** (unsupported or exaggerated distrust). Depression may also accompany dementia and will be discussed in more detail later in this chapter. Other psychological changes may lead to rummaging, hoarding items, and sundowning. *Sundowning* occurs at the end of the day and lasts into the evening. It is characterized by increased confusion, inability to follow directions, and anxiety (demonstrated by pacing and wandering). Residents may also become physically aggressive (demonstrated by hitting, pinching, scratching, biting, and hair pulling) and verbally aggressive (demonstrated by screaming, swearing, shouting, and making threats).

Aggression increases over the course of dementia and may be the result of insufficient sleep; pain; side effects from medications; a distracting, disorganized environment; loud noises; confusion from being asked too many questions or trying to understand something simple; and caregiver stress. *Perseveration* is another psychological change in which a resident has an uncontrollable need to repeat a word, phrase, or gesture for no apparent reason. Perseveration occurs due to organic changes in the brain.

Psychological changes during dementia also affect sexual behavior. For many older adults, including those living in long-term care facilities, sexuality remains an important part of life. Changes in sexual behavior result from organic changes in the brain and secondary issues such as physical discomfort. These changes may include less interest in sex; heightened libido; or inappropriate sexual behavior such as disrobing, exposure, masturbation, and fondling. These inappropriate sexual behaviors often occur as a result of confusion or disorientation. A resident may think he or she is at home in the privacy of a bedroom rather than in a public setting. Lack of control can also cause residents to act out their sexual urges with unwilling and inappropriate partners. Inappropriate sexual behaviors such as these can be embarrassing, frightening, and disturbing for a resident's family members, for other residents, and for caregivers.

As a nursing assistant, you may find that responding to inappropriate sexual behaviors is difficult. If a resident displays an inappropriate sexual behavior, be respectful, understanding, calm, and patient. Firmly but gently inform the resident that the behavior is inappropriate and guide the resident to a private area. Use distraction or redirect the resident to more positive activities, such as taking a walk or eating a favorite snack. Be sure to report any inappropriate sexual behaviors to the licensed nursing staff. These behaviors are important symptoms and signal changes in the resident's condition. Remember that these behaviors are not intentional, but are the result of organic brain changes.

As dementia progresses, more advanced psychological changes can develop. One of these advanced psychological changes is shadowing. *Shadowing* occurs when a resident follows a caregiver's every move due to growing feelings of dependency (Figure 24.21). The resident believes that staying close to the caregiver will fulfill his or her need for comfort and safety.

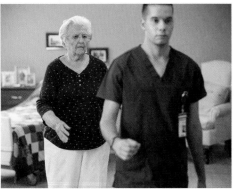

© *Tori Soper Photography*

Figure 24.21 As dementia progresses, residents may begin to shadow caregivers by following their every move.

Physical Changes

Physical changes also accompany dementia. Many of these changes have been discussed earlier (for example, trouble controlling bladder and bowel functions and alterations in sleep patterns). Issues related to nutrition develop from residents' inability to chew and swallow. Residents may also experience problems breathing if they choke on or aspirate food while eating. Choking and aspiration affect the respiratory system and may result in pneumonia. Falling is another physical challenge residents may encounter as they begin to lose their motor abilities. Maintaining a safe environment becomes a primary focus of care.

Treatment for Dementia

Treatment for dementia focuses on the management of symptoms; the restoration of as many daily functions as possible; and palliative care (providing relief and improving quality of life throughout a serious or life-threatening illness). The goal of care is to align with and support the capabilities of the resident. Many residents with dementia stay in long-term care facilities. Other residents are placed in special care or memory units, which deliver specialized care. Placement in a memory unit often occurs at later stages.

Prescribed medications have been shown to improve some symptoms of dementia. These medications often have side effects that result in GI system problems or dizziness.

Other approaches to the treatment of dementia include physical activity to help with sleep and reduce agitation; massage therapy; light therapy (exposure to bright light) for depression and sleep disorders; doll, cuddle, or toy therapy to bring back happy memories (reminiscence); and music and art therapy (including dance, drawing, and painting). Integrative medicine (IM) approaches include the use of aromatherapy and dietary and herbal supplements, though scientific evidence is limited. Pet assistive therapy (visits from specially trained animals) has been shown to improve mood and help promote appropriate behaviors in residents with dementia (Figure 24.22).

Care Considerations for Dementia

The greatest and ongoing benefit to residents with dementia is safe, quality care. As a holistic nursing assistant, you can take actions to help improve the daily life of a resident and help manage symptoms.

Understand Symptoms

As you care for residents with dementia, understand that dementia symptoms are caused by organic brain cell damage and secondary effects such as pain, infection, constipation, lack of sleep, and physical and psychological reactions to prescribed medications. Realize that many behaviors may result from unmet physical or social needs and always try to understand what might be causing behaviors.

Residents with dementia may not know *why* they are doing or feeling something, but will always know *how* they are feeling. When caring for a resident with dementia, try to determine if pain is the cause of a behavior. If it is, alert the licensed nursing staff.

Never take the behavior of residents with dementia personally, but be sure to protect yourself from personal danger and step back or stand away if residents are physically aggressive.

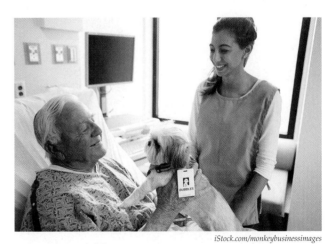

iStock.com/monkeybusinessimages

Figure 24.22 Specially trained animals can improve the mood of residents with dementia and encourage appropriate behaviors.

Respect Individuality

As a holistic nursing assistant, be sure to respect the individuality of residents and focus on them as people. Use the plan of care to guide activities and provide as much independence as is possible and safe, but understand that using reasoning and logic will not likely affect residents' behaviors, as residents cannot think or take action at that level of cognition.

Never try to restrain residents, even if they are physically aggressive. Instead, give adequate space and use distraction or redirection (for example, by affirming what they are saying and suggesting a different activity). For example, a resident may shout and start to move others out of the way, saying, "I am late to work, so I need to hurry!" To affirm, you can say, "I will drive you to work so you won't be late," and then use redirection by saying, "but let's eat breakfast first."

Be Calm and Professional

Maintain a calm, professional manner and approach and be positive and reassuring. Do not express anxiety, fear, or anger about a resident's behavior and keep an even tone of voice, as loud noises can cause aggressive responses. Maintain eye contact with residents and calmly explain why you are there and what is needed. Do not argue, criticize, or use punishing approaches or behavior. Use proper body language to demonstrate respect and listen carefully, particularly when the resident is losing language skills. Smile, touch gently, and hug, when appropriate.

Keep instructions simple, break them down into steps, and wait between questions for answers. Never rush, and use closed-ended questions such as "Would you like to wear this sweater today?" This approach can keep confusion and stress to a minimum. Offering open-ended choices is important if residents can still make independent decisions, however.

Provide Cues

Use **cues**, or actions that invite responses. Verbal cues might be simple words such as "Roll to the right" or "Stand up," followed with praise such as "Great job." If verbal cues are not successful, use visual and manual cues, such as demonstrating a step or touching an item (Figure 24.23). For example, you could point to or tap a drinking glass you want a resident to drink. Be sure the resident is paying attention to and can see the cue. You can use a *hand-over-hand cue* to help with ADLs in later stages of dementia. For example, with a light touch, you could place your hand over the resident's hand while holding a utensil and begin the act of feeding (Figure 24.24). Always give praise to show the resident he or she is doing a good job.

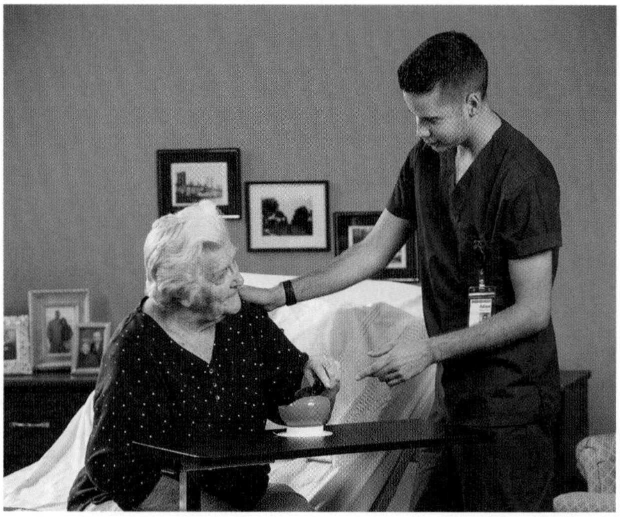

Ensure a Safe Environment

Maintain a safe, familiar, comfortable, organized, clutter-free, simple, and quiet environment to reduce overstimulation and help prevent agitation or aggression. Ensure the resident's personal items are easy to find. Label drawers and cabinets with easy-to-use memory cues to help residents find items. Pictures and words placed in clear sight can aid recognition. For example, a resident may need clear signs to safely find the toilet. Monitoring systems are used to alert caregivers when a resident is wandering out of bounds. Also, make sure personal care items that may be hazardous are removed. Mouthwash contains alcohol. A confused resident might easily drink a bottle of mouthwash.

© Tori Soper Photography

Figure 24.23 Using visual and manual cues can help residents understand you.

Maintain a routine schedule for ADLs to reduce confusion. Identify what time of day the resident is most alert so you can more easily communicate and perform tasks during this time.

Incorporate Positive Activities

Involving residents in cognitive and sensory stimulation can improve memory, communication skills, and social interaction and decrease boredom, inactivity, and sensory deprivation. Activities should be based on a resident's changing abilities and interests. You can also incorporate relaxing activities (such as turning on favorite music), particularly during the time of day a resident demonstrates more aggressive behaviors. Giving a hand massage can be very beneficial to residents who have delusions. Touch can provide grounding and comfort.

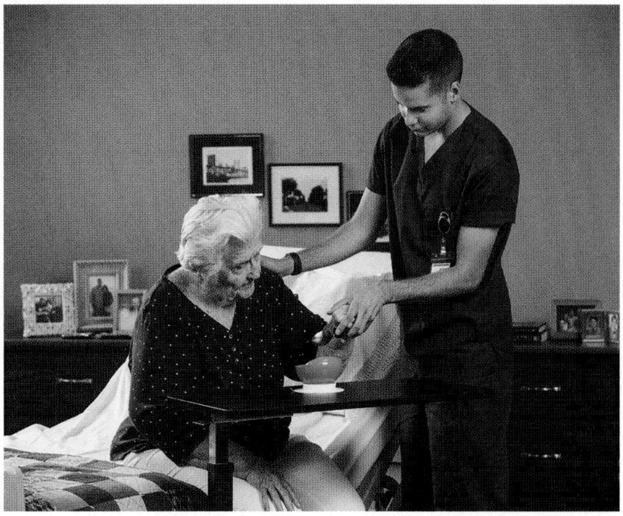

As a nursing assistant, you can use *reminiscence* (recollection of memories) to increase pleasurable experiences and improve mood. In dementia, long-term memories fade more slowly than short-term memories, so asking about past experiences can reduce stress. Conversations should be personal, positive, and significant to the resident. Sometimes making a memory box of photographs and other familiar items or a life story book can be helpful. Residents can review these by themselves or with family members.

Other treatment approaches may also be considered. For example, *validation therapy* has some evidence of success. In validation therapy, a resident's values, beliefs, and reality are validated. This approach focuses on agreeing with and then redirecting residents to reduce stress and maintain balance. Feelings and emotions are the primary consideration, even if they do not make sense. For example, if a resident is fearful of losing a precious picture, you might provide a box to store the item. If a resident states that she is angry after her deceased mother's visit last evening, you might say, "I understand why you might feel that way."

© Tori Soper Photography

Figure 24.24 Using the hand-over-hand cue can enable you to guide a resident's hand and promote eating.

Communicate with Family Members and the Licensed Nursing Staff

As a nursing assistant working under the direction of the plan of care and licensed nursing staff, you can help family members understand the changes they see in their loved one. As dementia progresses, you can ask family members to assist with activities and approaches (Figure 24.25). Always observe, report, and document behavioral changes (such as increased agitation and aggression, changes in memory loss or confusion, or increased wandering) and the effectiveness of actions taken. Observations and reports are important to maintaining and ensuring an appropriate, effective, and individualized plan of care. Caring for residents with dementia is not easy, particularly when residents are in late stages. Taking care of yourself is essential. To care for yourself, you should get good nutrition and exercise, find ways to relax at home, and talk about your feelings with appropriate people. This will ensure you have the energy and patience to care for others.

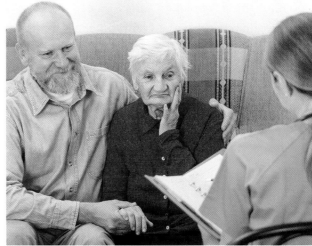

Ocskay Bence/Shutterstock.com

Figure 24.25 Communicating with the resident's family members and encouraging them to participate with certain activities may help residents manage dementia.

Using the Key Terms

Complete the following sentences using key terms in this section.

1. _____ is a condition caused by the overuse of a chemical substance.
2. A sideways curve of the spine is called _____.
3. One psychological change of dementia is _____, an unsupported or overblown distrust of others.
4. To help residents with dementia, nursing assistants use _____, or actions that invite responses.
5. People with dementia may experience irrational beliefs called _____.
6. _____ is a genetic disorder that changes how the body makes mucus and sweat.
7. _____ is a condition of fluid in the brain.

Know and Understand the Facts

8. Identify two types of vision impairment, hearing impairment, and speech impairment.
9. What is the difference between congenital and genetic disorders?
10. Explain three care considerations for helping those with TBI or SCI.
11. Identify two care considerations for a resident who is paralyzed.
12. Describe the different levels of consciousness.
13. Compare delirium and dementia.
14. Discuss two cognitive, psychological, and physical changes in dementia.

Analyze and Apply Concepts

15. Give one example of a method you could use to communicate with a patient on a mechanical ventilator.
16. Explain three important care guidelines for those in a coma.
17. Describe four specific actions a holistic nursing assistant can take when caring for residents with dementia.
18. How can a nursing assistant practice self-care while caring for a resident with dementia?

Think Critically

Read the following care situation. Then answer the questions that follow.

Mrs. K, an 84-year-old widow with seven children who live nearby, has been in the long-term care facility in which you work for one year. She was diagnosed with Alzheimer's disease (AD) and has functioned fairly well over the time you have cared for her. Lately, Mrs. K's memory loss and confusion have been increasing, and she seems much more restless. Mrs. K has had a few episodes of incontinence and is very embarrassed about it. She is also frustrated because she can't find things she is sure she put away. Mrs. K's children are very concerned and upset over the changes in their mother.

19. In what stage of AD do you think Mrs. K is?
20. How would you respond to Mrs. K's embarrassment?
21. What could you do to help with Mrs. K's continuing loss of memory and confusion?
22. What three actions could you take to care for and maintain Mrs. K's ADLs?
23. List three safety and comfort guidelines you could put in place when caring for Mrs. K.
24. In what ways might you support Mrs. K's children and ensure they are involved in her care?

Objectives

Mental and emotional health are essential for all human beings. Effectively functioning and being involved in all of life's activities requires not only physical abilities, but also mental capabilities and emotional balance. Mental health conditions interfere with daily living. In this section, you will explore mental and emotional health and associated mental health conditions. You will also learn about substance use disorders, violence, self-harm, and suicide and explore the care provided to those with mental health conditions. To achieve the objectives for this section, you must successfully

- **describe** the characteristics of mental and emotional health;
- **discuss** how mental health conditions are categorized;
- **explain** selected mental health conditions, including anxiety disorders, trauma- or stress-related disorders, substance use disorders, depressive disorders, personality disorders, and schizophrenia spectrum disorder;
- **examine** issues related to self-harm and suicide; and
- **identify** care guidelines for those who experience mental health conditions.

Key Terms

Learn these key terms to better understand the information presented in the section.

asylums	self-harm
bipolar disorder	stigma
post-traumatic stress disorder (PTSD)	suicide
schizophrenia spectrum disorder	

Questions to Consider

- What do you know about mental and emotional health? Do you believe you are mentally and emotionally healthy?
- If you had to describe mental health conditions, what terms would you use? What terms have other people used to describe someone who has a mental health condition? How did you feel about the use of these terms?
- Do you know someone diagnosed with a mental health condition? What symptoms does the person have, and how are these symptoms being treated?

What Are Mental and Emotional Health?

In chapter 6, you learned about the importance of satisfying human needs and the ways that people grow and develop physically, mentally, and emotionally. You also examined how the body, mind, and spirit are linked. In chapter 7, you explored wellness and illness and learned that they lie on a continuum and are open to individual interpretation. These are important concepts in exploring mental and emotional health, as mental and emotional health are built on needs; growth and development; links between the body, mind, and spirit; and levels of wellness and illness.

Mental health encompasses a person's ability to function productively by processing and storing information, shaping his or her environment to meet needs, making voluntary choices, taking action, initiating and maintaining satisfying and meaningful relationships, engaging in creative work, adapting to change, being flexible, having resilience, and coping with challenges. *Emotional health* involves feeling good about and having respect for one's self and others, enjoying life, giving and receiving love, and positively expressing and managing emotions. Mental and emotional health are important and interact with and help promote physical well-being. Mental and emotional health require a positive interaction among physical, social, family, psychological, and environmental factors throughout life.

There are times when mental and emotional health may be at risk. Life changes, aging, or limited coping mechanisms can lead to stress. As you learned in chapter 4, *stress* is a physical or psychological response to a situation that causes worry or tension.

Think About This

It is important to note that the presence of a mental health condition does not mean a person is legally *insane*. Insanity is a legal term and is not used by healthcare professionals. It is defined as the inability to manage one's affairs or understand the consequences of one's actions. A determination of insanity is made by a judge and jury based on an expert witness, such as a qualified psychiatrist. A person who is declared insane is not legally responsible for his or her actions and can be involuntarily committed to a psychiatric hospital.

Stress is normal, but it can affect each person differently and impacts a person's mental and emotional health.

As you learned in chapter 7, there are several signs and symptoms of stress. These signs and symptoms can affect mental, emotional, physical, and behavioral health:

- **Mental symptoms**: inability to concentrate, constant worry, or ability to see only the negative

- **Emotional symptoms**: moodiness, short temper, agitation, loneliness, or depression

- **Physical symptoms**: aches and pains, dizziness, nausea, rapid heartbeat, or frequent colds

- **Behavioral symptoms**: procrastination, isolation, nervous habits, or the use of alcohol or drugs to relax

It is not possible to completely eliminate all stress from your life. In fact, good stress (*eustress*) helps motivate people to learn or change. When stress becomes harmful, it is called *distress*. You can, however, determine what common sources of stress, or *stressors*, you may experience and deal with them. Specific strategies for coping, managing stress, and achieving a life balance are discussed in chapter 7. These strategies can be applied to yourself and are also helpful guidelines for caring for others.

Some people experience more than just everyday stressors. Changes in their thinking, mood, or behavior impair daily functioning. When learning about mental health conditions, remember that the goal of health and wellness is still possible.

What Are Mental Health Conditions?

Mental health conditions are the most common cause of disability in the United States. They are characterized by changes in thinking (cognition), mood (emotions), or behaviors and can cause distress and limited or impaired functioning. It is estimated that over 43 million or 18 percent of people in the United States have a diagnosed mental health condition, and over 9 million people have a severe disorder so incapacitating they are unable to function. Risk factors for these conditions include stressful living conditions, overcrowding, abuse, adverse childhood experiences (ACEs), learning disorders, congenital disorders, low birthweight, and chronic illnesses. Veterans who have experienced physical and mental trauma, people who have experienced large-scale trauma (such as natural disasters or violence), and older adults who have dementia are also at increased risk.

During the mid-1800s, US activist Dorothea Dix vigorously worked to improve living conditions for people with mental health conditions (Figure 24.26). By 1900, many government-funded psychiatric hospitals were available for those who needed care. Unfortunately, these hospitals were understaffed, were poorly funded, and offered most healthcare in **asylums** (shelters). In the late 1900s, people worked to move mental healthcare into the community as much as possible. This led to more community-based mental healthcare services, such as mental health centers and residential centers. In these centers, mental health treatment teams typically include a psychiatrist, psychologist, counselor, licensed social worker, psychiatric mental health nurse practitioner, and others.

Today, one in five US adults experience a mental health condition each year, and over one-half do not have available mental healthcare. In addition, many people with a mental health condition experience **stigma** (a negative perception from others), feel they are negatively labeled because of their conditions, and feel separated from others.

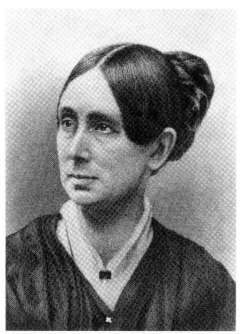

Everett Historical/Shutterstock.com

Figure 24.26 Dorothea Dix advocated for the effective treatment of people with mental health conditions. Born in 1802, she helped create the first mental health asylums.

What Are the Different Types of Mental Health Conditions?

Mental health conditions are categorized in several different ways. The categories most often used by psychiatrists, psychologists, and researchers come from the American Psychiatric Association's Diagnostic and Statistical Manual of Mental Disorders (DSM-5). This framework is used for discussing the different types of conditions in this section. Though mental health conditions are characterized by distinctive symptoms and risks, be aware that each person's experience will be unique. You learned about eating disorders in chapter 22. In this section, you will learn about anxiety disorders, trauma- and stress-related disorders, depressive disorders, personality disorders, substance use disorders, schizophrenia spectrum disorder, and self-harm.

Think About This

According to results recently published by a large insurance company, depression, anxiety, and other mood disorders were the top three conditions that affected longevity and quality of life. Substance use disorders were the fifth-ranking condition.

Anxiety Disorders

Anxiety disorders are more than normal anxiety. They are characterized by persistent, excessive worry or fear of nonthreatening situations. Symptoms of anxiety disorders include tension, apprehensiveness, irritability, a racing heart, shortness of breath, headaches, fatigue, an upset stomach, and diarrhea. Most people who have anxiety disorders develop them before age 21, and women experience anxiety disorders more often than men. Anxiety disorders are caused by genetics and by the environment (including stressful or traumatic events, such as abuse or violence).

Some anxiety disorders are characterized by *panic attacks*, which are sudden feelings of terror that happen without warning. People with panic attacks experience chest pain, heart palpitations, dizziness, shortness of breath, and stomach upset. Other anxiety disorders include *phobias*, which are strong, persistent, irrational fears. Some phobias include *claustrophobia* (fear of enclosed spaces) and *acrophobia* (fear of heights).

People can also have phobias of animals, needles, thunderstorms, and flying (Figure 24.27). Some people have more than one phobia. People with phobias experience difficulty functioning normally and do everything possible to avoid the item or situation that causes the fear.

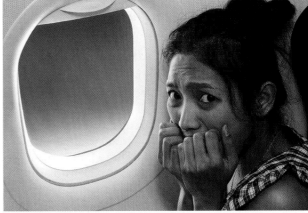

Milkovasa/Shutterstock.com

Figure 24.27 One example of a phobia is a strong, persistent fear of flying.

Another common, chronic anxiety disorder is *obsessive-compulsive disorder (OCD)*, which can interfere with daily living. OCD is characterized by uncontrollable, recurrent, and interfering thoughts and urges (*obsessions*) that result in repetitive behaviors (*compulsions*). Obsessions may range from a fear of germs to a fear that something bad will happen if everything is not in perfect order. Compulsions are the behaviors a person uses in response to an obsession. For example, a person may excessively clean or repeatedly arrange things in a particular way.

Trauma- and Stress-Related Disorders

Trauma- and *stress-related disorders* can develop after a person experiences or witnesses a traumatic or stressful event. One example of a stress-related disorder is **post-traumatic stress disorder (PTSD)**. PTSD can be caused by childhood neglect or physical abuse, sexual assault, physical attacks, or combat exposure. People with PTSD have a variety of symptoms, which may begin within three months after the event or not emerge until years later. Symptoms of PTSD can fluctuate in intensity over time, depending on life events and reminders of the trauma, and can include the following:

- reliving the event with unpleasant and disturbing memories, dreams, nightmares, and flashbacks (even a certain smell, touch, or noise can trigger these symptoms)
- avoiding thinking or talking about the trauma or visiting places associated with the trauma
- having intense, anxious feelings that disrupt daily living
- feeling emotionally numb and hopeless
- having negative feelings about self and others
- experiencing memory and concentration problems
- finding it difficult to maintain close relationships
- feeling angry and irritable
- participating in self-destructive behaviors such as drinking

A second trauma- and stress-related disorder is *acute stress disorder (ASD)*. In ASD, a person develops severe anxiety and dissociation (disconnection between thoughts, memories, feelings, and actions) within one month after an extreme traumatic event, such as a death or serious accident. If ASD lasts longer than one month and if severe symptoms continue, the person may be diagnosed with PTSD.

Another short-term condition is *adjustment disorder* or *stress-response syndrome*. This condition usually lasts no longer than six months. A person with this condition has extreme difficulty coping with or adjusting to a particular source of stress, such as a major life change, stressful workplace event, or loss of a job. Someone with this condition may become situationally depressed and be tearful, have feelings of hopelessness, and lose interest in daily activities.

Depressive Disorders

Depressive disorders are the most common type of mental health condition and include persistent depressive disorder (*dysthymia*), major or clinical depression, and perinatal depression. Seasonal affective disorder (SAD) and bipolar disorder are also included in this category. Depression can develop at any age and is caused by a combination of biological, genetic, environmental, and psychological factors. Risk factors can include a family history of depression; a major life change; certain illnesses, such as cancer or heart disease; or a reaction to a medication.

Depressive disorders are characterized by feelings of sadness, anxiety, hopelessness, helplessness, guilt, and worthlessness. They are also characterized by a sense of emptiness; irritability; and cognitive issues such as difficulty concentrating, memory loss, troubled sleep, and loss of interest in pleasurable activities (Figure 24.28). Physical symptoms of depressive disorders include decreased energy; fatigue; slow movements; appetite and weight changes; and pain, headaches, and GI upsets that do not originate from physiological illness. Typically, not all symptoms will occur at any one time.

Depressive disorders vary in duration, symptoms, and causes; however, for depression to be diagnosed, symptoms must be present daily for a minimum of two weeks. One example of diagnosed depression is *major depression*, a serious mood disorder with severe symptoms that profoundly affect daily life activities. In SAD, symptoms are present during the winter months when there is less sunlight, but disappear during spring and summer.

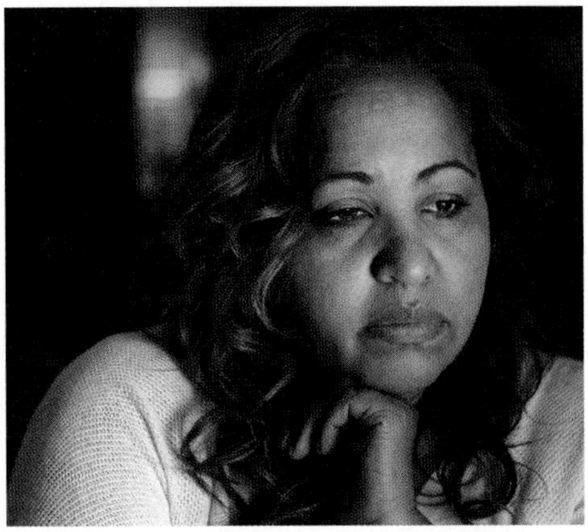

Bipolar disorder is a serious mental health condition characterized by manic and depressive episodes. There is no single cause of bipolar disorder, but risk factors may include family history and genetics. Women are more likely than men to develop bipolar disorder, and symptoms appear most often in the late teen years or early adulthood. There are four basic types of bipolar disorder, and each type is characterized by different changes in mood, energy, and activity levels. A person with bipolar disorder may swing from extreme happiness, increased energy, trouble sleeping, fast talking, agitation, and multitasking (mania) to sadness, fatigue, worry, memory loss, trouble concentrating, and confusion (depression). Some people experience mania and depression at the same time; other people are only manic and are not depressed. Some episodes may include hallucinations or delusions. People with bipolar disorder may also abuse substances such as alcohol or drugs.

iStock.com/pixelheadphoto

Figure 24.28 Depressive disorders are characterized by intense feelings of hopelessness, worthlessness, and helplessness.

Personality Disorders

Personality disorders are characterized by trouble sensing and relating to everyday situations and other people. These disorders can cause serious problems and limitations in relationships, social activities, and performance at work or school. Personality disorders usually develop during adolescence or early adulthood. There are different types of personality disorders with unique symptoms that can be mild or severe. People with personality disorders may have trouble realizing they have a problem.

Borderline personality disorder (BPD) is one example of a personality disorder. BPD affects how a person feels about himself or herself, relates to others, and behaves. BPD is a serious disorder characterized by ongoing instability in moods, self-image, actions, and relationships. A person with BPD may experience extreme swings in mood and be uncertain about his or her identity, leading to rapidly changing interests. Some signs and symptoms of BPD include an intense fear of abandonment; inappropriate anger; impulsive behavior, such as binge eating or quitting a good job; and a pattern of unstable and intense relationships. For example, a person with BPD might feel extremely close and loving toward someone one moment and then suddenly believe the other person doesn't care enough about him or her.

Substance Use Disorders

Substance use disorders are characterized by the excessive use of caffeine, alcohol, tobacco, cannabis (marijuana), hallucinogens, inhalants, opioids, sedatives, hypnotics (sleep medications), and stimulants such as cocaine. The most commonly abused substances are alcohol, tobacco, cannabis, stimulants, hallucinogens, and opioids.

Alcohol Use Disorder

More than one-half of people in the United States ages 12 and older drink alcohol. *Binge drinking* is defined as consuming five or more alcoholic drinks for males or consuming four or more alcoholic drinks for females in a short period of time. *Excessive alcohol use* is considered five or more drinks at the same event on five or more days in the past 30 days.

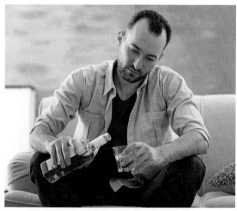
Africa Studio/Shutterstock.com

Figure 24.29 People with AUD continue consuming alcohol, even when alcohol assumption leads to negative health effects.

Alcohol use disorder (AUD) is more than just excessive drinking, although excessive drinking can lead to AUD. AUD is characterized by problems controlling alcohol intake, alcohol tolerance that leads to dangerous risks, withdrawal symptoms, and the continuation of drinking even with serious physical consequences (Figure 24.29). It is estimated that 16 million people in the United States (nearly 10 million adult men and over 5 million adult women) have AUD. A person's genetics influence the likelihood of developing AUD. AUD can be mild, moderate, or severe, depending on the number of symptoms displayed.

Stimulant Use Disorder

People with a *stimulant use disorder* consume amphetamines, methamphetamines, and cocaine orally, through nasal ingestion, or intravenously. Stimulants increase energy, alertness, attention, heart rate, blood pressure, and breathing. Stimulant use disorder is characterized by intense desire for a stimulant, the continuation of use even though it interferes with daily life, the use of larger amounts over time, and withdrawal symptoms.

Opioid Use Disorder

Opioid use disorder is characterized by the improper use or abuse of opioids and can have serious consequences. Opioids are a class of medications that includes the illegal drug heroin, synthetic opioids such as fentanyl, and pain relievers available legally by prescription (for example, codeine and morphine). Opioids relieve pain and can also lead to a sense of *euphoria* (joy and excitement). Consuming more opioids intensifies the feeling; however, opioid overdose can depress respirations and cause death. Approximately 1.9 million people in the United States have an opioid use disorder.

Schizophrenia Spectrum Disorder

Think About This

Schizophrenia spectrum disorder is an example of a psychotic disorder. Psychotic disorders are characterized by delusions, hallucinations, and a loss of touch with reality. Other examples of psychotic disorders are delusional disorder, brief psychotic disorder, and psychosis associated with substance use or medical conditions.

Schizophrenia spectrum disorder is a severe and chronic mental health condition that affects a person's entire life and ways of thinking, feeling, and behaving. Risk factors for schizophrenia spectrum disorder include genetics, the environment (including problems during pregnancy, such as increased stress, infections, and malnutrition), and possible chemical imbalances in the brain. Symptoms usually begin between the ages of 16 and 30. Most symptoms of schizophrenia spectrum disorder signify a loss of reality and include delusions such as persecution, hallucinations, thought disorders, and agitated body movements. Other symptoms interfere with emotions and behavior. For example, a symptom called the *flat affect* is characterized by the lowering of emotions, lack of facial expression, and a dull tone of voice. Symptoms that influence cognitive function include trouble with focus and attention and an inability to make decisions.

What Should Nursing Assistants Know About Self-Harm and Suicide?

In addition to understanding mental health conditions, nursing assistants must also familiarize themselves with the concepts of self-harm and suicide. Some people practice self-harm as a way to cope with emotional pain. Fatal, self-inflicted injuries, or suicide, may also be a sign of poor mental or emotional health. If a resident in your care practices self-harm or expresses suicidal thoughts, you must inform the licensed nursing staff immediately. Do not leave a resident who is considering suicide alone.

Self-Harm

When people inflict **self-harm**, they hurt themselves on purpose. Although practicing self-harm is not considered a mental health condition, it is a sign of emotional distress. For some people, self-harm is a coping mechanism used to lessen emotional pain or hard-to-express feelings. It is a way to provide emotional release or to create pain so the person feels something else.

Risk factors for self-harm include trauma, neglect, and abuse. Self-harm is practiced most often by adolescents and young adults. A common method is skin cutting; however, some people burn themselves, pull out their hair, or pick at wounds to prevent healing.

When people harm themselves, they have feelings of shame. If that shame leads to intense negative feelings, people may hurt themselves again, creating a temporary but habitual cycle of self-harm. While self-harm is not the same as attempting suicide, it may increase the risk of suicide.

There are effective treatments for self-harm. Psychotherapy is important to any plan of care and helps the person learn new coping mechanisms. Sometimes medications can also help.

Suicide

Suicide is also not a mental health condition in and of itself, but is a sign of poor mental and emotional health. **Suicide** is intentional death caused by fatal, self-inflicted injuries. Firearms are the most common method of suicide, accounting for almost one-half of suicide attempts. Suffocation and poisoning are also common methods, and poisoning is often used by females.

Some people may attempt suicide and inflict nonfatal injuries. Other people may have *suicidal ideation* and think about, consider, and plan suicide. Someone who survives a suicide attempt is likely to try again within the next three months and may succeed unless treated.

Risk factors for suicide include mental health conditions (such as depression), previous suicidal attempts, family history and violence, physical or sexual abuse, and chronic illness and pain. Traumatic life events may also lead to thoughts of suicide.

As a holistic nursing assistant, you must be aware of the warning signs of suicide. These warning signs include hopelessness, increased anxiety, agitation, uncontrolled anger, dramatic mood changes, risky behaviors, feelings of being trapped, increased use of drugs or alcohol, and sudden withdrawal and isolation. The following signs indicate that someone is seriously considering a suicide attempt and are an emergency:

- making threats of wanting to die or expressing a death wish
- looking for ways to die by suicide (such as taking risks or suddenly purchasing a firearm)
- talking or writing about suicide, putting affairs in order, or visiting or calling people to say goodbye

Always take people seriously when they are intent on suicide. If working in a facility, never leave a resident who threatens suicide alone. Call for help and stay with the resident. If working outside a facility, help the person in danger seek assistance from a trained professional as quickly as possible or call a suicide hotline. Do not leave the person alone. Instead, immediately seek help from the nearest emergency room and call 9-1-1.

While federal laws do not require people to report if a person intends to attempt suicide, some states do have laws about mandatory suicide reporting. Reporters must have reasonable cause to suspect a person will self-harm or attempt suicide. These reporters tend to be professionals such as teachers, social workers, healthcare providers, counselors or therapists, child care providers, or law enforcement officers. In some states, privileged communication that is considered confidential may complicate reporting. Privileged communication may include interactions between a doctor and patient, between an attorney and client, or with religious officials.

Think About This

Every 13 minutes, one person in the United States dies by suicide, making suicide the tenth leading cause of death overall and the second leading cause of death for people ages 10–34. Men die by suicide at a rate nearly four times that of women, accounting for 78 percent of suicides in the United States. The number of suicides in the United States is more than twice the number of homicides. In the United States, more than 19.4 million people over age 18 report having serious thoughts about killing themselves.

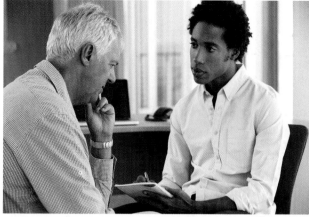
Monkey Business Images/Shutterstock.com

Figure 24.30 CBT is a type of therapy that involves mastering thoughts and feelings.

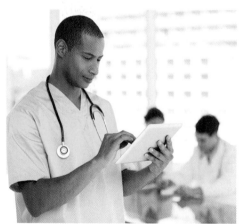
wavebreakmedia/Shutterstock.com

Figure 24.31 Documenting changes in health and behavior can help provide information to healthcare staff members who write the plan of care.

What Care Is Available for Residents with Mental Health Conditions?

Proper and accurate diagnosis is essential for the care of a person who has a mental health condition. Each person will have his or her own response to the condition, set of symptoms, and plan of care for treatment. The goal of treatment is to improve quality of life. Plans of care will be individual, but will likely involve one or more of the following:

- **Psychotherapy**: usually includes talk therapy as an individual, in a group, or with the family. *Cognitive behavioral therapy (CBT)* helps a person develop mastery over thoughts and feelings (Figure 24.30). *Exposure therapy* treats phobias with gradual, repeated exposure so the person can learn to manage associated anxiety and feelings.

- **Selected medications**: may include antianxiety medications, antidepressants, sedatives, mood stabilizers, or antipsychotics. These will have side effects that need to be monitored.

- **Integrative medicine (IM) health approaches**: include stress relief, relaxation techniques, and supplements.

Most treatments may be specific to the individual mental health condition. For example, brain stimulation therapies may be used to treat depression and sometimes mania. The brain stimulation therapy most often used is *electroconvulsive therapy (ECT)*. In ECT, a person is placed under general anesthesia, and electrodes are placed on the scalp. A controlled electric current causes a brief seizure, which results in symptom relief. ECT is usually performed three times a week for two to four weeks. Side effects include memory problems.

Holistic nursing assistants can take many actions to improve the daily lives of residents who have mental health conditions. Some of these actions include the following:

- Understand the symptoms of the mental health condition and recognize that they are very real to the resident.

- Never take a resident's behavior personally. Do, however, step back or stand away if a resident is physically aggressive.

- Respect the individuality of residents and focus on them as people, not on the behaviors they display. Use the plan of care as your guide and acknowledge that residents have rights.

- Be respectful, supportive, and caring. Understand that a mental health condition does not affect a resident's intelligence.

- Speak and act calmly to provide a peaceful and safe environment.

- Assist in providing proper nutrition and adequate exercise and activities.

- Observe, report, and document physical and behavioral changes, such as possible side effects of medications or alterations in behavior (Figure 24.31). These observations and reports are essential to maintaining and ensuring an appropriate and effective plan of care.

Using the Key Terms

Complete the following sentences using key terms in this section.

1. _____ is a mental health condition characterized by loss of reality, delusions, hallucinations, and thought disorders.
2. Skin cutting to release emotional pain is an example of _____.
3. People with mental health conditions often experience _____, or negative perceptions from others.
4. _____ is an example of a mental health condition that occurs after a traumatic or stressful event.
5. Intentional death by fatal, self-inflicted injuries is called _____.
6. Historically, much mental healthcare was delivered in _____, or shelters.
7. A person with _____ may swing between episodes of mania and depression.

Know and Understand the Facts

8. Explain four characteristics of mental and emotional health.
9. Describe how a mental health condition can affect a person's daily life.
10. Choose one mental health condition and identify its risks and symptoms.
11. List three symptoms that might indicate that a person has PTSD.
12. Identify two signs that a person may be seriously considering suicide.
13. Describe two types of treatment for a mental health condition.

Analyze and Apply Concepts

14. Describe two important pieces of information you learned that will help you provide care for residents with mental health conditions.
15. List three guidelines for caring for residents with mental health conditions.
16. What actions should you take if a resident expresses a death wish during morning care?
17. Why do you think opioid use disorder is so prevalent in the United States?

Think Critically

Read the following care situation. Then answer the questions that follow.

Mrs. O is a 75-year-old resident who was recently admitted to a long-term care facility. Mrs. O had a mild stroke, and her husband wants her to have full-time care while she is recuperating. She has minimal physical disabilities from the stroke, has a slight limp that requires a cane, and has some slurred speech. Mrs. O was diagnosed with clinical depression five years ago and has attempted suicide twice. She is taking antidepressants and has tried individual and group therapy. Both have helped some. Mrs. O feels sad and anxious and is sometimes irritable. She often has difficulty concentrating and trouble sleeping. Mrs. O is very thin and seems fatigued. She said yesterday that she feels very hopeless that she will ever recover from the stroke.

18. What would you say to Mrs. O about her feelings of hopelessness?
19. In what specific areas should you be particularly observant when caring for Mrs. O?
20. What two approaches could you take to support Mrs. O during her recuperation?
21. List three safety and comfort guidelines you could put in place when caring for Mrs. O.

Key Points

Reviewing the key points for this chapter will help you practice more safely and competently as a holistic nursing assistant and will help you prepare for the certification competency examination.

- Proper support and safe, quality care can help improve quality of life for residents with disabilities or cognitive disorders.

- A disability is a limitation of function due to aging, a disease process, a congenital or genetic disorder, injury, or trauma.

- Cognitive disorders are characterized by trouble thinking, remembering, learning, processing and understanding information, and displaying appropriate behavior in social settings.

- Mental health conditions are characterized by changes in thinking (cognition), mood (emotions), and behaviors and can cause distress and limited or impaired functioning.

- Observing, reporting, and documenting physical and behavioral changes are pivotal to maintaining and ensuring an appropriate and effective plan of care.

Action Steps to Holistic Care

Review the information in this chapter. Complete the following activities.

1. Select one disability you learned about in this chapter. Prepare a short paper or digital presentation that identifies and describes the top three most important issues surrounding care. Include one that promotes comfort and one that ensures safety.

2. With a partner, select one emotional health concern or mental health condition discussed in the chapter. Prepare a poster that illustrates at least four facts that residents and the public should know.

3. Research current scientific information about one physical disability, emotional health concern, or mental health condition not discussed in this chapter. Write a brief report that describes two current facts about the disability, concern, or condition.

4. Prepare a poster or digital presentation about caring for residents with dementia. Include a description of the disease, treatment options, and care considerations.

Preparing for the Certification Competency Examination

To prepare for the nursing assistant certification competency examination, you will need to know content found in this chapter. This content may be tested in the knowledge (written or oral) and skills (hands-on demonstration) portions of the exam. The following areas will be emphasized:

- vision, hearing, and speech impairments or loss
- levels of consciousness
- communication with comatose residents and ventilator care
- needs and behaviors of residents with cognitive disorders
- appropriate responses to difficult behaviors
- appropriate and inappropriate expressions of sexual behavior
- interventions used to reduce the effects of cognitive disorders
- the differences between mental health and illness
- appropriate care for common mental health conditions
- physical and verbal aggression
- mental status and behavior changes

These sample test questions are similar to ones you will find on the certification competency exam. See how well you can answer them. Be sure to select the *best* answer.

1. Someone who has achieved good mental and emotional health is
   A. overconfident
   B. balanced
   C. inactive
   D. unsure

2. A reversible cognitive disorder is called
   A. bipolar disorder
   B. dementia
   C. delirium
   D. depression

3. A new nursing assistant will be taking care of Mr. J, who has a hearing impairment, but will not wear his hearing aid. What is the best approach the nursing assistant could take?

    A. tell Mr. J he must wear his hearing aid
    B. talk as loudly as possible so Mr. J can hear her
    C. ask Mr. J's family to purchase him a new, more comfortable aid
    D. always face Mr. J when talking

4. While talking with Mr. L, you notice how depressed he has become. Mr. L asks you to call his daughter so she can see him. He wants to talk about his will and say goodbye to her. What should be your next action?

    A. He wants to put his affairs in order, so you should call his daughter immediately.
    B. He may be thinking about suicide, so you should alert the licensed nursing staff.
    C. He is a very organized man and wants to be sure all is settled, so you should do nothing.
    D. He is feeling sad and wants to see his daughter, so you should call her.

5. Mr. D knows what he wants to say, but just can't get the words out. What type of aphasia does he have?

    A. receptive   C. global
    B. anomic   D. expressive

6. Which of the following happens during sundowning?

    A. A resident becomes more confused at the end of the day.
    B. A resident is very tired and lethargic at the end of the day.
    C. A resident has more clarity at the end of the day.
    D. A resident is happier at the end of the day.

7. Mr. K had a car accident and suffered a TBI. He is still unconscious after 30 minutes. What level is this?

    A. moderate   C. severe
    B. mild   D. vegetative

8. When caring for a resident with vision impairment, what should a holistic nursing assistant do?

    A. tell the resident to be careful when going to the toilet
    B. keep the bed linens and towels in their proper place
    C. practice safety by making sure there are no obstacles
    D. keep the room clean and tidy at all times

9. Mrs. M is experiencing false and distorted sensory experiences that seem real to her. These are called

    A. delusions   C. depression
    B. hallucinations   D. phobias

10. A nursing assistant is taking care of a resident in a coma for the first time. What is one guideline she should keep in mind?

    A. talk loudly in case the resident can still hear
    B. never sing or read to an unresponsive resident
    C. never talk about, around, or above the resident
    D. keep looking for the resident's eyes to open

11. Which of the following is a cognitive change in dementia?

    A. inability to chew or swallow
    B. physical or verbal aggression
    C. memory loss and confusion
    D. delusions and phobias

12. What is a mental health condition?

    A. changes in thinking, mood, or behaviors that limit or impair function
    B. reversible changes to cognition that do not affect function
    C. irreversible impairments that change function and daily activities
    D. changes in the body systems that limit or impair the senses

13. Which is the most common mental health condition?

    A. anxiety disorder
    B. depression
    C. bipolar disorder
    D. suicide

14. If someone has an SCI and can move his arms, but not his legs, he has

    A. omniplegia
    B. quadriplegia
    C. paraplegia
    D. tetraplegia

15. Mrs. B has bipolar disorder. What symptoms might you see?

    A. hallucinations and then delusions
    B. rage and then irritability
    C. sadness and then phobias
    D. increased energy and then fatigue

Did you have difficulty with any of the questions? If you did, review the chapter to find the correct answer(s).

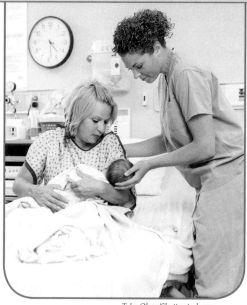

Tyler Olson/Shutterstock.com

Chapter Outline

Section 25.1
Mothers, Newborns, and Infants

Section 25.2
Surgery

Welcome to the Chapter

As a nursing assistant, you may work with several special populations, including mothers, newborns, infants, and patients who require surgery. In this chapter, you will learn about the normal changes women experience during pregnancy and childbirth, as well as possible complications. Caring for newborns and infants is also discussed, along with skills for feeding, bathing, diapering, and clearing an obstructed airway of a newborn or infant. In addition, you will explore the reasons patients have surgery, different types of surgery, and the care needed before and after surgery. Pre- and postoperative care may include care of drains and the use of antiembolism stockings and other devices to ensure proper blood circulation after surgery.

The information and procedures presented in this chapter will help you build the knowledge and skills needed to become a holistic nursing assistant. Check with your instructor to ensure these procedures are within your state's regulations for nursing assistant practice. The topics discussed in the chapter are highlighted on the Providing Holistic Care Framework.

You are now ready to start this chapter, *Caring for Special Populations and Needs*.

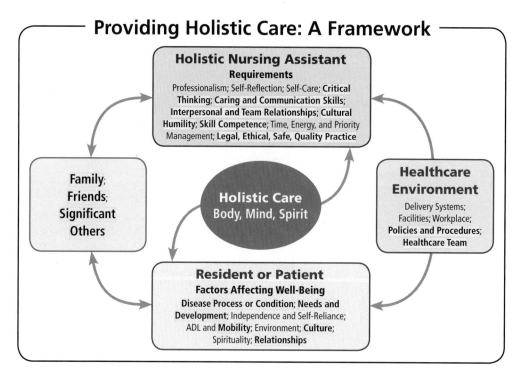

Providing Holistic Care: A Framework

Holistic Nursing Assistant
Requirements
Professionalism; Self-Reflection; Self-Care; **Critical Thinking; Caring and Communication Skills; Interpersonal and Team Relationships; Cultural Humility; Skill Competence;** Time, Energy, and Priority Management; **Legal, Ethical, Safe, Quality Practice**

Family; Friends; Significant Others

Holistic Care
Body, Mind, Spirit

Healthcare Environment
Delivery Systems; Facilities; Workplace; **Policies and Procedures; Healthcare Team**

Resident or Patient
Factors Affecting Well-Being
Disease Process or Condition; **Needs and Development;** Independence and Self-Reliance; ADL and **Mobility;** Environment; **Culture;** Spirituality; **Relationships**

Objectives

Having children is a normal part of the developmental process and is one many women and families choose to experience. In chapter 8, you learned about the anatomy of the male and female reproductive systems. In this section, preconception, conception, and pregnancy are discussed. You will examine labor and delivery and the importance of pre- and postnatal care. While having a baby is a safe and normal process, there can be complications. These complications may arise due to preexisting health issues in the mother, congenital and genetic disorders, viruses or infections, problems with the advancement of pregnancy, issues related to the growth of the fetus, and difficulties during delivery. You will explore the special care needs of newborns and infants and learn how to feed, bathe, and diaper infants. You will also learn the procedure for clearing the obstructed airway of a newborn or infant. To achieve the objectives for this section, you must successfully

- **describe** the process of childbearing, including preconception care, pregnancy, labor, delivery, and pre- and postnatal care;
- **discuss** possible complications of pregnancy and childbirth;
- **identify** the care needs of newborns and infants; and
- **demonstrate** how to feed, bathe, and diaper newborns and infants and how to clear an obstructed airway.

Key Terms

Learn these key terms to better understand the information presented in the section.

amniocentesis	miscarriage
antepartum	natal
colostrum	ovulation
ectopic pregnancy	placenta
embryo	placental abruption
fetus	placenta previa
hemophilia	postpartum
infertility	preeclampsia
intrapartum	stillbirth
lochia	

Questions to Consider

- Do you know someone who recently gave birth to a baby? What was her experience? Was the pregnancy smooth, or were there problems?
- What made the pregnancy smooth? If there were problems, how were they treated?
- What feelings and emotions did she have about becoming pregnant and having a baby? Did these feelings and emotions affect the pregnancy?

A woman who has a baby goes through three phases. The first **antepartum** phase happens prior to labor and delivery. This phase includes preconception and prenatal care, as well as the pregnancy itself. The second phase is called the **intrapartum** phase and includes labor and delivery. The final **postpartum** phase takes place after childbirth and includes postnatal care.

How Can Women Prepare for Pregnancy and Childbirth?

For some women, pregnancy may come as a surprise, but for others, it is a planned experience. In either case, it is important that the woman and developing fetus are as healthy and prepared as possible. The first step in ensuring a healthy mother and fetus is learning how the process of fertilization occurs and how pregnancy begins.

In chapter 8, you learned about the anatomy and physiology of the male and female reproductive systems. Familiarity with these structures and their functions is important to understanding fertilization, implantation, and pregnancy.

Fertilization, Implantation, and Pregnancy

Pregnancy most commonly occurs through vaginal intercourse. During this process, a man ejaculates sperm into a woman's vagina. Sperm then travel through the cervix and into the uterus and fallopian tubes. Between 40 million and 1.2 billion sperm can be released in a single ejaculation. A woman may also become pregnant through *artificial insemination*, in which sperm are inserted into a woman's vagina or uterus using a syringe or similar device. Another way to become pregnant is *in vitro fertilization (IVF)*. During IVF, ova are harvested from a woman's body and combined with sperm in a petri dish, allowing *fertilization*, or the union of an ovum and sperm, to occur. Then one or more fertilized ova are implanted into the uterus.

The conditions must be right for a woman to become pregnant through vaginal intercourse. **Ovulation**, or the release of an ovum from a woman's ovary, must have occurred (Figure 25.1). The ovum and sperm must meet to form a single cell. Then the fertilized ovum must travel down the fallopian tube and divide into additional cells. The ovum usually reaches the uterus approximately three to four days after fertilization and stays in the uterus for another two to three days. *Implantation* occurs if the fertilized ovum attaches to the lining of the uterus. Together, fertilization and implantation mark the moment of *conception*, and pregnancy has begun.

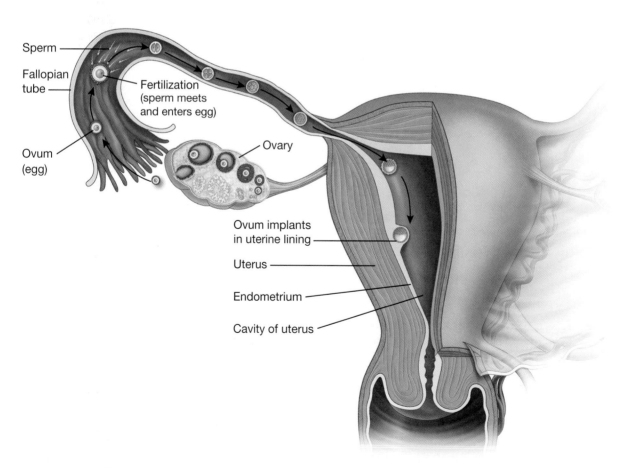

Sperm
Fallopian tube
Fertilization (sperm meets and enters egg)
Ovum (egg)
Ovary
Ovum implants in uterine lining
Uterus
Endometrium
Cavity of uterus

© Body Scientific International

Figure 25.1 During ovulation, an ovum is released from the ovary into the fallopian tube. This must occur for sperm to meet the ovum and for the ovum to be fertilized.

After implantation, the fertilized ovum becomes an **embryo**. Outside the embryo, an organ called the **placenta** forms from uterine and fetal tissue. The placenta, the umbilical cord, and the fluid-filled amniotic sac all provide life support for the growing embryo and **fetus** (fertilized ovum from the ninth week of pregnancy until birth). One side of the placenta is connected to the fetus via the *umbilical cord*. The other side of the placenta is connected to the wall of the uterus (Figure 25.2). The upper surface of the placenta is smooth, and the lower surface is rough. The placenta delivers oxygen and nutrients to the fetus through the umbilical cord. Waste products from the fetus also pass through the umbilical cord to the placenta. The placenta produces hormones that provide passive immunity for the fetus and help regulate the woman's responses to the pregnancy.

The *amniotic sac* is filled with a clear, slightly yellowish fluid that surrounds the growing fetus. During much of the pregnancy, the amniotic sac contains about 800 ml (3½ cups) of amniotic fluid, though this amount drops slightly before birth. Amniotic fluid cushions the fetus and gives it freedom to move. It regulates fetal temperature and helps the fetus's lungs develop. The fetus swallows and inhales the fluid, and fluid is then replaced through fetal exhalation and urination.

While the fetus is developing, the lining of the uterus becomes thicker. The cervix is sealed by a plug of mucus until the fetus is ready to be born. Just prior to birth, amniotic fluid may leak or gush from the vagina. After the delivery of the fetus, the placenta, or *afterbirth*, is also discharged from the vagina.

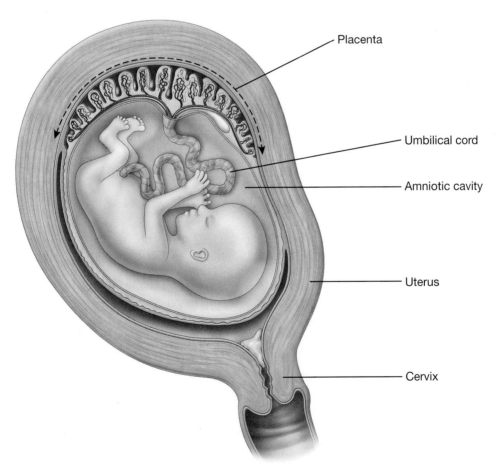

- Placenta
- Umbilical cord
- Amniotic cavity
- Uterus
- Cervix

© Body Scientific International

Figure 25.2 The placenta and umbilical cord help circulate nutrients, oxygen, and waste products between the mother and fetus. The amniotic sac, located in the amniotic cavity, also supports the developing fetus.

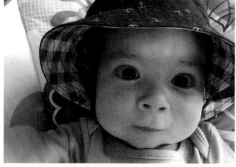

Mallory Dufek

A

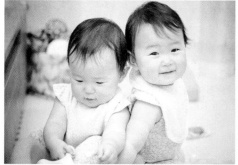

beeboys/Shutterstock.com

B

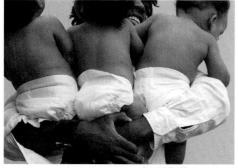

digitalskillet/Shutterstock.com

C

Figure 25.3 In a single pregnancy (A), a single fetus develops. In a multiple pregnancy, two (B) or three (C) fetuses may develop. Greater multiples are also possible.

Gestational Age

To determine when pregnancy begins, a measure called *gestational age* is used. Gestational age is calculated using the first day of the woman's last menstrual period (LMP). A woman's LMP is approximately three to four weeks before conception actually occurs, making a full-term pregnancy 40 weeks (approximately 10 months).

Sex Determination

The sex of the fetus depends on the sperm that fertilizes the ovum. If the sperm carries a male sex gene (Y chromosome), the developing fetus will be male. If the sperm carries the female sex gene (X chromosome), the fetus will be female. Statistics indicate that more boys than girls are born in the United States.

Multiple Pregnancy

A *multiple pregnancy* occurs when more than one fetus develops (Figure 25.3). Up until the fourth week of pregnancy, a fertilized ovum may divide in two, resulting in the development of identical twins. Fraternal twins develop if two ova are fertilized and implanted during the same cycle. In the United States, for every 1000 live births, 34 sets of twins are born. For every 100,000 live births, 104 sets of triplets or greater multiples are born.

Preconception Care

Women who plan their pregnancies often pursue *preconception care*, which is healthcare designed to help women and men have healthy babies. Preconception care is personalized for each woman or man and often includes discussions with a healthcare provider and plans to discontinue birth control. Partners may also consider whether they are emotionally and financially prepared to expand their family. During preconception care, it is helpful for women planning to become pregnant to review their lifestyle behaviors related to nutrition, exercise, consumption of caffeinated beverages, smoking, use of drugs and alcohol, and exposure to toxic substances (such as chemicals, fertilizers, or bug sprays).

Discontinuation of Birth Control

In preparation for pregnancy, partners discuss plans to discontinue the use of birth control. Forms of birth control include abstinence, natural family planning methods, barrier methods (for example, contraceptive sponges, diaphragms, cervical caps or shields, and female and male condoms), hormonal methods (oral contraceptives, patches, vaginal rings, and injections), or an implantable rod or intrauterine device (IUD). In some cases, birth control may be discontinued immediately, but some forms of birth control (such as an IUD or implantable rod) must be removed by a healthcare provider.

Discussions with Healthcare Providers

An important element of preconception care is discussing plans and concerns with a healthcare provider such as a doctor or nurse practitioner (Figure 25.4). During this discussion, partners and the healthcare provider will usually review health, family history, and medications and medical conditions that might affect the pregnancy (such as diabetes or hypertension). Genetic counseling may be advised to identify risk factors for congenital or genetic disorders. Screening or diagnostic tests may be performed using blood samples from each parent. Congenital or genetic disorders can cause a baby to have Down syndrome, **hemophilia** (a disorder characterized by the blood's inability to clot), or cystic fibrosis (CF). Any history of sexually transmitted infections (STIs) is also discussed. Older women may experience problems with fertility and have an increased risk for congenital disorders. If either partner has a history of **infertility**, or an inability to get pregnant, this would be discussed with the healthcare provider. Other items for discussion include issues regarding the sexual dysfunction of either partner, such as lack of desire or arousal, pain, or physical limitations.

Prenatal Care

The term **natal** means "related to birth." *Prenatal care* care occurs before a baby is born, or during pregnancy. Once a woman is pregnant, regular prenatal care is essential. The goal of prenatal care is to monitor the progress of the pregnancy and ensure early treatment for any problems that may arise. Prenatal care is important for the first-time mother as well as for the mother of several children.

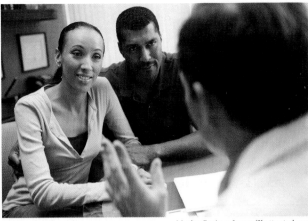

Monkey Business Images/Shutterstock.com

Figure 25.4 Discussions with a healthcare provider can help prepare partners for pregnancy.

During pregnancy, a woman should schedule regular visits with her doctor or another licensed healthcare provider. Visits should usually occur once a month between weeks 4 and 28, twice a month between weeks 29 and 36, and weekly between week 37 and birth. An older woman or a woman with a high-risk pregnancy may need more frequent visits.

At the first visit, health and family history will be discussed, and the healthcare provider will review any medications and supplements being taken by the woman. A physical and pelvic exam will be performed. Blood will be tested to determine Rh factor, and urine will be tested to determine presence of glucose or protein. The healthcare provider will calculate gestational age or due date. In addition, the healthcare provider will answer many of the woman's questions and share pregnancy guidelines (Figure 25.5).

During subsequent visits, blood pressure and weight are checked, the abdomen is measured for growth, and fetal heart rate is monitored. Any physical or emotional problems are discussed. Routine blood tests may also be performed for anemia, blood type, and other factors individual to the woman. Some partners also choose

Culture Cues
Pregnancy and Childbirth

Many cultural and religious beliefs exist about pregnancy and childbirth. Practicing cultural humility means being sensitive to these beliefs when providing care. In some cultures, older family members play an important role during pregnancy. They may offer the pregnant woman or new mother advice and support and expect their advice to be followed. Some cultures may also have certain customs or traditions that are practiced during pregnancy and childbirth. These customs often concern what a pregnant woman should do to positively influence the unborn baby. For example, the pregnant woman might read poetry, listen to music, and avoid any negative emotions. In some cultures, the role of the pregnant woman's husband is also vital. The husband may be directly involved in the pregnant woman's care and ensure that she eats correctly and has the services needed for an easy delivery.

Apply It

1. What cultural and religious customs and traditions does your family practice regarding pregnancy and childbirth?

2. How can you learn about patients' customs and traditions regarding pregnancy and childbirth?

3. In what ways do you think cultural and religious customs and traditions will affect the care you give?

Pregnancy Guidelines	
Dos	**Don'ts**
• Eat a nutrient-rich diet. • Drink plenty of water. • Take a prenatal vitamin with iron and folic acid. • Exercise appropriately. • Get a flu shot. • Get plenty of sleep. • Practice frequent hand hygiene to avoid infections.	• Do not consume fish heavy with mercury. • Do not smoke or be around secondhand smoke. • Do not drink alcohol or use drugs. • Do not have X-rays (unless required by a healthcare provider). • Do not take extremely hot baths or use a hot tub or sauna. • Do not use toxic chemicals.

Figure 25.5 Guidelines during pregnancy help ensure the health of the mother and fetus.

to have genetic testing performed. Genetic testing can include blood tests, ultrasounds, or a procedure called **amniocentesis** (in which a small amount of fluid is withdrawn from the amniotic sac and tested to identify any genetic abnormalities).

The woman's weight will be monitored to ensure she gains the appropriate amount. An average-sized woman should gain between 25 and 35 pounds during pregnancy. Most women gain 2 to 4 pounds during the first trimester and 1 pound per week thereafter (Figure 25.6). In addition, the healthcare provider will discuss healthy habits such as not smoking or drinking alcohol during pregnancy. Expectations for labor and delivery and signs and symptoms of possible complications are also discussed.

Healthcare Providers

Several healthcare providers can deliver prenatal care and care for the mother and child during labor and delivery. Partners may choose a desired healthcare provider during and after pregnancy and may also be able to choose where the baby will be born. Often, these decisions are based on preference, financial resources, and the woman's potential for a high-risk pregnancy or delivery. The healthcare provider's experience; recommendations from others; cultural traditions and customs; philosophies about pregnancy, delivery, or postnatal care; and the availability for appointments and delivery may also influence partners' decisions:

- **Obstetrician-gynecologist (OB/GYN)**: this licensed medical doctor is specially trained to provide care during pregnancy and address female medical and surgical issues. An obstetrician provides pregnancy care and delivers babies. Gynecologists offer female reproductive care, such as annual well-woman exams, postnatal care, and treatment for gynecological diseases and conditions. Gynecologists also perform surgeries such as hysterectomies. Usually, all of these services are performed by one healthcare provider.

- **Perinatologist**: this type of obstetrician specializes in caring for women who have high-risk pregnancies or problems during pregnancy.

- **Family practitioner (FP)**: this licensed medical doctor provides care for the whole family and may offer OB/GYN services.

- **Certified nurse midwife (CNM)**: this specially trained, licensed nurse is experienced in providing obstetric and newborn care and pre- and postnatal care through labor and delivery (Figure 25.7). CNMs work with obstetricians if complications occur during pregnancy, labor, or delivery.

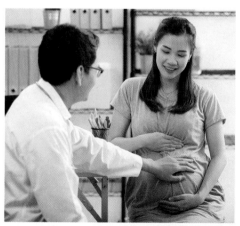

AnemStyle/Shutterstock.com

Figure 25.6 If a woman gains more or less weight than 25–35 pounds, her weight will be evaluated against her weight prior to pregnancy.

- **Certified midwife (CM)**: trained and certified in midwifery, a CM provides gynecological examinations, contraceptive counseling, labor and delivery care, and postnatal care. A *direct-entry midwife (DEM)* trains through an apprenticeship, self-study, midwifery school, or college or university program. A *lay midwife* is not certified or licensed, but has received informal training through self-study or apprenticeship.

- **Women's health nurse practitioner or family nurse practitioner**: this type of licensed nurse has advanced education and training and can provide pre- and postnatal care, family planning and screening services, reproductive health prevention, and treatment of female-specific diseases. Specific duties are regulated by the state board of nursing.

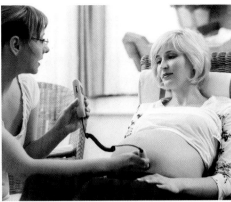

Kzenon/Shutterstock.com

Figure 25.7 A certified nurse midwife is experienced in providing prenatal care.

- **Doula**: this healthcare provider specializes in providing emotional, physical, and educational support before, during, and after childbirth. Doulas do not provide clinical care, and therefore, do not replace the obstetric healthcare provider. The purpose of a doula is to provide a safe and empowering birth experience. There are several different types of doulas. A *labor doula*, for example, answers questions a few months before birth. During delivery, the labor doula provides comfort and pain relief through breathing, relaxation, and massage. After birth, many doulas help with breastfeeding.

- **Pediatrician**: this licensed medical doctor specializes in the care of newborns, infants, children, and adolescents.

- **Pediatric nurse practitioner (PNP)**: this type of licensed nurse has advanced education and training in the care of newborns, infants, children, and adolescents. Specific duties are regulated by the state board of nursing.

Delivery Location

When selecting a healthcare provider, partners also consider the location of delivery. The preferred healthcare provider must have the appropriate privileges and be authorized to give care at the facility a couple chooses. Most women choose to give birth in a hospital, at a birthing center, or at home. When making this decision, partners consider their preferences, the nature of the delivery, and the policies and available services at each facility. For example, if a woman has a high-risk pregnancy, she may choose a hospital with a neonatal intensive care unit (NICU). Partners may also consider room layout (for example, if labor, delivery, and recovery can all occur in the same room and if the newborn can stay in the room with the mother). The woman may consider whether her partner, a family member, or another significant person can be in attendance during the entire delivery and whether her other children can visit after the delivery (Figure 25.8).

Birthing centers are usually located near a hospital. They are most often used by women with uncomplicated pregnancies. Centers may be run by doctors, nurse midwives, or both. They typically have all of the same birthing services as a hospital, but are not usually prepared to handle problems or complicated pregnancies.

Home births are an option if a pregnancy has been progressing well and if there are no risk factors. A home birth allows labor and delivery to occur in familiar surroundings, and partners have more control over the experience. The necessary supplies must be available, and all people involved in the home birth must commit to seeking sufficient and appropriate

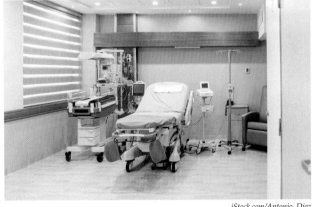

iStock.com/Antonio_Diaz

Figure 25.8 Room layout and facility policy may affect whether partners and children can visit mothers during and after labor and delivery.

support during the delivery and after birth. Home birth should be carefully considered for the first-time mother or if there are existing medical conditions. A nurse midwife or certified midwife is typically in attendance during a home birth.

What Are the Stages of Pregnancy?

Pregnancy typically lasts for 40 weeks and is divided into three stages, or *trimesters*. During this time, the fetus goes through significant development (Figure 25.9). The first trimester is the first 12 weeks of pregnancy. The second trimester spans week 13 to 28. The third and final trimester begins with week 29 and ends with birth at approximately week 40. After week 40, the fetus is usually considered overdue.

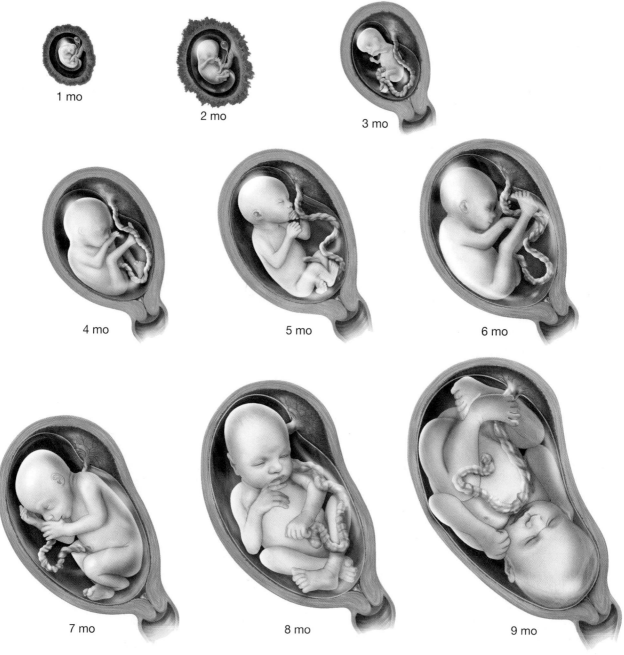

1 mo
2 mo
3 mo
4 mo
5 mo
6 mo
7 mo
8 mo
9 mo

© Body Scientific International

Figure 25.9 Month by month, the fetus grows larger and changes position. As the fetus grows, it is more able to sustain life outside the mother's body.

During pregnancy, a woman's body changes, and the woman must make adjustments to her daily routines. Some of these changes can cause discomfort. For example, some women do not feel well during the first trimester of pregnancy as their bodies get used to the changes. Pregnancy and the future responsibility of motherhood may also cause emotional and psychological changes. Common body changes that women experience during pregnancy are discussed in Figure 25.10.

What Happens During Labor and Delivery?

As pregnancy nears its end, certain signs indicate that labor will soon begin. For some women, these signs begin weeks before the due date. For others, these signs may not

Think About This

During pregnancy, the uterus grows up to 500 times larger than its normal size. It also becomes heavier, increasing from 2–4 ounces to 1–2 pounds. After delivery, the uterus slowly returns to its original size and weight.

Physical Changes During Pregnancy	
Trimester	**Changes in the Mother's Body**
First (weeks 1–12)	• Hormonal changes affect every body system and can trigger signs and symptoms, even in the first weeks of pregnancy. • Menstrual period stops. • The breasts may feel tender and swollen with nipples sticking out. • The mother may feel extremely tired. • The mother may experience an upset stomach and nausea with or without vomiting (*morning sickness*). • The mother may have cravings or distaste for certain foods and mood swings. • The mother may have trouble having bowel movements and experience increased urination. • The mother may have headaches and heartburn. • Weight may be gained or lost.
Second (weeks 13–28)	• Nausea and fatigue lessen. • The abdomen expands. • Fetal movement can be felt by the end of this trimester. • Body aches may increase. • Stretch marks may appear on the abdomen, breasts, and thighs. • The skin around the nipples may darken. • A line on the skin running from the bellybutton to the pubic hairline (*linea negra*) may become visible. • Dark patches may develop on both sides of the face over the cheeks, forehead, nose, or upper lip (sometimes called the *mask of pregnancy*). • The hands may feel numb or tingle. • The abdomen, palms, and soles of the feet may itch. • The ankles, fingers, and face may swell.
Third (weeks 29–40)	• Breathing may become difficult as the fetus grows and puts pressure on the organs. • The mother may experience increased urination and heartburn. • The ankles, fingers, and face may swell. • Hemorrhoids may develop. • Breast tenderness may increase, and *colostrum* (the earliest, protein-rich form of breastmilk) may leak out of the breasts. • The bellybutton may stick out due to the expanding abdomen. • The abdomen may lower due to the movement of the fetus.

Figure 25.10 During each trimester, physical changes in the mother can alter body shape and cause discomfort, requiring adjustments to daily routines.

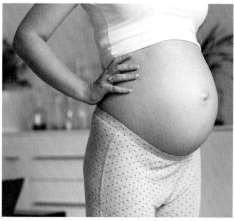

kryzhov/Shutterstock.com

Figure 25.11 In lightening, the fetus drops toward the pelvis, causing the abdomen to look lower.

begin until a week or two after the due date. Despite a woman's excitement for meeting her child, the period before labor is often a stressful and anxious time, particularly for the first-time mother. Providing support and comfort is helpful. Many women have attended childbirth education classes, and partners, parents, family members, and friends may help provide support.

Physical Signs of Labor

As labor approaches, the woman's body begins to show physical signs of impending labor. These signs include lightening, diarrhea, bloody show, ruptured membranes, effacement, and labor contractions:

- **Lightening**: the fetus starts to drop into the pelvis in preparation for delivery (Figure 25.11). The abdomen looks lower, and breathing is easier because the lungs are no longer crowded. Conversely, lightening puts pressure on the bladder, causing an increased need to urinate. Lightening can occur a few weeks or hours before delivery.

- **Diarrhea**: frequent and loose stools may mean labor will begin soon.

- **Bloody show**: the release of the mucus plug, which seals off the cervix to prevent infection, causes what is known as a *bloody show*. The bloody show appears as a blood-tinged or brownish discharge and can occur days before or at the beginning of labor.

- **Ruptured membranes**: when membranes of the amniotic sac tear, fluid will leak or flow from the vagina. This is commonly referred to as the *water breaking* and usually occurs hours before or during labor. If labor does not start soon after the membranes rupture, labor may be induced to prevent infection or delivery complications.

- **Effacement**: also known as the *thinning of the cervix*, effacement begins the birthing process. As the fetus drops closer to the cervix, the cervix gradually becomes softer, shorter, and thinner. During prenatal visits in the third trimester, the cervix is routinely checked for thinning because it will efface before it *dilates* (opens). Sometimes, if the woman has had previous children, dilation will occur before effacement. Effacement is measured in percentage, from 0 to 100 percent. The closer effacement is to 100 percent, the thinner the cervix is, and the sooner labor will begin.

- **Labor contractions**: before true labor begins, some women have false labor pains called *Braxton Hicks contractions*. These irregular uterine contractions cause a feeling of tightening and can start as early as the second trimester. Braxton Hicks contractions usually stop if the woman changes her position.

While different for each woman, true labor contractions cause a dull ache in the back and lower abdomen, along with pressure in the pelvis. Contractions come in a wavelike motion, starting at the top of the uterus and moving to the bottom. During a contraction, the abdomen becomes hard. Between contractions, the uterus relaxes, and the abdomen becomes soft. Regular intervals of 10 minutes between contractions mean labor has begun.

Stages of Labor

For vaginal deliveries, labor is divided into three stages (Figure 25.12). Each woman will have a different experience and time spent in labor. On average, labor lasts 12 to 14 hours for a first pregnancy. This may shorten for subsequent pregnancies.

Stage One

Stage one of labor contains three phases: latent, active, and transition. The *latent phase* is often the longest and least intense. Contractions become more frequent, allowing the cervix to dilate. If contractions become regular, frequent pelvic exams are typically performed to determine the extent of dilation. During the *active phase* of stage one, dilation progresses quickly, and contractions are more intense and occur in shorter intervals. The woman feels an urge to push, or bear down; however, pushing is discouraged, as the cervix is not yet fully dilated. In the *transition phase*, the cervix is fully dilated (10 centimeters, or approximately 4 inches). Contractions become strong and painful, occur every three to four minutes, and last 60–90 seconds.

Starting in stage one, the head of the fetus will press into the birth canal to help start the dilation of the cervix. The fetus will also twist and turn during labor.

The amount of pain a woman experiences is personal and is usually influenced by the strength of contractions and the size of the fetus. Many women manage their pain using breathing and relaxation techniques, change of position, and acupuncture (when permitted by the healthcare provider and available in the facility). Others achieve pain relief through medications. There are two categories of pain medications:

1. *analgesics*, which relieve pain without total loss of feeling or movement; and

2. *anesthetics*, which block all feeling and muscle movement.

If an anesthetic is used, vital signs will be checked frequently after delivery to guard against any post-anesthetic complications. See the next section of this chapter for more information about anesthetics. While using these medications is generally safe, medications may have potentially adverse side effects.

Stage Two

The second stage of labor begins when the cervix is completely dilated and ends with the expulsion of the fetus. Women are urged to push or bear down during contractions to move the fetus through the birth canal. The soft spots (*fontanels*) on the fetus's head allow it to fit through the narrow birth canal. When the head *crowns*, or can be seen, the newborn has reached the widest part of the vaginal opening. Once the head is delivered, amniotic fluid, blood, and mucus are suctioned from the nose and mouth of the newborn (*neonate*). Pushing continues to deliver the shoulders and the rest of the body. When the newborn is fully delivered, the umbilical cord is clamped and cut, usually 30 to 60 seconds after birth. This delay allows for a brief continued flow of oxygen-rich blood to the newborn. Some healthcare providers ask the woman's partner or designated significant other to help with the clamping and cutting.

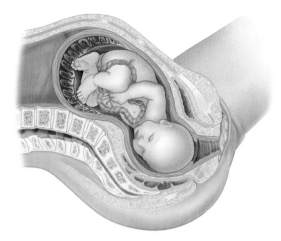

Stage 1

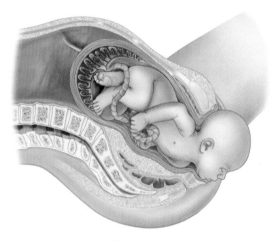

Stage 2

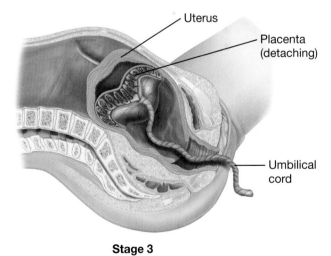

Uterus

Placenta (detaching)

Umbilical cord

Stage 3

© Body Scientific International

Figure 25.12 During the three stages of labor, the cervix dilates, the fetus is delivered, and the afterbirth is expelled.

Stage Three

During stage three, the placenta, or *afterbirth*, is delivered. This usually occurs after many small contractions, which signal that the placenta is separating from the uterine wall. Massaging the uterus and gently pulling the umbilical cord can help dislodge the placenta. Once the afterbirth is expelled, the new mother is observed for several hours to ensure that the uterus continues to contract and that there is no possibility of a hemorrhage.

Recovery

Recovery occurs after delivery as the mother transitions from the experience of childbirth. Recovery is marked by both physical and emotional changes.

One important change during recovery is *bonding*, or the creation of a connection between the mother and newborn. While bonding between the mother and newborn may have occurred during pregnancy, bonding is most intense after birth. Bonding not only gives the newborn a sense of security and self-esteem, but also creates a strong attachment between the parents and newborn. Bonding at this stage happens when the mother touches, feeds and cares for, rocks, and interacts with the newborn. The newborn responds to the mother by directly gazing back at the mother. Bonding is important. Children who were more securely attached to their mothers are better at resolving conflict and enjoy more stable, satisfying ties with partners in early adulthood.

Right after delivery and before the mother goes home, the mother's vital signs will be checked, and she will receive assistance with ambulation and toileting. Possible concerns may be inability to urinate, increased bleeding, trouble breathing, and dizziness.

At home, the following changes and issues may require attention:

- Contractions and pains may occur for a few days until the uterus goes back to its normal size.
- **Lochia** will occur for several weeks after birth. Lochia is vaginal discharge that is heavier than a menstrual period and is composed of blood, mucus, and uterine tissue. Eventually, lochia will fade to white or yellow and then disappear after four to six weeks.
- Vaginal birth sometimes requires a surgical cut called an *episiotomy* to be made in the perineum. This helps prevent tearing during the delivery. Stitches from this procedure may be uncomfortable, particularly when a mother is using the restroom, coughing, sneezing, sitting, or walking.
- Breasts may be painful and swollen, and nipples may be sore, until the milk comes in.
- Short-term hair loss may occur due to hormonal changes.
- Stretch marks that appeared during pregnancy will fade from reddish purple to silver or white. Other skin changes will also fade.
- Some women experience urinary or fecal incontinence when laughing or sneezing due to muscle stretching during delivery.
- Hemorrhoids and constipation may occur and are normal after delivery.
- Irritability, sadness, and crying, known as the *baby blues*, may occur within a few weeks after delivery. These symptoms are common for new mothers and may be the result of hormonal changes and exhaustion.

What Are Some Problems and Complications That Can Occur During Pregnancy and Childbirth?

Several problems can occur during pregnancy and childbirth. These problems include the following:

- **Placenta previa**: a condition in which the placenta covers part of, or the entire, opening of the cervix, causing severe bleeding for the mother

- **Placental abruption**: a condition in which the placenta separates from the uterine wall before delivery, resulting in a lack of oxygen and nutrients for the fetus and severe bleeding for the mother
- **Preeclampsia**: a condition characterized by high blood pressure and signs of organ damage during pregnancy; can result in *eclampsia* (seizures during pregnancy or birth)
- **Miscarriage**: spontaneous loss of a fetus before the twentieth week of pregnancy
- **Ectopic pregnancy**: a condition in which a fertilized ovum implants outside the uterus in the fallopian tube, abdominal cavity, ovary, or cervix (Figure 25.13)
- **Preterm labor**: labor that begins before the fetus can survive outside the mother's body
- **Stillbirth**: fetal death after 20 weeks of pregnancy

Complications that occur during pregnancy and childbirth can be the result of preexisting health issues with the woman, congenital and genetic disorders, viruses and infections, problems with the advancement of the pregnancy, issues related to the growth of the fetus (such as low birthweight), and difficulties during and after delivery (Figure 25.14). The need for a Cesarean delivery (C-section) and postpartum depression (PPD) are two other common complications.

Cesarean Delivery

A *Cesarean delivery*, or *C-section*, is the delivery of the fetus by means of a surgical incision into the woman's abdomen and uterus (Figure 25.15). Upon delivery, the newborn's mouth and nose are cleared of fluids, and the umbilical cord is clamped and cut. After the baby is delivered, the placenta is removed from the uterus, and surgical incisions are closed with sutures (*stitches*) or staples.

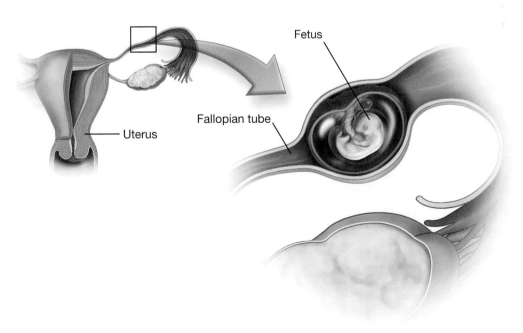

© *Body Scientific International*

Figure 25.13 In an ectopic pregnancy, a fertilized ovum implants outside the uterus. This condition usually leads to the termination of the pregnancy and can threaten the life of the mother.

Complications of Pregnancy and Childbirth		
Complication	**Example**	**Problems**
Preexisting health issues	Asthma; diabetes; eating disorders; hypertension; thyroid disease	Miscarriage; birth problems; other birthing issues
Congenital and genetic disorders	Rh incompatibility; cystic fibrosis (CF); hemophilia; sickle cell disease (CSD)	Newborn problems with lung function and digestion; newborn blood disorders and anemia; malfunctioning organs or limbs of the newborn
Viruses and infections	Influenza; parvovirus; urinary tract infection (UTI); sexually transmitted infection (STI); Zika virus	Ectopic pregnancy; low birthweight; early delivery; newborn brain malformation; pneumonia; eye problems; stillbirth
Problems during pregnancy	Anemia; gestational diabetes; placenta previa; placental abruption; preeclampsia	Bleeding and spotting; early delivery; high birthweight; miscarriage; newborn jaundice and breathing problems

Figure 25.14 Complications during pregnancy can affect both the mother and the baby.

In some cases, a C-section is planned ahead of time. The woman may be carrying multiples, the fetus may be in an abnormal position (for example, in a breech, the feet or buttocks enter the birth canal instead of the head), there may be a problem with the placenta or umbilical cord, it may be apparent the fetus is not receiving sufficient oxygen, or the woman may have had a previous C-section. Sometimes a C-section is not planned, but is performed if labor is prolonged, has stopped, or has complications.

Recovery from a C-section takes longer than recovery for a vaginal delivery. This is because a C-section is a surgical procedure that requires anesthesia and abdominal and uterine incisions. Some risks are associated with C-sections for the newborn and for the mother. For the newborn, one risk is breathing problems due to immature lungs. Potential complications for the mother are increased bleeding, blood clots, reactions to anesthesia, and wound infection.

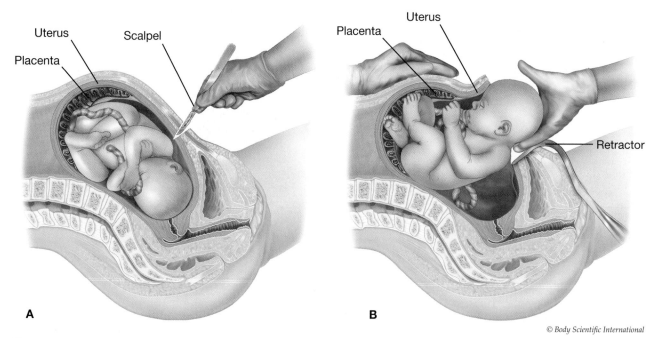

© Body Scientific International

Figure 25.15 In a C-section, an incision is made into the abdomen and uterus (A). Then the fetus is removed from the mother's body (B).

Postpartum Depression (PPD)

Postpartum depression (PPD) is more serious than a case of the baby blues. PPD can cause severe mood swings, intense irritability and anger, excessive crying, loss of appetite, overwhelming fatigue and insomnia, withdrawal, difficulty bonding with the newborn, and thoughts of harming one's self or the newborn. PPD is associated with the hormonal changes that occur after childbirth. Some women are at higher risk for PPD. Risk factors for PPD include depression or anxiety during pregnancy, a traumatic childbirth experience, an ill newborn, and lack of support. Treatment may include individual or family therapy and medications.

What Are Care Considerations for Mothers, Newborns, and Infants?

The arrival of a newborn marks a very busy time in a household. Some mothers find it challenging to set priorities, manage time, and maintain organization after bringing the newborn home. Often, mothers have help and support, but some do not. During this time, mothers and caregivers must attend to postnatal care, learn about infant growth and development, provide appropriate nutrition, and maintain mother and infant hygiene. They also continue to bond with the newborn and provide the love and care the newborn needs to grow and develop (Figure 25.16). As a holistic nursing assistant, you will find knowledge of these topics helpful as you assist the licensed nursing staff and mother.

Postnatal Care

Postnatal care refers to healthcare provided after childbirth. Approximately six weeks after delivery, a healthcare provider will examine the mother's vagina, cervix, and uterus to ensure proper healing. A breast exam may be performed, and blood pressure and weight may be measured. The healthcare provider and new mother also discuss progress related to breast-feeding or formula-feeding, sexual activity and birth control, any physical or emotional challenges the mother is experiencing, and any other issues regarding caring for the newborn. As you learned in chapter 19, the newborn will also receive well-baby exams to monitor his or her physical, developmental, and emotional growth throughout the first year of life. For the first year of life, a baby is known as an *infant.*

Infant Growth and Development

The first year of a baby's life is filled with joy, wonder, and significant growth. Infants learn to reach out and focus their vision, explore, and experience significant cognitive or brain development. Language becomes part of daily life, and infants begin to communicate by making simple sounds and progress as they connect sounds. During this year, the infant learns to love, trust, cuddle, and play.

Not all infants follow the same standard schedule of development, but certain behaviors are common to each age. In the first three months, the infant will raise his or her head and chest while lying on the tummy, open and shut his or her hands, and grip objects. By six months of age, the infant will roll over; sit up with support; and begin to babble, laugh, and reach for toys. Between seven and nine months of age, the infant may start to crawl and scoot, sit without support, and pull up to a standing position (Figure 25.17).

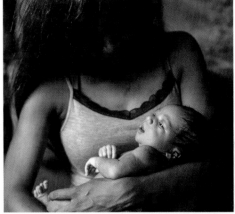

Ginny Filer/Shutterstock.com

Figure 25.16 Once a newborn enters the family, much attention and care are required. This is a time of recovery and adjustment.

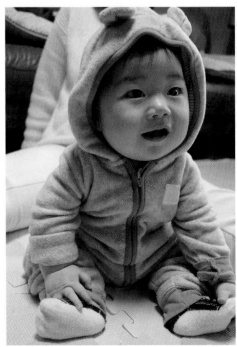

noranoranamona/Shutterstock.com

Figure 25.17 An infant learns to sit without support between seven and nine months of age.

The infant may respond to familiar words and play games such as peekaboo. In the remaining months of the first year, the infant may start walking by holding on to furniture, point at objects, say a few words, and begin self-feeding.

Infant Nutrition

During the first few months of life, an infant's diet consists solely of breast milk or formula. The mother or partners may decide prior to or after birth whether to breast-feed or bottle-feed. There are benefits to each choice.

Breast-Feeding

If a mother is able to produce enough breast milk to sustain her child, then breast-feeding is the best choice for the infant. During the first months of the infant's life, this is especially true, as breast milk is easily digestible and contains nutrients the infant needs. The first milk released from the breasts is **colostrum**, which contains antibodies that provide passive immunity for the newborn. Colostrum begins to be produced by the end of the third month of pregnancy and lasts a few days after the baby is born. In approximately two to four days, *transitional milk* replaces colostrum. Then, 10 to 15 days later, the production of *mature milk* begins. While breast-feeding, or *nursing*, is natural, it may not be comfortable for the mother. Some infants also have trouble *latching*, or connecting with the breast. A certified lactation consultant or licensed nursing staff member may help the mother and infant experience successful breast-feeding before they leave the healthcare facility. Some facilities offer continued lactation support in the weeks or months following birth.

Breast-feeding is convenient in that breast milk is free. Breast-feeding also provides increased protection against infections and releases a hormone that helps the mother's uterus contract and return to its normal size.

Exclusive breast-feeding is recommended for the first six months of an infant's life, at which point solid foods can be introduced into the infant's diet. Ideally, the mother is able to continue breast-feeding until the infant reaches one year of age.

Initially, most infants want to nurse 8–12 times in 24 hours, or about every two to three hours. The time between feedings may increase after solid foods are introduced and keep the infant full longer. Some infants like to breast-feed on both breasts during one feed, and others like to feed on only one breast. The timing and length of each breast-feeding session depend on the baby. A session might be 10–15 minutes or longer. It is important to breast-feed frequently to prevent the breasts from becoming *engorged*, or filled with milk.

A mother should look for hunger cues to determine when to feed her child. Infants show they are hungry by closing their fists, bringing their fingers to their mouths, and looking alert. Crying is a late sign of hunger. When feeding, infants will swallow quickly at first and slow down when satisfied. When full, infants will relax their arms and legs and close their eyes.

To ensure successful breast-feeding, a mother should use good hand hygiene before beginning. The mother should then bring her infant to her breast so the infant can feel the bare skin. This will trigger a reflex that causes the infant to latch on to the breast. The mother should cup her breast in her hand and stroke the infant's lower lip with the nipple. The infant will open his or her mouth wide. When this happens, the mother should aim the nipple toward the roof of the infant's mouth. The infant's chin should drive into the breast, and the infant's nose should be close to the breast (Figure 25.18).

The mother should be in a comfortable position with a back support. Provide a baby blanket to cover the infant and the breast. To remove the infant from the breast, the mother can push down on the breast tissue near the infant's mouth. She can break the suction

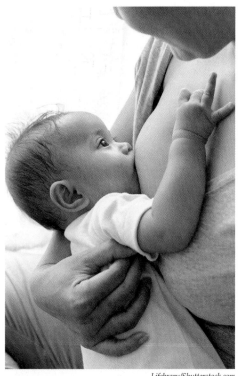

Lifebrary/Shutterstock.com

Figure 25.18 Infants have a reflex that helps them latch on to the breast for feeding.

by gently inserting her finger at the corner of the infant's mouth. The infant should be burped (to get rid of air that can cause cramping and discomfort) after feeding at each breast. Hold the infant to the shoulder, lay the infant on his or her stomach, or place the infant in a sitting position with a clean diaper or towel for protection (Figure 25.19). Gently rub or pat the infant's back in a circular motion for two to three minutes. If the infant's tongue needs to be cleansed of leftover milk, the mother should wet a clean washcloth with cool water and wrap it around one finger. She can use a gentle, circular motion to cleanse the infant's tongue and remove the milk.

Nutrition and hydration are particularly important for a breast-feeding mother. The mother will need extra nutrient-rich calories and plenty of fluids. Caffeine and alcohol should be consumed in moderation. Remember, alcohol leaves breast milk at the same rate it leaves the bloodstream. A doctor or healthcare provider should determine if prescribed medications are safe to take while breast-feeding.

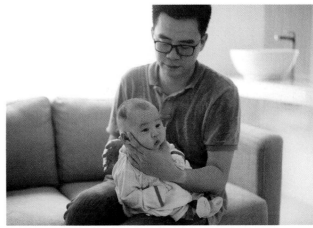

wong yu liang/Shutterstock.com

Figure 25.19 When burping an infant in a seated position, remember to gently support his or her head and neck with your opposite hand.

Bottle-Feeding

Some mothers decide that bottle-feeding with formula or with breast milk best fits their needs. Breast milk provides infants with immunities that lessen the risk for infection, but the majority of infants have passive immunity and are unlikely to get a serious infection in the first few months of life. Commercial formulas also have ingredients similar to breast milk. Infants should be bottle-fed every two to three hours or whenever they appear hungry. The infant will usually consume 2–3 ounces per feeding. Experts advise against encouraging the infant to finish the entire bottle. Infants should eat only as much as they want per feeding.

If the infant makes a noisy sucking sound, he or she may be taking in too much air. To remedy this, hold the infant at a 45° angle and tilt the bottle so the nipple and neck are always filled (Figure 25.20). The bottle should not be propped up, as this can cause choking. Using a clean washcloth, clean the infant's gums and tongue after every feeding.

Following are important bottle-feeding guidelines to consider:

- Select the type of formula that best suits the mother's and infant's needs. Powder, concentrate, and ready-to-feed formula are nutritionally the same.

- Prepare formula at room temperature.

- Discard formula that has not been consumed by the infant during a feeding. Unused formula that has not been prepared for a feeding can be saved.

- Wash your hands or use hand sanitizer when handling formula, breast milk, bottles, and other items to ensure infection control.

- Sterilize new bottles, nipples, and rings by immersing them in a pot of boiling water for a minimum of five minutes. Let them air-dry on a clean towel. After the initial sterilization, wash them with hot, soapy water or on the top shelf of the dishwasher.

- Look for BPA-free bottles or use bottles made of opaque plastic. Avoid clear plastic bottles with the letters *PC* for polycarbonate or the number seven on the bottom.

Think About This

There are several reasons mothers may have breast-feeding challenges. A mother may have sore nipples, low supply or an oversupply of milk, *engorgement* (buildup of milk in the breasts), or a breast infection (called *mastitis*) that can cause soreness or a lump in the breast. Other breast-feeding challenges relate to the newborn. Newborns with diseases or health conditions can have trouble breast-feeding, or a newborn may simply have problems latching on to the nipple.

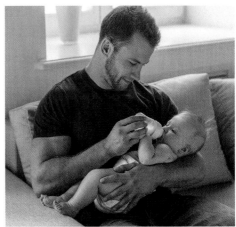

BlueSkyImage/Shutterstock.com

Figure 25.20 Holding the infant at a 45° angle can help prevent the infant from taking in too much air.

- When washing bottles, squeeze hot, soapy water through the nipples to remove the formula or breast milk. Rinse all bottles thoroughly with hot water. Run hot water through the nipples to remove soap.
- Wash the bottles and any other items used to prepare formula or breast milk for the feeding. Place all items on a clean towel on a flat surface or counter to dry.

Mother and Infant Hygiene

Hygiene is essential for both the mother and infant. New mothers often find themselves focusing on their infants and spending less time on themselves. This can cause stress and lead to poor hygiene. Maintaining proper hygiene is important for the mother.

Hygiene for the Mother

- **Hand washing**: proper hand washing or hand sanitizer use during daily activities helps prevent infection.
- **Hydration**: consuming the minimum recommended daily fluid intake reduces the risk of bladder infection and eliminates fluid accumulated during pregnancy (Figure 25.21).
- **Showers**: a daily shower is not only personal time, but is also an opportunity to clean the body of any perspiration and soiling. The warm water from the shower may also release tension and ease any aches and pains.
- **Breast hygiene**: if breast-feeding, the mother should wash her nipples lightly each day. Her bra should be changed daily or when it gets soiled or wet. Breast pads should also be changed often, particularly if they become wet, to prevent skin breakdown or possible infection. If a mother is not breast-feeding, her breasts will stop producing milk after approximately one week or more. Some mothers find a supportive bra comfortable during this transition. Cool compresses or ice packs are also helpful. Until milk production has ceased, a mother should avoid using warm water on her breasts when bathing, as this can stimulate milk production.
- **Toilet hygiene**: after childbirth, it is important to do more than just wipe the genital area after urination. Cleansing the area with warm water is necessary to prevent infection. A squirt bottle with warm water can be soothing. The water should flow from front to back. Using this same motion, gently pat the area dry with clean toilet paper or wipes.
- **Perineal care**: during healing from an episiotomy and stitches, consistent care of the perineum should be performed twice daily at minimum. Some mothers experience heavy bleeding following childbirth. Sanitary pads should be changed two or three times a day. A sitz bath can also be helpful.
- **Rest and exercise**: mothers are usually tired from the demands of caring for an infant. Getting adequate rest and sleep, accompanied with some postnatal exercise, is advised to ensure a healthy life balance.
- **Visitor hygiene**: when an infant comes home, there may be several visitors. Be sure visitors practice good hand hygiene and safety. Discourage potential visitors who are feeling unwell.

Infant Hygiene

Consistent hygiene not only cleans the infant, but also provides time for the mother to bond with her child. It can be a time to express loving emotion and create a playful environment.

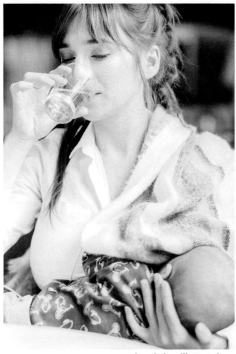
Iryna Inshyna/Shutterstock.com

Figure 25.21 Fluid consumption is important for health and helps prevent infections and other problems.

Bathing an infant around the same time each day establishes a good routine. Bath time for the infant should be comforting and fun. Some infants do not enjoy bathing early in their lives. For these infants, it is important to keep the diaper clean and use clean, warm water to wash key body areas such as the hands, face, axilla, perineum, and any folds of skin.

As a holistic nursing assistant, you may be asked to provide a full bath for or diaper a newborn or infant (or assist the mother with these procedures). Remember that a new mother may be inexperienced in bathing and diapering an infant. Provide support, assistance, and instruction, if needed.

Procedure   Bathing Infants

Rationale

Bathing maintains hygiene and provides an opportunity to observe the skin for possible irritation, rashes, or lesions. Bathing is also an excellent time to hold, touch, and talk to the baby, which promotes feelings of safety, security, and love.

Preparation

1. Ask the licensed nursing staff or the mother if there are any special instructions or precautions regarding the procedure.
2. Wash your hands or use hand sanitizer before entering the room.
3. Knock before entering the room.
4. Introduce yourself using your full name and title. Explain that you work with the licensed nursing staff and will be providing care.
5. Identify the infant by name and check the infant's identification bracelet. In some facilities, the baby's identification bracelet is compared with the mother's.
6. Explain the procedure to the mother in simple terms. Ask permission to perform the procedure.

> **Best Practice**
> Encourage the mother to do as much of the bathing as possible.

7. Bring the necessary equipment into the room. Place the following items in an accessible location:
   - infant-size bathtub (bath basin or sink)
   - tub liner (foam or towel)
   - 2 bath towels
   - paper towels
   - 2–3 washcloths
   - cotton balls
   - baby soap and shampoo
   - baby lotion or cream
   - baby nail scissors or clippers
   - clean diaper and clothes

The Procedure

8. Provide privacy by closing the curtains, using a screen, or closing the door to the room.

> **Best Practice**
> Make sure the room is warm and there are no drafts.

9. Wash your hands or use hand sanitizer to ensure infection control.
10. Fill the bathtub with no more than 1–2 inches of warm water. Check the water temperature. It should be 100–105°F. The water should feel comfortably warm to your elbow. Always check the temperature of the water before placing the infant in the tub.
11. Place a barrier such as a towel or paper towel on a hip-level counter or safe, flat surface. Place the bathtub on the towel or paper towel. Line the bottom of the bathtub with a foam liner or towel. This will help prevent the infant from slipping.
12. Lay a bath towel on the counter next to the tub.
13. Undress the infant and lay him on the clean towel. Always keep one hand on the infant for safety.

(continued)

14. Moisten a cotton ball with warm water and squeeze out the excess water. Wipe the infant's eyes and eyelids, moving from the nose out toward the ears (Figure 25.22). Use a clean cotton ball for each eye and eyelid.

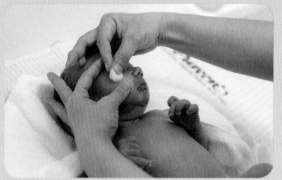

Figure 25.22

15. Wet the washcloth and squeeze out the excess water. Using a washcloth, wash and rinse the infant's face.

16. Gently lower the infant, feet first, into the tub.

Best Practice
Never leave an infant alone in a bath.

17. Support the infant in an upright position with the infant's head and chest out of the water. Make sure you support the infant's head at all times in the tub (Figure 25.23).

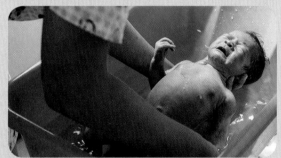

Figure 25.23

18. Wet a washcloth and put a small amount of baby shampoo on the infant's head. Squeeze a small amount of water from the washcloth onto the infant's head. Carefully wash the infant's hair and scalp using a circular motion. Rinse the infant's head and scalp thoroughly by squeezing water from the washcloth. Make sure soapsuds do not get into the infant's eyes.

19. Wash the infant's neck and behind his ears with a small amount of baby soap and a washcloth. Rinse.

Best Practice
Do not stick anything inside the infant's ears.

20. Using a clean washcloth, clean the infant's gums and tongue.

21. Continue by washing the infant's chest, arms, hands, and between the fingers. Wash the legs and between the toes. Pay special attention to washing all folds and creases. After washing with the soapy washcloth, rinse the washcloth. Thoroughly rinse the infant.

22. Clean the umbilical cord with a disposable wipe or cotton ball wet with soap and water (Figure 25.24). Make sure the umbilical cord is dry after cleaning.

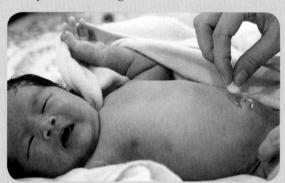

Figure 25.24

23. Using a clean washcloth, gently wash the perineal area. For female infants, gently spread the labia and wash from front to back. Use warm water and no soap. For male infants, gently wash from the urethra to the scrotum with warm water. If the infant is uncircumcised, do not pull back the foreskin, as it will gradually loosen on its own. If the infant has been circumcised, gently clean the penis with a disposable wipe or cotton ball wet with warm water. Follow the plan of care if a dressing is still needed for the circumcision.

24. Cleanse the anal area with soap and water.

25. Wash the infant's back and buttocks with a clean washcloth.

Best Practice
While bathing the infant, observe for signs of skin lesions, rashes, or irritations.

26. Lift the infant out of the tub and wrap him with a bath towel.

27. Using the bath towel, gently pat the infant dry. Be sure to carefully dry the folds and creases of the skin. Keep the infant covered and warm when wet.

28. Carefully trim the infant's fingernails and toenails using baby scissors or clippers. Nails should be trimmed once a week (or as needed), right after the bath, which softens nails. Trim the fingernails following the natural shape of the nail. Trim the toenails straight across.

29. Lightly apply lotion or cream to the skin, if appropriate.

30. Diaper and dress the infant. Make sure the infant is safe and comfortable.

31. Remove, clean, and store equipment in the proper location. Remove soiled linens and discard disposable equipment.

Follow-Up

32. Wash your hands to ensure infection control.

33. Conduct a safety check before leaving the room. The room should be clean and free from clutter or spills.

34. Wash your hands or use hand sanitizer before leaving the room.

Reporting and Documentation

35. Communicate any specific observations, complications, or unusual responses to the licensed nursing staff. Record this information, along with the care provided, in the chart or EMR.

Figure 25.22 Karkacheva Anna/Shutterstock.com;
Figure 25.23 Ivan Olianto/Shutterstock.com;
Figure 25.24 jirasak_kaewtongsorn/Shutterstock.com

Procedure | Diapering

Rationale

An infant's diaper must be changed whenever it becomes wet with urine or soiled with stool. Frequently changing the diaper helps reduce skin irritation.

Preparation

1. Ask the licensed nursing staff or the mother if there are any special instructions or precautions regarding the procedure.

2. Wash your hands or use hand sanitizer to ensure infection control.

3. Knock before entering the room.

4. Introduce yourself using your full name and title. Explain that you work with the licensed nursing staff and will be providing care.

5. Identify the infant by name and check the infant's identification bracelet. In some facilities, the baby's identification bracelet is compared with the mother's.

6. Explain the procedure to the mother in simple terms. Ask permission to perform the procedure.

> **Best Practice**
> Encourage the mother to do as much of the diapering as possible.

7. Bring the necessary equipment into the room. Place the following items in an accessible location:
   - disposable gloves
   - clean, prefolded cloth or disposable diaper
   - diaper cover
   - disposable protective pad
   - washcloth
   - disposable wipes or cotton balls
   - basin of warm water
   - baby soap
   - baby lotion or cream

The Procedure

8. Provide privacy by closing the curtains, using a screen, or closing the door to the room.

9. Wash your hands or use hand sanitizer to ensure infection control.

(continued)

Diapering (continued)

10. Put on disposable gloves.

11. Place a disposable protective pad under the infant.

12. Unfasten the tabs or pins on the dirty diaper. If diaper pins are used, place them out of reach.

13. Wipe the perineal area with the front of the diaper. Wipe from front to back. Remove as much stool as possible using the front of the diaper.

> **Best Practice**
> Note the amount and color of the urine and stool. Infants usually urinate about 6 to 8 times a day. Breast-fed infants have a yellow, soft, and runny stool. Bottle-fed infants have fewer stools, and stool is usually yellow to brown in color.

14. Roll the soiled diaper so the urine and stool are inside. Set the diaper aside.

15. Use disposable wipes or cotton balls wet with soap and water to clean the infant. If there is a large amount of stool, use a washcloth instead. Check for skin irritation, rashes, or lesions.

16. Rinse thoroughly and pat the area dry.

17. Remove and discard your gloves. Put on a new pair of disposable gloves.

18. Clean the umbilical cord with a disposable wipe or cotton ball wet with soap and water. If the infant is circumcised, gently clean the circumcision with a disposable wipe or cotton ball wet with soap and water.

19. Apply a small amount of cream or lotion to the perineal area and buttocks, if needed.

20. Raise the infant's legs. Slide a clean diaper under the infant's buttocks. Cloth diapers need to be folded before use. For a boy, fold the cloth diaper so there is extra thickness at the front. For a girl, fold the cloth diaper so there is extra thickness at the back.

21. Bring the diaper up between the legs to cover the lower abdomen. Make sure the diaper is snug around the hips and abdomen. If an infant's circumcision is not healed, make sure the diaper is loose near the penis. If the cord stump has not healed, the diaper should be below the umbilicus.

22. Secure the diaper in place. Use the tape strips on a disposable diaper to secure at the hips. If pins are used, insert the pins sideways, with points away from the infant's abdomen.

23. If using a cloth diaper, cover the diaper with a diaper cover.

24. Make sure the infant is safe and comfortable.

25. Rinse the stool from a cloth diaper into the toilet. Store the used cloth diaper in a covered pail or wet bag. Throw a disposable diaper in a covered waste container.

26. Remove and discard your gloves.

27. Wash your hands or use hand sanitizer to ensure infection control.

28. Put on a new pair of gloves.

29. Remove, clean, and store equipment in the proper location. Remove soiled linens and discard disposable equipment.

Follow-Up

30. Remove and discard your gloves.

31. Wash your hands to ensure infection control.

32. Conduct a safety check before leaving the room. The room should be clean and free from clutter or spills.

33. Wash your hands or use hand sanitizer before leaving the room.

Reporting and Documentation

34. Communicate any specific observations, complications, or unusual responses to the licensed nursing staff. Record this information, along with the care provided, in the chart or EMR.

Infant Safety

Infant safety is very important. Several actions can be taken to ensure safety, security, and comfort:

- Do not startle infants. Use smooth, not jerky, movements.
- When lifting an infant, use both hands. Use one hand to support the head and upper back and the other hand to support the legs. Never lift an infant by the arms.

- When laying an infant down for sleep, lay the infant on his or her back on a firm surface. Ensure proper chest expansion and breathing (Figure 25.25).
- Respond quickly if an infant cries (Figure 25.26). Crying can mean an infant is in discomfort or is hungry.
- Keep infants warm and away from drafts.
- Avoid clothing that will overheat the infant.

While playing, infants may put objects such as coins or buttons in their mouths out of natural curiosity. An infant should never be unsupervised, and all small objects should be put away to prevent any accidents. If an object does lodge in an infant's throat, it is important to know what to do.

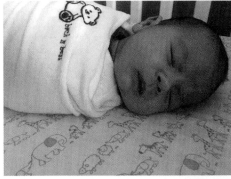

Mallory Dufek

Figure 25.25 Research has shown that lying a baby down to sleep on his or her back reduces the risk for Sudden Infant Death Syndrome (SIDS).

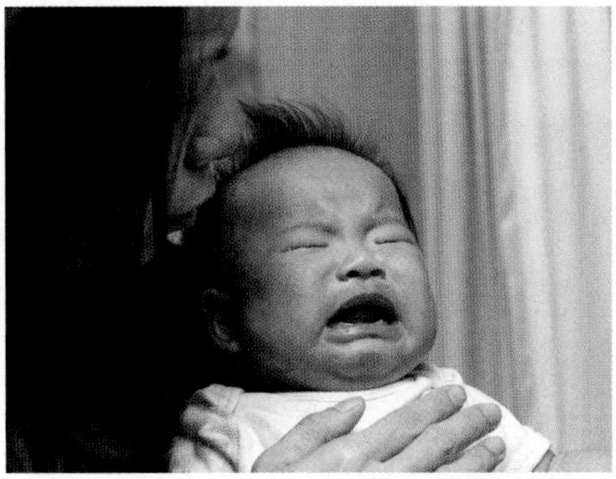

Kenishirotie/Shutterstock.com

Figure 25.26 A crying infant may be hungry, need to be changed, or crave comfort.

Procedure | Clearing an Infant's Obstructed Airway

Rationale

An obstructed airway blocks the flow of air to the lungs. It is not always easy to tell if an infant's or child's airway is obstructed. Removing the obstruction can help prevent further injury or death.

Preparation

1. If there is time, wash your hands or use hand sanitizer to ensure infection control.

The Procedure: Infant Is Conscious

2. Observe the infant. Note if the infant has difficulty breathing, a weak or absent cry, choking, or wheezing. Also note if the infant is unable to cough. Call for help. If there is an emergency system, activate it.

> **Best Practice**
> If you see a foreign object in the infant's mouth, remove it. Avoid pushing it farther down into the throat. Do not perform a finger sweep or attempt to remove an object you cannot see.

3. Expose the infant's upper body.
4. Position the infant over your forearm facedown with the infant's head lower than his trunk. Support the infant's head and neck with one hand. Rest your forearm on your thigh for support. Using the heel of your hand, deliver five back blows between the infant's shoulder blades (Figure 25.27). Check for the object obstructing the airway. Stop if the object has been dislodged.

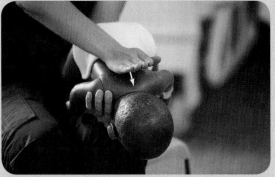

Figure 25.27

(continued)

5. Support the infant on your arm and turn the infant faceup. The infant should be in a back-lying position on your forearm. Rest your forearm on your thigh for support. The infant's head should be lower than his trunk. Using your index finger and middle finger, give five chest thrusts in the midsternal region (Figure 25.28). Give one thrust per second. Check for the object obstructing the airway. Stop if the object has been dislodged.

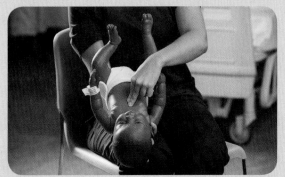

Figure 25.28

> **Best Practice**
> Do not use the Heimlich maneuver for an infant. Abdominal thrusts may injure the infant.

6. Repeat steps 4 and 5 until the foreign object is expelled or until the infant loses consciousness.

The Procedure: Infant Is Unconscious

7. Observe the infant. Note if the infant has difficulty breathing. Call for help. If there is an emergency system, activate it.

8. Place the infant on his back.

9. Open the infant's airway by tilting the head and lifting the chin. Do not hyperextend the infant's neck.

10. Breathe in, but not deeply. You will not need to blow much air into the infant's lungs.

11. Place your mouth over the infant's mouth and nose, making an airtight seal.

12. Blow one small puff of air into the infant's mouth and nose. Observe if the chest rises.

13. Remove your mouth to hear or feel an exhaled breath.

14. Replace your mouth over the infant's mouth and nose and blow another small puff of air.

15. If the infant's chest does not rise with each breath, reposition the infant's head by tilting it back slightly and lifting the infant's chin to open the airway.

> **Best Practice**
> If you see a foreign object in the infant's mouth, remove it. Avoid pushing it farther down into the throat. Do not perform a finger sweep or attempt to remove an object you cannot see.

16. Observe for breathing, coughing, or movement in response to the rescue breaths. Check the brachial pulse.

17. If the pulse is absent, begin CPR. CPR supports blood circulation and breathing. It will include manual external chest compressions (to make the heart pump) and rescue breaths.

18. Place two fingers on the sternum just below an imaginary line between the two nipples. Give 30 compressions to one-third the depth of the chest (about 1½ inches).

19. Open the infant's airway by tilting the head and lifting the chin. Do not hyperextend the infant's neck.

20. Give two breaths (1 second per breath) so the chest rises.

21. Continue the cycle of 30 compressions and two breaths.

22. If you see a foreign object in the infant's mouth, remove it.

23. Continue CPR until the object is expelled or until medical professionals arrive and take over.

Follow-Up

24. Wash your hands to ensure infection control.

25. Make sure the infant is safe and comfortable.

Reporting and Documentation

26. Communicate any specific observations, complications, or unusual responses to the licensed nursing staff or mother. If you are in a facility, record this information, along with the care provided, in the chart or EMR.

Images courtesy of © Tori Soper Photography

Using the Key Terms

Complete the following sentences using key terms in this section.

1. The _____ period occurs after childbirth.
2. The _____ period occurs during labor and delivery.
3. A(n) _____ is a fertilized ovum from implantation until the eighth week of pregnancy.
4. In a(n) _____, a fertilized ovum implants outside the uterus.
5. Vaginal discharge composed of blood, mucus, and uterine tissue is called _____.
6. After the ninth week of pregnancy, a fertilized ovum is known as a(n) _____.
7. The _____ period occurs before labor or childbirth.
8. The _____ transfers oxygen and nutrients from the mother to the fetus via the umbilical cord.

Know and Understand the Facts

9. List two physical changes that can occur in the mother during the second trimester of pregnancy.
10. Describe the stages of labor.
11. Discuss three important actions that mothers need to take during prenatal care.
12. Identify four possible complications of pregnancy and childbirth.
13. What are two reasons a mother might choose to breast-feed?

Analyze and Apply Concepts

14. Explain why proper hygiene is important for both the mother and the infant. Identify two actions for achieving proper postpartum hygiene.
15. Explain the steps for cleaning the umbilical cord.
16. What special actions are part of bathing a male infant?
17. Explain the procedure for diapering an infant.
18. What instructions would you give to a mother who is bottle-feeding her infant for the first time?
19. Describe the steps for responding to an infant with an obstructed airway.

Think Critically

Read the following care situation. Then answer the questions that follow.

Mrs. K is a 36-year-old new mother who just had her first baby. She had a difficult pregnancy and gestational diabetes, and her labor was very long. Mrs. K had a vaginal delivery and episiotomy. She is nervous about taking care of her baby, but she does have her husband and mother-in-law for support. The doctor would like Mrs. K to stay in the hospital for observation for three days. You have been asked to assist Mrs. K with breast-feeding, bathing, and diapering the baby.

20. What actions could you take to learn more about Mrs. K's nervousness concerning her baby?
21. How could you obtain the support and help of Mrs. K's mother-in-law and husband?
22. What instructions can you provide Mrs. K to help her breast-feed?
23. List the guidelines Mrs. K will need to know when she bathes her baby for the first time.
24. What care should you provide Mrs. K to help her maintain proper hygiene?

Questions to Consider

- Have you had a surgery? If not, did someone in your family or a friend have surgery? What was the experience like?
- If you underwent surgery, what were your feelings prior to the surgery? Did you feel frightened or anxious? How did you calm down? If a friend or family member had surgery, were you able to help the person prepare?
- How was the outcome of the surgery communicated?
- What could have made the experience more positive?

Objectives

Surgery is a major event in a person's life. A simple surgery might be the removal of a skin lesion, whereas a major surgery might be the removal of a body organ due to cancer. Whether simple or complex, surgery causes anxiety and stress and can be life changing. To achieve the objectives for this section, you must successfully

- **identify** different types of surgery, surgical staff members, and care considerations for surgical patients;
- **describe** surgical and postsurgical settings and safety precautions;
- **review** the phases of surgery and the care needed, including emotional support before and after surgery;
- **explain** common complications of surgery;
- **observe** and **report** the state of surgical dressings and wounds with drainage;
- **perform** care for drains and evacuators;
- **apply** flexible abdominal binders; and
- **put** on antiembolism stockings.

Key Terms

Learn these key terms to better understand the information presented in the section.

ablation	perioperative
gurney	polyp
hypovolemic shock	postoperative
intraoperative	preoperative
laparoscopic surgery	prolapse
meniscus	reservoir

Surgery may be planned (called *elective surgery*), performed as an emergency (called *emergency surgery*), performed because a patient is critically injured (called *trauma surgery*), or performed to obtain further information about a disease or condition (called *exploratory surgery*). Some surgeries occur in an *operating room (OR)* in a hospital, while others are performed in a hospital's outpatient surgical center or in a freestanding surgery center. Some simple procedures may be performed in a doctor's office. Various doctors and healthcare staff members are prepared and have credentials to perform surgeries and assist with surgical care.

What Types of Surgery May Be Performed?

There are many different types of surgeries. General surgeries can respond to a broad range of conditions and disorders (for example, the repair of a hernia). Specialized surgeries focus on one organ or body system (Figure 25.29). Surgeries can be fairly simple, as in surgeries that remove a **polyp** (growth or mass) or repair a **prolapse** (falling organ). More complex surgeries include the repair of the **meniscus** (cartilage pad) in a knee or the **ablation** (surgical removal) of tissue in the heart.

Specialized Surgeries

Type of Specialized Surgery	Examples
Vascular surgery	• Angioplasty and placement of stents • Aneurysm repair • Carotid endarterectomy
Colon and rectal surgery	• Removal of parts of the colon, anus, and rectum • Repair of a rectal prolapse • Removal of hemorrhoids or polyps
Neurosurgery	• Removal of a brain tumor • Removal of a cerebral aneurysm
Orthopedic and arthroscopic surgery	• Meniscus repair • Repair of a fractured shoulder • Knee replacement • Repair of open and closed fractures of the hand and wrist
Thoracic surgery	• Removal of pleural tumors • Pulmonary lobectomy
Endocrine surgery	• Removal of the thyroid or parathyroid glands
Gynecological surgery	• Endometrial ablation • Tubal ligation • Gynecological laparoscopy
Head and neck surgery	• Nasal and sinus obstruction surgery • Tonsillectomy • Removal of head and neck tumors • Repair of facial deformities
Ophthalmological surgery	• Removal of cataract • Corneal transplant
Urologic surgery	• Removal of kidney stones • Lithotripsy for bladder stones
Plastic and reconstructive surgery	• Abdominoplasty • Reconstruction of burned skin • Repair of complex wounds • Removal of skin cancer lesions • Carpal tunnel surgery • Breast reduction • Breast reconstruction surgery
Bariatric surgery	• Insertion of a gastric band or gastric sleeve • Gastric bypass

Figure 25.29 A specialized surgery targets a specific body system or organ.

Many traditional, open surgical techniques are very invasive. **Laparoscopic surgery** is an example of a surgery that is *minimally invasive*. Laparoscopic surgeries are performed using a *laparoscope* (a telescopic rod lens system connected to a video camera or digital camera). The laparoscope is inserted into the body through a small incision. Laparoscopic surgery results in less blood loss and scarring, which leads to quicker recovery and a reduced amount of pain (Figure 25.30). *Laser surgical procedures* are also available. In these procedures, light (*electromagnetic radiation*) is emitted to cut, burn, or destroy tissue, lesions, and tumors. The use of light minimizes bleeding, and light can easily reach difficult areas.

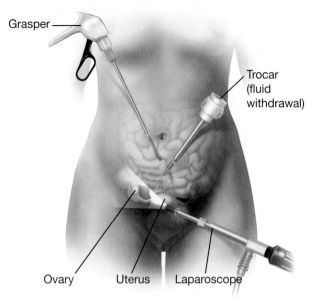

Grasper

Trocar (fluid withdrawal)

Ovary   Uterus   Laparoscope

© *Body Scientific International*

Figure 25.30 The laparoscopic hysterectomy (removal of the uterus) shown here is less invasive than a traditional hysterectomy. The use of a laparoscope leads to quicker recovery.

What Are the Phases of Surgery?

It is important to know the three phases of surgery, which are known collectively as **perioperative** (Figure 25.31). Each phase of surgery requires distinct care. When this care is well coordinated, the best possible outcomes can occur.

The first phase of a surgery or operation is **preoperative**. The preoperative phase starts with the decision to have surgery and ends when surgery begins. If surgery is needed immediately, the preoperative phase can be very short. It can be much longer when a surgery is planned ahead of time. The preoperative phase includes special testing, scheduling, screening, instruction (called *preoperative teaching*), and any preparation needed for the specific surgery.

The second phase is **intraoperative** and is the surgery itself. The intraoperative phase starts with the patient's arrival at the operating room and ends when the patient is moved to the recovery room. In a hospital, a recovery room is usually called a *post-anesthesia care unit (PACU)* because the patient is observed and cared for until the anesthesia wears off. At that time, patients are usually transferred to a hospital room. If patients are in an outpatient setting and are stable, they may return home. If a patient is in critical condition after surgery, he or she may be transferred directly to a specialized critical care unit.

The third and final stage of surgery is **postoperative**. The postoperative phase begins after surgery and lasts until the patient returns to his or her optimal level of health. This phase can last a few hours or several months, depending on the type of surgery, any complications, and the patient's ability to heal and recover. Rehabilitation therapies may be needed during the postoperative phase.

Who Are the Members of the Surgical Staff?

Specialized, trained surgical staff members oversee each phase of surgery and ensure it is performed well. These staff members may vary based on the surgical location (hospital OR, freestanding surgical center, or outpatient surgery setting). For minor procedures in a doctor's office, a doctor may have an RN or trained medical assistant. In some specialty offices, a physician assistant may perform minor surgical procedures under the supervision of a doctor. Common members of the surgical staff include general surgeons, specialty surgeons, the OR sterile team, the OR unsterile team, and registered nurses (RNs).

General Surgeons

General surgeons are licensed medical doctors who have advanced training in surgery. They can perform operations on almost any area of the body and are responsible for determining whether surgery is needed, performing surgery, and caring for the patient after surgery. General surgeons provide perioperative care through all of its phases.

Specialty Surgeons

Specialty surgeons pursue advanced training and credentials to specialize in surgeries on specific areas of the body. Some examples of specialty surgeons are *vascular surgeons* (who operate on blood vessels), *cardiac surgeons* (who operate on the heart and surrounding vessels), *thoracic surgeons* (who specialize in chest surgery),

Think About This

Surgical hand washing requires more time than routine hand hygiene, systematic scrubbing techniques, and the use of specific cleansing products. The intent is to remove microorganisms from the nails, hands, and forearms; reduce pathogens; and inhibit the rapid regrowth of bacteria under the gloved hand. Two systematic methods of scrubbing may be used. The first uses a brush to stroke the fingers, palms, backs of the hands, and arms a specific number of times. The second is a timed scrub lasting three to five minutes or longer. The method used depends on facility policy.

pediatric surgeons (who perform surgeries on children who are usually 16 years of age or younger), and *plastic* and *reconstructive surgeons* (who operate on the skin and soft tissues throughout the body).

The OR Sterile Team

Every OR has a *sterile team*, which is responsible for performing surgery within a limited area that must always be sterile. Because of this, members of the OR sterile team must perform surgical hand washing, don sterile gowns and gloves, wear masks, and handle only sterile items.

The surgeon is the principal member of the OR sterile team. The sterile team may also include assistants to the surgeon. For example, a surgeon may have one or two *assistant surgeons*, depending on the surgery. Other assistants may include a qualified medical doctor, medical resident, or a registered nurse or surgical technologist. Depending on their training, assistants arrange instruments for use, help maintain visibility of the surgical site, control bleeding, close wounds, and apply dressings. The sterile team also includes scrub persons, who may be RNs, LPNs/LVNs, or surgical technologists. These persons maintain the integrity, safety, and efficiency of the sterile field.

The OR Unsterile Team

In addition to the sterile team, the OR also has an *unsterile team* (Figure 25.32). Members of the unsterile team are not allowed to enter the sterile field but must still wear PPE, including a gown and gloves. The unsterile team includes the anesthesiologist or nurse anesthetist, the circulating nurse (an RN, or in some cases, a surgical technologist), and any other OR staff members required to operate specialized surgical machines or devices. The unsterile team helps maintain the sterile field, provides the sterile team with wrapped sterile supplies, touches unsterile surfaces and equipment, and provides patient care outside the sterile field.

An *anesthesiologist* is a licensed medical doctor with specialized training in the administration of anesthesia. A *nurse anesthetist* is an RN who has advanced credentials and training to administer anesthetics. The nurse anesthetist works under the supervision of an anesthesiologist or the surgeon. The responsibilities of the anesthesiologist and nurse anesthetist include positioning and moving the patient; preparing the patient for anesthesia; selecting and administering the appropriate anesthesia; monitoring vital signs; maintaining fluid and electrolyte balance; administering blood replacement, if needed; maintaining electrical and fire safety in the OR; and overseeing the status of the patient's recovery from anesthesia in the PACU until the patient is stable. The circulating nurse on the unsterile team monitors all activities in the OR, manages the care and comfort of the patient, and ensures the sterile field is strictly observed.

Registered Nurses (RNs)

In the PACU, *registered nurses (RNs)* help patients recover from anesthesia, monitor patients' vital signs, and provide postsurgical care. RNs and a full team of staff provide care after surgical patients are transferred to a hospital room.

How Is the OR Organized?

The OR environment is brightly lit and cool. It is air-conditioned and has special venting to help prevent infection and promote safety. The area around the patient

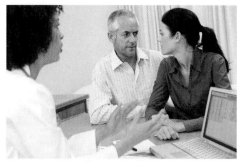

Preoperative
Monkey Business Images/Shutterstock.com

A

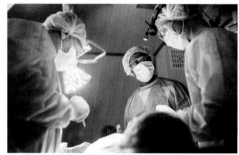

Intraoperative
LightField Studios/Shutterstock.com

B

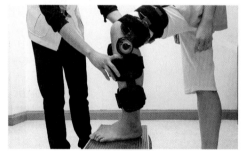

Postoperative
Praisaeng/Shutterstock.com

C

Figure 25.31 The three phases of surgery include preoperative (A), intraoperative (B), and postoperative (C). Unique care is required during each phase.

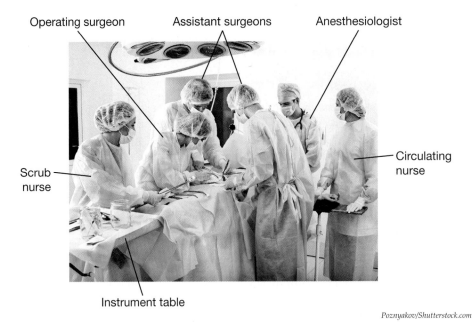

Operating surgeon　Assistant surgeons　Anesthesiologist

Scrub nurse

Circulating nurse

Instrument table

Poznyakov/Shutterstock.com

Figure 25.32 The sterile team works in the sterile field that surrounds the patient. The unsterile team stands outside the sterile field (as seen at the head of the operating table).

is sterile, and sterile drapes help establish the sterile field. These drapes cover the area on and around the patient to prevent contamination from unsterile surfaces. The general rule is that there should be a 12- to 24-inch barrier between the sterile and unsterile fields. OR staff members wear protective, sterile scrubs; sterile gowns; masks; caps; eye shields; and shoe covers to prevent the spread of pathogens. If lasers are used during the surgery, staff members will also need to wear eye protection.

The OR contains a variety of special equipment, including emergency devices such as a ventilator (*respirator*) and a portable *crash cart*, which holds devices and supplies in case the patient *codes* (experiences significant vital sign drop or cardiac arrest). The crash cart contains a defibrillator, airway intubation devices, a resuscitation bag or mask, and medications. The cart must be in an accessible location in the OR. During surgery, monitors also measure the patient's condition, such as electrical activity in the heart, respiratory rate, blood pressure, body temperature, and oxygen saturation. The OR may also contain mobile X-ray units used for bedside radiography and handheld, portable clinical laboratory devices (point-of-care analyzers) for blood analysis. Disposable equipment, such as urinary catheters, and supplies and equipment for wound closure and drainage are also available. Tables in the OR hold needed instruments (Figure 25.33).

Healthcare Scenario
Robotic Surgery

A local teaching hospital recently announced the installation of robotic surgery technology in two ORs. The equipment has enhanced 3-D imaging and can show a highly defined image of the operating field. It has the ability to mimic a surgeon's hand movements. The surgeon can sit at a computer console a few feet away from the operating table and use a joystick to guide a robotic arm that holds instruments and a camera to perform precise hand movements. The hospital is offering robotic surgery for minimally

invasive procedures such as cholecystectomies (gallbladder removals), hysterectomies, hernia repairs, and esophageal strictures.

Apply It

1. What surgical staff members will the hospital need to support this new system?

2. How will robotic surgery capabilities lead to better patient outcomes?

How Is Safety Maintained in the OR?

Safety in the OR is essential. OR equipment can cause several safety hazards, so it is important to follow all safety guidelines. In the OR, there are several areas of concern and strategies for prevention:

- Fires due to electrical units, high temperatures and smoke generated from lasers, and the oxygen-enriched atmosphere are one OR safety hazard. Never lay electrical or heat sources on surgical drapes. Maintain adequate ventilation and familiarize yourself with oxygen shutoffs.

- Electrical shocks are usually the result of faulty equipment. Never unplug equipment by pulling on the cord. Never operate equipment unless there is a ground. All electrical equipment and devices should be serviced and inspected regularly.

- The OR floor can be slippery; therefore, slipping, falling, and tripping are safety concerns. Wear slip-resistant footwear, report fluids on the floor for cleanup, and use caution signs consistently.

- There is a risk of hitting one's head on OR lights. To maintain safety, keep lights out of the way unless they are in use.

- Exposure to blood and body fluids from sharps is a risk when inserting IV lines, cutting, suturing, withdrawing needles, cleaning up, and disposing of equipment. Use protective gear, check for all sharps used, and immediately dispose of sharps in the proper container.

- Using lasers involves the risk of exposure to pathogenic particulates in the air. Wear tightly fitting goggles and keep particulates to a minimum by using lasers close to the laser beam's point of generation or origin.

- Another risk is exposure to waste anesthetic gases from leaks. All equipment connections should be checked carefully, and devices should be serviced regularly.

- Chemical cleaning agents can pose a risk in the OR. Protective gear should be used to eliminate the risk of exposure.

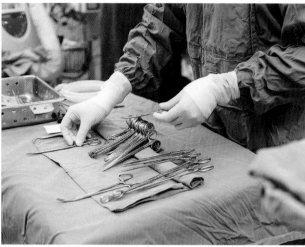

ChaNaWiT/Shutterstock.com

Figure 25.33 A variety of instruments are used for surgery. The exact instruments and their placement depend on the type of surgery and surgeon preference.

Think About This
Recent statistics indicate that there are more than 550 OR surgical fires in the United States each year.

What Do Patients Experience Before, During, and After Surgery?

The patient experience is different in each of the three perioperative phases of surgery. Every patient's experience is unique; however, there are some similarities in the healthcare staff members who provide care, facilities, and functions and processes in each phase.

Preoperative Care

The preoperative phase of surgery can vary significantly in length and includes several steps that must be completed to prepare for surgery. For example, urinalysis and blood tests (including blood typing, if replacement blood will be necessary) are done prior to surgery. Tests may also be performed to better understand the complexity of the surgery or the risk. For example, a surgeon might order cardiac testing to determine whether a patient is a good candidate for surgery.

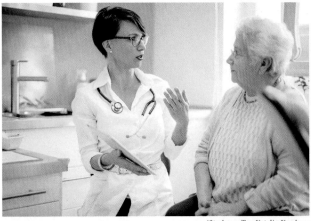
iStock.com/Eva Katalin Kondoros

Figure 25.34 During the visit with the surgeon, the patient will learn more about the surgery and sign a consent form confirming she understands the procedure and the risks.

Another important and required preoperative step is a visit with the surgeon. During this visit, the surgeon will explain the surgery and identify any risks associated with the procedure (including whether or not blood replacement will be necessary). The surgeon will review medications being taken to determine if any adjustments are necessary prior to surgery. For example, taking aspirin right before surgery can cause bleeding problems during surgery. The patient will be asked to sign an informed consent form confirming he or she understands this information (Figure 25.34).

If surgery is planned, a patient may modify his or her diet to gain or lose weight, increase exercise, and quit smoking (which helps reduce the risk for pneumonia after surgery). It is helpful for patients to check their insurance or medical benefits and determine if the surgery is covered. Surgery is usually expensive, and most insurance plans do not cover all of the charges, so determining financial resources is important. If patients are working, they should check the length of their sick leave or vacation time. Insurance forms and specific documents may be completed prior to the surgery or on the day of surgery.

If a patient is going to a surgical outpatient setting or freestanding surgical center, the patient will be admitted, and nursing staff members will help the patient into a gown and safely store personal items, if needed.

The day before surgery, patients will be asked not to eat or drink anything (*NPO*), usually starting around 5:00 p.m. NPO includes mints and chewing gum. On the day of surgery, patients take only medications advised by the surgeon with a sip of water. When brushing teeth, patients should not swallow any water.

The patient should bring his or her insurance card, personal identification, and medication list. The patient should not bring jewelry, credit cards, money, or other valuables. He or she will also be asked to remove nail polish so it does not interfere with oxygen delivery. For more information about the admission process, see chapter 5.

If a hospital stay is required, the patient should pack only essential items such as pajamas, loose comfortable clothing to wear home, and toiletries. If a patient is in the hospital, several additional tasks need to be completed prior to surgery. A nursing assistant will help with many of these needs:

- The patient will be asked to take a bath or shower.
- All jewelry must be secured with the family or according to facility policy.
- Makeup and nail polish must be removed if not removed prior to entering the hospital.
- Hairpins, clips, combs, wigs, and hairpieces must be removed.
- Contact lenses, hearing aids, and artificial eyes and limbs must be removed. Use the facility policy for proper storage.
- Dentures also must be removed and stored (see chapter 21).
- NPO signs should be posted per facility policy.
- The water pitcher should be removed from the hospital room.
- The surgical preoperative checklist must be completed and should include current vital signs and the time of the patient's last urination.
- If the patient is not in a hospital gown, a gown will need to be put on the patient.

Some patients may also need *surgical preparation*, which may require shaving the area of the surgery. This is usually done by the licensed nursing staff. Other types of surgical preparation may be an enema or vaginal douche. After checking the patient's identification bracelet or other patient identification used by the facility, transport staff members will take the patient, usually via a **gurney** (stretcher), to the preoperative section of the OR.

An IV catheter or needle will be inserted, if not already present, and medications may be given for specific health conditions and to relax the patient prior to surgery. The anesthesiologist or anesthetist will visit the patient to discuss the anesthesia being used, expectations for recovery, and any questions the patient might have. Vital signs are monitored, a head covering is put on the patient, and a final check ensures all paperwork and preoperative orders have been completed.

When the patient is ready, he or she is transported to the OR via a gurney or bed. The patient may be very drowsy from relaxation medications that were given, so safety is vital. The patient is carefully transferred from the gurney or bed to the operating table and positioned for surgery. The OR team now takes over. These team members are sensitive to the patient's privacy and follow protocols to ensure a safe experience during surgery.

Intraoperative Care

Prior to the start of surgery, surgical staff members have many preparations to make. They must communicate with one another and place equipment appropriately in the OR. Usually, the circulating nurse from the unsterile team will talk with the patient and address any comfort needs (for example, by putting a blanket on the patient if he or she is cold). If the patient is still awake when the surgeon comes in, the surgeon will say hello.

The anesthesiologist or nurse anesthetist will be at the head of the operating table and will talk with the patient while attaching a blood pressure cuff and ECG leads to monitor the heart. Monitoring equipment, infusion pumps that deliver anesthesia, and any necessary medications or blood are placed nearby. If the patient is receiving general anesthesia, the patient will become unconscious, and pain receptors to the brain will be blocked. A mask may be put over the patient's nose and mouth, and the patient may be asked to breathe deeply. The anesthetic can also be injected into an IV catheter, into the spine, or into another specific part of the body. Once the patient is asleep, an endotracheal tube (breathing tube) may be placed in the throat (Figure 25.35).

Just before surgery, the area where the surgery will take place is cleaned with an antiseptic solution and covered with a sterile drape. Only the site to be operated on is left uncovered. A *pause* or *time-out* occurs right before the surgery begins. During this pause, the OR team double-checks the patient's identity, the procedure and site, the side and position, and necessary equipment. If the surgery is long, compression boots or antiembolism stockings may be placed on the patient's lower legs to prevent blood clots.

The amount of time in the operating room will depend on the type of surgery and any complications encountered. OR staff members may call the patient's family or loved ones into a surgical waiting area to communicate progress and any delays. In some OR waiting areas, a surgical communication tracking board displays the patient's progress in surgery. When the surgery is over, the patient is moved to the recovery room or PACU for the next several hours (on average, one to three hours).

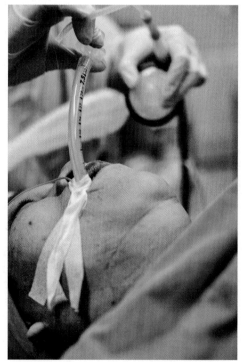

Chaikom/Shutterstock.com

Figure 25.35 An endotracheal tube helps a patient breathe during surgery.

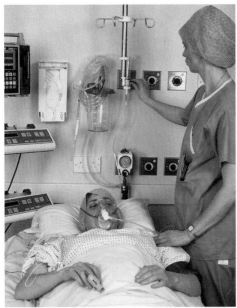

Simon Fraser/Science Source

Figure 25.36 After surgery, the patient recovers in the PACU.

Think About This

The specific criteria usually used in the recovery room or PACU to categorize a recovering patient includes

- **alert:** able to give appropriate responses to stimuli;
- **drowsy:** half-asleep and sluggish;
- **stupor:** lethargic, unresponsive, and unaware of surroundings;
- **comatose:** unconscious and unresponsive to stimuli.

A patient can only be removed from the PACU when he or she is categorized as alert.

Postoperative Care

Postoperative care begins in the recovery room or PACU. Here, patients recover from anesthesia with healthcare staff members who can detect any complications and provide support and comfort. Monitors are attached to the patient, and vital signs are taken every 5 to 15 minutes. An oxygen mask or nasal cannula helps with breathing, and PACU nursing staff will examine the surgical site and check the IV catheter. The endotracheal tube may have already been removed or may still be in the patient's throat to help with breathing. (Figure 25.36).

After awakening, some patients complain of a sore throat, aching muscles, and shivering. Some patients, especially older adults, may be confused. Warmed blankets are provided, if needed. Patients may also be nauseated and vomit. Medications can ease these feelings, and pain relief is key to comfort and healing. A pain scale is used to determine pain severity, and pain medications will be given, as needed. (See chapter 9 for more detailed information about pain relief.) The surgeon may come in to see the patient in the PACU or will discuss the patient's status with family members or loved ones by phone or in person.

The timing of discharge from the PACU depends on the surgery and the patient's recovery from anesthesia. While anesthesia stays in the body for approximately 24 hours, patients must meet the criteria for being awake. If patients are going home or will be transferred to another facility, they must have stable vital signs, manageable pain, and no nausea or vomiting. If patients have had spinal anesthesia, which wears off slowly, they will usually move their toes and feet before they first feel them. The ability to move, followed by sensations, first occurs in the toes and then moves up the legs. As feeling returns, patients often describe feeling like pins and needles are poking these areas. After spinal anesthesia, a patient is usually asked to remain in a supine position for six to eight hours. This prevents a headache that often occurs if the patient becomes active too soon.

If the patient is awake and has stable vital signs, the next step is transfer to a hospital room. If the patient did not have a hospital room prior to the surgery, a room will be assigned and prepared. The hospital bed must be made as a *surgical bed* (see chapter 20) so the patient can be easily transferred into the bed. An emesis basin and tissues should be placed on the bedside stand. Vital sign equipment, an IV pole, oxygen equipment, extra warm blankets, towels and washcloths, and any other equipment directed by the licensed nursing staff should be readily available in the room.

Once the patient arrives in the hospital room, a licensed nursing staff member confirms his or her identify by checking the identification bracelet. A nursing assistant often helps transfer the patient to the bed. Vital signs should be measured frequently per the doctor's order—as often as every 15 minutes upon arrival, with decreasing frequency as the patient becomes stable. Nursing assistants also help ensure the patient's airway is maintained and assist if the patient is still nauseous or vomiting. I&O must be accurately measured and recorded, and catheter care may also be required. If the patient does not have a catheter, the first urination after surgery is critical. The patient may need assistance with urination and may need a bedpan or urinal. Hand hygiene and standard precautions must be strictly maintained.

Patients will require different levels of postoperative care depending on their surgery, age, and preexisting health issues. Some patients will require more assistance after surgery than others. If patients are in a hospital or long-term care facility, their surgical needs will be included in the plan of care.

What Complications Are Possible During or After Surgery?

While the goal is always to have a complication-free surgery and postoperative period, this does not always happen. Potential surgical complications are numerous and can occur during or after surgery. Possible complications include the following:

- reaction to the anesthesia
- reactions to the insertion or removal of the endotracheal tube (for example, laryngospasm when the endotracheal tube is removed)
- changes in vital signs, such as the lowering of blood pressure or weak, rapid, or irregular pulse
- excessive bleeding during surgery, including hemorrhage, which may be followed by shock or cardiac arrest
- urinary retention due to anesthesia, which depresses the ability of the urinary bladder to contract
- slowing or stopping of intestinal peristalsis due to the anesthesia; can lead to nausea and vomiting, flatus, and constipation
- **hypovolemic shock**, or severe blood loss internally or externally after surgery; characterized by postoperative hypotension, rapid weak pulse, restlessness, and cool or moist skin
- *deep vein thrombosis (DVT)*, or blood clots that may break loose and travel through the bloodstream to cause a pulmonary embolus (PE) or a stroke; caused by inactivity during recovery and characterized by swelling in one or both legs, calf pain, shortness of breath, and chest pain
- difficulty breathing or shortness of breath after surgery; can cause a buildup of mucus in the lungs and lead to pneumonia
- infection of the skin at the surgical incision (especially antibiotic-resistant infection caused by methicillin-resistant *Staphylococcus aureus* or MRSA)

Becoming a Holistic Nursing Assistant
Caring for Surgical Patients

Planning for and recovering from surgery can create a significant amount of stress and anxiety. When caring for surgical patients, a holistic nursing assistant should remain observant during caregiving and support the patient during this challenging time. There are several actions a holistic nursing assistant can take to provide this care:

- Recognize the patient's anxiety and stress before and after surgery and give compassionate, supportive care. Family members will also feel anxious and may need support.
- Try to understand the patient's feelings, listen, and remind the patient that you are there to help.
- Talk with postoperative patients and ask supportive questions about how they feel.
- Pay special attention to the patient's pain, observe nonverbal communication, and report pain levels to the licensed nursing staff.

- Encourage questions and ask patients to share any changes or feelings they are experiencing.
- Create a relaxing and comfortable environment.
- Be very observant. Position patients often, pay special attention to tubing and dressings, and check for any signs of skin breakdown or infection.
- Reinforce information given by the surgeon, as appropriate and per direction from the licensed nursing staff.

Apply It

1. Consider how these guidelines fit into daily care. Which guidelines do you think will be most difficult to follow?
2. Brainstorm some questions you can ask a patient to demonstrate your support. Identify nonverbal communication strategies you can use to demonstrate care and compassion.

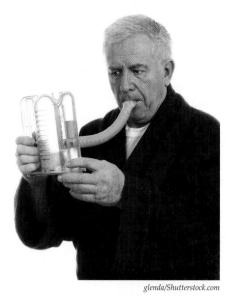

glenda/Shutterstock.com

Figure 25.37 Using an incentive spirometer helps prevent pneumonia in patients after surgery.

- delayed healing after surgery, which is more typical for patients who have a chronic disease or condition (such as diabetes), who have a problem with the immune system, or who were ill prior to surgery
- numbness and tingling around the surgical site due to the surgeon cutting through nerves to make the needed incision
- bruising, swelling, and scarring at the surgical site

There are several ways to prevent or help patients manage and overcome possible postsurgery complications. A nursing assistant may be responsible for taking the following actions based on the plan of care and direction by the licensed nursing staff:

- Observe consistent and thorough hand hygiene to prevent infection.
- Maintain safety at all times and be aware of any tangling or kinking of tubes.
- Check vital signs on the schedule ordered. The schedule is usually every 15 minutes for the first hour, every 30 minutes for one more hour, every hour for two hours, and every four hours for 24 hours, if the patient is stable. Also check circulation and observe the skin, lips, and fingernails for signs of cyanosis.
- Assist with pain relief. Frequently ask the patient about his or her level of pain.
- Observe the patient's level of consciousness, especially for the first 24 hours after surgery. Patients may remain sleepy.
- Monitor the patient's I&O accurately to ensure proper hydration. Note the time of the first urination.
- If the patient vomits, turn his or her head to the side to prevent aspiration. Hold the emesis basin in place. Provide hygiene and oral care.
- Encourage the patient to cough, turn frequently, and take deep breaths. Help the patient into a comfortable position (with the head elevated) and then ask the patient to take a few deep breaths and cough forcefully. If the patient has an abdominal incision, support the incision site with a small pillow or folded towel. Some patients use an *incentive spirometer* to breathe more deeply (Figure 25.37). This device measures how deeply the patient can inhale. Several times a day, the patient should use the device to take slow, deep breaths and then take out the mouthpiece and exhale normally. This helps prevent pneumonia.

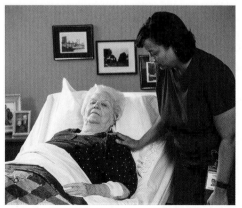

© Tori Soper Photography

Figure 25.38 To promote recovery, observe the patient's surgical dressing closely. Check for signs of bleeding and note the color of blood.

- Observe the patient's surgical dressing (Figure 25.38). If the patient has a large dressing, check under the patient, as blood may drain down the sides and pool under the patient (even if there is no evidence of bleeding on top of the dressing). Report the color and amount of blood to the licensed nursing staff. Bright red blood indicates fresh bleeding. Brownish blood indicates bleeding that is not fresh.
- Apply compression devices or antiembolism stockings, leg exercises, and early and frequent ambulation, as ordered, to prevent DVT. Initial ambulation after surgery can be challenging for the patient. Have the patient dangle prior to ambulation and provide safe care during ambulation (see chapter 17).
- Apply cold compresses, if ordered, to speed the healing process.
- Provide careful wound care to help minimize scarring.

What Surgical Care Considerations Should Be Observed?

In addition to care that prevents surgical complications, surgical patients also require specialized care that promotes recovery. Postoperative patients often have drains and evacuators to help remove exudate, or discharge such as blood or pus. Patients may also wear abdominal binders to keep dressings in place and compression devices such as antiembolism stockings to prevent DVT or PE. Nursing assistants must understand these important surgical care considerations to help maintain proper function, observe the patient's condition, and ensure patient comfort during associated procedures.

Drains and Evacuators

Drains promote healing by removing any accumulation of discharge or exudate. In some cases, drains are also used to empty air created by a removed organ. Drains help protect the skin by keeping exudate or discharge from seeping onto the skin surface. There are two types of drainage systems: open drainage and closed drainage (Figure 25.39).

In *open drainage*, a drain is placed within an incision, usually on an arm or leg. A dressing is also applied to capture exudate. The drain itself is a small, collapsible, plastic tube and is usually anchored with a safety pin so it does not slip down into the incision. The drawback of this system is that it is harder to measure the amount of drainage because of the way the drainage is absorbed by the dressing.

Closed drainage involves *evacuators* that use compression and suction to remove drainage. Evacuators collect drainage in a **reservoir** or drainage device. Closed drainage provides a more accurate measurement of drainage and reduces the risk of infection because drainage is removed.

The type of drainage system used depends on the needs of the patient, the type of surgery (for example, a mastectomy), the type of wound, the amount of drainage expected, and the surgeon's preference. No matter what system is used, nursing assistants should follow the following guidelines when caring for patients with drains or evacuators:

- Maintain strict standard precautions when handling drains. Wear disposable gloves.

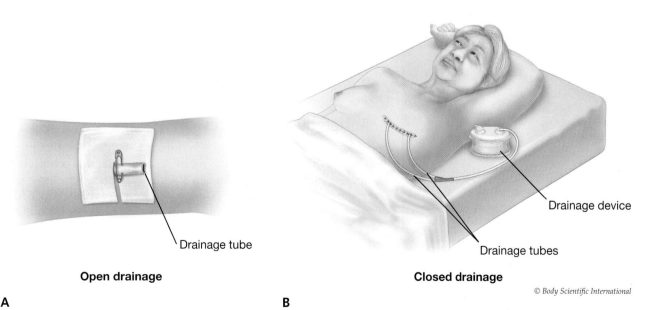

Drainage tube

Open drainage

A

Drainage device

Drainage tubes

Closed drainage

B

© Body Scientific International

Figure 25.39 In open drainage (A), exudate is absorbed by a dressing placed near the drain. In closed drainage (B), exudate is collected in a reservoir or drainage device.

- Prevent kinking and report any possible clogging, which can interfere with adequate drainage.
- Ensure the drain is properly secured, is located below the insertion site, and does not become tangled with other tubing (which can pull the drain out of place).
- Ensure drains are in place before assisting a patient with turning or ambulation.
- If a closed drainage system seems to have lost suction, immediately notify the licensed nursing staff.
- Observe and document the amount and type of fluid in the closed drainage system's reservoir or drainage device.
- Observe the drain insertion site for leakage, redness or oozing, and the condition of the skin. Report any concerns to the licensed nursing staff.
- Observe and report the type, amount, and odor of drainage. Drainage can be clear or bloody. It may also be *purulent* (filled with pus) and white, yellow, gray, green, or brown. Bloody drainage (in large amounts), purulent drainage, and foul-smelling drainage are causes for concern and should be reported immediately.
- Monitor the patient for signs of infection. Notify the licensed nursing staff immediately if the patient has a fever, if there is extreme tenderness at the drainage site, or if there is increased drainage.
- Help the patient understand the importance of the drain. Encourage the patient to take care when moving and ambulating so the drain is not dislodged.

Abdominal Binders

An *abdominal binder* is a wide, flat piece of fabric or elastic material applied to hold a dressing in place (Figure 25.40). Most binders have a Velcro™-like fastener. Any binder that is applied must be

- sized appropriately;
- applied firmly enough to hold dressings in place, but not tight enough to cause discomfort or constrict circulation;
  - fastened from the bottom up;
  - kept in place so that it does not slip up or down (as patient movement can loosen the binder); and
  - rewrapped often (at which point the dressing should be checked for the amount and type of drainage and the condition of the skin).

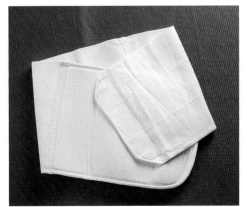

© *Tori Soper Photography*

Figure 25.40 An abdominal binder is made of fabric or an elastic material. It holds any dressings in place.

Antiembolic Measures

Risks for DVT and PE are high during the postoperative phase. The use of compression devices, including sequential compression devices (SCD) and antiembolism stockings, helps reduce these risks (Figure 25.41). If an SCD is used, follow the facility procedure. After the device is put in place, remain in the room for one full cycle (60–90 seconds) to be sure the device is working properly. The plan of care will determine the wearing schedule for antiembolism stockings. Some patients may continue to wear antiembolism stockings even after the postoperative phase is complete.

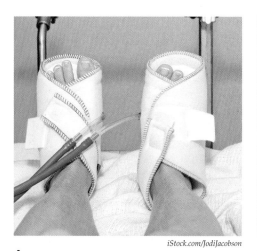

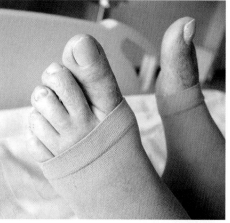

A   B

iStock.com/JodiJacobson   *Joe Prachatree/Shutterstock.com*

Figure 25.41 A sequential compression device (SCD), shown in A, inflates cuffs or wraps placed on the extremities to stimulate circulation. When the SCD is turned on, it inflates the chambers in the cuff or wrap in a sequential order. Shown in B, antiembolism stockings provide compression to promote circulation in the legs and feet.

Procedure Applying Antiembolism Stockings

Rationale

When a patient has had surgery and is not active, elastic stockings are applied to promote circulation in the legs and feet.

Preparation

1. Ask the licensed nursing staff how this procedure fits into the plan of care, if there are doctor's orders for the procedure, if there are any special instructions or precautions, and if the patient can be moved into the positions required for this procedure.

2. Wash your hands or use hand sanitizer before entering the room.

3. Knock before entering the room.

4. Introduce yourself using your full name and title. Explain that you work with the licensed nursing staff and will be providing care.

5. Greet the patient and ask the patient to state his full name, if able. Then check the patient's identification bracelet.

6. Use Mr., Mrs., or Ms. and the last name when conversing.

7. Explain the procedure in simple terms, even if the patient is not able to communicate or is disoriented. Ask permission to perform the procedure.

8. Bring the necessary equipment into the room. Place the following items in an accessible location:

   • compression stockings of the proper size and length (Figure 25.42)

   • disposable gloves, if needed

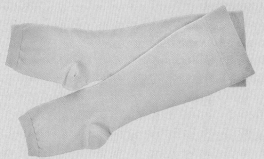

Figure 25.42

The Procedure

9. Provide privacy by closing the curtains, using a screen, or closing the door to the room.

10. Lock the bed wheels and then raise the bed to hip level.

11. Ensure safety during the procedure. If there are side rails, raise and secure the rails on the opposite side of the bed from where you will be working. Lower the rail on the side you are working.

(continued)

Applying Antiembolism Stockings
(continued)

12. Wash your hands or use hand sanitizer to ensure infection control.

> **Best Practice**
> Disposable gloves are worn only if required for infection prevention and control.

13. Assist the patient into a supine position.
14. Expose one leg by fanfolding the linens toward the opposite leg. Make sure the leg is dry and free from lotion, ointments, or oils.
15. Take one stocking. Gather or turn the stocking inside out to the heel.
16. Slip the foot of the stocking over the patient's toes, foot, and heel (Figure 25.43).

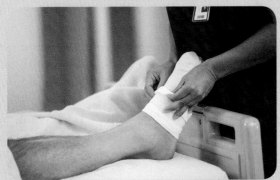

Figure 25.43

17. Roll the stocking up the leg to the knee or thigh, depending on the length ordered. Be sure the stocking is properly placed. The toes may be covered or uncovered, depending on the stocking.

18. Repeat steps 14–17 to apply a stocking to the other leg.

> **Best Practice**
> Check a patient's stockings often. Stockings should be smooth and wrinkle free and should not apply pressure to the toes. Also check circulation in the toes. Note sensation, if any swelling, and the temperature of the skin. Adjust the stockings as needed.

19. Check to be sure the bed wheels are locked, then reposition the patient and lower the bed.
20. Follow the plan of care to determine if the side rails should be raised or lowered.

Follow-Up

21. Wash your hands to ensure infection control.
22. Make sure the patient is comfortable and place the call light and personal items within reach.
23. Conduct a safety check before leaving the room. The room should be clean and free from clutter or spills.
24. Wash your hands or use hand sanitizer before leaving the room.

Reporting and Documentation

25. Communicate any specific observations, complications, or unusual responses to the licensed nursing staff. Record this information, along with the care provided, in the chart or EMR.

Figure 25.42 Geo-grafika/Shutterstock.com; Figure 25.43 © Tori Soper Photography

What Happens During and After Discharge

After surgery, some patients are discharged to another facility for rehabilitation or further care. Other patients return home. During the postoperative phase, following the discharge plan and instructions is vital. The *discharge plan* provides instructions concerning medications, activity levels, treatments that need to be continued, and follow-up appointments with the doctor. Chapter 5 provides detailed information about discharge. Depending on the complexity of surgery, patients will often need assistance at home and will likely become tired quickly. Patients may need regular visits from a home healthcare provider or nurse. Some patients will also require rehabilitation services such as physical therapy. The goal of this phase is always to help the patient return to his or her optimal level of health.

Using the Key Terms

Complete the following sentences using key terms in this section.

1. The three phases of surgery are known collectively as _____.
2. _____ care is provided after surgery until complete recovery.
3. _____ is a serious, life-threatening surgical complication characterized by decreased circulating blood volume.
4. The _____ phase of surgery occurs during the surgery and lasts until the patient arrives in the recovery room.
5. In _____, a laparoscope is inserted through a small incision and used to conduct a minimally invasive surgery.
6. _____ care is provided after the decision to have surgery is made, but before surgery begins.
7. Liquid or semisolid discharge from a wound is called _____.

Know and Understand the Facts

8. Identify three different members of the surgical staff.
9. What equipment should be present in the OR?
10. Describe two ways to maintain safety in the OR.
11. Explain the three phases of surgery.
12. How is a sterile field maintained in surgery?
13. Describe three common complications of surgery.
14. What conditions must be present for a patient to be transferred from a PACU?

Analyze and Apply Concepts

15. Identify three guidelines to follow when performing care for drains.
16. Describe what a nursing assistant should look for when observing drainage.
17. Explain three best practices for applying an abdominal binder.
18. Identify five guidelines for caring for a postoperative patient.
19. List the steps needed to put on antiembolism stockings.

Think Critically

Read the following care situation. Then answer the questions that follow.

Mr. A, a 62-year-old man, had a portion of his colon surgically removed early this morning. He was transferred to his hospital room from the PACU a few hours ago. Mr. A is alert and has an IV catheter, a urinary catheter, and a large bandage and gravity drain in his lower abdomen. He is wearing antiembolism stockings. When you answer Mr. A's call light, he tells you that he is in severe pain and that his antiembolism stockings feel very uncomfortable. You know he had pain medication two hours ago. During the change-of-shift report, you learned that Mr. A's wife died two years ago from breast cancer and that Mr. A has no children. He is alone in his room and has the lights out.

20. What is the first action you should take to assist Mr. A and respond to his complaint of severe pain?
21. You will need to observe Mr. A's dressing and drain. What should you look for, and how should you report and document your findings?
22. Describe what actions you should take to provide Mr. A with catheter care.
23. What should you do about Mr. A's antiembolism stockings?
24. How can you provide support for Mr. A during his postoperative period? What psychosocial and emotional issues might interfere with his healing?

Key Points

Reviewing the key points for this chapter will help you practice more safely and competently as a holistic nursing assistant and will help you prepare for the certification competency examination.

- Women who plan their pregnancies often pursue preconception care. Once pregnant, women need regular prenatal care to ensure a successful pregnancy and identify and treat problems as soon as possible.

- Pregnancy typically lasts 40 weeks and is divided into three trimesters, each characterized by specific changes in the woman's body and fetal developmental milestones.

- There are three phases of surgery: preoperative, intraoperative, and postoperative. Each phase requires distinct care.

- Specialized, surgical staff members are trained to ensure all phases of surgery are performed well. In the OR, this staff is divided into the sterile and unsterile teams.

- Complications such as reactions to anesthesia, difficulty breathing, and DVT may arise after surgery. After surgery, patients often have drains, pumps, and evacuators to help remove exudate. Patients may also need abdominal binders, compression devices, or antiembolism stockings.

Action Steps to Holistic Care

Review the information in this chapter. Complete the following activities.

1. Select one procedure in this chapter. Prepare a short paper or digital presentation that identifies and describes the top three most important steps in the procedure. Include one step that would promote comfort and one that assures safety.

2. With a partner, write a song or a poem about the stages of surgery. Discuss why this information is important.

3. With a partner, select one pregnancy- or surgery-related complication. Prepare a poster that illustrates at least four facts about the complication and explains why these complications are important to understand.

4. Research current scientific information about breast-feeding and formula-feeding. Write a brief report describing two new facts.

5. Create a poster or digital presentation to prepare first-time mothers for the postnatal period. Discuss what to expect when recovering from either a vaginal or cesarean delivery, the possibility of postpartum depression, and hygiene considerations. Research resources and support networks available for new mothers in your community and include this information as well.

Preparing for the Certification Competency Examination

To prepare for the nursing assistant certification competency examination, you will need to know content found in this chapter. This content may be tested in the knowledge (written or oral) and skills (hands-on demonstration) portions of the exam. The following areas will be emphasized:

- pre- and postoperative care
- physical and emotional needs before and after surgery
- common complications of surgery
- dressings and wounds with drainage
- care of open and closed drains
- abdominal binders
- antiembolism stockings

These sample test questions are similar to ones you will find on the certification competency exam. See how well you can answer them. Be sure to select the *best* answer.

1. Which of the following phases occurs before labor and delivery?
   - A. intrapartum
   - B. antepartum
   - C. peripartum
   - D. postpartum

2. After surgery, Mr. D has developed a blood clot. What is another name for his condition?
   - A. DVT
   - B. GERD
   - C. CAUTI
   - D. ABG

3. What is the most important action a nursing assistant should take to prevent postoperative infection?

   A. make sure the family visits often
   B. ambulate the patient as often as possible
   C. provide more lights in the room
   D. maintain excellent hand hygiene

4. Mrs. S has discussed her upcoming surgery with her surgeon. What form does she need to sign to give permission for the surgery?

   A. admission form
   B. insurance agreement
   C. informed consent
   D. informed admission

5. In the OR, the surgeon is a member of the

   A. unsterile team
   B. unclean team
   C. sanitary team
   D. sterile team

6. When a patient has difficulty breathing after surgery, what should a nursing assistant do to prevent or minimize the complication?

   A. have the patient ambulate often
   B. have the patient regularly cough and breathe deeply
   C. give a respiratory treatment
   D. provide a special medication

7. One sign of impending labor is

   A. lightening
   B. bleeding and spotting
   C. lochia
   D. vernix

8. When caring for a patient after surgery, what should a holistic nursing assistant *not* do?

   A. give a gentle bed bath
   B. keep the linens wrinkle free
   C. pay special attention to the patient's pain
   D. make sure the patient ambulates often

9. Mrs. R has noticed darkening of the skin around her nipples and dark patches on her face. Which trimester of her pregnancy is she in?

   A. first
   B. second
   C. third
   D. fourth

10. A nursing assistant is helping a new nursing assistant care for a patient with a drain. What is one guideline the nursing assistant should share?

    A. keep the drain tied down with other tubing
    B. put a blanket over the tubing to keep it safe
    C. always keep the drain below the incision site
    D. do not change the dressing too often

11. When an infant has had enough to eat, what sign indicates he is full?

    A. straight arms and legs and alertness
    B. eyes closed and kicking legs
    C. relaxed arms and legs and eyes closed
    D. relaxed arms and legs and eyes open

12. The primary purpose of time in the PACU is to let the patient

    A. recover from anesthesia
    B. have dressings changed
    C. communicate with the family
    D. get up and ambulate

13. Drainage needs to be reported immediately if there is

    A. a large amount of clear, yellow fluid
    B. a large amount of blood and pus
    C. a small amount of tissue
    D. a small amount of clear, yellow fluid

14. Mr. J is now NPO and is having an IV catheter inserted. What phase of surgery is he experiencing?

    A. postoperative
    B. intraoperative
    C. preoperative
    D. perioperative

15. Mrs. J was diagnosed with an STI at the beginning of her pregnancy. For which complication might she be at risk?

    A. sore breasts
    B. genetic disorder
    C. bleeding and spotting
    D. ectopic pregnancy

Did you have difficulty with any of the questions? If you did, review the chapter to find the correct answer(s).

26 Emergencies and Disasters

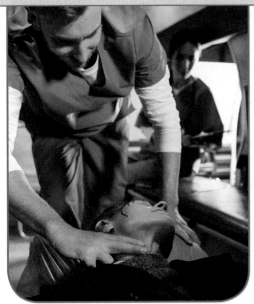

LightField Studios/Shutterstock.com

Chapter Outline

Section 26.1
Medical Emergencies

Section 26.2
Disasters, Terrorism,
and Bioterrorism

Welcome to the Chapter

This chapter provides information about the different types of medical emergencies you may encounter as a nursing assistant, as well as the best ways to respond to them. Medical emergencies include anaphylaxis, asphyxia, burns, chest pain, choking, fainting, heart attack (*myocardial infarction*), hemorrhage, poisoning, shock, and stroke (*cerebrovascular accident*). You will learn about first aid, first-responder responsibilities, cardiopulmonary resuscitation (CPR), and automated external defibrillators (AEDs). This chapter also discusses important issues concerning disasters, disaster preparedness, terrorism, bioterrorism, and violent attacks.

The information and procedures presented in this chapter will help you build the knowledge and skills needed to become a holistic nursing assistant. Check with your instructor to ensure these procedures are within your state's regulations for nursing assistant practice. The topics discussed in the chapter are highlighted on the Providing Holistic Care Framework.

You are now ready to start this chapter, *Emergencies and Disasters*.

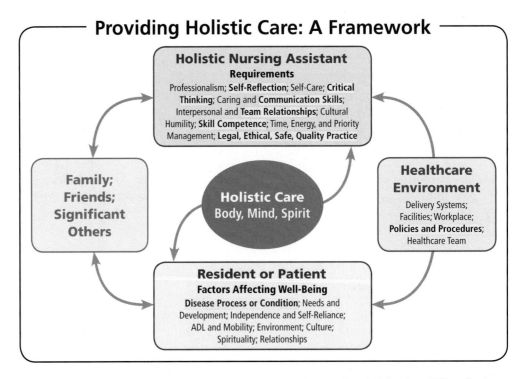

Providing Holistic Care: A Framework

Holistic Nursing Assistant
Requirements
Professionalism; **Self-Reflection**; Self-Care; **Critical Thinking**; Caring and **Communication Skills**; Interpersonal and **Team Relationships**; Cultural Humility; **Skill Competence**; Time, Energy, and Priority Management; **Legal, Ethical, Safe, Quality Practice**

Holistic Care
Body, Mind, Spirit

Family; Friends; Significant Others

Healthcare Environment
Delivery Systems; Facilities; Workplace; **Policies and Procedures**; Healthcare Team

Resident or Patient
Factors Affecting Well-Being
Disease Process or Condition; Needs and Development; Independence and Self-Reliance; ADL and Mobility; Environment; Culture; Spirituality; Relationships

Section 26.1 Medical Emergencies

Objectives

Medical emergencies can happen every day and often happen more frequently for older adults. As a nursing assistant, you must be able to respond confidently and effectively when emergencies occur. In this section, you will learn how best to respond to anaphylaxis, asphyxia, burns, chest pain, choking, fainting, heart attacks, hemorrhage, poisoning, shock, and strokes. You will learn guidelines for all of these medical emergencies and will learn specific procedures for choking, fainting, seizures, and bleeding. To achieve the objectives for this section, you must successfully

- **describe** the nursing assistant's responsibilities during medical emergencies;
- **recognize** when it is appropriate to act as a first responder;
- **explain** guidelines for giving first aid, performing CPR, and applying an AED; and
- **demonstrate** procedures for responding to choking, fainting, seizures, and hemorrhage.

Key Terms

Learn these key terms to better understand the information presented in the section.

allergen
anaphylaxis
angina
antihistamine
asphyxia
automated external defibrillator (AED)
basic life support (BLS)
cardiopulmonary resuscitation (CPR)
fibrillation

grand mal seizure
Hands-Only™ CPR
Heimlich maneuver
hemorrhage
petit mal seizure
rule of nines
seizures
shock

Questions to Consider

- Have you ever experienced a medical emergency? Have you broken a leg, severely burned yourself, or cut yourself so badly you bled a lot? What did you do? How did you feel? Were you scared?
- Did someone help you during or after the emergency? If so, what did the person do? Did the person's actions help make you feel better?
- Has someone you know experienced a medical emergency? If so, what did you do? If you did not know what to do, how did you feel?

What Is a Medical Emergency?

A *medical emergency* is a sudden, acute, and serious illness or injury. Many medical emergencies have long-lasting effects. Medical emergencies can result from trauma (such as severe cuts, burns, and broken bones) or medical conditions (such as strokes and heart attacks). No matter the origin or cause of the medical emergency, response and care must be immediate. Many areas in the United States have *emergency medical services (EMS)*, which are accessible by calling 9-1-1.

First responders are people who first arrive at an emergency. The immediate actions of first responders depend on the location of the emergency. Within a healthcare facility, nursing assistants should

- immediately turn on the emergency call light to alert staff if there is an emergency; and
- always follow facility policy and consider safety and comfort during and after procedures.

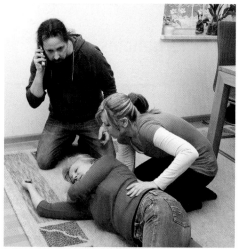
Miriam Doerr Martin Frommherz/Shutterstock.com

Figure 26.1 If you witness an emergency situation, call 9-1-1 immediately.

Outside a healthcare facility, your first actions should be to call for help using the emergency number 9-1-1 and provide basic first aid. When giving first aid, recognize the limits of your knowledge and skills. Do not try to perform a procedure if you do not feel prepared. First responders may do more if they have special education and training (certification or licensure). Examples of first responders who have specialized training might be emergency medical technicians, paramedics, licensed nursing staff members, and doctors. When responding outside a healthcare facility, a first responder should give his or her name and location to the 9-1-1 operator.

If you work as a nursing assistant in a healthcare facility, you will have the duty to respond to any medical emergencies. If a medical emergency occurs while you are outside a healthcare facility, respond according to your basic understanding of first aid and help within the limits of your knowledge and ability.

What Are Good Samaritan Laws?

Good Samaritan laws protect people who voluntarily help during a medical emergency outside a healthcare facility. In many states, laws outline the scope of what can be done. In some states, at a minimum, a person who witnesses a medical emergency must call for help. In other states, a person does not need to provide care unless it is part of his or her job description. As a result, people who respond to medical emergencies must be very careful when giving care. Many Good Samaritan laws protect a person against charges of negligence, unless reckless actions were taken that resulted in injury or worsened a situation. As a nursing assistant, you need to know the emergency care laws in your state.

Good Samaritan laws do not apply to emergency services in a healthcare facility. In a healthcare facility, it is your duty and responsibility to help in an emergency.

What First Aid Guidelines Are Important?

First aid is the process of observing and responding to a medical emergency, such as an injury, poisoning, burn, or medical issue (for example, a heart attack or stroke). First aid is performed at the onset of and during an emergency. It begins with determining the extent of the emergency and involves taking the correct and best course of action based on standards of care.

Every emergency situation is different, but in all instances, timing is crucial. Trained healthcare providers should always be sought immediately. Until help arrives, you should follow general first aid guidelines that can make the difference between a person's life and death.

If you witness an emergency situation, first and foremost, do not panic. Call for help (9-1-1) immediately (Figure 26.1). When speaking with a 9-1-1 dispatcher, remember the following first aid guidelines:

1. Provide as much factual information as possible.
2. Give the dispatcher the person's name (if you know it), gender, and approximate age.
3. Describe the symptoms, but only the symptoms you see or are told. Symptoms might include bleeding and location, the site of burns, or complaints of chest pain.
4. Describe your exact location and how trained healthcare providers can get there.
5. Answer any questions you are asked to the best of your ability.

Remember

There is nothing so strong or safe in an emergency of life as the simple truth.
Charles Dickens, English novelist

Pay attention to your own safety. Notice your surroundings and evaluate the situation. For example, never jump into a pool to save a drowning person if you are not a good, strong swimmer.

Always consider infection control. If you suspect a person may have a communicable disease, wear gloves and a mask, if possible. Avoid direct contact with the person's blood. If contact does occur, clean the blood off you as soon as possible.

Do not move the person except for safety reasons, such as fire. Moving the person may increase the chance of paralysis or death due to spinal cord damage.

If a person's condition or situation is *not* getting worse, always wait for trained healthcare providers to arrive. Remember to *do no harm*. You can further injure a person who is stable by performing a procedure for which you have no training. Be honest with yourself about what you are able to do.

Reassure the person that trained healthcare providers have been called and that you will stay until they arrive so the person will not be alone (Figure 26.2). As much as possible and appropriate, keep the area free from distractions such as onlookers, noise, or other disturbances. This type of support can help the person remain calm and promote safety.

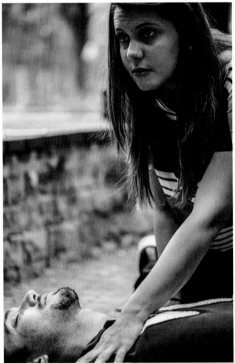

Figure 26.2 After calling for emergency help, stay with the person and perform basic life support depending on your level of training until help arrives.

What Is Basic Life Support?

As a nursing assistant, you will be asked to become certified in **basic life support (BLS)** and therefore will be expected to administer CPR, if needed. Certification is earned by satisfactorily completing a course offered by the American Heart Association, the American Red Cross, or other approved agencies or providers. Topics learned in basic life support typically include the *chain of survival* (Figure 26.3); CPR techniques for adults, children, and infants; bag-mask techniques for adults, children, and infants; rescue breathing for adults, children, and infants; choking relief for adults, children, and infants; and CPR with an advanced airway.

Cardiopulmonary Resuscitation (CPR)

In many emergencies, one of the first actions you can take to help someone is to perform cardiopulmonary resuscitation (CPR). **Cardiopulmonary resuscitation (CPR)** is an emergency, lifesaving procedure for a person whose breathing or heartbeat has stopped. The term *cardiopulmonary* means "pertaining to the heart and lungs," while *resuscitation* means "to revive." CPR supports blood circulation and breathing. It includes manual external chest compressions (to make the heart pump) and rescue breaths (to restore breathing until trained healthcare providers arrive). CPR may be necessary after a person suffers an electric shock; drowning; or *cardiac arrest* (when the heart stops beating), which can be caused by a heart attack.

According to the American Heart Association, more than 350,000 sudden, out-of-hospital cardiac arrests occur in the United States each year. Of those cardiac arrests, 70 percent happen at home. During cardiac arrest, the heart stops suddenly without warning. The person becomes unconscious, stops breathing, and has no pulse. The skin will be cool, pale, and gray. The person often appears healthy right before cardiac arrest.

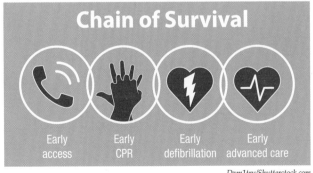

Figure 26.3 The chain of survival includes early access, early CPR, early defibrillation, and early advanced care. All of these links in the chain increase the chance of survival.

Responding quickly to cardiac arrest can help prevent death. A person's chance for survival drops 7 to 10 percent for every minute a normal heartbeat is not restored. CPR performed immediately can double or triple a person's chance of survival.

The American Heart Association identifies the best approach for CPR based on the amount of training a person has:

- People *not* trained in CPR should provide **Hands-Only™ CPR**. This involves performing chest compressions at a rate of around 100–120 compressions per minute until trained healthcare providers arrive. Chest compressions force blood through the cardiovascular system.
- People trained in CPR and confident in their ability should conduct *conventional CPR*. Conventional CPR begins with chest compressions and also includes clearing the airway and performing rescue breathing. The acronym *CAB* will help you remember these steps: Compressions, Airway, and Breathing.

Hands-Only™ CPR

Hands-Only™ CPR is CPR *without* rescue, or mouth-to-mouth, breathing. Hands-Only™ CPR can be used for teens or adults who suddenly collapse and are not breathing. Conventional CPR with compressions and rescue breathing is recommended for infants and children.

The steps for Hands-Only™ CPR include the following:

1. Call 9-1-1 (or send someone to do so) and follow the first aid guidelines discussed earlier in this section.

2. Before starting, check to see if the person is conscious. You can tap or shake the person's shoulder and ask, "Are you okay?" (Figure 26.4). Also look at the person's chest to see if he or she is breathing (if the chest is rising and falling). If the person is unconscious and is not breathing or is gasping, proceed. You can also check the carotid pulse located on the side of the person's neck (Figure 26.5). Place your index finger and middle finger on the neck to the side of the windpipe to feel the pulse. Check pulse for no more than 10 seconds. If there is no pulse, proceed.

3. Be sure the person is lying on his or her back (in the supine position), and if possible, on a hard surface. Get on your knees and bend over one side of the person.

4. Expose the chest. Move clothing out of the way so you can see the skin.

5. Place the heel of one hand on the lower half of the person's sternum. Place your other hand on top and interlock your fingers. Keep your fingers off the chest and do not lean on the person.

6. With your arms straight and your shoulders directly over your hands, use your body weight to push hard and fast in the center of the person's chest on the sternum (Figure 26.6).

7. Time your compressions to the beat of the disco song "Stayin' Alive" or use some other familiar method to help you give 100–120 chest compressions per minute with no interruptions. The chest should be compressed to a depth of 2 inches and then released back. Do not remove your hands from the sternum. It is helpful to count out loud each time you allow the chest to move back to its normal position between compressions. Continue chest compressions until the person starts to breathe, until an AED becomes available, or until trained healthcare providers arrive.

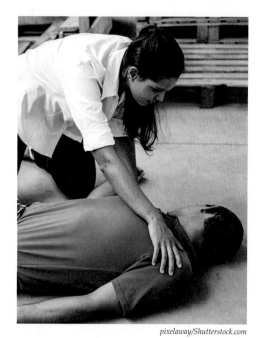

pixelaway/Shutterstock.com

Figure 26.4 Always check level of consciousness and breathing before beginning CPR.

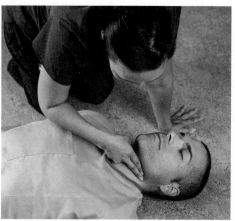

© *Tori Soper Photography*

Figure 26.5 Use your index finger and middle finger to check the carotid pulse.

Hands-Only™ CPR improves a person's chance of survival and is simple enough it should not be feared.

Conventional CPR

Conventional CPR includes chest compressions, airway clearing, and rescue breathing (CAB). Clearing the airway and performing rescue breathing should never be attempted without formal training. The steps of conventional CPR will be different for infants and children. You learned about CPR for infants in chapter 25. When giving CPR to children, use the same steps as for adults, but only compress the chest 1½ inches. If the child's chest is very small, use only one hand. Following are the steps of conventional CPR:

Chest Compressions—C

1. Check the carotid pulse located on the side of the person's neck. Place your index finger and middle finger on the neck to the side of the windpipe to feel the pulse. Check pulse for no more than 10 seconds.

2. If there is no pulse, prepare to start chest compressions. Be sure the person is lying on his or her back (in the supine position), and if possible, on a hard surface. Get on your knees and bend over one side of the person.

3. Using the heels of your hands, place one hand on top of the other. Interlock your fingers. Your dominant hand should touch the person's chest. With your arms straight and your shoulders directly over your hands, use your body weight to push hard and fast in the center of the person's chest on the sternum. Perform 30 chest compressions with no interruptions. For teens and adults, compress the chest to a depth of 2 inches. For children, compress the chest 1½ inches. It is helpful to count out loud each time you allow the chest to move back to its normal position between compressions.

Airway—A

4. After 30 chest compressions, clear the airway by tilting the head and lifting the chin. Put your palm on the person's forehead and gently tilt the head back. With your other hand, gently lift the person's chin forward to open the airway (Figure 26.7).

Rescue Breathing—B

5. After clearing the airway, quickly check for normal breathing for no more than 10 seconds. Assess breathing by looking for chest motion, listening for normal breath sounds, and feeling the person's breath on your cheek and ear. Gasping is not normal breathing. If the person is not breathing or is gasping, then begin rescue breathing.

6. Give mouth-to-mouth breathing or mouth-to-nose breathing if the mouth is injured or cannot be opened. If possible, use a barrier device to prevent contact with the person's mouth, secretions, and other body fluids (Figure 26.8). After clearing the airway and covering the mouth to form a seal, give two rescue breaths, each lasting one second. After the first breath, watch to see if the chest rises. Then give the second breath and resume chest compressions. Follow a cycle of 30 chest compressions, followed by two rescue breaths.

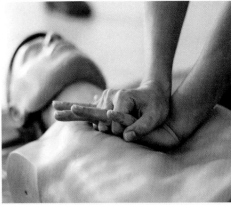

Nodty/Shutterstock.com

Figure 26.6 To perform chest compressions, interlock your fingers over the person's sternum. Push hard and fast in the center of the person's chest.

Think About This

As a holistic nursing assistant, you must respect the wishes of others when responding to a medical emergency. The CDC has indicated that *do-not-resuscitate (DNR) orders* are one of the most common *advance directives* (legal documents that specify what actions can be taken if a person is incapacitated) among home healthcare patients, residents, and discharged hospice patients. A DNR instructs healthcare providers not to attempt CPR or apply an AED if a person's heart and breathing stop.

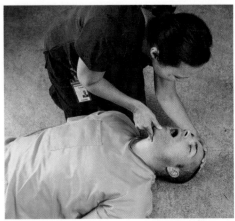

© *Tori Soper Photography*

Figure 26.7 Clear the airway by tilting the person's head back and lifting the chin.

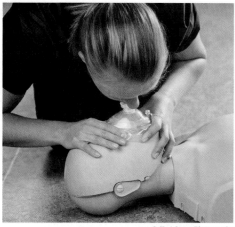

© Tori Soper Photography

Figure 26.8 Sometimes barrier devices are used to help ensure infection control.

7. Perform five cycles of CPR (lasting a total of two minutes) before using an available automated external defibrillator (AED). An AED is used if a person is not responding to CPR. It can be used twice between a set of five CPR cycles. If an AED is not available, continue CPR until the person starts to move, until an AED becomes available, or until trained healthcare providers arrive.

Automated External Defibrillator (AED)

The rate and rhythm of a person's heartbeat is controlled by an internal electrical system in the heart. Some people have problems with heart rhythm. The heart can beat too fast or too slow, beat irregularly, or stop due to cardiac arrest.

An **automated external defibrillator (AED)** is a medical device that delivers an electrical shock through the chest to the heart (Figure 26.9). This shock to the heart can stop **fibrillation** (irregular heart rhythm) and allow a normal heart rhythm to resume. Using an AED is an important part of responding to a medical emergency.

AEDs are located in a variety of places, such as ambulances, police cars, and public and private locations (doctors' offices, airports, and sports arenas). AEDs are lightweight, battery operated, and easy to use. Voice prompts inform the user if and when a shock should be delivered to the heart. Visual and vocal prompts from an AED also provide step-by-step instructions based on the person's heart rhythm.

To use an AED, follow these guidelines:

1. Provide two minutes of CPR at your level of training. After the two minutes of CPR, use an AED.

2. Always practice safety when using an AED. An AED emits an electrical shock, so check for any water nearby. Water conducts electricity, so using an AED in or near water poses a risk of shock. If there is water nearby, carefully move the person, if needed.

3. Turn on the AED's power.

4. Expose the person's chest, if it is not already exposed. Remove any metal necklaces or underwire bras and check for body piercings that may get in the way. Metal can conduct electricity and cause burns. To remove a bra, you can cut the center and pull the bra away from the skin. If the person has a lot of chest hair, use the tools provided with the AED to trim or shave it quickly.

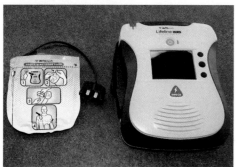

Goodheart-Willcox Publisher

Figure 26.9 An AED is an emergency medical device that shocks the heart to restore normal rhythm.

5. AEDs have sticky pads with sensors called *electrodes*. Apply the pads to the person's chest (Figure 26.10). The AED should also have extra pads available. Be sure the person's chest is dry. Lean over the person and place one pad on the right center of the person's chest above the nipple. Place the other pad slightly below the other nipple and to the left of the rib cage. Make sure the sticky pads make a good connection with the skin. If the connection is not good, a *Check electrodes* message will appear on the AED's screen.

6. Check for a medical alert bracelet to see if the person has any implanted devices, such as a pacemaker. Implanted devices are also visible under the skin of the chest or abdomen. Move the defibrillator pads at least 1 inch away from any implanted devices or piercings so the electrical current can flow freely between the pads. Also remove any medication patches on the chest and wipe the skin.

7. Check that the wires of the electrodes are connected to the AED. Make sure no one is touching the person and then press the AED's *Analyze* button. Stay clear while the machine checks the person's heart rhythm. The AED will determine if a shock can help restore normal heart rhythm. If a shock is needed, the AED will prompt you. The shock may be delivered automatically by the AED, or you may be prompted to press the *Shock* button.

8. Stand clear of the person and make sure others are clear before you push the AED's *Shock* button.

9. After the shock, resume CPR.

10. The AED will automatically reanalyze the person's heart rhythm to determine if another shock is needed.

11. If a shockable heart rhythm is not detected, the AED will prompt you to check the person's pulse and continue performing CPR.

12. If the person is still not responding, continue CPR until the person moves or until trained healthcare providers arrive. Stay with the person until help arrives. Report all the information you know.

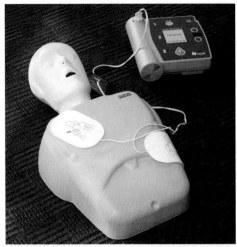

Goodheart-Willcox Publisher

Figure 26.10 One pad should lie on the right center of the person's chest over the nipple. The other pad should lie to the left of the ribcage below the other nipple.

How Should Chest Pain, Heart Attacks, and Strokes Be Handled?

In chapter 9, you learned about the causes, signs, and symptoms of chest pain (angina), heart attacks, and strokes. These diseases and conditions are medical emergencies and require quick response. There are actions you can take to respond to these medical emergencies outside a healthcare facility. If these medical emergencies occur within a healthcare facility, follow the facility's policy.

Chest Pain

Angina, or chest pain, is any major discomfort around the chest. Angina may or may not be caused by heart disease and is a common complaint. While chest pain may be located in the chest area, it can easily radiate to the back, neck, lungs, esophagus, or abdomen.

Until the cause of angina has been determined, angina should be considered a sign of a heart-related problem. Seek immediate help, either by calling 9-1-1 or transporting the person to an emergency department. If angina is caused by a heart attack, trained healthcare providers can determine how to proceed to increase the odds of survival.

Heart Attack

A *heart attack*, or *myocardial infarction*, occurs when blood flow to part of the heart muscle is blocked. Plaque ruptures within the coronary artery, causing a thrombus to form and cause blockage. The heart muscle becomes severely damaged and dies. Heart attacks can cause cardiac arrest.

Many heart attacks begin with hardly noticeable symptoms, such as discomfort or pain that comes and goes. Other initial symptoms may include lightheadedness; cold sweats; or mild, spreading pain (which some people mistakenly think will improve through rest or sleep). Women may experience different symptoms from men. Women are more likely to have generalized chest pain; pain in the arms, back, or jaw; sweating; nausea; or fatigue. Some people have a *silent heart attack* with no symptoms. A silent heart attack is more common among women and people with diabetes.

Think About This

According to the CDC, about 790,000 Americans have a heart attack every year. Of these, 580,000 experience their first heart attack, and 210,000 suffer a subsequent heart attack.

In general, a person experiencing a heart attack may have some or all of these signs and symptoms:

- discomfort or pain that is described as a tight ache, pressure, fullness, severe and crushing feeling, or squeezing in the chest
- pain that lasts more than a few minutes in the left, right, or both arms or below the breastbone
- pain, numbness, or tingling down the left arm (Figure 26.11)
- discomfort radiating to the back, jaw, or throat
- fullness, indigestion, or a choking feeling that may feel like heartburn
- sweating, nausea, vomiting, or dizziness
- extreme weakness or shortness of breath during exercise or at rest
- rapid or irregular heartbeats
- anxiety or a feeling of impending doom

If possible, call 9-1-1 within five minutes of experiencing these symptoms. The quicker treatment occurs, the better the outcome will be. If a person is not allergic to aspirin, he or she can chew and swallow one noncoated aspirin (325 mg) since chewing works faster than swallowing aspirin whole. Aspirin slows down the activity of platelets, inhibiting the growth of a blood clot. This helps blood flow through the coronary artery and keeps heart muscle cells from dying.

Above all, keep the person who is experiencing these symptoms calm and quiet, loosen the person's clothing if it is tight, and have the person sit or lie down and raise his or her head to breathe better. Check the person's respirations and pulse frequently. If the person stops breathing, start CPR based on your level of training.

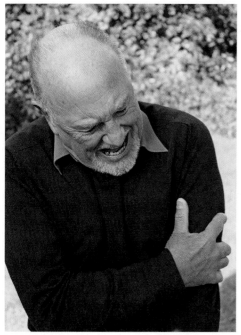

Giideon/Shutterstock.com

Figure 26.11 Pain in the left arm is one sign of a heart attack.

Stroke

A *stroke*, or *cerebrovascular accident (CVA)*, is the fifth leading cause of death in the United States and is also a leading cause of disability. A stroke occurs when a blood vessel carrying oxygen and nutrients to the brain becomes blocked by a clot or ruptures. When this happens, a part of the brain cannot get the blood and oxygen it needs. As you learned in chapter 9, there are three types of strokes: ischemic strokes, hemorrhagic strokes, and transient ischemic attacks (TIAs).

Some signs of a stroke include

- a severe headache;
- weakness and tingling in the arms, legs, or face;
- paralysis on one side;
- difficulty waking;
- sudden confusion and disorientation;
- slurred speech and drooping eyelids;
- facial drooping;
- drooling;
- change in vision;
- difficulty with speech; and
- change in vital signs.

If a person shows signs of a stroke, seek immediate help by calling 9-1-1 or transport the person to the emergency department. Keep the person warm, do not offer food or fluids, and provide CPR at your level of training, if needed.

What Is Anaphylaxis?

Many people have allergies to medications (such as aspirin or antibiotics), foods (such as nuts, fish, and shellfish), and insect stings. Some people respond with mild to moderate allergic reactions, and others experience **anaphylaxis**, a severe allergic reaction that can affect the whole body. An allergic reaction usually occurs within minutes of exposure to an **allergen**, or substance (often a protein) that causes an allergic reaction (Figure 26.12). Anaphylaxis, however, can occur 30 or more minutes after exposure to an allergen.

Not everyone has the same allergic reactions. Symptoms of an allergic reaction may include

- skin reactions such as hives, itching, and flushed or pale skin;
- swelling of the face, eyes, lips, or throat;
- a feeling of warmth throughout the body;
- the sensation of a lump in the throat;
- constriction of airways, which can cause wheezing and troubled breathing;
- a weak, rapid pulse;
- nausea, vomiting, or diarrhea; and
- dizziness, fainting, or unconsciousness.

If someone is experiencing moderate-to-severe symptoms of an allergic reaction or anaphylaxis, do not wait to see if the person gets better. Seek emergency treatment right away. In severe cases, untreated anaphylaxis can lead to death within 30 minutes. Be aware that an oral **antihistamine** (medication that reduces inflammation) will not work fast enough to treat anaphylaxis. Symptoms of anaphylaxis must be acted on immediately, and emergency treatment is needed even if symptoms start to improve.

Take the following actions to help someone having an allergic reaction:

1. Call 9-1-1 immediately and follow the first aid guidelines discussed earlier in this section.

2. Determine if the person has an epinephrine auto-injector to treat the allergic reaction. If the person does, ask if the person needs help with the injection. If help is needed, press the auto-injector against the middle of the person's upper leg (outer thigh). Inject into the skin or muscle. In an emergency, the injection can be given through clothing (Figure 26.13).

Common Allergens	
Type	**Examples**
Skin contact	• Poisonous plants • Pollen • Animal scratches • Latex
Inhalation	• Mold and mildew • Animal dander • Dust • Pollen
Ingestion	• Medications • Nuts and shellfish
Injection	• Bee stings

Figure 26.12 There are many types of allergens that can be inhaled, ingested, injected, or touched.

Culture Cues
Risk Factors for Heart Disease and Stroke

Members of particular ethnic groups are at higher risk for heart disease than others. Individuals from these groups may be more likely to experience a medical emergency. Heart disease is the leading cause of death for African-Americans and Hispanics. American Indians, Alaska Natives, Asians, and Pacific Islanders face heart disease as the second leading cause of death.

According to the American Stroke Association, compared to Caucasians, African-Americans are nearly twice as likely to suffer a stroke, and Hispanics also have an increased risk. African-Americans and Hispanics are more likely to die following a stroke than Caucasians.

Apply It

1. For what medical emergencies does your culture have increased risk?

2. How can you be respectful of a person's culture when responding to a medical emergency?

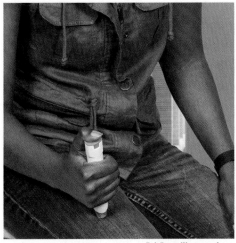

Rob Byron/Shutterstock.com

Figure 26.13 The epinephrine auto-injector should be placed against the middle of the outer thigh.

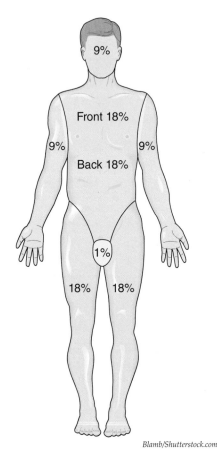

Blamb/Shutterstock.com

Figure 26.14 The rule of nines estimates the percentage of body surfaces burned using multiples of nine.

3. Have the person lie still on his or her back and loosen tight clothing. Cover the person with a blanket, if available.

4. Do not give the person anything to drink. If the person is vomiting or bleeding from the mouth, turn the person to the side to prevent choking.

5. If there are no signs of breathing, coughing, or movement, begin CPR depending on your level of training until the person starts moving or until trained healthcare providers arrive.

What Is the Best Method for Responding to Burns?

Burns pose a serious threat to a person's health. Remember that the skin is the body's first line of defense against infection. A *burn* is a break in the skin, so it increases the risk of infection at the burn site and potentially throughout the body.

The amount of damage a burn causes depends on its location, its depth, and the body surface it covers. The **rule of nines**, usually used for adults, provides a guide to assess the percentage of the body burned (Figure 26.14). It helps determine what treatment is needed (for example, if fluid replacement is necessary). The rule of nines applies only to second- and third-degree burns. It estimates the body surface area (BSA) burned using multiples of nine. For example, according to the rule of nines, a burn affecting the head and neck would be reported as 9 percent.

Burns are also classified by depth. There are three depth classifications: first degree, second degree, and third degree. The degree of a burn can change over time. For example, a sunburn that was originally considered a first-degree burn can blister and become a second-degree burn over a few hours.

First-Degree Burns

First-degree burns are superficial, meaning they exist only on the surface or outer layer of the skin. They are the least serious burns and usually take a few days to a week to heal. For example, touching a hot pan can give you a first-degree burn. First-degree burns are characterized by redness, mild swelling, skin that is tender to the touch, and pain.

As minor burns, most first-degree burns are easily treated using these guidelines:

- Hold the burned area under cool (not cold) running water for 10 to 15 minutes or until the pain eases. You can also apply a clean towel dampened with cool tap water to the burned area.

- Remove any jewelry or tight items from the burned area. Do this quickly and gently before swelling occurs.

- Apply moisturizer, aloe vera lotion or gel, or low-dose hydrocortisone cream to the burned area. These products may provide relief.

- Over-the-counter pain medications may also help.

If the burn affects a large portion of the hands, feet, face, groin, buttocks, or a major joint, emergency medical attention should be sought.

Second-Degree Burns

Second-degree burns (also called *partial-thickness burns*) are more serious than first-degree burns because they are deeper. These burns may cause permanent injury and scarring. If they are not too deep, second-degree burns will usually take two to three weeks to heal. Signs of a second-degree burn include red, white, or splotchy skin; swelling; pain; and blistering of the skin.

If a second-degree burn is fewer than 3 inches (7.6 centimeters) in diameter, treat it the same way you would a first-degree burn. If the burned area is larger or covers the hands, feet, face, groin, buttocks, or a major joint, treat it as you would a third-degree burn. Do not break small blisters (blisters no bigger than a small fingernail). If blisters break on their own, gently clean the area with mild soap and water, apply an antibiotic ointment, and cover the area with a nonstick gauze bandage.

Seek medical help if large blisters develop, as these are best removed by a medical professional. Do not attempt to remove these blisters on your own. Also seek medical help if there are signs of infection, such as oozing from the burned area, increased pain, redness, and swelling.

Third-Degree Burns

The most serious burn, a *third-degree burn* (also called a *full-thickness burn*), involves all layers of the skin and underlying fat. Nerves, blood vessels, muscle, and bone can also be affected. Third-degree burns will likely result in permanent injury (such as contractures) and scarring and usually take months or years to heal. Surgery is usually needed, and infection is a risk.

Burned areas may be charred black or white and become leathery. The person may experience difficulty breathing, and if smoke inhalation has occurred, may experience other toxic effects as well.

Because third-degree burns are major burns, the affected person needs medical attention as soon as possible. If someone has a third-degree burn, call 9-1-1 immediately and use the guidelines provided earlier in this section. Stay with the person. Until help arrives, you may also take these actions:

- Protect the affected person by safely checking that there is no further contact with smoldering materials or exposure to smoke or heat.

- Check for signs of breathing, coughing, or movement. If the person is unconscious, perform CPR depending on your level of training until trained healthcare providers arrive.

- If possible, remove jewelry, belts, and other restrictive items (especially from around burned areas and the neck), as swelling will occur rapidly. Do *not* remove burned clothing that is stuck to the skin.

Healthcare Scenario
Degrees of Burns

Yesterday's news covered a fire that partially burned a home next to yours. You know several family members who were involved in the fire. It was reported that two little girls had blistering burns on both of their hands. They were trying to save their cat. The father was coughing severely, was lying on the ground, and had very charred pants. The mother was rubbing her face, which was very red, as she cried.

Apply It

1. If you were a first responder in this situation, what would you do first?

2. Given the information in the news report, what level of burn do you think each family member has?

3. Based on the levels of the burns you identified, what actions should you take?

- Elevate burned areas above the heart, if possible.
- Do not use cold water for large, severe burns. This may cause a serious loss of body heat (known as *hypothermia*) or a drop in blood pressure and decreased blood flow (shock). Rather, cover the burned area with a cool, moist bandage or clean cloth.

What Should Be Done If Poisoning Is Suspected?

People are injured or die as a result of poisoning every day. Most poisons, such as cyanide, paint thinners, or household cleaning products, are ingested, but poisons can also enter the body through the skin, by inhalation, intravenously (by injection), through radiation exposure, or through the consumption of spoiled food. Residents with dementia and Alzheimer's disease are at increased risk for poisoning.

Poisoning is categorized as either

- unintentional or accidental (such as a child ingesting a cleaning product); or
- intentional (deliberate self-poisoning).

A person can be poisoned and not show symptoms for hours, days, or even months. For example, a person may take a large dose of aspirin for extreme pain, which seems harmless. Over a long period of time, however, the prolonged effects of the aspirin can slowly poison the person and cause an overdose. The delay in seeking medical help can result in long-term or permanent damage.

When a person has been poisoned, it can be difficult to determine what type of poisoning has occurred. Some signs and symptoms of poisoning are similar to those of common illnesses such as strokes, seizures, and head injuries. Typical signs and symptoms of poisoning include

- abnormal skin color;
- burns or redness around the mouth and lips;
- breath that smells like chemicals such as gasoline or paint thinner;
- nausea and vomiting;
- difficulty breathing;
- restlessness and agitation;
- seizure; and
- confusion or disorientation.

If you suspect that someone has been poisoned, look for clues, such as empty pill bottles; scattered pills; and burns, stains, or odors on the person or nearby objects. Children may have applied medicated patches to their skin or swallowed small batteries. If a person has no symptoms, but may have taken a potentially dangerous poison, call the US National Poison Control Center at 1-800-222-1222 or the Regional Poison Control Center to ask questions about possible poisoning. Have the pill bottle, medication, cleaning product, or other suspected container or material available so you can talk about it.

Call 9-1-1 or go to a local emergency department if a person displays active signs of poisoning, if an infant or toddler has been poisoned, or if the poisoning was intentional (even if the substance itself is not harmful). After calling 9-1-1, take the following actions until trained healthcare providers arrive:

- If a person has swallowed poison, check the person's mouth and remove any poison that remains. If the person ingested household cleaner or another chemical, read the container's label and follow instructions for accidental poisoning.
- If poison is on a person's skin, remove any contaminated clothing with gloves. Rinse the skin for 15 to 20 minutes in a shower or with a hose.

- If poison is in a person's eye, gently flush the eye with cool or lukewarm water for 20 minutes or until help arrives. If an eye needs to be flushed in a healthcare facility, use an eyewash station, if available. (Figure 26.15).

- If a person has inhaled poison, move the person into fresh air as soon as possible.

- If the poisoned person is vomiting, turn his or her head to the side to prevent choking.

- If the poisoned person is not breathing or has no pulse, begin and continue CPR depending on your level of training until trained healthcare providers arrive.

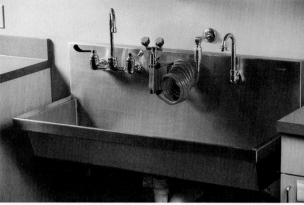

© *Tori Soper Photography*

Figure 26.15 Eyewash stations are usually available in healthcare facilities. These stations help flush the eyes.

Before trained healthcare providers arrive, gather any pill or vitamin bottles, packages or containers with labels, plants, or other information about the suspected poison. Be ready to describe the person's symptoms, the age and weight of the person, any medications being taken, and any information about the suspected poisoning (for example, the amount ingested and the time since the poisoning occurred).

What Should Be Done If Someone Is Choking?

Choking is a medical emergency that blocks the flow of oxygen to the lungs and the rest of the body. Lack of oxygen causes **asphyxia**, a condition in which the body is deprived of oxygen, leading to the loss of consciousness or death. If you witness someone choking, you must act quickly. For adults, the aspiration of a piece of food usually causes choking. For children, swallowing a small object usually causes choking. Older adults who have a weakened swallowing reflex are more at risk of choking.

Blockages that cause choking can be partial or complete:

- **Partial blockage**: the person is coughing vigorously, can speak, and can breathe. Encourage the person to continue coughing. Stay with the person and call 9-1-1 for help. Do not strike the person on the back or perform abdominal thrusts. If the person is coughing, his or her body is doing its job of trying to expel the object.

——— Becoming a Holistic Nursing Assistant ———
Responding to Medical Emergencies

Medical emergencies are frightening for everyone involved. Your first action when responding to a medical emergency should always be to get help. Whether the emergency is happening to you or someone else, always remain calm. If you are aiding another, focus on that person. Listen carefully and use your observation skills. Only do what you know how to do. Never try to be a hero. Instead, be helpful, supportive, and comforting. Remember that, when you are calm and reassuring, the victim will be able to sense your emotional state. A fast response and calmness during an emergency can make a positive difference in recovery.

Apply It

1. Think about an emergency situation you witnessed in the past. What was your first reaction and action? Did you effectively help yourself or another person?

2. Were you able to stay calm in the situation? If so, how did you do that? If you were not calm, what might you have done differently to become calm?

- **Complete blockage**: the person cannot speak and makes high-pitched sounds or clutches at the throat with his or her hands (Figure 26.16). These are universal signs of distress. Take quick action using the **Heimlich maneuver**, or abdominal thrusts using your fist.

The Heimlich maneuver may be combined with a series of back blows to help the choking person. When giving a back blow, lean the choking person forward and strike his or her back between the shoulder blades five times using the heel of your hand (Figure 26.17). The American Red Cross suggests using the *five-and-five method*, in which five back blows are followed by five abdominal thrusts. The American Heart Association's recommended response to choking does not include back blows, but focuses on the use of abdominal thrusts.

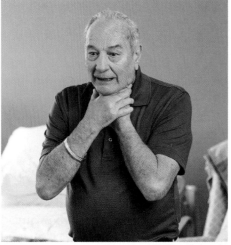

© Tori Soper Photography

Figure 26.16 Clutching the throat with the hands is a universal sign of distress.

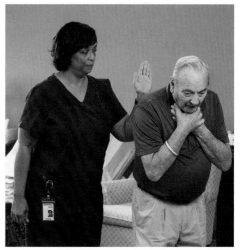

© Tori Soper Photography

Figure 26.17 Back blows should be given between the shoulder blades of the choking person using the heel of your hand.

| **Procedure** | **Responding to Choking Using the Heimlich Maneuver** |

Rationale

Foreign objects can obstruct a person's airway and cause choking. Relieving choking can prevent injury or death. The following procedure should be used with adults and children over one year of age. It should not be used with children under one year of age. The procedure for clearing the obstructed airway of an infant is found in chapter 25.

Preparation

1. Follow first aid guidelines and remain calm.
2. Call for help or have someone else call for help. If you are in a healthcare facility, press the emergency call light. Otherwise, call 9-1-1.

The Procedure: Choking—Conscious Adult or Child (Over One Year of Age)

3. Reassure the choking person that you are there to help. Check the person's ability to breathe.
4. If the person is coughing, wait to see if coughing dislodges the object.
5. If coughing does not dislodge the object, stand or kneel behind the person. Wrap your arms around the person's waist.

> **Best Practice**
> If possible, let the person's arms hang free. Many people will continue to clutch their throat.

6. Make a fist with one hand.

7. Place the thumb side of your fist against the person's abdomen, slightly above the navel and well below the sternum.

8. Grasp your clenched fist with your other hand. Do not tuck your thumb inside your fist. Avoid pressing on the person's ribs with your forearms.

9. Press forcefully into the abdomen with the thumb side of your fist. Use quick, inward and upward thrusts to dislodge the object (Figure 26.18).

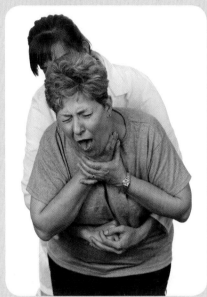

Figure 26.18

10. Perform five abdominal thrusts and then check to see if the object is visible or has been expelled.

11. Remove the foreign object only if you see it. To open the person's airway, tilt the person's head back and lift the chin. Look into the person's mouth for the object. Grasp and remove the object if it is within reach.

Best Practice
Do not perform a finger sweep or attempt to remove an object you cannot see. Make sure you can reach the object. Trying to remove an object you cannot reach or see may push the object farther into the throat and cause more distress.

12. If the object is not visible or has not been expelled, keep performing abdominal thrusts until the object is expelled or the person loses consciousness (stops responding). If the person loses consciousness, follow the steps for an unconscious, choking adult or child (over one year of age).

The Procedure: Choking—Unconscious Adult or Child (Over One Year of Age)

13. Put on disposable gloves, if available.

14. Turn the person so he or she is lying in the supine position.

15. Check for a pulse. If there is a pulse, open the airway by tilting the head back and lifting the chin. Deliver one breath and watch to see if the chest rises. If the chest does not rise, try one more time.

16. If rescue breaths do not cause the chest to rise, begin conventional or Hands-Only™ CPR depending on your level of training.

17. Every 30 compressions, open the person's airway and look for the foreign object in his or her mouth.

18. If you can see the foreign object, remove it, but do not push it farther down into the throat.

19. Continue performing CPR and checking for the object until the object is expelled or until trained healthcare providers arrive.

Follow-Up

20. If you are not in a healthcare facility, report your observations and actions to the trained healthcare providers when they arrive.

21. If you are in a healthcare facility, take the person's vital signs once the object has been expelled and alert the licensed nursing staff.

22. Remove and discard your gloves, if used.

23. Wash your hands to ensure infection control.

24. If you are in a healthcare facility, make sure the person is comfortable once the object has been expelled. Place the call light and personal items within reach.

25. Conduct a safety check before leaving the room. The room should be clean and free from clutter or spills.

26. Remove, clean, and store equipment in the proper location. Remove soiled linens and discard disposable equipment.

27. Wash your hands or use hand sanitizer before leaving the room.

Reporting and Documentation

28. Update a licensed nursing staff member with the person's vital signs.

29. If you are in a healthcare facility, communicate any specific observations, complications, or unusual responses to the licensed nursing staff. Record this information, along with the care provided, in the chart or EMR.

What Happens When a Person Faints?

Fainting is a brief loss of consciousness and is considered a medical emergency. Fainting is also called *syncope* or *passing out*. It is caused by a drop in blood flow to the brain.

Reasons for fainting include fatigue, hunger, certain medications, dehydration, heart conditions, age, or the temperature or ventilation in a room. Signs that a person may faint include

- a pale face;
- skin that feels cold and clammy (moist);
- perspiration;
- a weak pulse;
- shallow breathing;
- trembling and shaking; and
- complaints of dizziness or blurred vision.

To help prevent fainting when a resident gets out of bed, allow the resident to sit on the side of the bed for a few minutes, dangle the legs to increase circulation, and breathe deeply to promote oxygenation. If a resident is dizzy or faint, do not let him or her stand. Have the resident lie back down until a member of the licensed nursing staff arrives. Consider any signs of fainting a medical emergency and reportable, even if the person only says he or she feels faint. This prevents possible injury.

Procedure | Responding to Fainting

Rationale

Fainting is a sudden loss of consciousness due to an inadequate supply of blood to the brain. When consciousness is lost, a person is likely to fall, and injuries can occur.

Preparation

1. Follow first aid guidelines and remain calm.
2. Call for help or have someone else call for help. If you are in a healthcare facility, press the emergency call light. Otherwise, call 9-1-1.

The Procedure

3. Reassure the person that you are there to help.
4. If you have observed signs that the person is about to faint, assist her to a safe position using proper body mechanics. Help her sit or lie down before fainting occurs. Do not leave the person unattended.
5. If the person is sitting and feels like she is about to faint, have her bend forward and place her head between her knees for at least 5 minutes (Figure 26.19). If the person is lying down and there are no contraindications, place her on her back and raise or elevate her legs approximately 12 inches so they are above the heart, which increases blood circulation to her brain.

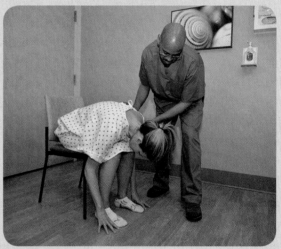

Figure 26.19

6. Check the clothing around the person's neck, chest, and abdomen. Loosen any tight clothing that may restrict breathing.
7. If fainting occurs when the person is not lying down, slowly lower the person to the floor using your body as an incline.
8. Turn the person's head to the side in case of vomiting. Check breathing and pulse. Call for help. Do not leave the person.

9. Do not let the person get up for at least five minutes after the fainting.

10. Do not give the person anything to eat or drink, unless directed by a trained healthcare provider.

11. Do not leave the person alone as you wait for trained healthcare providers to arrive.

Follow-Up

12. If you are not in a healthcare facility, report your observations and actions to the trained healthcare providers when they arrive.

13. Wash your hands to ensure infection control.

14. If you are in a healthcare facility, alert the licensed nursing staff. Make sure the person is comfortable and place the call light and personal items within reach.

15. Conduct a safety check before leaving the room. The room should be clean and free from clutter or spills.

16. Remove, clean, and store equipment in the proper location. Remove soiled linens and discard disposable equipment.

17. Wash your hands or use hand sanitizer before leaving the room.

Reporting and Documentation

18. If you are in a healthcare facility, communicate any specific observations, complications, or unusual responses to the licensed nursing staff. Record this information, along with the care provided, in the chart or EMR.

Image courtesy of Wards Forest Media, LLC

What Is the Appropriate Way to Respond to a Seizure?

Seizures are sudden changes in the brain's normal electrical activity that cause an altered or loss of consciousness. A seizure may be the result of a disease, such as epilepsy, tumors, or nervous system disorders. Seizures can also be the result of a head injury, so you should act quickly if you witness someone experiencing a seizure. Seizures can occur at any age and generally last from a few seconds to several minutes.

There are two different types of seizures: partial seizures and generalized seizures. *Partial seizures* include motor seizures, sensory seizures, and autonomic seizures. *Motor seizures* occur in the muscles and cause the hands and fingers to jerk. *Sensory seizures* are tingling sensations. *Autonomic seizures* cause changes in respiratory rate, sweating, and heart rate.

Generalized seizures can be one of two types: petit mal seizures and grand mal seizures. A person experiencing a **petit mal seizure** will have impaired awareness and responsiveness, may stare, and may have facial or body twitches.

A person having a **grand mal seizure** will experience tonic and clonic phases. In the *tonic phase*, muscles stiffen, and air is forced out of the lungs. A person usually groans and then loses consciousness. The person may also fall to the floor, turn blue, and bite his or her tongue. In the *clonic phase*, muscles contract and relax, which causes jerking and rhythmic movements of the arms and legs. Bowel and bladder control may be lost. Consciousness returns slowly and gradually after a grand mal seizure. This type of seizure may last a few seconds or as long as 10 minutes.

Procedure   Responding to a Seizure

Rationale

Preventing injury and maintaining an open airway are primary goals when responding to a seizure.

Preparation

1. Follow first aid guidelines and remain calm.

2. Call for help or have someone else call for help. If you are in a healthcare facility, press the emergency call light. Otherwise, call 9-1-1.

The Procedure

3. Reassure the person that you are there to help.

4. Never try to stop a seizure.

5. Note the time the seizure started.

6. Lower the person to the floor using your body as an incline (if the person is not already lying down) to protect the person from falling.

(continued)

7. Maintain an open airway. Turn the person onto her side and make sure her head is also turned to promote the drainage of any saliva or vomit.

8. Protect the person's head by placing something soft under her head. This will help prevent the head from striking the floor during the seizure. Use a pillow, chair cushion, folded jacket, blanket, or towel. You may also cradle the person's head in your lap.

9. Loosen tight clothing and jewelry around the person's neck. Clear the area of equipment or sharp objects. The person may strike these objects during the seizure.

10. Do not force the mouth open. Do not put any objects or your fingers between the teeth. Do not try to restrain or control movements.

11. Note the time the seizure ends and place the person in a recovery position (lying on her side). The head should be turned to the side to allow saliva to drain from the mouth (Figure 26.20).

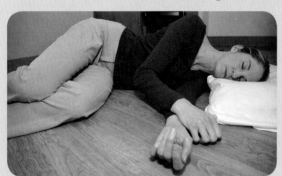

Figure 26.20

Follow-Up

12. If you are not in a healthcare facility, report your observations and actions to the trained healthcare providers when they arrive.

13. Wash your hands to ensure infection control.

14. If you are in a healthcare facility, alert the licensed nursing staff. Make sure the person is comfortable and place the call light and personal items within reach.

15. Conduct a safety check before leaving the room. The room should be clean and free from clutter or spills.

16. Remove, clean, and store equipment in the proper location. Remove soiled linens and discard disposable equipment.

17. Wash your hands or use hand sanitizer before leaving the room.

Reporting and Documentation

18. If you are in a healthcare facility, communicate any specific observations, complications, or unusual responses to the licensed nursing staff. Record this information, along with the care provided, in the chart or EMR.

What Is a Hemorrhage, and How Can It Be Controlled?

A **hemorrhage**, which is excessive blood loss over a short period of time, is a medical emergency. You must act quickly if hemorrhage occurs.

There are two types of hemorrhages: internal hemorrhages, which you cannot see, and external hemorrhages, which you can see. *Internal hemorrhages* occur inside the body's tissues and cavities. Signs of an internal hemorrhage are pain, shock, vomiting, coughing up blood, and loss of consciousness. In *external hemorrhage*, blood may spurt or flow steadily out of the body. Spurting blood usually comes from an artery. A steady flow usually comes from a vein.

When a person loses a large amount of blood, he or she may go into **shock**. In shock, there is not enough oxygen available to the organs and tissues of the body. When a person is in shock, blood pressure drops; the pulse is rapid and weak; the skin is cool, clammy, and pale; and the person may lose consciousness. Immediate treatment by trained medical professionals who can replace needed fluids is essential to prevent death.

The signs and symptoms of a hemorrhage include

- a pale or cyanotic (blue and discolored) face;
- low blood pressure;

- increased, but weak, heart rate;
- rapid, shallow respirations;
- feelings of weakness and helplessness;
- restlessness;
- complaints of thirst; and
- coldness, shaking, or trembling.

To control the bleeding of an external hemorrhage, you can use direct or indirect pressure. Direct pressure is applied to the bleeding wound. Indirect pressure is applied to a pressure point near or on top of the wound. Pressure points exist where blood vessels are located close to the surface of the skin (Figure 26.21). When these points are pressed, blood flow to the wound slows. Combined with direct pressure, this will help stop bleeding. Pressure can be applied using the fingers, thumb, or heel of the hand.

Pressure points, especially the carotid artery, should be used with extreme caution. Sometimes indirect pressure can cause tissue damage.

Pressure Points

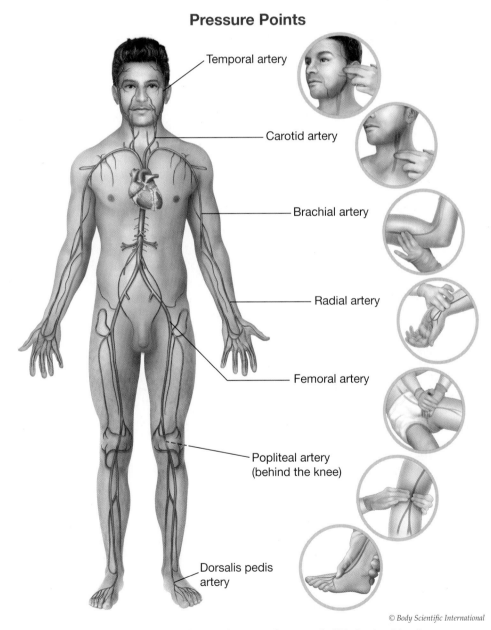

Temporal artery

Carotid artery

Brachial artery

Radial artery

Femoral artery

Popliteal artery (behind the knee)

Dorsalis pedis artery

© Body Scientific International

Figure 26.21 Applying pressure to these points near the wound will help slow bleeding.

Rationale

A hemorrhage can be life threatening if not stopped. Hemorrhages can occur internally or externally, and they are often caused by an injury.

Preparation

1. Follow the first aid guidelines and remain calm.
2. Call for help or have someone else call for help. If you are in a healthcare facility, press the emergency call light. Otherwise, call 9-1-1.

The Procedure: Internal Hemorrhage

3. Reassure the person experiencing a hemorrhage that you are there to help.
4. Keep the person flat, warm, and quiet.
5. Do not give the person any fluids.
6. Do not remove any objects that may have caused the hemorrhage.
7. Wait calmly with the person for trained healthcare providers to arrive.

The Procedure: External Hemorrhage

8. Reassure the person experiencing the hemorrhage that you are there to help.
9. Do not remove any objects that may have caused the hemorrhage.
10. Put on disposable gloves, if available.
11. Apply firm, steady, direct pressure to the bleeding site (Figure 26.22). Do not stop applying pressure until the bleeding stops.

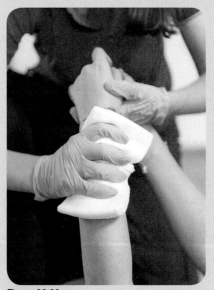

Figure 26.22

12. Use a sterile dressing, if available. If a sterile dressing is not available, apply a clean material, such as a towel or cloth, and secure it with a bandage or tape.
13. If possible, elevate the affected area of the body (hand, arm, foot, or leg). This will help minimize blood flow to the area. Bind the wound when the bleeding stops.
14. Watch for bleeding through the bandage. If you have the knowledge to do so, apply indirect pressure on a pressure point to try to slow the bleeding.
15. Keep the person warm by covering him with a blanket.
16. Do not give the person anything to eat or drink.
17. Wait calmly with the person for trained healthcare providers to arrive.

Follow-Up

18. If you are not in a healthcare facility, report your observations and actions to the trained healthcare providers when they arrive.
19. Remove and discard your gloves, if used.
20. Wash your hands to ensure infection control.
21. If you are in a healthcare facility, alert the licensed nursing staff. Make sure the person is comfortable and place the call light and personal items within reach.
22. Conduct a safety check before leaving the room. The room should be clean and free from clutter or spills.
23. Remove, clean, and store equipment in the proper location. Remove soiled linens and discard disposable equipment.
24. Wash your hands or use hand sanitizer before leaving the room.

Reporting and Documentation

25. If you are in a healthcare facility, communicate any specific observations, complications, or unusual responses to the licensed nursing staff. Record this information, along with the care provided, in the chart or EMR.

Using the Key Terms

Complete the following sentences using key terms in this section.

1. An irregular heart rhythm is called _____.
2. _____ refers to the excessive loss of blood over a short period of time.
3. CPR that uses only chest compressions is called _____.
4. A severe allergic reaction that can affect the whole body is _____.
5. _____, or lack of oxygen in the body, may be caused when breathing stops due to an obstruction in the trachea.
6. The _____ is a method of calculating the surface area of the body affected by burns.
7. A sudden change in the brain's normal electrical activity that causes an altered or loss of consciousness is called a(n) _____.
8. One complication of blood loss is _____, a condition in which the organs and tissues of the body lack sufficient oxygen.
9. During _____, air is exhaled into a person's mouth or nose to provide ventilation and external chest compressions are performed to help oxygenated blood flow to the heart and brain.
10. _____ is characterized by a sensation of squeezing, pressure, heaviness, or tightness in the center of the chest.

Know and Understand the Facts

11. What are three responsibilities nursing assistants have during medical emergencies?
12. Describe the role of the first responder.
13. What specific actions should you take to help someone experiencing anaphylaxis?
14. How can you tell if someone has been poisoned?
15. What should you do if a person has a second-degree burn?

Analyze and Apply Concepts

16. Explain the importance of following Hands-Only™ CPR guidelines.
17. List the steps required to effectively use an AED.
18. Explain the procedures for responding to choking in adults and children over one year of age.
19. Describe the actions a nursing assistant should take if a resident has a seizure.

Think Critically

Read the following care situation. Then answer the questions that follow.

Jean, your best friend's grandmother, became very pale, clutched her chest, and started to collapse like she was fainting while she was making you and your friend lunch. You know that Jean had been sick last month and that she takes medication. She had been fine just a few minutes before and had been laughing and telling a great story. You are sitting closest to Jean.

20. What signs should you look for to determine if Jean might be having a heart attack?
21. What should you do to keep Jean safe?
22. What is the first action you should take?

Questions to Consider

- Have you ever experienced a disaster, such as a hurricane or tornado? If you have, what was it like? Did you know about the disaster ahead of time? If you did, what precautions did you take?
- If you have not experienced a disaster, have you watched or read news coverage about one? During the disaster, what actions were taken by emergency response personnel? What happened after the disaster? How did watching the disaster feel?

Objectives

Although you may have never experienced a major fire, earthquake, tornado, or other disaster, you need to know how to respond to one effectively and appropriately. In today's world, the threat of terrorism, bioterrorism, and violent attacks also exists. As a nursing assistant, you need to understand and be ready in case a disaster or attack occurs in a healthcare facility. To achieve the objectives for this section, you must successfully

- **identify** types of disasters, terrorism, and bioterrorism; and
- **explain** how a nursing assistant can respond to a disaster, terrorist attack, or other violent attack appropriately.

Key Terms

Learn these key terms to better understand the information presented in the chapter.

bioterrorism   evacuation

cyberattacks

Medical emergencies have a small scope. For example, only one person suffers from a heart attack. A disaster's scope is much bigger, affects many people, and can potentially cause large-scale destruction of life and property. Both medical emergencies and disasters demand quick action and preparation to improve recovery.

What Are Disasters, Terrorism, and Bioterrorism?

Think About This

The United States ranks second in the world for its number of natural disasters. Natural disasters tend to be *meteorological*, or related to the weather. For example, tornados are more common in the United States than in any other country. Other natural disasters include heat waves, cyclones, earthquakes, and floods. Wildfires also destroy property and threaten lives.

According to the World Health Organization (WHO), a *disaster* causes human, material, economic, and environmental loss and limits a community's ability to function. Disasters can range from natural disasters (such as earthquakes, hurricanes, avalanches, wildfires, and tornados) to aircraft crashes, *arson* (fires set intentionally to cause damage), explosions, and epidemics.

Terrorism is violence that is politically motivated. Examples of terrorism include the September 11, 2001, attacks in New York and the Boston Marathon bombing, which were politically motivated. Terrorist attacks can also include biological and chemical threats, the use of nuclear weapons, **cyberattacks** (illegal attempts to gain access to a digital device or network to cause harm), and bombings. Violent attacks that are not politically motivated (for example, mass shootings) can also have devastating consequences. Terrorism and violent attacks are disasters and often cause significant casualties (deaths or injuries), damage to buildings, the need for heavy law enforcement, extensive media coverage, work and school closures, travel restrictions, and possible evacuation.

Bioterrorism is the intentional use of pathogens such as viruses and bacteria to cause illness or death in people, animals, or plants. Bioterrorism agents can be spread by air, through water, or in food. They are categorized based on their ability to spread and the severity of illness or death they cause.

What Is the Best Way to Respond to a Disaster?

If a natural disaster or terrorist attack occurs while you are working as a nursing assistant, follow the healthcare facility's policies, procedures, and disaster plans (Figure 26.23). Disaster plans are typically discussed with staff members during orientation, and specific training and practice ensure that staff members are ready for a disaster. Your most important responsibility as a nursing assistant is to maintain your preparedness.

It is also helpful to be prepared for disasters that may occur outside a healthcare facility. To prepare, consider creating a supply kit and disaster and communication plan. Disaster and communication plans should include responsibilities, emergency contacts, pet safety guidelines, procedures, safe spots for different types of emergencies, **evacuation** routes (routes for the removal of people or objects from a dangerous area), and a shelter location. Practicing these plans twice a year will improve your ability to execute them. It is also important to familiarize yourself with emergency plans for the places you and your family spend time (for example, schools, faith organizations, and sporting events). Further preparation includes

- teaching children how and when to call 9-1-1 for help;
- learning your community's warning signals;
- showing family members how and when to turn off the water, gas, and electricity (Figure 26.24);
- teaching family members how to use and where to find fire extinguishers; and
- checking your emergency supplies throughout the year to replace batteries, food, and water as needed.

If a disaster occurs in your community, follow these steps to respond:

1. Remain calm.
2. Follow the advice of local emergency officials.
3. Listen to your radio or television for news and instructions.
4. If the event occurs near you, check for injuries. Give first aid and get help for seriously injured people.
5. Check and shut off damaged utilities.
6. Check on your neighbors, especially older adults or people with disabilities.

Agencies and organizations in the United States typically collaborate and coordinate their efforts to prepare for and respond to disasters. The primary organizations include the following:

- **American Red Cross**: a nonprofit, volunteer organization that responds to disasters regardless of size or scope (Figure 26.25). The American Red Cross is responsible for mass care, including food, shelter, bulk distribution of disaster relief supplies, first aid, and disaster welfare information.
- **Centers for Disease Control and Prevention (CDC)**: a federal agency that focuses on preparedness to support the US Department of Homeland Security. The CDC protects the public from health threats and assists with public health and medical preparedness.

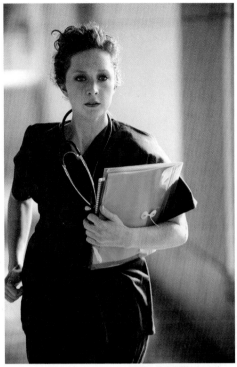

EHStockphoto/Shutterstock.com

Figure 26.23 All healthcare facilities have disaster plans that clearly lay out what staff members should do before, during, and after an emergency or disaster.

> **Remember**
>
> *Preparation doesn't assure victory, it assures confidence.*
>
> Amit Kalantri, American author

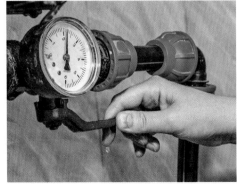

iStock.com/Grigorev_Vladimir

Figure 26.24 Knowing the location of a water shutoff valve like this one can help prepare you for an emergency situation.

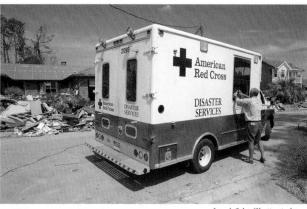

Joseph Sohm/Shutterstock.com

Figure 26.25 The American Red Cross responds to disasters of any scale.

- **Federal Emergency Management Agency (FEMA)**: a federal agency that helps in disasters recognized by the US president. Some of FEMA's work involves community recovery tasks such as rebuilding bridges, roads, and public buildings.

- **US Department of Homeland Security**: a federal agency responsible for the National Response Framework and Plan. This agency supports citizen and community preparedness and ensures first responders have the resources needed to respond to a violent attack or natural disaster.

The Food and Drug Administration (FDA) and the Environmental Protection Agency (EPA) also provide protection against bioterrorism and ensure water security.

Section 26.2 Review and Assessment

Using the Key Terms

Complete the following sentences using key terms in this section.

1. A(n) _____ is an illegal attempt to gain access to a digital device or network to cause harm.
2. The intentional removal of people from a dangerous area is called _____.
3. _____ uses harmful agents and products with biological origins as weapons.

Know and Understand the Facts

4. Describe three different types of disasters.
5. Explain why bioterrorism and terrorist attacks are considered disasters.
6. Describe the roles and responsibilities of three different agencies or organizations in preparing for and responding to disasters.

Analyze and Apply Concepts

7. Why are disaster plans so important?
8. What is the most important thing a nursing assistant can do to be prepared for a disaster?
9. Identify three important actions a person can take to be prepared for a disaster.

Think Critically

Read the following care situation. Then answer the questions that follow.

Bianca works in a long-term care facility. She is a relatively new nursing assistant and recently moved from a city in which annual tornados were common. While she lived there, she had to evacuate her home three times due to a tornado, and her home was damaged significantly once. She is very frightened of tornados and wants to be prepared to help residents if one strikes.

10. What is the most important thing Bianca can do to ensure she is ready if a disaster occurs?
11. How can Bianca decrease her fears about disasters?
12. If Bianca prepares a personal disaster plan, what should she include?

Key Points

Reviewing the key points for this chapter will help you practice more safely and competently as a holistic nursing assistant and will help you prepare for the certification competency examination.

- First aid is the initial process of evaluating and responding to a medical emergency. First responders arrive first at an emergency, and their immediate actions are to call 9-1-1 and provide basic first aid. When responding to an emergency in a healthcare facility, turn on the emergency call light immediately.

- Nursing assistants need to be certified in conventional CPR, which includes chest compressions and rescue breaths. A person who is not certified in conventional CPR should use Hands-Only™ CPR. Using an AED can stop an irregular heart rhythm and restore normal rhythm.

- If you witness a person choking, fainting, having a seizure, or hemorrhaging, remain calm and respond appropriately.

- Natural disasters, bioterrorism, and terrorism cause the loss of life and property damage.

- As a nursing assistant, one of the best ways to respond to a disaster is to become familiar with your healthcare facility's policies, procedures, and disaster plans. Maintaining preparedness is your most important responsibility.

Action Steps to Holistic Care

Review the information in this chapter. Complete the following activities.

1. Select one medical emergency discussed in this chapter. Prepare a short paper or digital presentation that identifies and describes the three most important practices when responding to the emergency.

2. Create a poster or digital presentation explaining how to use an automated external defibrillator (AED). For each step, include both a visual and written description.

3. With a partner, prepare a poster that lists at least four facts about emergency care for strokes and heart attacks. Include how these actions can slow down or reduce injuries and complications.

4. Research current scientific information about the impact of a recent disaster or emergency. Write a brief report describing two current facts you did not know about how the disaster or emergency influenced people's short- and long-term health.

5. Create a supply kit and disaster and communication plan for your family in the event of a natural disaster that is possible in your area. Discuss your preparations with your family, ensure each person knows their role, identify evacuation routes, and practice your plans. Then write a brief report about your experience.

Preparing for the Certification Competency Examination

To prepare for the nursing assistant certification competency examination, you will need to know content found in this chapter. This content may be tested in the knowledge (written or oral) and skills (hands-on demonstration) portions of the exam. The following areas will be emphasized:

- principles and goals of basic emergency care
- basic first aid principles
- signs of medical emergencies such as anaphylaxis, asphyxia, burns, choking, fainting, hemorrhage, poisoning, shock, and stroke
- CPR and the Heimlich maneuver
- responses to and documentation of emergency situations according to standards of care

These sample test questions are similar to ones you will find on the certification competency exam. See how well you can answer them. Be sure to select the *best* answer.

1. An AED is used to help during
   A. the control of bleeding
   B. CPR
   C. the Heimlich maneuver
   D. a seizure

2. A second-degree burn is characterized by
   A. slight redness
   B. white, leathery skin
   C. blistering
   D. charred white skin

(continued)

3. What is the most important responsibility of the US Department of Homeland Security?

   A. evacuating people from their homes
   B. maintaining the National Response Framework and Plan
   C. rebuilding towns and highways
   D. making sure the water is safe during a disaster

4. What is a first responder?

   A. the first person who knows the victim
   B. the first person who hears about an emergency
   C. the first person who knows what to do in an emergency
   D. the first person to arrive at an emergency

5. When giving Hands-Only™ CPR, you should

   A. perform chest compressions with your hands
   B. perform rescue breaths, but not chest compressions
   C. perform rescue breaths and chest compressions
   D. do nothing, but call for help

6. Mrs. G is clutching at her throat with her hands. She is most likely

   A. having a seizure
   B. having a stroke
   C. choking
   D. having a heart attack

7. How is the Heimlich maneuver performed?

   A. using rhythmic breathing
   B. using abdominal thrusts
   C. using chest compressions
   D. using a firm back slap

8. On which type of burn should you *not* use cool water?

   A. first-degree burn
   B. fourth-degree burn
   C. second-degree burn 2 inches in diameter
   D. third-degree burn

9. What is the difference between a disaster and a medical emergency?

   A. A disaster requires fewer resources than a medical emergency.
   B. A disaster does not require the help of organizations and agencies.
   C. A disaster affects larger groups of people than a medical emergency.
   D. A disaster is not as serious as a medical emergency.

10. Mr. D was recently admitted to a long-term care facility. When you give him morning care, you notice that his right eyelid is drooping and that he is having trouble speaking. These symptoms most likely indicate

    A. stroke
    B. heart attack
    C. seizure
    D. anaphylaxis

11. After arriving at a medical emergency, what is the first thing a nursing assistant should do?

    A. check for consciousness
    B. take vital signs
    C. reassure the person
    D. call for help

12. When responding to a medical emergency in a healthcare facility, nursing assistants should

    A. always use basic first aid principles
    B. always consult with a supervisor first
    C. always follow facility policy
    D. always wait until a licensed nursing staff member arrives

13. Ms. C is eating lunch in the dining room and is exhibiting signs of fainting. What should you do after calling for help?

    A. continue to talk with Ms. C to divert her attention
    B. have Ms. C bend forward and place her head between her knees
    C. offer Ms. C a glass of water and some crackers
    D. move Ms. C to her bed so she is lying flat

14. Jody has a severe allergic reaction that affects her whole body when she eats nuts. This is called

    A. anaphylaxis
    B. aphagia
    C. asphyxia
    D. angina

15. Which of the following is an important principle in giving first aid?

    A. stand back and let others help
    B. take control and tell others what to do
    C. push yourself to perform challenging tasks
    D. know your limits when helping

Did you have difficulty with any of the questions? If you did, review the chapter to find the correct answer(s).

CHAPTER 27 End-of-Life Care

Welcome to the Chapter

This chapter will provide you with information about the views and attitudes people have about dying and death and about the decisions people make about the end of their life. Family traditions and spiritual and religious beliefs have a significant impact on these decisions. As a holistic nursing assistant, you will need to understand how you view dying and death and how your views influence the care you give. You must treat residents and their families with dignity, offer compassion, and provide resources that may be needed. In this chapter, you will also learn about the signs of dying and impending death, loss, the stages of grief, advance directives, and organ donation. You will learn how to provide personal care and support during the process of dying and after death (postmortem care).

The information and procedures presented in this chapter will help you build the knowledge and skills needed to become a holistic nursing assistant. Check with your instructor to ensure these procedures are within your state's regulations for nursing assistant practice. The topics discussed in the chapter are highlighted on the Providing Holistic Care Framework.

You are now ready to start this chapter, *End-of-Life Care*.

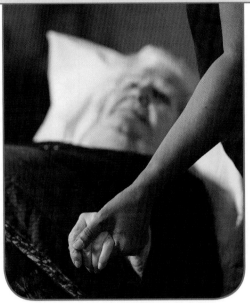
© Tori Soper Photography

Chapter Outline

Section 27.1
Dying, Death, and Grief

Section 27.2
Family Support and Postmortem Care

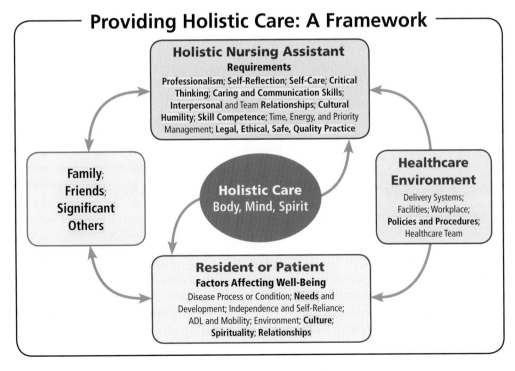

Providing Holistic Care: A Framework

Questions to Consider

- Think about an experience you have had with dying and death. Has a family member, friend, or pet passed away? Was the death sudden or prolonged?
- What feelings did you have, and how did you express them? Was it difficult for you? What did you do to accept the death? Were any rituals, traditions, and decisions important to you or the deceased person?
- What resources provided comfort during this experience? Were the resources helpful, and in what ways?

Objectives

To provide the best possible care, you must reflect on your own feelings, attitudes, and experiences surrounding dying and death. You must also understand the different traditions and beliefs held by others. Understanding your own feelings and the feelings of others will help you express compassion and preserve the dignity of others as you care for them. In this section, you will learn about the rights of dying residents, the process of dying, preparations such as advance directives, and ways in which people deal with loss and grief. You will also become familiar with changes preceding death and will learn how to provide holistic care for those who are dying. To achieve the objectives for this section, you must successfully

- **examine** your feelings and beliefs about dying and death;
- **describe** different traditions and beliefs about dying and death;
- **identify** behaviors associated with loss and grief;
- **explain** the purpose and categories of advance directives;
- **recognize** the changes that occur during the process of dying;
- **summarize** how to provide holistic care to those who are dying;
- **examine** ways to support the family of the person who is dying; and
- **describe** how to pay attention to yourself as a caregiver of those who are dying.

Key Terms

Learn these key terms to better understand the information presented in the section.

advance directives

dignity

do-not-resuscitate (DNR) order

grief

incapacitation

living will

mourn

palliative care

power of attorney

Remember

Death, the one appointment we all must keep, and for which no time is set.

Charlie Chan, fictional
US Chinese detective

We all experience the end of life. Death may come after an extended illness, after a long life, or suddenly. When death is impending, a person is considered *terminally ill*. A person with a terminal illness can be reasonably expected to die in 24 months or less. Someone may be terminally ill due to old age or due to an illness or condition such as end-stage cancer or kidney disease, heart failure, stroke, or chronic respiratory problems. Death is something we all have in common and all must face.

What Are My Feelings About Dying and Death?

Examining your own feelings about dying and death will prepare you to assist others in their journeys at the end of life. Your feelings about dying and death are influenced by the experiences you had growing up and the beliefs you currently have. Your own family traditions and spiritual and religious beliefs will also impact your feelings.

It can be helpful to write down the experiences you've had with dying and death. When you consider your experiences with dying and death, do you feel comforted or do you feel fearful or angry? If you experience feelings of fear or anger, think about what might be causing these feelings. Do you believe it is not "your time?" Do you fear the unknown, dying alone, or severe pain? Can you bear the thought of leaving your loved ones? Feelings of fear and anger are natural. We all have them.

It is important to reflect on your feelings about dying and death, as strong feelings can transfer to those in your care. If you are fearful, you may communicate fear to residents and their families through nonverbal behaviors such as not holding a resident's hand or avoiding the resident's room. You may also communicate these feelings verbally by not listening or responding to residents and their families when they share **grief** (distress) about their impending loss. As a result of your feelings, you may also have inappropriately strong responses to death and may not be able to separate your feelings from those of a resident's family (Figure 27.1).

One way to resolve feelings of fear and anger is to talk about them with someone you feel comfortable with, such as a friend or other healthcare staff member. Your feelings need to be resolved or managed so they do not influence or interfere with the lives and feelings of those in your care. Another way to resolve these feelings is to learn more about the death-related beliefs and traditional practices of others. Being aware of how people **mourn** (express grief) will help you make them feel better understood and respected.

How Do Family Traditions and Spiritual and Religious Beliefs Influence Dying and Death?

Different beliefs, traditions, and practices impact a person's experience of dying and death. They can help those who are dying feel at peace and can also help mourners come to terms with death.

In chapter 11, you learned about how beliefs affect health and healthcare. You learned that having *cultural humility* means recognizing differences among all people and assessing one's own culture to understand its limitations, barriers, and gaps in knowledge. Cultural humility and sensitivity are especially important during end-of-life care. Giving end-of-life care requires you to understand and respect the beliefs and traditional practices of different cultures and religious groups.

The following sections provide a general overview of some traditions, beliefs, and practices you may encounter when delivering end-of-life care. These traditions, beliefs, and practices are discussed in a general way because individuals respond differently to dying and death and may have different levels of adherence to particular traditional practices.

Some residents' traditions, beliefs, and practices may be unfamiliar to you, and you may not believe in them. It is still essential, however, that you respect these traditions, beliefs, and practices. The more you know about residents' beliefs, the better you will be able to provide support and care.

Family Traditions

Each family has unique traditions surrounding dying and death. Often, these traditions are influenced by a family's cultural background and dynamics. Following are some traditions you may observe in families facing dying and death:

- Some families do not discuss bad things such as death and believe that talking about bad things makes them happen.
- Some families believe that one should live intensely until death arrives. When people die, they move to a different phase of life, and the death should be accepted by all.

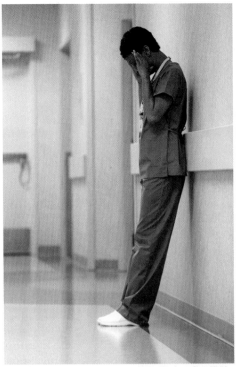

iStock.com/FangXiaNuo

Figure 27.1 If you have strong feelings about dying and death, these feelings could overwhelm you as you give care to residents who are terminally ill. Understanding and managing your feelings can help prevent this.

Remember

Life and death are one thread, the same line viewed from different sides.

Lao Tzu, philosopher and poet of ancient China

Think About This

A person's stage of life has a significant influence on his or her perceptions of dying and death individually and in the family. For example, parents may think it is too soon for their child to face dying, but the child may accept death more readily. An older adult may feel he or she has lived a fulfilling life and see death as just another phase, while a mother may feel she does not want to die and leave her young children.

- In some families, a strong sense of community accompanies loss. Extended family members gather at the time of death.
- In some families, females typically provide the majority of care for a person who is terminally ill.
- Some families believe that an older family member (sometimes the son or closest relative) must be present at the time of death.
- Some families may resist leaving a loved one in a healthcare facility and prefer that the person die at home with family members close.
- Some family members may cry and wail, while others may remain quiet and resigned.

Spiritual and Religious Beliefs

Many people rely on spirituality to understand death. For example, some people believe in the sacredness of life and consider the soul eternal. They may believe the souls of the dead pass into a spirit world. Thus, death is part of nature, is not to be feared, and is a journey to another world. Some people also believe the soul of the deceased travels safely, with adequate provisions, to the afterlife. Spiritual beliefs and religious practices often influence perspectives about burial, cremation, organ donation, and autopsy.

Every religion has its own unique practices and beliefs related to death and dying. Some religions teach that there is an *afterlife*, or a life after death, potentially in another world. Other religions teach *reincarnation*, or the rebirth of the soul in another body. Residents who believe these teachings may find comfort in thinking they will continue to live in some capacity after death. Residents may seek comfort from a religious leader, complete specific predeath rituals, or find solace in knowing loved ones will perform specific tasks after the moment of death. Prayers—either the resident's own or those of others—may also ease this difficult time.

Whatever a resident's religious beliefs may be, it is important to deliver respectful care. Special accommodations may be needed to help family members, friends, or religious leaders to complete religious practices and rituals. Some religions also dictate how the body should be treated after death. There are many resources that can help you understand the various religious practices associated with death and dying. You may also ask the resident, a family member, or a licensed nursing staff member any questions you may have. Remember to always be respectful.

If you are ever uncomfortable discussing something with a resident or find that your beliefs conflict with what you are asked to do, you must discuss this with a licensed nursing staff member to work out a resolution.

How Are Loss and Grief Expressed?

Throughout our lives, we all experience loss and grief. For example, you may experience sadness or grief after missing an important event, losing a piece of jewelry, being fired from a favorite job, ending a friendship, experiencing the realization you are going to die soon, or experiencing the death of a loved one. When people lose something important, they often feel sad, frustrated, or even angry. They may believe they should have been more careful, planned better, or been more sensitive to others. Whatever its reason, loss is personal, causes change, and brings feelings that need to be resolved. The most important thing to remember about loss is that it creates change in a person's life. What once was is no longer, and when this occurs, most of us grieve.

Stages of Grief

Elisabeth Kübler-Ross, a Swiss-American psychiatrist, discovered in her practice that all people experience five stages, or patterns, of grief and mourning. These stages were denial, anger, bargaining, depression, and acceptance and were unique to each individual. The stages were not all experienced in the same order or intensity. Since Kübler-Ross' discovery, the five stages have been expanded to seven stages that describe the grief of the person who is dying and the grief of those left behind (Figure 27.2). These seven stages are the following:

1. **Shock and denial**: people experience complete disbelief and describe themselves as being numb. They may become withdrawn, detached, and disoriented. This reaction helps people protect themselves from being completely overwhelmed. When the initial shock wears off, people may deny the reality of the situation or bad news by temporarily blocking it out or hiding from the facts. This allows people to push the news away and carries them through the first wave of pain.

2. **Pain and guilt**: when denial no longer works, pain (which may be emotional or physical) worsens, and guilt may appear. People may have guilty feelings about what they have or should have done for themselves and others. People might say, "If only I had had those tests done sooner," or "If I had been nicer to my mother, this would not have happened to her."

3. **Anger and bargaining**: pain is now expressed as anger. People may say, "Why me?" People may direct anger at themselves or at the person who is dying and leaving them. They are reacting to feelings of helplessness and vulnerability and are trying to find a way to regain control. People may seek second and third medical opinions. They may try to make deals with a higher spiritual power to postpone the unavoidable.

4. **Depression**: in this stage, the true extent of loss is realized, and feelings of depression develop. People understand that they or their loved ones won't get better, which brings feelings of sadness, despair, or regret. People may say, "I have not done all I wanted," or "I did not spend enough time with my family." People may also quietly prepare to say goodbye.

5. **Upward turn**: depression is not as intense at this stage, and a feeling of calmness begins. Physical signs of pain and depression have become more manageable, and one's "spirits have lifted."

Stages of Grief

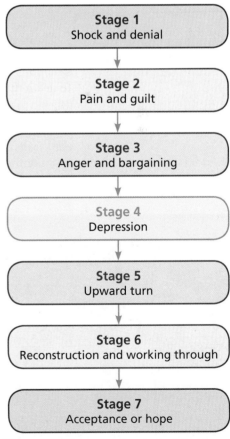

Stage 1
Shock and denial

Stage 2
Pain and guilt

Stage 3
Anger and bargaining

Stage 4
Depression

Stage 5
Upward turn

Stage 6
Reconstruction and working through

Stage 7
Acceptance or hope

Figure 27.2 The seven stages of grief address the grief of both the person who is dying and grieving family members.

6. **Reconstruction and working through**: as depression continues to lift, acceptance becomes more of a reality, and things left undone or unsaid are more readily addressed. People who are left behind become more in touch with their daily lives without their loved ones. They begin to think more about practical and financial concerns.

7. **Acceptance or hope**: some people experience this stage faster than others. They may have come to peace with any concerns or issues about dying long ago. Others do not experience acceptance at all. Death may be sudden, or a person may never leave the denial or depression stage. When acceptance or hope does occur, time has passed, and the pain has lessened. People sense a new reality. What was can never be again, but there is a way to move forward. People who are dying can accept death, and those left behind can go on.

Holistic Care for Grieving Residents

Holistic nursing assistants can provide support through all seven stages of grief. First, as a nursing assistant, recognize that residents' reactions are normal responses. Second, accept residents as they cope with the reality of the end of life. If a resident expresses anger toward you, do not take that anger personally. The resident is not angry at you, but with the situation. Reflect on the anger by saying, "Mrs. J, you seem very angry today." Then be prepared to talk with the resident about his or her anger.

When caring for grieving residents, use communication techniques such as mindfulness, active listening, open-ended questions, and reflection. These techniques will help support residents as they deal with grief. Also offer support by reassuring residents they will receive care. Use gentle touch and silence to provide a sense of calmness and comfort, particularly during the depression stage (Figure 27.3). If a resident refuses food or medication, alert the licensed nursing staff so that guidance can be provided. If appropriate, have the family bring in the resident's favorite foods.

Remember that, while all people experience dying and death, each person goes through the stages of grief in his or her own time and way. No two people or situations will be the same. For example, a younger person will respond differently to death than someone who is older and has experienced a long life.

Anticipatory Grief

Anticipatory grief is a reaction to impending loss, as a person faces his or her own death or the death of a loved one. This type of grief is different from grief that occurs after death. Not everyone experiences anticipatory grief; however, anticipatory grief does provide the opportunity to resolve feelings prior to death and find closure. Anticipatory grief might include feelings of sadness, fear, anger, guilt, and denial. Feelings of anticipatory grief are difficult, but are preparatory. They do not substitute the grief felt after a loved one dies.

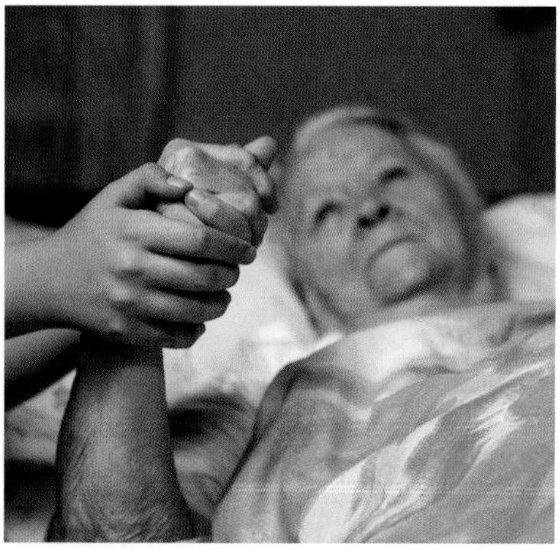

Prolonged Grief

Prolonged grief, or *unresolved grief*, is grief that lasts more than one year after the death of a loved one and strongly influences a person's daily life and relationships. Prolonged grief may result from feelings of guilt about the loss. For example, a person may feel he or she did not do something important for the person or may believe it was his or her fault the person died. Prolonged grief may also result from a violent, traumatic loss. Prolonged grief may be characterized by refusing to talk about the loved one after death, becoming consumed by the memory of the person lost, being overly involved with work, showing excessive concern about health, and starting or increasing addictive habits (such as drinking alcohol

Volodymyr Baleha/Shutterstock.com

Figure 27.3 Gentle touch can help comfort a resident and provide a sense of calmness.

or smoking cigarettes). Children may express prolonged grief by having behavior problems or being afraid to be alone, particularly at night. People who experience prolonged grief may need help from a trained healthcare professional to break grief's cycle, move forward to acceptance, and resume life after the death of a loved one.

What Preparations Do People Make Before Death?

The *Patient Self-Determination Act (PSDA)* of 1990 gives people the control and autonomy to make decisions about end-of-life care. The PSDA also

- requires that rights to control and autonomy be communicated in writing by the healthcare facility;
- specifies that **advance directives** (legal documents containing medical and healthcare instructions) must be recognized and honored;
- states that healthcare facilities must offer advance directives if people do not have them; and
- requires that people be told they have the right to refuse treatment.

The PSDA does not usually affect doctors' offices, but does affect hospitals, long-term care facilities, and home healthcare agencies that receive Medicare and Medicaid reimbursement.

The PSDA requires that healthcare facilities follow people's advance directives. Advance directives are legal documents under the jurisdiction of state law. They provide instructions for medical treatment, healthcare, and preferences at the end of life. Advance directives may be handwritten or written and stored electronically. Some doctors and healthcare facilities provide advance directive forms that people can complete, sometimes with the help of an attorney.

Advance directives are legal documents that must adhere to specific requirements outlined in state law (for example, they must include the right to accept or refuse medical or surgical treatment). These documents should be kept in a safe, accessible place, and copies should be given to a doctor and to the agent or representative in case of **incapacitation** (lack of ability to make decisions). A copy of the advance directive should also reside in the person's health record.

Four categories of advance directives are a living will, a do-not-resuscitate (DNR) order, power of attorney, and the Five Wishes. These directives provide instructions about end-of-life care and identify a representative or agent to carry out the instructions if the person who is dying is unable.

Think About This

The average life expectancy in the United States for all races and both sexes is 78.8 years. While most people prefer to die at home, the majority of deaths occur in hospitals.

Living Will

A **living will** details the medical treatment a person desires in the event of incapacitation during a terminal illness or permanent unconsciousness (Figure 27.4). The living will specifies what types of *life-prolonging medical treatments* (treatments that extend life, such as tube feeding to maintain nutrition or measures that prolong dying) are desired. The living will does not become effective until the person is certified by a doctor to be incapacitated and until recovery is not possible.

Common statements in a living will might be, "I direct all life-prolonging procedures be withheld or withdrawn," or "I do not want any of the following life-prolonging procedures," followed by specific information regarding treatment decisions. Treatment decisions might specify guidelines about the types of pain relief desired, the use of antibiotics and life-sustaining medications, enteral or parenteral feeding, ventilator use, and organ and tissue donation.

Living wills must be dated and signed by the person and two witnesses. If you are asked to be a witness as a nursing assistant, explain that witnessing this or any other similar document is not within your scope of practice.

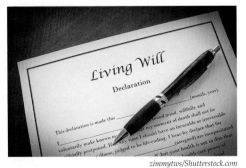

zimmytws/Shutterstock.com

Figure 27.4 A living will takes effect when a person is certified to be incapacitated by a doctor.

Do-Not-Resuscitate (DNR) Order

A **do-not-resuscitate (DNR) order** is an advance directive that instructs healthcare providers not to attempt resuscitation if a person's heart and breathing stop (for example, if the person has a cardiac arrest or has an advanced stage of cancer). Prohibited resuscitation efforts include performing CPR, applying an AED, inserting breathing tubes to open the airway, and giving rescue medications. A doctor may write a DNR order, or a *No Code*. Another order is a *do-not-intubate order*, which ensures an airway is not provided if a person's breathing stops. The doctor writes the order only after talking with the person (if possible), the healthcare proxy, or the family. DNR orders must be signed and dated.

Power of Attorney

A medical or healthcare **power of attorney** (also called a *healthcare proxy* or *durable power of attorney for healthcare*) is another advance directive. A power of attorney gives a designated person the authority to make healthcare decisions on behalf of another person. This authority only takes effect if the person who writes the power of attorney becomes unable to make his or her own decisions.

Often, the person designated to receive authority is a spouse, family member, friend, lawyer, or member of a faith community. This person may be called an *agent*, *proxy*, *surrogate*, *representative*, or *advocate* and must meet the state's requirements. The person selected may not be a member of the healthcare team delivering care and must be trusted to make decisions that adhere to declared wishes and to advocate if there are disagreements between the healthcare provider and those wishes. According to the person's wishes, the power of attorney must either follow all instructions in the advance medical directive or use them as guidance.

Five Wishes

Think About This

Some cultures avoid discussing the end of life and resist completing advance directives. For example, some think advance directives violate their beliefs. As a result, you should always be sensitive to differing beliefs if you are asked to inquire about advance directives.

The *Five Wishes* is another advance directive you may encounter. This document meets the legal requirements for an advance directive in 42 states and the District of Columbia. In the other eight states, the Five Wishes can be attached to the state's required form.

The Five Wishes is unique because it addresses medical needs, personal needs, emotional needs, and spiritual needs. Unlike other advance directives, this document addresses how a person wants to be treated and what the person wants his or her loved ones to know.

What Care Is Available to People Who Are Dying?

People who are in the process of dying can benefit from **palliative care**. The goal of palliative care is to relieve the symptoms of a disease or condition and improve quality of life for the person who is dying and his or her family. Palliative care does *not* aim to cure or treat a disease or condition, but is supportive. Palliative care relieves symptoms such as pain, nausea, fatigue, breathing problems, and anxiety and promotes comfort when an active treatment program is no longer possible. This type of care should be provided holistically and should be specifically designed to meet the needs of the person.

Palliative care, which can be provided at any time during a person's illness, is often provided through *hospice* during the last six months of a person's life. Hospice is a model and philosophy for the quality, compassionate care of people with terminal illnesses. Hospice care was first seen in the eleventh century during the Crusades, and its intent was to provide care and comfort for people with incurable diseases. This concept of specialized care for people with terminal illnesses endured over time and was fully established in the United States by the 1970s. Today, more than 1.3 million people in the United States receive care through hospice facilities and services.

Ninety-four percent of people receiving hospice care are 65 years of age or older, and 27 percent have been diagnosed with cancer. In the United States, hospice services are a part of Medicare benefits and can be made available through a referral or request.

Hospice care can be delivered in a person's home, in a long-term care facility, in an inpatient hospice facility, or in an acute care hospital. The hospice team consists of staff members who provide medical and nursing services focused on pain relief, emotional support, counseling, and guidance (Figure 27.5). The hospice team also provides social services and spiritual resources.

In addition to supporting the person who is dying, hospice also helps family members deal with emotional and practical issues related to the death of a loved one, provides respite care to give family caregivers a break, and directs families to volunteer services that can help with preparing meals and running errands. As a nursing assistant, you will participate in hospice care by being familiar with the plan of care and assisting in any way appropriate.

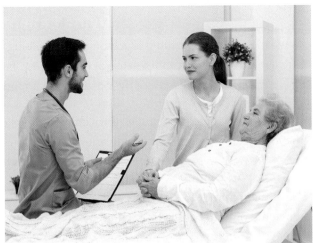

Africa Studio/Shutterstock.com

Figure 27.5 Hospice care aims to help meet people's physical and emotional needs by providing pain relief and support.

How Do Nursing Assistants Provide Holistic Care for Those Who Are Dying?

Caring for residents at the ends of their lives is a special privilege and honor. As a holistic nursing assistant, you will be with residents during one of the most important times of their lives, and your actions will make a difference in residents' journeys.

Respecting the Dying Patient's Bill of Rights

Patients and residents who are dying still have all the rights outlined in the Patient Bill of Rights and Nursing Home Resident Rights. Additional rights are included in the *Dying Patient's Bill of Rights*, which is a useful guide to the expectations of those near death (Figure 27.6). As a nursing assistant, you will not be able to help in all of the areas described in these rights. If you encounter areas you cannot help, such as pain relief, you are responsible for alerting the licensed nursing staff.

Meeting Physical, Emotional, and Spiritual Needs

Except in the case of sudden death, the process of dying begins before death itself. Dying is a personal journey, and people approach death in their own ways. Specific symptoms are associated with the natural dying process and the "shutting down" of a person's body. People typically do not experience all the symptoms of dying. The process of dying may be very quick for some and slow for others.

Residents who are dying have specific physical, emotional, and spiritual needs. As a nursing assistant, you must be aware of these needs and respond appropriately and effectively. The goal of care will not be to promote recovery, and treatment procedures may be discontinued. Instead, care focuses on promoting comfort for the resident. When providing this care, be gentle, use appropriate touch and communication, and treat the resident with **dignity** (value or worth) at all times. Pay attention to the safety of the resident and of the environment. Always follow the plan of care and facility policy.

I have the right to be treated as a living human being until I die.

I have the right to maintain a sense of hopefulness, however changing its focus may be.

I have the right to be cared for by those who maintain a sense of hopefulness, however changing its focus may be.

I have the right to express my feelings and emotions about approaching death in my own way.

I have the right to participate in decisions concerning my care.

I have the right to expect continuing medical and nursing attention, even though "cure" goals must be changed to "comfort" goals.

I have the right not to die alone.

I have the right to be free from pain.

I have the right to have my questions answered honestly.

I have the right not to be deceived.

I have the right to receive help accepting my death from and for my family.

I have the right to die in peace and dignity.

I have the right to retain my individuality and not to be judged for my decisions, even if they are contrary to the beliefs of others.

I have the right to discuss and enlarge my religious and spiritual experiences, no matter what they mean to others.

I have the right to expect that the sanctity of my human body will be respected after death.

I have the right to be cared for by caring, sensitive, and knowledgeable people who will attempt to understand my needs and will gain some satisfaction in helping me face my death.

Created at a workshop, "The Terminally Ill Patient and the Helping Person," in Lansing, Michigan sponsored by the South Western Michigan Inservice Education Council and conducted by Amelia Barbus (1975), Associate Professor of Nursing, Wayne State University

Figure 27.6 Even when patients and residents are dying, they still have rights that need to be respected.

Responding to Physical Needs

The process of dying is characterized by specific changes in the body. When someone begins to die, certain signs of impending death appear. As a nursing assistant, you will provide care that addresses the physical changes in the resident's body:

- **Respiratory changes**: breathing will be more difficult and rapid. Congestion may cause a rattling sound and cough. Pay attention to and record breathing patterns. Oxygen therapy may be used to improve breathlessness. If not contraindicated, a Fowler's position can be helpful and lower the risk of the possible aspiration of phlegm.

- **Cardiovascular changes**: the nose, lips, fingers, nail beds, and extremities may become pale, gray, or blue due to slowed blood circulation. The legs and ankles may swell, and wounds and infections may not heal well. Check the body's extremities for discoloration (Figure 27.7). When you take the resident's vital signs, blood pressure will likely be lower than normal, and pulse will be irregular.

- **Temperature changes and increased perspiration**: body temperature often lowers by one degree or more and may be accompanied by sweating. Keep the resident's body dry and change linens, if needed. Pay attention to the room environment. Maintain a comfortable temperature. Sometimes the resident who is dying has a high temperature due to a primary or secondary disease or condition (such as pneumonia caused by limited mobility in the advanced stages of cancer). If the resident has a high temperature, use cold compresses on the forehead and neck according to the plan of care.

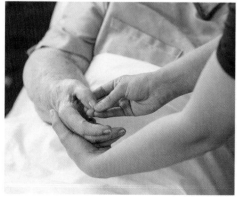

© Tori Soper Photography

Figure 27.7 Checking the body's extremities for discoloration can help you determine a resident's level of blood circulation.

- **Decreased appetite**: the need for food declines. A resident may refuse meals and beverages or consume only small amounts. Even favorite foods may be rejected. Residents who are dying may experience weight loss as their bodies begin to slow down. Continue to offer a variety of soft foods as long as the resident is conscious. Don't ever force-feed. The resident may experience nausea and vomiting due to bowel obstruction, constipation, and certain medications. Periodically offer the resident ice chips or sips of water, if tolerated.

- **Dry mouth and nose**: gently wipe a moistened washcloth around the mouth and nose. Lubricate the lips and nose with lip swabs or balm to prevent cracking (Figure 27.8). Moisten the mouth with a few drops of water from a straw or wet toothette.

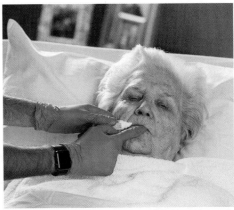

© *Tori Soper Photography*

Figure 27.8 Lubricating the lips can help prevent them from cracking.

- **Fatigue and increased sleep**: residents who are dying tend to sleep more, sometimes for a good portion of the day. Fatigue is usually the result of limited food intake and possible dehydration, which cause the metabolism to slow down. Residents may not seem to enjoy or desire activities due to fatigue. Let residents sleep. Always avoid jostling a resident awake. Due to increased sleep, the resident's eyes may not blink as often, causing the eyes to become dry. Mucus may crust on the eyelids. Use a warm, wet washcloth to cleanse the eyes and eyelids.

- **Decubitus ulcers**: residents who are dying often have limited mobility, increasing their risk for decubitus ulcers. Check the skin often and provide skin care (see chapter 21). Gently reposition the resident every two hours (see chapter 17). Provide needed padding around bony parts of the body and use pillows and other positioning devices to maintain comfort and protect the skin.

- **Changes in elimination**: constipation is common due to immobility, poor diet, dehydration, and weakness. Stool softeners and medications may be given by the licensed nursing staff.

- **Pain**: check on and report a resident's pain levels. If the resident sleeps a great deal or is semiconscious, observe for signs such as grimacing, moaning, guarding an area, and having an increased heart and respiratory rate. Pain relief medications do not shorten the life span, but can make the resident more comfortable during the process of dying. Sometimes a back rub can be comforting (see chapter 20).

As you provide care, be aware that the sense of hearing continues even if a resident is not communicating with you. Therefore, always assume that everything you say can be heard clearly.

Responding to Emotional and Spiritual Needs

Physical changes in the body affect a resident's emotional health, and residents will have emotional and spiritual needs that need to be met during dying. Many of these needs are related to the emotional changes that accompany dying:

- **Concerns**: conscious residents may fear death or be worried about dying and things they have not done or said. They may know they are dying or want to start the process of saying goodbye. You can ask residents if anything is worrying them. Listen actively and carefully, and encourage residents to share their worries with their families. It is not your role to give advice; however, you can ask if a resident would like to talk with a licensed nursing staff member or spiritual leader. Be sure to report any information to the licensed nursing staff.

- **Restlessness, confusion, and anxiety**: residents may feel restless, confused, or anxious due to an inability to relax and due to staying in one position. Change residents' positions frequently. Some residents may try to climb out of bed. Maintain safety precautions for these residents.
- **Hallucinations or visions**: do not be alarmed if a resident who is dying starts speaking with someone who is not there. Many times, the resident is talking with someone dear who is already dead. Hallucinations may be caused by medications, changes in metabolism, an infection, the disease itself, or brain metastases.
- **Withdrawal from active participation in social activities**: as residents who are dying start to accept their mortality, they may separate themselves from their surroundings. They may desire visits from significant people in their lives, but not show an interest or willingness to talk. Continue to speak to the resident while giving care, even if the resident does not respond. Don't try to make the resident talk with you or with the family.

Providing Family Support

The family is an important part of a resident's care. As a holistic nursing assistant, you can help with communication between the family and resident, the doctor, and the healthcare staff by making sure questions or concerns are answered, particularly as the resident nears death. Families may become frightened when they see their loved one's condition worsen. They may be upset by the changes in breathing, confusion, or extreme drowsiness associated with dying. Provide comfort by assuring the family you are there to help care for the resident and keep him or her safe and comfortable. Always alert a licensed nursing staff member to any changes.

Many family members will want to stay with their loved one and provide care. The family's presence and touch can help the resident who is dying feel calmer and more at peace. Remind the family that their loved one may be able to hear them up until the moment of death.

Maintain a calm and comfortable environment. Keep lights dim and be slow and patient when giving care. Be sure to give family members an opportunity to help with care if they want to and are able.

Help make family members and visitors feel welcome and comfortable and provide them with information about the facility, facility policy regarding meals, and areas of rest outside the room.

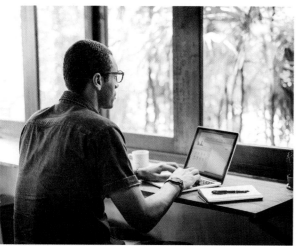

Figure 27.9 Journaling about your feelings can help you acknowledge and express them so they do not interfere with your care.

Caring for One's Self

The time of dying is challenging and is filled with emotions and feelings, including your own feelings, the feelings of the family, and the feelings of staff members and other healthcare providers. As a holistic nursing assistant, you can use the following guidelines to manage your own emotions as a caregiver:

- Keep in touch with your emotions so they do not influence the care you give (Figure 27.9).
- If you are ever uncomfortable caring for a resident, let a licensed nursing staff member know.
- Talk about your feelings with other appropriate staff.
- Always use your resources. Consult with the charge nurse about any care issues and ask for assistance from the palliative care team.

Always maintain professional boundaries and understand what is and is not within your scope of practice. Be particularly aware of what you say to the resident and his or her family. If you are doing any of the following, you may be crossing boundaries:

- You begin to think a lot about the resident when you are not at work.
- You visit or spend extra time with a resident who is not part of your work assignment.
- You take sides with the resident against his or her family or other staff members.
- You share inappropriate personal information.
- You act in a verbally or physically abusive way or use touch inappropriately.
- You accept personal gifts from the resident or family.

Section 27.1 Review and Assessment

Using the Key Terms

Complete the following sentences using key terms in this section.

1. _____ is care that provides relief from the symptoms of a disease or condition.
2. A(n) _____ is also called a *healthcare proxy* or *durable power of attorney for healthcare*.
3. To _____ is to express grief.
4. It is important to treat residents with _____, or value or worth.
5. A(n) _____ is a written legal document that describes a person's medical and healthcare instructions.
6. A medical and legal request that lifesaving measures not be administered if a person's heart stops is called a(n) _____.
7. _____ is experienced in seven stages.
8. An advance directive that details the life-prolonging treatments a person desires in the event of incapacitation is called a(n) _____.

Know and Understand the Facts

9. Explain three actions nursing assistants can take to provide holistic care for grieving residents.
10. Briefly describe the seven stages of grief.
11. Identify three physical changes that signal someone is dying and explain how a nursing assistant can deliver care that addresses each change.
12. Describe two different types of advance directives.

Analyze and Apply Concepts

13. Describe the behaviors associated with the seven stages of grief.
14. Explain how nursing assistants can give care that meets the emotional and spiritual needs of a resident who is dying.
15. Identify two ways nursing assistants can perform self-care when caring for residents who are dying.

Think Critically

Read the following care situation. Then answer the questions that follow.

You have been assigned to care for Mr. O, an 80-year-old Hispanic man. Mr. O has end-stage kidney disease and had been receiving hospice care at home. He was admitted one week ago due to a serious bladder infection and pneumonia. Mr. O has been sleeping a great deal and is irritable when awakened for meals. He usually refuses meals and does not have an IV or feeding tube. He says he hates being in this facility and would rather go home. His large family visits regularly. Mr. O has advance directives, and his oldest daughter is his agent. By the end of the week, Mr. O is more inactive and withdrawn. He does not want to eat or drink anything.

16. What are Mr. O's signs of impending death?
17. How can you support Mr. O's family?
18. How might Mr. O's advance directives affect his care?

Questions to Consider

- How do you feel when you think about caring for people who are dying or near death? Do you feel uncomfortable, frightened, or distressed?
- How can you deal with or overcome negative feelings about death?
- How might your care be affected if you don't feel comfortable providing care for those who are dying or near death?

Objectives

When death is close or has occurred, respectful, compassionate care is of utmost importance. The family's beliefs and rituals must be honored. As a nursing assistant, you will need to assist with carrying out any special instructions regarding care of the person's body (such as cultural practices, organ donation, cremation, or burial). You will also need to know how to provide appropriate and effective postmortem care. To achieve the objectives for this section, you must successfully

- **recognize** signs of death;
- **describe** ways to provide holistic family support at the time of death;
- **explain** decisions residents may make at or before death concerning organ donation, cremation, and burial; and
- **identify** the steps in performing postmortem care.

Key Terms

Learn these key terms to better understand the information presented in the section.

Cheyne-Stokes respiration
coroner
cremation
crypt
forensic
mausoleum

moribund
pathologist
postmortem care
rigor mortis
transplants

What Are the Signs of Approaching Death?

Death arrives on its own schedule; however, certain changes in the body signal that death is imminent and that a person is **moribund**, or near death. There are two phases of dying: the *pre-active phase* of dying and the *active phase* of dying. Most people are in the pre-active phase for approximately two weeks, while others last a month or longer in this phase.

The active phase of dying typically lasts approximately three days, although some people experience this phase for two weeks or longer. The exact length of the dying process will vary from person to person, as will the signs of death. Signs of death can be seen in the respiratory, cardiovascular, nervous, musculoskeletal, gastrointestinal, and urinary systems.

Respiratory System

The breathing of the person who is dying becomes irregular and slow. The person breathes in a pattern called **Cheyne-Stokes respiration**, which is characterized by periods of rapid breathing followed by periods of *apnea*, or no breathing (Figure 27.10). Secretions collect in the throat, causing congestion and a loud, rattling sound during breathing. Toward the end of the dying process, a person will experience much longer periods of apnea and other abnormal breathing patterns, such as breathing that is very slow, speeds up, and then slows again and breathing that is very fast and becomes very slow. At the very end, the person breathes through a wide-open mouth and can no longer speak, even if awake. Providing comfort and care during approaching death is essential.

Cardiovascular System

Because blood circulation decreases, the skin of a person who is dying becomes pale and cool to the touch. The person's hands and feet may appear blotchy and purplish (*mottled*) and feel numb. Discoloration may affect the arms and legs as well. The person's lips and nail beds will become bluish or purple, and due to the decrease in blood circulation, blood pressure will drop 20–30 points from the person's normal range.

Nervous System

As a person dies, less blood circulates through the brain, and the person may drift in and out of consciousness. The person's eyes may be open or semiopen, but will not focus on the surroundings. The person may become agitated or restless due to cognitive impairment (called *terminal delirium*). The person will eventually become unresponsive and move into a *coma*, or state of unconsciousness.

Musculoskeletal System

A person who is dying may experience a short burst of energy. As death approaches, however, the person will not move his or her extremities as much, and the body will start to become more rigid. The jaw will no longer be held straight and may droop to the side.

Gastrointestinal System

The person who is dying will not eat and typically will be unable to swallow. Lack of eating during the dying process is actually protective and causes chemical changes that lead to a sense of well-being. The person will experience bowel incontinence.

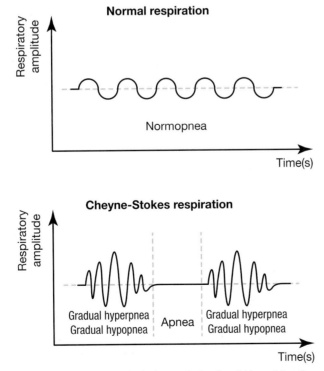

Figure 27.10 Cheyne-Stokes respiration includes periods of rapid breathing (hyperpnea), slow breathing (hypopnea), and no breathing (apnea).

Urinary System

As the body slows down and the person who is dying stops drinking fluids, urine output decreases, and urine darkens (to red or brown). Like lack of eating, lack of fluids and dehydration also cause chemical changes that increase a sense of well-being. The person will experience urinary incontinence.

At Death

At the moment of death, breathing will cease, and the heart will stop (leading to no heartbeat or pulse). The pupils will be fixed and dilated, and the eyes will remain open unless the person is sleeping. The skin will be pale, bluish, and cool to the touch, and the jaw will become slack and drop open. These signs will be used to determine death.

When a person dies, all of his or her muscles relax completely and then stiffen. The stiffening of muscles after death is called **rigor mortis**. Rigor mortis's onset depends on age, gender, physical condition, and muscular build, but typically begins two to six hours after death and starts with the eyelids, neck, and jaw. After four to six hours, rigor mortis spreads to all other muscles.

The pronouncement of death can be made by a variety of healthcare providers, including doctors, coroners, medical examiners or deputy medical examiners, or licensed nursing staff members. Each state has its own laws regarding who can pronounce death. The termination of vital signs must be documented and can be included in the person's health record. Once death occurs, the focus of your care should shift from the deceased person to the family (Figure 27.11).

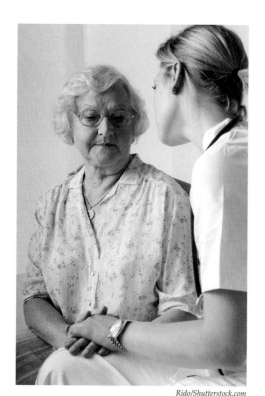

Rido/Shutterstock.com

Figure 27.11 As a nursing assistant, you should provide holistic care to the family of the deceased after a person's passing.

What Decisions Affect Care After Death?

When a person dies, the care you deliver will depend on arrangements in several areas. For example, a person may have volunteered for organ or tissue donation or may require an autopsy. The person or family will also have made decisions about burial and cremation.

Organ Donation

Donated organs and tissues are used for **transplants**, or surgeries in which organs or body tissues are removed from one person and transferred into another. There are several ways an organ can be donated. Before death, a person can decide whether to donate organs or tissues. The person can become an organ or tissue donor by registering with a state donor agency or placing the decision on a driver's license. It is important that the donor lets his or her family or a significant individual know about this decision.

If a person is dying and is not already an organ donor, a healthcare facility, doctor, or licensed nursing staff member can provide special instructions prior to and upon the person's death, so that if a decision is made, organs can be secured quickly. If the person has not made a decision about organ donation before death, the family may be consulted and asked if they would like their loved one's organs donated.

Organ donation can only occur after a person has been declared dead by an approved healthcare provider who is not in any way connected to the donation or transplant recovery team. Quick action ensures that organs are still usable and smooths the way for the family to proceed with burial or cremation.

Autopsy

Sometimes, after a person dies, an autopsy is performed on the person's body. An *autopsy* is a specialized surgical procedure performed by a **pathologist** (disease specialist) for legal or medical reasons. Autopsies are **forensic** when the cause of death is suspected to be criminal. A *clinical autopsy* is performed to find the medical cause of death.

Autopsies are ordered by a **coroner**, a government official who also certifies death. In an *external autopsy*, a person's body is fingerprinted and photographed, but not opened, and blood and fluid samples are taken. In an *internal autopsy*, organs are removed and examined.

The family or a legally responsible party must give permission for an internal autopsy. A consent form will need to be signed. A medical examiner can order an autopsy without the family's permission if the cause of death is unclear or suspicious.

After an internal autopsy, a person's body is sewn back together. If an autopsy has been ordered, a healthcare facility, doctor, or licensed nursing staff member will provide special instructions prior to and upon death so that special arrangements can be made.

Burial and Cremation

When a person is dying, decisions are made concerning burial and cremation. A person and his or her family can select either an *in-ground burial* or an *above-ground burial*. An in-ground burial uses a casket or coffin. A *casket* is rectangular and is the most common shape used in the United States. A *coffin* is six sided. Caskets can be made of metal, wood, or an ecofriendly material such as cardboard, bamboo, willow, wicker, pressed paper, or wool. Some caskets are made to accommodate religious practices.

An above-ground burial is burial inside a **mausoleum** (freestanding building) or **crypt** (vault or chamber). These arrangements are usually made with a funeral home.

A person and his or her family can also choose cremation. During **cremation**, a person's body is subjected to extreme heat (usually 1800–2000°F) for two or more hours. This process normally yields 3–9 pounds of remains. Cremations are done in a special facility called a *crematorium*. After cremation, a person's remains are placed in a container and given to the family or responsible party. At that time, the family or responsible party will carry out any instructions related to the burial or spreading of the remains.

How Do Nursing Assistants Assist with Postmortem Care?

Care provided after the death of a patient or resident is **postmortem care**. The purposes of postmortem care include

- preparing the resident's body for viewing by the family;
- providing appropriate care and disposition of belongings; and
- ensuring proper identification prior to transport to the morgue or funeral home.

Of primary importance in postmortem care is preparing the resident to ensure a clean environment and peaceful and comforting atmosphere for family members who want to say goodbye before transport. Caring for the resident's body shows the family that you have empathy and concern for the deceased.

Religious or cultural practices that have been requested must be accommodated. Practices might relate to the way the body is washed and dressed. For example, upon death, body openings may be filled with gauze or cotton, and the deceased may be dressed in his or her finest clothes. According to some religions, the body should not be left unattended. A family member, designated person, or religious official may stay in the room.

The death of a loved one is a challenging and emotional time for a family. If appropriate, you may invite the family to participate in the preparation of the body and provide instructions.

When delivering postmortem care, you can use a *postmortem kit*, which includes a shroud or body bag for transport, identification tags, gauze squares, ties to hold the hands together, safety pins, and tape to secure the shroud. Some kits have a chin strap to secure the jaw (Figure 27.12).

Keep in mind that rigor mortis and other bodily changes after death can impact the postmortem procedure. Because of this, postmortem care should be completed as soon as possible after death. When you are delivering postmortem care, a resident's body may make unexpected sounds or movements. Do not be alarmed. Bodies hold air, and when the body relaxes at death, air often escapes through the mouth or anus. Sometimes a resident's body may appear to be breathing again, as air trapped in the lungs leaves the body and makes a noise like a moan or cry. The bowels and bladder also relax, so stool and urine may be expelled. Remember that these sounds and actions are normal after death. Respect and dignity should be maintained at all times.

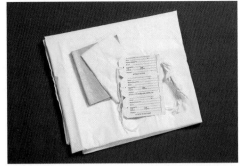

© Tori Soper Photography

Figure 27.12 A postmortem kit contains the supplies necessary for delivering postmortem care.

Procedure   Providing Postmortem Care

Rationale

Postmortem care must be provided as soon as possible after death to keep the resident's body in proper alignment (preceding rigor mortis) and prevent skin damage. Postmortem care also prepares the resident's body for family viewing, if appropriate, and transport.

Preparation

1. Ask the licensed nursing staff how this procedure fits into the plan of care, if there are doctor's orders for the procedure, and if there are any special instructions or precautions (such as organ donation or autopsy). A licensed nursing staff member will provide instructions about the maintenance or removal of equipment such as IV or urinary catheters.

2. Wash your hands or use hand sanitizer before entering the room.

3. Knock before entering the room if the deceased resident's family is in the room.

4. Introduce yourself to the deceased resident's family using your full name and title. Explain that you work with the licensed nursing staff and will be providing care.

5. Check the deceased resident's identification bracelet.

6. Use Mr., Mrs., or Ms. and family members' last names when conversing.

7. Determine if the family will be staying in the room for the procedure. If the family wants to stay, explain the procedure in simple terms.

8. Bring the necessary equipment into the room. Place the following items in an accessible location:
   - postmortem kit
   - an envelope or bag for personal belongings and valuables
   - several pairs of disposable gloves
   - several washcloths
   - several towels
   - disposable protective pad
   - bath blanket
   - cotton balls
   - gauze bandages and tape
   - clean gown
   - washbasin
   - labeled denture cup

The Procedure

9. Provide privacy by closing the curtains, using a screen, or closing the door to the room.

> **Best Practice**
> If instructed by the licensed nursing staff, turn off all medical equipment.

10. Lock the bed wheels and then raise the bed to hip level.

11. Ensure safety during the procedure. If there are side rails, raise and secure the rails on the opposite side of the bed from where you will be working. Lower the rail on the side you are working.

(continued)

Providing Postmortem Care *(continued)*

> **Best Practice**
> Always follow facility policy and consider your own safety during and after the postmortem procedure.

12. Wash your hands or use hand sanitizer to ensure infection control.
13. Put on disposable gloves.
14. Make sure the bed is flat. Place a pillow under the resident's head and shoulders to keep the body aligned.
15. Fanfold the linens to the foot of the bed.
16. Straighten the resident's arms and legs and place the arms at the side of the body.
17. Undress the resident and cover the resident with a bath blanket.

> **Best Practice**
> Always show an attitude of respect while quickly and calmly providing care.

18. Gently close the resident's eyes if they are open by grasping the eyelashes and pulling the eyelids down. Hold the eyes shut for a few seconds. Place moistened cotton balls over the eyelids if the eyelids will not stay closed over the eyes.
19. If appropriate, clean and insert dentures into the resident's mouth to maintain a normal appearance. If dentures are not to be worn, clean and place them in a labeled denture cup.
20. Close the resident's mouth. If the mouth will not stay closed, request instructions from the charge nurse. A rolled washcloth under the chin can help keep the mouth closed.
21. Remove all jewelry, except for a wedding ring, unless instructed to do otherwise. If a ring is left in place, put a cotton ball over it and tape it in place.
22. Place the resident's jewelry and personal belongings (such as eyeglasses) into an envelope or bag designated for valuables. Attach an identification tag to the envelope or bag. All valuables should remain in the facility safe until they are claimed and signed for by an approved relative or person.
23. Empty and replace any drainage bags, such as a colostomy bag. If instructed, remove tubing and appliances. Ask for guidance from the licensed nursing staff if the resident is wearing a prosthetic.

24. Remove and discard your gloves.
25. Wash your hands or use hand sanitizer to ensure infection control.
26. Put on a new pair of disposable gloves.
27. Fill the washbasin with warm water. Place the washbasin on the overbed table.
28. Wash the resident's body. Dry the body thoroughly. Place and tape gauze bandages on areas that may need drainage absorbed.
29. Change any wet or soiled linens on the bed.

> **Best Practice**
> Always ask for help if you need it. This may be necessary if you are caring for overweight residents.

30. Place a disposable protective pad under the resident's buttocks.
31. If the family has requested to view the resident, put a clean gown on the resident's body. Comb or brush the hair as needed.
32. Keep a pillow behind the resident's head and raise the bed to a supine or low Fowler's position. Cover the resident's body up to the shoulders with a sheet. *Never* cover the resident's face.
33. Before the family arrives, dispose of any soiled linens, dressings, and tubing. Straighten the room, lower the lights, and provide chairs for the family.
34. Remove and discard your gloves.
35. Wash your hands or use hand sanitizer to ensure infection control.

> **Best Practice**
> Maintain the family's privacy and provide sufficient time for the viewing.

36. When the family leaves, close the door and remove the sheet covering the resident's body.
37. Put on disposable gloves.
38. Fill out the identification tags. Tie one identification tag on the resident's ankle or right big toe.
39. Position the shroud or body bag under the resident's body.
40. If using a shroud, bring the top of the shroud over the resident's head and fold the bottom of the shroud up over the resident's feet. Fold the sides of the shroud over the resident's body and pin or tape the shroud in place.

41. Attach one identification tag to the shroud.

42. Gather all personal belongings and the denture cup, if used. List and label these items, as they will stay with the resident's body.

43. Ask the licensed nursing staff if the resident's body should stay in the room until transport to the funeral home or if the resident's body should be moved to the morgue. If the resident's body should be transported to the morgue, check facility transport policy.

44. Remove, clean, and store equipment in the proper location. Remove soiled linens and discard disposable equipment.

45. If the resident's body is still in the room, pull the privacy curtain around the bed or close the door.

Follow-Up

46. Remove and discard your gloves.

47. Wash your hands or use hand sanitizer before leaving the room.

48. After the resident's body has been removed from the room, follow the steps for cleaning a room after discharge (found in chapter 15).

Reporting and Documentation

49. Report to the licensed nursing staff and communicate the date and time the resident's body was transported to the funeral home or moved to the morgue. Report how the resident's personal belongings and valuables were handled and secured and if dentures and any other artificial body parts accompanied the resident. Record this information, along with the care provided, in the chart or EMR.

Section 27.2 Review and Assessment

Using the Key Terms

Complete the following sentences using key terms in this section.

1. A(n) _____ is a government official who can certify death.

2. Surgeries that remove organs from one person's body and transfer them into another are called _____.

3. After death, _____ causes the body's muscles to stiffen several hours after death.

4. A doctor who specializes in the study of disease is a(n) _____.

5. _____ is care provided after the death of a patient or resident.

6. _____ is a pattern of breathing that indicates death is near.

Know and Understand the Facts

7. Identify four signs of death.

8. Explain how a nursing assistant's caregiving role shifts at the time of death.

9. Which actions have to occur for organ donation to take place?

10. Name two ways a person can be buried.

Analyze and Apply Concepts

11. Identify three ways a nursing assistant can provide holistic family support.

12. Describe the purposes of postmortem care.

13. List the steps needed to perform postmortem care.

Think Critically

Read the following care situation. Then answer the questions that follow.

Janie, a new nursing assistant, has just witnessed the death of Mrs. L and was asked to provide postmortem care. Janie became close with Mrs. L, her husband, and son while caring for Mrs. L. When Mrs. L passed, her family cried, and now they do not want to leave Mrs. L's body. Janie knows she has to provide postmortem care quickly, but also does not want to cause the family more grief.

14. What can Janie do to support Mrs. L's family at this difficult time?

15. What three postmortem care steps should Janie be sure to complete when preparing Mrs. L's body?

Key Points

Reviewing the key points for this chapter will help you practice more safely and competently as a holistic nursing assistant and will help you prepare for the certification competency examination.

- Examining your own feelings about dying and death can help you deliver effective and appropriate end-of-life care. Strong feelings about dying and death can be transferred to those in your care.

- The seven stages of grief are shock and denial, pain and guilt, anger and bargaining, depression, upward turn, reconstruction and working through, and acceptance or hope.

- The natural dying process is characterized by signs of the body "shutting down." Providing holistic family support is important at this time.

- Advance directives are legal documents that provide instructions about treatment and care preferences at the end of life.

- People who are dying and families often face difficult decisions about organ donation, autopsy, and burial or cremation.

- Postmortem care must be performed as soon as possible after death to keep the person in proper alignment and prevent skin damage. Postmortem care prepares a person's body for family viewing, if appropriate, and transport.

Action Steps to Holistic Care

Review the information in this chapter. Complete the following activities.

1. Prepare a short paper or digital presentation that identifies and describes the three most important practices of postmortem care. Include one that promotes comfort for the family and one that assures safety.

2. With a partner, prepare a poster that illustrates at least four facts about advance directives that residents and the public should know. Include the legal requirements for these documents in your state.

3. Find two pictures in a magazine, in a newspaper, or online that represent different stages of grief. Describe each image and why it was selected.

4. Research current scientific information about the dying process. Write a brief report that describes two current facts you did not know.

5. Create a poster or digital presentation that discusses the emotional challenges associated with death and dying. Discuss how to provide emotional support for a resident who is dying, strategies to support a grieving family, and self-care techniques to help other nursing assistants deal with their own feelings during this time.

Preparing for the Certification Competency Examination

To prepare for the nursing assistant certification competency examination, you will need to know content found in this chapter. This content may be tested in the knowledge (written or oral) and skills (hands-on demonstration) portions of the exam. The following areas will be emphasized:

- the impact of death on self and others
- influence of attitudes, beliefs, and cultural and spiritual practices on dying and death
- signs of impending death, stages of grief, and the dying process
- care of the dying resident and support for family members
- the role of the nursing assistant in hospice care
- legal and ethical standards in end-of-life care
- requirements of advance directives
- postmortem personal care

These sample test questions are similar to ones you will find on the certification competency exam. See how well you can answer them. Be sure to select the *best* answer.

1. Which of the following is an advance directive?
   - A. cremation
   - B. patient rights
   - C. living will
   - D. PSDA

2. A person who says, "If only I had had those tests done sooner," is in the stage of grief known as
   - A. shock and denial
   - B. pain and guilt
   - C. upward turn
   - D. depression

3. Which of the following is a sign of imminent death?

   A. increased activity
   B. bluish tinge of the nail beds
   C. increased appetite
   D. increased urine output

4. A nursing assistant is assigned to care for Mr. B, who is dying. Which symptom is Mr. B most likely to have?

   A. increased activity
   B. hunger and thirst
   C. fatigue and sleep
   D. decreased pain

5. Palliative care is care that focuses on

   A. treatments that cure
   B. aggressive action
   C. no medications
   D. the relief of symptoms

6. A physical sign of impending death is

   A. depression
   B. withdrawal from family and friends
   C. increased appetite
   D. difficult and rapid breathing

7. A nursing assistant has been asked by Mrs. J's doctor to witness a DNR order. The nursing assistant should respond by saying,

   A. "Of course. I would be happy to."
   B. "I am not able. It is not in my scope of practice."
   C. "Let me ask the charge nurse if it is okay."
   D. "Did you check with the family to see if it is okay?"

8. When a resident is dying, a nursing assistant should

   A. help the resident ambulate to prevent constipation
   B. help the resident eat as much as possible
   C. observe and record breathing patterns, as they will change
   D. encourage the resident to talk with family as much as possible

9. When providing postmortem care, how should a nursing assistant handle valuables?

   A. place them in a labeled bag and give them to a family member
   B. place them in a labeled bag and give them to the charge nurse
   C. place them in a labeled bag and put them in the facility safe
   D. place them in a labeled bag and give them to the unit clerk

10. A nursing assistant who recently lost his mother to cancer has been asked to take care of Mrs. G, who has end-stage cancer. What might the nursing assistant do to be sure he does not overstep his boundaries?

    A. use Mrs. G's experience to process his mother's death
    B. never talk with Mrs. G about her feelings about dying
    C. share his experience with Mrs. G
    D. talk with the charge nurse about his feelings

11. During the last viewing of Mrs. D's body, Mrs. D's daughter tells the nursing assistant that her mother would not have died if the nurses had taken better care of her. What should the nursing assistant do?

    A. tell the daughter the charge nurse will talk with her
    B. apologize
    C. ignore the daughter and console other members of the family
    D. tell the daughter there is nothing more to do

12. Which stage of grief is characterized by someone asking, "Why me?"

    A. pain and guilt
    B. anger and bargaining
    C. shock and denial
    D. depression

13. Which of the following is true of organ donation?

    A. It can only occur after death is pronounced by an approved healthcare provider.
    B. It does not affect the care given during or after death.
    C. Everyone has to make a decision about it before death.
    D. Only the charge nurse needs to know about it.

14. Mr. F's family has decided to request hospice services. Why might they make this decision?

    A. Mr. F needs to increase his mobility and activity.
    B. Mr. F has withdrawn and needs companionship.
    C. Mr. F has a special diet and needs guidance.
    D. Mr. F has a terminal illness and needs special care.

15. How can a nursing assistant best deal with her own feelings about dying and death?

    A. exercise as a way to be more active
    B. spend more time with family and friends
    C. hold feelings in so they don't interfere with her work
    D. talk with someone with whom she is comfortable

Did you have difficulty with any of the questions? If you did, review the chapter to find the correct answer(s).

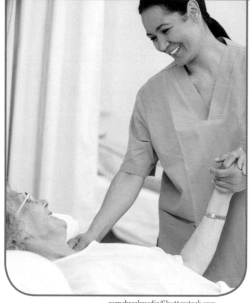

wavebreakmedia/Shutterstock.com

Welcome to the Chapter

You are now ready to prepare for and take the nursing assistant certification competency examination. This chapter provides information about studying for the exam and using test-taking strategies. You will also explore ways to search for employment as a nursing assistant and learn how to best interview for a position. This chapter will emphasize beginning and advancing your nursing career and becoming a lifelong learner.

What you learn in this chapter will help you build the knowledge and skills needed to become a holistic nursing assistant. The topics discussed in the chapter are highlighted on the Providing Holistic Care Framework.

You are now ready to start this chapter, *Certification, Employment, and Lifelong Learning.*

Chapter Outline

Section 28.1
The Certification Competency Examination

Section 28.2
Your Nursing Career

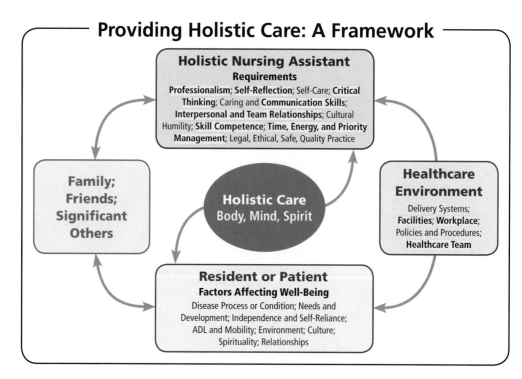

Providing Holistic Care: A Framework

Holistic Nursing Assistant
Requirements
Professionalism; **Self-Reflection**; Self-Care; **Critical Thinking**; Caring and **Communication Skills**; **Interpersonal and Team Relationships**; Cultural Humility; **Skill Competence; Time, Energy, and Priority Management**; Legal, Ethical, Safe, Quality Practice

Family; Friends; Significant Others

Holistic Care
Body, Mind, Spirit

Healthcare Environment
Delivery Systems; **Facilities; Workplace;** Policies and Procedures; **Healthcare Team**

Resident or Patient
Factors Affecting Well-Being
Disease Process or Condition; Needs and Development; Independence and Self-Reliance; ADL and Mobility; Environment; Culture; Spirituality; Relationships

Objectives

To successfully take and pass the nursing assistant certification competency examination, you will need to prepare and adopt effective study habits and skills. Familiarity with successful test-taking strategies will help you feel more comfortable when taking the exam. To achieve the objectives for this section, you must successfully

- **describe** the skills needed to study effectively and prepare for the certification competency examination; and
- **demonstrate** successful test-taking strategies.

Key Terms

Learn these key terms to better understand the information presented in the section.

auditory

concentration

cramming

flash cards

procrastination

Questions to Consider

- Describe your experience taking tests. Do you know how to prepare for tests? Are you calm when getting ready for a test?
- How do you feel when you are taking a test? Do you feel relaxed? anxious? nervous?
- How well do you score on tests? If you do not score well, what areas of studying and preparation can you strengthen? If you do score well, what actions do you take to get a good score?

What Is the Certification Competency Examination?

As you learned in chapter 1, the *certification competency examination* is a test that nursing assistants must take and pass to become certified. Each state is responsible for making sure nursing assistant education and training programs meet the OBRA (*Omnibus Reconciliation Act*) standards set by the federal government and for establishing the minimum age people can enter a program. States also determine how nursing assistant certification is granted, which certification competency examination will be used, and when and where the exam will occur. Each state has different fees for taking the exam, requirements for application, and exam schedules. Each state also determines how many times a person can attempt the exam (from three times within a two-year period to three attempts within six months of completing training).

The length of instruction in a training program ranges from a minimum of 75 hours to more than 150 hours. Requirements for supervised clinical training may be 24 hours or more in long-term care facilities. Some programs also include hospital and other related clinical experiences.

Upon completion of a state-approved nursing assistant education and training program, graduates take the certification competency examination required by the states in which they reside. The certification competency exam tests knowledge (in a written or oral exam) and skills (in a hands-on demonstration). The written exam may be completed electronically or by hand. The written exam usually consists of 50 or more multiple-choice questions covering such areas as safety, infection control, personal care, communication, and basic nursing skills. Each state has a test *blueprint* detailing the content areas covered and the number of questions on the exam. Information about a state's exam may be found in a handbook on the state's board of nursing website, on the Department of Health and Human Services website, or through the state's exam administrator.

The skills demonstration portion of the exam requires applicants to perform specified procedures on a model in front of a test observer or evaluator. Skills demonstrations are timed, and only skills that are performed (not verbalized or explained) count. Generally, the list of required skills is provided ahead of time. Some states provide specific procedures for performing each skill. Other states randomly draw skills to test from the list of skills provided. Examples of skills that may be tested include hand washing, providing oral care or perineal care, dressing a resident, performing a partial bed bath, or providing range-of-motion exercises.

To become certified as a nursing assistant, a person must meet the exam application requirements, verify completion of a state-approved training program, pay the fees, schedule the exam, and pass both parts with a state-determined score. In some states, the application process occurs online. In others, there is a paper application. In addition to the completion of a state-approved nursing assistant training program, other requirements might include photo identification, documentation that shows legal presence in the United States, and a fingerprint background check.

It is often best to take the exam right after completing the training program, as the knowledge and skills learned are most current at this time. Be sure to check state standards regarding test-taking requirements and time lines.

How Can You Prepare for the Certification Competency Exam?

Knowing what to expect is an important part of successfully taking the certification competency exam. Reviewing the certification competency exam handbook will provide information not only about how to apply for the exam, but also about what to prepare for and bring on the day of the exam.

To start your preparation, focus on what you need to know. Read your state's handbook and review the end of each chapter in this textbook to find a list of topics that might be covered on the written test and hands-on demonstrations. You can also complete the practice test questions at the end of each chapter.

Having the correct knowledge and skills is not the only preparation you need. You also need to have good *test-taking skills*. For some people, test taking causes a lot of anxiety. Other people are not nervous at all. Often, what makes the difference is the amount of test preparation and past test-taking experiences. A person who has done poorly taking tests in the past may find that negative memories influence future test taking. The person may have done poorly because he or she did not prepare well, felt nervous, or faced a challenging test. Whatever the reason for the poor performance, it can make test taking a stressful experience to be avoided, if possible.

Learning how to study and prepare for the exam can make a difference in the outcome (Figure 28.1). The more prepared and comfortable you feel with the exam content and process, the more likely you will succeed. Building excellent study habits and skills is essential.

Do you know how to study to your best advantage? Think about how you study now as you read these helpful study habits and skills. Determine which habits or skills you already possess. Keep using these skills. Then select new habits or skills you want to try as you study for the certification competency exam.

Know Your Learning Style

Are you aware of the way you learn best? The way you learn best is your *learning style*. For example, if you are a *visual learner*, you must see material to learn it best. If you are an **auditory** learner, your learning is related to your sense of hearing, and you may prefer to listen to material to learn it best. You might also be a *kinesthetic learner* and need to feel or experience material to learn it best.

Instead of being one type of learner, you may use a combination of these styles. Even so, one style will be dominant. When you know your learning style, you can use it to your advantage. For example,

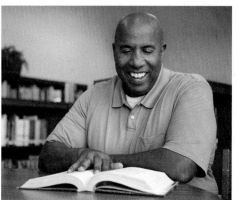

Figure 28.1 Study skills and exam preparation can improve your chances of passing the certification competency exam.

if you are a visual learner, you can use **flash cards** for studying. By taking notes on and reviewing the flash cards, you will "see" the important information you want to learn and remember.

Concentrate

Once you know your learning style, identify the best place to study. Some people like to study at a desk or table. Some people like to study indoors, and other people like to study outdoors. Wherever you choose to study, make sure you can use the place consistently. You will want to associate the place with studying so your brain switches into "study mode" as soon as you sit down. This will help with your **concentration**, or ability to direct your complete attention toward a particular object or task.

Your selected study place should be quiet, well lit, and devoted to studying (Figure 28.2). An easy chair and your bed are not the most suitable locations for serious studying. While studying, avoid distractions such as your phone, video games, or other activities you like to do. Let others know you are studying so they do not disturb you. Be sure your study area is clutter free, is organized, and has the resources you need. Getting up to get additional supplies will divert you from your main purpose: studying.

Schedule Study Time and Breaks

How motivated are you to study? Are you willing to spend the time needed and sacrifice other activities in your life to learn what you need to know? One way to increase motivation and focus on studying is to set a realistic daily study schedule that includes both study time and activities you like to do. Setting a realistic schedule will help you do "fun" things and also study. Scheduling time can help avoid **procrastination** (the purposeful postponement of a task) and **cramming** (studying a lot of material in a short amount of time) before a test.

The study time you schedule need not be long. In fact, it is good to start with a shorter amount of time and then build from there. First, schedule 15 minutes to study one particular subject or content area in which you are having difficulty. You can then add time from there. As you increase your study time, be sure to include breaks. This will help you divide the material into smaller portions that are more manageable. Do not waste your valuable time. If you are not able to concentrate, are tired, or do not want to study, stop. Schedule another study time during that same day.

Scheduling time to study is essential, but using your time to your best advantage is even more important. How well do you concentrate when you are studying? Concentration is a learned skill and develops over time. The time between when you start studying and when your mind wanders is called your *concentration span*. To determine your concentration span, note how long it takes for your mind to wander when you are reading something you do not find interesting. This is your *minimum concentration span*. Then read something of interest. Again, note how long it takes for your mind to wander. This is your *maximum concentration span*. Concentration spans can range between 10 and 20 minutes. Once you know your concentration span, do not study beyond it. Rather, take a break. Watch a video, take a walk, or have a snack, but keep thinking about what you were studying. This gives your brain time to organize the information. When you return to studying, you will find the information clearer and easier to recall.

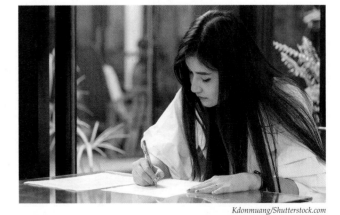

Kdonmuang/Shutterstock.com

Figure 28.2 A good study location is well lit and quiet. It is devoted to studying and has needed supplies.

Build Short- and Long-Term Memories

Concentration is related to how the brain stores information for memory. Two types of memory are short-term memory and long-term memory. *Short-term memory* allows you to temporarily remember information for a brief period of time. If this information is not stored, it is forgotten. For example, if you cram right before a test, the information may be recorded in your short-term memory and remembered for the test, but will disappear quickly after that. To be retained on a permanent basis, information must pass into *long-term memory*. Long-term memories are formed through rehearsal, repetition, and association with information. Committing information to long-term memory actually requires physical changes in the brain. Long-term memory allows you to readily retrieve information, such as the steps for performing your nursing assistant skills. To improve your long-term memory, you can do the following:

- Keep material you want to memorize well defined. Focus your studying on one section at a time (for example, only vital signs or only infection control). Study these topics on different days.

- Practice active reading by asking yourself questions such as "What does this term mean?" or "Why is this important?" while you read. Look for answers to these questions while you are reading (Figure 28.3). When you finish reading, ensure all of your questions have been answered.

- Take good notes, but don't write down everything. Keep your notes short and focus on the main points. Write the main points in your own words so you can remember them later. Review your notes often.

- Use *acronyms*, or abbreviations formed from the first letters of a series of words. Acronyms can help you recall information you need to memorize. For example, when you need to determine a resident's pain, you can use the acronym *ELR* to remember to consider how the resident **E**xpresses pain, the **L**evel of pain, and any specific aspects of pain you should **R**eport.

- Draw, find, or imagine a picture of a topic you are studying. Mentally refer to the picture when you are studying or taking a test.

- Use certain smells to improve memory. Rosemary, lemon, lavender, and peppermint are scents that provide a calming effect and increase memory. Essential oils of these scents can be purchased at local health food markets. Look for bottles that have the Latin botanical name and list the properties desired. You can put one drop on a cotton ball and place it where you can smell it, such as in your pocket.

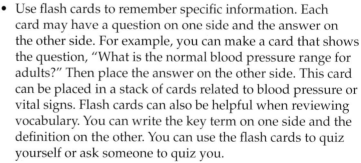

- Use flash cards to remember specific information. Each card may have a question on one side and the answer on the other side. For example, you can make a card that shows the question, "What is the normal blood pressure range for adults?" Then place the answer on the other side. This card can be placed in a stack of cards related to blood pressure or vital signs. Flash cards can also be helpful when reviewing vocabulary. You can write the key term on one side and the definition on the other. You can use the flash cards to quiz yourself or ask someone to quiz you.

- Form a study group (Figure 28.4). Select other students who are as motivated as you. Make sure each student contributes to the group's learning and keep the group focused on studying. Use the group to practice skills. Set up a simulated setting in which you and your group members perform the required skills. Exchange roles periodically (with one person as the nursing assistant, one as the resident, and one as the observer and evaluator). Use the information provided in your state's handbook to guide the steps and evaluation.

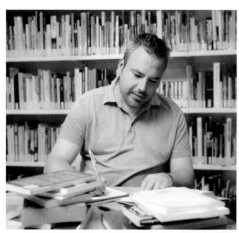

iStock.com/Maica

Figure 28.3 Reading to answer your questions will help you focus on what you are learning.

- Reward yourself for your studying efforts. When you reach a studying milestone, such as learning a particularly difficult concept, reward yourself by spending time with friends or playing a video game. If you set rewards for yourself, you will be more motivated to continue studying.

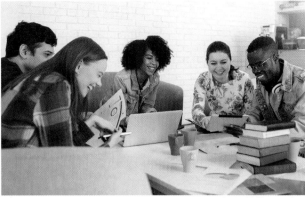

Figure 28.4 Study groups can help you review information and practice important skills.

What Should You Do on the Day of the Exam?

There are several steps you can take to prepare shortly before an exam. The night before the exam, quickly review the material and make a checklist of items to bring with you the next day. For example, many states require that you bring a watch with a second hand. Organize the needed items so you will remember to collect them the next morning. If there are specific instructions about the exam, review them. Then go to bed early and try to get your normal amount of sleep. Remember that cramming will not help. If you have been studying consistently, you have learned what you need to know. It is important to give your brain and body the rest they need to function well during the exam.

On the day of the exam, set your alarm so you get up early enough to eat a healthy breakfast. Have a meal that includes starch from cereal, waffles, or any kind of bread. This type of breakfast will release a steady supply of sugar to your brain during the exam. Stay away from candy, soda, or fruit juice, which will cause your sugar levels to rise too quickly and then drop so you feel sleepy. If you exercise regularly, do so before the exam. You might consider quickly reviewing any materials you still find challenging.

When you go to the exam, take all of the items and materials you will need, such as sharpened #2 pencils to complete the test answer sheet. If you are asked to dress in a particular way (wearing scrubs or some other type of clothing), make sure your clothes are clean and neat. Exam sites typically do not permit personal electronic devices such as cell phones. Personal belongings such as extra books, backpacks, and study materials are also not permitted. Arrive at the exam site early so you do not feel rushed. Late arrivals are not admitted to the exam. Go to the bathroom before walking into the exam room. Visualize yourself as being successful, and it will be easier to achieve success (Figure 28.5).

Remember

Before anything else, preparation is the key to success.

Alexander Graham Bell, Scottish scientist, inventor, and engineer

Successfully Preparing for Your Exam

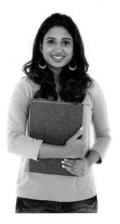

Review material the night before.

Make a list of items to bring to the exam.

Go to bed early.

Eat a healthy breakfast.

Quickly review any challenging materials.

Dress appropriately for the exam.

Gather all items you need for the exam.

Arrive at the exam early.

Use the restroom before the exam.

Visualize yourself as being successful.

Figure 28.5 Successful preparation can help you do your best on the exam.

What Are Successful Test-Taking Strategies?

When taking the nursing assistant certification competency exam, you want to be successful. One of the first issues you may need to overcome to be successful is test anxiety. *Test anxiety* is an exaggerated worry about doing well. Anxiety can negatively influence your performance and can cause extreme nervousness and memory lapses during the exam. The following strategies can help you reduce or overcome test anxiety and be successful:

- Be familiar with specific instructions found in your state's handbook.
- Make sure you have everything you need at hand.
- Listen closely to verbal directions and read instructions slowly and carefully.
- Ask for explanations of any instructions you do not understand.
- Stay relaxed. If you feel nervous, take two or three slow, deep breaths to relax yourself. Do this as often as you need to.
- Be positive. Visualize yourself completing the exam successfully.

The following are test-taking strategies specific to the written portion of the certification competency exam:

- Budget your time so you don't have to rush. If taking a paper test, quickly scan the questions to determine how you will spend your time. If taking an electronic test, know how long you have to complete the exam and the number of test items (Figure 28.6). Wear a watch to help pace yourself.
- Focus on your own test and on each question. Do not let your mind wander and don't be concerned if others finish before you do.
- If possible, answer all of the questions you are sure about first. This will help build your confidence.
- If you don't know the answer to a question, reread it. If you still cannot answer it, move on and come back to it later. You don't have to answer every question correctly to do well on the written exam.

The written exam will be comprised of multiple-choice questions. When answering multiple-choice questions, use the following strategies:

- Read the whole question.
- Think of the answer before looking at the options listed.

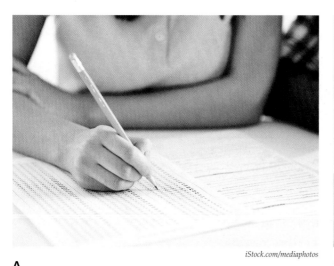

iStock.com/mediaphotos

A

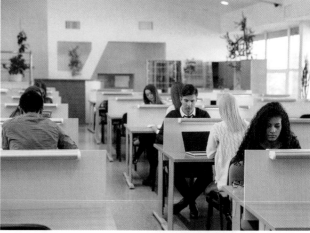

ESB Professional/Shutterstock.com

B

Figure 28.6 The written exam may be a paper test (A) or a computerized test (B).

- Read all of the answer options and choose the one that most closely matches your answer.
- If you are unsure of the answer, eliminate any answer options that appear totally wrong. Select the option that seems like the best choice.
- If you are forced to guess, choose the longest, most detailed answer.
- Don't keep changing your answer. Your first choice is usually the correct answer.
- If you finish with time left, review your answers. Be sure you answered all of the questions you can. Review questions you were not sure of, but only change an answer if you did not correctly interpret the question or misread it.

Section 28.1 Review and Assessment

Using the Key Terms
Complete the following sentences using key terms in this section.

1. _____ learners rely primarily on the sense of hearing.
2. _____ is the act of purposely postponing a task.
3. Focusing your complete attention toward a particular object or task is _____.
4. _____ are a set of cards used for studying.
5. A student who spends a short period of time studying large amounts of information is _____.

Know and Understand the Facts

6. Identify three skills needed to study effectively.
7. What types of testing are part of the certification competency exam?
8. Describe two ways to prepare for taking the certification competency exam.
9. List three ways to increase your concentration span.
10. Explain two ways you can improve your memory.

Analyze and Apply Concepts

11. In what two ways can people reduce test-taking anxiety?
12. What are three actions you can take to be successful answering multiple-choice questions?
13. Identify three actions you can take to prepare you to be successful on the skills portion of the certification competency exam.

Think Critically
Read the following situation. Then answer the questions that follow.

Mario is ready to take his nursing assistant certification competency exam. He has done well in school, but is always nervous before taking exams. Sometimes he does well, and other times he gets so anxious that he feels physically ill. When this happens, his grades are lower than usual. He does not want this to happen when he takes the certification competency exam.

14. What can Mario do to study for the exam?
15. What actions can Mario take before the exam to remain calm?
16. If Mario does start to get anxious, what strategies can he use during the exam to decrease these feelings?

Questions to Consider

- What has been your experience looking for and getting a job? Have you had an easy time finding and applying for the perfect job, or was the process challenging? Did you get the job or were you turned down? How did that feel?
- If you got the job, what was it like? Was it what you expected, or did it not turn out as you had hoped? What did you do about that?

Objectives

Starting your career as a nursing assistant is a very exciting time. In this section, you will learn how to search for a nursing assistant position, develop a cover message and résumé, complete an employment application, and be successful at employment interviews. In addition, you will explore how to prepare for your first position, what further career goals you may have in nursing, and what it will take to realize these goals. To achieve the objectives for this section, you must successfully

- **identify** the steps and strategies for finding nursing assistant positions;
- **develop** a cover message and résumé;
- **complete** employment applications;
- **demonstrate** successful employment interview skills;
- **design** a nursing or healthcare career plan; and
- **explain** strategies for becoming a lifelong learner.

Key Terms

Learn these key terms to better understand the information presented in the section.

bullying   network
cover message   résumé
job campaign

What Are the Best Ways to Find a Nursing Assistant Position?

Finding your first nursing assistant position can be exciting, but it does require work. As a soon-to-be nursing assistant, you will want to explore which facilities you are most interested in and want to pursue. You may have the opportunity to secure a position in the facility where you did your clinical training. You will have experienced the culture and organization of the facility, the types of patients or residents, and the delivery of care. The facility staff members there will have also had the chance to observe your professional behaviors and attitudes, skills, abilities, and approach to care. If staff members like what they see, they may offer you a position.

If this does not occur or if you would rather work in another facility, you will need to develop and implement a **job campaign**, or organized activities needed to find a desired job. A job campaign can include the following strategies:

- Visit school or college job-placement centers and job fairs.
- Look for open position ads in newspapers, online, and on job boards.
- Search the websites of federal, state, and local government offices; job career centers; community organizations; and schools and colleges (posted ads and placement offices).
- Search websites of local healthcare facilities or visit or call facilities' human resources departments.
- **Network**, or communicate, with friends, relatives, members of religious institutions, and participants in social activities to ask if anyone is aware of job openings (Figure 28.7).

- Identify facilities in which you would like to work and contact them about a position. You can ask to talk with the human resources department to find out if there are any open positions. Career opportunities may also be posted on the facility's website.

- If you identify a facility in which you would like to work, ask to talk with the supervisor of the department in which you are interested, even if there are no open positions. You can ask the supervisor about his or her expectations of nursing assistants and about the experience of working in the facility and on that unit.

- Review the descriptions of jobs of interest to be sure they fit your interests and qualifications. Many times, job descriptions can usually be found on a facility's website. They may also be retrieved from the human resources department.

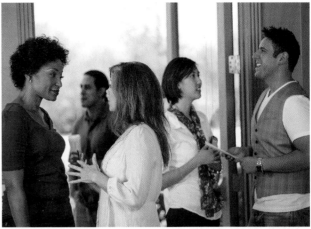
pixelheadphoto digitalskillet/Shutterstock.com

Figure 28.7 Networking allows you to connect with people who have similar interests and aspirations. It can help you learn about job openings and opportunities.

Applying directly to a facility, networking, and answering employment ads are the most common strategies for finding nursing assistant positions. You might also ask friends about opportunities or use school placement offices to secure a position.

Remember
You might well remember that nothing can bring you success but yourself.
Napoleon Hill, American author

What Tools Are Needed to Find and Obtain a Position?

To obtain a position as a nursing assistant, you first need to develop a cover message and résumé. Once you have identified a position of interest, you will likely also be required to complete an employment application.

A cover message and résumé provide an opportunity for you to show a potential employer your education, skills, experience, and abilities. Each document should be a factual representation of you and should give enough information that the employer can decide if you are a good fit.

Cover Message

A **cover message** precedes a résumé and introduces you, your capabilities, and your skills to a prospective employer. If written in letter format, a cover message should include your return address, the current date, and the mailing address of the employer. The greeting should be directed at the person responsible for hiring. In large facilities, this person might be the human resources manager. In small facilities, this person might be the director of nursing. Often, the information of the person responsible can be found on the facility website. You can also call the facility to ask who should receive this material. Many facilities request hiring information electronically and require that a cover message be inputted or uploaded.

When writing a cover message, start with a greeting such as "Dear Mrs. Jones" or the correct contact in the facility. If you do not have a specific name, use "To Whom It May Concern." The body of the letter should have an opening paragraph, in which you indicate the position you are applying for and how you heard about it. The next paragraph should briefly describe why you believe your education, skills, and experience relate to the position. For example, you could write, "I just completed a nursing assistant program and received my certification. I am enclosing my résumé, which provides more information about my experiences in helping others." The final paragraph should request a personal interview to discuss the position and your qualifications. Always thank the recipient for his or her time and indicate you look forward to hearing back soon. If using a letter format, write your signature following a closing of "Sincerely." Be sure to also print or type your name below the signature so the recipient can see the spelling of your name. If you are submitting the cover message electronically, a signature is usually not necessary.

A cover message should always be formal, clear, and to the point (Figure 28.8). If printed, it should appear on letter-size, white or off-white paper.

Résumé

The **résumé** follows a cover message. A résumé goes into more detail than a cover message and should be brief (one page, if possible). Great résumés quickly grab the reader's attention and sell the applicant's accomplishments and strengths. They show why the applicant is a good fit and match for the position (Figure 28.9). A well-crafted résumé will take you to your desired next step: a personal interview for the position.

Jamelle Thompson
765 State Street
Lansing, Michigan 48906
517-776-8321
jthomp2@e-mail.com

January 8, 20XX

Natalie Smith
Manager
Briar Senior Living Center
533 Pat Street
Lansing, Michigan 48906

Dear Ms. Smith,

I am writing to express my interest in the opening your facility has for a certified nursing assistant. I found out about this position when I contacted your human resources department.

I am eager to work at your facility because of my interest in and experience with working with older adults. I discovered through weekend and summer volunteer work at the community Senior Citizen Center that I have a special ability to motivate others to become more active and independent. I also enjoy assisting others. I am responsible for helping my two great aunts, who need transportation to and from their doctors and extra help shopping. I always enjoy the times I spend with them.

I just completed a nursing assistant program and received my certification. My plans are to go back to school and become a registered nurse. My career goal is another reason I am interested in this position. My research about your facility has shown that there are many opportunities for motivated people such as myself.

I am enclosing my résumé, which provides more information about my experiences helping others. I look forward to talking with you further about my interest in the position and experience. Thank you for your time and consideration.

Sincerely,

Jamelle Thompson

Figure 28.8 A good cover message has an introduction, body paragraphs that highlight your interests and skills, and a closing that requests a desired next step.

There is no best way to write a résumé; however, several important items should always be included:

- **Personal information**: list your full name, address, telephone number, and e-mail address.

- **A brief employment objective or goal**: in one or two sentences, state what you would like to do at the facility or accomplish in your nursing career. For example, you could write, "My goal is to provide the best possible care for older adults," "My passion is to help others be as healthy as possible," or "I would like to begin my nursing career as a nursing assistant so I can someday be an RN."

- **Work experience**: start with the most recent experience and include dates employed, position title, organization, and address. You may want to provide a short sentence describing your primary responsibilities.

- **Education**: include the school, college, and program; time attended; and diploma, degree, or certificates earned. In some résumés, education precedes work experience.

- **Additional information**: this section can include licenses and certifications earned (with their identification numbers), organizations to which you belong, and volunteer experiences.

- **References**: you can simply say "Furnished upon request" or you can list no more than three *references*, or people who can speak to your skills and abilities. Include each reference's name, address, job title, and telephone number or e-mail address. Do not put a reference on your résumé without the reference's permission.

The cover message and résumé should always have correct spelling, grammar, and sentence structure. Carefully proofread these documents to ensure they are free from errors. Use a 12-point font. If printed, the résumé should be letter size on white or off-white paper. It should not include a photo.

Employment Application

Most positions will require you to fill out and submit an *employment application* (Figure 28.10). A paper copy of the application may be filled out in person or the application may be available to complete and submit online. The following information will likely be needed to complete the application:

- **Your address and phone number**: include your current address and the number of a phone you will answer.

- **Work experience**: include organization names, addresses, dates of employment, positions, and contact information. If you have limited work experience, you can include part-time positions, summer jobs, and volunteer work.

- **Education**: include the names and addresses of schools and dates attended.

- **References**: list the names, addresses, and phone numbers of people who can speak to your knowledge and skills. You should usually include three references. Be sure you have asked these references for permission.

- **Salary expectations**: provide the minimum salary you require or indicate you are open to negotiations.

- **Reason for applying**: provide an answer that shows how you are a good fit for the position and facility.

Answer all of the questions on the application. If you do not answer a question, have a reason why, as you will likely be asked about unanswered questions at the interview.

Think About This

As you look for a position, have your driver's license and copies of your certifications or licenses on hand. Once you are employed, you may need to complete an I-9 (Employment Eligibility Verification), which will ask you to certify your identity using a combination of items (such as your driver's license, Social Security card, US passport, or birth certificate). You may also need to complete a background check and fingerprinting. You will likely be required to show evidence of specific immunizations (such as for hepatitis B) and have signed documentation from a healthcare provider that you have no communicable diseases and are able to perform the required job duties.

Jamelle Thompson
765 State Street
Lansing, Michigan 48906
Cell Phone: 517-776-8321
E-mail: jthomp2@e-mail.com

Employment Goal:

My goal is to help older adults be as healthy, active, and independent as possible.

Work Experience:

Call Desk Representative, June 2016 to August 2017

Basic Credit Card Company, 17 Broadway, Lansing, Michigan 48909

My primary job responsibility was to gather basic customer information and direct the call to the appropriate department.

Clerk, June 2015 to May 2016

City Pharmacy, 4 Main Avenue, Lansing, Michigan 48909

My primary job responsibility was to help customers with their desired purchases. I also helped stock inventory.

Education:

Michigan Community College, Fall 2018

Completed Nurse Assisting Program

East Lansing Community College, Spring 2017

Completed Anatomy and Physiology and Chemistry courses

Lansing High School, 2011 to 2015

College preparatory program

Additional Information:

Nursing Assistant Certification, Michigan, #75443

Volunteer Experiences:

Volunteer, Arts and Music Program, during high school (summers and weekends)
Community Senior Citizen Center, 17 Lakewood Avenue, Lansing, Michigan 48906
Helped older adults become involved with arts, music, and reading programs.

References:

Jade Johnson, supervisor

Community Senior Citizen Center, 17 Lakewood Avenue, Lansing, Michigan 48906

Phone: 517-776-2323

Jim Sims, supervisor

Basic Credit Card Company, 17 Broadway, Lansing, Michigan 48909

Phone: 517-798-5421

John Lane, pharmacy manager

City Pharmacy, 4 Main Avenue, Lansing, Michigan 48909

Phone: 517-798-6655

Figure 28.9 A résumé should always have correct spelling, grammar, and sentence structure. Carefully proofread before sending it out.

Employment Application

Date

January 8, 20XX

Which position(s) are you applying for?

- ○ RN
- ○ LPN
- ○ Home Health Aide
- ● CNA

- ○ Speech Therapist
- ○ Administrative Staff
- ○ Social Worker

- ○ Physical Therapist
- ○ Occupational Therapist
- ○ Data Entry

Name

First

Jamelle

Last

Thompson

Type/License #

Certified Nursing Assistant, License #75443

Issued by the State of

Michigan ▼

Expiration

November 30, 20XX

Address

Street Address

765 State Street

City

Lansing

State

Michigan ▼

Zip Code

48906

Phone Number

517-776-8321

E-mail

jthomp2@e-mail.com

Do you have a valid driver's license?

● Yes ○ No

Have you ever been convicted of a criminal offense other than a traffic violation?

○ Yes ● No

What days/hours are you available to work?

- ● Sunday
- ● Monday
- ● Tuesday
- ● Wednesday

- ● Thursday
- ○ Friday
- ● Saturday

Please tell us about any experience you feel may qualify you for this position.

When I was in high school, I volunteered during the summers and weekends at a community Senior Citizen Center. I helped with arts, music, and reading programs. I also worked for two years as a call desk representative for a credit card company. My primary responsibility was to gather basic customer information and direct the call to the appropriate department. I also spent one year working as a clerk in a local pharmacy. There, I helped customers with their desired purchases. For the past five years, I have assisted two of my older family members who have chronic illnesses. I transport them to the doctor, help them with their meals, accompany them to the store and church, and often read to them.

Figure 28.10 Always answer the questions on an employment application completely and honestly.

How Can You Be Successful When Interviewing for a Position?

After reviewing your cover message, résumé, and employment application, the hiring manager at the facility to which you applied will decide whether or not to seek a phone or in-person interview. The purpose of an interview is for the facility to find the right person for a position, but the interview is also an opportunity for you to determine if the position and facility are good fits. The outcome of a successful interview is an offer of a position from the facility.

A *phone interview* is often conducted before an in-person interview. A phone interview is a screening tool and allows the hiring manager to determine which candidates to meet in person. During a phone interview, speak clearly and confidently and be prepared to answer questions about your skills and experience.

Several skills can help you have a successful in-person interview. It is often helpful to practice your interviewing skills with a friend or family member. Follow these guidelines to be prepared and professional during your interview:

- Be on time and come alone. Do not bring family members or friends.
- Enter the interview prepared and with a positive attitude. Research the facility before the interview. Know the facility's leadership, mission, and values. You may want to determine how the facility is unique compared to others.
- Wear clothing that establishes you as a professional person (Figure 28.11). Dress in clean, neat business attire. Be sure that you have bathed and that your hair is groomed. Do not wear cologne or perfume. Remove body jewelry, such as lip, nose, and eyebrow rings and studs. Cover body art, if possible.
- Turn off your cell phone.
- Politely greet the interviewer(s). There may be more than one interviewer. An interviewer may be a supervisor from the area in which you would be working, a person from the human resources department, or another supervisor or director.
- Establish eye contact and smile. Try to be as relaxed as possible without slouching in the chair.
- Actively listen and be friendly.
- Speak clearly and with respect.
- Do not chew gum or communicate nonverbally that you are nervous or disinterested.
- Answer questions honestly to the best of your ability. If you do not understand a question, politely ask the interviewer to repeat it or ask it in another way. If you do not have an answer for a question, say you don't know the answer.
- Be prepared to answer several different kinds of questions related to your work history, relationships with coworkers, conflicts and resolutions at work, desires for a position in the facility, career goals, strengths, and areas or skills that need development. You will also be asked questions related to being a nursing assistant in the facility (Figure 28.12).
- When answering questions, emphasize your strengths. Explain why you think you are the best person for the position.

Remember

Confidence is the companion of success.

Unknown

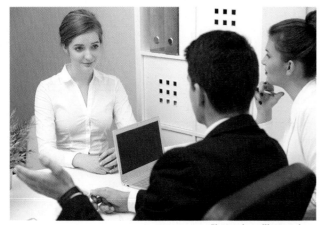

Photographee.eu/Shutterstock.com

Figure 28.11 When attending an interview, wear professional clothes that are clean and neat.

Commonly Asked Interview Questions

Why have you chosen nurse assisting as a career?

What do you like and dislike about being a nursing assistant?

What motivates you to work in healthcare and with residents or patients?

Describe a time you were very satisfied in a job you were doing.

What are your strengths, and what areas do you think you need to develop?

What do you find most stressful in a workplace? How do you handle your stress?

With what type of manager do you work best?

Talk about a difficult person you worked with and how you handled the situation.

If you noticed a nurse, doctor, or nursing assistant not doing his or her job properly, what would you do?

What would you do if a resident became agitated?

What would you do if a resident refused care?

How would you spend your time if all of your work was done and you had a few minutes to spare before completing your shift?

What are your nursing career goals?

Figure 28.12 Formulating answers to questions like these before the interview can help you feel more prepared.

- Do not prolong the interview, but do ask questions, if appropriate. Ask questions that will help you understand and make a decision about the position. You can ask such questions as "What are you looking for in a successful nursing assistant?" or "What is the best thing about working in this facility?"
- Do not bring up salary yourself, but if the interviewer mentions it, you can ask about the salary and benefits of the position.

At the close of the interview, emphasize your accomplishments and ask if you can provide any additional information to show your abilities and interest in the position. Also ask when you will be notified about the position.

After the interview, you may want to send a thank-you message to the interviewer. The thank-you message should be brief and express appreciation for the interviewer's time and consideration. Offer again to provide any further information and reinforce that you are excited about the possibility of working at the facility.

After the interview, you may receive a job offer immediately or after several weeks. Generally, you should contact the facility about the position two weeks after the interview if you have not heard back. A job offer may come from the human resources department, the hiring supervisor, or some other administrative staff member. If you receive a job offer, always request it in writing. If salary, wages, and benefits (such as health insurance) were not discussed at the interview, be sure they are outlined and agreed to in the job offer. You should also know your start date, any other requirements (such as a physical examination), the location where you will be working, and the name of your supervisor. When you receive a job offer, express your appreciation and ask any remaining questions you have. If you are not sure whether you want to accept the offer, ask for time (usually 24 hours) to think it over before accepting.

What Will Your Work Environment Be Like?

Starting your first position as a nursing assistant can be very exciting and motivating. When you begin your job, you will be oriented to the facility and learn what is expected of you. You will be provided with on-the-job training, usually an employee handbook, and guidance from the licensed nursing staff. The first few weeks will be a learning experience, and as time passes, the environment and care will become more familiar.

Think About This

Equal employment opportunity (EEO) laws, both federal and state, help prevent discrimination against an applicant or employee based on race, color, religion, sex (including pregnancy, gender identity, and sexual orientation), national origin, age (40 or older), disability, or genetic information. As a result, only job-related questions may be asked during an interview. For example, an interviewer may not ask an applicant about his or her marital status or children. Any questions about family status must center on any responsibilities or commitments that may prevent the applicant (regardless of sex) from meeting a work schedule.

Determining If a Job Is Right for You

Most facilities have a 60–90 day *probationary period*, during which time an employee is evaluated for fit in the facility. The employee is evaluated on whether he or she demonstrates the behaviors, attitudes, skills, and capabilities needed to provide safe, quality care. When you start a new position, pay attention to whether the position is a good fit for you, too. You may not know this until you are well into the position, but you can start by considering whether you are excited to come to work each day, enjoy the people you work with, can take advantage of the educational programs provided, and feel supported in providing safe, quality care. If you feel supported, you will be able to help others feel supported and motivated.

Managing Stress and Dealing with Workplace Violence

For a nursing assistant, the goal of each and every day at work is to provide safe, quality care. Healthcare today, however, is very fast paced, and those in your care will have needs and demands that can create a great deal of stress. Sometimes this stress can lead patients, residents, family members, other healthcare providers, and coworkers to act aggressively. Aggressive acts may range from violent or physical acts (such as assault) to verbal abuse, threats, hostility, **bullying** (repeated and harmful verbal, physical, social, or psychological behavior), or harassment. The Occupational Safety and Health Administration (OSHA) reports that incidents of serious workplace violence (incidents requiring days off work for the injured worker) are four times more common in healthcare than in other industries. Patients and residents can act aggressively toward healthcare workers, and worker-to-worker violence can also occur.

Being aware of violence in the workplace is essential. Some strategies to deal with workplace violence include the following:

- Understand the facility's workplace violence policy and safety and security procedures.
- Immediately report incidents.
- Recognize the warning signs of possible violence. Verbal cues include speaking loudly or yelling, swearing, or using a threatening tone of voice. Nonverbal cues include holding the arms tight across the chest, clenching the fists, or pacing with agitation.
- Remember to use effective communication techniques and skills to resolve conflicts (see chapter 10).
- Use stress-management and relaxation techniques (see chapter 7).
- Be aware that fatigue can lower your alertness and ability to respond appropriately to a challenging situation.
- Practice personal security measures. Dress for safety, keep long hair tucked away so it can't be grabbed, and avoid wearing earrings or necklaces that can be pulled. Avoid overly tight clothing that can restrict movement and overly loose clothing or scarves that can be caught. Do not leave anything dangling from cords or chains and use breakaway safety cords or lanyards.

Resigning a Position

The goal of every professional should be to make the work and work environment as positive as possible. Remember, however, that if a position is not a good fit, it is best to look for another. If you wait to look for another position, you may become frustrated, depressed, or angry, and this can affect the care being delivered. It is helpful to talk with your supervisor first. There may be another position available in the same facility. If you decide to leave the facility, be professional by giving adequate notice (at least two weeks) and providing a letter of resignation. You do not have to provide a reason, but try to leave with a positive impression in case you want to come back to the facility in the future. Do not share negative comments about your experience. Rather, say you are leaving for another opportunity.

How Do You Advance Your Nursing or Healthcare Career?

In addition to career development, advancing your career also means gaining further education, training, and experience. In nursing, advancement might mean becoming a registered nurse. If you are interested in another field in healthcare, you might become a dietitian, physical therapist, or doctor. Thinking about your future career now is helpful and gives you a chance to determine your short- and long-term career goals. There are four stages in career planning for advancement.

Stage One: Examination

The first stage in career planning is examination. In the examination stage, you determine your present values, skills, and abilities. You might complete career or job strength assessments or talk with a counselor. Often, you are aware which careers will best suit you. For example, you might know that you really like working with and taking care of people. On the other hand, perhaps you are more interested in discovering how things work, but do not like communicating with people. Recognizing these qualities will help you determine if you should seek a career of service to people or of working with machines or technology.

Stage Two: Exploration and Preparation

The second stage of career planning is exploration and preparation. In this stage, you research careers of interest. Once you select these careers, research what is required. Learn about the career's education, training, certification, experience, salaries and benefits, employment possibilities, and career advancement. You might interview someone who has this career or ask to spend a day observing to see what an average day in the career is like. If possible, you might volunteer with an organization or facility related to your career of interest.

Stage Three: Commitment to a Career

The third stage of career planning is commitment to a career. You are aware of what you want to do and feel confident that you have found your life's work. Some people reach this stage very quickly. They have known what they were meant to do since they were young. Others need to complete the first two stages of career planning to make this decision. Either way, commitment requires setting goals, focusing on the expectations of the career, and fulfilling the career's requirements. If you wish to pursue a nursing career, completing a nursing assistant training program is an effective first step.

Stage Four: Transformation

The final stage of career planning is transformation. This stage occurs after an initial career is launched. Many times, a person decides to advance further in a career (for example, by going from a staff nurse to a nurse manager or nurse practitioner). A person may also decide to pursue a related career. For example, a registered nurse working in acute care might decide to transition into a role promoting health and wellness education in the community. Other times, people decide to change careers completely and may go from healthcare to a position in business. Changes usually require further education, training, certification, and experience.

The way to implement career planning is to establish an action plan that helps guide you through each stage. Your action plan should include all four stages and identify your goals.

How Can You Become a Lifelong Learner?

A key part of developing as a nursing assistant and building your healthcare career is becoming a person who desires and seeks learning. Further learning improves competence throughout life and makes a lifelong learner. There are several qualities and characteristics of lifelong learners. These include

- curiosity;
- flexibility, adaptability, and comfort with change;
- accountability and self-reliance;
- innovation and creativity in problem solving;
- quality and excellence;
- education to promote self-development, well-being, and care; and
- workplaces that promote lifelong learning.

Section 28.2 Review and Assessment

Using the Key Terms

Complete the following sentences using key terms in this section.

1. A(n) _____ quickly grabs the reader's attention and sells the applicant's accomplishments and strengths.
2. People who are searching for a job should _____ with an interconnected group of people to learn about available positions.
3. A(n) _____ is a series of organized activities needed to find a desired job.
4. Repeated and harmful verbal, physical, social, or psychological behavior is called _____.
5. A(n) _____ introduces you, your capabilities, and your skills to a prospective employer.

Know and Understand the Facts

6. Identify two different methods of finding a nursing assistant position.
7. List two important items to include in a cover message.
8. List two important items to include in a résumé.
9. Identify two important pieces of information to include on an employment application.
10. Describe four successful interviewing skills.
11. Identify two follow-up actions to take after an interview.

Analyze and Apply Concepts

12. How can you best determine if a nursing assistant position will be a good or bad fit for you?
13. Complete a career planning action plan for your future career.
14. List two strategies for becoming a lifelong learner.

Think Critically

Read the following situation. Then answer the questions that follow.

LoriAnne has just completed her nursing assistant training program and has successfully passed the nursing assistant certification competency exam. She applied for a position at the facility in which she did her clinical training. LoriAnne was asked to submit a cover message and résumé and complete the employment application. She was told the director of nursing would like to interview her next week. She really wants this position.

15. What type of information should LoriAnne include in her cover message and résumé to best represent her qualifications?
16. What advice would you give LoriAnne about conducting herself during the interview?
17. What questions should LoriAnne ask during the interview?
18. List four attitudes and behaviors LoriAnne can demonstrate to help her get this position.

Key Points

Reviewing the key points for this chapter will help you practice more safely and competently as a holistic nursing assistant and will help you prepare for the certification competency examination.

- Using excellent study habits and skills can help you pass the nursing assistant certification competency exam.

- Curb test anxiety by listening closely to instructions and breathing deeply if nervous. Budget your time, answer the questions you know, and eliminate incorrect options.

- To find a nursing assistant position, search online, network, and apply to desired facilities.

- A cover message and résumé are opportunities to show a potential employer your education, skills, experience, and abilities.

- An employment application is a requirement for all positions, and each facility will have its own form for completion.

- When interviewing, be prepared, professional, answer questions honestly and fully, and ask questions to better understand the position and facility.

- Being a lifelong learner means desiring and seeking learning to improve competence throughout your life.

Action Steps to Holistic Care

Review the information in this chapter. Complete the following activities.

1. Prepare a short paper or digital presentation that identifies your three most effective test-taking strategies. Explain why these strategies work for you.

2. With a partner, prepare a poster that lists at least eight actions you can take to effectively prepare for the certification competency exam.

3. Write a song or a poem about short- and long-term memories. Discuss why this information is important.

4. Research current scientific information about how people concentrate. Write a brief report describing two current facts you did not know.

5. Prepare a one-page résumé that outlines your employment objective, education, work experience, and any additional information you think wise to include. Identify three references and seek permission to use them on your résumé. Carefully proofread and format your résumé. Then exchange résumés with a partner. Critique his or her résumé, offering constructive criticism. Review their feedback on your résumé and implement any changes you deem appropriate.

 Preparing for the Certification Competency Examination

This chapter provides information to help you prepare for the nursing assistant certification competency exam and find your first position as a nursing assistant. As you get ready to accomplish these tasks, reflect on and answer the following questions about preparing for the certification competency exam and finding your first nursing assistant position.

Consider the following questions about preparing for the certification competency exam:

1. Describe where you study best.

2. Can you make any changes to your study space to improve the quality and time of your studying?

3. How do you handle distractions when studying?

4. What is the length of your concentration span?

5. What have you done to improve your memory skills in the past?

6. After reading this chapter, do you want to use any new skills to improve your memory?

7. Draft a plan of action you can use to prepare the night before and the day of the certification competency exam.

8. Which of the test-taking strategies discussed in this chapter do you think you will use? Why?

Consider the following questions about pursuing your first nursing assistant position:

9. How will you go about getting your first nursing assistant position? What specific strategies will you use in your job campaign?

10. What information should you include in a cover message and résumé to secure your first nursing assistant position?

11. Are any parts of the employment application unclear? If so, what can you do to clarify these questions?

12. Describe the most important steps in having a successful interview.

Metric Conversion Table

Conversion Table: US Customary to SI Metric*		
When You Know ⬇	**Multiply By:** ⬇	**To Find** ⬇
Length		
inches	25.4	millimeters
inches	2.54	centimeters
feet	0.3048	meters
feet	30.48	centimeters
yards	0.9	meters
miles	1.6	kilometers
Weight		
ounces	28.0	grams
ounces	0.028	kilograms
pounds	0.45	kilograms
short tons	0.9	tonnes
Volume		
teaspoons	5.0	milliliters
tablespoons	15.0	milliliters
fluid ounces	30.0	milliliters
cups	0.24	liters
pints	0.47	liters
quarts	0.95	liters
gallons	3.8	liters
cubic inches	0.02	liters
cubic feet	0.03	cubic meters
cubic yards	0.76	cubic meters
Area		
square inches	6.5	square centimeters
square feet	0.09	square meters
square yards	0.8	square meters
square miles	2.6	square kilometers
acres	0.4	hectares
Temperature		
Fahrenheit	$5/9 \times (F - 32)$	Celsius
Celsius	$(9/5 \times C) + 32$	Fahrenheit

*Note: For all but temperature, when you know the metric measurement, divide by the same numbers given above to determine the US customary measurement.

BMI Calculation	US Customary	SI Metric
	$BMI = \dfrac{wt\ (lb)}{ht\ (in^2)} \times 703$	$BMI = \dfrac{wt\ (kg)}{ht\ (m^2)}$

Sexually Transmitted Infections (STIs)

Sexually Transmitted Infection (STI)	Cause	Signs and Symptoms	Treatment
Chlamydia	• Caused by bacteria (*Chlamydia trachomatis*) • Spread during vaginal and anal intercourse	• Symptoms begin 5–10 days after exposure. • Symptoms are often mild, particularly for men. • In women, symptoms include abdominal pain, abnormal vaginal discharge, bleeding between menstrual periods and after intercourse, low-grade fever, painful intercourse, burning during urination, swelling in vagina, and itching and swelling around anus. • In men, symptoms include pain or burning during urination, pus or watery/milky discharge from the penis, swollen or tender testicles, and itching and swelling around the anus.	• Antibiotics are taken to resolve the infection. • Both partners must be treated and remain abstinent until treatment is completed. • Condoms should be used to prevent future infection.
Gonorrhea	• Caused by bacteria (*Neisseria gonorrhoeae*) transmitted during sexual contact • Spread by vaginal and anal intercourse and oral sex • May also be passed from a woman to her fetus during childbirth • May not be passed through kissing or hugging • Often accompanied by chlamydia	• Some people do not show symptoms or only have minor symptoms. • Symptoms begin 1–14 days after exposure. • In women, symptoms include abdominal pain, bleeding between menstrual periods, menstrual irregularities, fever, painful intercourse, painful or frequent urination, swelling or tenderness of the vulva, vomiting, and yellow or yellow-green vaginal discharge. • In men, symptoms include puslike discharge from the penis, pain or burning during urination, and frequent urination. • In both sexes, symptoms include anus itchiness, discharge and pain during bowel movements, and itching and soreness of the throat (with trouble swallowing if the infection is oral).	• Antibiotics are used to treat infection. The full course of antibiotics must be taken, even if symptoms resolve early. • Pregnant women and teens should not be given certain antibiotics. • Both partners must be treated and remain abstinent until treatment is completed. • Untreated gonorrhea in pregnant women can cause premature labor and stillbirth. • Condoms should be used to prevent future infection.

Sexually Transmitted Infection (STI)	Cause	Signs and Symptoms	Treatment
Herpes	• Caused by herpes simplex virus type 1 (HSV-1) and herpes simplex virus type 2 (HSV-2) • Spread by touching, kissing, and sexual contact (including vaginal, anal, and oral sex) • Can also be spread from a woman to her fetus during childbirth • Is most contagious when sores are open, moist, or leaking, but can be spread when no symptoms are present	• Some people do not show symptoms or only have minor symptoms. • Symptoms may last several weeks and then go away for weeks, months, or years. The initial outbreak has the worst symptoms. • Symptoms typically begin 2–20 days after exposure, but may take years. • Symptoms include a cluster of blistery sores on the vagina, vulva, cervix, penis, buttocks, or anus; a burning feeling if urine flows over sores; inability to urinate if severe swelling blocks the urethra; and itching and pain in the infected area. • During the initial outbreak, symptoms include swollen, tender glands in the pelvic area, throat, and underarms; fever or chills; headache; general rundown feelings; and achy, flulike feelings.	• There is no cure, but certain medications help manage the infection. Treatment is usually very effective in speeding the healing of sores and preventing them from returning frequently. • Warm baths give some pain relief, as do cold compresses or ice packs. • Pain medications such as aspirin, acetaminophen, or ibuprofen may help relieve discomfort and fever. • Partners must stop all sexual activity as soon as they feel warning signs of an outbreak. • A small, daily dose of antiherpes medication (called *suppressive therapy*) can reduce the risk of transmission and the frequency and duration of recurrences. • Other antiherpes medications treat individual outbreaks. • Good diet, adequate rest and sleep, and effective stress management may help prevent herpes recurrences.
Human papillomavirus (HPV)	• Transferred through skin-to-skin contact, usually during vaginal, anal, or oral sex	• Some types of HPV do not cause any noticeable signs or symptoms. • One possible symptom is genital warts. • Some types of HPV cause cell changes that may lead to cervical cancer and other genital and throat cancers.	• There is currently no cure for HPV. • Some HPV infections are harmless, do not require treatment, and go away within 8–13 months. • Colposcopy, cryotherapy, and LEEP procedures may be used to remove abnormal cells from the cervix. • Condoms reduce the risk of transmitting HPV during vaginal or anal intercourse, but are not as effective as against other STIs.

(continued)

Sexually Transmitted Infection (STI)	Cause	Signs and Symptoms	Treatment
Pelvic inflammatory disease (PID)	• Usually caused by bacteria from other STIs such as chlamydia or gonorrhea • Sometimes caused by normal bacteria found in the vagina	• The early stages of PID may not produce noticeable symptoms. • Later stages are characterized by unusually long or painful periods, unusual vaginal discharge, spotting and pain between menstrual periods or during urination, pain in the lower abdomen and back, fever, chills, nausea, vomiting, and pain during vaginal intercourse.	• Infections are treated with antibiotics, bedrest, and lots of fluids. • Surgery may be needed to repair or remove reproductive organs in advanced cases. • Pain medications such as aspirin, acetaminophen, or ibuprofen may help relieve discomfort. • A heating pad on the stomach may reduce discomfort. • Both partners must be treated and remain abstinent until treatment is completed.
Syphilis	• Caused by bacteria (*Treponema pallidum*) introduced through direct contact with a syphilis sore (during unprotected vaginal, anal, or oral sex) • Can be transferred from an infected mother to her unborn baby	• The primary stage is characterized by a single or multiple firm, round, painless sores at the location bacteria entered the body. The sore lasts three to six weeks. • The secondary stage starts with a rough and red, itch-free body rash on the palms or soles of the feet. Other symptoms are mucous membrane lesions, fever, swollen lymph glands, sore throat, muscle aches, and fatigue. • The late stage is characterized by numbness, blindness, difficult coordination, and dementia. The stage may result in death.	• A single dose of penicillin will usually treat syphilis in the first year of infection. • Additional doses may be required for those who have had untreated syphilis for longer than one year.

Glossary

12-hour clock: a method of indicating time that splits the day into two 12-hour periods: the 12 hours from midnight to noon (called *a.m. hours*) and the 12 hours from noon to midnight (called *p.m. hours*); each hour is numbered consecutively and labeled as *a.m.* or *p.m.*

24-hour clock: a method of indicating time that divides the day into 24 hours, from midnight to midnight and numbered from 0 to 24; does not use *a.m.* or *p.m.* designations; also called *military time*.

A

ablation: the surgical removal of body tissue.

abrasion: a scraping of the outer layer of skin.

abscess: an enclosed collection of pus in any part of the body; usually causes swelling and inflammation.

abuse: a deliberate action (physical, verbal, financial, or sexual) that causes harm.

accountable: responsible; able to explain any actions taken.

accreditation: an official recognition that a healthcare facility meets predetermined professional and community standards that promote safety and quality.

acronyms: words formed from the first letters or groups of letters in a phrase.

active listening: the process of showing interest in what a person is saying; includes paying attention, making eye contact, clarifying, and summarizing what a person has said.

activities of daily living (ADLs): actions that people take during a typical day; includes such actions as bathing, walking, eating, dressing, and toileting.

acuity: clearness.

acute care: serious, critical, or surgical care; typically delivered in hospitals.

acute disease: a short-term disease or condition that usually has an abrupt onset.

acute pain: an intense discomfort, often the result of trauma, that goes away within six months with treatment.

addendum: a type of amendment in which an item is added to a health record to correct an error.

advance directives: written legal documents signed by a living, competent person; describe that person's medical and healthcare instructions in the event of incapacitation.

aerobic: needing oxygen to live.

alcohol-based hand sanitizer: a liquid, gel, or foam preparation containing alcohol; kills most bacteria and fungi and destroys some viruses found on the skin.

alimentary canal: a muscular tube of organs that starts in the mouth and leads down to the anus; a part of the gastrointestinal system; also called the *gastrointestinal (GI) tract*.

allergen: any substance that the body perceives as a threat, causing an allergic reaction.

alternative feeding therapy: the practice of delivering food intravenously or through a gastrointestinal tube due to a resident's inability to ingest food through the mouth.

always events: routine activities and processes that are so important they must be performed reliably and consistently; result in effective admissions, transfers, discharges, and handoffs.

Alzheimer's disease (AD): a degenerative brain disease and the most common form of dementia; results in progressive memory loss, impaired thinking, disorientation, and changes in personality and mood; advanced cases lead to decline in cognitive and physical functioning.

ambulating: moving about or walking.

amendments: corrections to a health record.

amniocentesis: a diagnostic procedure in which a small amount of fluid is withdrawn from the amniotic sac to identify genetic abnormalities or determine the sex of a fetus.

anaerobic: able to live without oxygen.

analgesic: a type of pain medication that does not cause loss of consciousness.

anaphylaxis: a severe allergic reaction that can affect the whole body; is characterized by skin reactions, swelling, trouble breathing, rapid pulse, nausea, and dizziness.

anatomy: the study of the body's structure and parts.

anesthetic: a medication that produces a loss of sensation.

aneurysm: a distended and weak area in the wall of an artery supplying blood to the brain.

anger: a strong feeling or emotion that develops from frustration, displeasure, or a threat.

angina: chest pain or discomfort; is characterized by a sensation of squeezing, pressure, heaviness, or tightness in the center of the chest.

ankylosis: the stiffening or immobility of a joint.

antepartum: before labor or childbirth.

antibodies: blood proteins that reduce the effects of bacteria and viruses by identifying and attacking red blood cells marked with antigens.

anticoagulants: medications that prevent the formation of blood clots.

antigens: substances foreign to the body that trigger the production of antibodies as part of the immune response.

antihistamine: a medication that slows or stops the actions of *histamine*, a substance that causes inflammation.

antiseptics: fluids or substances that prevent the growth of microorganisms on the body.

anxiety: a feeling of worry, uneasiness, or nervousness.

aphasia: a condition in which a person cannot understand or use words.

apical pulse: a measurement of heartbeat taken by listening to the apex of the heart (to the left of the sternum slightly under the left breast) with a stethoscope.

apnea: a lack of breathing.

appendicular skeleton: the skeletal structure that enables the body to move; includes bones in the body's appendages (arms and legs).

arrhythmias: abnormal heart rhythms.

arteriosclerosis: a condition in which arteries thicken, harden, and lose elasticity.

asepsis: the absence of infection or infectious material; also called *sterility*.

asphyxia: a lack of oxygen in the body; may be caused when breathing stops due to an obstruction or swelling in the trachea.

aspirate: to inhale a foreign object or substance, such as food or liquid, when eating.

assault: any words or actions that a person finds threatening or that cause a person to fear harm.

assertive: bold and clear.

assessing: examining a situation so it can be evaluated.

asylums: places offering safety and shelter.

atherosclerosis: a condition in which arteries narrow due to plaque buildup.

atony: a lack of sufficient muscular strength.

atrophy: to shrink or decrease in size.

attitudes: ways of thinking or feeling about a person, situation, or object.

auditory: related to the sense of hearing.

aural: relating to the ear or the sense of hearing.

auscultation: the act of listening to the internal sounds of the body with a stethoscope.

automated external defibrillator (AED): a medical device that delivers an electric shock to the heart to stop irregular heart rhythm and allow normal heart rhythm to resume.

autonomic nervous system (ANS): the part of the peripheral nervous system that controls involuntary, unconscious body functions.

autonomy: the personal independence and freedom to determine one's own actions and behavior.

autopsies: examinations conducted to determine cause of death.

axial skeleton: the skeletal structure that provides stability for the body; includes bones in the body's trunk.

axilla: the armpit.

axillary temperature: a measurement of body temperature taken by placing a thermometer under the axilla.

B

bacteria: single-celled, microscopic pathogens that can cause infection.

ballistic: moving under one's own momentum against external forces of gravity and air resistance.

basic life support (BLS): care given to a person experiencing respiratory arrest, cardiac arrest, or airway obstruction; includes giving cardiopulmonary resuscitation (CPR), using an automated external defibrillator (AED), and relieving an obstructed airway.

bath blanket: a blanket, usually made from cotton or another absorbent material, that keeps a resident warm during a bed bath; may also be used as a protective covering to maintain resident modesty and warmth during various procedures.

battery: the act of touching a person without his or her permission.

behavior: a manner of acting; the way a person responds to stimulation.

beliefs: ideas that a person or group of people accepts to be true.

beneficence: the moral obligation to do good.

benign: not cancerous.

bias: an unfair belief that some people, objects, or situations are better than others.

biopsy: the removal of a small piece of tissue from a tumor using a special needle; the sample is tested for cancer cells.

bioterrorism: the use of harmful agents and products with biological origins (including pathogens or toxins) as weapons.

bipolar disorder: a serious mental health condition characterized by changes in mood, energy, and activity levels; a person with bipolar disorder may swing from mania to depression.

bloodborne pathogens: infectious microorganisms in the blood; can cause disease.

body alignment: the optimal placement of all body parts such that bones are in their proper places and muscles are used efficiently.

body cavities: spaces in the human body that contain organs.

body language: gestures, posture, and movements that communicate a person's thoughts and feelings.

body mass index (BMI): a number that uses height and weight to determine whether a person is a healthy weight, overweight, or underweight; is determined by dividing weight in kilograms (kg) by height in meters (m) squared.

body mechanics: actions that promote safe, efficient movement without straining any muscles or joints.

botanicals: plant-based substances.

boundaries: accepted and expected limits on behavior or actions.

bradycardia: an abnormally slow pulse (fewer than 60 beats per minute).

bradypnea: abnormally slow breathing.

bullying: repeated and harmful verbal, physical, social, or psychological behavior toward others.

C

calories: units of energy.

carbohydrates: the body's main source of energy; includes three types: starches, sugars, and fiber.

cardiopulmonary resuscitation (CPR): an emergency procedure in which air is exhaled into a person's mouth or nose to provide ventilation; external chest compressions help oxygenated blood flow to the brain and heart.

care conferences: routinely scheduled meetings that bring together all members of the healthcare staff who deliver care to a particular resident; during the meeting, the resident's plan of care is discussed.

caring: providing assistance and comfort to affect the health and well-being of a resident positively.

carotid pulse: a measurement of heartbeat taken by feeling the carotid artery, which is located on the neck by the trachea below the angle of the jaw.

catheter: a flexible tube that is inserted through a narrow opening into a body cavity.

cell: the smallest and most basic structural and functional unit of the human body.

Celsius (C): a temperature measurement scale in which the freezing point of water is 0° and the boiling point is 100° under normal atmospheric pressure; also called *centigrade*.

census: the number of patients or residents on a nursing unit.

Centers for Disease Control and Prevention (CDC): a US federal agency responsible for preventing and controlling the spread of infectious diseases and responding to health threats; also provides information and research to the healthcare community.

central nervous system (CNS): the part of the nervous system that consists of the brain and spinal cord.

cerebral palsy (CP): a disability that affects movement, muscle tone, and posture; is typically caused by damage to the developing fetal brain.

certification: a credential earned when a person has completed the designated education, training, and testing that prepares him or her for a specific field, discipline, or professional advancement.

certified nursing assistant (CNA): a person who has successfully completed the education and training needed to take and pass the CNA state certification competency examination; scope of practice is regulated by the state, and CNAs are supervised by registered nurses (RNs) or licensed practical/vocational nurses (LPNs/LVNs); in some states, CNAs are called *nurse aides, licensed nursing assistants,* or *registered nursing assistants*.

chain of command: the levels of staff in a facility with regard to authority; from top to bottom, staff members at each level have direct authority over staff members below them.

change-of-shift report: a verbal report that transfers essential information about residents from one shift to the next.

charge nurse: the RN or LPN/LVN who leads a particular nursing unit; is responsible for supervising the staff of that nursing unit.

Cheyne-Stokes respiration: a pattern of breathing that indicates death is near; characterized by hyperpnea (rapid breathing) followed by periods of no breathing (apnea).

chlorophyll: a green substance found in plants; absorbs light and transfers it through the plant during photosynthesis.

chronic care: care given to those who have long-term diseases or illnesses; is given in a variety of healthcare facilities, including doctors' offices, outpatient clinics, rehabilitation centers, or long-term care facilities.

chronic disease: a long-term or recurring disease or condition.

chronic pain: a persistent, uncomfortable feeling that does not go away over time.

circadian rhythm: the physical, mental, and behavioral changes that occur in a person in a roughly 24-hour cycle; influenced primarily by light and darkness in a person's environment.

civil law: a type of law that deals with disagreements between individuals and organizations; money is awarded to the victim for injuries or damages.

clarification: the process of restating what you believe was said to make sure you heard the message correctly.

clinically adverse events: medical errors.

closed-ended question: a question that requires only a one-word answer, such as *yes* or *no*.

cognitive status: the ability to understand, think clearly, and remember.

collaboration: the process by which people work together to resolve conflict in a way that satisfies everyone.

colostrum: a thin, milky fluid discharged from the breasts; contains antibodies that provide passive immunity for the newborn; develops by the end of the third month of pregnancy.

coma: a state of deep and prolonged unconsciousness.

commode: a chair that contains a chamber pot; can be used as a toilet by residents with mobility challenges.

communicable diseases: diseases that can be transmitted from one person, object, or animal to another; also called *contagious diseases* or *infectious diseases*.

communication barriers: any actions, behaviors, or situations that block or interfere with a person's ability to successfully send and receive communication messages.

compassion: the desire to help another person who is suffering or in pain.

competence: possession of the knowledge and skills needed to do something well.

complementary and alternative medicine (CAM): treatments that are performed in addition to conventional medicine or that are entirely separate and serve as replacements for conventional medicine.

compresses: pads of material; can be warm, cold, dry, or moist.

compromise: the process by which two sides of a conflict make concessions to find the best resolution.

concentration: complete attention directed toward a particular object or task.

condition: a state of poor physical or mental health.

confidentiality: the act of keeping personal information that has been shared with the healthcare staff private.

conflict: a disagreement between two or more people.

congruent communication: a type of communication in which the sender's words, facial expressions, and body language all send the same message.

connective tissue: a type of body tissue that connects or supports other body tissues, structures, and organs; is composed of collagen fibers that provide strength and elastic fibers that enable flexibility.

conscious: aware of feelings, actions, and outside surroundings.

constipation: a condition in which bowel movements occur fewer than three times a week and contain hard, dry stools that are difficult to evacuate; can be an acute or chronic condition.

consultations: meetings with a healthcare expert; the expert gives advice or information.

contaminated: soiled or dirty as a result of contact or mixture with something that is not clean.

continuity: an uninterrupted connection or sequence of events.

contracture: the tightening or shortening of a body part (such as a muscle, a tendon, or the skin) due to lack of movement.

contraindicate: to advise against or point out the possible dangers of a particular medication or treatment.

contusions: bruises caused by damaged or broken blood vessels; may cause swelling.

conventional medicine: treatments performed by medical doctors, nurses, and other healthcare providers who use evidence-based scientific data to diagnose and treat diseases; also called *Western medicine* or *allopathic medicine*.

co-payment: a fixed fee for specific medical services covered partially by health insurance; the patient is required to pay this fee.

coronal plane: a body plane that divides the body into front and back halves; also called the *frontal plane*.

coroner: a government official who can certify death and order an autopsy.

cover message: a formal, written introduction that outlines a person's capabilities and skills to a prospective employer.

covert: not shown openly; concealed.

cramming: studying large amounts of information in a short period of time.

cremation: a process in which a deceased person's body is subjected to extreme heat (1800–2000°F) for two or more hours, yielding 3–9 pounds of ashes.

criminal law: a type of law that punishes criminal offenses; includes imposing a fine or a prison sentence to keep offenders and others from acting unlawfully again.

critical observation: the appropriate use of both objective and subjective observation.

cross-cultural communication: the use of practices and approaches that promote and improve relationships between people from different cultures.

cryotherapy: the use of cold applications to reduce swelling and ease pain.

crypt: a vault or chamber used for burial.

cues: actions that invite a response; may be verbal or manual and can guide resident behavior.

cultural humility: awareness and understanding of one's own culture, as well as the cultures of others; includes knowledge of personal limitations, barriers, and gaps in knowledge and provides the openness needed to be sensitive to and respectful of other cultures.

culture: (1) a set of traditions, beliefs, rituals, customs, and values that are learned over time and are specific to a group of people; (2) the process of cultivating living tissue cells in a substance favorable to their growth.

culture of safety: the shared commitment of a healthcare facility's leadership and staff to ensure a safe work environment.

customs: established practices and beliefs that are followed by a group of people over multiple generations.

cyanotic: discolored and bluish due to insufficient oxygen.

cyberattacks: illegal attempts to gain access to a digital device or network to cause harm.

cystic fibrosis (CF): a genetic disorder that changes how the body makes mucus and sweat; is characterized by congestion, difficult digestion, and salty sweat.

D

decubitus ulcer: a skin condition caused when continuous pressure on the skin and on bony areas restricts blood flow and creates a sore; also called a *bedsore* or *pressure ulcer*.

deductible: the amount of money that a health insurer, program, or employer requires people to pay out of pocket as their share of the cost for health insurance coverage.

deduction: the use of specific assumptions to reach a conclusion.

defamation of character: false statements made about a person that damage his or her reputation.

defecate: to have a bowel movement.

defense mechanisms: unconscious behaviors that enable people to ignore or forget situations or thoughts that cause fear, anxiety, and stress.

deformity: the distortion of a body part.

dehydration: a lack of adequate fluids in the body tissues.

delegate: to transfer duties to another competent person; the person who delegates the responsibility is still accountable for the proper completion of the tasks involved.

delusions: irrational beliefs that something is true, even when there is overwhelming proof that it is not.

dementia: a progressive, permanent, severe loss of mental capacity that interferes with a person's ability to lead a normal life.

deoxyribonucleic acid (DNA): a chemical compound that contains instructions for developing and directing the growth and activities of living organisms.

dermis: the inner, thick layer of the skin; contains sensory nerve receptors, hair and nail follicles, and sweat and sebaceous glands.

diabetes mellitus: a disorder in which there are excessive amounts of glucose (sugar) in a person's blood due to insufficient production of insulin (the hormone that regulates glucose) or insulin resistance; commonly referred to as *diabetes*.

dialysis: the process of removing waste products and excess fluid from the body.

diarrhea: a condition in which bowel movements have stools with excess water and occur frequently; can be an acute or chronic condition.

diastolic blood pressure: the pressure of blood against the arteries when the heart muscle relaxes.

dietary fats: lipids; provide energy for and insulate the body; include saturated fat, *trans* fat, and unsaturated fat.

dignity: value or worth.

dilemma: a choice between two difficult options; options may be desirable or undesirable.

discharge plan: a set of instructions given to the patient at the time of discharge; may include the doctor's instructions about activity level, medications, continued treatment, important changes in condition, and follow-up appointments with the doctor.

disease: a condition in which an organ or body system functions incorrectly and exhibits particular signs and symptoms.

disinfectants: chemicals used to destroy or slow the growth of microorganisms to prevent them from spreading.

disposable protective pad: a pad that is small, often multilayered, leakproof, and highly absorbent; can be placed under the buttocks of incontinent residents, used to absorb drainage, or used during procedures to prevent the bed from becoming soiled; also called an *incontinence pad*.

distress: bad stress; causes bodily symptoms that can lead to disease and poor coping and decision making.

diversity: the presence of differences among people.

do-not-resuscitate (DNR) order: a medical and legal request that lifesaving measures such as CPR not be administered if a person's heart or breathing stops.

dormant: having slowed or stopped functions.

double pendulum: the action of ambulation; the leg swings forward from the hip, and the heel touches and rolls forward to the toe.

draw sheet: a small, flat sheet or a regular-size flat sheet folded in half and placed lengthwise over the middle of the bottom sheet of the bed; is used to help turn a resident in bed; also called a *pull sheet*, *turning sheet*, or *lift sheet*.

dressing: a protective material placed on a wound; also called a *bandage*.

ducts: tubes for conveying substances in the body.

dysphagia: difficulty or discomfort when swallowing.

dyspnea: difficult breathing or shortness of breath.

dysrhythmia: an irregular or abnormal heart rhythm.

E

eating disorder: an abnormal pattern of eating that leads to serious and often fatal medical consequences.

ectopic pregnancy: a condition in which a fertilized ovum implants outside the uterus in the fallopian tube, abdominal cavity, ovary, or cervix.

edema: the retention of fluid in body tissues.

elder abuse: a deliberate action (physical, verbal, financial, or sexual) that causes harm to a senior.

electrolytes: substances in the blood and body fluids that carry electrical charges when dissolved in water.

electronic health record (EHR): an electronic record that includes information about a resident's entire medical history and all healthcare experiences.

electronic medical record (EMR): a component of an EHR that includes administrative and clinical information about a single stay in a healthcare facility.

embolus: a mass (most commonly a blood clot) that travels through the blood and can become lodged in a blood vessel and obstruct blood flow.

embryo: the fertilized ovum from implantation to the end of the eighth week of pregnancy.

emesis basin: a small, kidney-shaped bowl often used for oral care or if the resident needs to vomit.

empathy: understanding for another person's feelings and emotions.

empower: to give a person the power to control his or her own destiny and decision making.

endocrine glands: ductless glands that secrete hormones directly into the bloodstream.

enema: a procedure in which liquid is inserted into the rectum to clean the lower intestine.

energy: the power and drive to make decisions and complete tasks.

energy rhythm: the sequence of energy peaks a person experiences over a certain time period.

engagement: the practice of being fully involved and committed to the task at hand.

enteral: by way of the gastrointestinal system.

entrapment: a harmful event in which a resident falls between the bed and side rails.

enzymes: chemical agents that can cause specific biochemical reactions.

epidemic: an outbreak of an infectious disease that spreads quickly and makes many people sick.

epidermis: the outermost layer of the skin; contains keratin and melanin.

ethics: principles that guide behavior with respect to what is right and wrong.

ethnicity: identification with common social, cultural, and traditional practices that are shared within a group.

ethnocentrism: an outlook in which one judges another culture based on the beliefs and standards of one's own culture.

eustress: good stress; helps people become motivated and productive.

evacuation: the intentional removal of people or objects from a dangerous area.

evidence-based practice: the process of locating and using research findings to guide decisions made about care delivery.

excretions: waste products expelled from the body.

exocrine glands: glands with ducts that transport substances to other organs or to the surface of the skin.

exudate: a liquid or semisolid discharge from body tissues or a blood vessel; drains from a wound and is caused by tissue damage.

F

Fahrenheit (F): a temperature measurement scale in which the freezing point of water is 32° and the boiling point is 212° under normal atmospheric pressure.

false imprisonment: illegal confinement in which a person is held against his or her will by another, resulting in restraint of movement; the person can be confined using force or threats.

fatigue: a feeling of extreme tiredness or exhaustion.

fear: an unpleasant feeling or emotion resulting from the threat or presence of danger.

fetus: the fertilized ovum from the ninth week of pregnancy until birth.

fibrillation: an irregular heart rhythm.

fibrous: composed of tough, thin threads.

fidelity: the quality of being faithful and not abandoning those who need care.

fire triangle: the three elements—fuel, oxygen, and heat—needed to start a fire.

fistula: an abnormal and permanent opening between an organ and the exterior of the body.

flares: sudden intensifications or escalations of a disease.

flash cards: a set of cards used for studying; cards typically have a question on one side and an answer on the other.

flatus: gas or air in the gastrointestinal tract; is expelled via the anus.

flow meter: a medical device used to make sure a resident receives the prescribed amount of oxygen.

follicles: small sacs or cavities.

foot drop: a condition of paralysis or weakness in the dorsiflexion muscles of the foot and ankle; results in the dragging of the foot and toes.

forensic: related to the methods used for investigating and solving crimes.

formed elements: the solid component of blood; consists of red blood cells, platelets, and white blood cells.

Fowler's position: a body position in which a patient lies with legs extended on an examining table or bed; the head of the bed is raised to a 45° angle.

friction: the resistance between two objects or surfaces rubbing against each other.

frostbite: a condition in which extremely cold temperatures cause freezing and damage to body tissues, such as the skin on the fingers, toes, nose, ears, cheeks, and chin.

G

gait: a manner of walking.

gait belt: a belt worn around a resident's waist that serves as a safety device when a resident stands and ambulates; also called a *transfer belt* when used for moving a resident.

gangrene: a condition characterized by the death and decay of body tissue due to lack of blood supply.

generation: a group of people who are born and who live during the same time.

generation gap: a lack of communication between one generation and another; is often due to differences in customs, attitudes, and beliefs.

genuine: honest, open, and sincere in communication and relationships.

giving of self: the quality of putting a resident's health and wellness needs before one's own needs as a caregiver.

gland: a group of specialized cells that secrete substances.

glucometer: a medical device that measures blood sugar levels.

graduate: a container used to measure intake and output.

grand mal seizure: a generalized seizure in which a person may experience loss of consciousness and violent muscle contractions; is caused by abnormal electrical activity in the brain.

grief: an emotional response to or distress about a physical or personal loss.

guaiac test: a diagnostic procedure used to detect fecal occult blood.

gurney: a flat, padded table with wheels; also called a *stretcher*.

H

hallucinations: visual, verbal, or physical perceptions of objects that are not real, but are mistaken for reality.

Hands-Only™ CPR: an emergency procedure in which uninterrupted chest compressions restore heartbeat and promote blood circulation; is a procedure for those not trained in conventional CPR.

harm: unintended physical injury that requires additional monitoring, treatment, or hospitalization; may result in death.

health: the condition of a person's physical, mental, social, and spiritual self.

healthcare: the prevention, diagnosis, and treatment of diseases; the management of acute and chronic illnesses; and the promotion of wellness.

healthcare facility: a building in which healthcare is delivered.

healthcare services: screening, diagnostic, and evaluation activities that assist and support the restoration, maintenance, or improvement of health.

health literacy: a person's ability to understand fully and use information about health, diseases, conditions, or treatments.

health promotion: the process of making efforts to help people improve or increase control over their health and wellness.

Heimlich maneuver: an emergency procedure in which a person places his or her fist just above the navel of a choking person, covers his or her fist with the other hand, and performs abdominal thrusts inward and upward.

hemiplegia: a condition of paralysis on one side of the body.

hemoglobin: the component of a red blood cell that allows the cell to transport oxygen and that gives the cell its red color.

hemophilia: a blood disorder caused by changes in a gene on the X chromosome; is characterized by the inability of the blood to clot.

hemorrhage: the excessive loss of blood over a short period of time due to internal or external injury.

hemorrhoids: swollen, inflamed veins found under the skin around the anus (external) or inside the rectum (internal); are caused by pressure from straining during bowel movements or labor in childbirth; may be itchy or painful at times and can cause rectal bleeding.

herbals: substances containing herbs.

hernia: a protrusion or bulge of an organ through the wall of the body cavity or structure that contains it.

holistic care: care that is sensitive to a person's values and desires and that integrates a person's physical (body), emotional (mind), and spiritual (spirit) needs to help achieve the highest level of well-being possible.

homeostasis: the constant or stable state of the human body and its complex body systems; allows self-healing of the body.

hormones: chemical substances that are produced in the body and that control and regulate specific body processes.

hospice: a healthcare facility or service that provides supportive care for those who are terminally ill and their families; is available on-site at healthcare facilities or in private homes.

humility: modesty; the quality of not putting one's self first.

hydrated: having sufficient fluids in the body tissues over a 24-hour period.

hydration: a sufficient amount of fluid in the body tissues.

hydrocephalus: a condition of fluid in the brain.

hygiene: routine actions such as bathing that promote and maintain cleanliness and health.

hypertension: a condition of high blood pressure.

hyperventilation: deep, rapid breathing.

hypotension: low blood pressure.

hypothermia: a condition of abnormally low body temperature.

hypoventilation: slow, shallow breathing.

hypovolemic shock: a life-threatening condition resulting from the loss of 15 to 30 percent of circulating blood volume.

hypoxia: a lack of adequate oxygen supply in the body.

I

ideal body weight (IBW): the healthiest weight for an individual; is determined primarily by height, but also takes gender, age, build, and muscular development into account using adjusted statistical tables.

illness: a feeling of poor health; is not always caused by a disease.

immobility: an inability to move on one's own.

immunization: a method of providing protection against diseases such as influenza, pneumonia, measles, tetanus, and polio; a weakened or killed antigen is introduced to prompt the body to develop antibodies specific to that antigen; usually given by injection.

impaction: a blockage of hard stool in the rectum.

incapacitation: the lack of ability to make decisions.

incident report: a document that records information about an unusual event, such as a resident injury; also called an *accident report* or *occurrence report*.

incontinence: a lack of bowel or bladder control.

infection: the invasion and growth of harmful pathogens in the body; leads to disease.

infection control: policies and procedures used to minimize the risk of diseases and infections spreading.

infertility: a continued inability to reproduce after trying to conceive for one year or experiencing repeated miscarriages.

inflammation: the protective response of body tissue to irritation, injury, or infection; is characterized by swelling and redness.

informed consent: the legal process of securing written permission prior to giving care or conducting procedures.

inspection: the visual examination of a body part.

integrative medicine (IM): treatments that take a coordinated approach to the diagnosis, treatment, and prevention of diseases; IM providers see people as whole individuals and focus on the energy of the body; formerly known as *complementary and alternative medicine (CAM)*.

integrity: strong moral principles and professional standards.

international units (IUs): units of measurement based on international standards; one IU results in a specific biological effect.

interpersonal relationships: relationships between two or more people who share similar interests or goals; meet physical and emotional needs.

interpreter: a person who translates written or spoken words into another language.

intimate relationships: relationships between two people who have romantic feelings of love for each other.

intoxication: a condition of reduced control caused by the overuse of a chemical substance.

intraoperative: during surgery, up until the patient's arrival in the recovery room.

intrapartum: during labor and delivery.

intuition: a feeling that is not based on facts or evidence, but that guides actions.

intuitive: perceptive about a situation; having insight.

ischemia: an insufficient supply of blood to a tissue or organ.

isolation: specific preventive measures that limit or eliminate the spread of pathogens from an infected person to others.

J

jargon: words, phrases, and language used by a specific group of people or culture.

job campaign: a series of organized activities needed to find a desired job.

job description: a written document that describes the duties, responsibilities, and qualifications required for a particular position.

joints: locations where two or more bones connect.

journal: a written record of observations and experiences.

K

kinship: a feeling of being close or of having an association or connection.

L

labeling: describing someone using a specific word or phrase.

lacerations: wounds that tear body tissue and result in ragged edges.

laparoscopic surgery: a minimally invasive surgical technique in which an operation is performed through a small incision in the body; uses a *laparoscope* (a telescopic rod lens system connected to a video camera or digital camera).

laryngeal mirror: a medical instrument used to examine the mouth, tongue, and teeth.

lateral position: a body position in which a patient lies on his or her side with arms free and knees slightly bent.

legal blindness: a refractive error of 20/200, even after vision correction.

legumes: plants with pods (long cases) that contain edible seeds.

lesions: abnormal spots or areas of damaged body tissue.

level of care: the type of care needed for a particular patient or resident; is typically higher for a patient with a serious illness and lower for a resident who needs assistance only with ADLs.

liability: legal responsibility.

libel: false written statements made about a person that damage his or her reputation; a type of defamation of character.

licensed nursing staff: nursing staff members who have passed state licensing examinations that allow them to perform healthcare tasks within their scope of practice; RNs and LPNs/LVNs.

licensed practical/vocational nurse (LPN/LVN): a person who has successfully completed the education and training needed to take and pass an LPN/LVN state licensing examination; scope of practice is regulated by the state, and LPNs/LVNs provide care under the supervision of an RN; care can include monitoring and reporting, preparing and giving medications, inserting catheters, and performing wound care.

licensure: recognition that a person or facility has permission to deliver care; is based on meeting standards set by law.

ligaments: fibrous cords of tissue that attach bone to bone and support organs.

living will: an advance directive that details the life-prolonging treatments a person desires in the event of incapacitation during a terminal illness or permanent unconsciousness.

lochia: a vaginal discharge composed of blood, mucus, and uterine tissue.

lubricants: natural substances that reduce friction between surfaces.

M

malabsorption: the reduced ability of the intestine to take in essential nutrients and fluids and transfer them to the bloodstream.

malignant: cancerous.

malnutrition: lack of proper nourishment due to inadequate or unbalanced intake of vitamins, minerals, and other nutrients or due to the body's inability to use nutrients.

malpractice: a form of negligence in which a caregiver in a healthcare discipline does not comply with the standards set by his or her discipline's regulatory body, resulting in injury.

managed care: a form of insurance in which there are contracts with specific healthcare providers who will deliver care at a reduced cost.

manually: by hand.

mausoleum: a freestanding building in which a deceased person is buried.

Medicaid: a US law passed in 1965 that provides a combination of federal and state financing to offer healthcare at the state level for those with low incomes; participants must meet certain income requirements to qualify.

medical terminology: medical terms related to body systems, diseases, diagnostic procedures, and treatments; the language used in healthcare.

Medicare: a US law passed in 1965 that supplies federal funds to deliver healthcare to people who are 65 years of age or older, who are under 65 years and have disabilities, or who have end-stage renal disease.

meditation: the practice of emptying the mind of thoughts, feelings, and emotions to reach a state of relaxation through concentration.

membranes: thin, soft, flexible structures that cover, line, or act as boundaries for cells or organs.

memory: the storage and remembrance of past experiences.

meniscus: a cartilage pad that creates a smooth surface for a joint such as the knee to move.

metabolism: the chemical process by which nutrients are converted into energy in the body.

metastasis: the spread of cancer cells to other locations in the body.

microorganisms: living things, or *organisms*, that are so small they can only be seen through a microscope.

mindfulness: the practice of being aware and mentally present in every situation by focusing on what is being said, what is being done, or what is happening in the environment; requires a nonjudgmental attitude.

minerals: inorganic substances in the body that regulate and assist in metabolism.

miscarriage: the spontaneous loss of a fetus before the twentieth week of pregnancy.

monotone: flat-sounding with no change in pitch.

morbidity: the number of people who have a disease.

moribund: about to die.

mortality: the number of deaths due to a disease.

motility: movement; in the gastrointestinal system, the contraction of muscles that moves substances through the gastrointestinal tract.

motivation: a person's prompting to act in a particular way; results from an emotional response to a stimulus or a conscious decision that directs behavior.

mourn: to express feelings and behaviors that signify grief.

mucus: a thick, slippery fluid that moistens and protects parts of the body.

N

nasal cannula: a narrow, flexible, plastic tube used to deliver oxygen through the nostrils using nasal breathing.

natal: relating to birth.

near misses: unplanned health outcomes that do not cause harm, even though they have the potential to; considered *close calls*.

necrosis: the death of body tissue.

needlesticks: puncture wounds caused by needles.

neglect: the failure to provide necessary care that meets a resident's daily needs.

negligence: the unintentional failure to act or provide care that a reasonably prudent or sensible person would; can result in injury.

network: to communicate with an informal, interconnected group of people.

neural tube: the prenatal structure from which the nervous system develops; consists of the brain and spinal cord.

neurons: cells of the nervous system that transmit information throughout the body in the form of electrochemical messages (neural impulses); each neuron is composed of a cell body, dendrites, and axons.

never events: actions or errors that result in harm, death, or significant disability; are usually preventable.

nodules: small, round, or knotlike collections of body tissue; can be felt by touch.

noncommunicable diseases: diseases that are not contagious and cannot be transmitted between people, objects, and animals.

nonmaleficence: the moral obligation to avoid harm.

nonpenetrating wounds: wounds that do not enter into or through the skin; are caused by rubbing or friction on the surface of the skin.

nonpharmacological: without the use of medication.

nonverbal communication: the use of gestures, facial expressions, tone of voice, or body movements to convey a message.

numbness: an inability to feel sensations due to changes in nerve function.

nursing diagnosis: the identification of a health problem or the cause of a health problem; does not identify a specific disease.

nursing orders: instructions outlining the actions that should be taken to achieve stated goals of care; are written by the RN.

nursing process: a method of problem solving that includes assessing, identifying, and organizing nursing knowledge, judgments, and actions to provide safe, quality care.

nursing unit: an area in a healthcare facility in which care is delivered; is typically designated by a floor name, area, or type of illness (as in an *Alzheimer's* or *surgical unit*).

nutrients: substances the body needs to function normally; include water, protein, carbohydrates, fats, minerals, and vitamins.

nutrition: the ingestion of foods that provide nutrients to maintain the health of the body.

O

obesity: a health condition characterized by a body weight much greater than what is considered healthy for a certain height.

objective observations: descriptions based on the facts about a situation.

occult blood: the presence of very small amounts of blood in the stool.

open-ended question: a question that requires more than a one-word answer.

ophthalmoscope: a medical instrument used to examine the eyes.

organs: collections of tissues that have specific structures and functions.

orientation: introduction and training given to new employees; addresses a facility's mission, structure, policies, and procedures.

orthostatic hypotension: a condition in which blood pressure falls when a person stands.

orthotic: a device that supports, aligns, or corrects a weakened, immobile, injured, or deformed part of the body.

osteoporosis: a condition of porous bones; characterized by low bone density.

ostomy: a surgical procedure that creates an opening in the abdominal wall so that stool can be eliminated from the intestines to the outside of the body.

otoscope: a medical instrument used to examine the ears.

overt: open to view; easy to observe.

ovulation: the process by which a mature ovum is released from an ovary.

P

pain scales: devices used to measure the perception of the severity of pain.

palliative care: care that provides relief from the symptoms of a disease or condition; does not aim to cure the disease or condition.

pallor: an unusually pale color of the skin.

palpation: the act of using the hands to examine the body.

paralysis: the loss of function and feeling in one or more muscle groups.

paranoia: an unsupported or exaggerated distrust of others.

parasympathetic nervous system (PNS): a component of the autonomic nervous system; controls the automatic daily functions of the cardiovascular, respiratory, and gastrointestinal systems and helps the body return to a homeostatic state after experiencing pain or stress.

parenteral: by way of the veins or intravenous infusion.

patent: open.

pathogens: disease-causing microorganisms.

pathologist: a doctor who specializes in studying diseases; conducts autopsies to determine causes of death.

pathology: a collection of changes to the body's tissues or organs; can trigger a disease or can be caused by a disease.

patients: people who visit a healthcare facility, such as a hospital, for a physical examination or for the treatment of an illness or disease.

payroll: the amount of money an organization pays its staff.

penetrating wounds: wounds that enter into or through the skin.

perception: the ability to notice or recognize something using the senses (sight, hearing, or touch).

percussion: the act of placing one hand on the surface of the body and striking or tapping a finger on that hand with the index finger or middle finger of the other hand.

perineal care: hygiene care that involves cleansing the area between the thighs (the coccyx, pubis, anus, urethra, and external genitals).

perineum: the area between the thighs; includes the coccyx, pubis, anus, urethra, and external genitals.

perioperative: relating to the three phases of surgery (preoperative, intraoperative, and postoperative).

peripheral nervous system (PNS): the part of the nervous system that consists of 12 pairs of cranial nerves and 31 pairs of spinal nerves.

peristalsis: the involuntary, wavelike constriction and relaxation of smooth muscles; moves contents through the gastrointestinal system.

personal protective equipment (PPE): specialized clothing and accessories, such as gloves, gowns, masks, goggles, and other pieces of equipment, that are worn to protect against infection or injury.

petit mal seizure: a generalized seizure in which a person has impaired awareness and responsiveness and may lose consciousness; is caused by abnormal electrical activity in the brain.

phagocytosis: the process by which a white blood cell engulfs and destroys foreign antigens.

phenol: an acid that can be used as a disinfectant in dilute form.

philosophy: fundamental beliefs and values.

phobias: unsupported, exaggerated fears that sometimes interfere with daily life.

photosynthesis: the process by which plants and other organisms convert light energy from the sun into chemical energy; allows plants and other organisms to function.

physiology: the study of how the body functions.

placenta: a temporary, disk-shaped organ that develops and attaches to the uterus during pregnancy; transfers oxygen and nutrients from the woman to the fetus via the umbilical cord.

placental abruption: a condition in which the placenta separates from the uterine wall before delivery; results in a lack of oxygen and nutrients for the fetus and severe bleeding for the mother.

placenta previa: a condition in which the placenta covers part of or the entire opening of the cervix; can cause the mother to have severe vaginal bleeding or hemorrhage.

plan of care: a written plan that provides directions and serves as a guide to delivering individualized, holistic care; also called a *service plan*.

plaques: superficial, solid, elevated lesions.

plasma: the liquid component of blood; is composed of water, hormones, protein, sugar, and waste products.

platelets: flat, circular cells in the blood that assist in the clotting process.

podiatrist: a doctor who specializes in diagnosing and treating diseases and conditions that affect the feet.

point-of-care testing (POCT): specimen collection at the place in which a resident is receiving care.

polyp: a growth or mass bulging from a mucous membrane.

positive regard: an attitude that is supportive and accepting of others.

postmortem care: care performed shortly after death; prepares the body for burial or cremation, puts the body in alignment, and prevents skin damage.

postoperative: after surgery, until the patient has completely recovered from the surgery.

postpartum: after childbirth.

post-traumatic stress disorder (PTSD): a stress-related mental health condition that develops after a person experiences or witnesses a traumatic or stressful event.

posture: the way in which a person holds his or her body; the manner in which the body remains upright against gravity when sitting down, lying down, or standing up.

power of attorney: an advance directive that gives a designated person the authority to make healthcare decisions on behalf of another person; authority only takes effect if the person who writes the power of attorney becomes unable to make his or her own decisions; also called a *healthcare proxy* or *durable power of attorney for healthcare*.

predisposition: a tendency to suffer from a particular condition.

preeclampsia: a condition characterized by high blood pressure and signs of organ damage during pregnancy; usually occurs after 20 weeks.

prejudice: an opinion or feeling that is formed without facts and that often leads to unfair feelings of dislike for a person or group because of race, sex, or religion.

premium: the amount of money paid, usually on a schedule, to an insurance company for a specific insurance policy.

preoperative: before surgery, from the decision to have surgery until the surgery begins.

primary care provider (PCP): a doctor, nurse practitioner, or physician assistant whose legal scope of practice allows him or her to be the first contact for a person's healthcare needs; is responsible for monitoring a person's overall healthcare needs and coordinates care across healthcare services when necessary.

priorities: items or actions that are ranked as having high importance.

prioritizing: organizing responsibilities or tasks so that the most important tasks are completed first.

private insurance: a plan for the payment of healthcare services; may be purchased by an employer on the employee's behalf or by an individual.

probe: a long, thin, medical instrument used to measure temperature.

probiotics: oral dietary supplements that contain live bacteria; restore beneficial bacteria to the body.

procrastination: the act of purposely postponing a task.

professional: demonstrating an expected level of excellence and competence.

prognosis: a projection of the likely course and outcome of a disease and the potential for recovery.

prolapse: a condition in which an organ or body part sinks or falls out of place.

prone position: a body position in which a patient lies on his or her abdomen with arms and hands at each side, feet comfortably positioned, and head turned to the side.

prosthetic: an artificial device designed to replace a missing body part.

proteins: strings of amino acids that are vital to cell structure, contribute to energy production, build body tissue, and promote growth and repair; eight are acquired through diet.

pulse: the beat of the heart measured through the walls of a peripheral artery.

pulse oximeter: a medical device, usually applied to a fingertip, that indirectly measures the amount of oxygen in the blood; oxygen content is recorded as a percentage.

R

race: a set of inherited physical characteristics, such as skin, eye, and hair color.

RACE: an acronym for the process of responding to a fire; stands for *rescue*, *activate alarm*, *confine the fire*, and *extinguish*.

racism: intolerance, discrimination, or prejudice based on race.

radial pulse: a measurement of heartbeat taken by feeling the radial artery, which is located on the inside of the thumb side of the wrist.

range of motion (ROM): the amount that a person can move a joint voluntarily.

rapport: mutual understanding in a relationship.

ratio: the number of patients or residents in a healthcare facility or unit assigned to each member of the healthcare staff.

rational: having the ability to think clearly and make decisions based on facts.

rationale: the research- and science-based reasoning behind a specific nursing action.

receptors: sensory nerve endings on or within a cell that react to various stimuli and produce an effect.

Recommended Dietary Allowances (RDAs): daily levels of nutritional intake needed to maintain good health.

red blood cells: the components of the blood that contain hemoglobin; are responsible for oxygen and carbon dioxide exchange; also called *erythrocytes*.

registered nurse (RN): a person who has successfully completed the education and training needed to take and pass an RN state licensing examination; delivers nursing care, assesses residents, and provides nursing diagnoses; also plans, implements, and evaluates care.

regulation: in healthcare, a rule or requirement that healthcare facilities and staff members must follow; is usually enforced by an authority, such as the federal or state government.

rehabilitation: a period of recovery in which healthcare staff members help patients regain their strength and mobility with the goal of learning to function independently.

reservoir: a place in which fluid can collect.

residents: people staying in a long-term care facility due to age, illness, or inability to care for themselves at home.

respect: a feeling of appreciation and admiration for another person.

restorative care: care that assists with any modifications and adjustments residents must make to live as independently as possible.

restraint: any physical equipment or chemical substance that prevents a resident from moving freely.

résumé: a formal, written representation of a person's experience, skills, and credentials.

retinal detachment: the separation of the retina from the back of the eye; is a medical emergency.

rigor mortis: the stiffening of the body's muscles several hours after death.

rituals: actions that are always done in the same way, often for religious purposes or as part of a ceremony.

rounds: opportunities to monitor and discuss the status of a resident's condition or disease; are conducted inside or right outside the resident's room.

rule of nines: a method of calculating the surface area of the body affected by burns.

S

safety data sheet (SDS): a document found in the facility safety plan; contains information about the potential hazards of a chemical product and use, storage, handling, and emergency procedures; also called a *material safety data sheet (MSDS)*.

sagittal plane: a body plane that divides the body into left and right sides; also called the *vertical plane*.

saliva: a watery mixture found in the mouth that contains enzymes, lubricates the mouth, and breaks down food.

schizophrenia spectrum disorder: a severe and chronic mental health condition in which a person experiences a loss of reality; has delusions, hallucinations, and thought disorders; and displays agitated body movements.

sclerosis: the thickening or hardening of a body part.

scoliosis: a condition in which the spine is curved sideways.

scope of practice: the specific responsibilities, procedures, and actions of a healthcare provider, as permitted by state regulations; actions within the scope of practice are allowed only when special educational requirements have been met and when knowledge and skill competency are demonstrated.

secretion: the release of chemical substances, such as mucus or saliva, that are manufactured by cells.

secretions: substances produced and released by cells or organs.

sedentary: inactive.

seizures: sudden changes in the brain's normal electrical activity; cause an altered or loss of consciousness.

self-actualization: a state in which someone has become everything he or she hopes to be; the fulfillment of a person's potential.

self-determination: the process of making choices and decisions based on one's own preferences and interests.

self-esteem: a person's confidence and regard for himself or herself.

self-harm: the act of hurting one's self on purpose.

self-image: the way a person thinks about his or her self, abilities, and appearance.

self-reflection: the practice of looking at one's self in an honest and truthful way and being open to any changes that may be needed.

self-respect: a person's appreciation and acceptance of himself or herself.

sharps: objects such as needles, razors, broken glass, and scalpels that can penetrate the skin.

shift: a period of time that a staff member works; is usually described as a *day*, *evening*, or *night shift*; typically lasts 8, 10, or 12 hours.

shock: a condition in which the organs and tissues of the body do not have sufficient oxygen.

sign: a piece of objective or factual information about a disease or condition.

sitz bath: a type of therapeutic bath that soaks a person's perineum, buttocks, and sometimes hips in warm water.

skin integrity: the condition of the skin; healthy skin is whole or intact without irritation, inflammation, or damage.

slander: false spoken statements made about a person that damage his or her reputation; a type of defamation of character.

sleep deprivation: a loss or deficiency of the recommended hours of sleep.

Social Security: a US law established in 1935 that provides retirement benefits, disability coverage, dependent coverage, and survivor benefits; is funded by mandatory payments by employers and employees.

software applications: software programs with different uses; also called *apps*.

somatic nervous system: the part of the peripheral nervous system that controls voluntary body functions and the movement of skeletal muscle.

specimens: samples of a bodily substance.

speculum: a medical instrument used to examine the vagina or other body cavities.

sperm: the male reproductive cell; fertilizes the ovum during reproduction.

sphincter: a circular muscle that can open or close; found in the heart and gastrointestinal system.

sphygmomanometer: a medical device used to measure blood pressure; includes a cuff that wraps around a person's upper arm and a measuring device.

spina bifida (SB): a congenital disorder resulting in incomplete development of the spinal cord.

sputum: a blend of saliva and mucus; also called *phlegm*.

staffing: the process of determining the numbers and types of healthcare staff needed to take care of a group of patients or residents on a nursing unit.

staffing plan: a formal document that outlines the mix and types of healthcare staff members who will work on each shift in the nursing unit; changes are based on the needs of the facility and the care requirements of particular patients or residents.

standards of care: reasonable and sensible processes or actions healthcare providers follow when addressing certain medical conditions.

stem cell: a human cell capable of renewing, dividing, and changing to become a specific tissue or organ cell.

stereotypes: simplifications or biases about a group that shape the treatment of all group members.

sterile: free of living microorganisms.

sterile field: an area that is free from living pathogenic microorganisms.

stertorous breathing: a type of breathing that sounds like snoring.

stethoscope: a medical device used to listen to body sounds such as breathing, heartbeat, and lung and bowel sounds; has two earpieces connected by flexible tubing and a diaphragm at the end.

stigma: a negative perception that causes others to think less of an idea or person.

stillbirth: the death of a fetus after 20 weeks of pregnancy.

stoic: detached from emotion or feeling.

stoma: a surgically created abdominal opening, through which stool are eliminated.

stress: a physical or psychological response to a situation that causes worry or tension.

stress management: the process of taking actions to lessen or remove reactions to stress and stressful events.

stroke: a sudden blockage or rupture of a blood vessel in the brain; can cause a loss of consciousness, partial loss of movement, and speech impairment; also called a *cerebrovascular accident (CVA)*.

subacute care: care provided to a person who has a moderate-to-severe illness, injury, or recurrence of a disease, but who does not require acute care in a hospital.

subconscious: not fully aware of feelings, actions, and outside surroundings.

subjective observations: descriptions based on feelings or opinions about a situation.

suicide: the intentional self-infliction of fatal injuries.

supine position: a body position in which a patient lies flat on his or her back with the arms at each side.

suppositories: small, meltable, solid cones or cylinders that may be medicated; are inserted into a body passage such as the rectum or vagina.

sympathetic nervous system (SNS): a component of the autonomic nervous system; initiates the fight-or-flight response.

symptom: a piece of subjective information about a disease or condition; is based on a person's feelings or opinions.

syncope: temporary unconsciousness; fainting.

systematic: using a specific method; orderly.

systolic blood pressure: the pressure of blood against the arteries when the heart muscle contracts and pushes blood out to the body.

T

taboos: practices determined by society or religion to be improper, unacceptable, or forbidden.

tachycardia: an abnormally fast pulse (more than 100 beats per minute).

tachypnea: rapid, shallow breathing.

temporal arteries: arteries located on each side of the head.

tendons: bands of fibrous tissue that connect muscle to bone.

tepid: slightly warm.

The Joint Commission (TJC): a private regulatory agency that accredits various healthcare facilities, such as hospitals, behavioral health agencies, home healthcare services, and nursing and rehabilitation centers; facilities that pursue accreditation by TJC must meet specific guidelines and standards for safety and quality.

therapeutic: having a healing effect on the body and mind.

therapeutic diets: eating plans that promote healing.

thermotherapy: the use of heat applications to increase circulation and ease pain.

thrombus: a blood clot that forms within a blood vessel and does not travel through the blood.

tingling: a sensation that feels like sharp points digging into the skin due to changes in nerve function.

tissue: a collection of specialized cells that act together to perform specific functions.

topical: on the surface of the skin.

toxins: poisons.

tracheostomy: a surgical opening in the trachea; a tube is inserted into the opening to help people experiencing difficulty breathing.

traction: weights, pulleys, and tape used to exert a slow, gentle pull; used to treat a muscular or skeletal disorder, such as a fracture, and to bring displaced bones back into place.

traditions: behaviors or practices that have special meanings or symbolism and that are handed down from one generation to another.

trait: a distinctive physical quality or characteristic.

transparency: lack of secretive or hidden information; honesty.

transplants: surgeries in which organs or body tissues are removed from one person and transferred into another.

transverse plane: a body plane that divides the body into upper and lower halves; also called the *horizontal plane*.

trauma: a serious or life-threatening injury or shock to a person's body.

triglycerides: calories stored in a person's fat cells.

trochanter rolls: soft rolls that are placed along the body and that span from above the hip to above the knee; prevent external rotation of the hips; are usually premade or made from a towel or bath blanket and are usually 12–14 inches long.

tumor: an abnormal growth of tissue that has no function in the body; can be benign (noncancerous) or malignant (cancerous).

turnover: the number of staff members who leave a healthcare facility and are replaced by new employees during a specific period of time.

tympanic temperature: a measurement of body temperature taken by placing a thermometer into the ear.

U

ultrasound: a test that uses ultrasonic waves to view the internal structures of the body.

unethical: not in line with accepted rules of conduct.

V

vaccine: a mixture that is given by injection or taken orally to protect a person against a specific disease; contains a weakened or killed antigen, which prompts the body to develop antibodies specific to that antigen, increasing immunity.

values: beliefs or ideals; set a standard for what is good or bad and significantly influence attitude and behavior; may be shared by people of the same culture.

ventilator: a device used to mechanically aid breathing.

veracity: honesty; the act of providing full disclosure to enable residents to make informed decisions.

verbal communication: the use of spoken words to convey a message.

vital signs: the rates or values of a person's body temperature, pulse, respirations, and blood pressure.

vitamins: organic compounds needed for cell development and growth; must be ingested from foods in a person's diet or from vitamin supplements.

voided: expelled from the body.

W

ward: a room in which several patients are given care in a healthcare facility.

well-being: the state of a person's health; is influenced by balancing one's diet, exercise, relationships, financial resources, work, education, and leisure.

wellness: a state of health and well-being that includes all aspects of health; is achieved by making conscious life choices that improve health and well-being.

whirlpool: a type of bathtub used for therapeutic purposes; has small spray jets that swirl water.

white blood cells: components of the blood that fight infection and provide protection; also called *leukocytes*.

work ethic: a belief in the importance of work; can strengthen a person's character.

work-life balance: the state of a person's time and energy contributions to career, work, and family commitments.

World Health Organization (WHO): an agency of the United Nations that focuses on international public health.

wound: an injury to body tissue; can be caused by a cut, blow, or other force.

Index

antiembolism stockings, 744–746
antigens, 321
antihistamines, 759
antiseptics, 325
antiviral medications, 202, 328
anus, 179
anxiety, 70, 270–271, 697–698
    anxiety disorders, 697–698
    easing during admission, 90
    in residents and caregivers,
        270–271
apex, of the heart, 170, 467
aphasia, 224, 260, 679
apical pulse, 467, 470–471
apnea, 471, 538–539, 790
appearance, professional, 13–14
appendicular skeleton, 157–158
applications (employment forms),
    811
applications (of heat and cold),
    581–590
applications (software), 310
apps, 310
aquathermia pad, 581–582
arrhythmias, 222
arteriosclerosis, 223
arthritis, 206–207
ASD (acute stress disorder), 698
ASD (autism spectrum disorder),
    682–683
asepsis, 338–339. *See also* infection
    control
ASL (American Sign Language),
    677
asphyxia, 763
aspiration, 616, 618
assault, 50
assertiveness, 275
assessing, step of nursing process,
    84–85
assignment sheets, 296–297
assisted living, 28, 80
assistive devices and equipment,
    428–438, 449–450, 617, 676, 679
asthma, 226–227
asylums, 696
atherosclerosis, 220
atony, 440
atrophy, of cells, muscles, and
    tissues, 148, 187, 209
attitudes, 109
    generational differences, 109–111
    professional, 12–16
AUD (alcohol use disorder), 699–700
auditory canal, 166
auditory learner, 802

aural blood vessels, 463
auscultation, 491
authentication, of a document
    addendum or amendment, 316
autism spectrum disorder
    (ASD), 682–683
autoimmune disorders, 230
automated external defibrillator
    (AED), 756–757
autonomic nervous system
    (ANS), 163–164
autonomy, 52, 115, 783
autopsies, 326, 793
axial skeleton, 157–158
axilla, 425
axillary temperatures, 456, 458,
    461–462
Ayurvedic medicine, 134

B

B cells, 175
baby blues, 718
baby boomers, 111
back belts, 403
back blows, 764
back rubs, 540–542
bacteria, 320, 326–328
bacterial pneumonia, 327
bag bath, 549
balance scale, 480, 482–483
Barnard, Dr. Christiaan, 24
basic life support (BLS), 753–757
    automated external
        defibrillator (AED), 756–757
    cardiopulmonary resuscitation
        (CPR), 753–756
    chain of survival, 753
basic needs, 102–103
bath blanket, 526
bathing, 547–553, 725–727
    bed baths, 548–552
    infants, 725–727
    residents with limited
        mobility, 548
    therapeutic, 548–549
    traditions, 553
battery, 50
beats per minute (bpm), 468
bed baths, 548–552
bed board, 405
bed making, 526–534
bedpans, 635–636, 639–641
bedridden residents
    caring for, 202–204, 422
    making occupied beds, 526,
        529–531

measuring height and weight
    of, 481, 483–486
turning and positioning, 408–415
beds, 525–534
    controls, 525
    making, 526–534
    types of, 525
bed scales, 481, 484–486
bedside stand, 518
bedsores. *See* decubitus ulcers
behavior, 109–111
    generational differences,
        109–111
    professional, 12–16
beliefs, 280, 295, 779–780
belonging, human need for, 103
beneficence, 52
benign prostate hypertrophy
    (BPH), 238–239
benign tumor, 149, 241
bias, 71, 282
bills of rights, 47–49, 785
binders, abdominal, 744
binge drinking, 699
binge-eating disorder, 607
biohazard waste bags, 350–351
biopsy, 238
bioterrorism, 772
bipolar disorder, 699
birth. *See* childbirth
birth control, discontinuation of, 710
birthing centers, 713
bladder, urinary, 182
    overactive, 650
    retraining, 665–667
bland diet, 613
bleeding, 768–770
blindness, 674
blood, 170–172
bloodborne pathogens, 332,
    353–354
blood oxygenation, 471, 473
blood pressure, 170–171, 473–478
    factors affecting, 474
    measuring, 475–478
    normal ranges, 473
blood vessels, 171
    aneurysm, 223
    arteriosclerosis, 223
    atherosclerosis, 220
    coronary artery disease, 220,
        222–223
    peripheral vascular disease
        (PVD), 225–226, 566–567
BLS. *See* basic life support
BMI (body mass index), 480,
    605–606, 821

E

ear infection, 214–215
ears
    anatomy, 166–167
    diseases and conditions, 214–215
eating. *See also* nutrition
    assisting residents, 617–618, 620–622, 676
    assistive devices, 617
    optimal experience, 609–611
    problems, 604–607, 618
    traditions, 596
eating disorders, 606–607
eating patterns, 595
Ebola virus, 322, 328, 354
eclampsia, 719
ectopic pregnancy, 719
edema, 222, 480, 586, 627
education, 4, 801
EEO (equal employment opportunity) laws, 815
EHR (electronic health record), 306, 308, 315–316
elder abuse, 50
elective admission, 90
electrical burns, 359
electrical safety, 392–393
electric beds, 525
electrolytes, 599
electronic communication, 9–10, 54, 75, 309–312
electronic health record (EHR), 306, 308, 315–316
electronic medical record (EMR), 9, 306–308, 315–316
electronic records
    advantages of, 308
    confidentiality, 54, 75, 309
    correcting errors, 315–316
    devices, 309–310
    documentation, 314–315
    electronic health record (EHR), 306, 308, 315–316
    electronic medical record (EMR), 9, 306–308, 315–316
elimination, 635–667
    assisting residents, 636–643, 666
    bowel, 636–641, 652–665
    cultural habits and customs, 653
    retraining the bladder or bowel, 665–667
    specimen collection, 505–511
    urinary, 635–651
embolus, 441, 741
embryo, 709

emergencies. *See* disasters; emergency procedures; medical emergencies
emergency admission, 90
emergency procedures, 10
    anaphylaxis, 759–760
    automated external defibrillator (AED), 756–757
    basic life support (BLS), 753–757
    bleeding, 768–770
    burns, 760–762
    cardiopulmonary resuscitation (CPR), 753–756
    chest pain, 757
    choking, 729–730, 764–765
    disasters, 772–774
    fainting, 766
    fire, 389–391
    first aid, 752–770
    heart attack, 757–758
    Heimlich maneuver, 764–765
    poisoning, 762–763
    seizure, 767–768
    stroke, 758
emesis basin, 559
emotional abuse, 50
emotional health. *See* mental and emotional health
emotional support, 243, 267–269
emotions
    and stress, 124, 696
    managing, 71–72, 270–275
empathy, 103, 267
emphysema, 229
employment
    application, 811
    cover message, 809–810
    equal opportunity laws, 815
    finding a position, 808–809
    interviewing, 814–815
    orientation, 815
    resigning from a position, 816–817
    résumé, 810–811
EMR (electronic medical record), 9, 306–308, 315–316
endocrine glands, 167. *See also* endocrine system
endocrine system
    anatomy, 167–170
    diseases and conditions, 215–220
end-of-life care, 80, 245, 778–797
    cancer patients, 245
    emotional and spiritual needs, 787–788
    family support, 788, 793

    grief, 780–783
    holistic care, 782, 785–789
    palliative care, 784–785
    physical needs, 786–787
    postmortem care, 794–797
    preparations and decisions, 783–784, 792–794
    signs of approaching death, 790–792
    self-care, 788
    traditions and beliefs, 779–780
enemas, 659–662
energy, managing, 126–127
energy balance, 597
energy rhythm, 126
engagement, 70–73
    critical thinking, 72–73
    mindfulness, 71–72
    self-reflection, 71–72
enteral feeding, 615–617
enteric precautions, 353
entrapment, 373, 382–383
environment, maintaining a safe, 10, 517–542. *See also* safety
    bed making, 525–534
    call light systems, 518–521
    emergencies and disasters, 751–774
    ensuring safety, 372–374, 377–379, 389–396
    healing environment, 522, 524, 535–542
    infection control, 338–357
    noise exposure, 539
    personal items of residents, 521–522
    resident rooms, 517–518
    restraint-free care, 382–385
Environmental Protection Agency (EPA), 604, 774
enzymes, 169
EPA (Environmental Protection Agency), 604, 774
epidemics, 23, 322, 326, 772
epidemiology, 326. *See also* communicable diseases
epidermis, 153–154, 320
epiglottis, 173, 178
episiotomy, 718
epithelial membranes, 150
epithelial tissue, 149
equal employment opportunity (EEO) laws, 815
Erikson, Erik, 106
errors, documentation, 315–316
erythrocytes. *See* red blood cells
esophageal ulcer, 233

essential amino acids, 599
ethical practice. *See* ethics
ethics, 52–57
    abuse, 50
    boundaries, 16–17, 548, 789
    caregiving principles, 52–53
    codes of, 53–54
    committees, 56–57
    confidentiality, 46–47, 52,
      308–309
    decision making, 54–56
    dilemmas, 56–57
    neglect, 49–50
    problem solving, 54–56
    respecting rights, 47–49, 785
ethics committees, 56–57
ethnicity, 279
ethnocentrism, 282
eustress, 123, 696
evacuation, 773
evacuators, 743–744
evaluation, plan of care, 293
evening care, 539–540
evidence-based practice, 84
exchange. *See* Health Insurance
  Marketplace
excretion, 344
exercise
    ambulation, 424–438
    impact on disease risk, 186–187,
      216, 218, 223, 243
    importance of, 14, 121
    range-of-motion exercises,
      440–448
    weight management, 596–597
exocrine glands, 167. *See also*
  endocrine system
exposure control plan, 356–357
exposure therapy, 702
extremities. *See* appendicular
  skeleton
extrinsic motivation, 101
exudate, 361. *See* drainage
eyeglasses, 673, 675
eyes
    anatomy, 164–166
    diseases and conditions,
      213–214, 673–674
eyesight, 164–166, 213–215, 260,
  673–676

F

face masks, 344, 348–349
face protection, 344–345, 348–349
face shield, 344, 349

facilities, healthcare, 26–29
    accreditation, 44
    culture, 37–39
    facility safety plan, 374
    history of, 25, 517, 596
    licensure, 44
    organizational structure, 35–37
    policies, 9, 86–88
    room equipment and features,
      517–518
    types of, 26–29
Fahrenheit (F) scale, 455
fainting, 415, 766–767
fallopian tubes, 185
falls, 376–380
    causes of, 376–377
    prevention, 377–379
    responding to, 379–380, 425
    risk program, 377
false imprisonment, 48
family nurse practitioner, 713
family practitioner (FP), 712
family relationships, 265, 280,
  284–285
family support, 788, 793
family types, 280
fatigue, in residents, 536
fatigue, personal. *See* self-care
fats, dietary, 598
fat-soluble vitamins, 599
FDA (Food and Drug
  Administration), 597, 600,
  603–604, 774
fear, in residents and caregivers,
  271–272
fecal incontinence, 655
fecal occult blood test (FOBT),
  512–513
feces. *See* stool
Federal Emergency Management
  Agency (FEMA), 774
feeding tubes, 615–617
feelings. *See* emotions
FEMA (Federal Emergency
  Management Agency), 774
female catheter care, 646–647
female perineal care, 569–570
female reproductive system
    anatomy, 184–185
    diseases and conditions,
      239–241
    pregnancy and childbirth,
      707–721
fertilization, 708
fetus, 709
fever, 455
fiber, dietary, 597

fibrillation, 756
fidelity, 53
fight-or-flight response, 114,
  123–124, 164, 272
financial abuse, 50
fingernails, 154, 564–566
fire extinguishers, 390–391
fire safety, 389–392
    fire prevention, 391–392
    fire triangle, 389
    responding to fires, 389–391
first aid
    anaphylaxis, 759–760
    basic life support (BLS),
      753–757
    burns, 760–762
    chest pain, 757
    choking, 729–730, 763–765
    fainting, 766–767
    first aid, 752–753
    Good Samaritan laws, 752
    heart attack, 757–758
    hemorrhage, 768–770
    poisoning, 762–763
    seizures, 767–768
    stroke, 758
first-degree burns, 760
first responders, 751–752
fistula, 235
five-and-five method, 764
five rights of delegation, 82–83
Five Wishes, 784
flash cards, 803
flatus, 653
Fleming, Sir Alexander, 23
flexibility, 15
flow meter, 393
flu, 328
fluid intake, 600–601, 630, 632
FOBT (fecal occult blood test),
  512–513
food
    alternative feeding therapies,
      615–617
    Dietary Guidelines for Americans,
      602
    eating disorders, 606–607
    labels, 602–603
    MyPlate, 601–602
    nutrients, 597–601
    preferences, 595
    safety, 604
    therapeutic diets, 612–615
    traditions, 596
    weight management, 604–606
Food and Drug Administration
  (FDA), 597, 600, 603–604, 774

foodborne illnesses, 604
food labels, 602–603
food safety, 604
footboard, 405
foot care, 566–568
foot drop, 405
forensic autopsy, 793
Fowler's position, 144, 406, 497
FP (family practitioner), 712
fracture bedpans, 635–636, 639–641
fractures, 207–208
fragile X syndrome (FXS), 683
freedom, 52
friendships, 265–266
frontal plane. *See* coronal plane
frostbite, 359, 587
fruits, 601
full liquid diet, 613
functional nursing, 81
funding, healthcare, 30–34
fungi, 328–329
FXS (fragile X syndrome), 683

G

gait, 377, 435–436
gait belt, 379, 417
gallbladder, 180, 234–235
gallstones, 234
gangrene, 587
gas. *See* flatus
gas exchange, 172–173
gastric ulcer, 233
gastroesophageal reflux disease
   (GERD), 232–233
gastrointestinal (GI) system
   accessory organs, 179–180
   alimentary canal, 177–179
   diseases and conditions,
      232–235
   signs of approaching death, 791
gastrointestinal (GI) tract. *See*
   alimentary canal
gender identity, 281–282
general surgeons, 734
generations, 109–111
   diversity, 280
   generation gap, 110
generation X, 111
generation Z, 111
genes, 185–186
genetic disorders, 198, 680–682,
   710–711
genome, 185–186
geographic diversity, 280
GERD (gastroesophageal reflux
   disease), 232–233

germs. *See* pathogens
germ theory, 326
gestational age, 710
gestational diabetes, 216
GI system. *See* gastrointestinal
   system
GI tract. *See* alimentary canal
giving of self, 267
glaucoma, 213–214, 674
glucometer, 501
gluten sensitivity and intolerance,
   601
glycated hemoglobin (A1C) test,
   217
glycemic index, 614
glycosuria, 505
goggles, 344, 349
goiter, 219
Good Samaritan laws, 752
gowns, PPE, 344, 347–348
gowns, resident, 575–576
graduate (container), 630
grains, 601
grand mal seizure, 767
Graves' disease, 219
grief, 779–783
   anticipatory, 782
   prolonged, 782–783
   stages of, 780–782
   support, 782
   ways of expressing, 781
grooming. *See* hygiene
growth and development
   newborns and infants, 721–722
   physical, 104–105
   psychosocial, 106
growth charts, 104
guaiac test, 512–513
gurney, 739

H

hair, 154
hair care, 553–557
HAIs (healthcare-associated
   infections), 323, 330
hallucinations, 537, 690, 700
hand hygiene, 9, 339–343, 724
hand-over-hand cue, 692
hand sanitizer, 339–340, 342–343
Hands-Only™ CPR, 754–755
hand washing, 9, 339–342, 724
harm, 371
Hashimoto's thyroiditis, 219
hazards. *See* safety
head-to-toe examination, 491

healing environment, 522–524,
   535–542
health and wellness
   body, mind, and spirit, 113–116
   mental and emotional health,
      71–72, 271–273, 695–696
   nutrition, 595–607
   stress management, 123–129
   wellness and illness, 120–122
healthcare-associated infections
   (HAIs), 323, 330
healthcare facilities
   accreditation, 44
   culture, 37–39
   facility safety plan, 374
   history of, 25, 517, 596
   licensure, 44
   organizational structure, 35–37
   policies, 9, 86–88
   room equipment and features,
      517–518
   types of, 26–29
healthcare funding
   managed care, 32–33
   Medicaid, 30–32
   Medicare, 30–31
   Patient Protection and
      Affordable Care Act
      (ACA), 32
   private insurance, 33–34
healthcare history, 22–25, 517, 596
healthcare laws and regulations,
   43–50, 308–309, 752, 783, 785
healthcare proxy. *See* power of
   attorney
healthcare services
   healthcare facilities, 26–29
   home healthcare, 29
   hospice, 29
   maternity, 707–730
   physical examinations, 490–495
   residential care, 28
   surgery, 732–746
healthcare team, 62–68, 111
healthcare technology. *See*
   technology
health information, 46–47, 308–309
Health Insurance Marketplace,
   30, 32
Health Insurance Portability and
   Accountability Act (HIPAA),
   46–47, 308–309
health literacy, 263–264
health maintenance organization
   (HMO). *See* managed care
health promotion, 130–132
health records. *See* records

health unit coordinator (HUC), 64
hearing aids, 677–679
hearing impairment and loss
    aids, 677–679
    care considerations, 678–679
    communication, 259–260
    signs and symptoms, 677
heart, 170–171
heart attack, 221, 757–758
heart disease, 220–226, 759
heart-healthy diet, 614
heat applications, 581–586
height, measuring, 480–484
Heimlich, Dr. Henry, 24
Heimlich maneuver, 764–765
hematopoiesis, 156
hematuria, 505
hemiplegia, 224, 686
Hemoccult kit, 512–513
hemoglobin, 172
hemophilia, 710
hemorrhage, 768–770
hemorrhagic stroke, 223–225
hemorrhoids, 549, 656
herbals, 133, 600
hernia, 232, 494, 656
high-fiber diet, 615
high Fowler's position, 406
HIPAA (Health Insurance
    Portability and Accountability
    Act), 46–47, 308–309
hip abduction wedge, 405
history of healthcare, 22–25, 517,
    596
HIV (human immunodeficiency
    virus), 230–232
HMO (health maintenance
    organization). See managed care
Hoffmann, Felix, 23
holistic care
    body, mind, and spirit, 113–116
    end-of-life care, 785–789
    framework, 5–7
    holistic communication,
        255–264, 274
    skills, 13, 16, 37, 54, 67, 72, 90,
        115, 125, 187, 199, 263, 287,
        299, 314, 333, 356, 378, 422,
        474, 498, 521, 548, 610, 666,
        685, 741, 763, 793, 818
home healthcare
    ambulation, 425
    definition, 29
    hospice, 785
    staff, 63
homeopathy, 135
homeostasis, 102

honesty, 15
horizontal plane. See transverse
    plane
hormones, 123, 167–170
hospice care, 4, 29, 245, 784–785
hospital gowns, resident, 575–576
hospitals, 26–27
HUC (health unit coordinator), 64
huddles. See change-of-shift reports
human behavior. See behavior
human body. See anatomy; body
    cavities; body planes; body
    positions; body structures; body
    systems; physiology
Human Genome Project, 148
human immunodeficiency virus
    (HIV), 230–232
humanistic theory of motivation,
    102
human needs. See needs
humility, 73
hydration, 582, 600–601, 627–634
    importance of, 627–628
    intake and output (I&O),
        630–634
    parenteral intravenous (IV)
        infusion, 628–630
    water, 600–601
hydraulic digital body lift, 481,
    484–485
hydrocephalus, 681
hygiene
    bathing, 547–553
    catheter care, 643–647
    changing a hospital gown,
        575–576
    denture care, 558–559, 562–563
    dressing and undressing,
        572–574
    fingernail care, 564–566
    foot care, 566–568
    hair care, 553–557
    hand hygiene, 9, 339–343, 724
    infants, 724–728
    mothers, 724
    oral care, 558–561
    perineal care, 569–572
    shaving, 557–558
    skin care, 578–590
hyperglycemia, 216, 218
hyperplasia, 149
hypertension, 224, 473
hyperthyroidism, 219–220
hypertrophy, 148
hyperventilation, 471
hypnotherapy, 133
hypodermis, 154

hypoglycemia, 218
hypotension, 473
hypothalamus, 162, 168
hypothermia, 376
hypothyroidism, 219–220
hypoventilation, 471
hypovolemic shock, 741, 768

I

I&O (intake and output), 618–619,
    630–634
IBW (ideal body weight), 480
ice packs, 586, 589–590
ideal body weight (IBW), 480
ileostomy, 663. See also ostomy care
illness, 120–121
IM (integrative medicine), 132–135,
    691, 702
immediate-care centers. See urgent-
    care centers
immobile residents
    caring for, 202–204, 422
    making occupied beds, 526,
        529–531
    measuring height and weight
        of, 481, 483–486
    turning and positioning,
        408–415
immune system
    anatomy, 175–176
    diseases and conditions,
        229–232
    immune response, 321
immunity
    autoimmune disorders, 230
    HIV/AIDS, 230–232
    immune response, 321
    types of, 175
    vaccines, 23, 321–322
immunization, 23, 321–322
impaction, 653
implantation, 708
incapacitation, 783
incentive spirometer, 742
incident report, 379–380
incontinence
    definition, 202
    fecal (bowel), 655
    urinary, 650–651
incontinence pad, 526
independence, promoting, 10, 12,
    81, 115, 399, 546, 665, 676
independent living, 28
individually identifiable health
    information, 46–47, 308–309

infants
    bathing, 725–727
    care considerations, 721–730
    choking, 729–730
    diapering, 727–728
    growth and development,
        721–722
    hygiene, 724–728
    nutrition, 722–724
    postnatal care, 721
    safety, 728–730
infection
    chain of, 331
    defenses against, 320–323
    identification, 333
    pathogens, 325–329
    risk factors, 323
    transmission, 332
    types of, 329–330
infection control
    cleaning and disinfection,
        350–352
    cultural aspects, 323
    definition, 9, 338–339
    exposure control plan,
        356–357
    hand hygiene, 9, 339–343, 724
    isolation, 354–355
    personal protective equipment
        (PPE), 9, 344–349, 364–365
    respiratory hygiene, 349–350
    standard precautions, 339–352
    transmission-based
        precautions, 352–356
    wound care, 358–365
infection prevention. See infection
    control
infectious diseases. See
    communicable diseases
infertility, 711
infiltration, 629
inflammation, 199, 322
inflammatory response, 322
influenza, 328
informed consent, 49
infusion, intravenous (IV), 628–630
inguinal hernia, 494
inner ear, 167
insomnia, 538
inspection, examination method,
    491
intake and output (I&O), 618–619,
    630–634
integrative medicine (IM), 132–135,
    691, 702
integrity, 15

integumentary system. See also
    skin; skin care
        anatomy, 153–154
        diseases and conditions, 201–204
intermediate care, 80
internal hemorrhage (bleeding),
    768, 770
international units (IUs), 599
interpersonal relationships, 265–267
interpreters, 258, 260
intersex, 282
interviews, employment, 814–815
intimate relationships, 266
intimate space, 257
intoxication, 673, 699–670
intraoperative care, 734, 739
intrapartum, 707, 715–721
intravenous (IV) catheters, 628–630
intravenous (IV) pump, 628
intrinsic motivation, 101
intuition, 73, 130–131
invasion of privacy, 47, 308–309
involuntary muscles, 149–150, 160
iris, 165
ischemia, 221
ischemic strokes, 223–225, 758
isolation, 350–351, 354–356
IUs (international units), 599
IV. See intravenous catheters;
    intravenous pump

J

jargon, 258–259
Jenner, Edward, 23
job campaign, 808
job description, 7–8, 809
job orientation, 36–37, 773
Joint Commission, The (TJC), 44
joints, 156, 206–207, 401
journaling, 71–72
justice, 53

K

K-pad. See aquathermia pad
Kegel exercises, 667
keratosis, 201
kidney failure, 237–238
kidneys, 180–181
kidney stones, 236–237
kinship, 285
knee-chest position, 497
Koch, Robert, 326
Kolcaba, Katharine, 535
Kübler-Ross, Elisabeth, 780–781

L

labia, 184
labor, 715–721
laboratories, 29
laboratory staff, 64
lacerations, 358
lactose intolerance, 602
laparascopic surgery, 733–734
large intestine, 179
laryngeal mirror, 496
lateral position, 144, 407
laws
    accreditation, 44
    Americans with Disabilities
        Act (ADA), 673
    equal employment opportunity
        (EEO), 815
    Good Samaritan, 752
    healthcare regulations, 43–50
    Health Insurance Portability
        and Accountability Act
        (HIPAA), 46–47, 308–309
    licensure, 44
    Occupational Safety and
        Health Administration
        (OSHA), 332, 353–354, 356,
        374, 392–393, 816
    Omnibus Budget
        Reconciliation Act (OBRA),
        4, 44, 48, 801
    Patient Protection and
        Affordable Care Act (ACA), 32
    Patient Self-Determination Act
        (PSDA), 783
    rights of patients and residents,
        46–50, 785
    scope of practice, 44–46
learning styles, 802–803
legal blindness, 674
legal practice. See laws; scope of
    practice
legal scope of practice. See scope
    of practice
leg bags, 649–650
legumes, 597
lesions, 199
leukocytes. See white blood cells
level-of-care assignment, 79–80
levels of care, 66, 79–80
liability, 45
libel, 50
liberalized diets, 612
lice, 553–554
licensed beds, 26, 30
licensed nursing assistant. See
    certified nursing assistant

gastrointestinal, 177
immune and lymphatic, 175
integumentary, 153
muscular, 160
nervous, 161
reproductive, 183
respiratory, 173
sensory, 165
skeletal, 155
urinary, 181
Medicare, 30–31
medication administration record
(MAR), 307
medication assistant, 45
medications
antibiotics, 327–328
anticoagulants, 557, 579
antihistamines, 759
antiviral, 202, 328
bronchodilators, 229
chemical restraints, 381
for HIV/AIDS, 231–232
for mental health conditions,
702
for pain, 202, 212, 717, 739
observation, 200
penicillin, 23
tolerance, 248
medication technician, 45
medicine. *See* medications
meditation, 71, 133
membranes, 150
memory, 299, 804–805
memory loss. *See* cognitive disorders
Ménière's disease, 215
meninges, 150, 162
meniscus, 732
mental abuse, 50
mental and emotional health
body, mind, and spirit, 113–116
care considerations, 702
definition, 695
managing emotions, 270–272
mental health conditions,
696–700
mindfulness, 71–72, 782
self-harm, 700–701
self-reflection, 71–72
stress management, 123–129,
696
suicide, 700–701
wellness and illness, 120–122
mental health conditions, 696–700
mesenteries, 150
metabolic rate, 596
metabolism, 595–597
metastasis, 241

metric system and units, 599–600,
821
microbes. *See* microorganisms
microorganisms, 320, 325–329
bacteria, 326–328
fungi, 328–329
parasites, 329
viruses, 328
middle ear, 167
midstream urine specimen, 505,
508–509
midwife, 712–713
millennials, 111
mind, component of holistic care,
113–116
mind and body practices, 133–134
mindfulness, 71–72, 782
mindful eating, 610–611
mindful presence, 536
minerals, 133, 600
minimally invasive surgery, 733
minimum data sets (MDSs), 370
miscarriage, 719
mistreatment, 49–50
mitered corners, 526
mobility
abbreviations and acronyms,
425
ambulation, 424–438
assistive devices and
equipment, 428–438, 449
body mechanics, 400–403
importance of, 405, 424
moving and positioning
residents, 404–422
range-of-motion (ROM)
exercises, 440–448
rehabilitation and restorative
care, 439–448
modes of communication, 256
modesty, 285–286
monotone speech, 211
morbidity, 198
moribund, 790
morning care, 546–547
morning sickness, 714
mortality, 197
mothers. *See* maternity
motility, 655
motivation, 101–102
mourning, 779. *See* grief
mouth, 177–178. *See also* oral care
movement. *See* mobility
movements, of the body, 147, 442
MS (multiple sclerosis), 210–211
MSDs (musculoskeletal disorders),
374–375, 400

MSDS. *See* safety data sheet
mucous membranes, 150, 320–321
mucus, 150, 320–321
multidrug-resistant organisms
(MDROs), 328
multiple pregnancy, 710
multiple sclerosis (MS), 210–211
muscle fibers, 160
muscles. *See* muscular system
muscle tissue, 149
muscular dystrophy (MD), 208
muscular system
anatomy, 158–160
diseases and conditions,
208–209, 374–375, 400
signs of approaching death, 791
musculoskeletal disorders (MSDs),
374–375, 400
musculoskeletal system. *See*
muscular system; skeletal system
myelin sheath, 161
myelomeningocele, 681
myocardial infarction, 221, 757–758
MyPlate, 601–602

N

nails. *See* fingernails; toenails
narcolepsy, 539
nasal cannula, 229, 394–396
National Institute of Occupational
Safety and Health (NIOSH), 353
National Prevention Strategy, 131
natural products, 133
naturopathy, 135
near misses, 372
necrosis, 203, 587
needlesticks, 332, 354, 374
needs
at the end of life, 785–788
body, mind, and spirit, 113–116
eating, 617–618, 620–622, 676
elimination, 635–667
holistic care, 5–7
hygiene, 546–576, 578–590
Maslow's hierarchy of, 102–104
mobility, 405, 424
nutrition, 595–607
safety, 372–374, 377–379,
389–396
sleep, 536–537
neglect, 49–50
negligence, 46
nerves. *See* nervous system;
neurons
nerve tissue, 150

nervous system
    anatomy, 160–164
    diseases and conditions, 210–213
    divisions of, 114, 162–164
    signs of approaching death, 791
network, healthcare. *See* managed care
networking, 808
neural impulses, 160–161
neural tube, 681
neurons, 150, 160–161
neuropathy, 212, 566
never events, 372
newborns
    bathing, 725–727
    care considerations, 721–730
    choking, 729–730
    diapering, 727–728
    growth and development, 721–722
    hygiene, 724–728
    nutrition, 722–724
    postnatal care, 721
    safety, 728–730
Nightingale, Florence, 23
NIOSH (National Institute of Occupational Safety and Health), 353
nodules, 219
noise exposure, 539
noncontagious diseases. *See* noncommunicable diseases
noncommunicable diseases
    acute or chronic, 198–200
    chronic pain, 247–248
    definition, 332
    effect of lifestyle choices, 121–122, 186–187, 204, 216, 219–220, 223, 225, 242, 594
    types of, 201–230, 232–245
nondigital thermometers, 457–458
noninfectious diseases. *See* noncommunicable diseases
nonmaleficence, 52
nonpenetrating wounds, 358–359
nonpharmacological pain relief, 249–250
nonREM (NREM) sleep, 537
nonsterile dressings, 361–363
nonverbal communication, 16, 74, 257
normal flora, 321, 325, 606
nose, 167, 173
nosocomial infections. *See* healthcare-associated infections (HAIs)

NREM (nonREM) sleep, 537
numbness, 300
nurse aide. *See* certified nursing assistant
nurse anesthetist, 735, 739
nurse managers, 36. *See also* licensed nursing staff
nursing assistant. *See* certified nursing assistant
nursing care
    care conferences, 293–294
    change-of-shift reports, 295–296
    delegation, 82–83
    levels of, 79–80
    nursing assistant responsibilities, 7–10
    nursing process, 84–86
    plan of care, 291–293
    policies, 86–88
    rounds, 294
    teamwork, 62–68
    types of, 80–82
nursing diagnosis, 85, 292
nursing goal, 292
Nursing Home Reform Act, 48
Nursing Home Resident Rights, 48–49, 785
nursing homes. *See* long-term care facilities
nursing orders, 291–293
nursing process, 84–86
nursing rounds, 294, 520
nursing unit, 35–37
nutrients, 148, 597–601
nutrition
    alternative feeding therapies, 615–617
    assisting residents, 609–611, 618, 620–622, 676
    assistive eating devices, 617–618
    Dietary Guidelines for Americans, 602
    eating disorders, 606–607
    food labels, 602–603
    food preferences, 595
    food safety, 604
    metabolism, 595–597
    MyPlate, 601–602
    newborns and infants, 722–724
    nutrients, 597–601
    nutritional support, 611–612
    therapeutic diets, 612–615
    weight management, 604–606
nutritional status assessment, 611
Nutrition Facts labels, 602–603

O

OAB (overactive bladder), 650
obesity, 604–606
OB/GYN (obstetrician-gynecologist), 712
objective observations, 258, 298–300
OBRA (Omnibus Budget Reconciliation Act), 4, 44, 48, 801
observation, 9, 258, 298–300
obsessive-compulsive disorder (OCD), 698
obstetrician-gynecologist (OB/GYN), 712
obstructive sleep apnea, 538–539
occult blood, 510, 512–513
Occupational Safety and Health Administration (OSHA), 332, 353–354, 356, 374, 392–393, 816
occupational therapist, 65, 440
occupied beds, 526, 529–531
occurrence report, 379–380
OCD (obsessive-compulsive disorder), 698
ocular prostheses, 675
OIs (opportunistic infections), 330
Omnibus Budget Reconciliation Act (OBRA), 4, 44, 48, 801
online portals, 310
open beds, 526, 532
open drainage, 743
open-ended questions, 262, 692
operating room (OR), 732, 735–737
operation. *See* surgery
ophthalmoscope, 496
opioid use disorder, 700
opportunistic infections (OIs), 330
optic nerve, 166
OR (operating room), 732, 735–737
oral care, 558–561
oral cavity, 177–178
oral temperatures, 456–460, 463
organ donation, 792, 794
organelles, 147
organizational structure, of a healthcare facility, 35–37
organs, 146, 187. *See* body systems
organ systems. *See* body systems
orientation, job, 36–37, 773
orientation, sexual, 281–282
orthostatic hypotension, 415, 424
orthotics, 450, 682
OSHA (Occupational Safety and Health Administration), 332, 353–354, 356, 374, 392–393, 816
osteoporosis, 204, 206, 376
ostomy bag, 662–663

ostomy care, 662–665
otitis media, 214–215
otoscope, 496
outer ear, 166
outpatient clinics, 27
output, fluid, 630–634
ovaries, 169, 185, 708
overactive bladder (OAB), 650
overbed table, 518
overt behaviors, 109
overweight, 604–606
ovulation, 185, 708
oxygen, exchange during respiration, 172–173
oxygenation, of blood, 471, 473
oxygen therapy, 394–396

P

PACU (post-anesthesia care unit), 734, 740
pain, 246–250
    chest pain, 757
    cycle of chronic pain, 247–248
    experience of, 246, 248–249
    in comatose patients, 685
    observing and reporting, 249–250, 299
    pain scales, 249–250
    relief, 250, 536
    types of, 247
pain management. See pain relief
pain management clinics, 27
pain relief, 250, 536
    at the end of life, 787
    cold applications, 207, 586–590
    heat applications, 207, 581–586
    integrative medicine (IM), 250
    medications, 202, 212, 248, 717
    pain scales, 249–250
    techniques, 207, 250, 536
pain scales, 249–250
palliative care, 784–785. See also hospice care
pallor, 580
palpation, 491
pancreas, 169, 179
panic attacks, 697
paperwork. See records
Pap smears, 493
paralysis, 225, 685–688
paranoia, 690
paraplegia, 686
parasites, 329
parasympathetic nervous system, 114, 164
parathyroid glands, 169

parenteral feeding, 615
parenteral intravenous (IV) infusion, 628–630
Parkinson's disease, 211–212
partial bed bath, 548–552
Pasteur, Louis, 23, 326
pathogens, 172, 325–329, 604. See also communicable diseases
pathologist, 793
pathology, 200. See diseases and conditions
patience, 268
Patient Bill of Rights, 47–48, 785
patient care. See eating; environment; holistic care; hygiene; mobility; procedures
Patient Care Partnership, 48
patient-centered care, 81–82
patient culture. See culture
Patient Protection and Affordable Care Act (ACA), 32
patient records. See records
patient rights, 46–50, 785
patient safety. See safety
Patient Self-Determination Act (PSDA), 783
payroll records, 308
PCPs (primary care providers), 27, 62
PE. See physical examinations
pediatrician, 713
pediatric nurse practitioner (PNP), 713
pelvic examinations, 493
penetrating wounds, 358
penis, 183, 494
peptic ulcers, 233–234
percent Daily Value (DV), 603
percussion, 491
perinatal depression, 698–699
perinatologist, 712
perineal care, 546, 569–572
perioperative care, 734, 737–746
peripheral nervous system, 161, 163–164
peripheral neuropathy, 212, 566
peripheral vascular disease (PVD), 225–226, 566–567
peristalsis, 149, 177
perseveration, 690
personal boundaries, 16–17, 548, 789
personal care, 14–15, 71–72, 114–115
personal care homes. See residential care
personal hygiene. See hygiene
personal items, of residents, 521–522

personality disorders, 699
personal protective equipment (PPE)
    definition, 9, 339, 344
    disposable gloves, 345–346
    face protection, 344–345, 348–349
    gowns, 344, 347–348
    sterile gloves, 363–365
personal space, 257–258, 522, 548
petit mal seizure, 767
phagocytosis, 321
pharmacies, 29
pharmacogenomics, 186
pharmacology. See medications
pharynx, 173, 178
phenol, 326
PHI (protected health information), 46–47, 308–309
philosophy, of a healthcare facility, 80
phlegm. See sputum
phobias, 270
photosynthesis, 328
physical abuse, 50
physical activity. See exercise
physical examinations (PEs), 490–500
physical growth and development, 104–105
physical restraints, 381–382, 385–388
physical stamina, 14
physical therapist (PT), 65, 440
physician, 62
physiological needs, 102–103
physiology, 152–153. See also body systems
Piaget, Jean, 106
pillowcases, 526–527
pill rolling, 211
pineal gland, 162, 169
pituitary gland, 168
placenta, 709
placental abruption, 719
placenta previa, 718–719
planes, of the body, 144
plan of care, 85, 291–294
plan of care conferences, 293–294
plaques, 201
plasma, 172
platelets, 156, 172
p.m. care, 539–540
pneumonia, 327
PNP (pediatric nurse practitioner), 713
POCT (point-of-care testing), 501, 505, 512

prostate-specific antigen (PSA) serologic assay, 494
prosthetics, 449–450, 675
protected health information (PHI), 46–47, 308–309
proteins, 598–599, 601
PSA (prostate-specific antigen) serologic assay, 494
PSDA (Patient Self-Determination Act), 783
psoriasis, 201–202
psychosocial development, 106–107
psychotherapy, 702
PT (physical therapist), 65, 440
PTSD (post-traumatic stress disorder), 698
public space, 257
pull sheet, 405, 526
pulse
    locations, 466–467
    measuring, 468–471
    normal rates, 171, 468
    rhythm and quality, 468
    stethoscope use, 467–468
pulse oximeter, 90, 473
pump, intravenous (IV), 628
pupil, 165
purging, 607
pus, 322
PVD. See peripheral vascular disease
pyrexia, 455

Q

qigong, 134, 250
quadriplegia, 686

R

race, 279–280
RACE system, 390
racism, 282
radial pulse, 467–469
radiation, cancer treatment, 243–244
RAI (resident assessment instrument), 370
range of motion (ROM), 387
range-of-motion (ROM) exercises, 7, 147, 440–449
rapid eye movement (REM) sleep, 537–538
rapport, 115–116
rate of respiration, 471
ratio, staff and patients or residents, 66

rationale, 293
RBCs (red blood cells), 156, 172
RDAs (Recommended Dietary Allowances), 599–600
receptors, 153–154, 167
Recommended Dietary Allowances (RDAs), 599–600
reconstructive memory, 299
records
    confidentiality, 46–47, 308–309
    correcting errors, 315–316
    documentation, 314–315
    electronic records, 306–308
    importance of, 313
    information sources, 313–314
    observation, 258, 298–299
    types of, 305–308
    use of technology, 309–312
recovery room. See post-anesthesia care unit
rectal suppositories, 657–658
rectal temperatures, 456, 458, 460–461
rectal tube, 654–655
rectovaginal examinations, 493
rectum, 179
red blood cells (RBCs), 156, 172
reflection, 262
refractive errors, 673–674
registered nurse (RN), 3–4, 63, 735. See also licensed nursing staff
registered nursing assistant. See certified nursing assistant
registration, 5
regular diet, 612
regulations
    accreditation, 44
    Americans with Disabilities Act (ADA), 673
    equal employment opportunity (EEO), 815
    Good Samaritan, 752
    healthcare, 43–50
    Health Insurance Portability and Accountability Act (HIPAA), 46–47, 308–309
    licensure, 44
    Occupational Safety and Health Administration (OSHA), 332, 353–354, 356, 374, 392–393, 816
    Omnibus Budget Reconciliation Act (OBRA), 4, 44, 48, 801
    Patient Protection and Affordable Care Act (ACA), 32

Patient Self-Determination Act (PSDA), 783
    rights of patients and residents, 46–50, 785
    scope of practice, 44–46
regulator. See flow meter
rehabilitation, 44, 439–448
relationships
    building, 15, 266–267
    communication, 9–10, 15–16, 73–75, 255–262
    conflict resolution, 274–275
    family, 265
    holistic, 113–116
    interpersonal, 265–267
    intimate, 266
    managing emotions, 270–273
    types of, 265–266
relaxation techniques, 133, 536, 702
reliability, 14, 268
religious customs, 285, 553, 596, 780
religious diversity, 280
reminiscence, 693
REM (rapid eye movement) sleep, 537–538
renal diet, 614
renal failure, 237–238
reporting
    importance of, 9, 300–301
    incidents and accidents, 379–380
    mandatory reporting, 50, 701
    observation, 258, 298–300
    transparency, 15, 371
reproductive systems
    anatomy, 182–186
    diseases and conditions, 238–241
    female, 184–185, 707–710, 714–720
    male, 182–183, 708
    pregnancy and childbirth, 707–721
rescue breaths, 730, 755–756
reservoir, 743
resident assessment instrument (RAI), 370
resident care. See eating; environment; holistic care; hygiene; mobility; procedures
resident councils, 49
resident culture. See culture
residential care, 28
resident records. See records
resident rights, 46–50, 785

supplemental nutrition drinks, 611–612

supplements, dietary, 600

supportive care, 80

support network, 125–126

suppositories, rectal, 657–658

surgeons, 734–735

surgery
    care considerations, 741, 743–746
    complications, 741–742
    discharge plan, 746
    intraoperative care, 739
    operating room (OR), 735–736
    phases of, 734
    postoperative care, 740
    preoperative care, 737–739
    safety guidelines, 736
    staff members, 734–735
    types of, 732–733

surgical asepsis, 339

surgical beds, 526, 533–534, 740

surgical centers (surgicenters), 28

sweat glands, 154

sympathetic nervous system (SNS), 114, 123, 163–164, 272

symptoms, of diseases or conditions. *See* diseases and conditions

synapses, 161

syncope, 415, 766–767

synovial membranes, 150, 156

systemic infections, 330

systems, of the body. *See* body systems

systolic blood pressure, 473

T

taboos, 110

tachycardia, 219, 229, 468

tachypnea, 471

tai chi, 134–135, 250

taste, sense of, 167, 178

TB (tuberculosis), 327

TBI. *See* traumatic brain injury

TCM (traditional Chinese medicine), 134–135

T cells, 175

team nursing, 81

teamwork
    communication, 9–10, 15–16, 73–75, 255–262
    conflict resolution, 274–275
    effective, 67–68
    functions of, 66–67
    healthcare team members, 62–65

    importance of, 15
    surgical team, 735
    team life cycle, 67–68

technology
    apps, 310
    communication devices, 309–312
    digital ROM exercise, 449
    electronic records, 306–308, 315–316
    robotics, 24, 687, 736
    social media, 9–10, 54, 75
    telephones, 310–312

teeth, 178. *See also* oral care

telephone communication, 310–312

temperature
    locations for taking, 456–457
    measuring, 458–466
    normal ranges, 457
    thermometers, 457–466

temporal artery temperatures, 456, 465–466

tendons, 156

terminal cleaning, 351–352

terminal delirium, 791

terminal illness, 199, 778. *See also* end-of-life care

terms. *See* medical terminology

terrorism, 772

tertiary care, 26

testes, 170, 183, 494

test strip, 505

test-taking strategies, 806–807

tetraplegia, 686

thalamus, 162

Theory of Comfort, 535

theories
    Erikson's theory of psychosocial development, 106–107
    germ theory, 326
    Maslow's hierarchy of human needs, 102–104
    Piaget's theory of cognitive development, 106
    Theory of Comfort, 535

therapeutic baths, 547–549

therapeutic diets, 610, 612–615

thermal burns, 359

thermometers
    axillary, 458, 461–462
    digital, 458–466
    disposable oral, 463
    nondigital, 457–458
    oral, 458–460
    rectal, 458, 460–461
    temporal artery, 465–466
    tympanic, 463–464

thermotherapy, 581–586

third-degree burns, 761–762

throat, 173, 178

thrombocytes. *See* platelets

thrombus, 441

thrush, 227

thymus, 169, 176, 219–220

thyroid gland, 169, 219–220

TIA (transient ischemic attack), 224

time management, 126–127

tingling, 300

tinnitus, 215, 677

tissues, body, 149–150, 187

TJC (The Joint Commission), 44

to-do lists, 127

toenails, 219, 564, 566–568

toe pleat, 528

To Err is Human, 370

toilet, 636–638

toileting. *See* elimination

tongue, 167, 177–178

tonsils, 176

topical treatments, 201

torts, 46

total bed bath, 548–552

total blindness, 674

total carbohydrate, 603

total patient care, 81

touch contamination, 338

touch, sense of, 153–154, 167

towel bath, 548

toxins, 321

trachea, 173

tracheostomy, 80

traction equipment, 518

traditional Chinese medicine (TCM), 134–135

traditions, 280, 553, 596, 779–780

training, 4, 801

traits, 279

trans fats, 598

transfer
    bed to chair or wheelchair, 418–420
    bed to stretcher, 420–421
    between units or facilities, 93–95

transfer belt. *See* gait belt

transgender, 282

transient ischemic attack (TIA), 224

transmission, 332

transmission-based precautions
    airborne precautions, 353
    bloodborne pathogen precautions, 353
    contact precautions, 353
    droplet precautions, 353

enteric, wound, and skin precautions, 353
    exposure control plan, 356–357
    isolation, 354–355
transparency, in reporting, 15, 371
transplants, 792
transverse plane, 144
trauma, 26, 698
traumatic brain injury (TBI), 683–684, 687–688
Trendelenburg position, 407
triglycerides, 597
trimesters, of pregnancy, 714–715
trochanter rolls, 405
trustworthiness, 14–15
tuberculosis (TB), 327
tubes, feeding, 615–617
tumors, 149, 241–245
turning a resident in bed, 411–415
turning sheet, 405, 526
turnover, 68
tympanic temperatures, 456–457, 463–464
type 1 and type 2 diabetes mellitus, 216

U

ULs (upper intake levels), 599
ultrasound, 212, 712
umbilical cord, 709
underweight, 604–606
undressing, 572, 574
unethical conduct, 17–18, 45–46, 50, 789
unit clerk. *See* health unit coordinator
unit secretary. *See* health unit coordinator
unoccupied beds, 526, 531–533
unsaturated fats, 598
unsterile team, 735
upper intake levels (ULs), 599
upper respiratory tract, 173
ureters, 182
urethra, 182
urgent-care centers, 28
urinals, 636, 642–643
urinary bladder, 182, 650, 665–667
urinary catheters, 643–647
urinary drainage bags, 647–650
urinary elimination
    assisting residents, 636–643, 666
    bladder retraining, 666–667
    catheter care, 643–647
    drainage bags, 647–649

incontinence, 650–651
    intake and output (I&O), 632–634
    leg bags, 649–650
    urinary incontinence, 650–651
urinary system
    anatomy, 180–182
    diseases and conditions, 235–238
    signs of approaching death, 791
urinary tract infections (UTIs), 235–236, 643
urine
    formation, 180–182
    hydration level, 628
    specimen collection, 506–510
    straining, 510
    testing, 505
    types of specimens, 505–506
US customary units, 599–600, 821
US Department of Homeland Security, 774
uterine prolapse, 240–241
uterus, 185, 708–709, 714–718
UTIs. *See* urinary tract infections

V

vaccines, 23, 321–322
vagina, 185, 708–709, 714–718
vaginitis, 229–230
validation therapy, 693
values, 14, 37–38, 49, 52
vascular dementia, 688–689
vasoconstriction, 586
vector transmission, 332
vegetables, 601
vehicle transmission, 332
ventilation, 172–173
ventilator, 683, 686, 736
veracity, 53
verbal abuse, 50
verbal communication, 74, 257
vertebrae, 158
vertigo, 215
vestibular nerve, 167
vestibulocochlear nerve, 167
violence
    abuse, 50
    assault, 50
    battery, 50
    in residents, 384, 690–692, 702
    terrorism, 772
    workplace violence, 816
visceral muscle tissue. *See* smooth muscle tissue

vision impairment and loss
    care considerations, 675–676
    communication, 260
    low vision, 674
    refractive errors, 673–674
    vision-correction devices, 673–675
vital signs, 9, 454–478
    blood pressure, 473–478
    importance of, 9, 454–455
    pulse, 466–471
    resident anxiety about taking, 455
    respirations, 471–473
    temperature, 455–466
vitamins, 133, 599–600
voluntary muscles, 149, 160
vulva, 184

W

walkers, 431–433
walking. *See* ambulation
wards, 517
warm compresses, 582–584
warm soaks, 584–586
waste. *See* bowel elimination; urinary elimination
waste, infectious, 350–351
water, 600–601, 627–634
water-soluble vitamins, 599
WBCs. *See* white blood cells
weight, measuring, 480–486
weight loss, in seniors, 611
weight management, 604–606
well-baby examinations, 494–495
well-being, 120–121. *See also* health and wellness
well-man examinations, 494
wellness, 26, 120–122. *See* health and wellness
well-woman examinations, 27, 492–494
wheelchairs, 417–420
whirlpools, 548–549
white blood cells (WBCs), 147, 156, 172, 175
white-coat syndrome, 492
WHO. *See* World Health Organization
whole person, 113–116, 132. *See also* holistic care
Wilson, Bill, 24
windpipe, 173
womb. *See* uterus
women's health nurse practitioner, 713

word parts. *See* medical word parts
work ethic, 14
work-life balance, 128–129
workplace violence, 816
work schedules, 15, 36, 65–66,
    296–297
World Health Organization
    (WHO), 339, 371, 772
wound care, 358–365
wound precautions, 353
wounds
    categories of, 358–359
    dressings, 361–365
    observation and reporting,
        359–360
written communication, 74

Y

yoga, 134–135

Z

Zika virus, 332, 720